Red Book®:

2012 REPORT OF THE COMMITTEE ON INFECTIOUS DISEASES
TWENTY-NINTH EDITION

Author: Committee on Infectious Diseases
American Academy of Pediatrics

Larry K. Pickering, MD, FAAP, Editor

Carol J. Baker, MD, FAAP, Associate Editor
David W. Kimberlin, MD, FAAP, Associate Editor
Sarah S. Long, MD, FAAP, Associate Editor

American Academy of Pediatrics
141 Northwest Point Blvd
Elk Grove Village, IL 60007-1098

D1469072

Suggested Citation: American Academy of Pediatr   ɛr CJ,
Kimberlin DW, Long SS, eds. *Red Book: 2012 Repor*   ʳove
Village, IL: American Academy of Pediatrics; 2012:[page numbers]

29th Edition
1st Edition – 1938
2nd Edition – 1939
3rd Edition – 1940
4th Edition – 1942
5th Edition – 1943
6th Edition – 1944
7th Edition – 1945
8th Edition – 1947
9th Edition – 1951
10th Edition – 1952
11th Edition – 1955
12th Edition – 1957
13th Edition – 1961
14th Edition – 1964
15th Edition – 1966
16th Edition – 1970
16th Edition Revised – 1971
17th Edition – 1974
18th Edition – 1977
19th Edition – 1982
20th Edition – 1986
21st Edition – 1988
22nd Edition – 1991
23rd Edition – 1994
24th Edition – 1997
25th Edition – 2000
26th Edition – 2003
27th Edition – 2006
28th Edition – 2009

ISSN No. 1080-0131
ISBN No. 978-1-58110-703-6
MA0625

Quantity prices on request. Address all inquiries to:
American Academy of Pediatrics
141 Northwest Point Blvd
Elk Grove Village, IL 60007-1098

or Phone:
1-888-227-1770 Publications

3-230/0512   1 2 3 4 5 6 7 8 9 10

Committee on Infectious Diseases 2010–2012

Joseph A. Bocchini, Jr, MD
Michael T. Brady, MD
John S. Bradley, MD
Carrie L. Byington, MD
H. Dele Davies, MD
Kathryn M. Edwards, MD
Mary P. Glode, MD
Mary Anne Jackson, MD
Harry L. Keyserling, MD

Yvonne A. Maldonado, MD
Walter A. Orenstein, MD
Gordon E. Schutze, MD
Rodney E. Willoughby, MD
Theoklis E. Zaoutis, MD
Margaret C. Fisher, MD, Section on Infectious Diseases
Dennis L. Murray, MD, Section on Infectious Diseases

Ex Officio
Carol J. Baker, MD, *Red Book* Associate Editor
Henry H. Bernstein, DO, *Red Book* Online Associate Editor
David W. Kimberlin, MD, *Red Book* Associate Editor
Sarah S. Long, MD, *Red Book* Associate Editor
H. Cody Meissner, MD, *Visual Red Book* Associate Editor
Larry K. Pickering, MD, *Red Book* Editor

Consultants
Edgar O. Ledbetter, MD
Lorry G. Rubin, MD

Liaisons

Beth Bell, MD, MPH	Centers for Disease Control and Prevention
Robert Bortolussi, MD	Canadian Paediatric Society
Richard D. Clover, MD	American Academy of Family Physicians
Marc A. Fischer, MD	Centers for Disease Control and Prevention
Bruce Gellin, MD	National Vaccine Program Office
Richard L. Gorman, MD	National Institutes of Health
Lucia Lee, MD	Food and Drug Administration
R. Douglas Pratt, MD	Food and Drug Administration
Jennifer S. Read, MD	National Vaccine Program Office
Joan Robinson, MD	Canadian Paediatric Society
Marco Aurelio Palazzi Safadi, MD	Sociedad Latinoamericana de Infectologia Pediatrica (SLIPE)
Jane Seward, MBBS, MPH	Centers for Disease Control and Prevention
Jeffrey R. Starke, MD	American Thoracic Society
Geoffrey Simon, MD	Committee on Practice Ambulatory Medicine
Jack Swanson, MD	Committee on Practice Ambulatory Medicine
Tina Q. Tan, MD	Pediatric Infectious Diseases Society

Staff
Jennifer Frantz, MPH

Collaborators

Mark Abramowicz, MD, *The Medical Letter,* New Rochelle, NY

Mark J. Abzug, MD, University of Colorado, Denver School of Medicine, and the Children's Hospital, Aurora, CO

Angela Ahlquist, MPH, Centers for Disease Control and Prevention, Atlanta, GA

Iyabode Akinsanya-Beysolow, MD, MPH, Centers for Disease Control and Prevention, Atlanta, GA

Renata Albrecht, MD, Food and Drug Administration, Silver Spring, MD

John J. Alexander, MD, MPH, Food and Drug Administration, Silver Spring, MD

Upton D. Allen, MBBS, MSc, FRCPC, Hospital for Sick Children, University of Toronto, Toronto, Ontario, Canada

Manual R. Amieva, MD, PhD, Stanford University School of Medicine, Palo Alto, CA

Alicia Anderson, DVM, MPH, Centers for Disease Control and Prevention, Atlanta, GA

Paul M. Arguin, MD, Centers for Disease Control and Prevention, Atlanta, GA

Stephen S. Arnon, MD, California Department of Public Health, Richmond, CA

David M. Asher, MD, Food and Drug Administration, Kensington, MD

Chintamani D. Atreya, PhD, Food and Drug Administration, Rockville, MD

Carol J. Baker, MD, Baylor College of Medicine, Houston, TX

Robert S. Baltimore, MD, Yale University School of Medicine, New Haven, CT

Casey Barton Behravesh, DVM, DrPH, MS, Centers for Disease Control and Prevention, Atlanta, GA

Erza J. Barzilay, MD, US Centers for Disease Control and Prevention, Atlanta, GA

Margaret Bash, US Public Health Service, Rockville, MD

Melisse S. Baylor, MD, Food and Drug Administration, Rockville, MD

Michael J. Beach, PhD, Centers for Disease Control and Prevention, Atlanta, GA

Judy A. Beeler, MD, Food and Drug Administration, Bethesda, MD

Ermias Belay, MD, Centers for Disease Control and Prevention, Atlanta, GA

Ozlem A. Belen, MD, MPH, Food and Drug Administration, Silver Spring, MD

Yodit Belew, MD, Food and Drug Administration, Silver Spring, MD

Latanya T. Benjamin, MD, Stanford University School of Medicine, Palo Alto, CA

Jay E. Berkelhamer, MD, Children's Healthcare of Atlanta, Atlanta, GA

Frank E. Berkowitz, BSc, MBBCh, MPH, Emory University School of Medicine, Atlanta, GA

Caryn Bern, MD, MPH, Centers for Disease Control and Prevention, Atlanta, GA

Henry H. Bernstein, DO, Dartmouth Medical School, Hanover, NH

Stephanie R. Bialek, MD, MPH, Centers for Disease Control and Prevention, Atlanta, GA

Robin M. Biswas, MD, Food and Drug Administration, Rockville, MD

Adam Bjork, PhD, Centers for Disease Control and Prevention, Atlanta, GA

David D. Blaney, MD, MPH, Centers for Disease Control and Prevention, Atlanta, GA

Margaret J. Blythe, MD, Indiana University School of Medicine, Indianapolis, IN

Joesph A. Bocchini, MD, Louisiana State University Health Sciences Center-Shreveport, Shreveport, LA

Elizabeth A. Bolyard, RN, MPH, Centers for Disease Control and Prevention, Atlanta, GA

Cheryl A. Bopp, MS, Centers for Disease Control and Prevention, Atlanta, GA

Robert Bortolussi, MD, Dalhousie University, Halifax, Nova Scotia, Canada

Anna Bowen, MD, MPH, Centers for Disease Control and Prevention, Atlanta, GA

Kenneth M. Boyer, MD, Rush University Medical Center, Chicago, IL

John S. Bradley, MD, Children's Hospital San Diego, San Diego, CA

Michael T. Brady, MD, Nationwide Children's Hospital, The Ohio State University, Columbus, OH

Mary E. Brandt, PhD, Centers for Disease Control and Prevention, Atlanta, GA

Joseph Bresee, MD, Centers for Disease Control and Prevention, Atlanta, GA

Meghan Brett, MD, Centers for Disease Control and Prevention, Fort Collins, CO

Elizabeth C. Briere, MD, MPH, Centers for Disease Control and Prevention, Atlanta, GA

Karen Broder, MD, Centers for Disease Control and Prevention, Atlanta, GA

June Brown, MS, Centers for Disease Control and Prevention, Atlanta, GA

Gary Brunette, MD, MS, Centers for Disease Control and Prevention, Atlanta, GA

Joan Brunkard, PhD, Centers for Disease Control and Prevention, Atlanta, GA

Ellen Buerk, MD, Oxford Pediatrics and Adolescents, Oxford, OH

Jane L. Burns, MD, Seattle Children's Hospital/University of Washington, Seattle, WA

Carrie L. Byington, MD, University of Utah, Salt Lake City, UT

Grant Campbell, MD, PhD, Centers for Disease Control and Prevention, Fort Collins, CO

Paul T. Cantey, MD, MPH, Centers for Disease Control and Prevention, Atlanta, GA

Michael Cappello, MD, Yale School of Medicine, New Haven, CT

Mary T. Caserta, MD, University of Rochester Medical Center, Rochester, NY

Tom Chiller, MD, MPHTM, Centers for Disease Control and Prevention, Atlanta, GA

Lance A. Chilton, MD, University of Mexico, Albuquerque, NM

Thomas A. Clark, MD, MPH, Centers for Disease Control and Prevention, Atlanta, GA

Eleanor S. Click, MD, PhD, Centers for Disease Control and Prevention, Atlanta, GA

Amanda Cohn, MD, Centers for Disease Control and Prevention, Atlanta, GA

Laura Conklin, MD, Centers for Disease Control and Prevention, Atlanta, GA

Margaret M. Cortese, MD, Centers for Disease Control and Prevention, Atlanta, GA

James E. Crowe, Jr, MD, Vanderbilt University Vaccine Center, Nashville, TN

Therese Cvetkovich, MD, Food and Drug Administration, Silver Spring, MD

Lee (Toni) A. Darville, MD, University of Pittsburgh, Children's Hospital of Pittsburgh of UPMC, Pittsburgh, PA

Gregory A. Dasch, PhD, Centers for Disease Control and Prevention, Atlanta, GA

Barry Dashefsky, MD, New Jersey Medical School, University of Medicine and Dentistry of New Jersey, Newark, NJ

Jon R. Daugherty, PhD, Food and Drug Administration, Rockville, MD

Whitni Davidson, MPH, Centers for Disease Control and Prevention, Atlanta, GA

Alma C. Davidson, MD, Food and Drug Administration, Silver Spring, MD

Michael Deming, MD, MPH, Centers for Disease Control and Prevention, Atlanta, GA

Penelope H. Dennehy, MD, Alpert Medical School of Brown University and Hasbro Children's Hospital, Providence, RI

Kenneth L. Dominguez, MD, MPH, Centers for Disease Control and Prevention, Atlanta, GA

Benjamin D. Gold, MD, Children's Center for Digestive Healthcare, LLC, Atlanta, GA

Richard L. Gorman, MD, National Institutes of Health, National Institute of Allergy and Infectious Disease, Bethesda, MD

Rachel Gorwitz, MD, MPH, Centers for Disease Control and Prevention, Atlanta, GA

Sami L. Gottlieb, MD, MSPH, Centers for Disease Control and Prevention, Atlanta, GA

L. Hannah Gould, PhD, MS, Centers for Disease Control and Prevention, Atlanta, GA

Carolyn Gould, MD, MSCR, Centers for Disease Control and Prevention, Atlanta, GA

Kim Y. Green, PhD, National Institutes of Health, Bethesda, MD

Patricia M. Griffin, MD, Centers for Disease Control and Prevention, Atlanta, GA

Kevin Griffith, MD, MPH, Centers for Disease Control and Prevention, Fort Collins, CO

Charles F. Grose, MD, University of Iowa, Iowa City, IA

Marta Guerra, DVM, MPH, PhD, Centers for Disease Control and Prevention, Atlanta, GA

Penina Haber, MPH, Centers for Disease Control and Prevention, Atlanta, GA

Jeffrey Hageman, MHS, Centers for Disease Control and Prevention, Atlanta, GA

Aron J. Hall, DVM, MSPH, DACVPM, Centers for Disease Control and Prevention, Atlanta, GA

Caroline B. Hall, MD, University of Rochester School of Medicine and Dentistry, Rochester, NY

Scott A. Halperin, MD, Dalhousie University, Halifax, Nova Scotia, Canada

Lee Hampton, MD, MSc, Centers for Disease Control and Prevention, Atlanta, GA

Julie R. Harris, PhD, MPH, Centers for Disease Control and Prevention, Atlanta, GA

Christopher J. Harrison, MD, Children's Mercy Hospital and Clinics, Kansas City, MO

C. Mary Healy, MD, Baylor College of Medicine, Houston, TX

Thomas W. Hennessy, MD, MPH, Centers for Disease Control and Prevention, Anchorage, AK

Barbara L. Herwaldt, MD, MPH, Centers for Disease Control and Prevention, Atlanta, GA

Beth Hibbs, RN, MPH, Centers for Disease Control and Prevention, Atlanta, GA

Sheila M. Hickey, MD, University of New Mexico, Albuquerque, NM

Lauri A. Hicks, DO, Centers for Disease Control and Prevention, Atlanta, GA

Michele C. Hlavsa, RN, MPH, Centers for Disease Control and Prevention, Atlanta, GA

Scott D. Holmberg, MD, MPH, Centers for Disease Control and Prevention, Atlanta, GA

Karen W. Hoover, MD, MPH, Centers for Disease Control and Prevention, Atlanta, GA

Peter J. Hotez, MD, PhD, Baylor College of Medicine, Houston, TX

Christine Hughes, MPH, Centers for Disease Control and Prevention, Atlanta, GA

Dmitri E. Iarikov, MD, PhD, Food and Drug Administration, Silver Spring, MD

Joseph P. Icenogle, PhD, Centers for Disease Control and Prevention, Atlanta, GA

Martha Iwamoto, MD, MPH, Centers for Disease Control and Prevention, Atlanta, GA

Mary Anne Jackson, MD, University of Missouri-Kansas City School of Medicine, Kansas City, MO

Ruth A. Jajosky, DMD, MPH, Centers for Disease Control and Prevention, Atlanta, GA

John A. Jereb, MD, Centers for Disease Control and Prevention, Atlanta, GA

Robert Jerris, PhD, Children's Healthcare of Atlanta, Atlanta, GA

Robert E. Johnson, MD, MPH, Centers for Disease Control and Prevention, Atlanta, GA

Jeffrey L. Jones, MD, MPH, Centers for Disease Control and Prevention, Atlanta, GA

John M. Kelso, MD, Scripps Clinic, San Diego, CA

Gilbert J. Kersh, PhD, Centers for Disease Control, Atlanta, GA
David L. Kettl, MD, Food and Drug Administration, Silver Spring, MD
Henry L. Keyserling, MD, Emory University School of Medicine, Atlanta, GA
Tina Khoie, MD, MPH, Food and Drug Administration, Rockville, MD
Peter W. Kim, MD, MS, Food and Drug Administration, Silver Spring, MD
David W. Kimberlin, MD, University of Alabama at Birmingham, Birmingham, AL
Robert D. Kirkcaldy, MD, MPH, Centers for Disease Control and Prevention,
    Atlanta, GA
Martin B. Kleiman, MD, Indiana University School of Medicine, Indianapolis,
    Indianapolis, IN
Keith P. Klugman, MD, PhD, Emory University/Rollins School of Public Health,
    Atlanta, GA
Emilia Koumans, MD, MPH, Centers for Disease Control and Prevention, Atlanta, GA
Athena P. Kourtis, MD, PhD, MPH, Centers for Disease Control and Prevention,
    Atlanta, GA
Phyllis E. Kozarsky, MD, Centers for Disease Control and Prevention, Atlanta, GA
Philip R. Krause, MD, Food and Drug Administration, Bethesda, MD
Andrew T. Kroger, MD, MPH, Centers for Disease Control and Prevention, Atlanta, GA
Matthew J. Kuehnert, MD, Centers for Disease Control and Prevention, Atlanta, GA
David T. Kuhar, MD, Centers for Disease Control and Prevention, Atlanta, GA
Preeta K. Kutty, MD, MPH, Centers for Disease Control and Prevention, Atlanta, GA
Nicole M. Le Saux, MD, FRCPC, University of Ottawa, Ottawa, Canada
John A. D. Leake, MD, MPH, Rady Children's Hospital San Diego/University of
    California San Diego, San Diego, CA
Lucia H. Lee, MD, Food and Drug Administration, Rockville, MD
Mark Lehman, DVM, MS, MPH, Centers for Disease Control and Prevention,
    Atlanta, GA
Zanie C. Leroy, MD, MPH, Centers for Disease Control and Prevention, Atlanta, GA
Myron M. Levine, MD, DTPH, Center for Vaccine Development, University of
    Maryland School of Medicine, Baltimore, MD
Linda L. Lewis, MD, Food and Drug Administration, Silver Spring, MD
Jennifer L. Liang, DVM, MPVM, Centers for Disease Control and Prevention,
    Atlanta, GA
Sue Lim, MD, Food and Drug Administration, Silver Spring, MD
Jill A. Lindstrom, MD, Food and Drug Administration, Silver Spring, MD
Mark N. Lobato, MD, Centers for Disease Control and Prevention, Hartford, CT
Anagha Loharikar, MD, Centers for Disease Control and Prevention, Atlanta, GA
Sarah S. Long, MD, Drexel University College; St Christopher Hospital for Children,
    Section of Infectious Diseases, Philadelphia, PA
Benjamin A. Lopman, PhD, MSc, Centers for Disease Control and Prevention,
    Atlanta, GA
Benjamin D. Lorenz, MD, Food and Drug Administration, Silver Spring, MD
Taranisia MacCannell, PhD, Centers for Disease Control and Prevention, Atlanta, GA
Adam MacNeil, PhD, MPH, Centers for Disease Control and Prevention, Atlanta, GA
Jessica MacNeil, MPH, Centers for Disease Control and Prevention, Atlanta, GA
Yvonne A. Maldonado, MD, Stanford University, Stanford, CA
Nina Marano, DVM MPH, Centers for Disease Control and Prevention, Atlanta, GA

Harold Margolis, MD, Centers for Disease Control and Prevention, San Juan,
     Puerto Rico
Paulina E. Mariki, MD, Food and Drug Administration, Rockville, MD
Mona Marin, MD, Centers for Disease Control and Prevention, Atlanta, GA
Lauri E. Markowitz, MD, Centers for Disease Control and Prevention, Atlanta, GA
Els Mathieu, MD, MPH, Centers for Disease Control and Prevention, Atlanta, GA
Gerald H. Mazurek, MD, Centers for Disease Control and Prevention, Atlanta, GA
Anne E. McCarthy, MD, Ottawa Hospital, Division of Infectious Diseases, Ottawa,
     Ontario, Canada
Shasta D. McClenahan, PhD, Food and Drug Administration, Bethesda, MD
Linda J. McKibben, MD, DrPH, MPH, Food and Drug Administration, Rockville, MD
Huong McLean, PhD, MPH, Centers for Disease Control and Prevention, Atlanta, GA
Julia A. McMillan, MD, Johns Hopkins University School of Medicine, Baltimore, MD
Meredith L. McMorrow, MD, MPH, Centers for Disease Control and Prevention,
     Atlanta, GA
Jennifer McQuiston, DVM, MS, Centers for Disease Control and Prevention,
     Atlanta, GA
Paul Mead, MD, MPH, Centers for Disease Control and Prevention, Fort Collins, CO
Felicita Medalla, MD, MS, Centers for Disease Control and Prevention, Atlanta, GA
H. Cody Meissner, MD, Tufts Medical Center and Tufts University School of Medicine,
     Boston, MA
Heather J. Menzies, MD, MPH, Centers for Disease Control and Prevention, Atlanta, GA
Nancy Messonnier, MD, Centers for Disease Control and Prevention, Atlanta, GA
Joette M. Meyer, PharmD, Food and Drug Administration, Silver Spring, MD
Marian G. Michaels, MD, MPH, University of Pittsburgh School of Medicine,
     Department of Pediatrics, Pittsburgh, PA
Elaine R. Miller, BSN, MPH, Centers for Disease Control and Prevention, Atlanta, GA
Eric Mintz, MD, MPH, Centers for Disease Control and Prevention, Atlanta, GA
John F. Modlin, MD, Dartmouth Medical School, Lebanon, NH
Rajal K. Mody, MD, MPH, Centers for Disease Control and Prevention, Atlanta, GA
Nasim R. Moledina, MD, Food and Drug Administration, Silver Spring, MD
Susan P. Montgomery, DVM, MPH, Centers for Disease Control and Prevention,
     Atlanta, GA
Jose G. Montoya, MD, Stanford University School of Medicine, Palo Alto, CA
Anne Moore, MD, PhD, Centers for Disease Control and Prevention, Atlanta, GA
Matthew Moore, MD, MPH, Centers for Disease Control and Prevention, Atlanta, GA
Dennis L. Murray, MD, Medical College of Georgia, Augusta, GA
Oidda I. Museru, MSN, MPH, Centers for Disease Control and Prevention, Atlanta, GA
Sumathi Nambiar, MD, MPH, Food and Drug Administration, Silver Spring, MD
Santosh Nanda, DVM, PhD, Food and Drug Administration, Rockville, MD
Roger S. Nasci, PhD, Centers for Disease Control and Prevention, Fort Collins, CO
James P. Nataro, MD, PhD, MBA, School of Medicine at the University of Virginia,
     Division of Infectious Disease and Tropical Pediatrics, Charlottesville, VA
Eileen Navarro, MD, Food and Drug Administration, Silver Spring, MD
George E. Nelson, MD, Centers for Disease Control and Prevention, Atlanta, GA
Steven R. Nesheim, MD, Centers for Disease Control and Prevention, Atlanta, GA

William L. Nicholson, PhD, MS, Centers for Disease Control and Prevention, Atlanta, GA

Cynthia J. Nolletti, MD, Food and Drug Administration, Rockville, MD

Ryan T. Novak, MSc, PhD, Centers for Disease Control and Prevention, Atlanta, GA

Steve Oberste, PhD, Centers for Disease Control and Prevention, Atlanta, GA

Paul A. Offit, MD, The Children's Hospital of Philadelphia, Philadelphia, PA

Gloria E. Oramsionwu, MD, MPH, Centers for Disease Control and Prevention, Atlanta, GA

Walter A. Orenstein, MD, Emory University School of Medicine, Atlanta, GA

Miguel G. O'Ryan, MD, Programa de Microbiologia, ICBM, Facultad de Medicina, Universidad de Chile, Santiago, Chile

Elizabeth M. O'Shaughnessy, MB, BCh, Food and Drug Administration, Silver Spring, MD

Christopher D. Paddock, MD, MPHTM, Centers for Disease Control and Prevention, Atlanta, GA

Umesh Parashar, MBBS, MPH, Centers for Disease Control and Prevention, Atlanta, GA

Monica Parise, MD, Centers for Disease Control and Prevention, Atlanta, GA

Benjamin J. Park, MD, Centers for Disease Control and Prevention, Atlanta, GA

Sarah K. Parker, MD, University of Colorado School of Medicine, Aurora, CO

Amy Parker Fiebelkorn, MSN, MPH, Centers for Disease Control and Prevention, Atlanta, GA

Manish Patel, MD, MSc, Centers for Disease Control and Prevention, Atlanta, GA

Thomas Peterman, MD, MSc, Centers for Disease Control and Prevention, Atlanta, GA

Brett W. Petersen, MD, MPH, Centers for Disease Control and Prevention, Atlanta, GA

Larry K. Pickering, MD, Centers for Disease Control and Prevention, Atlanta, GA

Emily Piercefield, MD, DVM, MPH, Centers for Disease Control and Prevention, Atlanta, GA

Joseph Piesman, DSc, Centers for Disease Control and Prevention, Fort Collins, CO

Andreas Pikis, MD, Food and Drug Administration, Silver Spring, MD

Ariel R. Porcalla, MD, MPH, Food and Drug Administration, Silver Spring, MD

Susan M. Poutanen, MD, MPH, FRCPC, Mount Sinai Hospital, Toronto, ON, Canada

Dwight A. Powell, MD, The Ohio State University College of Medicine and Nationwide Children's Hospital, Columbus, OH

R. Douglas Pratt, MD, Food and Drug Administration, Kensington, MD

Charles G. Prober, MD, Stanford School of Medicine, Stanford, CA

Conrad P. Quinn, PhD, Centers for Disease Control and Prevention, Atlanta, GA

Octavio Ramilo, MD, The Ohio State University and Nationwide Children's Hospital, Columbus, OH

Anuja Rastogi, MD, MHS, Food and Drug Administration, Rockville, MD

Jennifer S. Read, MD, National Institutes of Health, Rockville, MD

Joanna Regan, MD, MPH, Centers for Disease Control and Prevention, Atlanta, GA

Neil G. Rellosa, MD, Food and Drug Administration, Silver Spring, MD

Frank O. Richards, Jr, MD, The Carter Center, Atlanta, GA

Jeffrey N. Roberts, MD, Food and Drug Administration, Rockville, MD

Joan Robinson, MD, Canadian Paediatric Society, Edmonton, Alberta, Canada

Lance E. Rodewald, MD, Centers for Disease Control and Prevention, Atlanta, GA

Pierre E. Rollin, MD, Centers for Disease Control and Prevention, Atlanta, GA

Lisa Rotz, MD, Centers for Disease Control and Prevention, Atlanta, GA

Monika Roy, MD, Centers for Disease Control and Prevention, Atlanta, GA

Sharon Roy, MD, MPH, Centers for Disease Control and Prevention, Atlanta, GA

Steven A. Rubin, PhD, Food and Drug Administration, Bethesda, MD

Lorry G. Rubin, MD, Schneider Children's Hospital of the North Shore-Long Island
  Jewish Health System, Albert Einstein College of Medicine, New Hyde Park, NY

Charles Rupprecht, VMD, PhD, MS, Centers for Disease Control and Prevention,
  Atlanta, GA

Hugh A. Sampson, MD, Mount Sinai School of Medicine, New York, NY

Pablo J. Sanchez, MD, University of Texas Southwestern Medical Center, Dallas, TX

Jason B. Sauberan, PharmD, University of California San Diego Medical Center, San
  Diego, CA

Mark H. Sawyer, MD, University of California San Diego School of Medicine, Rady
  Children's Hospital San Diego, San Diego, CA

Melissa Schaefer, MD, Centers for Disease Control and Prevention, Atlanta, GA

D. Scott Schmid, PhD, MS, Centers for Disease Control and Prevention, Atlanta, GA

Eileen Schneider, MD, MPH, Centers for Disease Control and Prevention, Atlanta, GA

Lawrence B. Schonberger, MD, MPH, Centers for Disease Control and Prevention,
  Atlanta, GA

Gordon E. Schutze, MD, Baylor College of Medicine, Houston, TX

Ann T. Schwartz, MD, Food and Drug Administration, Rockville, MD

Steven M. Schwarz, MD, Children's Hospital at Downstate, Brooklyn, NY

David M. Scollard, MD, PhD, National Hansen's Disease Programs, Health Resources
  and Services Administration, Baton Rouge, LA

Dorothy E. Scott, MD, Food and Drug Administration, Bethesda, MD

James Sejvar, MD, Centers for Disease Control and Prevention, Atlanta, GA

Jane F. Seward, MBBS, MPH, Centers for Disease Control and Prevention, Atlanta, GA

Sean V. Shadomy, DVM, MPH, Centers for Disease Control and Prevention, Atlanta, GA

Hala H. Shamsuddin, MD, Food and Drug Administration, Silver Spring, MD

Andi L. Shane, MD, MPH, MSc, Emory University School of Medicine, Atlanta, GA

Alan M. Shapiro, MD, PhD, Food and Drug Administration, Silver Spring, MD

Craig A. Shapiro, MD, Emory University School of Medicine, Atlanta, GA

Eugene D. Shapiro, MD, Yale University Department of Pediatrics, New Haven, CT

Umid M. Sharapov, MD, MSc, Centers for Disease Control and Prevention, Atlanta, GA

Devindra Sharma, MSN, MPH, Centers for Disease Control and Prevention,
  Atlanta, GA

Sharmila Shetty, MD, Centers for Disease Control and Prevention, Atlanta, GA

Tom Shimabukuro, MD, MPH, MBA, Centers for Disease Control and Prevention,
  Atlanta, GA

Tim R. Shope, MD, MPH, Naval Medical Center Portsmouth, Portsmouth, VA

Stanford T. Shulman, MD, Northwestern University, Feinberg School of Medicine,
  Children's Memorial Hospital-Chicago, Chicago, IL

Benjamin J. Silk, PhD, MPH, Centers for Disease Control and Prevention, Atlanta, GA

Barbara Slade, MD, MS, Centers for Disease Control and Prevention, Decatur, GA

Theresa L. Smith, MD, MPH, Centers for Disease Control and Prevention, Atlanta, GA

Thomas D. Smith, MD, Food and Drug Administration, Silver Spring, MD

Paul W. Spearman, MD, Emory University and Children's Healthcare of Atlanta,
  Atlanta, GA
Arjun Srinivasan, MD, Centers for Disease Control and Prevention, Atlanta, GA
Mary Allen Staat, MD, MPH, Cincinnati Children's Hospital Medical Center,
  Cincinnati, OH
J. Erin Staples, MD, PhD, Centers for Disease Control and Prevention, Fort Collins, CO
Jeffrey R. Starke, MD, Baylor College of Medicine, Houston, TX
William J. Steinbach, MD, Duke University, Durham, NC
John L. Sullivan, MD, University of Massachusetts Medical School, North Worcester, MA
Anil G. Suryaprasad, MD, Centers for Disease Control and Prevention, Atlanta, GA
Jack T. Swanson, MD, McFarland Clinic, Ames, IA
Deborah F. Talkington, PhD, MS, Centers for Disease Control and Prevention,
  Atlanta, GA
Tina Q. Tan, MD, Children's Memorial Hospital, Chicago, IL
Shuang Tang, PhD, Food and Drug Administration, Bethesda, MD
Jacqueline E. Tate, PhD, MSPH, Centers for Disease Control and Prevention,
  Atlanta, GA
Eyasu Teshale, MD, Centers for Disease Control and Prevention, Atlanta, GA
Rosemary Tiernan, MD, MPH, Food and Drug Administration, Rockville, MD
Tejpratap Tiwari, MD, Centers for Disease Control and Prevention Atlanta, GA
Kay M. Tomashek, MD, MPH, DTM&H, Centers for Disease Control and Prevention,
  San Juan, Puerto Rico
Suxiang Tong, PhD, Centers for Disease Control and Prevention, Atlanta, GA
Rita Traxler, MHS, Centers for Disease Control and Prevention, Atlanta, GA
James R. Treat, MD, Children's Hospital of Philadelphia, Philadelphia, PA
Christine Uhlenhaut, PhD, Federal Information Centre for Biological Security,
  Berlin, Germany
Elizabeth R. Unger, PhD, MD, Centers for Disease Control and Prevention, Atlanta, GA
Gary A. Urquhart, MPH, Centers for Disease Control and Prevention, Atlanta, Ga
Julienne M. Vaillancourt, RPh, MPH, Food and Drug Administration, Rockville, MD
Chris Van Beneden, MD, MPH, Centers for Disease Control and Prevention,
  Atlanta, GA
John A. Vanchiere, MD, PhD, Louisiana State University, Health Sciences Center,
  Shreveport, LA
Tafadzwa S. Vargas-Kasambira, MD, MPH, Food and Drug Administration, Silver
  Spring, MD
Claudia Vellozzi, MD, MPH, Centers for Disease Control and Prevention, Atlanta, GA
Jennifer R. Verani, MD, MPH, Centers for Disease Control and Prevention, Atlanta, GA
Govinda S. Visvesvara, PhD, Centers for Disease Control and Prevention, Atlanta, GA
Prabha Viswanathan, MD, Food and Drug Administration, Silver Spring, MD
Debra Wagner, MSPH, Centers for Disease Control and Prevention, Atlanta, GA
Gregory S. Wallace, MD, MS, MPH, Centers for Disease Control and Prevention,
  Atlanta, GA
Elaine Wang, MD, CM, MS, University of Toronto, The Hospital for Sick Children,
  Ridgefield, CT
Michelle Weinberg, MD, MPH, Centers for Disease Control and Prevention, Atlanta, GA
Richard J. Whitley, MD, The University of Alabama at Birmingham, Birmingham, AL

Patricia Wilkins, PhD, Centers for Disease Control and Prevention, Atlanta, GA

Rodney E. Willoughby, Jr, MD, Medical College of Wisconsin, Milwaukee, WI

Emily Jane Woo, MD, MPH, Food and Drug Administration, Rockville, MD

Kimberly A. Workowski, MD, Centers for Disease Control and Prevention, Atlanta, GA

Alexandra S. Worobec, MD, Centers for Disease Control and Prevention, Rockville, MD

Fujie Xu, MD, PhD, Centers for Disease Control and Prevention, Atlanta, GA

Albert C. Yan, MD, Children's Hospital of Philadelphia, University of Pennsylvania
  School of Medicine, Philadelphia, PA

Sixun Yang, MD, PhD, Food and Drug Administration, Rockville, MD

Yuliya I. Yasinskaya, MD, Food and Drug Administration, Silver Spring, MD

Jonathan Yoder, MSW, MPH, Centers for Disease Control and Prevention, Atlanta, GA

Emily C. Zielinski-Gutierrez, DrPH, MPH, Centers for Disease Control and Prevention,
  Fort Collins, CO

Committee on Infectious Diseases, 2010–2012

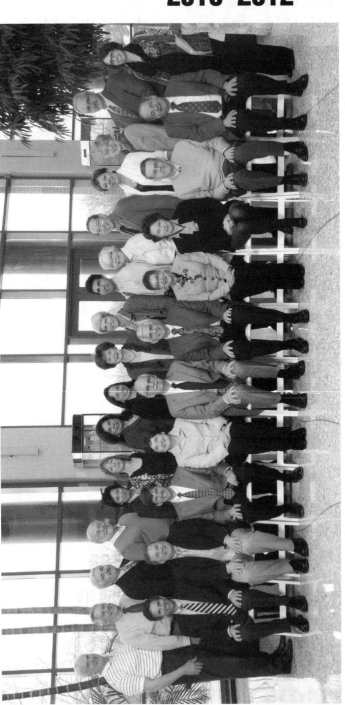

SEATED, LEFT TO RIGHT: Lorry G. Rubin, Henry H. Bernstein, David W. Kimberlin, Carol J. Baker, Larry K. Pickering, Michael T. Brady, Carrie L. Byington, Sarah S. Long, H. Cody Meissner, Harry L. Keyserling

STANDING, LEFT TO RIGHT: Rodney E. Willoughby, Jr, Jack T. Swanson, Richard L. Gorman, Joseph A. Bocchini, Jr, Lucia Lee, Joan Robinson, Yvonne A. Maldonado, Tina Q. Tan, Mary P. Glode, Jane Seward, Marc A. Fischer, Margaret C. Fisher, Walter A. Orenstein, Mary Anne Jackson, Kathryn M. Edwards, Gordon E. Schutze, Jennifer Frantz

NOT PICTURED: Beth Bell, John S. Bradley, Robert Bortolussi, H. Dele Davies, Richard D. Clover, Bruce Gellin, Dennis L. Murray, Jennifer S. Read, Marco Aurelio Palazzi Safadi, Geoffrey Simon, Jeffrey R. Starke, Theoklis Zaoutis

2012 *Red Book* Dedication For Samuel L. Katz, MD, FAAP

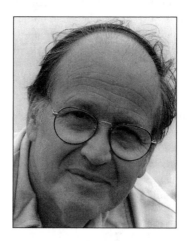

This edition of the *Red Book* is dedicated to Samuel L. Katz, MD, FAAP, who served on the American Academy of Pediatrics (AAP) Committee on Infectious Diseases for 12 years and who was chairman of this committee from 1969 to1976.

Sam began his career in Boston where he trained in pediatrics at Children's Hospital and where he was a research fellow in virology and infectious diseases with Nobel Laureate John F. Enders. He worked alongside Dr. Enders for 12 years, and together, they developed the attenuated measles virus vaccine, which was licensed in the United States in 1963 and which has resulted in a dramatic decline in the incidence of measles. Once the measles vaccine was proven to be effective domestically, Sam was eager to see its success taken globally, and currently it is used worldwide. By 2011, more than a billion children had received the measles vaccine as a key part of the initiative to eliminate measles worldwide. In addition to his investigations of measles, Sam has been involved in studies of smallpox, polio, rubella, influenza, pertussis, and *Haemophilus influenzae* type b vaccines. He is a giant in the field of immunizations and has served on virtually every committee or panel in the United States and internationally dealing with vaccine development, licensure, and policy. His wisdom and advice are valued by all.

Sam served as Chairman of the Department of Pediatrics at Duke University School of Medicine from 1968 to 1990. He was the Wilburt C. Davison Professor of Pediatrics from 1972 to 1997, and he currently is the Wilburt C. Davison Professor and Chair of Pediatrics Emeritus. During his time at Duke, Sam has inspired countless medical students, pediatric residents, and infectious diseases fellows with his passion for clinical excellence, knowledge both in the lecture hall and at the bedside, compassion for ill children, and wisdom as mentor and counselor. He has an enviable memory, both for medical facts and for names and attributes of his generation of "medical children," and he often is seen at meetings giving handshakes, hugs, smiles, and personal greetings. He is the essence of a teacher and mentor and is a consummate professional.

Sam has received too many honors and awards to list in full, but several notable accolades include the Jacobi Award from the AAP and American Medical Association, the first St. Geme Award from the Federation of Pediatric Organizations, the Bristol Award and a Society Citation from the Infectious Diseases Society of America, the Howland Award from the American Pediatric Society, the Gold Medal from the Albert Sabin Vaccine Institute, the Alfred I. duPont Award for Excellence in Children's Health Care, and the Hilleman Award from the American Society for Microbiology. In addition, he has been elected to the Institute of Medicine of the National Academy of Sciences.

Sam has shared his personal and medical pursuits with his wife of many years, Dr. Catherine Wilfert, an internationally renowned pediatric infectious disease physician who has devoted the past decade of her life to improving the care of HIV-infected children in Africa. Sam and Cathy raised 8 sons and daughters and now share the joys of spending time with their many grandchildren. Sam is devoted to his family, his students, his patients, and his friends and is a true gentleman and scholar.

Dr. Sam Katz has left a huge mark on the field of pediatrics and vaccinology and is a giant of 20th century medicine. This edition of the *Red Book* is dedicated to Sam to thank him on behalf of all the children and pediatricians whose lives are better through his contributions.

PREVIOUS RED BOOK DEDICATION RECIPIENTS:
2009 Ralph Feigin, MD
2006 Caroline Breese Hall, MD
2003 Georges Peter, MD
2000 Edgar O. Ledbetter, MD
1997 Georges Peter, MD

Preface

The *Red Book* is a unique source of information on immunizations and infectious diseases for practitioners. The practice of pediatric infectious diseases is changing rapidly. With the limited time available to the practitioner, the ability to quickly obtain up-to-date information about new vaccines and vaccine recommendations, emerging infectious diseases, new diagnostic modalities, and treatment recommendations is essential. The Committee on Infectious Diseases of the American Academy of Pediatrics (AAP) and the editors of the *Red Book* are dedicated to providing the most current and accurate information available in the concise, practical format for which the *Red Book* is known.

The value of the *Red Book* is further enhanced by the *Red Book* Online (**www.aapredbook.org**), where statements and recommendations from the AAP and other important information that becomes available during the 3 years between editions of Red Book are provided. Another important resource is the visual library of *Red Book* Online, which has been updated and expanded to include more images of infectious diseases, examples of classic radiologic and other findings, and recent epidemiology of infectious diseases.

The Committee on Infectious Diseases relies on information and advice from many experts, as evidenced by the lengthy list of contributors to *Red Book*. We especially are indebted to the many contributors from other AAP committees, the Centers for Disease Control and Prevention, the Food and Drug Administration, the National Institutes of Health, the Canadian Paediatric Society, the World Health Organization, and many other organizations and individuals who have made this edition possible. In addition, suggestions made by individual AAP members to improve the presentation of information on specific issues and on topic selection have been incorporated into this edition.

Most important to the success of this edition is the dedication and work of the editors, whose commitment to excellence is unparalleled. Under the able leadership of Larry K. Pickering, MD, editor, with associate editors Carol J. Baker, MD, David W. Kimberlin, MD, and Sarah S. Long, MD, this new edition was made possible. We also are indebted to Edgar O. Ledbetter, MD, and H. Cody Meissner, MD, for their invaluable and untiring efforts to gather and organize the slide materials that make up the visual library of *Red Book* Online and are part of the electronic versions of the *Red Book*, and to Henry H. Bernstein, MD, for his continuous efforts to maintain up-to-date content as editor of *Red Book* Online.

As noted in previous editions of the *Red Book*, some omissions and errors are inevitable in a book of this type. We ask that AAP members continue to assist the committee actively by suggesting specific ways to improve the quality of future editions.

Michael T. Brady, MD, FAAP
Chairperson, Committee on Infectious Diseases

Introduction

The Committee on Infectious Diseases (COID) of the American Academy of Pediatrics (AAP) is responsible for developing and revising guidelines for the AAP for control of infectious diseases in infants, children, and adolescents. Every 3 years, the committee issues the *Red Book: Report of the Committee on Infectious Diseases*, which contains a composite summary of current AAP recommendations on various aspects of infectious diseases, including updated vaccine recommendations for the most recent US Food and Drug Administration (FDA)-licensed vaccines for infants, children, and adolescents. These recommendations represent a consensus of opinions developed by members of the COID in conjunction with liaison representatives from the Centers for Disease Control and Prevention (CDC), the FDA, the National Institutes of Health, the National Vaccine Program Office, the Canadian Paediatric Society, the American Thoracic Society, *Red Book* consultants, and numerous collaborators. All COID recommendations become AAP policy following approval by the AAP Board of Directors. This edition of the *Red Book* is based on information available as of February 2012. Policy updates between editions will be posted on *Red Book* Online (**www.aapredbook.org**). Information is provided in hard copy and as digital versions, which can be downloaded to mobile devices and contain links to supplemental information, including visual images, graphs, maps, and tables.

The COID endeavors to provide current, relevant, science-based recommendations for prevention and management of infectious diseases in infants, children, and adolescents. Seemingly unanswerable scientific questions, the complexity of medical practice, ongoing innovative technology, continuous new information, and inevitable differences of opinion among experts all are addressed when preparing the *Red Book*. In some cases, other committees and experts may differ in their interpretation of data and resulting recommendations. In certain instances, no single recommendation can be made because several options for management are equally acceptable.

In making recommendations in the *Red Book*, the committee acknowledges differences in viewpoints by use of the phrases "most experts recommend..." and "some experts recommend..." Both phrases indicate valid recommendations, but the first phrase signifies more agreement and support among the experts. Inevitably in clinical practice, questions arise that cannot be answered easily on the basis of currently available data. When this happens, the COID still provides guidelines and information that, coupled with clinical judgment, will facilitate well-reasoned, clinically relevant decisions. For many conditions, an expert in the field of infectious diseases should be consulted. The COID appreciates receiving questions, different perspectives, and alternative recommendations that will improve future editions of the *Red Book*. Through this process of lifelong learning, the committee seeks to provide a practical and authoritative guide for physicians and other health care professionals in their care of infants, children, and adolescents.

To aid physicians and other health care professionals in assimilating current changes in recommendations in the *Red Book*, a list of major changes has been compiled (see Summary of Major Changes, p XXXI). However, this list only begins to cover the many in-depth changes that have occurred in each chapter and section. Therefore, health care professionals should consult individual chapters and sections of the book for current guidelines. New data inevitably will outdate current information in the *Red Book*, so health care professionals need to remain informed of ongoing developments and resulting changes in recommendations. Throughout the Red Book, Web site addresses enable rapid access to new information. In order to ensure widespread dissemination between editions, the AAP publishes new recommendations from the COID in *Pediatrics* and in *AAP News*. In addition, all AAP policies concerning infectious diseases published between editions of the Red Book will be posted on *Red Book* Online (**www.aapredbook.org**). Use of *Red Book* Online enables AAP members to enroll to receive e-mail alerts automatically when new information becomes available.

When using antimicrobial agents, physicians should review the package inserts (product labels) prepared by manufacturers, particularly for information concerning contraindications and adverse events. No attempt has been made in the *Red Book* to provide this information, because it is available readily in the *Physicians' Desk Reference*, online (**www.pdr.net**), and in package inserts. As in previous editions of the *Red Book*, recommended dosage schedules for antimicrobial agents are provided (see Section 4, Antimicrobial Agents and Related Therapy) and may differ from those of the manufacturer as provided in the package insert. Physicians also should be familiar with information in the package insert for vaccine use as licensed by the FDA (which also may differ from COID and ACIP/CDC recommendations for use) and immune globulins as well as recommendations of other committees (see Sources of Vaccine Information, p 3), many of which are included in the *Red Book*.

This book could not have been prepared without the dedicated professional competence of many people. Jay Berkelhamer, MD, Joseph A. Bocchini, MD, and Ellen Buerk, MD, served as *Red Book* reviewers appointed by the AAP Board of Directors. H. Cody Meissner, MD, and Henry H. Bernstein, MD, led the charge in gathering and organizing the visual materials for the electronic versions of the *Red Book*. The AAP staff has been outstanding in its committed work and contributions, particularly Jennifer Frantz, manager, who served as the administrative director for the committee and coordinated preparation of the *Red Book;* Jennifer Shaw, senior medical copy editor, who improved every aspect of the *Red Book;* Barbara Drelicharz, division assistant; Peg Mulcahy, graphic designer; Jeff Mahony, Mark Grimes, and Mark Ruthman, who devoted hours of time to insert the visual images into the electronic version of the *Red Book*; and the staff of the Department of Marketing, all of whom make the *Red Book* Online and other *Red Book* products possible. Marc Fischer, MD, of the CDC, and R. Douglas Pratt, MD, and Lisa Lee, MD, of the FDA, devoted time and effort in providing significant input from their organizations. Special appreciation is given to Tanya Lennon, assistant to the editor, for her work, patience, and support. I am especially indebted to the associate editors Carol J. Baker, MD, Sarah S. Long, MD, and David W. Kimberlin, MD, for their expertise, tireless work, good humor, and immense contributions in their editorial and committee work. Members of the COID contributed countless hours and deserve appropriate recognition for their patience, dedication, revisions, and reviews. The COID appreciates the guidance and dedication of the past and current COID chairpersons, Joseph A. Bocchini, MD, and Michael Brady, MD, whose respective knowledge, dedication, insight, and leadership are reflected in the quality and productivity of the committee's work. I thank Mimi for always being there and for her patience, understanding, and never-ending support.

There are many other contributors whose professional work and commitment have been essential in the committee's preparation of the *Red Book*. Of special note is the person to whom this edition of the *Red Book* is dedicated, Samuel L. Katz, MD, an exceptional leader, a constant inspiration, and a good friend. Sam serves as a role model for all of us.

Larry K. Pickering, MD, FAAP
Editor

Table of Contents

SECTION 2
RECOMMENDATIONS FOR CARE OF CHILDREN
IN SPECIAL CIRCUMSTANCES

SECTION 3
SUMMARIES OF INFECTIOUS DISEASES

SECTION 4
ANTIMICROBIAL AGENTS AND RELATED THERAPY

SECTION 5
ANTIMICROBIAL PROPHYLAXIS

APPENDICES

Summary of Major Changes in the 2012 *Red Book*

MAJOR CHANGES: GENERAL

1. Throughout the *Red Book,* the number of Web sites where additional current and future information can be obtained has increased. All Web sites are in bold type for ease of reference, and all have been verified for accuracy and accessibility.
2. Direct links to visual images have been added throughout the electronic version of the *Red Book.* These include images of clinical manifestations, maps showing geographic locations of specific diseases, graphs and tables of disease rates, and microbiologic findings.
3. Reference to evidence-based policy recommendations from the American Academy of Pediatrics (AAP), the Advisory Committee on Immunization Practices (ACIP) of the Centers for Disease Control and Prevention (CDC), and other select professional organizations have been updated throughout the *Red Book.*
4. Standardized approaches to disease prevention through immunizations, antimicrobial prophylaxis, and infection-control practices have been updated throughout the *Red Book.*
5. Reference to use of tetracycline and fluoroquinolone agents in children has been standardized throughout the book, with reference to a standardized approach to use in children.
6. Policy updates released after publication of this edition of the *Red Book* will be posted on *Red Book* Online.
7. Appropriate chapters throughout the *Red Book* have been updated to be consistent with AAP and CDC 2012 vaccine recommendations, CDC sexually transmitted disease guidelines, CDC recommendations for immunization of health care personnel, drug recommendations from *Nelson's Pediatric Antimicrobial Therapy* and the *Handbook of Antimicrobial Therapy* from the *Medical Letter,* and recommendations for treatment and prevention of opportunistic infections among children infected with or exposed to human immunodeficiency virus (HIV) from the CDC, National Institutes of Health, and Infectious Diseases Society of America.
8. Several tables and figures have been added for ease of information retrieval.

SECTION 1. ACTIVE AND PASSIVE IMMUNIZATION

1. Table 1.1, showing baseline **20th century annual morbidity and current morbidity from vaccine-preventable diseases,** has been updated to include 2010 data.
2. A new Table (1.2), titled **Comparison of Prevaccine Era Estimated Annual Morbidity With Current Estimates of Vaccine-Preventable Diseases,** has been added. The table includes hepatitis A, hepatitis B, invasive pneumococcal disease, rotavirus hospitalizations, and varicella.
3. Web sites for access to Interactive Web-based **immunization schedulers** for children, adolescents, and adults have been added.

4. Table 1.5, **Vaccines Licensed for Immunization and Distribution in the United States and Routes of Administration,** has been updated to include indications for use of PCV13, MCV4, influenza, Tdap, HPV, JE vaccines, and rabies vaccines.

5. The **2012 childhood and adolescent immunization schedules** (Fig 1.1–1.3) have been added with a Web site for access to future childhood and adolescent immunization schedules.

6. Table 1.9, Suggested Intervals Between Immune Globulin Administration and Measles Immunization (MMR or MMRV), has been moved from the measles chapter to Section 1.

7. Information about the Health Information Technology for the Economic and Clinical Health Act (NITECH) has been added to the **Immunization Records of Physicians** section.

8. A summary of and reference to the **Institute of Medicine (IOM) Reviews of Adverse Events After Immunization** titled "Adverse Effects of Vaccines: Evidence and Causality" findings are provided. Eight vaccines covered by the Vaccine Injury Compensation Program were reviewed, using 158 causality conclusions.

9. **Vaccine Contraindications and Precautions.** Breastfeeding is a precaution to yellow fever vaccine administration.

10. The **Allergic Reactions to Egg Protein** section has been updated to state that trivalent inactivated influenza vaccine is well tolerated by nearly all recipients who have an egg allergy. Specific recommendations are provided in the Influenza chapter.

11. **Common Misconceptions About Immunizations.** The approach to vaccine-hesitant parents has been updated and Web sites where educational material that can be provided to parents have been added.

12. In the **Pregnancy** section, recommendations for immunization of pregnant women with influenza and Tdap vaccines have been updated. Other vaccines, including yellow fever vaccine, with potential use in pregnancy, are reviewed.

13. **Pregnancy.** Information on the varicella pregnancy registry and where to report instances of inadvertent immunization with a varicella/zoster-containing vaccine during pregnancy is provided. Information on 2 HPV vaccine registries for reporting inadvertent exposure to HPV vaccine during pregnancy is provided.

14. **Varicella postexposure prophylaxis.** Varicella-Zoster Immune Globulin or Immune Globulin Intravenous may be considered for certain people up to 10 days (previously 96 hours) after exposure to a person with varicella or zoster.

15. Table 1.16, **Immunization of Children and Adolescents With Primary and Secondary Immune Deficiencies,** has been updated to include new vaccine contraindications and recommendations. Two conditions, asplenia and chronic renal disease, have been added to the secondary immune deficiencies category.

16. The section on **Health Care Personnel (HCP)** was updated to include current ACIP immunization recommendations that might be indicated in certain circumstances for HCP and diseases for which immunization or documentation of immunity is recommended because of risks to HCP in their work settings for acquiring disease or transmitting to patients.

17. **Required or Recommended Travel Related-Related Immunizations.** A table of contraindications and precautions for use of yellow fever vaccine has been added. Recommendations for use of Japanese encephalitis virus vaccine have been updated to reflect availability of Japanese encephalitis Vero cell (JE-VC) vaccine, which was licensed in 2009 for people 17 years of age or older and is the only JE vaccine available in the United States.

18. A new section titled **Biologic Response Modifiers (BRMs) Used to Decrease Inflammation** provides recommendations to prevent infections in children receiving biologic response modifiers including tumor necrosis alpha inhibitors as well as recommendations for screening before therapy with a BRM is begun.

19. Table 1.11 has been updated to include bone marrow transplantation and chronic inflammatory demyelinating polyneuropathy as **Uses of Immune Globulin Intravenous (IGIV) for Which There is Approval by the US Food and Drug Administration.**

SECTION 2. RECOMMENDATIONS FOR CARE OF CHILDREN IN SPECIAL CLINICAL CIRCUMSTANCES

1. Table 2.1, **Bioterrorism Agents and Categories,** has been added to clarify the 3 categories into which potential bioterrorism agents are classified.

2. Table 2.2, **Emergency Contacts and Educational Resources,** has been updated to include new emergency contact and Web site information.

3. **Blood Safety.** Current blood screening procedures have been updated as have strategies implemented to further decrease the risk of transmission of infectious agents through blood and blood products. All blood donations are tested routinely for syphilis, human immunodeficiency virus, hepatitis C virus, hepatitis B virus, human T-lymphotropic virus types 1 and 2, West Nile virus, and Chagas disease, and selected donations are tested for other potential pathogens.

4. **Human Milk: Effect of Maternal Immunization.** Women who have not received recommended immunizations before or during pregnancy, especially Tdap and influenza, may be immunized postpartum regardless of lactation status.

5. In **Children in Out-of-Home Child Care,** updates to all vaccines in the recommended immunization schedule and how they have decreased disease rates in children attending child care have been added.

6. **School Health: Diseases Preventable by Routine Childhood Immunization.** Susceptible people exposed to measles, varicella, or hepatitis A may be protected if immunized within 72 hours (measles or varicella) or 14 days (hepatitis A) of exposure.

7. Respiratory hygiene/cough etiquette has been added to **Standard Precautions** and to Table 2.8.

8. **Strategies to Prevent Health Care-Associated Infections.** A section has been added and includes practice improvements used to prevent health care-associated infections. An approach referred to as a "bundle" implements several multidisciplinary practice improvements simultaneously. A "bundled" approach to prevention of central line-associated bloodstream infections is highlighted.

9. **Occupational Health.** Guidelines from the Centers for Disease Control and Prevention for immunization of health care personnel are provided in which updates to hepatitis B, influenza, measles-mumps-rubella, pertussis, varicella, and meningococcal vaccine recommendations are provided.

10. Immunization recommendations for health care personnel have been updated in the **Infection Control and Prevention in Ambulatory Settings** section, as has guidance regarding training, avoiding reinserting a needle into a medication vial, and avoiding use of single-dose vials for multiple patients.

11. Recommendations for management of sexually transmitted infections have been updated in the **Sexually Transmitted Infections in Adolescents and Children** section to include expanded diagnostic evaluation for cervicitis and trichomoniasis, new treatment recommendations for bacterial vaginosis and genital warts, and the increasing prevalence of antimicrobial-resistant Neisseria gonorrhoeae.

12. Recommendations for use of HPV vaccine to include males as well as females from 9 through 26 years of age have been updated in the **Sexually Transmitted Infections in Adolescents and Children** section.

13. Table 2.16, **Screening Tests for Infectious Diseases,** has been updated to include current recommendations for hepatitis C and lymphatic filariasis in children from countries with endemic infection.

14. **Prevention of Illnesses Associated With Recreational Water Use** has been updated to include current CDC data on etiologic agents, adequacy of regulations, public awareness, and public health priorities. Of reported outbreaks, 60% involved the intestinal tract, 18% were dermatologic, and 18% involved the respiratory tract.

15. Table 2.19, **Antimicrobial Agents for Human or Animal Bite Wounds,** has been modified to clarify antimicrobial use depending on the source of the bite.

16. Recommendations for prevention of diseases transmitted by animals have been updated in the **Diseases Transmitted by Animals (Zoonoses)** section to include a mnemonic for appropriate pet selection from the Black Pine Animal Park.

SECTION 3. SUMMARIES OF INFECTIOUS DISEASES

1. **Adenovirus Infections.** A live, oral adenovirus vaccine for types 4 and 7 was approved in 2011 by the US Food and Drug Administration (FDA) for prevention of febrile acute respiratory tract disease and is being used in military personnel.

2. **Arboviruses.** New recommendations for use of Vero cell culture-derived Japanese encephalitis vaccine (JE-VC) are included. JE-VC was licensed in 2009 for use in people $\geq$17 years of age. Information about clinical trials in children is provided.

3. **Human Calicivirus Infections (Norovirus and Sapovirus).** Updates on epidemic strains, outbreaks in specific situations, guidelines for outbreak management and disease prevention, and diagnostic testing have been added.

4. **Candidiasis.** Guidelines for management of candidiasis from the Infectious Diseases Society of America and chemoprophylaxis with fluconazole for infants with birth weights of $\leq$1000 g have been added.

5. **Clostridial Infections—Botulism and Infant Botulism.** In 2010, equine-derived heptavalent botulinum antitoxin (HBAT), available through the CDC, became the only botulinum toxin available in the United States for treatment of noninfant forms of botulism. HBAT contains antitoxin against of 7 (A-G) botulinum toxin types. Human-derived Baby BIG is licensed for treatment of infant botulism.

6. ***Clostridium difficile.*** Diagnosis and treatment have been updated. The AAP Committee on Infectious Diseases is preparing guidelines for *C difficile* infection in children.

7. **Coronaviruses, Including SARS.** This chapter was rewritten extensively to update epidemiology.

8. **Cyclosporiasis.** Epidemiology and diagnosis have been updated, including the role of travel in acquisition of this organism and the role in foodborne and water-borne outbreaks.

9. **Cytomegalovirus Infection.** A positive polymerase chain reaction (PCR) assay result from a neonatal dried blood spot confirms congenital infection, but because of low sensitivity, a negative PCR assay result does not rule out congenital infection. Valganciclovir administered orally to young infants provides a therapeutic option for treatment of infants with symptomatic congenital cytomegalovirus infection involving the central nervous system.

10. **Dengue.** Dengue has been expanded into a separate chapter and removed from the Arboviruses chapter.

11. **Enterovirus (Nonpoliovirus) and Parechovirus Infections.** Echoviruses 22 and 23 are classified as human parechovirus, which cause febrile illness, exanthema, sepsis-like syndromes, and respiratory and intestinal tract infections.

12. ***Escherichia coli* Diarrhea.** Recommendations for diagnosis of Shiga toxin-pro-ducing *Escherichia coli* (STEC), specifically non O157:H7 strains, are included, as is an update on the epidemiology of infection with STEC.

13. **Hepatitis A.** For people 12 months through 40 years of age for postexposure prophylaxis and international travel, HAV vaccine is recommended. Updates for vaccination now include people traveling from the U.S. to countries with high or intermediate HAV endemicity, and household members and other close personal contacts (e.g. regular child sitters) of adopted children newly arriving from countries with high or intermediate HAV endemicity.

14. **Hepatitis B.** The epidemiology and treatment sections have been updated; recom-mendations for immunization of adults with diabetes mellitus and a figure showing stages of acute hepatitis B virus infection and recovery has been added.

15. **Herpes Simplex.** Recommendations that all infants surviving neonatal herpes receive 6 months of oral acyclovir suppressive therapy and addition of whole blood PCR and ALT for diagnosis of neonatal HSV in addition to surface and lesion cul-tures and PCR of CSF have been added. For diagnosis of neonatal herpes, swab specimens from mouth, nasopharynx, conjunctivae and anus can be obtained with a single swab ending with the anus and placed in one viral transport media tube.

16. **Human Immunodeficiency Virus Infection.** HIV infection is an area of medicine that is changing rapidly. The epidemiology, diagnosis, and therapy sections have been updated. Table 3.28 has been modified to clarify dosing of zidovudine by gestational age of the infant. The AAP recommends that routine screening be offered at least once to all adolescents at 16 through 18 years of age who live in high-risk set-tings where HIV prevalence in the patient population is >0.1% and is encouraged for all sexually active adolescents and adolescents with risk factors for HIV infection.

17. **Influenza.** Recommendations have been updated to include new vaccines, an algorithm recommending an approach to immunization of children with egg allergy has been added, and the current status of antiviral recommendations has been updated. Information about occurrence of febrile seizures following coadministration of TIV and PCV13 to children 12 through 23 months has been added, but vaccine recommendations remain the same. Quadrivalent influenza vaccine(s) are expected to be available for the 2013–2014 influenza season.

18. **Isosporiasis** nomenclature has been changed to **Cystoisosporiasis.**

19. **Measles.** The outbreak of measles in the United States in 2011 is highlighted, as is the need to immunize infants 6 through 11 months of age who travel internationally.

20. **Meningococcal Infections.** Recommendations for routine use of meningococcal vaccines for adolescents, and for children and adolescents at high risk of disease have been updated and placed into 2 tables. Specific changes include guidance for adolescents and people in high-risk groups, need for booster doses, and vaccine interchangeability.

21. **Microsporidia Infections.** Microsporidia have been reclassified from protozoa to fungi.

22. **Mumps.** Vaccine recommendations using MMR or MMRV vaccines have been updated.

23. **Human Papillomaviruses.** Tests that detect high-risk types of HPV DNA in exfoliated cervical cells are available for clinical use for screening females for HPV infection. Guidance for cancer screening from professional societies is provided. Recommendations for immunizing females and males from 9 through 26 years of age with HPV vaccine are provided.

24. **Pediculosis Capitis.** The head lice chapter has been updated to reflect the 2010 AAP clinical report, which provides a therapeutic update, including new products for treatment.

25. **Pelvic Inflammatory Disease.** This chapter has been updated to be consistent with the 2010 CDC Sexually Transmitted Diseases Treatment Guidelines.

26. **Pertussis (Whooping Cough).** Diagnostic and antimicrobial prophylaxis after exposure have been updated, as have recommendations for Tdap use in children 7 through 10 years of age, pregnant women, and adults of all ages.

27. **Pinworm Infection *(Enterobius vermicularis).*** Mebendazole no longer is available to treat pinworm and other parasitic infections, including giardiasis, ascariasis, trichuriasis, and hookworm infection.

28. **Pneumococcal Infections.** Immunization recommendations using PCV13 for all children, including children at increased risk of invasive pneumococcal disease, have been updated.

29. **Poliovirus Infections.** Recommendations for vaccine administration were updated to state that the final dose in the IPV series should be administered at 4 years of age or older and at least 6 months after the last dose, regardless of the number of previous doses.

30. **Polyomaviruses (BK virus and JC virus).** There are now 9 human polyomaviruses associated with a variety of diseases, generally in immunocompromised people. Diseases include renal diseases and progressive multifocal leukoencephalopathy.

31. **Rabies.** The postexposure prophylaxis regimen of rabies vaccine has been reduced from 5 to 4 doses given at 0, 3, 7, and 14 days following exposure. Other postexposure recommendations remain the same.

32. **Rotavirus.** History of intussusception and severe combined immune deficiency (SCID) have been added as contraindications to administration of rotavirus vaccine. The epidemiology of rotavirus disease showing the marked reduction in hospitalization following licensure of rotavirus vaccine has been updated.

33. ***Staphylococcus aureus.*** Table 3.64 showing treatment of bacteremia and other serious *Staphylococcus aureus* infections has been updated, as has Fig 3.5, an algorithm for initial management of skin and soft tissue infections caused by *S aureus*.

34. **Group B Streptococcal Infections.** Guidelines for prevention of group B streptococcal disease have been updated according to the 2011 revised guidelines from the CDC. Changes to management of newborn infants include use of lumbar puncture in infants who have signs of sepsis, change in use of intrapartum prophylaxis and inclusion of a revised algorithm for management of newborn infants with possible risk of early-onset group B streptococcal disease.

35. **Syphilis.** Reaffirms that nontreponemal antibody tests (VFRL and RPR) are used for screening and treponemal tests are used to establish a diagnosis of syphilis. The algorithm (Fig 3.7) for evaluation and treatment of infants born to mothers with reactive serologic tests for syphilis has been clarified and harmonized with the text.

36. **Tuberculosis.** A table (3.78) providing recommendations for use of the tuberculin skin test and interferon gamma release assay (IGRA) in children by age has been added. Isoniazid and rifapentine, a long-acting rifamycin, have been added, but because evaluation in children younger than 13 years of age has been limited, this therapeutic option is not recommended for this age group.

37. **Varicella-Zoster Infections.** Updates on disease prevention following 1 and 2 doses of varicella vaccine, recommendations for use of MMRV vaccine, and an update on herpes-zoster vaccine in adults have been added. The FDA has extended the period for administration of Varicella-Zoster Immune Globulin from 96 hours to 10 days after exposure for people without evidence of immunity.

SECTION 4. ANTIMICROBIAL AGENTS AND RELATED THERAPY

1. The **Introduction** has been updated to clarify the FDA approval process for antimicrobial agents, to clarify use of fluoroquinolones and tetracyclines in children, and to provide Web sites for additional information. Use of systemic and topical fluoroquinolones in children has been updated to reflect COID recommendations. The benefits of therapy with doxycycline for serious infections, including those caused by *Rickettsia*, *Ehrlichia*, and *Anaplasma* organisms, has been clarified.

2. The **Antimicrobial Stewardship** section highlights appropriate use of antimicrobial agents in children with the aim of decreasing inappropriate use that leads to resistance and toxicity.

3. The **Drugs for Parasitic Infections** section is reproduced with permission from the 2010 edition of *The Medical Letter*. A new table titled Principal Adverse Effects of Antiparasitic Drugs has been added, and the table titled Principal Adverse Effects of Antiparasitic Drugs in Pregnancy has been updated.

4. **Antibacterial Drugs** for neonates and pediatric patients (Tables 4.1 and 4.2) were adapted from the AAP publication, *2012–2013 Nelson's Pediatric Antimicrobial Therapy*.
5. Table 4.3, **Guidelines for Treatment of Sexually Transmitted Infections,** has been updated to be consistent with the 2010 CDC Sexually Transmitted Diseases Treatment Guidelines to include revised diagnostic and treatment options.

SECTION 5. ANTIMICROBIAL PROPHYLAXIS

1. **Antimicrobial Prophylaxis** for prevention of urinary tract infections has been updated to be consistent with the 2011 AAP clinical practice guideline on urinary tract infections.
2. Table 5.1, **Antimicrobial Prophylaxis.** *Haemophilus influenzae* and *Bacillus anthracis* have been added to the Exposed Host column, and rheumatic fever has been added to the Vulnerable Host (Pathogen) column.

APPENDICES

1. Appendix III. **The ICD-9-CM Codes for Commonly Administered Pediatric Vaccines/Toxoids and Immune Globulins** has been updated to reflect changes and to add new products.
2. Appendix IV. A summary of **Selected Vaccine Safety Resources** has been added as a new Appendix.
3. Appendix V. The **National Childhood Vaccine Injury Act Reporting and Compensation Table** has been restructured to include adverse events and intervals from vaccination to onset of event for reporting and for compensation. In addition, vaccines licensed since the last edition have been added.
4. Appendix VI. The table of **Nationally Notifiable Infectious Diseases in the United States** has been updated to include diseases notifiable in 2012.
5. Appendix VII, **Guide to Contraindications and Precautions to Immunizations,** has been updated to include new vaccines and to reflect the new format of showing conditions that are not contraindications as well as accepted contraindications and precautions.
6. Appendix VIII. **Clinical Practice Guidelines for Immunization Programs for Infants, Children, Adolescents, and Adults** from the Infectious Diseases Society of America (IDSA) have been added as an Appendix.

Active and Passive Immunization

....
PROLOGUE

The ultimate goal of immunization is eradication, elimination, or control of disease; the immediate goal is prevention of disease in people or groups. To accomplish these goals, physicians must make timely immunization, including active and passive immunoprophylaxis, a high priority in the care of infants, children, adolescents, and adults. The global eradication of smallpox in 1977, elimination of poliomyelitis disease from the Americas in 1991, elimination of ongoing measles transmission in the United States in 2000 and in the Americas in 2002, and elimination of rubella and congenital rubella syndrome from the United States in 2004 serve as models for fulfilling the promise of disease control through immunization. These accomplishments were achieved by combining a comprehensive immunization program providing consistent, high levels of vaccine coverage with intensive surveillance and effective public health disease control measures. Future success in the worldwide elimination of polio, measles, rubella, and hepatitis B is possible through implementation of similar prevention strategies.

High immunization rates, in general, have reduced dramatically the incidence of all vaccine-preventable diseases (see Tables 1.1 and 1.2, p 2) in the United States. Yet, because organisms that cause vaccine-preventable diseases persist in the United States and elsewhere around the world, continued immunization efforts must be maintained and strengthened. Discoveries in immunology, molecular biology, and medical genetics have resulted in burgeoning vaccine research. Licensing of new, improved, and safer vaccines; anticipated arrival of additional combination vaccines; establishment of an adolescent immunization platform; and application of novel vaccine-delivery systems promise a new era of preventive medicine. The advent of population-based postlicensure studies of new vaccines facilitates detection of rare adverse events temporally associated with immunization that were undetected during prelicensure clinical trials. Identification of the rare occurrence of intussusception after administration of the first licensed oral rhesus rotavirus vaccine confirmed the value of such surveillance systems. Physicians must regularly update their knowledge about specific vaccines, including information about their recommended use, safety, and effectiveness.

Each edition of the *Red Book* provides recommendations for immunization of infants, children, and adolescents. These recommendations, which are harmonized among the American Academy of Pediatrics (AAP), the Advisory Committee on Immunization Practices of the Centers for Disease Control and Prevention, and the American Academy of Family Physicians, are based on careful analysis of disease epidemiology, benefits and risks of immunization, feasibility of implementation, and cost-benefit analysis. Whereas immunization recommendations represent the best approach to disease prevention on a population basis, in rare circumstances, individual considerations may warrant a different approach.

Use of trade names and commercial sources in the *Red Book* is for identification purposes only and does not imply endorsement by the AAP. Internet sites referenced in the

Table 1.1. Comparison of 20th Century Annual Morbidity and Current Morbidity: Vaccine-Preventable Diseases[a]

Disease	20th Century Annual Morbidity[b]	2010 Reported Cases[c]	Percent Decrease
Smallpox	29 005	0	100
Diphtheria	21 053	0	100
Measles	530 217	63	>99
Mumps	162 344	2612	98
Pertussis	200 752	27 550	86
Polio (paralytic)	16 316	0	100
Rubella	47 745	5	>99
Congenital rubella syndrome	152	0	100
Tetanus	580	26	96
Haemophilus influenzae	20 000	246[d]	99

[a]National Center for Immunization and Respiratory Diseases. Historical Comparisons of Vaccine-Preventable Disease Morbidity in the U.S. Atlanta, GA: Centers for Disease Control and Prevention
[b]Roush SW, Murphy TV, Vaccine-Preventable Disease Table Working Group. Historical comparisons of morbidity and mortality for vaccine-preventable diseases in the United States. *JAMA*. 2007;298(18):2155–2163
[c]Centers for Disease Control and Prevention. Notice to readers: final 2010 reports of nationally notifiable infectious diseases. *MMWR Morb Mortal Wkly Rep*. 2011;60(32):1088–1101
[d]23 type b and 223 unknown serotype (<5 years of age).

Table 1.2. Comparison of Prevaccine Era Estimated Annual Morbidity With Current Estimates: Vaccine-Preventable Diseases[a]

Disease	Prevaccine Era Annual Estimate	2010 Reported Cases	Percent Decrease
Hepatitis A	117 333[b]	9670[c]	92
Hepatitis B (acute)	66 232[b]	3374[c]	95
Pneumococcus (invasive)			
All ages	63 067[b]	16 569[c]	84
<5 years of age	16 069[b]	1877[c]	88
Rotavirus (hospitalizations, <3 years of age)	62 500[d]	28 125[e]	55
Varicella	4 085 120[b]	9920[c]	99.8

[a]National Center for Immunization and Respiratory Diseases. Historical Comparisons of Vaccine-Preventable Disease Morbidity in the U.S. Atlanta, GA: Centers for Disease Control and Prevention
[b]Roush SW, Murphy TV, Vaccine-Preventable Disease Table Working Group. Historical comparisons of morbidity and mortality for vaccine-preventable diseases in the United States. *JAMA*. 2007;298(18):2155–2163
[c]Centers for Disease Control and Prevention. Notice to readers: final reports of nationally notifiable infectious diseases. *MMWR Morb Mortal Wkly Rep*. 2011;60(32):1088–1101
[d]Centers for Disease Control and Prevention. Prevention of rotavirus gastroenteritis among infants and children: recommendations of the Advisory Committee on Immunization Practices (ACIP). *MMWR Recomm Rep*. 2009;58(RR-02):1–25
[e]New Vaccine Surveillance Network (unpublished data).

Red Book are provided as a service to readers and may change without notice; citation of Web sites does not constitute AAP endorsement.

Sources of Vaccine Information

In addition to the *Red Book*, which is published every 3 years, physicians should use evidence-based literature and other sources for data to answer specific vaccine questions encountered in practice. Such sources include the following:

- **Pediatrics.** Policy statements developed by the Committee on Infectious Diseases (COID) providing updated recommendations are published in *Pediatrics* between editions of the *Red Book*. Policy statements also may be accessed via the American Academy of Pediatrics (AAP) Web site **(http://aappolicy.aappublications.org/).** Recommendations of the COID are not official until approved by the Board of Directors of the AAP.

- The updated recommended childhood and adolescent immunization schedules for the United States are published annually in the February issue of *Pediatrics* and elsewhere (see Scheduling Immunizations, p 25). This is a harmonized schedule developed by the Centers for Disease Control and Prevention (CDC), AAP, and American Academy of Family Physicians.

- **AAP News.** Policy statements (or statement summaries) from the COID often are published initially in *AAP News*, the monthly newsmagazine of the AAP **(http://aapnews.aappublications.org),** to inform the membership promptly of new recommendations.

- **Red Book Online.** The AAP has developed an information page **(http://aapredbook.aappublications.org/news/vaccstatus.dtl)** to provide current information about the vaccine licensure process and AAP recommendations about vaccines listed in the table. This table is updated when changes occur.

- **Morbidity and Mortality Weekly Report (MMWR).** Published weekly by the CDC, the *MMWR* contains current vaccine recommendations, reports of specific disease activity, alerts concerning vaccine availability, changes in vaccine formulations, vaccine safety issues, policy statements, and other infectious disease and vaccine information. Recommendations of the Advisory Committee on Immunization Practices (ACIP) of the CDC are published periodically, as policy notes or as supplements in the *MMWR*, and are posted on the CDC Web site **(www.cdc.gov/mmwr).** Recommendations of the ACIP are not official until approved by the CDC director and the Department of Health and Human Services and published in the *MMWR*.

- **Manufacturers' prescribing information (product inserts).** Manufacturers provide product-specific information with each vaccine product. The product label must be in full compliance with US Food and Drug Administration (FDA) regulations pertaining to labeling for prescription drugs, including indications and usage, dosage and administration, contraindications, warnings and precautions, adverse reactions, use in specific populations, and clinical studies. Each product insert lists contents of the vaccine, including preservatives, stabilizers, antimicrobial agents, adjuvants, and suspending fluids. Health care professionals should be familiar with the label for each product they administer. Vaccine prescribing information is accessible through the

FDA Web site (**www.fda.gov/cber/vaccines.htm**). Most manufacturers maintain Web sites with current information concerning new vaccine releases and changes in labeling. Additionally, 24-hour contact telephone numbers for medical questions are available in the *Physicians' Desk Reference* (**www.pdr.net**).

- *Health Information for International Travel (The Yellow Book).* This useful monograph is published approximately every 2 years by the CDC as a guide to requirements of various countries for specific immunizations. The monograph also provides information about other vaccines recommended for travel in specific areas and other information for travelers. This document can be purchased from the Superintendent of Documents, US Government Printing Office, Washington, DC 20402–9235. This information also is available on the CDC Web site (**wwwn.cdc.gov/travel/default. aspx**). For additional sources of information on international travel, see International Travel (p 103).

- *CDC materials.* The National Center for Immunization and Respiratory Diseases (NCIRD) of the CDC maintains a comprehensive Web site (**www.cdc.gov/vaccines**) that includes a section for health care professionals that facilitates immunization delivery. The CDC has partnered with the AAP and American Academy of Family Physicians to develop "Provider Resources for Vaccine Conversations with Parents." For up-to-date resources, see **www.cdc.gov/vaccines/conversations.** All current and past ACIP/CDC vaccine recommendations are listed at **www.cdc.gov/vaccines/ recs/acip**. A CDC textbook, *Epidemiology and Prevention of Vaccine-Preventable Diseases,* also referred to as the Pink Book, is available online (**www.cdc.gov/vaccines/ pubs/pinkbook/default.htm**) and provides comprehensive information on use and administration of childhood vaccines as well as selected ACIP statements and other vaccine-related information (for purchase of the Pink Book, contact the Public Health Foundation at 877-252-1200 or visit **www.cdc.gov/vaccines/pubs/#text**). A CDC publication titled *Manual for Surveillance of Vaccine-Preventable Diseases* provides insight into principles used to investigate and control outbreaks of disease. The NCIRD publishes a series of brochures on immunization topics and produces a CD-ROM that contains a wide range of resources, including vaccine information statements (VISs) and the complete text of the Pink Book. To obtain CDC materials, contact the CDC information center at 1-800-CDC-INFO (1-800-232-4636) or visit NCIRD's publication Web site (**www.cdc.gov/vaccines/pubs/default.htm**).

- **Satellite broadcasts and Web-based training courses.** The NCIRD conducts several immunization-related "train the trainer" courses that are available on DVD, live via satellite and through the Internet via Webcast, Web-on-demand, or self-study sessions each year. Annual course offerings include the Immunization Update, Vaccines for International Travel, Influenza, and a 9-module introductory course on the Epidemiology and Prevention of Vaccine-Preventable Diseases. The course schedule, slide sets, and written materials can be accessed online (**www.cdc.gov/ vaccines/ed/default.htm**). In addition, each meeting of the ACIP in February, June, and October is Webcast for viewing. See **www.cdc.gov/vaccines/recs/ acip/default.htm** for details and specific dates.

- **Immunization information e-mail–based inquiry system.** This system responds to immunization-related questions submitted from health care professionals and members of the public. Individualized responses to inquiries typically are sent within 24 hours. Inquiries should be sent by completing a form available at **www.cdc.gov/vaccines/about/contact/nipinfo_contact_form.htm.**
- **CDC telephone hotline.** The hotline is a telephone-based resource available to answer immunization-related questions from health care professionals and members of the public. The hotline can be reached at 1-800-CDC-INFO (1-800-232-4636) and is available in English and Spanish.
- **Independent sources of reliable immunization information.** Appendix I (p 883) provides a list of reliable immunization information resources, including facts concerning vaccine efficacy, clinical applications, schedules, and unbiased information about safety. Two resources comprehensively address concerns of practicing physicians: the National Network for Immunization Information (**www.immunizationinfo. org**) and the Immunization Action Coalition (**www.immunize.org**). State-specific requirements for immunizations are available at **www.immunize.org.**
- **Vaccine price list.** Information about pediatric and adolescent vaccines, types of packaging, and CDC and private-sector costs are available at **www.cdc.gov/ vaccines/programs/vfc/cdc-vac-price-list.htm.**
- **Other resources**[1] include the FDA and the Institute of Medicine; infectious disease and vaccine experts at university-affiliated hospitals, at medical schools and children's hospitals, and in private practice; and state immunization programs and local public health departments. Information can be obtained from state and local health departments about current epidemiology of diseases; immunization recommendations; legal requirements; public health policies; and nursery school, child care, and school health concerns or requirements. Information regarding global health matters can be obtained from the World Health Organization (**www.who.int/**).
- **Immunization schedulers.** Online catch-up immunization schedulers are available for use by parents, other care providers, and health care professionals. The schedulers are based on the recommended immunization schedules for children, adolescents, and adults. The schedulers, which can be downloaded, allow the user to determine vaccines needed by age and are useful for viewing missed or skipped vaccines quickly according to the recommended childhood and adult immunization schedules. The interactive vaccine schedules are available at the following sites:
  - catch-up scheduler: **https://www.vacscheduler.org;**
  - adolescent scheduler: **www.cdc.gov/vaccines/recs/Scheduler/ AdolescentScheduler.htm;** and
  - adult scheduler: **www.cdc.gov/vaccines/recs/Scheduler/AdultScheduler. htm.**

---

[1] Appendix I, Directory of Resources, p 883.

INTERNET RESOURCES FOR ACCURATE IMMUNIZATION INFORMATION (ALSO SEE APPENDIX I, P 883, FOR ADDITIONAL INFORMATION)

Several health care professional associations, nonprofit groups, universities, and government organizations provide Internet resources containing immunization information.

HEALTH PROFESSIONAL ASSOCIATIONS

American Academy of Family Physicians (AAFP)
  www.familydoctor.org
American Academy of Pediatrics (AAP)
  www.aap.org/immunization
  www.cispimmunize.org (AAP Childhood Immunization Support Program)
American Medical Association (AMA)
  www.ama-assn.org
American Nurses Association (ANA)
  www.nursingworld.org
Association of State and Territorial Health Officials (ASTHO)
  www.astho.org
Association for Prevention Teaching and Research
  www.atpm.org/prof_dev/ed.html
National Medical Association (NMA)
  www.nmanet.org

NONPROFIT GROUPS AND UNIVERSITIES

Albert B. Sabin Vaccine Institute
  www.sabin.org
Allied Vaccine Group (AVG)
  www.vaccine.org
Every Child By Two (ECBT)
  www.ecbt.org
  www.vaccinateyourbaby.org
GAVI Alliance
  www.gavialliance.org
Health on the Net Foundation (HON)
  www.hon.ch
History of Vaccines, The College of Physicians of Philadelphia
  www.historyofvaccines.org
National Healthy Mothers, Healthy Babies Coalition (HMHB)
  www.hmhb.org
Immunization Action Coalition (IAC)
  www.immunize.org
Institute for Vaccine Safety (IVS), Johns Hopkins University
  www.vaccinesafety.edu
Institute of Medicine (IOM)
  www.iom.edu/?ID=4705
National Alliance for Hispanic Health
  www.hispanichealth.org

National Network for Immunization Information (NNii)
www.immunizationinfo.org
Parents of Kids with Infectious Diseases (PKIDS)
www.pkids.org
Texas Children's Hospital Vaccine Center
www.texaschildrens.org/Locate/Departments-and-Services/Vaccine/
University of Pennsylvania
www.vaccineethics.org
Vaccine Education Center at the Children's Hospital of Philadelphia
www.vaccine.chop.edu
Vaccine Page
www.vaccines.com
World Health Organization
www.who.int/topics/immunization/en/

GOVERNMENT ORGANIZATIONS

Centers for Disease Control and Prevention (CDC)
www.cdc.gov/vaccines
www.cdc.gov/vaccinesafety
Food and Drug Administration (FDA)
www.fda.gov/cber/vaccines.htm
National Vaccine Program Office (NVPO)
www.hhs.gov/nvpo/
National Institute of Allergy and Infectious Diseases (NIAID)
www3.niaid.nih.gov/topics/vaccines/default.htm

INFORMING PATIENTS AND PARENTS

Patients, parents, and/or legal guardians should be informed about benefits to be derived from vaccines in preventing diseases in immunized people and in the community where they live and about possible risks of disease-preventive and therapeutic procedures, including immunizations. Questions should be encouraged, and adequate time should be allowed so that information is understood (**www.cdc.gov/vaccines/conversations**).

The National Childhood Vaccine Injury Act (NCVIA) of 1986 included requirements for notifying *all* patients and parents about vaccine benefits and risks. Whether vaccines are purchased with private or public funds, this legislation mandates that a vaccine information statement (VIS) be provided *each* time a vaccine covered under the National Vaccine Injury Compensation Program (VICP), established by the NCVIA, is administered (see Table 1.3, p 8). This applies in all settings, including clinics, offices, hospitals (eg, for the birth dose of hepatitis B vaccine), and pharmacies. Providing this information before the day of immunization is desirable. For vaccines not yet included in the VICP, VISs are available but are not mandated unless the vaccine is purchased through a contract with the Centers for Disease Control and Prevention (CDC [ie, the Vaccines for Children Program, state immunization grants, or state purchases through the CDC]). Copies of current VISs are available online from the CDC (**www.cdc.gov/vaccines/pubs/vis/default.htm**) and the Immunization Action Coalition Web

Table 1.3. Guidance in Using Vaccine Information Statements (VISs)[a]

Distribution

Must be provided each time a VICP-covered vaccine is administered[b]

Must be given to patient (nonminor), parent, and/or legal guardian[b,c]

Must be the current version[d]

Can provide (not substitute) other written materials or audiovisual aids in addition to VISs[e]

VICP indicates Vaccine Injury Compensation Program.
[a] VISs are available at **www.cdc.gov/vaccines/pubs/vis/default.htm**.
[b] Required under the National Childhood Vaccine Injury Act.
[c] Consenting adolescent may vary by state.
[d] Required by Centers for Disease Control and Prevention (CDC) regulations for vaccines purchased through CDC contract. See the VIS Web site for current versions.
[e] An electronic version of the VIS can be uploaded to the patient (nonminor), parent, and/or legal guardian.

site (**www.immunize.org**) in English and many other languages. Copies also can be obtained from the American Academy of Pediatrics (AAP), state and local health departments, and vaccine manufacturers or by calling the CDC telephone hotline (1-800-232-4636). Information is available in English and in Spanish. Physicians need to ensure that the VIS provided is the current version by noting the date of publication. The latest version can be determined by calling the CDC telephone hotline or viewing the CDC VIS Web site.

The NCVIA requires physicians administering vaccines covered by the VICP, whether purchased with private or public funds, to record in the patient's medical record information shown in Tables 1.3 and 1.4 as well as confirmation that the relevant VIS was provided at the time of each immunization (see Record Keeping and Immunization Information Systems, p 39). For vaccines purchased through CDC contract, physicians are required to record the VIS date of publication as well as the date on which the VIS was provided to the patient, parent, and/or legal guardian. Although VIS distribution and vaccine record-keeping requirements do not apply to privately purchased vaccines not covered by the VICP, the AAP recommends following the same record-keeping practices for all vaccines. The AAP also recommends recording the site and route of administration and vaccine expiration date when administering any vaccine. Health care professionals also should be aware of local confidentiality laws involving adolescents.

Parents' or patients' signatures are not required to indicate that they have read and understood material in the VIS. However, the health care professional has the option to obtain a signature. Health care professionals should be familiar with requirements of the state in which they practice. Whether or not a signature is obtained, health care professionals should document in the chart that the VIS has been provided and discussed with the patient, parent, and/or legal guardian.

Parental Concerns About Immunization

Health care professionals should anticipate that some parents will question the need for or the safety of immunizations, want to space out vaccines, refuse certain vaccines, or even decide to reject all immunizations for their child. Some parents may have religious or philosophic objections to immunization, which are permitted by some states. Other

Table 1.4. Documentation Requirements Under the National Childhood Vaccine Injury Act

Documentation in the patient's medical record

Vaccine manufacturer, lot number, and date of administration[a]

Name and business address of the health care professional administering the vaccine[a]

Date that VIS is provided (and VIS publication date[b])

Site (eg, deltoid area) and route (eg, intramuscular) of administration and expiration date of the vaccine[c]

[a]Required under the National Childhood Vaccine Injury Act.
[b]Required by Centers for Disease Control and Prevention (CDC) regulations for vaccines purchased through CDC contract. See the VIS Web site for current versions.
[c]Recommended by the American Academy of Pediatrics.

parents want only to enter into a dialogue with their child's physician about the risks and benefits of one or more of the vaccines. Several factors contribute to parental vaccine concerns or lack of understanding of the benefits of vaccines, including: (1) lack of information about the vaccine being given and about immunizations in general; (2) opposing information from other sources (eg, alternative medicine practitioners, antivaccination organizations, some religious groups, and alternative Web sites); (3) mistrust of the source of information (eg, vaccine manufacturer); (4) perceived risk of serious vaccine adverse events; (5) concern regarding number of injections or the vaccine schedule; (6) information being delivered in a way that does not recognize cultural differences or that is not tailored to individual concern; (7) information being delivered at an inconvenient time; (8) not perceiving risk of vaccines accurately; and (9) lack of appreciation of the severity of vaccine-preventable diseases. One important aspect physicians can control is their relationship with patients and their parents. Physicians are the most trusted source of health information for parents. If parents trust their child's physician, information presented to them by the physician in support of vaccines is accepted more readily. A nonjudgmental approach is best for parents who question the need for immunizations. Ideally, health care professionals should determine in general terms what parents understand about vaccines their children will be receiving, the nature of their concerns, their health beliefs, and what information they find credible.

People understand and react to vaccine information on the basis of a variety of factors, including previous experiences, attitudes, health beliefs, personal values, and education. The method in which data are presented about immunizations as well as a person's perceptions of the risks of disease, perceived ability to control those risks, and risk preference also contribute to understanding of immunizations. For some people, the risk of immunization can be viewed as disproportionately greater than the risk of disease so that immunization is not perceived as beneficial, in part because of the relative infrequency of vaccine-preventable diseases in the United States. Others can dwell on sociopolitical issues, such as mandatory immunization, informed consent, and the primacy of individual rights over that of societal benefit.

Parents may be aware through the media or information from alternative Web sites about alleged controversial issues concerning vaccines their child is scheduled to receive. Many issues about childhood vaccines communicated by these means are presented incompletely or inaccurately. When a parent initiates discussion about an alleged vaccine controversy, the health care professional should listen carefully and then calmly and non-judgmentally discuss specific concerns. Health care professionals always should provide factual information and use language appropriate for parents and other care providers. Through direct dialogue with parents and use of available resources, health care professionals can help reduce and possibly prevent acceptance of inaccurate media reports and information from nonauthoritative sources. Encouraging a dialogue may be the most important step to eventual vaccine acceptance.

Helpful information sources that can be provided to parents or to which parents can be directed include the National Center for Immunization and Respiratory Diseases' "Parent's Guide to Childhood Immunization" (**www.cdc.gov/vaccines** or contact the CDC telephone hotline at (1-800-232-4636), the Vaccine Education Center at Children's Hospital of Philadelphia (**www.vaccine.chop.edu**), and the AAP Immunization Initiatives Web site (**Healthychildren.org**).

Parents who refuse vaccines should be advised of state laws pertaining to school or child care entry, which can require that unimmunized children not attend school during disease outbreaks. Documentation of such discussions in the patient's record may help to decrease any potential liability should a vaccine-preventable disease occur in an unimmunized patient. This *informed refusal* documentation should note that the parent was informed why the immunization was recommended, the risks and benefits of immunization, and the possible consequences of not allowing the vaccine to be administered. A sample Refusal to Vaccinate form can be found on the AAP Web site at **www.cispimmunize.org/pro/ParentalRefusaltoVaccinate.html.**

···

PARENTAL REFUSAL OF IMMUNIZATION

The approach of a health care professional to a parent who refuses immunization of his or her child is complex and should be based on the reason for refusal and knowledge of the parent. Suggested responses to parental refusals of immunization of children are outlined as follows[1]:

- The pediatrician should listen carefully and respectfully to the parent's concerns, recognizing that parents may not use the same decision criteria as physicians and may weigh evidence differently than physicians.
- The pediatrician should share honestly what is and is not known about risks and benefits of the vaccine in question and attempt to correct any misperceptions and misinformation.
- The pediatrician should assist parents in understanding that risks of any vaccine should not be considered in isolation but in comparison with risks to the child and community should the child remain unimmunized.
- Parents can be referred to one of several accurate and data-based Web sites for additional information on specific immunizations and the diseases they prevent (**www. healthychildren.org**; see Internet Resources for Immunization Information, p 6).

---

[1] Diekema DS; American Academy of Pediatrics, Committee on Bioethics. Responding to parental refusals of immunization of children. *Pediatrics.* 2005;115(5):1428–1431 (Reaffirmed October 2008)

Physicians can access information on this topic at **www.aap.org/immunization/** and at **www.cdc.gov/vaccines/spec-grps/hcp/conversations.htm.**

- Many parents have concerns related to 1 or 2 specific vaccines. Pediatricians and nurses should discuss benefits and risks of each vaccine, because a parent who is reluctant to accept administration of 1 vaccine may be willing to accept others.
- Parents who have concerns about administering multiple vaccines to a child in a single visit may have their concerns addressed by using methods to reduce the pain of injection (see Managing Injection Pain, p 23) or by using combination vaccines. Any schedule should adhere to age ranges of vaccine administration provided for many vaccines in the Recommended Childhood and Adolescent Immunization schedules (p 27–31).
- Physicians also should explore the possibility that cost is a reason for refusing immunization and assist parents by helping them obtain recommended immunizations for their children.
- For all cases in which parents refuse vaccine administration, pediatricians should take advantage of their ongoing relationship with the family and revisit the immunization discussion on subsequent visits.
- Continued refusal after adequate discussion should be acknowledged unless the child is put at significant risk of serious harm (eg, during an epidemic). Only then should state agencies be involved to override parental discretion on the basis of medical neglect.
- Physician concerns about liability should be addressed by appropriate documentation of the discussion of benefits of immunization and risks to the child and risks to others (eg, children too young to be immunized or children who are immune compromised) associated with remaining unimmunized. Physicians also may wish to consider having the parents sign a refusal waiver. A sample refusal-to-vaccinate waiver can be found at **www.aap.org/immunization/pediatricians/refusaltovaccinate.html.**
- When significant differences in philosophy of care emerge, a substantial level of distrust develops, or poor quality of communication persists, the pediatrician can choose to encourage the family to find another physician or practice after providing sufficient advance notice in writing to the patient or custodial parent or legal guardian to permit another health care professional to be secured.

ACTIVE IMMUNIZATION

Active immunization involves administration of all or part of a microorganism or a modified product of a microorganism (eg, a toxoid, a purified antigen, or an antigen produced by genetic engineering) to evoke an immunologic response that mimics that of natural infection but usually presents little or no risk to the recipient. Immunization can result in antitoxin, anti-adherence, anti-invasive, or neutralizing activity or other types of protective humoral or cellular responses in the recipient. Some immunizing agents provide nearly complete and lifelong protection against disease, some provide partial protection, and some must be readministered at regular intervals to maintain protection. The immunologic response to vaccination is dependent on the type and dose of antigen, the effect of adjuvants and host factors related to age, preexisting antibody, nutrition, concurrent disease, or drug effect and genetics of the host. The effectiveness of a vaccine is assessed by evidence of protection against the natural disease. Induction of antibodies is an indirect measure of protection (eg, antitoxin against *Clostridium tetani* or neutralizing antibody against measles virus), but for some infectious diseases, an immunologic response that correlates with protection is understood poorly, and serum antibody concentration does not always predict protection.

Vaccines incorporating an intact infectious agent may contain live-attenuated, inactivated, or genetically engineered subunits. Vaccines licensed for use in the United States are listed in Table 1.5 (p 13). The US Food and Drug Administration (FDA) maintains and updates a Web site listing vaccines licensed for immunization and distribution in the United States with supporting documents (**www.fda.gov/ BiologicsBloodVaccines/vaccines/ApprovedProducts/ucm093830.htm**). Appendix II shows the years of licensure of vaccines available in the United States, and Appendix III provides the *Current Procedural Terminology* (CPT) and *International Classification of Diseases* (ICD-9) codes used for vaccine administration. Among currently licensed vaccines in the United States, there are 2 live-attenuated bacterial vaccines (oral typhoid and bacille-Calmette Guérin vaccines) and several live-attenuated viral vaccines. Although active replication (with bacterial or viral replication) ensues after administration of these vaccines, infection is modified, and little or no adverse host effect is expected. Vaccines for some viruses (eg, hepatitis A and hepatitis B, human papillomavirus) and most bacteria are inactivated, component, subunit (purified components) preparations or inactivated toxins. Some vaccines contain purified bacterial polysaccharides conjugated chemically to immunobiologically active proteins (eg, tetanus toxoid, nontoxic variant of mutant diphtheria toxin, meningococcal outer membrane protein complex). Viruses and bacteria in inactivated, subunit, and conjugate vaccine preparations are not capable of replicating in the host; therefore, these vaccines must contain a sufficient antigen content to stimulate a desired response. In the case of conjugate polysaccharide vaccines, the protein linkage between the polysaccharide and the protein enhances vaccine immunogenicity. Maintenance of long-lasting immunity with inactivated viral or bacterial vaccines and toxoid vaccines may require periodic administration of booster doses. Although inactivated vaccines may not elicit the range of immunologic response provided by live-attenuated agents, efficacy of licensed inactivated vaccines is high. For example, an injected inactivated viral vaccine may evoke sufficient serum antibody or cell-mediated immunity but evoke only minimal mucosal antibody in the form of secretory immunoglobulin (Ig) A. Mucosal protection after administration of inactivated vaccines generally is inferior to mucosal immunity induced by live-attenuated vaccines. Nonetheless, the demonstrated efficacy for such vaccines against invasive infection is high. Bacterial polysaccharide conjugate vaccines (eg, *Haemophilus influenzae* type b and pneumococcal conjugate vaccines) reduce nasopharyngeal colonization through exudated IgG. Viruses and bacteria in inactivated vaccines cannot replicate in or be excreted by the vaccine recipient as infectious agents and, thus, do not present the same safety concerns for immunosuppressed vaccinees or contacts of vaccinees as might live-attenuated vaccines.

Recommendations for dose, vaccine storage and handling (see Vaccine Handling and Storage, p 16), route and technique of administration (see Vaccine Administration, p 20), and immunization schedules should be followed for predictable, effective immunization (see also disease-specific chapters in Section 3). Adherence to recommended guidelines is critical to the success of immunization practices.

Table 1.5. Vaccines Licensed for Immunization and Distributed in the United States and Their Routes of Administration[a]

Vaccine	Type	Route of Administration
BCG	Live bacteria	ID (preferred) or SC
Diphtheria-tetanus (DT, Td)	Toxoids	IM
DTaP	Toxoids and inactivated bacterial components	IM
DTaP, hepatitis B, and IPV	Toxoids and inactivated bacterial components, recombinant viral antigen, inactivated virus	IM
DTaP-IPV	Toxoids and inactivated bacterial components, inactivated virus	IM
DTaP-IPV/Hib (PRP-T reconstituted with DTaP-IPV)	Toxoids and inactivated bacterial components, polysaccharide-protein conjugate, inactivated virus	IM
Hepatitis A	Inactivated virus	IM
Hepatitis B	Recombinant viral antigen	IM
Hepatitis A-hepatitis B	Inactivated virus and recombinant viral antigens	IM
Hib conjugate (tetanus toxoid)[b]	Bacterial polysaccharide-protein conjugate	IM
Hib conjugate (PRP-OMP[b]) hepatitis B	Bacterial polysaccharide-protein conjugate with recombinant viral antigen	IM
Human papillomavirus (HPV2 and HPV4)	Recombinant viral antigens	IM
Influenza	Inactivated viral components	IM
Influenza	Live-attenuated viruses	Intranasal
Japanese encephalitis	Inactivated virus	SC or IM
Meningococcal polysaccharide (MPSV4)	Bacterial polysaccharide	SC
Meningococcal conjugate (MCV4)	Bacterial polysaccharide-protein conjugate	IM
MMR	Live-attenuated viruses	SC
MMRV	Live-attenuated viruses	SC
Pneumococcal polysaccharide (PPSV)	Bacterial polysaccharide	IM or SC
Pneumococcal conjugate (PCV)	Bacterial polysaccharide-protein conjugate	IM

Table 1.5. Vaccines Licensed for Immunization and Distributed in the United States and Their Routes of Administration,[a] continued

Vaccine	Type	Route of Administration
Poliovirus (IPV)	Inactivated viruses	SC or IM
Rabies	Inactivated virus	IM
Rotavirus (RV1 and RV5)	Live-attenuated virus	Oral
Tdap	Toxoids and inactivated bacterial components	IM
Tetanus	Toxoid	IM
Typhoid	Bacterial capsular polysaccharide	IM
Typhoid	Live-attenuated bacteria	Oral
Varicella	Live-attenuated virus	SC
Zoster	Live-attenuated virus	SC
Yellow fever	Live-attenuated virus	SC

BCG indicates bacille Calmette-Guérin; ID, intradermal; SC, subcutaneous; DT, diphtheria and tetanus toxoids (for children 7 years of age or older and adults); IM, intramuscular; DTaP, diphtheria and tetanus toxoids and acellular pertussis; IPV, inactivated poliovirus; Hib, *Haemophilus influenzae* type b; PRP-T, polyribosylribitol phosphate-tetanus toxoid; PRP-OMP, polyribosylribitol phosphate-meningococcal outer membrane protein; HPV, human papillomavirus; MMR, live measles-mumps-rubella; MMRV, live measles-mumps-rubella-varicella (monovalent measles, mumps, and rubella components are not being produced in the United States); Tdap, tetanus toxoid, reduced diphtheria toxoid, and acellular pertussis.

[a] Other vaccines licensed in the United States but not distributed include anthrax, smallpox, oral poliovirus (OPV), and H5N1 influenza vaccines. The FDA maintains a Web site listing currently licensed vaccines in the United States. (**http://www.fda.gov/BiologicsBloodVaccines/Vaccines/ApprovedProducts/ucm093830.htm**). The AAP maintains a Web site (**http://aapredbook. aappublications.org/news/vaccstatus.dtl**) showing status of licensure and recommendations for newer vaccines.

[b] See Table 3.11, p 350.

Immunizing Antigens

Physicians should be familiar with major constituents of vaccines used. Major constituents, including cell line derivation or animal derivatives, as relevant, are listed in package inserts. Sometimes multiple vaccines, each made by a different manufacturer, are licensed for similar indications and use. When this is the case, physicians should be aware that such products may have different active and/or inert ingredients. Major constituents of vaccines include the following:

- *Active immunizing antigens/agents.* Some vaccines consist of a single antigen that is a highly defined constituent (eg, tetanus or diphtheria toxoid). Other vaccines consist of multiple antigens, which can vary substantially in chemical composition and number (eg, acellular pertussis components, *Haemophilus influenzae* type b, and pneumococcal and meningococcal products). Vaccines containing live-attenuated viruses (eg, measles-mumps-rubella [MMR], measles-mumps-rubella-varicella [MMRV], varicella, oral poliovirus [OPV], live-attenuated influenza vaccine, oral rotavirus vaccine), killed viruses or portions of virus (eg, enhanced inactivated poliovirus [IPV], hepatitis A, and inactivated influenza vaccines), or viral proteins incorporated into a vaccine through recombinant technology (eg, hepatitis B vaccine, human papillomavirus [HPV] vaccine) produce both humoral and cellular-mediated responses to ensure long-term protection.

- *Conjugating agents.* Carrier proteins of proven immunologic potential (eg, tetanus toxoid, nontoxic variant of diphtheria toxin, meningococcal outer membrane protein complex), when chemically bound to less immunogenic polysaccharide antigens (eg, *H influenzae* type b, meningococcal and pneumococcal polysaccharides), enhance the type and magnitude of immune responses, particularly in children younger than 2 years of age, who have immature immune systems.

- *Suspending fluid.* Sterile water for injection or saline solution is used commonly as a vaccine vehicle or suspending fluid. Some vaccine products use a complex tissue-culture fluid, which may contain proteins or other constituents derived from the medium and biological system in which the vaccine is produced (eg, egg antigens, gelatin, or cell culture-derived antigens).

- *Preservatives, stabilizers, and antimicrobial agents.* Some vaccines and immune globulin preparations contain added substances (eg, preservatives or stabilizers) or residual materials from the manufacturing process (eg, antibiotic agents or other chemicals, including trace amounts of thimerosal). Allergic reactions may occur if the recipient is sensitive to one or more of these additives. Whenever feasible, these reactions should be anticipated by screening the potential vaccinee for known severe allergy to specific vaccine components. Standardized forms are available to assist clinicians in screening for allergies and other potential contraindications to immunization (**www.immunize.org/catg.d/p4060.pdf**).

- *Thimerosal.* Thimerosal has been the most commonly used preservative in vaccines, added to multidose vaccine vials specifically to kill or inhibit growth of microorganisms. All routinely recommended vaccines for infants and children in the United States are available only as thimerosal-free formulations or contain only trace amounts of thimerosal, with the exception of some inactivated influenza vaccines. Inactivated influenza vaccines for pediatric use are available as thimerosal preservative-containing formulation, trace thimerosal-containing formulation, and thimerosal-free formulation. Information about the thimerosal content of vaccines is available from the FDA (**www.fda.gov/cber/vaccine/thimerosal.htm**). Thimerosal does not cause harm, other than rare allergic reactions. Institute of Medicine safety reviews regarding thimerosal-containing vaccines as well as vaccines and autism are available[1] (**www. iom.edu/CMS/**).

- The only nonvaccine biologic agents that contain thimerosal in production and distributed in the United States are certain antivenins. Immune Globulin Intravenous (IGIV) does not contain thimerosal or other preservatives, and none of the Rho (D) Immune Globulin (Human) products contain thimerosal (**www.fda.gov/BiologicsBlood Vaccines/SafetyAvailability/BloodSafety/ucm095529.htm**).

ADJUVANTS. An aluminum salt commonly is used in varying amounts to increase immunogenicity and to prolong the stimulatory effect, particularly for vaccines containing inactivated microorganisms or their products (eg, hepatitis B vaccine and diphtheria and tetanus toxoids). New adjuvants include molecules that stimulate innate immune responses to enhance immunogenicity of vaccine antigens (eg, deacylated monophosphoryl lipid A plus aluminum hydroxide [ASO4], as used in HPV2 vaccine) or spare the amount of antigen required when vast numbers of doses are needed (eg, pandemic influenza).

Vaccine Handling and Storage

Vaccines should be transported and stored at recommended temperatures. Inattention to vaccine handling and storage conditions can contribute to vaccine failure. Live-virus vaccines, including MMR, MMRV, varicella, yellow fever, live-attenuated influenza, rotavirus, and OPV vaccines, are heat sensitive. Vaccines licensed for refrigerator storage should be stored at 35°F–46°F (2°C–8°C). Inactivated vaccines may tolerate limited exposure to elevated temperatures but are damaged rapidly by freezing (cold sensitive). Examples of cold-sensitive vaccines include diphtheria and tetanus-containing vaccines (DT, Td) and pertussis-containing vaccines (DTaP, Tdap); IPV vaccine; *H influenzae* type b (Hib) vaccine; pneumococcal polysaccharide and conjugate vaccines; hepatitis A and hepatitis B vaccines; inactivated influenza vaccine; meningococcal polysaccharide and conjugate vaccines; and HPV vaccines. Some vaccines must be protected from light, which can be accomplished by keeping each vial or syringe in its original carton while in recommended storage and until immediate use. Some products may show physical evidence of altered integrity, and others may retain their normal appearance despite a loss of potency. Physical appearance is not an appropriate basis for determining vaccine acceptability. Therefore, all personnel responsible for handling vaccines in an office or clinic setting should be familiar with standard procedures designed to minimize risk of vaccine failure.

Recommendations for handling and storage of selected biologics are summarized in several areas, including the package insert for each product and in a publication titled *Vaccine Management*, available from the Centers for Disease Control and Prevention (CDC)[2] at **www.cdc.gov/vaccines/pubs/downloads/bk-vac-mgt.pdf.** The most current information about recommended vaccine storage conditions and handling instructions can be obtained directly from manufacturers; their telephone numbers are listed

---

[1] Institute of Medicine. *Adverse Effects of Vaccines: Evidence and Causality*. Washington, DC: National Academies Press; 2011

[2] Centers for Disease Control and Prevention. *Vaccine Management: Recommendations for Handling and Storage of Selected Biologicals*. Atlanta, GA: US Department of Health and Human Services, Public Health Service; 2007

in product labels (package inserts) and in the *Physicians' Desk Reference*, which is published yearly. The following guidelines are suggested as part of a quality-control system for safe handling and storage of vaccines in an office or clinic setting.

PERSONNEL

- Designate one person as the vaccine coordinator, and assign responsibility for ensuring that vaccines and other biologic agents and products are handled and stored in a careful, safe, recommended, and documentable manner. Assign a backup person to assume these responsibilities during times of illness or vacation.
- Inform all people who will be handling vaccines about specific storage requirements and stability limitations of the products they will encounter. The details of proper storage conditions should be posted on or near each refrigerator or freezer used for vaccine storage or should be readily available to staff.

  Receptionists, mail clerks, and other staff members who may receive shipments also should be educated.

EQUIPMENT

- Ensure that refrigerators and freezers in which vaccines are to be stored are working properly and are capable of meeting storage requirements.
- Do not connect refrigerators or freezers to an outlet with a ground-flow circuit interrupter or one activated by a wall switch. Use plug guards and warning signs to prevent accidental dislodging of the wall plug. Post **"Do Not Unplug"** warning signs on circuit breakers.
- Avoid using compact refrigerators intended for dormitory use to store vaccines. Instead, refrigerator-freezers with separate external doors and well-sealed compartments for refrigeration and freezing should be used. Alternatively, separate refrigerator and freezer units can be used.
- Equip each refrigerator and freezer compartment with a certified thermometer located away from the walls of the storage compartment. A certified thermometer has been individually tested against a reference standard, such as the National Institute of Standards and Technology or ASTM International. These thermometers are sold with an individually numbered certificate documenting this testing. A calibrated, constant-recording thermometer with graphical readings or a thermometer that indicates upper and lower extremes of temperature during an observation period ("minimum-maximum" thermometer) will provide more information as to whether vaccines have been exposed to potentially harmful temperatures than will single-reading thermometers. Placement of vaccine cold-chain monitor cards[1] in refrigerators and freezers can serve to detect potentially harmful increases in temperature but should not be a substitute for use of certified thermometers.
- Maintain a logbook in which temperature readings are recorded at the beginning and end of each clinic day and in which the date, time, and duration of any mechanical malfunctions or power outages are noted. The current temperature log should be posted on the door to remind staff to monitor and record temperatures. Previous logs should be stored for a minimum of 3 years.

---

[1] Available from 3M Pharmaceuticals.

- Place all opened vials of vaccine in a refrigerator tray. To avoid mishaps, do not store other pharmaceutical products in the same tray. Store unopened vials in the original packaging, which facilitates inventory management and rotation of vaccine by expiration date. Store opened vials of light-sensitive vaccines, such as MMR and MMRV, in original packaging, and mark the outside with a large "X" to indicate that it has been opened.
- Equip refrigerators with several bottles of chilled water and freezers with several ice trays or ice packs to fill empty space, which will help to minimize temperature fluctuations during brief electrical or mechanical failures.

PROCEDURES

- A vaccine log should be maintained and include vaccine name, number of doses, arrival condition of the vaccine, manufacturer and lot numbers, and expiration date.
- Acceptance of vaccine on receipt of shipment:
  - Ensure that the expiration date of the delivered product has not passed.
  - Examine the merchandise and its shipping container for any evidence of damage during transport.
  - Consider whether the interval between shipment from the supplier and arrival of the product at its destination is excessive (more than 48 hours) and whether the product has been exposed to excessive heat or cold that might alter its integrity. Review vaccine time and temperature indicators, both chemical and electronic, if included in the vaccine shipment.
  - Do not accept the shipment if reasonable suspicion exists that the delivered product may have been damaged by environmental insult or improper handling during transport.
  - Contact the vaccine supplier or manufacturer when unusual circumstances raise questions about the stability of a delivered vaccine. Store suspect vaccine under proper conditions and label it **"Do Not Use"** until the viability has been determined.
- Refrigerator and freezer inspection:
  - Determine which area of the storage unit maintains a constant temperature and place the thermometer in this location.
  - Measure the temperature of the central part of the storage compartment twice a day, and record this temperature on a temperature log. A minimum-maximum thermometer is preferred to record extremes in temperature fluctuation and reset to baseline. Consider use of an alarm system to monitor temperature fluctuations. The refrigerator temperature should be maintained between 2°C and 8°C (35°F and 46°F) with a target temperature of 40°F, and the freezer temperature should be −15°C (5°F) or colder. A **"Do Not Unplug"** sign should be affixed directly next to the refrigerator electrical outlet.
- Train and designate staff to respond immediately to temperature recordings outside the recommended range and to document response and outcome.
  - Inspect the unit weekly for outdated vaccine and either dispose of or return expired products appropriately.

- Routine procedures:
  - Store vaccines according to temperatures recommended in the package insert.
  - Rotate vaccine supplies so that the shortest-dated vaccines are in front to reduce wastage because of expiration.
  - Promptly remove expired (outdated) vaccines from the refrigerator or freezer and dispose of them appropriately or return to manufacturer to avoid accidental use.
  - Keep opened vials of vaccine in a tray so that they are readily identifiable.
  - Indicate on the label of each vaccine vial the date and time the vaccine was reconstituted or first opened.
  - Unless immediate use is planned, avoid reconstituting multiple doses of vaccine or drawing up multiple doses of vaccine in multiple syringes. Predrawing vaccine increases the possibility of medication errors and causes uncertainty of vaccine stability.
  - Because different vaccines can share similar components/names (eg, DTaP and Tdap or meningococcal polysaccharide vaccine [MPSV4] and meningococcal conjugate vaccine [MCV4]), care should be taken during storage to ensure that the different products are stored separately in a manner to avoid confusion and possible medication errors.
  - When feasible, use prefilled unit-dose syringes supplied by the vaccine manufacturer to prevent contamination of multidose vials and errors in labeling syringes or dosing.
  - Discard reconstituted live-virus and other vaccines if not used within the time interval specified in the package insert. Examples of discard times following reconstitution include varicella vaccine after 30 minutes and MMR vaccine after 8 hours. All reconstituted vaccines should be refrigerated during the interval in which they may be used.
  - Always store vaccines in the refrigerator or freezer as indicated, including throughout the office day.
  - Do not open more than 1 vial of a specific vaccine at a time.
  - Store vaccine where temperature remains constant.
  - Do not keep food or drink in refrigerators in which vaccine is stored; this will limit frequent opening of the unit that leads to thermal instability.
  - Do not store radioactive materials in the same refrigerator in which vaccines are stored.
  - Discuss with all clinic or office personnel any violation of protocol for handling vaccines or any accidental storage problem (eg, electrical failure), and contact vaccine suppliers for information about disposition of the affected vaccine.
  - Develop a written plan for emergency storage of vaccine in the event of a catastrophic event. Office personnel should have a written and easily accessible procedure that outlines vaccine packing and transport. Vaccines that have been exposed to temperatures outside the recommended storage range may be ineffective. Vaccines should be packed in an appropriate insulated storage box and moved to a location where the appropriate storage temperatures can be maintained. Office personnel need to be aware of alternate storage sites and trained in the correct techniques to store and transport vaccines to avoid warming vaccines that need to be refrigerated or frozen and to avoid freezing vaccines that should be refrigerated. Recommended

storage conditions for commonly used vaccines can be found at **www.cdc.gov/ vaccines/pubs/downloads/bk-vac-mgt.pdf.** After a power outage or mechanical failure, do not assume that vaccine exposed to temperature outside the recommended range is unusable. Contact the vaccine manufacturer for guidance before discarding vaccine.

Other resources on vaccine storage and handling are available, including a video from the CDC National Immunization Program, "How to Protect Your Vaccine Supply" (available at **www.cdc.gov/vaccines/pubs/videos-webcasts.htm#satbrd**). Additional materials are available at **www.cdc.gov/vaccines/recs/default.htm.**

Vaccine Administration

GENERAL INSTRUCTIONS FOR VACCINE ADMINISTRATION

Personnel administering vaccines should take appropriate precautions to minimize risk of spread of disease to or from patients. Hand hygiene should be used before and after each new patient contact. Gloves are not required when administering vaccines unless the health care professional has open hand lesions or will come into contact with potentially infectious body fluids. Syringes and needles must be sterile and disposable. To prevent inadvertent needlesticks or reuse, a needle should **not** be recapped after use, and disposable needles and syringes should be discarded promptly in puncture-proof, labeled containers placed in the room where the vaccine is administered. Changing needles between drawing a vaccine into a syringe and injecting it into the child is not necessary. A patient should be restrained adequately if indicated before any injection. Different vaccines should not be mixed in the same syringe unless specifically licensed and labeled for such use.

Because of the rare possibility of a severe allergic reaction to a vaccine component, people administering vaccines or other biologic products should be prepared to recognize and treat allergic reactions, including anaphylaxis (see Hypersensitivity Reactions After Immunization, p 51). Facilities and personnel should be available for treating immediate allergic reactions. This recommendation does not preclude administration of vaccines in school-based or other nonclinic settings.

Syncope may occur following any immunization, particularly in adolescents and young adults. Personnel should be aware of presyncopal manifestations and take appropriate measures to prevent injuries if weakness, dizziness, or loss of consciousness occurs. The relatively rapid onset of syncope in most cases suggests that health care professionals should consider observing adolescents for 15 minutes after they are immunized. Having vaccine recipients *sit or lie down for at least 15 minutes* after immunization could avert many syncopal episodes and secondary injuries. If syncope develops, patients should be observed until symptoms resolve.[1] Syncope following receipt of a vaccine is not a contraindication to subsequent doses.

[1] Centers for Disease Control and Prevention. Syncope after immunization—United States, January 2005–July 2007. *MMWR Morb Mortal Wkly Rep.* 2008;57(17):457–460

SITE AND ROUTE OF IMMUNIZATION (ACTIVE AND PASSIVE)

ORAL VACCINES. Breastfeeding does not interfere with successful immunization with OPV or rotavirus vaccines. Vomiting within 10 minutes of receiving an oral dose is an indication for repeating the dose of OPV but not rotavirus vaccine. If the repeated dose of OPV vaccine also is not retained, neither dose should be counted, and the vaccine should be readministered. OPV is not available for use in the United States.

INTRANASAL VACCINE. Live-attenuated influenza vaccine is the only vaccine licensed for intranasal administration. This vaccine is licensed for healthy, nonpregnant people 2 through 49 years of age. With recipient in the upright position, approximately 0.1 mL (ie, half of the total sprayer contents) is sprayed into one nostril. An attached dose-divider clip is removed from the sprayer to administer the second half of the dose into the other nostril. If the recipient sneezes after administration, the dose should not be repeated. The vaccine can be administered during minor illnesses. However, if clinical judgment indicates that nasal congestion might impede delivery of the vaccine to the nasopharyngeal mucosa, vaccine deferral should be considered until resolution of the illness.

PARENTERAL VACCINES.[1] Injectable vaccines should be administered using aseptic technique in a site as free as possible from risk of local neural, vascular, or tissue injury. Data do not warrant recommendation of a single preferred site for all injections, and product recommendations of many manufacturers allow flexibility in the site of injection. Preferred sites for vaccines administered via the subcutaneous (SC) or intramuscular (IM) route include the anterolateral aspect of the upper thigh (SC or IM); upper, outer triceps area of the upper arm (SC); and the deltoid area of the upper arm (IM).

Recommended routes of administration are included in package inserts of vaccines and are listed in Table 1.5 (p 13). The recommended route is based on studies designed to demonstrate maximum safety and immunogenicity. To minimize untoward local or systemic effects and ensure optimal efficacy of the immunizing procedure, vaccines should be given by the recommended route.

For IM injections, the choice of site is based on the volume of the injected material and size of the muscle. The needle should be directed at a 90° angle. In children younger than 1 year of age (ie, infants), the anterolateral aspect of the thigh provides the largest muscle and is the preferred site. In older children, the deltoid muscle usually is large enough for IM injection.

Ordinarily, the upper, outer aspect of the buttocks should not be used for active immunization, because the gluteal region is covered by a significant layer of subcutaneous fat and because of the possibility of damaging the sciatic nerve. However, clinical information on use of this area is limited. Because of diminished immunogenicity, hepatitis B and rabies vaccines should not be given in the buttocks at any age. People, especially adults, who were given hepatitis B vaccine in the buttocks should be tested for immunity and reimmunized if antibody concentrations are inadequate (see Hepatitis B, p 369).

When the upper, outer quadrant of the buttocks is used for large-volume passive immunization, such as IM administration of large volumes of Immune Globulin (IG), care must be taken to avoid injury to the sciatic nerve. The site selected should be well

---

[1] For a review on intramuscular injections, see Centers for Disease Control and Prevention. *Epidemiology and Prevention of Vaccine-Preventable Diseases (Pink Book).* Atlanta, GA: Centers for Disease Control and Prevention; 2011. For copies, contact the Public Health Foundation at 877-252-1200 or visit **www.cdc.gov/vaccines/pubs/pinkbook/index.html.**

into the upper, outer quadrant of the gluteus maximus, away from the central region of the buttocks, and the needle should be directed anteriorly—that is, if the patient is lying prone, the needle is directed perpendicular to the table's surface, not perpendicular to the skin plane. The ventrogluteal site may be less hazardous for IM injection, because it is free of major nerves and vessels. This site is the center of a triangle for which the boundaries are the anterior superior iliac spine, the tubercle of the iliac crest, and the upper border of the greater trochanter.

Vaccines containing adjuvants (eg, aluminum present in vaccines recommended for IM injection) must be injected deep into the muscle mass. These vaccines should not be administered subcutaneously or intracutaneously, because they can cause local irritation, inflammation, granuloma formation, and tissue necrosis. IG, Rabies Immune Globulin (RIG), Hepatitis B Immune Globulin (HBIG), palivizumab, and other similar products administered for passive immunoprophylaxis also are injected intramuscularly, except that as much of the RIG as possible should be is infiltrated around the site of a bite wound.

Needles used for IM injections should be long enough to reach the muscle mass to prevent vaccine from seeping into subcutaneous tissue and, therefore, minimize local reactions and not so long as to involve underlying nerves, blood vessels, or bone. Suggested needle lengths are shown in Table 1.6, below. Appropriate needle length depends on body mass. For most children up to 70 kg, a $5/8$–inch-long needle is sufficient for IM injections.

Serious complications resulting from IM injections are rare. Reported adverse events include broken needles, muscle contracture, nerve injury, bacterial (staphylococcal, streptococcal, and clostridial) abscesses, sterile abscesses, skin pigmentation, hemorrhage, cellulitis, tissue necrosis, gangrene, local atrophy, periostitis, cyst or scar formation, and inadvertent injection into a joint space. For patients with a known bleeding disorder or

Table 1.6. Site and Needle Length by Age for Intramuscular Immunization

Age Group	Needle Length, inches (mm)[a]	Suggested Injection Site
Newborns (preterm and term) and infants <1 mo of age	$5/8$ (16)[b]	Anterolateral thigh muscle
Term infants, 1–12 mo of age	1 (25)	Anterolateral thigh muscle
Toddlers and children	$5/8$–1 (16–25)[b]	Deltoid muscle of the arm
	1–1¼ (25–32)	Anterolateral thigh muscle
Adults		
Female and male, weight <60 kg	1 (25)[c]	Deltoid muscle of the arm
Female and male, weight 60–70 kg	1 (25)	Deltoid muscle of the arm
Female, weight 70–90 kg	1 (25)–1½ (38)	Deltoid muscle of the arm
Male, weight 70–118 kg	1 (25)–1½ (38)	Deltoid muscle of the arm
Female, weight >90 kg	1½ (38)	Deltoid muscle of the arm
Male, weight >118 kg	1½ (38)	Deltoid muscle of the arm

[a] Assumes that needle is inserted fully.
[b] If the skin is stretched tightly and subcutaneous tissues are not bunched.
[c] Some experts recommend a $5/8$-inch needle for men and women who weigh less than 60 kg.

people receiving anticoagulant therapy, bleeding complications following IM immunization can occur. Such events can be minimized by administration immediately after the patient's receipt of replacement factor if relevant, by utilization of a finer needle (23-gauge or less of appropriate length), and by applying firm pressure at the immunization site for at least 2 minutes. Scheduling vaccines after replacement therapy, if feasible, may be considered.

SC injections can be administered at a 45° angle into the anterolateral aspect of the thigh or the upper, outer triceps area by inserting the needle in a pinched-up fold of skin and tissue. A 23- or 25-gauge needle of $\frac{5}{8}$ inch length is recommended. Immune responses after SC administration of hepatitis B or recombinant rabies vaccine are decreased compared with those after IM administration of either of these vaccines; therefore, these vaccines should not be given subcutaneously. Quadrivalent meningococcal polysaccharide vaccine (MPSV4) is administered subcutaneously, whereas quadrivalent meningococcal conjugate vaccine (MCV4) is administered intramuscularly. Intradermal injections usually are given on the volar surface of the forearm. Because of the decreased antigenic mass administered with intradermal injections, attention to technique is essential to ensure that material is not injected subcutaneously. A 25- or 27-gauge needle is recommended.

When multiple vaccines are administered, separate sites should be used. When necessary, 2 or more vaccines can be given in the same limb at a single visit. The anterolateral aspect of the thigh is the preferred site for multiple simultaneous IM injections because of its greater muscle mass. The distance separating the injections is arbitrary but should be at least 1 inch, if possible, so that local reactions are unlikely to overlap. Multiple vaccines should not be mixed in a single syringe unless specifically licensed and labeled for administration in 1 syringe. A different needle and syringe should be used for each injection.

Aspiration before injection of vaccines or toxoids (ie, pulling back on the syringe plunger after needle insertion, before injection) is not recommended, because no large blood vessels are located at the preferred injection sites, and the process of aspiration has been demonstrated to increase pain.

A brief period of bleeding at the injection site is common and usually can be controlled by applying gentle pressure.

Managing Injection Pain

A planned approach to managing the child before, during, and after immunization is helpful for children of any age.[1] Parents should be educated about techniques for reducing injection pain or distress. Truthful and empathetic preparation for injections is beneficial, using words that are explanatory without evoking anxiety—for example, "pressure," "squeezing," and "poking" rather than "pain," "hurt," and "shot." If possible, parents should have a role in comforting rather than restraining their child. Parents should be advised not to threaten children with injections or use them as a punishment for inappropriate behavior. Techniques for minimizing pain can be divided into physical, psychological, and pharmacologic. Combinations of techniques are useful. Routine preemptive administration of acetaminophen is not recommended.

[1] Schechter NL, Zempsky WT, Cohen LL, McGrath PJ, McMurtry CM, Bright NS. Pain reduction during pediatric immunizations: evidence-based review and recommendations. *Pediatrics.* 2007;1119(5):e1184–e1198

PHYSICAL TECHNIQUES FOR MINIMIZING INJECTION PAIN

Skin-to-skin contact between mothers and their infants has been shown to reduce crying and decrease heart rate significantly during heel sticks. In addition, breastfeeding is a potent analgesic intervention in newborn infants during blood collection. Nonnutritive sucking on a pacifier also may have analgesic properties. Infants may exhibit less pain behavior when held on the lap of a parent or other caregiver. Older children may be more comfortable sitting on a parent's lap or examination table edge and hugging their parent chest to chest, while an immunization is administered. Stroking or rocking a child after an injection decreases crying and other pain behaviors.

The limb should be positioned to allow relaxation of the muscle to be injected. For the deltoid, some flexion of the arm may be required. For the anterolateral thigh, some degree of internal rotation may be helpful. A rapid plunge of the needle through the skin without aspirating and rapid injection may decrease discomfort.

If multiple injections are to be given, having different health care professionals administer them simultaneously at multiple sites (eg, right and left anterolateral thighs) may lessen anticipation of the next injection. In this circumstance, a parent or guardian should assist in comforting the child. It may be helpful to give older children a degree of control by allowing some choice in selecting the injection site.

PSYCHOLOGICAL TECHNIQUES FOR MINIMIZING INJECTION PAIN

For younger children, parents may soothe, stroke, and calm the child. For older children, parent demeanor affects the child's pain behavior. Humor and distraction techniques tend to decrease distress, whereas excessive parental reassurance, concern, or apology tends to increase distress. Breathing and distraction techniques, such as "blowing the pain away," use of pinwheels or soap bubbles, telling children stories, reading books, or use of music, are effective. Techniques that involve the child in a fantasy or reframe the experience with the use of suggestion ("magic love" or "pain switch") also are effective but may require training.

PHARMACOLOGIC TECHNIQUES FOR MINIMIZING INJECTION PAIN

Topically applied agents may reduce the pain of injection. Topical anesthetics (eg, lidocaine/pilocaine) have been evaluated in placebo-controlled, randomized clinical trials and have been demonstrated to provide pain relief. Because currently available topical anesthetics require 30 to 60 minutes to provide adequate anesthesia, planning is necessary, such as applying the cream before an office visit or immediately on arrival. Additional studies need to be performed on the use of local anesthetic agents to better establish their safety and effectiveness when used to manage injection pain and to ensure that their use does not interfere with the immune response, particularly to SC injections. Oral administration of a small volume of a 25% to 75% sucrose solution (eg, dissolving 1 packet of sugar in 10 mL water) or dipping a pacifier into a sucrose solution just before the injection reduces crying time in infants younger than 6 months of age.

Scheduling Immunizations

A vaccine is intended to be administered to a person who is capable of an appropriate immunologic response and who likely will benefit from the protection given. However, optimal immunologic response for the person must be balanced against the need to achieve timely protection against disease. For example, pertussis-containing vaccines may be less immunogenic in early infancy than in later infancy, but the benefit of conferring protection in young infants—who experience the highest morbidity and mortality from pertussis—mandates that immunization should be given early, despite a lessened serum antibody response. For this reason, in some developing countries, oral polio vaccine is given at birth, in accordance with recommendations of the World Health Organization.

With parenterally administered live-virus vaccines, the inhibitory effect of residual specific maternal antibody determines the optimal age of administration. For example, live-virus measles-containing vaccine in use in the United States provides suboptimal rates of seroconversion during the first year of life, mainly because of interference by transplacentally acquired maternal antibody. If a measles-containing vaccine is administered before 12 months of age, the child should receive 2 additional doses of measles-containing vaccine at the recommended ages and interval (see Fig 1.1, p 27).

An additional factor in selecting an immunization schedule is the need to achieve a uniform and regular response. With some products, a response is achieved after 1 dose. For example, live-virus rubella vaccine evokes a predictable response at high rates after a single dose. With many inactivated or component vaccines, a primary series of doses is necessary to achieve an optimal initial response in recipients. Some people require multiple doses to respond to all included antigens. For example, some people respond only to 1 or 2 types of poliovirus after a single dose of poliovirus vaccine, so multiple doses are given to produce antibody against all 3 types, thereby ensuring complete protection for the person and maximum response rates for the population. For some vaccines, periodic booster doses (eg, with tetanus and diphtheria toxoids and acellular pertussis antigen) are administered to maintain protection.

Vaccines are safe and effective when administered simultaneously. This information is particularly important for scheduling immunizations for children with lapsed or missed immunizations and for people preparing for international travel (see Simultaneous Administration of Multiple Vaccines, p 33). Data indicate possible impaired immune responses when 2 or more parenterally administered live-virus vaccines are not given simultaneously but within 28 days of each other; therefore, live-virus vaccines not administered on the same day should be given at least 28 days (4 weeks) apart whenever possible. An exception is made for certain orally administered live vaccines (Table 1.7, p 26). No minimum interval is required between administration of different inactivated vaccines.

The recommended childhood (0 through 6 years of age), adolescent (7 through 18 years of age), and catch-up immunization schedules in Fig 1.1–1.3 (p 27–31) represent a consensus of the American Academy of Pediatrics (AAP), the Advisory Committee on Immunization Practices (ACIP) of the CDC, and the American Academy of Family Physicians (AAFP). These schedules are reviewed regularly, and updated national schedules are issued annually in February; schedules are available at **www.cdc.gov/vaccines/recs/schedules/default.htm** and are posted at *Red Book* Online. Interim recommendations occasionally may be made when issues such as a shortage of a product or a safety concern arise or a new recommendation may be made to incorporate a new

Table 1.7. Guidelines for Spacing of Live and Inactivated Antigens

Antigen Combination	Recommended Minimum Interval Between Doses
2 or more inactivated[a]	None; can be administered simultaneously or at any interval between doses
Inactivated plus live	None; can be administered simultaneously or at any interval between doses
2 or more live injectable[b]	28-day minimum interval if not administered simultaneously

[a] Some experts recommend a 28-day interval between Tdap and MCV4-D if not administered simultaneously.
[b] An exception is made for some live oral vaccines (ie, Ty21a typhoid vaccine, oral poliovirus vaccine, oral rotavirus vaccine) that can be administered simultaneously or at any interval before or after inactivated or live parenteral vaccines.

vaccine or vaccine indication. Special attention should be given to footnotes on the schedule, which summarize major recommendations for routine childhood immunizations.

Combination vaccine products may be given whenever any component of the combination is indicated and its other components are not contraindicated, provided they are licensed by the FDA for that dose in the schedule for each component and for the child's age. The use of a combination vaccine generally is preferred over separate injections of its equivalent component vaccines. Considerations should include provider assessment, patient preference, and the potential for adverse events. The provider assessment should include the number of injections, vaccine availability, the likelihood of improved coverage, the likelihood of patient return, and storage and cost considerations.

Fig 1.3 (p 31) gives the recommended catch-up schedule for children who were not immunized appropriately during the first year of life. Web-based childhood immunization schedulers using the current vaccine recommendations are available for parents, caregivers, and health care professionals to make instant immunization schedules for children, adolescents, and adults (see Immunization Schedulers, p 5, or **www.cdc.gov/vaccines**).

For children in whom early or rapid immunization is urgent or for children not immunized on schedule, simultaneous immunization with multiple products allows for more rapid protection. In addition, in some circumstances, immunization can be initiated earlier than at the usually recommended time or schedule, or doses can be given at shorter intervals than are recommended routinely (for guidelines, see the disease-specific chapters in Section 3). Physicians or localities using such a compressed schedule should be certain to observe the 6-month minimum interval between doses 3 and 4 of DTaP vaccine as well as other minimal interval recommendations. The final dose of the hepatitis B vaccine series should be administered at least 16 weeks after the first dose and no earlier than 24 weeks of age.

Influenza vaccine should be administered before the start of influenza season but provides benefit if administered at any time during the influenza season (ie, usually through March) (see Influenza, Timing of Vaccine Administration, p 450).

The immunization schedule issued by the AAP, ACIP, and AAFP primarily is intended for children and adolescents in the United States. In many instances, the guidelines will be applicable to children in other countries, but individual pediatricians and recommending committees in each country are responsible for determining the appropriateness of the recommendations for their setting. The schedule recommended by the Expanded Programme on Immunization of the World Health Organization should be

FIGURE 1.1 RECOMMENDED IMMUNIZATION SCHEDULE FOR PERSONS AGED 0 THROUGH 6 YEARS

FIGURE 1: Recommended immunization schedule for persons aged 0 through 6 years—United States, 2012 (for those who fall behind or start late, see the catch-up schedule [Figure 1.3])

Vaccine ▼ Age ►	Birth	1 month	2 months	4 months	6 months	9 months	12 months	15 months	18 months	19–23 months	2–3 years	4–6 years
Hepatitis B[1]	Hep B	HepB			HepB							
Rotavirus[2]			RV	RV	RV[2]							
Diphtheria, tetanus, pertussis[3]			DTaP	DTaP	DTaP		see footnote[3]	DTaP				DTaP
Haemophilus influenzae type b[4]			Hib	Hib	Hib[4]		Hib					
Pneumococcal[5]			PCV	PCV	PCV		PCV				PPSV	
Inactivated poliovirus[6]			IPV	IPV		IPV						IPV
Influenza[7]					Influenza (Yearly)							
Measles, mumps, rubella[8]							MMR		see footnote[8]			MMR
Varicella[9]							Varicella		see footnote[9]			Varicella
Hepatitis A[10]							Dose 1[10]				HepA Series	
Meningococcal[11]							MCV4 — see footnote[11]					

Range of recommended ages for all children

Range of recommended ages for certain high-risk groups

Range of recommended ages for all children and certain high-risk groups

This schedule includes recommendations in effect as of December 23, 2011. Any dose not administered at the recommended age should be administered at a subsequent visit, when indicated and feasible. The use of a combination vaccine generally is preferred over separate injections of its equivalent component vaccines. Vaccination providers should consult the relevant Advisory Committee on Immunization Practices (ACIP) statement for detailed recommendations, available online at http://www.cdc.gov/vaccines/pubs/acip-list.htm. Clinically significant adverse events that follow vaccination should be reported to the Vaccine Adverse Event Reporting System (VAERS) online (http://www.vaers.hhs.gov) or by telephone (800-822-7967).

FIGURE 1.1 RECOMMENDED IMMUNIZATION SCHEDULE FOR PERSONS AGED 0 THROUGH 6 YEARS, CONTINUED

1. **Hepatitis B (HepB) vaccine.** (Minimum age: birth)

   At birth:
   - Administer monovalent HepB vaccine to all newborns before hospital discharge.
   - For infants born to hepatitis B surface antigen (HBsAg)–positive mothers, administer HepB vaccine and 0.5 mL of hepatitis B immune globulin (HBIG) within 12 hours of birth. These infants should be tested for HBsAg and antibody to HBsAg (anti-HBs) 1 to 2 months after completion of at least 3 doses of the HepB series, at age 9 through 18 months (generally at the next well-child visit).
   - If mother's HBsAg status is unknown, within 12 hours of birth administer HepB vaccine for infants weighing ≥2,000 grams, and HepB vaccine plus HBIG for infants weighing <2,000 grams. Determine mother's HBsAg status as soon as possible and, if she is HBsAg-positive, administer HBIG for infants weighing ≥2,000 grams (no later than age 1 week).

   Doses after the birth dose:
   - The second dose should be administered at age 1 to 2 months. Monovalent HepB vaccine should be used for doses administered before age 6 weeks.
   - Administration of a total of 4 doses of HepB vaccine is permissible when a combination vaccine containing HepB is administered after the birth dose.
   - Infants who did not receive a birth dose should receive 3 doses of a HepB-containing vaccine starting as soon as feasible (Figure 3).
   - The minimum interval between dose 1 and dose 2 is 4 weeks, and between dose 2 and 3 is 8 weeks. The final (third or fourth) dose in the HepB vaccine series should be administered no earlier than age 24 weeks and at least 16 weeks after the first dose.

2. **Rotavirus (RV) vaccines.** (Minimum age: 6 weeks for both RV-1 [Rotarix] and RV-5 [Rota Teq])
   - The maximum age for the first dose in the series is 14 weeks, 6 days; and 8 months, 0 days for the final dose in the series. Vaccination should not be initiated for infants aged 15 weeks, 0 days or older.
   - If RV-1 (Rotarix) is administered at ages 2 and 4 months, a dose at 6 months is not indicated.

3. **Diphtheria and tetanus toxoids and acellular pertussis (DTaP) vaccine.** (Minimum age: 6 weeks)
   - The fourth dose may be administered as early as age 12 months, provided at least 6 months have elapsed since the third dose.

4. **Haemophilus influenzae type b (Hib) conjugate vaccine.** (Minimum age: 6 weeks)
   - If PRP-OMP (PedvaxHIB or Comvax [HepB-Hib]) is administered at ages 2 and 4 months, a dose at age 6 months is not indicated.
   - Hiberix should only be used for the booster (final) dose in children aged 12 months through 4 years.

5. **Pneumococcal vaccines.** (Minimum age: 6 weeks for pneumococcal conjugate vaccine [PCV]; 2 years for pneumococcal polysaccharide vaccine (PPSV))
   - Administer 1 dose of PCV to all healthy children aged 24 through 59 months who are not completely vaccinated for their age.
   - For children who have received an age-appropriate series of 7-valent PCV (PCV7), a single supplemental dose of 13-valent PCV (PCV13) is recommended for:
     — All children aged 14 through 59 months
     — Children aged 60 through 71 months with underlying medical conditions.
   - Administer PPSV at least 8 weeks after last dose of PCV to children aged 2 years or older with certain underlying medical conditions, including a cochlear implant. See *MMWR* 2010;59(No. RR-11), available at http://www.cdc.gov/mmwr/pdf/rr/rr5911.pdf.

6. **Inactivated poliovirus vaccine (IPV).** (Minimum age: 6 weeks)
   - If 4 or more doses are administered before age 4 years, an additional dose should be administered on or after the fourth birthday and at least 6 months after the previous dose.

7. **Influenza vaccines.** (Minimum age: 6 months for trivalent inactivated influenza vaccine [TIV]; 2 years for live, attenuated influenza vaccine [LAIV])
   - For most healthy children aged 2 years and older, either LAIV or TIV may be used. However, LAIV should not be administered to some children, including 1) children with asthma, 2) children 2 through 4 years who had wheezing in the past 12 months, or 3) children who have any other underlying medical conditions that predispose them to influenza complications. For all other contraindications to use of LAIV, see *MMWR* 2010;59(No. RR-8), available at http://www.cdc.gov/mmwr/pdf/rr/rr5908.pdf.
   - For children aged 6 months through 8 years:
     — For the 2011–12 season, administer 2 doses (separated by at least 4 weeks) to those who did not receive at least 1 dose of the 2010–11 vaccine. Those who received at least 1 dose of the 2010–11 vaccine require 1 dose for the 2011–12 season.
     — For the 2012–13 season, follow dosing guidelines in the 2012 ACIP influenza vaccine recommendations.

8. **Measles, mumps, and rubella (MMR) vaccine.** (Minimum age: 12 months)
   - The second dose may be administered before age 4 years, provided at least 4 weeks have elapsed since the first dose.
   - Administer MMR vaccine to infants aged 6 through 11 months who are traveling internationally. These children should be revaccinated with 2 doses of MMR vaccine, the first at ages 12 through 15 months and at least 4 weeks after the previous dose, and the second at ages 4 through 6 years.

9. **Varicella (VAR) vaccine.** (Minimum age: 12 months)
   - The second dose may be administered before age 4 years, provided at least 3 months have elapsed since the first dose.
   - For children aged 12 months through 12 years, the recommended minimum interval between doses is 3 months. However, if the second dose was administered at least 4 weeks after the first dose, it can be accepted as valid.

10. **Hepatitis A (HepA) vaccine.** (Minimum age: 12 months)
    - Administer the second (final) dose 6 to 18 months after the first.
    - Unvaccinated children 24 months and older at high risk should be vaccinated. See *MMWR* 2006;55(No. RR-7), available at http://www.cdc.gov/mmwr/pdf/rr/rr5507.pdf.
    - A 2-dose HepA vaccine series is recommended for anyone aged 24 months and older, previously unvaccinated, for whom immunity against hepatitis A virus infection is desired.

11. **Meningococcal conjugate vaccines, quadrivalent (MCV4).** (Minimum age: 9 months for Menactra [MCV4-D], 2 years for Menveo [MCV4-CRM])
    - For children aged 9 through 23 months 1) with persistent complement component deficiency; 2) who are residents of or travelers to countries with hyperendemic or epidemic disease; or 3) who are present during outbreaks caused by a vaccine serogroup, administer 2 primary doses of MCV4-D, ideally at ages 9 months and 12 months or at least 8 weeks apart.
    - For children aged 24 months and older with 1) persistent complement component deficiency who have not been previously vaccinated; or 2) anatomic/functional asplenia, administer 2 primary doses of either MCV4 at least 8 weeks apart.
    - For children with anatomic/functional asplenia, if MCV4-D (Menactra) is used, administer at a minimum age of 2 years and at least 4 weeks after completion of all PCV doses.
    - See *MMWR* 2011;60:72–6, available at http://www.cdc.gov/mmwr/pdf/wk/mm6003.pdf, and Vaccines for Children Program resolution No. 6/11-1, available at http://www.cdc.gov/vaccines/programs/vfc/downloads/resolutions/06-11mening-mcv.pdf, and *MMWR* 2011;60:1391–2, available at http://www.cdc.gov/mmwr/pdf/wk/mm6040.pdf, for further guidance, including revaccination guidelines.

This schedule is approved by the Advisory Committee on Immunization Practices (http://www.cdc.gov/vaccines/recs/acip/), the American Academy of Pediatrics (http://www.aap.org), and the American Academy of Family Physicians (http://www.aafp.org/).
Department of Health and Human Services • Centers for Disease Control and Prevention

FIGURE 1.2 RECOMMENDED IMMUNIZATION SCHEDULE FOR PERSONS AGED 7 THROUGH 18 YEARS

Recommended immunization schedule for persons aged 7 through 18 years — United States, 2012 (for those who fall behind or start late, see the schedule below and the catch-up schedule [Figure 1.3])

Vaccine ▼ / Age ▶	7–10 years	11–12 years	13–18 years
Tetanus, diphtheria, pertussis[1]	1 dose (if indicated)	1 dose	1 dose (if indicated)
Human papillomavirus[2]	See footnote[2]	3 doses	
Meningococcal[3]	See footnote[3]	Dose 1	Booster at age 16 years / Complete 3-dose series
Influenza[4]	Influenza (yearly)		
Pneumococcal[5]		See footnote[5]	
Hepatitis A[6]		Complete 2-dose series	
Hepatitis B[7]		Complete 3-dose series	
Inactivated poliovirus[8]		Complete 3-dose series	
Measles, mumps, rubella[9]		Complete 2-dose series	
Varicella[10]		Complete 2-dose series	

Legend:
- Range of recommended ages for all children
- Range of recommended ages for catch-up immunization
- Range of recommended ages for certain high-risk groups

This schedule includes recommendations in effect as of December 23, 2011. Any dose not administered at the recommended age should be administered at a subsequent visit, when indicated and feasible. The use of a combination vaccine generally is preferred over separate injections of its equivalent component vaccines. Vaccination providers should consult the relevant Advisory Committee on Immunization Practices (ACIP) statement for detailed recommendations, available online at http://www.cdc.gov/vaccines/pubs/acip-list.htm. Clinically significant adverse events that follow vaccination should be reported to the Vaccine Adverse Event Reporting System (VAERS) online (http://www.vaers.hhs.gov) or by telephone (800-822-7967).

FIGURE 1.2 RECOMMENDED IMMUNIZATION SCHEDULE FOR PERSONS AGED 7 THROUGH 18 YEARS, CONTINUED

1. **Tetanus and diphtheria toxoids and acellular pertussis (Tdap) vaccine.** (Minimum age: 10 years for Boostrix and 11 years for Adacel)
   - Persons aged 11 through 18 years who have not received Tdap vaccine should receive a dose followed by tetanus and diphtheria toxoids (Td) booster doses every 10 years thereafter.
   - Tdap vaccine should be substituted for a single dose of Td in the catch-up series for children aged 7 through 10 years. Refer to the catch-up schedule if additional doses of tetanus and diphtheria toxoid–containing vaccine are needed.
   - Tdap vaccine can be administered regardless of the interval since the last tetanus and diphtheria toxoid–containing vaccine.

2. **Human papillomavirus (HPV) vaccines (HPV4 [Gardasil] and HPV2 [Cervarix]).** (Minimum age: 9 years)
   - Either HPV4 or HPV2 is recommended in a 3-dose series for females aged 11 or 12 years. HPV4 is recommended in a 3-dose series for males aged 11 or 12 years.
   - The vaccine series can be started beginning at age 9 years.
   - Administer the second dose 1 to 2 months after the first dose and the third dose 6 months after the first dose (at least 24 weeks after the first dose).
   - See *MMWR* 2010;59:626–32, available at http://www.cdc.gov/mmwr/pdf/wk/mm5920.pdf.

3. **Meningococcal conjugate vaccines, quadrivalent (MCV4).**
   - Administer MCV4 at age 11 through 12 years with a booster dose at age 16 years.
   - Administer MCV4 at age 13 through 18 years if patient is not previously vaccinated.
   - If the first dose is administered at age 13 through 15 years, a booster dose should be administered at age 16 through 18 years with a minimum interval of at least 8 weeks after the preceding dose.
   - If the first dose is administered at age 16 years or older, a booster dose is not needed.
   - Administer 2 primary doses at least 8 weeks apart to previously unvaccinated persons with persistent complement component deficiency or anatomic/functional asplenia, and 1 dose every 5 years thereafter.
   - Adolescents aged 11 through 18 years with human immunodeficiency virus (HIV) infection should receive a 2-dose primary series of MCV4, at least 8 weeks apart.
   - See *MMWR* 2011;60:72–76, available at http://www.cdc.gov/mmwr/pdf/wk/mm6003.pdf; and Vaccines for Children Program resolution No. 6/11–1, available at http://www.cdc.gov/vaccines/programs/vfc/downloads/resolutions/06-11mening-mcv.pdf, for further guidelines.

4. **Influenza vaccines (trivalent inactivated influenza vaccine [TIV] and live, attenuated influenza vaccine [LAIV]).**
   - For most healthy, nonpregnant persons, either LAIV or TIV may be used, except LAIV should not be used for some persons, including those with asthma or any other underlying medical conditions that predispose them to influenza complications. For all other contraindications to use of LAIV, see *MMWR* 2010;59(No.RR-8), available at http://www.cdc.gov/mmwr/pdf/rr/rr5908.pdf.
   - Administer 1 dose to persons aged 9 years and older.
   - For children aged 6 months through 8 years:
     — For the 2011–12 season, administer 2 doses (separated by at least 4 weeks) to those who did not receive 1 dose of the 2010–11 vaccine. Those who received at least 1 dose of the 2010–11 vaccine require 1 dose for the 2011–12 season.
     — For the 2012–13 season, follow dosing guidelines in the 2012 ACIP influenza vaccine recommendations.

5. **Pneumococcal vaccines (pneumococcal conjugate vaccine [PCV] and pneumococcal polysaccharide vaccine [PPSV]).**
   - A single dose of PCV may be administered to children aged 6 through 18 years who have anatomic/functional asplenia, HIV infection or other immunocompromising condition, cochlear implant, or cerebral spinal fluid leak. See *MMWR* 2010;59(No. RR-11), available at http://www.cdc.gov/mmwr/pdf/rr/rr5911.pdf.
   - Administer PPSV at least 8 weeks after the last dose of PCV to children aged 2 years or older with certain underlying medical conditions, including a cochlear implant. A single revaccination should be administered after 5 years to children with anatomic/functional asplenia or an immunocompromising condition.

6. **Hepatitis A (HepA) vaccine.**
   - HepA vaccine is recommended for children older than 23 months who live in areas where vaccination programs target older children, who are at increased risk for infection, or for whom immunity against hepatitis A virus infection is desired. See *MMWR* 2006;55(No. RR-7), available at http://www.cdc.gov/mmwr/pdf/rr/rr5507.pdf.
   - Administer 2 doses at least 6 months apart to unvaccinated persons.

7. **Hepatitis B (HepB) vaccine.**
   - Administer the 3-dose series to those not previously vaccinated.
   - For those with incomplete vaccination, follow the catch-up recommendations (Figure 3).
   - A 2-dose series (doses separated by at least 4 months) of adult formulation Recombivax HB is licensed for use in children aged 11 through 15 years.

8. **Inactivated poliovirus vaccine (IPV).**
   - The final dose in the series should be administered at least 6 months after the previous dose.
   - If both OPV and IPV were administered as part of a series, a total of 4 doses should be administered, regardless of the child's current age.
   - IPV is not routinely recommended for U.S. residents aged 18 years or older.

9. **Measles, mumps, and rubella (MMR) vaccine.**
   - The minimum interval between the 2 doses of MMR vaccine is 4 weeks.

10. **Varicella (VAR) vaccine.**
    - For persons without evidence of immunity (see *MMWR* 2007;56[No. RR-4], available at http://www.cdc.gov/mmwr/pdf/rr/rr5604.pdf), administer 2 doses if not previously vaccinated or the second dose if only 1 dose has been administered.
    - For persons aged 7 through 12 years, the recommended minimum interval between doses is 3 months. However, if the second dose was administered at least 4 weeks after the first dose, it can be accepted as valid.
    - For persons aged 13 years and older, the minimum interval between doses is 4 weeks.

This schedule is approved by the Advisory Committee on Immunization Practices (http://www.cdc.gov/vaccines/recs/acip), the American Academy of Pediatrics (http://www.aap.org), and the American Academy of Family Physicians (http://www.aafp.org). p://www.aafp.org).

FIGURE 1.3 CATCH-UP IMMUNIZATION SCHEDULE FOR PERSONS AGED 4 MONTHS THROUGH 18 YEARS WHO START LATE OR WHO ARE MORE THAN 1 MONTH BEHIND

Catch-up immunization schedule for persons aged 4 months through 18 years who start late or who are more than 1 month behind —United States • 2012
The figure below provides catch-up schedules and minimum intervals between doses for children whose vaccinations have been delayed. A vaccine series does not need to be restarted, regardless of the time that has elapsed between doses. Use the section appropriate for the child's age. **Always use this table in conjunction with the accompanying childhood and adolescent immunization schedules (Figures 1 and 2) and their respective footnotes.**

Vaccine	Minimum Age for Dose 1	Persons aged 4 months through 6 years			
		Minimum Interval Between Doses			
		Dose 1 to dose 2	Dose 2 to dose 3	Dose 3 to dose 4	Dose 4 to dose 5
Hepatitis B	Birth	4 weeks	8 weeks and at least 16 weeks after first dose; minimum age for the final dose is 24 weeks		
Rotavirus[1]	6 weeks	4 weeks	4 weeks[1]		
Diphtheria, tetanus, pertussis[2]	6 weeks	4 weeks	4 weeks	6 months	6 months[2]
Haemophilus influenzae type b[3]	6 weeks	4 weeks if first dose administered at younger than age 12 months / 8 weeks (as final dose) if first dose administered at age 12–14 months / No further doses needed if first dose administered at age 15 months or older	4 weeks[3] if current age is younger than 12 months / 8 weeks (as final dose)[3] if current age is 12 months or older and first dose administered at younger than age 12 months and second dose administered at younger than 15 months / No further doses needed if previous dose administered at age 15 months or older	8 weeks (as final dose) This dose only necessary for children aged 12 months through 59 months who received 3 doses before age 12 months	
Pneumococcal[4]	6 weeks	4 weeks if first dose administered at younger than age 12 months / 8 weeks (as final dose for healthy children) if first dose administered at age 12 months or older or current age 24 through 59 months / No further doses needed for healthy children if first dose administered at age 24 months or older	4 weeks if current age is younger than 12 months / 8 weeks (as final dose for healthy children) if current age is 12 months or older / No further doses needed for healthy children if previous dose administered at age 24 months or older	8 weeks (as final dose) This dose only necessary for children aged 12 months through 59 months who received 3 doses before age 12 months or for children at high risk who received 3 doses at any age	
Inactivated poliovirus[5]	6 weeks	4 weeks	4 weeks	6 months[5] minimum age 4 years for final dose	
Meningococcal[6]	9 months	8 weeks[6]			
Measles, mumps, rubella[7]	12 months	4 weeks			
Varicella[8]	12 months	3 months			
Hepatitis A	12 months	6 months			
		Persons aged 7 through 18 years			
Tetanus, diphtheria/ tetanus, diphtheria, pertussis[9]	7 years[9]	4 weeks	4 weeks if first dose administered at younger than age 12 months / 6 months if first dose administered at 12 months or older	6 months if first dose administered at younger than age 12 months	
Human papillomavirus[10]	9 years	Routine dosing intervals are recommended[10]			
Hepatitis A	12 months	6 months			
Hepatitis B	Birth	4 weeks	8 weeks (and at least 16 weeks after first dose)		
Inactivated poliovirus[5]	6 weeks	4 weeks	4 weeks[5]	6 months[5]	
Meningococcal[6]	9 months	8 weeks[6]			
Measles, mumps, rubella[7]	12 months	4 weeks			
Varicella[8]	12 months	3 months if person is younger than age 13 years / 4 weeks if person is aged 13 years or older			

1. **Rotavirus (RV) vaccines (RV-1 [Rotarix] and RV-5 [Rota Teq]).**
   - The maximum age for the first dose in the series is 14 weeks, 6 days; and 8 months, 0 days for the final dose in the series. Vaccination should not be initiated for infants aged 15 weeks, 0 days or older.
   - If RV-1 was administered for the first and second doses, a third dose is not indicated.
2. **Diphtheria and tetanus toxoids and acellular pertussis (DTaP) vaccine.**
   - The fifth dose is not necessary if the fourth dose was administered at age 4 years or older.
3. **Haemophilus influenzae type b (Hib) conjugate vaccine.**
   - Hib vaccine should be considered for unvaccinated persons aged 5 years or older who have sickle cell disease, leukemia, human immunodeficiency virus (HIV) infection, or anatomic/functional asplenia.
   - If the first 2 doses were PRP-OMP (PedvaxHIB or Comvax) and were administered at age 11 months or younger, the third (and final) dose should be administered at age 12 through 15 months and at least 8 weeks after the second dose.
   - If the first dose was administered at age 7 through 11 months, administer the second dose at least 4 weeks later and a final dose at age 12 through 15 months.
4. **Pneumococcal vaccines.** (Minimum age: 6 weeks for pneumococcal conjugate vaccine [PCV]; 2 years for pneumococcal polysaccharide vaccine [PPSV])
   - For children aged 24 through 71 months with underlying medical conditions, administer 1 dose of PCV if 3 doses of PCV were received previously, or administer 2 doses of PCV at least 8 weeks apart if fewer than 3 doses of PCV were received previously.
   - A single dose of PCV may be administered to certain children aged 6 through 18 years with underlying medical conditions. See age-specific schedules for details.
   - Administer PPSV to children aged 2 years or older with certain underlying medical conditions. See *MMWR* 2010:59(No. RR-11), available at http://www.cdc.gov/mmwr/pdf/rr/rr5911.pdf.
5. **Inactivated poliovirus vaccine (IPV).**
   - A fourth dose is not necessary if the third dose was administered at age 4 years or older and at least 6 months after the previous dose.
   - In the first 6 months of life, minimum age and minimum intervals are only recommended if the person is at risk for imminent exposure to circulating poliovirus (i.e., travel to a polio-endemic region or during an outbreak).
   - IPV is not routinely recommended for U.S. residents aged 18 years or older.
6. **Meningococcal conjugate vaccines, quadrivalent (MCV4).** (Minimum age: 9 months for Menactra [MCV4-D]; 2 years for Menveo [MCV4-CRM])
   - See Figure 1 ("Recommended immunization schedule for persons aged 0 through 6 years") and Figure 2 ("Recommended immunization schedule for persons aged 7 through 18 years") for further guidance.
7. **Measles, mumps, and rubella (MMR) vaccine.**
   - Administer the second dose routinely at age 4 through 6 years.
8. **Varicella (VAR) vaccine.**
   - Administer the second dose routinely at age 4 through 6 years. If the second dose was administered at least 4 weeks after the first dose, it can be accepted as valid.
9. **Tetanus and diphtheria toxoids (Td) and tetanus and diphtheria toxoids and acellular pertussis (Tdap) vaccines.**
   - For children aged 7 through 10 years who are not fully immunized with the childhood DTaP vaccine series, Tdap vaccine should be substituted for a single dose of Td vaccine in the catch-up series; if additional doses are needed, use Td vaccine. For these children, an adolescent Tdap vaccine dose should not be given.
   - An inadvertent dose of DTaP vaccine administered to children aged 7 through 10 years can count as part of the catch-up series. This dose can count as the adolescent Tdap dose, or the child can later receive a Tdap booster dose at age 11–12 years.
10. **Human papillomavirus (HPV) vaccines (HPV4 [Gardasil] and HPV2 [Cervarix]).**
    - Administer the vaccine series to females (either HPV2 or HPV4) and males (HPV4) at age 13 through 18 years if patient is not previously vaccinated.
    - Use recommended routine dosing intervals for vaccine series catch-up; see Figure 2 ("Recommended immunization schedule for persons aged 7 through 18 years").

Clinically significant adverse events that follow vaccination should be reported to the Vaccine Adverse Event Reporting System (VAERS) online (http://www.vaers.hhs.gov) or by telephone (800-822-7967). Suspected cases of vaccine-preventable diseases should be reported to the state or local health department. Additional information, including precautions and contraindications for vaccination, is available from CDC online (http://www.cdc.gov/vaccines) or by telephone (800-CDC-INFO [800-232-4636]).

consulted (**www.who.int**). Modifications may be made by the ministries of health in individual countries on the basis of local considerations. Recommendations for vaccine schedules in Europe are available at the European Center for Disease Prevention and Control (**www.ecdc.europa.eu**).

Minimum Ages and Minimum Intervals Between Vaccine Doses

Immunizations are recommended for members of the youngest age group at risk of experiencing the disease for whom efficacy, immunogenicity, and safety have been demonstrated. Most vaccines in the childhood and adolescent immunization schedule require 2 or more doses for stimulation of an adequate and persisting antibody response. Studies have demonstrated that the recommended age and interval between doses of the same antigen(s) provide optimal protection. Fig 1.3 (p 31) lists recommended minimum ages and intervals between immunizations for vaccines in the childhood and adolescent immunization schedules. Administering doses of a multidose vaccine at intervals shorter than those in the childhood and adolescent immunization schedules might be necessary in circumstances in which an infant or child is behind schedule and needs to be brought up to date quickly or when international travel is pending. In these cases, an accelerated schedule using minimum age or interval criteria can be used. These accelerated schedules should not be used routinely.

Vaccines should not be administered at intervals less than the recommended minimum or at an earlier age than the recommended minimum (eg, accelerated schedules). Two exceptions to this may occur. The first is for measles vaccine during a measles outbreak, in which case the vaccine may be administered as early as 6 months of age. However, if a measles-containing vaccine is administered before 12 months of age, the dose is not counted toward the 2-dose measles vaccine series, and the child should be reimmunized at 12 through 15 months of age with a measles-containing vaccine. A third dose of a measles-containing vaccine is indicated at 4 through 6 years of age but can be administered as early as 4 weeks after the second dose (see Measles, p 489). The second consideration involves administering a dose a few days earlier than the minimum interval or age, which is unlikely to have a substantially negative effect on the immune response to that dose. Although immunizations should not be scheduled at an interval or age less than the minimums listed in Fig 1.3 (p 31), a child may be in the office early or for an appointment not specifically for immunization (eg, recheck of otitis media). In this situation, the clinician can consider administering the vaccine before the minimum interval or age. If the child is known to the clinician, rescheduling the child for immunization closer to the recommended interval is preferred. If the parent or child is not known to the clinician or follow-up cannot be ensured (eg, habitually misses appointments), administration of the vaccine at that visit rather than rescheduling the child for a later visit is preferable. Vaccine doses administered 4 days or fewer before the minimum interval or age can be counted as valid. This 4-day recommendation does not apply to rabies vaccine because of the unique schedule for this vaccine. Doses administered 5 days or more before the minimum interval or age should not be counted as valid doses and should be repeated as age appropriate. The repeat dose should be spaced after the invalid dose by at least 4 weeks (Fig 1.3 [p 31]). Health care professionals need to be aware of local or state requirements to be certain that doses of selected vaccines (in particular, MMR) administered within 4 days of the minimal interval will be accepted as valid.

Interchangeability of Vaccine Products

Similar vaccines made by different manufacturers can differ in the number and amount of their specific antigenic components and formulation of adjuvants and conjugating agents, thereby eliciting different immune responses. However, such vaccines have been considered interchangeable by most experts when administered according to their recommended indications, although data documenting the effects of interchangeability are limited. Licensed vaccines that may be used interchangeably during a vaccine series from different manufacturers, according to recommendations from AAP or ACIP, include diphtheria and tetanus toxoids vaccines, hepatitis A vaccines, hepatitis B (HepB) vaccines for infants, and rabies vaccines (see Rabies, p 600). An example of similar vaccines used in different schedules that are not recommended as interchangeable is the 2-dose HepB vaccine option currently available for adolescents 11 through 15 years of age. Adolescent patients begun on a 3-dose HepB regimen are not candidates to complete their series with HepB vaccine used in the 2-dose protocol, and the 2-dose schedule is applicable only to Recombivax HB (see Hepatitis B, p 369).

Licensed *Haemophilus influenzae* type b (Hib) conjugate vaccines are considered interchangeable for primary as well as for booster immunization as long as recommendations concerning conversion from a 3-dose regimen (polyribosylribitol phosphate-meningococcal outer membrane protein [PRP-OMP]) to a 4-dose regimen (all other conjugated polyribosylribitol [PRP] preparations) are followed (see *Haemophilus influenzae* Infections, p 345). Licensed rotavirus (RV) vaccines are considered interchangeable as long as recommendations concerning conversion from a 2-dose regimen (RV-1) to a 3-dose regimen (RV-5) are followed (see Rotavirus, p 626).

Minimal data on safety and immunogenicity and no data on efficacy are available for interchangeability of DTaP vaccines from different manufacturers. When feasible, DTaP from the same manufacturer should be used for the primary series (see Pertussis, p 553). However, in circumstances in which the DTaP product received previously is not known or the previously administered product is not readily available, any of the DTaP vaccines may be used according to licensure for dose and age. Matching of booster doses of DTaP and adolescent Tdap by manufacturer is not necessary. Whenever possible, the same HPV vaccine product should be used for the 3-dose series, particularly since the 2 vaccines differ in serotype content (see Human Papillomaviruses, p 524). However, if the product previously received is not known or is not readily available, either HPV vaccine can be used to continue the series in females and should provide protection for HPV types 16 and 18. HPV2 vaccine is not licensed or recommended for use in males. Single-component vaccines from the same manufacturer of combination vaccines, including DTaP-HepB-IPV and DTaP-IPV/Hib are interchangeable (see Combination Vaccines, p 34).[1]

Simultaneous Administration of Multiple Vaccines

Simultaneous administration of most vaccines is safe, effective and recommended. Infants and children have sufficient immunologic capacity to respond to multiple vaccines. No contraindications to the simultaneous administration of multiple vaccines routinely

---

[1] Centers for Disease Control and Prevention. General recommendations on immunization—recommendations of the Advisory Committee on Immunization Practices (ACIP). *MMWR Recomm Rep.* 2011;60(RR-02):1–64

recommended for infants and children are known. Immune response to one vaccine generally does not interfere with responses to other vaccines. Simultaneous administration of IPV, MMR, varicella, or DTaP vaccines results in rates of seroconversion and of adverse effects similar to those observed when the vaccines are administered at separate visits. MMRV is associated with a higher rate of fever and febrile seizures after the recommended first dose than MMR and varicella administered separately at the same visit. Because simultaneous administration of routinely recommended vaccines is not known to affect the effectiveness or safety of any of the recommended childhood vaccines, simultaneous administration of all vaccines that are appropriate for the age and immunization status of the recipient is recommended.[1] When vaccines are administered simultaneously, separate syringes and separate sites should be used, and injections into the same extremity should be separated by at least 1 inch so that any local reactions can be differentiated. Simultaneous administration of multiple vaccines can increase immunization rates significantly. Some vaccines administered simultaneously may be more reactogenic than others (see disease-specific chapters). Individual vaccines should never be mixed in the same syringe unless they are specifically licensed and labeled for administration in one syringe. If an inactivated vaccine and an immune globulin product are indicated concurrently (eg, hepatitis B vaccine and HBIG, rabies vaccine and RIG), they should be administered at separate anatomic sites.

Combination Vaccines

Combination vaccines represent one solution to the issue of increased numbers of injections during single clinic visits and generally are preferred over separate injections of equivalent component vaccines. Combination vaccines can be administered instead of separately administered vaccines if licensed and indicated for the patient's age. Table 1.8 lists combination vaccines licensed for use in the United States. Separately administered vaccines also are available. Health care professionals who provide immunizations should stock combination and monovalent vaccines needed to immunize children against all diseases for which vaccines are recommended, but all available types or brand-name products do not need to be stocked. It is recognized that the decision of health care professionals to implement use of new combination vaccines involve complex economic and logistical considerations. Factors that should be considered by the provider, in consultation with the parent, include the potential for improved vaccine coverage, the number of injections needed, vaccine safety, vaccine availability, interchangeability, storage and cost issues, and whether the patient is likely to return for follow-up.

When patients have received the recommended immunizations for some of the components in a combination vaccine, administering the extra antigen(s) in the combination vaccine is permissible if they are not contraindicated and doing so will reduce the number of injections required. Excessive doses of toxoid vaccines (diphtheria and tetanus) may result in extensive local reactions. To overcome the potential for recording errors and ambiguities in the names of vaccine combinations, systems that eliminate error are needed to enhance the convenience and accuracy of transferring vaccine-identifying information into medical records and immunization information systems.

---

[1] Centers for Disease Control and Prevention. General recommendations on immunization. Recommendations of the Advisory Committee Immunization Practices. *MMWR Recomm Rep.* 2011;60(RR-02):1–64

Table 1.8. Combination Vaccines Licensed by the US Food and Drug Administration (FDA)[a]

Vaccine[b]	Trade Name (Year Licensed)	Age Group	Use in Immunization Schedule
		FDA Licensure	
Hib-HepB	Comvax (1996)	6 wk through 71 mo	Three-dose series administered at 2, 4, and 12 through 15 mo of age.
HepA-HepB	Twinrix (2001)	≥18 y	Three doses on a 0-, 1-, and 6-mo schedule.
DTaP-HepB-IPV	Pediarix (2002)	6 wk through 6 y	Three-dose series at 2, 4, and 6 mo of age.
MMRV	ProQuad (2005)	12 mo through 12 y	Two doses (see Varicella-Zoster Infections, p 774).
DTaP-IPV	Kinrix (2008)	4 y through 6 y	Booster for fifth dose of DTaP and fourth dose of IPV.
DTaP-IPV/Hib	Pentacel (2008)	6 wk through 4 y	Four-dose series administered at 2, 4, 6, and 15 through 18 mo of age.

Hib indicates *Haemophilus influenzae* type b vaccine; HepB, hepatitis B vaccine; DTaP, diphtheria and tetanus toxoids and acellular pertussis vaccine; HepA, hepatitis A vaccine; IPV, inactivated poliovirus vaccine; MMRV, measles-mumps-rubella-varicella vaccine.

[a]Excludes measles-mumps-rubella (MMR), DTaP, Tdap, Td, and IPV vaccines, for which individual components are not available. DTaP/Hib (TriHIBit) no longer is manufactured.

[b]Dash (-) indicates products are supplied in their final form by the manufacturer and do not require mixing or reconstitution by user; slash (/) indicates products are mixed or reconstituted by user.

Lapsed Immunizations

A lapse in the immunization schedule does not require reinitiation of the entire series or addition of doses to the series for any vaccine in the recommended schedule. If a dose of vaccine is missed, subsequent immunizations should be given at the next visit as if the usual interval had elapsed. For RV vaccine, the doses to be administered are age limited, so catch-up may not be possible (see Rotavirus Infections, p 626). See specific influenza vaccine recommendations for children younger than 9 years of age whose first 2 doses were not administered in the same season. The medical charts of children for whom immunizations have been missed or postponed should be flagged to remind health care professionals to resume the child's immunization regimen at the next available opportunity. Minimum age and interval recommendations should be followed for administration of all doses (see Fig 1.3, p 31). A computer-based tool is available for downloading and can be used to determine which vaccines a child 6 years of age and younger needs according to the childhood immunization schedule, including timing of missed or skipped vaccines (**https://www.vacscheduler.org**).

Unknown or Uncertain Immunization Status

Many children, adolescents, and young adults do not have adequate documentation of their immunizations. Parent or guardian recollection of a child's immunization history may not be accurate. Only written, dated records should be accepted as evidence of immunization. In general, when in doubt, a person with unknown or uncertain immunization status should be considered disease susceptible, and recommended immunizations should be initiated without delay on a schedule commensurate with the person's current age. An alternative approach in appropriate circumstances would be to perform specific serologic testing to evaluate immunity. No evidence suggests that administration of most vaccines to already immune recipients is harmful. In general, initiation of revaccination with an age-appropriate schedule of pertussis, diphtheria, and tetanus toxoid-containing vaccine is appropriate, with performance of serologic testing for specific IgG antibody only if a severe local reaction occurs.[1] Tdap, rather than DTaP, should be given to people 7 years of age or older, and Tdap should be used for a tetanus-diphtheria-containing vaccine for people 11 through 64 years of age who previously have not received Tdap (see Pertussis, p 553, for specific recommendations for different Tdap vaccines). People 7 through 64 years of age should receive a dose of Tdap if they did not receive complete age-appropriate DTaP schedule of pertussis immunization and have not already received Tdap. Adults 65 years of age and older who previously have not received Tdap should receive a single dose of Tdap.

Immunizations Received Outside the United States

People immunized in other countries, including internationally adopted children, refugees, and exchange students, should be immunized according to recommended schedules (including minimal ages and intervals) in the United States for healthy infants, children, and adolescents (see Fig 1.1–1.3, p 27–31). In general, only written documentation should be accepted as evidence of previous immunization. Written records may be considered valid if the vaccines, dates of administration, numbers of doses, intervals between doses, and age of the patient at the time of immunization are comparable with those of the current US or World Health Organization schedules (**http://apps.who.int/ immunization_monitoring/en/globalsummary/countryprofileselect.cfm**). Although some vaccines with inadequate potency have been produced in other countries, most vaccines used worldwide are produced with adequate quality-control standards and are reliable. However, immunization records for certain children, especially children from orphanages, may not accurately reflect protection because of inaccuracies, fraudulent data, lack of vaccine potency, or other problems, such as recording MMR vaccine but giving a product that did not contain one or more of the components (eg, mumps and/ or rubella). Therefore, serologic testing or reimmunization may be reasonable for these children (see Unknown or Uncertain Immunization Status, p 36). If serologic testing is not available and receipt of immunogenic vaccines cannot be ensured, the prudent course is to repeat administration of the immunizations in question (see Medical Evaluation of Internationally Adopted Children, p 191).

---

[1] Centers for Disease Control and Prevention. General recommendations on immunization: recommendations of the Advisory Committee on Immunization Practices (ACIP). *MMWR Recomm Rep.* 2011;60(RR-02):1–64

Vaccine Dose

Reducing or dividing doses of DTaP or any other vaccine, including vaccines given to preterm or low birth weight infants, is never recommended and can result in inadequate immune response. A diminished antibody response in both term and preterm infants to reduced doses of diphtheria and tetanus and whole-cell pertussis (DTP) has been documented. A previous immunization with a dose that was less than the standard dose or one administered by a nonstandard route should not be counted, and the person should be reimmunized as recommended for age. However, doses of vaccine administered by the IM route rather than by the SC route do not need to be repeated. Exceeding a recommended dose volume is never recommended, because it may result in theoretical but unproven risks of adverse events.

Active Immunization of People Who Recently Received Immune Globulin and Other Blood Products

Live-virus vaccines may have diminished immunogenicity when given within 2 weeks before or during the several months after receipt of IG (both standard and hyperimmune globulins following intramuscular or intravenous administration). In particular, IG administration has been demonstrated to inhibit the response to measles vaccine for a prolonged period. Inhibition of immune response to rubella vaccine also has been demonstrated. The appropriate interval between IG administration and measles immunization varies with the dose of IG and the specific product; suggested intervals are given in Table 1.9. The effect of administration of IG on antibody response to varicella vaccine is not known. Because of potential inhibition, varicella vaccine administration should be delayed after receipt of an IG preparation or a blood product (except washed Red Blood Cells), as recommended for measles vaccine (see Table 1.9). If IG must be given within 14 days after administration of measles- or varicella-containing vaccines, these live-virus vaccines should be administered again after the interval period specified in Table 1.9. One exception to this rule is when serologic testing at an appropriate interval after IG administration indicates that adequate serum antibodies were produced.

Administration of IG preparations does not interfere with antibody responses to yellow fever, OPV, or oral rotavirus vaccines and is not expected to affect response to live-attenuated influenza vaccine. Hence, these vaccines can be administered simultaneously with or at any time before or after administration of IG.

In contrast to some live-virus vaccines, administration of IG preparations has not been demonstrated to cause significant inhibition of the immune responses to inactivated vaccines and toxoids. Concurrent administration of recommended doses of HBIG, Tetanus Immune Globulin, or RIG and the corresponding inactivated vaccine or toxoid for postexposure prophylaxis provides immediate protection and long-term immunity and does not impair the efficacy of the vaccine. Standard doses of the corresponding vaccines are recommended. Increases in vaccine dose volume or number of immunizations are not indicated. Vaccines should be administered at a separate body site from that of intramuscularly administered IG. For additional information, see chapters on specific diseases in Section 3.

Table 1.9. Suggested Intervals Between Immune Globulin Administration and Measles Immunization (MMR or MMRV)

Indications or Product	Route	Dose U or mL	Dose mg IgG/kg	Interval, mo[a]
Tetanus prophylaxis (as TIG)	IM	250 U	10	3
Hepatitis A prophylaxis (as IG)				
Contact prophylaxis	IM	0.02 mL/kg	3.3	3
International travel	IM	0.06 mL/kg	10	3
Hepatitis B prophylaxis (as HBIG)	IM	0.06 mL/kg	10	3
Rabies prophylaxis (as RIG)	IM	20 IU/kg	22	4
Varicella prophylaxis (as VariZIG)	IM	125 U/10 kg (maximum 625 U)	20–40	5
Measles prophylaxis (as IG)				
Standard	IM	0.25 mL/kg	40	5
Immunocompromised host	IM	0.50 mL/kg	80	6
RSV prophylaxis (palivizumab monoclonal antibody)[b]	IM	...	15 mg/kg (monoclonal)	None
Cytomegalovirus Immune Globulin	IV	3 mL/kg	150	6
Blood transfusion				
Washed RBCs	IV	10 mL/kg	Negligible	0
RBCs, adenine-saline added	IV	10 mL/kg	10	3
Packed RBCs	IV	10 mL/kg	20–60	5
Whole blood	IV	10 mL/kg	80–100	6
Plasma or platelet products	IV	10 mL/kg	160	7
Replacement (or therapy) of immune deficiencies (as IGIV)	IV	...	300–400	8
Therapy for ITP (as IGIV)	IV	...	400	8
Therapy for ITP	IV	...	1000	10
Therapy for ITP or Kawasaki disease (as IGIV)	IV	...	1600–2000	11

MMR indicates measles-mumps-rubella; MMRV, measles-mumps-rubella-varicella; TIG, Tetanus Immune Globulin; IM, intramuscular; IG, Immune Globulin; HBIG, Hepatitis B Immune Globulin; RIG, Rabies Immune Globulin; VariZIG, Varicella-Zoster Immune Globulin; RSV, respiratory syncytial virus; IV, intravenous; RBCs, Red Blood Cells; IGIV, Immune Globulin Intravenous; ITP, immune (formerly termed "idiopathic") thrombocytopenic purpura.

[a] These intervals should provide sufficient time for decreases in passive antibodies in all children to allow for an adequate response to measles vaccine. Physicians should not assume that children are protected fully against measles during these intervals. Additional doses of IG or measles vaccine may be indicated after exposure to measles (see text).

[b] Monoclonal antibodies, such as palivizumab, do not interfere with the immune response to vaccines.

Administration of hepatitis A vaccine generally is preferred to IG (with or without vaccine) for postexposure prophylaxis of most hepatitis A contacts (see Hepatitis A, p 361). Specific monoclonal antibody products (eg, respiratory syncytial virus monoclonal antibody [palivizumab]) do not interfere with response to inactivated or live vaccines.

Testing for *Mycobacterium tuberculosis* Infection

Recommendations for screening with a tuberculin skin test (TST) or interferon gamma release assay (IGRA) (see Tuberculosis, p 736) are independent of those for immunization. Testing for *Mycobacterium tuberculosis* infection at any age is not required before administration of live-virus vaccines. A TST or IGRA can be performed at the same visit during which these vaccines are administered, but the testing should be deferred at least 6 weeks after administration of measles-containing vaccine (including MMR and MMRV), because the vaccine temporarily can suppress tuberculin sensitivity for at least 4 to 6 weeks. The effect of live-virus varicella, mumps, rubella, yellow fever, and live-attenuated influenza vaccines on TST reactivity is not known. The effect of live-virus vaccines on IGRA results has not yet been studied but, in theory, could be similar to the effect on the TST. In the absence of data, the same spacing recommendation for TST and IGRA should be applied to these vaccines as is described for measles, which means waiting at least 6 weeks after administration of vaccine before testing. Inactivated vaccines, polysaccharide vaccines, and recombinant or subunit vaccines and toxoids do not interfere with interpretation of the TST.

Record Keeping and Immunization Information Systems

The National Vaccine Advisory Committee in 1993 recommended a set of standards to improve immunization practices for health care professionals serving children and revised the standards in 2002. The standards include the recommendation that immunizations of patients be documented through use of immunization records that are accurate, complete, and easily accessible. In addition, the standards also recommend use of tracking systems to provide reminder/recall notices to parents/guardians and physicians when immunizations are due or overdue. Immunization information systems address record-keeping needs and tracking functions and have additional capacities, such as vaccine inventory management; generation of reports on vaccine usage, including those required for vaccines provided through the Vaccines for Children program; vaccine forecasting; adverse event reporting; interoperability with electronic medical records; emergency preparedness functions; and linkage with other public health programs. Additional information about immunization information systems can be found at **www.cdc.gov/vaccines/programs/iis/default.htm.**

PERSONAL IMMUNIZATION RECORDS OF PATIENTS

The AAP and state health departments have developed an official immunization record. This record should be given to parents of every newborn infant and should be handled like a birth certificate or passport and retained with vital documents for subsequent referral. Physicians should cooperate with this endeavor by recording immunization data in this record and by encouraging patients not only to preserve the record but also to present it at each visit to a health care professional.

The immunization record especially is important for people who frequently move or change health care professionals. The record facilitates maintaining an accurate patient medical history, enables the physician to evaluate a child's immunization status, and fulfills the need for documentation of immunizations for child care and school attendance and for admission to other institutions and organizations.

Although still used, paper-based immunization records are not always kept up-to-date and may be misplaced or destroyed. The absence of an immunization card can result in missed opportunities, extra immunizations, or inability to meet legal requirements.

Almost all states and some large metropolitan areas are developing population-based computerized immunization information systems to record and track immunizations regardless of where in the state or metropolitan area the immunization services are provided. Most immunization information systems can consolidate records from physician offices, help remind parents and health care professionals when immunizations are due or overdue, help health care professionals determine the immunization needs of their patients at each visit, and generate official immunization records to meet child care or school requirements. Immunization information systems also can provide measurements of immunization coverage by age, immunization series, and physician or clinic practice. The AAP urges physicians to cooperate with state and local health officials in providing immunization data for state or local immunization information systems. Parents also have access to Web-based immunization schedulers where immunization data can be maintained (see Immunization Schedulers, p 5).

IMMUNIZATION RECORDS OF PHYSICIANS

Every physician should ensure that the immunization history of each patient is maintained in a permanent, confidential record that can be reviewed easily and updated when subsequent immunizations are administered. The medical record maintained by the primary health care professional and in some states by the Immunization Information Systems (see Record Keeping and Immunization Information Systems, p 39) should document all vaccines received, including vaccines received in another health care setting. The format of the record should facilitate identification and recall of patients in need of immunization and if maintained in a hard copy medical chart record should be kept as a single summary sheet of all immunizations administered.

Records of children whose immunizations have been delayed or missed should be flagged to indicate the need to complete immunizations. For data that are required by the National Childhood Vaccine Injury Act of 1986 as well as data recommended by the AAP to be recorded in each patient's medical record for each immunization, see Informing Patients and Parents (p 7).

Interest in use of electronic health record (EHR) systems prompted the AAP to issue a revised statement in 2007 outlining functions that would need to be performed in a pediatric practice for EHR systems to be useful.[1]

Congress passed the Health Information Technology for Economic and Clinical Health Act (HITECH) in 2009 to support adoption and use of EHRs. The purpose of HITECH is to achieve significant improvements in care through meaningful use of EHRs by health care professionals. HITECH established incentive payments to eligible professionals and hospitals to promote adoption and meaningful use of interoperable health information technology systems and qualified EHRs. Under HITECH, there are 2 regulations: the first defines the "meaningful use" objectives that providers must meet to qualify for Medicare and Medicaid incentive payments, and the other identifies the technical capabilities required for certified EHR technology. Public health objectives for

---

[1] American Academy of Pediatrics, Council on Clinical Information Technology. Special requirements of electronic health record systems in pediatrics. *Pediatrics*. 2007;119(3):631–637

use of EHRs are to use HL7 messaging standards to send data electronically in the following 3 areas: immunization registries (IRs)/immunization information systems (IISs); syndromic surveillance systems; and reportable laboratory results. Approval by the US Food and Drug Administration for use of 2-dimensional bar codes on individual vaccines will facilitate improved efficacy and safety in entering vaccine data, including manufacturer, vaccine lot number, and expiration date, into the EHR.

Vaccine Shortages

When vaccine shortages occur, temporary changes in childhood or adolescent immunization recommendations by the AAP and CDC may be necessary, including temporary deferral of certain vaccines or specific doses in the schedule for those vaccines, establishment of vaccine priorities for high-risk children, and suspension of school and child care entry immunization requirements in some states. Several national committees and organizations, including the National Center for Immunization and Respiratory Diseases, National Vaccine Advisory Committee, and the US Government Accountability Office, have proposed comprehensive strategies to prevent future shortages and encourage key stakeholders to work together to develop corrective action.

When vaccines are in short supply, physicians and other health care professionals should maintain lists of children and adolescents who do not receive vaccines at the recommended time or age so they can be recalled when the vaccine supply becomes adequate. For current information about vaccine shortages and resulting recommendations, see the Web sites of the CDC (**www.cdc.gov/vaccines/vac-gen/shortages/default.htm**), FDA (**www.fda.gov/BiologicsBloodVaccines/SafetyAvailability/Shortages/default.htm**), or *Red Book* online (**http://aapredbook.aappublications.org**). The FDA Web site also provides information on other biologic products in short supply (eg, Immune Globulin products) as well as products permanently discontinued. For analyses of vaccine shortages and recommended solutions, see the published recommendations from the National Vaccine Advisory Committee.[1]

Vaccine Safety[2]

RISKS AND ADVERSE EVENTS

All vaccines licensed in the United States have been shown to be safe and effective. However, adverse events after vaccination occasionally occur, and some immunized people still acquire disease despite vaccination. The most effective vaccines achieve the highest degree of protection with the lowest rate of adverse events. Adverse events following immunization include both true vaccine events, such as local pain and tenderness at the injection site, and coincidental events that occur after vaccination but are unrelated. Highly effective vaccines have reduced the threat of infectious diseases, and now some families worry more about the vaccines than the illnesses vaccines prevent. As immunizations successfully eliminate their target diseases, providers need to commu-

---

[1] Santoli JM, Peter G, Arvin AM, et al. Strengthening the supply of routinely recommended vaccines in the United States: recommendations from the National Vaccine Advisory Committee. *JAMA.* 2003;290(23):3122–3128

[2] A table summarizing select vaccine safety resources can be found in Appendix IV (p 895).

nicate benefits and risks of immunizations (see Appendix IV, p 895) to a population whose first-hand experience with vaccine-preventable diseases increasingly is rare.

Adverse events after vaccination vary from more common minor and inconvenient reactions to rare, severe, or life-threatening events. Vaccine risk and benefit must be weighed, and immunization recommendations must be based on this assessment. Recommendations are made to maximize protection and minimize risk by providing specific advice on dose, route, and timing and by identifying precautions or contraindications to immunization.

Common vaccine adverse events usually are mild to moderate in severity (eg, fever or injection site reactions, such as swelling, redness, and pain) and have no permanent sequelae. Examples include local inflammation after administration of DTaP, Td, or Tdap vaccines and fever and rash 1 to 2 weeks after administration of MMR or MMRV vaccines.

The occurrence of an adverse event following immunization does not mean that the vaccine caused the symptoms or signs. Because chance temporal association of an adverse event to the timing of administration of a specific vaccine can occur, a true causal association usually requires that the event occur at a significantly higher rate in vaccine recipients than in unimmunized groups of similar age and residence or that the event may have been reported earlier in prelicensure or postlicensure epidemiologic studies. Although extremely rare, recovery of a vaccine virus from an ill child with compatible symptoms may provide support for a causal link with a live-virus vaccine (eg, rotavirus vaccine-associated diarrhea in a patient with severe combined immunodeficiency). Clustering in time of unusual adverse events following immunizations or the recurrence of the adverse event with subsequent dose of the same vaccine (eg, rare but well-documented instances of recurrent Guillain-Barré syndrome after administration of tetanus toxoid-containing vaccines) also suggest a causal relationship.

Reporting of any clinically significant adverse event following immunization to the Vaccine Adverse Event Reporting System (VAERS, see p 45) is imperative, because when analyzed in conjunction with other VAERS reports, this information can provide signals of unanticipated potentially causally related adverse events. Health care professionals are mandated by law to report serious adverse events (those that are reported as fatal, disabling, life-threatening, requiring hospital admission, prolonging a hospital stay, potentially resulting in a congenital anomaly, or requiring medical intervention to prevent such an outcome). The Reportable Events Table (Appendix V, p 897) is a list of such events. However, VAERS is not designed to assess whether a vaccine caused an adverse event but as a system to generate hypotheses to be tested in other vaccine safety monitoring systems, such as the Vaccine Safety Datalink (**www.cdc.gov/vaccinesafety/Activities/vsd. html**) or the Clinical Immunization Safety Assessment Network (**www.cdc.gov/ vaccinesafety/Activities/cisa.html**). A nationally notifiable vaccine-preventable disease that occurs in a child or adolescent at any time, including after immunization (vaccine failure), should be reported to the local or state health department (see Appendix VI, p 902).

INSTITUTE OF MEDICINE REVIEWS OF ADVERSE EVENTS AFTER IMMUNIZATION

The US Health Resources and Services Administration (HRSA) of the US Department of Health and Human Services, with support provided by the CDC and the National Vaccine Program Office, commissioned the National Academy of Sciences' Institute of Medicine (IOM) to convene a committee of experts to review the epidemiologic, clinical, and biological evidence regarding adverse health events associated with specific vaccines covered by the Vaccine Injury Compensation Program (VICP). This committee was composed of people with expertise in pediatrics, internal medicine, neurology, immunology, immunotoxicology, neurobiology, rheumatology, epidemiology, biostatistics, and law. It is expected that the report will provide the scientific basis for review and adjudication of claims of vaccine injury by VICP.[1]

Eight different vaccines covered by VICP were reviewed: varicella zoster vaccines, influenza vaccines, hepatitis B vaccine, human papillomavirus virus vaccines, tetanus toxoid-containing vaccines other than those containing whole-cell pertussis component, hepatitis A vaccines, meningococcal vaccines, and measles-mumps rubella vaccine. The benefit and effectiveness of vaccines were not assessed during the study. On the basis of scientific evidence, the IOM committee developed 158 causality conclusions and assigned each one of 4 relationships (categories) showing the vaccine and its adverse events.

A summary of the IOM committee causality conclusions are as follows:

Category 1: Evidence convincingly supports a causal relationship between vaccines and some adverse events:

- Varicella vaccine and 5 specific adverse events:
  - disseminated varicella-zoster virus (VZV) infection without other organ involvement
  - disseminated VZV infection with subsequent infection resulting in pneumonia, meningitis, or hepatitis
  - vaccine-strain viral reactivation without other organ involvement
  - vaccine-strain viral reactivation with subsequent infection resulting in meningitis or encephalitis
  - anaphylaxis
- MMR vaccine and measles inclusion body encephalitis, febrile seizures, and anaphylaxis.
- Influenza vaccine and anaphylaxis.
- Hepatitis B vaccine and anaphylaxis.
- Tetanus toxoid vaccine and anaphylaxis.
- Meningococcal vaccine and anaphylaxis.
- Injection-related events and deltoid bursitis.
- Injection-related events and syncope.

Category 2: Evidence favors acceptance of a vaccine-adverse event relationship (evidence is strong and generally suggestive but not firm enough to be described as convincing):

- Influenza vaccine and oculorespiratory syndrome.
- HPV vaccine and anaphylaxis.
- MMR vaccine and transient arthralgia in women and in children.

---

[1] Institute of Medicine. *Adverse Effects of Vaccines: Evidence and Causality.* Washington, DC: National Academies Press; 2011

Category 3: Evidence favors rejection of a vaccine-adverse event relationship:
- MMR vaccine and autism.
- MMR vaccine and type 1 diabetes mellitus.
- DT, TT, or acellular pertussis-containing vaccines and type 1 diabetes mellitus.
- Inactivated influenza vaccine and Bell palsy.
- Inactivated influenza vaccine and exacerbation of asthma or reactive airways disease episodes in children and adults.

Category 4: Evidence is inadequate to accept or reject a causal relationship for the vast majority (135 vaccine-adverse event pairs).

THE BRIGHTON COLLABORATION

The Brighton Collaboration is an international voluntary collaboration formed to develop globally accepted and standardized case definitions for adverse events following immunization, known as the Brighton Standardized Case Definitions for use in surveillance and research. The project began in 2000 with formation of a steering committee and creation of work groups, composed of international volunteers with expertise in vaccine safety, patient care, pharmaceuticals, regulatory affairs, public health, and vaccine delivery. The guidelines for collecting, analyzing, and presenting safety data developed by the collaboration will facilitate sharing and comparison of vaccine data among vaccine safety professionals worldwide. Additional information, including current definitions and updates of progress, can be found online (**https://brightoncollaboration.org/public/resources.html**). As of January 2012, a total of 25 case definitions have been completed, and all definitions can be accessed online.

Reporting of Adverse Events

Before administering a dose of any vaccine, health care professionals should ask parents and patients if they have experienced adverse events following immunization with previous doses. Although extensive safety testing is required before vaccine licensure, these prelicensure studies may not be large enough to detect rare adverse events or determine the rate of adverse events previously linked with the vaccine. Unexpected events after administration of any vaccine, particularly events judged to be clinically significant, should be described in detail in the patient's medical record and subsequently submitted to VAERS (**http://vaers.hhs.gov**). There is no time limit for reporting an adverse event. The FDA and CDC encourage health care professionals to report any clinically significant adverse event following an immunization, even if it is uncertain that the event was caused by the vaccine. Adverse events are evaluated on a continuous basis by VAERS. If unexpected adverse events are reported, a more comprehensive evaluation of possible causation is pursued.

The National Childhood Vaccine Injury Act of 1986 requires physicians and other health care professionals who administer vaccines covered under the National Vaccine Injury Compensation Program to maintain permanent immunization records and to report to the VAERS any condition listed on the reportable events table (see Appendix V, p 897) or listed in the manufacturer's package insert as a contraindication to additional doses of vaccine. The antigens to which these requirements apply, as of September 2010, are measles, mumps, rubella, varicella, poliovirus, hepatitis A, hepatitis B, pertussis, diphtheria, tetanus, rotavirus, Hib, pneumococcal conjugate, meningococcal (conjugate and polysaccharide), human papillomavirus, and influenza (inactivated and live intranasal) vaccines (see Record Keeping and Immunization Information Systems, p 39).

VACCINE ADVERSE EVENT REPORTING SYSTEM (VAERS)

VAERS is a national passive surveillance system that monitors vaccines licensed for use in the United States. Jointly administered by the CDC and the FDA, VAERS accepts reports of suspected adverse events after administration of any vaccine. The strength of VAERS is its ability to detect previously unrecognized adverse events that might be causally related to vaccines, monitor known reactions, identify possible risk factors for adverse events, and evaluate lot-specific frequencies of adverse events. Like all passive surveillance systems, VAERS is subject to limitations, including underreporting, reporting of temporal (but not causal) associations or unconfirmed diagnoses, lack of denominator data, and absence of an unimmunized control group. Because of these limitations, determining causal associations between vaccines and adverse events from VAERS reports usually is not possible.

Vaccine providers are required by law to report certain adverse events that occur after immunization with vaccines covered under the National Vaccine Injury Compensation Program to VAERS (Appendix V, p 897). Health care professionals are encouraged to report to VAERS any clinically significant adverse event that occurs after administration of any vaccine licensed for use in the United States. Reports may be submitted by anyone who considers that an adverse event occurred after immunization. Submission of a report does not necessarily indicate that the vaccine caused the adverse event. All patient-identifying information is kept confidential. Written notification that the report has been received is provided to the person submitting the form or the electronic report. In addition to adverse events, vaccine failures (disease in an immunized person who received one or more doses of vaccine) and vaccine administration errors may be reported. VAERS forms (see Fig 1.4, p 46) are available by calling 1-800-822-7967 or downloading from the Web site (**http://vaers.hhs.gov**) or by sending an e-mail to **info@vaers.org**. Reports can be submitted online through a secure system at **https://vaers.hhs.gov/ esub/index** or by mail or facsimile. VAERS data, excluding personal identifiers, are made available to the public and are made accessible through the VAERS Web site or CDC's Wide-ranging Online Data for Epidemiologic Research (WONDER) Web site at **http://wonder.cdc.gov/vaers.html**.

Information in VAERS reports is evaluated and analyzed by VAERS staff to determine whether there are unusual patterns of adverse events associated with vaccines or concerns about specific vaccine lots. Reports are coded as serious when at least one of the following outcomes results: death, hospitalization, prolongation of hospitalization, life-threatening illness, disability, or congenital anomaly. Medical records are obtained, when available, by VAERS staff for serious reports, and these reports are reviewed by FDA and CDC medical officers when received. Vaccine and adverse event-specific surveillance summaries, which describe reported adverse events and look for unexpected patterns ("signals") that would generate an hypothesis of a possible causal link between a vaccine and an adverse event, periodically are prepared by VAERS staff. These summary reports also may provide reassurance of the safety of a vaccine. Vaccine

FIGURE 1.4 VAERS FORM

FOR DIRECTIONS FOR COMPLETING FORM AND FOR A NEW ELECTRONIC
REPORTING FORM, SEE HTTP://VAERS.HHS.GOV/ESUB/INDEX.

WEBSITE: www.vaers.hhs.gov   E-MAIL: info@vaers.org   FAX: 1-877-721-0366

VACCINE ADVERSE EVENT REPORTING SYSTEM	For CDC/FDA Use Only
VAERS 24 Hour Toll-Free Information 1-800-822-7967 P.O. Box 1100, Rockville, MD 20849-1100 PATIENT IDENTITY KEPT CONFIDENTIAL	VAERS Number _____ Date Received _____

Patient Name: _____

Last   First   M.I.

Address
_____
_____
_____

City   State   Zip

Telephone no. (___) _____

Vaccine administered by (Name): _____

Responsible
Physician _____
Facility Name/Address
_____
_____
_____

City   State   Zip

Telephone no. (___) _____

Form completed by (Name): _____

Relation   ☐ Vaccine Provider   ☐ Patient/Parent
to Patient   ☐ Manufacturer   ☐ Other
Address (if different from patient or provider)
_____
_____
_____

City   State   Zip

Telephone no. (___) _____

1. State	2. County where administered	3. Date of birth __/__/__ mm dd yy	4. Patient age	5. Sex ☐ M ☐ F	6. Date form completed __/__/__ mm dd yy

7. Describe adverse events(s) (symptoms, signs, time course) and treatment, if any

8. Check all appropriate:
☐ Patient died   (date __/__/__ mm dd yy)
☐ Life threatening illness
☐ Required emergency room/doctor visit
☐ Required hospitalization (_____days)
☐ Resulted in prolongation of hospitalization
☐ Resulted in permanent disability
☐ None of the above

9. Patient recovered ☐ YES ☐ NO ☐ UNKNOWN	10. Date of vaccination __/__/__ mm dd yy Time _____ AM PM	11. Adverse event onset __/__/__ mm dd yy Time _____ AM PM
12. Relevant diagnostic tests/laboratory data		

13. Enter all vaccines given on date listed in no. 10

	Vaccine (type)	Manufacturer	Lot number	Route/Site	No. Previous Doses
a.					
b.					
c.					
d.					

14. Any other vaccinations within 4 weeks prior to the date listed in no. 10

	Vaccine (type)	Manufacturer	Lot number	Route/Site	No. Previous doses	Date given
a.						
b.						

15. Vaccinated at: ☐ Private doctor's office/hospital ☐ Military clinic/hospital ☐ Public health clinic/hospital ☐ Other/unknown	16. Vaccine purchased with: ☐ Private funds ☐ Military funds ☐ Public funds ☐ Other/unknown	17. Other medications
18. Illness at time of vaccination (specify)	19. Pre-existing physician-diagnosed allergies, birth defects, medical conditions (specify)	

20. Have you reported this adverse event previously? ☐ No ☐ To health department ☐ To doctor ☐ To manufacturer	**Only for children 5 and under**
	22. Birth weight _____ lb. _____ oz.	23. No. of brothers and sisters

21. Adverse event following prior vaccination (check all applicable, specify)

	Adverse Event	Onset Age	Type Vaccine	Dose no. in series	**Only for reports submitted by manufacturer/immunization project**
☐ In patient					24. Mfr./imm. proj. report no.	25. Date received by mfr./imm.proj.
☐ In brother or sister					26. 15 day report? ☐ Yes ☐ No	27. Report type ☐ Initial ☐ Follow-Up

Health care providers and manufacturers are required by law (42 USC 300aa-25) to report reactions to vaccines listed in the Table of Reportable Events Following Immunization. Reports for reactions to other vaccines are voluntary except when required as a condition of immunization grant awards.

Form VAERS-1(FDA)

safety concerns identified through VAERS nearly always require further studies for confirmation using established systems, such as the Vaccine Safety Datalink.

VACCINE SAFETY DATALINK PROJECT

To supplement the VAERS program, which is a passive surveillance system, the CDC in 1990 formed partnerships with several large managed-care organizations to establish the Vaccine Safety Datalink (VSD) project, an active surveillance system designed to evaluate vaccine safety continuously. The VSD project includes comprehensive medical and immunization histories on more than 9 million people. Data from the study population can be monitored for potential adverse events resulting from immunization. The VSD project allows for both retrospective and prospective observational vaccine safety studies as well as for timely investigations of newly licensed vaccines or emerging vaccine safety concerns. The VSD allows calculation of rates of adverse events following immunization that can be compared with rates in other time periods or unvaccinated populations when available. The VSD concept to evaluate vaccine safety has been proven to be valuable for many vaccines. Information about the VSD can be found at **www.cdc.gov/vaccinesafety/Activities/vsd.html.**

CLINICAL IMMUNIZATION SAFETY ASSESSMENT (CISA) NETWORK

Serious and other uncommon clinically significant adverse events following immunization rarely occur in prelicensure clinical trials, and health care professionals see them too infrequently to be able to provide standardized evaluation, diagnosis, and management. The CISA Network was established by the Centers for Disease Control and Prevention (CDC) in 2001 with primary goals including: (1) developing research protocols for clinical evaluation, diagnosis, and management of adverse events following immunization; (2) improving understanding of adverse events following immunization at the individual level, including determining possible genetic and other risk factors to identify predisposed people and high-risk subpopulations; (3) developing evidence-based guidelines for immunization of people at risk of serious adverse events following immunization; and (4) serving as an expert resource for clinical vaccine safety inquiries. The CISA Network is comprised of 6 academic centers with expertise in neurology, infectious diseases, virology, allergy and immunology, biostatistics, epidemiology, computer programming, pediatrics, internal medicine, health economics, preventative medicine, genetics, dermatology, and gastroenterology. Patients with rare and serious adverse events following immunization can be referred to the CISA Network for inclusion in the CISA Vaccine Safety BioRepository so that clinical samples from patients with these rare events may be accrued and used in future vaccine safety studies (eg, genetic and immunologic studies using newly developed assays).

The CISA Network advises clinicians on evaluation, diagnosis, and management of adverse events after immunization. The network conducts research on clinically significant adverse events following immunization through identification of specific cases through its consultative service and creation of standardized protocols for evaluation of specific events. CISA Network data will be used to improve scientific understanding of these adverse events and to develop protocols or guidelines for health care professionals that will assist in evaluation, diagnosis, and management of similar events in affected people. In addition, the CISA Network provides regional clinical vaccine safety resources for clinicians. Current information about the CISA Network can be found online (**www.cdc.gov/vaccinesafety/Activities/CISA.html**).

VACCINE INJURY COMPENSATION

The national Vaccine Injury Compensation Program (VICP) is a no-fault system in which compensation may be sought if people are thought to have suffered death or other injury as a result of administration of a covered vaccine. The VICP was developed as an alternative to civil litigation and has been operational since 1988. Claims must be filed within 36 months after the first symptom appeared after immunization, and death claims must be filed within 24 months of the death and within 48 months after onset of the vaccine-related injury from which death occurred. People seeking compensation for alleged injuries from covered vaccines must first file claims with the VICP before civil litigation against manufacturers or vaccine providers. Legal fees are paid by the program regardless of the outcome of the case, provided that the claim is filed in good faith. If the claimant accepts the judgment of the VICP, neither vaccine providers nor manufacturers can be sued in civil litigation. If the claimant rejects the VICP judgment, he or she could file a claim against the health care professional on such grounds as failure to adequately warn, negligent vaccine administration, or negligent postvaccination care. Experience to date has shown that the program has decreased the number of lawsuits against health care professionals and vaccine manufacturers and has assisted establishing a stable vaccine supply and marketplace while ensuring access to compensation for vaccine-associated injury and death. Vaccine Information Statements (VISs), which are required to be used by the National Childhood Vaccine Injury Act, are designed to provide adequate information to parents and guardians regarding vaccine benefits and risks.

The program is based on the Vaccine Injury Table (VIT [see Appendix V, p 897] or **www.hrsa.gov/vaccinecompensation/vaccinetable.html**), which lists the vaccines covered by the program, as well as injuries, disabilities, illnesses, and conditions (including death) for which compensation may be awarded. The VIT defines the time during which the first symptoms or significant aggravation of an injury must appear after immunization. If an injury listed in the VIT is proven, claimants receive a "legal presumption of causation," thus avoiding the need to prove causation in an individual case. If the claim pertains to conditions not listed in the VIT, claimants may prevail if they prove causation. Any vaccine that is recommended by the CDC for routine use in children and has an excise tax placed on it by Congress is eligible for coverage by the program.

Program and contact information about the National Vaccine Injury Compensation Program and the VIT are in Appendix I (p 883):

Parklawn Building
5600 Fishers Lane
Room 11C-26
Rockville, MD 20857
Telephone: 800-338-2382
Web site: **www.hrsa.gov/vaccinecompensation**

People wishing to file a claim for a vaccine injury should telephone or write to the following:

United States Court of Federal Claims
717 Madison Place, NW
Washington, DC 20005-1011
Telephone: 202-357-6400

Information on the VICP is available to parents or guardians through Vaccine Information Statements (**www.cdc.gov/vaccines/pubs/vis/default.htm**), which are required to given prior to administering each dose of vaccines covered through the program.

VACCINE CONTRAINDICATIONS AND PRECAUTIONS

A **contraindication** to immunization is a condition in a recipient that increases the risk of a serious adverse reaction. For example, a history of anaphylactic allergy to a dose of influenza vaccine is a contraindication to further doses of influenza vaccine (unless the person has undergone desensitization), because it could cause serious illness or death in the vaccinee. A vaccine should not be administered when a contraindication is present. In contrast, a **precaution** is a condition in a recipient that might increase the risk of a serious adverse reaction or that might compromise the ability of the vaccine to produce immunity. However, immunization might be recommended in the presence of a precaution, because the benefit of protection from the vaccine outweighs the risk of an adverse reaction or incomplete response. Most precautions are the result of temporary conditions (eg, moderate or severe illness), and a vaccine can be administered at a later time. Failure to understand true contraindications and precautions can result in administration of a vaccine when it should be withheld (see Immunocompromised Children, p 74). Misconceptions about vaccine contraindications can result in missed opportunities to provide vaccines and protect people from serious diseases. Contraindications, precautions, and reasons for deferral of immunizations are addressed in pathogen-specific chapters and are listed in Appendix VII (p 905).

Common conditions or circumstances that are NOT contraindications, precautions, or reasons for deferral include (with exceptions noted):

- Recent exposure to an infectious disease.
- Mild acute illness with low-grade fever (eg, upper respiratory tract illness, otitis media) or mild diarrheal illness in an otherwise well child. Most evidence does not indicate an increased risk of adverse events or decrease in effectiveness associated with use of inactivated, subunit, or live-attenuated vaccines administered during a minor illness with or without fever. For optimal safety, vaccines should not be administered if an adverse reaction to the vaccine could affect severity of illness or be confused with an intercurrent illness. A child with frequent febrile illnesses that are moderate or severe, leading to deferrals of immunization, should be asked to return as soon as the illness subsides so that missed vaccines can be administered and the child can remain on the usual schedule.
- Receipt of blood products or immunoglobulins and use of inactivated vaccines. However, live vaccines (except yellow fever, oral typhoid vaccine, rotavirus, and live-attenuated influenza vaccine) should be delayed until passive antibody concentrations have declined. See Table 1.9, p 38.
- The convalescent phase of an illness.

- Currently receiving antimicrobial therapy (in most situations). Administration of certain antimalaria drugs can reduce efficacy of oral typhoid vaccine, and certain antiviral drugs reduce efficacy of live varicella virus or live-attenuated influenza virus vaccines. Certain antimicrobial agents can inhibit oral typhoid vaccine and bacille Calmette-Guérin (BCG) vaccine (see pathogen-specific chapters in Section 3).
- Preterm birth. The appropriate age for initiating most immunizations in the preterm infant is the recommended chronologic age; vaccine doses should not be reduced for preterm infants (see Preterm and Low Birth Weight Infants, p 69, and Hepatitis B, p 369). Birth weight and size are not factors in deciding whether to postpone routine vaccinations of a clinically stable preterm infant, except for Hepatitis B vaccine.
- Pregnancy in a household contact. Pregnancy in a household contact is not a contraindication to administration of any routinely recommended live-virus vaccines, including MMR, MMRV, varicella, rotavirus, or live-attenuated influenza vaccine, to a child or other nonpregnant household contact. Vaccine viruses in MMR vaccine are not transmitted by vaccine recipients, and although varicella vaccine virus and influenza vaccine virus (in live-virus vaccines only) can be transmitted by healthy vaccine recipients to contacts, the frequency is low, and only mild or asymptomatic infection has been reported (see Varicella-Zoster Infections, p 774, and Influenza, p 439).
- Pregnancy. Women who are pregnant generally should not receive live vaccines.
- Breastfeeding. The only vaccine virus that has been isolated from human milk is rubella; no evidence indicates that human milk from women immunized against rubella is harmful to infants. If rubella infection does occur in an infant as a result of exposure to the vaccine virus in human milk, infection likely would be well tolerated, because the vaccine virus is attenuated. Breastfeeding is a precaution to yellow fever vaccine administration.[1]
- Immunosuppression of a household contact. Immunosuppression of a household contact is not a contraindication to administration of most routinely recommended live-virus vaccines, including MMR, MMRV, varicella, and rotavirus. Live-attenuated influenza vaccine (LAIV) should not be administered to close contacts of people with immunosuppression who require a protective environment (eg, recipients of hematopoietic stem cell transplants and patients with severe combined immunodeficiency) but may be administered to others.
- History of nonspecific allergies or relatives with allergies, including history of a nonanaphylactic allergy to a vaccine component (such as egg). Only anaphylactic allergy to a vaccine component is a true contraindication to immunization.
- History of allergies to penicillin or any other antimicrobial agent, except anaphylactic reactions to neomycin, gentamicin, or streptomycin (see Hypersensitivity Reactions After Immunization, p 51). Product inserts can be consulted to determine specific vaccines that contain these ingredients (**www.fda.gov/BiologicsBloodVaccines/Vaccines/ApprovedProducts/ucm093830.htm**). These reactions occur rarely, if ever. No vaccine licensed for use in the United States contains penicillin.
- Allergies to duck meat or duck feathers. No vaccine licensed for use in the United States is produced in substrates containing duck antigens.
- For Children With a Personal or Family History of Seizures, see p 90.

---

[1] Centers for Disease Control and Prevention. Yellow fever vaccine: recommendations of the Advisory Committee on Immunization Practices (ACIP). *MMWR Recomm Rep.* 2010;59(RR-7):1–26

- Family history of sudden infant death syndrome.
- Family history of an adverse event following immunization.
- Malnutrition.

HYPERSENSITIVITY REACTIONS AFTER IMMUNIZATION

Hypersensitivity reactions to constituents of vaccines are rare; however, facilities and health care professionals should be available for treating immediate hypersensitivity reactions (anaphylaxis) in all settings in which vaccines are administered. This recommendation includes administration of vaccines in school-based, pharmacy, or other complementary or nontraditional settings. Children should be observed for 15 minutes following vaccine administration to intervene if a reaction including syncope occurs.

Children who have experienced an apparent allergic reaction to a vaccine or vaccine constituent should be evaluated by an allergist prior to receiving subsequent doses of the suspect vaccine or other vaccines containing common ingredients. This evaluation and appropriate allergy testing will determine whether the child currently is allergic, which vaccines pose a risk, and whether alternative vaccines (without the allergen) are available. Even when the child truly is allergic and no alternative vaccines are available, in almost all cases, the risk of remaining unimmunized exceeds the risk of careful vaccine administration, under observation in a facility with personnel and equipment prepared to recognize and treat anaphylaxis, should it occur.

Hypersensitivity reactions related to vaccine constituents can be immediate or delayed and are more often attributable to an excipient rather than the immunizing agent itself.

IMMEDIATE-TYPE ALLERGIC REACTIONS

As with most IgE-mediated, immediate-type allergic reactions, the allergens usually are proteins. The proteins most often implicated in vaccine reactions are egg and gelatin, with perhaps rare reactions to yeast or latex. On rare occasions, nonprotein antimicrobial agents present in some vaccines can be the cause of an allergic reaction.

ALLERGIC REACTIONS TO EGG PROTEIN (OVALBUMIN). Current measles and mumps vaccines (and some rabies vaccines) are derived from chicken embryo fibroblast tissue cultures and do not contain significant amounts of egg proteins. Studies indicate that children with egg allergy, even children with severe hypersensitivity, are at low risk of anaphylactic reactions to these vaccines, singly or in combination (eg, MMR or MMRV), and that skin testing with the vaccine is not predictive of an allergic reaction to immunization. Most immediate hypersensitivity reactions after measles or mumps immunization appear to be reactions to other vaccine components, such as gelatin. Therefore, children with egg allergy may be given MMR or MMRV vaccines without special precautions.

The approach to a patient who may be allergic to eggs and requires influenza vaccine should be distinguished from the approach to a patient who has had an apparent allergic reaction to influenza vaccination described previously under "Hypersensitivity Reactions After Immunization." People who can eat egg directly (such as scrambled egg) without reaction are not allergic. Although both TIV and LAIV are produced in eggs, data have shown that TIV vaccine administration in a single, age-appropriate dose is well tolerated by nearly all recipients who have an egg allergy. LAIV has not been evaluated in egg-allergic people. More conservative approaches, such as skin testing or a 2-step graded challenge, no longer are recommended.[1] For recommendations regarding administration of influenza vaccine to people with egg allergy, see Influenza (p 439).

Yellow fever vaccine may contain a larger amount of egg protein than influenza vaccines, and there are fewer reports on administering the vaccine to egg-allergic patients. The package insert for the vaccine describes a protocol involving skin testing the patient with the vaccine and if positive, giving the vaccine in graded doses. Such a procedure would best be performed by an allergist.

ALLERGIC REACTIONS TO GELATIN. Some vaccines, such as MMR, MMRV, varicella, yellow fever, zoster, and some influenza and rabies vaccines contain gelatin as a stabilizer. The Vero cell culture-derived Japanese encephalitis (JE-VC) vaccine available in the United States does not contain gelatin stabilizers. People with a history of food allergy to gelatin may develop anaphylaxis after receipt of gelatin containing vaccines. Additionally, people who experience an immediate hypersensitivity reaction following receipt of a vaccine containing gelatin may, in fact, be allergic to gelatin, despite not having a known gelatin food allergy. In either case, such a patient should be evaluated by an allergist prior to receiving gelatin-containing vaccines to confirm the gelatin allergy and to administer the vaccine under observation and in accordance with established protocols.

ALLERGIC REACTIONS TO YEAST. Hepatitis B and quadrivalent human papillomavirus (HPV4) vaccines are manufactured using recombinant technology in yeast cells. In theory, vaccine recipients with hypersensitivity to yeast could experience an allergic reaction to these vaccines. Allergy to yeast is rare; however, patients claiming such an allergy should be evaluated by an allergist prior to receiving yeast-containing vaccines to confirm the yeast allergy and administer the vaccine under observation and in accordance with established protocols.

ALLERGIC REACTIONS TO LATEX. Dry natural rubber latex contains naturally occurring proteins that may be responsible for allergic reactions. Some vaccine vial stoppers and syringe plungers contain latex. Other vaccine vials and syringes contain synthetic rubber that poses no risk to the latex-allergic child. Information about latex used in vaccine packaging is available in the manufacturer's package inserts or at **www.cdc.gov/vaccines/ pubs/pinkbook/downloads/appendices/B/latex-table.pdf**. Hypersensitivity reactions to latex after immunizations are rare; however, latex-allergic patients should be evaluated by an allergist prior to receiving vaccines with natural rubber latex in the packaging to confirm the latex allergy and to administer the vaccine under observation and in accordance with established protocols.

DELAYED-TYPE ALLERGIC REACTIONS

As with most cell-mediated, delayed-type allergic reactions, the allergens usually are small molecules. The small molecules present in vaccines include thimerosal, aluminum, and antimicrobial agents.

ALLERGIC REACTIONS TO THIMEROSAL. Most patients with localized or delayed-type hypersensitivity reactions to thimerosal tolerate injection of vaccines containing thimerosal uneventfully or with only temporary swelling at the injection site. This is not a contraindication to receive a vaccine that contains thimerosal.

---

[1] American Academy of Pediatrics, Committee on Infectious Diseases. Recommendations for prevention and control of influenza in children, 2011-2012. *Pediatrics.* 2011;128(4):813–825

ALLERGIC REACTIONS TO ALUMINUM. Sterile abscesses or persistent nodules have occurred at the site of injection of certain inactivated vaccines. These abscesses may result from a delayed-type hypersensitivity response to the vaccine adjuvant, aluminum (alum). In some instances, these reactions may be caused by inadvertent SC inoculation of a vaccine intended for IM use. Alum-related abscesses recur frequently with subsequent dose(s) of vaccines containing alum. Only if such reactions were severe would they constitute a contraindication to further vaccination with aluminum-containing vaccines.

ALLERGIC REACTIONS TO ANTIMICROBIAL AGENTS. Many vaccines contain trace amounts of streptomycin, neomycin, and/or polymyxin B. Some people have delayed-type allergic reactions to these agents and may develop an injection site papule 48 to 96 hours after vaccine administration. This minor reaction is not a contraindication to future doses of vaccines containing these agents. People with a history of an anaphylactic reaction to one of these antimicrobial agents should be evaluated by an allergist prior to receiving vaccines containing them. No vaccine currently licensed for use in the United States contains penicillin or its derivatives.

OTHER VACCINE REACTIONS

People who have high serum concentrations of tetanus IgG antibody, usually as the result of frequent booster immunizations, may have an increased incidence of large injection site swelling after vaccine administration, presumed to be immune complex mediated (Arthus reaction). These reactions are self-limited and do not contraindicate future doses of vaccines at appropriate intervals. Such reactions had been thought to be common with tetanus-containing vaccines, but studies suggest that the reactions are uncommon, even with short intervals between immunizations. Therefore, when indicated, Tdap should be administered regardless of interval since the last tetanus-containing vaccine.

Reactions resembling serum sickness have been reported in approximately 6% of patients after a booster dose of human diploid rabies vaccine, probably resulting from sensitization to human albumin that had been altered chemically by the virus-inactivating agent. Such patients should be evaluated by an allergist but likely will be able to receive additional vaccine doses.

Reporting of Vaccine-Preventable Diseases

Most vaccine-preventable diseases are reportable throughout the United States (see Appendix VI, p 902). Public health officials depend on health care professionals to report promptly to state or local health departments all suspected cases of vaccine-preventable disease. These reports are transmitted weekly to the CDC and are used to detect outbreaks, monitor disease-control strategies, and evaluate national immunization practices and policies. Reports provide useful information about vaccine efficacy, changing or current epidemiology of vaccine-preventable diseases, and possible epidemics that could threaten public health. Reporting confirmed and suspected vaccine-preventable diseases is a legal obligation of the physician.

Clinical Practice Guidelines for Immunization Programs

See Appendix VIII (p 913) for evidence-based guidelines from the Infectious Diseases Society of America.

Common Misconceptions About Immunizations

Misconceptions about the need for and safety of recommended childhood and adolescent immunizations are associated with delayed immunization, underimmunization, or both. Table 1.10 (p 55) outlines several of these misconceptions.

The concerns about potential associations of MMR vaccine and autism, as well as thimerosal-containing vaccines and autism, have been evaluated. Evidence from many studies examining trends in vaccine use and changes in the frequency of autism does not support such an association. In addition, the Institute of Medicine (IOM) convened experts to review evidence regarding adverse health events associated with specific vaccines, including the hypothesis that MMR vaccine and thimerosal-containing vaccines are associated with autism. In May 2004, the IOM Immunization Safety Review Committee published several conclusions and recommendations, including the following:

- Scientific evidence favors rejection of a causal relationship between thimerosal-containing vaccines and autism.
- Scientific evidence favors rejection of a causal relationship between MMR vaccine and autism.
- Available funding for autism research should be channeled to more promising areas of inquiry.
- Risk-benefit communication requires attention to the needs of both the scientific community and the public.

In 2011, the IOM issued a report on 158 causality conclusions for 8 different vaccines (see Institute of Medicine Reviews of Adverse Events After Immunization, p 43).

Each person understands and reacts to information regarding vaccines on the basis of many factors, including past experience, education, perception of risk of disease and vaccine offered, perception of his or her ability to control risk, and personal values. Although parents receive information from multiple sources, they consider health care professionals their most trusted source of health information. Health care professionals should obtain and distribute copies of available immunization documents from the AAP and CDC as well as the required VISs to parents to address their questions and concerns. These materials are written in understandable language and can help parents make informed decisions about immunizing their children. Other sources of objective vaccine information are available (see Internet Resources for Accurate Immunization Information, p 6) that can help health care professionals respond to questions and misconceptions about immunizations and vaccine-preventable diseases. Various approaches to informing patients and parents about the benefits and risks of disease prevention, including immunizations (see Informing Patients and Parents, p 7), and approaches to parents who refuse immunizations for their child (see Parental Refusal of Immunization, p 10) are available. The CDC, AAP, and AAFP have developed provider resources for vaccine conversations with parents, which are available at no charge at **www.cdc.gov/vaccines/conversations.**

ADDRESSING PARENTS' CONCERNS ABOUT VACCINES, VACCINE-PREVENTABLE DISEASES, AND VACCINE SAFETY

To help health care professionals address parent's questions and concerns about vaccines, vaccine-preventable diseases, and vaccine safety, the CDC, the AAP, and the American Academy of Family Physicians developed *Provider Resources for Vaccine Conversations with Parents*. These reproducible resources provide strategies to assist health care professionals

Table 1.10. Common Misconceptions About Immunizations[a]

Claims	Facts
Natural methods of enhancing immunity are better than vaccinations.	The only "natural way" to be immune is to have the disease. Immunity from a preventive vaccine provides protection against disease when a person is exposed to it in the future. That immunity is usually similar to what is acquired from natural infection, although several doses of a vaccine may have to be given for a child to develop an adequate immune response.
Epidemiology—often used to establish vaccine safety—is not science but number crunching.	Epidemiology is a well-established scientific discipline that, among other things, identifies the cause of diseases and factors that increase a person's risk of acquiring a disease.
Giving multiple vaccines at the same time causes an "overload" of the immune system.	Vaccination does not overburden a child's immune system; the recommended vaccines use only a small portion of the immune system's "memory."
Vaccines are ineffective.	Vaccines have spared millions of people the effects of devastating diseases.
Prior to the use of vaccinations, these diseases had begun to decline because of improved nutrition and hygiene.	In the 19th and 20th centuries, some infectious diseases began to be better controlled because of improvements in sanitation, clean water, pasteurized milk, and pest control. However, vaccine-preventable diseases decreased dramatically after the vaccines for those diseases were licensed and were given to large numbers of children.
Vaccines cause poorly understood illnesses or disorders, such as autism, sudden infant death syndrome (SIDS), immune dysfunction, diabetes, neurologic disorders, allergic rhinitis, eczema, and asthma.	Scientific evidence does not support these claims. See IOM reports.
Vaccines weaken the immune system.	Vaccinated children are not at greater risk of infection, regardless of cause. Importantly, natural infections like influenza, measles, and chickenpox do weaken the immune system, increasing the risk of other infections.
Giving many vaccines at the same time is untested.	Concomitant use studies require all new vaccines to be tested with existing vaccines. These studies are performed to ensure that new vaccines do not affect the safety or effectiveness of existing vaccines given at the same time and that existing vaccines administered at the same time do not affect the safety or effectiveness of new vaccines.
Vaccines can be delayed, separated, and spaced out without consequences.	Many vaccine-preventable diseases occur in early infancy. Optimal vaccine-induced immunity may require a series of vaccines over time. Any delay in receiving age-appropriate immunization would increase the risk and severity of diseases that vaccines are administered to prevent.

Adapted from: Myers MG, Pineda D. *Do Vaccines Cause That? A Guide for Evaluating Vaccine Safety Concerns.* Galveston, TX: Immunizations for Public Health; 2008:79

[a] Institute of Medicine. *Adverse Effects of Vaccines: Evidence and Causality.* Washington, DC: National Academies Press; 2011

in conveying vaccine information to parents. These educational materials build on the latest research in vaccine and communication science and are designed to help health care professionals remain current on vaccine topics; strengthen communication and trust between health care professionals and parents; and share up-to-date, easy-to-use information about vaccines and vaccine-preventable diseases with parents. The materials include the following:

- Strategies on talking with parents about vaccines for infants.
- Current vaccine safety topics, such as Understanding MMR Vaccine Safety, Ensuring the Safety of US Vaccines, The Childhood Immunization Schedule, and more.
- Basic and in-depth fact sheets on 14 vaccine-preventable diseases for parents. Fact sheets are available in English and Spanish and are written for a variety of reading levels, and many include stories of families whose children have experienced a vaccine-preventable disease.
- If You Choose Not to Vaccinate Your Child, Understand the Risks and Responsibilities shares the possible risks for parents who choose to delay or decline a vaccine and offers steps for parents to take to protect their child, family, and others.
- Interactive, online childhood immunization scheduler and waiting room videos, such as Get the Picture: Childhood Immunization Video.

People can download these materials and enroll for e-mail updates when new resources are posted at **www.cdc.gov/conversations.htm.** Feedback can be provided on these materials to the CDC at **www.cdc.gov/vaccines/tellus/.**

PASSIVE IMMUNIZATION

Passive immunization entails administration of preformed antibody to a recipient and, unlike active immunization, achieves protection for only a short period of time. Passive immunization is indicated in the following general circumstances for prevention or amelioration of infectious diseases:

- When people are deficient in synthesis of antibody as a result of congenital or acquired B-lymphocyte defects, alone or in combination with other immunodeficiencies.
- Prophylactically, when a person susceptible to a disease is exposed to or has a high likelihood of exposure to that infection, especially when that person has a high risk of complications from the disease or when time does not permit adequate protection by active immunization alone.
- Therapeutically, when a disease already is present, antibody may ameliorate or aid in suppressing the effects of a toxin (eg, foodborne, wound, or infant botulism; diphtheria; or tetanus) or suppress the inflammatory response (eg, Kawasaki disease).

Passive immunization can be accomplished with several types of products. The choice is dictated by the types of products available, the type of antibody desired, the route of administration, timing, and other considerations. These products include standard Immune Globulin (IG) for intramuscular use; hyperimmune globulins, some of which are for intramuscular use (eg, hepatitis B, rabies, tetanus, varicella) and some of which are for intravenous use (eg, cytomegalovirus [CMV], vaccinia, botulism); standard Immune Globulin Intravenous (IGIV); and antibodies of animal origin and monoclonal antibodies. Immune Globulin Subcutaneous (Human) has been approved for treatment of patients with primary immune deficiency states.

Indications for administration of IG preparations other than those relevant to infectious diseases are not reviewed in the *Red Book*.

Whole blood and blood components for transfusion (including plasma) from US registered blood banks are released only after appropriate donor screening and testing for presence of bloodborne pathogens, including syphilis, hepatitis B virus, hepatitis C virus (HCV), human immunodeficiency virus (HIV)-1, HIV-2, human T-lymphotropic virus (HTLV)-1, and HTLV-2. Most donations also are screened for *Trypanosoma cruzi* (Chagas disease), and selected donations are screened for CMV. Whole blood and blood components also are batch tested for West Nile virus; during an outbreak in a particular geographic area, units may be tested by individual unit nucleic acid amplification testing (see Blood Safety, p 114; and West Nile Virus, p 792). A similar array of tests is performed by US-licensed establishments that collect plasma used only to manufacture plasma derivatives, such as IGIV, IG, and specific immune globulins. Current IG and specific immune globulin preparations licensed in the United States have not been associated with transmission of any of these diseases. HCV transmission in 1993 was associated with administration of IGIV produced by a single manufacturer, which at the time did not have a specific viral inactivation step. The US Food and Drug Administration (FDA) now requires that IGIV and other IG preparations for intravenous (IV) or intramuscular (IM) administration undergo additional manufacturing procedures that inactivate or remove viruses.

Immune Globulin (Intramuscular)

IG (IM) is derived from pooled plasma of adults by a cold ethanol fractionation procedure (Cohn fraction II). IG consists primarily of the immunoglobulin (Ig) fraction (at least 90% IgG and trace amounts of IgA and IgM), is treated with solvent/detergent to inactivate viruses, is sterile, and is not known to transmit any virus or other infectious agent. IG is a concentrated protein solution (approximately 16.5% or 165 mg/mL) containing specific antibodies that reflect the infectious and immunization experience of the population from whose plasma the IG was prepared. Many donors (1000 to 60 000 donors per lot of final product) are used to include a broad spectrum of antibodies.

IG is licensed and recommended for IM administration. Therefore, IG should be administered deep into a large muscle mass (see Site and Route of Immunization, p 21). Ordinarily, no more than 5 mL should be administered at one site in an adult, adolescent, or large child; a lesser volume per site (1–3 mL) should be given to small children and infants. Health care professionals should refer to the package insert for total maximal dose at one time. Peak serum levels usually are obtained 2 to 3 days after IM administration.

Human IG should not be administered intravenously. Intradermal use of IG is not recommended. Specific preparations of subcutaneous IG have been shown to be safe and effective in children and adults with primary immune deficiencies (see Immune Globulin Subcutaneous, p 63).

INDICATIONS FOR THE USE OF IG

REPLACEMENT THERAPY IN ANTIBODY DEFICIENCY DISORDERS. The usual dose (limited by muscle mass and the volume that should be administered) is 100 mg/kg (equivalent to 0.66 mL/kg) per month, intramuscularly. Customary practice is to administer twice this dose initially and to adjust the interval between administration of the doses (2–4 weeks) on the basis of trough IgG concentrations and clinical response (absence of or decrease in infections). For most cases, IG administered intramuscularly has been replaced by IGIV or subcutaneously administered IG, because higher plasma IgG concentrations and greater efficacy can be achieved.

HEPATITIS A PROPHYLAXIS. In people 12 months through 40 years of age, hepatitis A immunization is preferred over IG for postexposure prophylaxis against hepatitis A virus infection and for protection of travelers going to areas with endemic hepatitis A infection. For people younger than 12 months or older than 40 years of age, immunocompromised people of all ages, and people who have chronic liver disease, IG is preferred (see Hepatitis A, p 361). IG is not indicated for people with clinical manifestations of hepatitis A infection or for people exposed more than 14 days earlier.

MEASLES PROPHYLAXIS. IG administered to exposed, measles-susceptible people will prevent or attenuate infection if given within 6 days of exposure (see Measles, p 489). Measles vaccine and IG should not be given at the same time. The appropriate interval between IG administration and measles immunization varies with the dose of IG and the specific product (see Table 1.9, p 38).

RUBELLA PROPHYLAXIS. IG administered to rubella-susceptible pregnant women after rubella exposure may decrease the risk of fetal infection but should only be offered to women who decline a therapeutic abortion (see Rubella, p 629).

ADVERSE REACTIONS TO IG

- Most recipients experience local discomfort, and some experience pain at the site of IG administration (which are lessened if the preparation is at room temperature at the time of injection). Less common reactions include flushing, headache, chills, and nausea.
- Serious reactions are uncommon; these reactions may involve chest pain or constriction, dyspnea, anaphylaxis, or hypotension and shock. An increased risk of systemic reaction results from inadvertent IV administration. People requiring repeated doses of IG have been reported to experience systemic reactions, such as fever, chills, sweating, and shock.
- IG should not be administered to people with IgA deficiency. Because IG contains trace amounts of IgA, people who have IgA deficiency can develop anti-IgA antibodies on rare occasions and react to a subsequent dose of IG. These reactions include systemic symptoms such as chills, fever, and shock-like symptoms. In rare cases in which reactions related to anti-IgA antibodies have occurred, use of a licensed IGIV preparation with a low IgA concentration (IgA <1 μg/mL) may decrease the likelihood of further reactions. Because these reactions are rare, routine screening for IgA deficiency is not recommended.

PRECAUTIONS FOR THE USE OF IG

- Caution should be used when giving IG to a patient with a history of adverse reactions to IG.
- Although systemic reactions to IG are rare (see Adverse Reactions to IG), epinephrine and other means of treating serious acute reactions should be available immediately. Health care professionals administering IG should have training to manage emergencies appropriately.
- IG should not be used in patients with severe thrombocytopenia or any coagulation disorder that would preclude IM injection. In such cases, use of IGIV is recommended.

Specific Immune Globulins

Specific immune globulins differ from other preparations in selection of donors and may differ in number of donors whose plasma is included in the pool from which the product is prepared. These include preparations for which random plasma donations are selected for high titers against certain pathogens (such as CMV), or for which donors are vaccinated to produce high titers ("hyperimmune" globulins). Specific human plasma-derived immune globulins are prepared by the same types of procedure as other immune globulin preparations. Specific immune globulin preparations for use in infectious diseases include Hepatitis B Immune Globulin, Rabies, Immune Globulin, Tetanus Immune Globulin, Vari-ZIG, CMV-IGIV, Vaccinia IGIV, and Botulism IGIV (to treat infant botulism). Recommendations for use of these immune globulins are provided in the discussions of specific diseases in Section 3. The precautions and adverse reactions for IG intramuscular and IGIV are applicable to specific immune globulins. An intramuscularly administered humanized mouse monoclonal antibody preparation (palivizumab) for prevention of respiratory syncytial virus is available.

Immune Globulin Intravenous

IGIV is a highly purified preparation of IgG antibodies prepared from pooled plasma of qualified adult donors. Various methods are used by different manufacturers to prepare a product for intravenous use. The FDA recommends that the number of donors contributing to a pool used for IGIV be greater than 15 000 but no more than 60 000. IGIV consists of more than 95% IgG and trace amounts of IgA and IgM. IGIV is available as a lyophilized powder or as a formulated liquid solution, with final concentrations of IgG ranging from 3% to 12%, depending on the product. IGIV does not contain thimerosal. IGIV products vary in their sodium content, type of stabilizing excipients (sugars, amino acids), osmolarity/osmolality, pH, IgA content, and recommended infusion rate. Each of these factors may contribute to tolerability. The FDA specifies that all IGIV preparations must have a minimum concentration of antibodies to measles virus, *Corynebacterium diphtheriae*, poliovirus, and hepatitis B virus. Antibody concentrations against other pathogens, such as *Streptococcus pneumoniae*, vary widely among products and even among lots from the same manufacturer.

INDICATIONS FOR THE USE OF IGIV

Initially, IGIV was developed as an infusion product that allowed patients with primary immunodeficiencies to receive enough IgG at monthly intervals to protect them from infection until their next infusion. IGIV is approved by the FDA for 7 conditions

(Table 1.11, p 61). IGIV products may be useful for other conditions, although demonstrated efficacy from controlled trials is not available for many conditions.

FDA licensure of specific indications for a manufacturer's IGIV product is based on availability of data from one or more clinical trials demonstrating that the product is safe and effective for that indication. All IGIV products are licensed to prevent serious infections in primary immunodeficiency, and many are licensed to treat immune-mediated thrombocytopenia, but not all licensed products are approved for the other indications listed in Table 1.11. In some cases, only a single product has certain indications. Therapeutic differences among IGIV products from different manufacturers may exist, but comparative clinical trials generally have not been undertaken. Among the licensed IGIV products, but not necessarily for each product individually, indications for prevention or treatment of infectious diseases in children and adolescents include the following:

- *Replacement therapy in antibody-deficiency disorders.* The typical dose of IGIV in primary immune deficiency 400 to 600 mg/kg, administered approximately every 21 to 28 days by infusion. Effective dosages have ranged from 200 to 800 mg/kg monthly. Maintenance of a trough IgG concentration of at least 500 mg/dL (5 g/L) has been demonstrated to correlate with clinical response, but individual patient dosing should be optimized to decrease the frequency of serious infections. Studies in children with agammaglobulinemia suggest that IgG trough concentrations maintained at greater than 800 mg/dL prevented serious bacterial illnesses and enteroviral meningoencephalitis. Dosage and frequency of infusions should be based on clinical effectiveness in an individual patient and in conjunction with an expert on primary immune deficiency disorders.

- *Kawasaki disease.* Administration of IGIV at a dose of 2 g/kg as a single dose within the first 10 days of onset of fever decreases the frequency of coronary artery abnormalities and shortens the duration of symptoms. IGIV treatment for children with symptoms of Kawasaki disease for more than 10 days is recommended, although data on efficacy are not available (see Kawasaki Disease, p 454).

- *Pediatric HIV infection.* In children with HIV infection and hypogammaglobulinemia, IGIV may be used to prevent serious bacterial infection. IGIV also might be considered for HIV-infected children who have recurrent serious bacterial infection[1] (see Human Immunodeficiency Virus Infection, p 418).

- *Hypogammaglobulinemia in chronic B-cell lymphocytic leukemia.* Administration of IGIV to adults with this disease has been demonstrated to decrease the incidence of serious bacterial infections.

- *Varicella postexposure prophylaxis.* If Varicella-Zoster Immune Globulin (VariZIG) is not available, IGIV may be considered for certain people up to 10 days after exposure to a person with varicella or zoster (see Varicella-Zoster Infections, p 774). For maximum benefit, it should be administered as soon as possible after exposure.

IGIV has been used for many other conditions, some of which are listed below.

---

[1] Centers for Disease Control and Prevention. Guidelines for prevention and treatment of opportunistic infections among HIV-exposed and HIV-infected children. Recommendations from CDC, the National Institutes of Health, the HIV Medical Association of the Infectious Diseases Society of America, the Pediatric Infectious Diseases Society, and the American Academy of Pediatrics. *MMWR Recomm Rep.* 2009;58(RR-11):1–166

Table 1.11. Uses of Immune Globulin Intravenous (IGIV) for Which There is Approval by the US Food and Drug Administration[a]

Primary immunodeficiency disorders

Kawasaki disease, for prevention of coronary aneurysms

Immune-mediated thrombocytopenia, to increase platelet count

Pediatric human immunodeficiency virus infection, for replacement therapy

Secondary immunodeficiency in B-cell chronic lymphocytic leukemia

Bone marrow transplantation

Chronic inflammatory demyelinating polyneuropathy (CIDP)

[a]Not all IGIV products are approved by the FDA for all indications.

- **_Low birth weight infants._** Results of most clinical trials have indicated that IGIV does not decrease the incidence or mortality rate of late-onset infections in infants who weigh less than 1500 g at birth. Trials have varied in IGIV dosage, time of administration, and other aspects of study design. IGIV is not recommended for routine use in preterm infants to prevent late-onset infection.
- **_Guillain-Barré syndrome and chronic inflammatory demyelinating polyneuropathy._** In Guillain-Barré syndrome and chronic inflammatory demyelinating polyneuropathy, IGIV treatment has been demonstrated to have efficacy equivalent to that of plasmapheresis.
- **_Toxic shock syndrome._** IGIV has been administered to patients with severe staphylococcal or streptococcal toxic shock syndrome and necrotizing fasciitis. Therapy appears most likely to be beneficial when used early in the course of illness.
- **_Other potential uses._** IGIV may be useful for severe anemia caused by parvovirus B19 infection and for neonatal autoimmune thrombocytopenia that is unresponsive to other treatments, immune-mediated neutropenia, decompensation in myasthenia gravis, dermatomyositis, polymyositis, and severe thrombocytopenia that is unresponsive to other treatments.

Periodic shortages of IGIV have occurred in the United States for various reasons, including manufacturing compliance issues, product withdrawals for theoretical or actual safety concerns, plasma availability, increased usage, or decreased production. Clinicians should review their IGIV use to ensure consistency with current recommendations. Off-label use of IGIV should be limited until there is adequate scientific evidence of effectiveness. The FDA monitors supply issues and can take actions to ameliorate shortages partially. Supply shortages can be reported to the FDA online.

An outbreak of HCV infection occurred in the United States in 1993 among recipients of IGIV lots from a single domestic manufacturer. Changes in the preparation of IGIV, including additional viral inactivation steps (such as solvent/detergent exposure, pH 4 incubation, and heat treatment), subsequent to this episode have been instituted to prevent transmission of HCV and other enveloped viruses by IG preparations. All products currently available in the United States are believed to be free of known pathogens. HIV infection never has been transmitted by IGIV.

ADVERSE REACTIONS TO IGIV

Reactions such as fever, headache, myalgia, chills, nausea, and vomiting often are related to the rate of IGIV infusion and usually are mild to moderate and self-limited. These reactions may result from formation of IgG aggregates during manufacture or storage. There may be product-to-product variations in adverse effects among individual patients. Isoimmune hemolytic reactions can occur, especially if large doses of IGIV (≥ 2 g/kg) are infused. Less common but severe reactions include hypersensitivity and anaphylactoid reactions marked by flushing, changes in blood pressure, and tachycardia; thrombotic events; aseptic meningitis; noncardiogenic pulmonary edema; and renal insufficiency and failure. Renal failure occurs mainly in patients with preexisting renal dysfunction receiving sucrose-containing products and, in such cases, likely is attributable to sucrose-mediated acute tubular necrosis. Many thrombotic adverse events could be linked to presence of trace amounts of clotting factors that copurify with IgG and occur more commonly (but not exclusively) in patients with risk factors for thrombosis. Determining the precise cause and how to prevent thrombotic complications is an area of active investigation. Aseptic meningitis syndrome beginning several hours to 2 days following IGIV treatment may be associated with severe headache, nuchal rigidity, fever, nausea, and vomiting. Pleocytosis frequently is present.

Anaphylactic reactions induced by anti-IgA can occur in patients with primary immune deficiency who have a total absence of circulating IgA and develop IgG antibodies to IgA. These reactions are rare in patients with panhypogammaglobulinemia and potentially are more common in patients with selective IgA deficiency and subclass IgG deficiencies. Infusion of a licensed IGIV product with a low concentration of IgA (IgA <1 µg/mL) may reduce the likelihood of further reactions. Because of the extreme rarity of these reactions, however, screening for IgA deficiency and anti-IgA antibodies is not recommended routinely.

PRECAUTIONS FOR THE USE OF IGIV

- Caution should be used when giving IGIV to a patient with a history of adverse reactions to IG.
- Because anaphylactic or anaphylactoid reactions to IGIV may occur (see Adverse Reactions to IGIV, above), epinephrine and other means of treating acute reactions should be available immediately.
- Infusion-related nonallergic adverse reactions often can be alleviated by reducing either the rate or the volume of infusion. For patients with repeated severe reactions unresponsive to these measures, hydrocortisone (Solu-Cortef, 5–6 mg/kg in children or 100–150 mg in adults; or Solu-Medrol, 2 mg/kg) can be given intravenously 30 minutes before infusion. Using a different IGIV preparation or pretreatment with prednisone, diphenhydramine, acetaminophen, a nonsteroidal anti-inflammatory agent, or aspirin may modify or relieve symptoms.
- Seriously ill patients with compromised cardiac function who are receiving large volumes of IGIV may be at increased risk of vasomotor or cardiac complications manifested by elevated blood pressure, cardiac failure, or both.
- Screening for IgA deficiency is not recommended routinely for potential recipients of IGIV (see Adverse Reactions to IGIV, above).

Immune Globulin Subcutaneous (IGSC)

Subcutaneous (SC) administration of IG using battery-driven pumps has been shown to be safe and effective in adults and children with primary immunodeficiencies. Smaller doses, administered more frequently (ie, weekly), result in less fluctuation of serum IgG concentrations over time. Systemic reactions are less frequent than with IV therapy, and some parents or patients can be taught to infuse at home. The most common adverse effects of IGSC are injection-site reactions, including local swelling, redness, itching, soreness, induration, and local heat. The most common systemic reaction is headaches. Three products are licensed in the United States for SC use (Hizentra, Vivaglobin, and Gammunex-C). There are no data on administration of IgG by the SC route for conditions requiring high-dose Immune Globulin, such as Kawasaki disease and immune-mediated thrombocytopenic purpura.

Antibodies of Animal Origin (Animal Antisera)

Products of animal origin used for neutralization of toxins or prophylaxis of infectious diseases are derived from serum of horses or sheep immunized with the agent/toxoid of interest. These animal-derived immunoglobulin products are referred to here as "serum," for convenience. Experimental products prepared in other species also may be available. These products are derived by concentrating the serum globulin fraction with ammonium sulfate. Some, but not all, products are subjected to an enzyme digestion process to decrease clinical reactions to administered foreign proteins.

Use of the following products is discussed in the disease-specific chapters in Section 3:

- Heptavalent Botulism Antitoxin (Equine), available from the Centers for Disease Control and Prevention (CDC), contains antitoxin against all 7 (A–G) botulinum toxin types (see Clostridial Infections, Botulism and Infant Botulism, p 281).
- Diphtheria Antitoxin (Equine) can be obtained only from CDC and is used under an investigational new drug protocol.

INDICATIONS FOR USE OF ANIMAL ANTISERA

Antibody-containing products prepared from animal sera pose a special risk to the recipient, and the use of such products should be limited strictly to certain indications for which specific IG preparations of human origin are not available (eg, diphtheria and botulism, other than infant botulism of the A or B serotypes).

REACTIONS TO ANIMAL SERA

Before any animal immune globulin is injected, the patient must be questioned about his or her history of asthma, allergic rhinitis, and urticaria after previous exposure to animals or injections of animal sera. Patients with a history of asthma or allergic symptoms, especially from exposure to horses, can be dangerously sensitive to equine sera and should be given these products with the utmost caution. People who previously have received animal sera are at increased risk of developing allergic reactions and serum sickness after administration of sera from the same animal species.

SENSITIVITY TESTS FOR REACTIONS TO ANIMAL SERA

Patients who need animal serum immune globulin should be skin tested before administration of the therapeutic products. Intradermal (ID) skin tests have resulted in fatalities, but the scratch test usually is safe. Therefore, scratch tests always should precede ID tests. Nevertheless, any sensitivity test must be performed by trained personnel familiar with treatment of acute anaphylaxis; necessary medications and equipment should be available readily (see Treatment of Anaphylactic Reactions, p 67).

SCRATCH, PRICK, OR PUNCTURE TEST.[1] Apply 1 drop of a 1:100 dilution of serum in preservative-free isotonic sodium chloride solution to the site of a superficial scratch, prick, or puncture on the volar aspect of the forearm. Positive (histamine) and negative (physiologic saline solution) control tests for the scratch test also should be applied. A positive test result is a wheal with surrounding erythema at least 3 mm larger than the negative control test area, read at 15 to 20 minutes. The histamine control must be positive for valid interpretation. If the scratch test result is negative, an ID test is performed.

INTRADERMAL TEST.[1] A dose of 0.02 mL of a 1:1000 dilution of serum in preservative-free isotonic saline-diluted serum (enough to raise a small wheal) is administered. Positive and negative control tests, as described for the scratch test, also should be applied. If the test result is negative, it should be repeated using a 1:100 dilution. For people with negative history for both animal allergy and previous exposure to animal serum, the 1:100 dilution may be used initially if a scratch, prick, or puncture test result with the serum is negative. Interpretation is the same as for the scratch test.

Positive test results not attributable to an irritant reaction indicate sensitivity, but a negative skin test result is not an absolute guarantee of lack of sensitivity. Therefore, animal sera should be administered with caution even to people whose test results are negative. Immediate hypersensitivity testing is performed to identify IgE-mediated disease and does not predict other immune reactions, such as serum sickness.

If the ID test result is positive or if the history of systemic anaphylaxis after previous administration of serum is highly suggestive in a person for whom the need for serum is unquestioned, desensitization can be undertaken (see Desensitization to Animal Sera).

If history and sensitivity test results are negative, the indicated dose of serum can be given intramuscularly. The patient should be observed afterward for at least 30 minutes. IV administration may be indicated if a high concentration of serum antibody is imperative, such as for treatment of diphtheria or botulism. In these instances, serum should be diluted and slowly administered intravenously according to the manufacturer's instructions. The patient should be monitored carefully for signs or symptoms of anaphylaxis.

DESENSITIZATION TO ANIMAL SERA

Tables 1.12 (p 65) and 1.13 (p 65) serve as guides for desensitization procedures for administration of animal sera. IV (Table 1.12) or ID, SC, or IM (Table 1.13) regimens may be chosen. The IV route is considered safest, because it offers better control. The desensitization procedure must be performed by trained personnel familiar with treatment of anaphylaxis and with appropriate drugs and available equipment (see Treatment of Anaphylactic Reactions, p 67). Some physicians advocate concurrent use of an oral or parenteral antihistamine (such as diphenhydramine) during the procedure, with or

---

[1] Antihistamines may inhibit reactions in the scratch, prick, or puncture test and in the ID test; hence, testing should not be performed for at least 24 hours or, preferably, 48 hours after receipt of these drugs.

Table 1.12. Desensitization to Serum—Intravenous (IV) Route

Dose Number[a]	Dilution of Serum in Isotonic Sodium Chloride	Amount of IV Injection, mL
1	1:1000	0.1
2	1:1000	0.3
3	1:1000	0.6
4	1:100	0.1
5	1:100	0.3
6	1:100	0.6
7	1:10	0.1
8	1:10	0.3
9	1:10	0.6
10	Undiluted	0.1
11	Undiluted	0.3
12	Undiluted	0.6
13	Undiluted	1.0

[a] Administer consistently at 15-minute intervals.

Table 1.13. Desensitization to Serum—Intradermal (ID), Subcutaneous (SC), and Intramuscular (IM) Routes

Dose Number[a]	Route of Administration	Dilution of Serum in Isotonic Sodium Chloride	Amount of ID, SC, or IM Injection, mL
1	ID	1:1000	0.1
2	ID	1:1000	0.3
3	SC	1:1000	0.6
4	SC	1:100	0.1
5	SC	1:100	0.3
6	SC	1:100	0.6
7	SC	1:10	0.1
8	SC	1:10	0.3
9	SC	1:10	0.6
10	SC	Undiluted	0.1
11	SC	Undiluted	0.3
12	IM	Undiluted	0.6
13	IM	Undiluted	1.0

[a] Administer consistently at 15-minute intervals.

without IV hydrocortisone or methylprednisolone. If signs of anaphylaxis occur, aqueous epinephrine should be administered immediately (see Treatment of Anaphylactic Reactions, p 67). Administration of sera during a desensitization procedure must be continuous, because if administration is interrupted, protection achieved by desensitization will be lost.

TYPES OF REACTIONS TO ANIMAL SERA

The following reactions can occur as the result of administration of animal sera. Of these, only anaphylaxis is mediated by IgE antibodies, and thus, occurrence can be predicted by previous skin testing results.

ACUTE FEBRILE REACTIONS. These reactions usually are mild and can be treated with antipyretic agents. Severe febrile reactions should be treated with antipyretic agents or other safe, available methods to decrease temperature physically.

SERUM SICKNESS. Manifestations, which usually begin 7 to 10 days (occasionally as late as 3 weeks) after primary exposure to the foreign protein, consist of fever, urticaria, or a maculopapular rash (90% of cases); arthritis or arthralgia; and lymphadenopathy. Local edema can occur at the serum injection site a few days before systemic signs and symptoms appear. Angioedema, glomerulonephritis, Guillain-Barré syndrome, peripheral neuritis, and myocarditis also can occur. However, serum sickness may be mild and resolve spontaneously within a few days to 2 weeks. People who previously have received serum injections are at increased risk after readministration; manifestations in these patients usually occur shortly (from hours to 3 days) after administration of serum. Antihistamines can be helpful for management of serum sickness for alleviation of pruritus, edema, and urticaria. Fever, malaise, arthralgia, and arthritis can be controlled in most patients by administration of aspirin or other nonsteroidal anti-inflammatory agents. Corticosteroids may be helpful for controlling serious manifestations that are controlled poorly by other agents; prednisone or prednisolone in therapeutic dosages (1.5–2 mg/kg per day; maximum 60 mg/day) for 5 to 7 days are appropriate regimens.

ANAPHYLAXIS. The rapidity of onset and overall severity of anaphylaxis may vary considerably. Anaphylaxis usually begins within minutes of exposure to the causative agent, and in general, the more rapid the onset, the more severe the overall course. Major symptomatic manifestations include (1) cutaneous: pruritus, flushing, urticaria, and angioedema; (2) respiratory: hoarse voice and stridor, cough, wheeze, dyspnea, and cyanosis; (3) cardiovascular: rapid weak pulse, hypotension, and arrhythmias; and (4) gastrointestinal: cramps, vomiting, diarrhea, and dry mouth. Anaphylaxis is a medical emergency.

Treatment of Anaphylactic Reactions

Health care professionals administering biologic products or serum must be able to recognize and be prepared to treat systemic anaphylaxis. Medications, equipment, and competent staff necessary to maintain the patency of the airway and to manage cardiovascular collapse must be available.[1]

The emergency treatment of systemic anaphylactic reactions is based on the type of reaction. In all instances, epinephrine is the primary drug. Mild symptoms, such as skin reactions alone (eg, pruritus, erythema, urticaria, or angioedema), may be the first sign of an anaphylactic reaction but intrinsically are not dangerous and can be treated with antihistamines (Table 1.14, p 68). However, using clinical judgment, an injection of epinephrine may be given depending on the clinical situation (Table 1.15, p 68). Epinephrine should be injected promptly for anaphylaxis, which is likely (although not exclusively) occurring if the patient has: (1) skin symptoms (generalized hives, itch-flush, swollen lips/tongue/uvula) and respiratory compromise (dyspnea, wheeze, bronchospasm, stridor, or hypoxemia); or (2) 2 or more organ systems involved, including skin symptoms or respiratory compromise as described above, *plus* gastrointestinal tract symptoms (eg, persistent gastrointestinal tract symptoms, such as crampy abdominal pain or vomiting) or cardiovascular symptoms (eg, reduced blood pressure, syncope, collapse, hypotonia, incontinence). If a patient is known to have had a previous severe allergic reaction to the biologic product/serum, onset of skin, cardiovascular, or respiratory symptoms alone may warrant treatment with epinephrine.[2] Aqueous epinephrine, 0.01 mg/kg (maximum dose, 0.5 mg), usually is administered intramuscularly every 5 to 15 minutes as necessary to control symptoms and maintain blood pressure (because measurement is clear and accurate). Injections can be given at shorter than 5-minute intervals if deemed necessary. Because concentrations of epinephrine are higher and achieved more rapidly after IM administration, SC administration no longer is recommended. When the patient's condition improves and remains stable, oral antihistamines and possibly oral corticosteroids (1.5–2.0 mg/kg per day of prednisone; maximum 60 mg/day) can be given for an additional 24 to 48 hours.

Severe or potentially life-threatening systemic anaphylaxis involving severe bronchospasm, laryngeal edema, other airway compromise, shock, and cardiovascular collapse necessitates additional therapy. Maintenance of the airway and administration of oxygen should be instituted promptly. Epinephrine is administered intramuscularly immediately while IV access is being established. IV epinephrine may be indicated; for this use, the epinephrine must be diluted from 1:1000 aqueous base to a dilution of 1:10 000 using physiologic saline solution (see Table 1.15, p 68). Administration of epinephrine intravenously can lead to lethal arrhythmia; cardiac monitoring is recommended. A slow, continuous, low-dose infusion is preferable to repeated bolus administration, because the dose can be titrated to the desired effect, and accidental administration of large boluses of epinephrine can be avoided. Nebulized albuterol is indicated for bronchospasm (see

---

[1] Hegenbarth MA; American Academy of Pediatrics, Committee on Drugs. Preparing for pediatric emergencies: drugs to consider. *Pediatrics.* 2008;121(2):433–443

[2] Sampson HA, Munoz-Furlong A, Campbell RL, Adkinson NF, Jr, Bock SA, Branum A, et al. Second Symposium on the Definition and Management of Anaphylaxis: Summary Report-Second National Institute of Allergy and Infectious Disease/Food Allergy and Anaphylaxis Network Symposium. *J Allergy Clin Immunol.* 2006;117(2):391–397

Table 1.14. Dosages of Commonly Used Secondary Drugs in the Treatment of Anaphylaxis

Drug	Dose
H$_1$ receptor-blocking agents (antihistamines)[a]	
Diphenhydramine	Oral, IM, IV: 1–2 mg/kg, every 4–6 h (100 mg, maximum single dose)
Hydroxyzine	Oral, IM: 0.5–1 mg/kg, every 4–6 h (100 mg, maximum single dose)
H$_2$ receptor-blocking agents (also antihistamines)	
Cimetidine	IV: 5 mg/kg, slowly over a 15-min period, every 6–8 h (300 mg, maximum single dose)
Ranitidine	IV: 1 mg/kg, slowly over a 15-min period, every 6–8 h (50 mg, maximum single dose)
Corticosteroids	
Methylprednisolone	IV: 1.5–2 mg/kg, every 4–6 h (60 mg, maximum single dose)
Prednisone	Oral: 1.5–2 mg/kg, single morning dose (60 mg, maximum single dose); use corticosteroids as long as needed
B$_2$-agonist	
Albuterol	Nebulizer solution: 0.5% (5 mg/mL), 0.05–0.15 mg/kg per dose in 2–3 mL isotonic sodium chloride solution, maximum 5 mg/dose every 20 min over a 1-h to 2-h period, or 0.5 mg/kg/h by continuous nebulization (15 mg/h, maximum dose)
Other	
Dopamine	IV: 5–20 µg/kg per minute. Mixing 150 mg of dopamine with 250 mL of saline solution or 5% dextrose in water will produce a solution that, if infused at the rate of 1 mL/kg/h, will deliver 10 µg/kg/min. The solution must be free of bicarbonate, which may inactivate dopamine.

IM indicates intramuscular; IV, intravenous.

[a]Cetirizine may be considered for oral use, because it is less sedating and, therefore, less likely to lead to confusion about the mental status of the patient.

Table 1.15. Epinephrine in the Treatment of Anaphylaxis[a]

Intramuscular (IM) administration

Epinephrine 1:1000 (aqueous): IM (anterolateral thigh), 0.01 mL/kg per dose, up to 0.5 mL, repeated every 5–15 min, up to 3 doses.[b]

Intravenous (IV) administration

An initial bolus of IV epinephrine is given to patients not responding to IM epinephrine using a dilution of 1:10 000 rather than a dilution of 1:1000. This dilution can be made using 1 mL of the 1:1000 dilution in 9 mL of physiologic saline solution. The dose is 0.01 mg/kg or 0.1 mL/kg of the 1:10 000 dilution. A continuous infusion should be started if repeated doses are required. One milligram (1 mL) of 1:1000 dilution of epinephrine added to 250 mL of 5% dextrose in water, resulting in a concentration of 4 µg/mL, is infused initially at a rate of 0.1 µg/kg per minute and increased gradually to 1.5 µg/kg per minute to maintain blood pressure.

[a]In addition to epinephrine, maintenance of the airway and administration of oxygen are critical.

[b]If agent causing anaphylactic reaction was given by injection, epinephrine can be injected into the same site to slow absorption.

Table 1.14, p 68). Rapid IV infusion of physiologic saline solution, lactated Ringer solution, or other isotonic solution adequate to maintain blood pressure must be instituted to compensate for the loss of circulating intravascular volume.

In some cases, the use of inotropic agents, such as dopamine (see Table 1.14, p 68), may be necessary for blood pressure support. The combination of histamine H_1 and H_2 receptor-blocking agents (see Table 1.14, p 68) may be synergistic in effect and could be used as adjunctive therapy. Corticosteroids should be used in all cases of anaphylaxis except cases that are mild and have responded promptly to initial therapy (see Table 1.14, p 68). However, no data support the usefulness of corticosteroids in treating anaphylaxis, and therefore, they should not be administered in lieu of treatment with epinephrine and should be considered as adjunctive therapy.

All patients showing signs and symptoms of systemic anaphylaxis, regardless of severity, should be observed for several hours in an appropriate facility, even after remission of immediate symptoms. Although a specific period of observation has not been established, a period of observation of 4 hours would be reasonable for mild episodes, and as long as 24 hours would be reasonable for severe episodes.

Anaphylaxis occurring in people who already are taking beta-adrenergic–blocking agents can be more profound and significantly less responsive to epinephrine and other beta-adrenergic agonist drugs. More aggressive therapy with epinephrine may override receptor blockade in some patients. Some experts recommend use of IV glucagon for cardiovascular manifestations and inhaled atropine for management of bradycardia or bronchospasm.

....
IMMUNIZATION IN SPECIAL CLINICAL CIRCUMSTANCES

Preterm and Low Birth Weight Infants

Preterm infants born at less than 37 weeks' gestation and infants of low birth weight (less than 2500 g) should, with few exceptions, receive all routinely recommended childhood vaccines at the same chronologic age as term infants. Gestational age and birth weight are not limiting factors when deciding whether a clinically stable preterm infant is to be immunized on schedule. Although studies have shown decreased immune responses to several vaccines given to neonates with very low birth weight (less than 1500 g) and neonates of very early gestational age (less than 29 weeks), most preterm infants, including infants who receive dexamethasone for chronic lung disease, produce sufficient vaccine-induced immunity to prevent disease. Vaccine dosages given to term infants should not be reduced or divided when given to preterm or low birth weight infants.

Preterm and low birth weight infants tolerate most childhood vaccines as well as term infants. Apnea with or without bradycardia was reported to have occurred in some extremely low birth weight (less than 1000 g) infants after use of diphtheria and tetanus toxoids and whole-cell pertussis vaccine (DTP). More recent reports demonstrate that apnea episodes were neither more frequent nor more severe in extremely low birth weight infants immunized with acellular pertussis-containing vaccines (DTaP) compared with matched controls. However, cardiorespiratory events, including apnea and bradycardia with oxygen desaturation, frequently increase in very low birth weight infants given the combination diphtheria and tetanus toxoids and acellular pertussis (DTaP), inactivated poliovirus, hepatitis B, and *Haemophilus influenzae* b conjugate vaccine. Apnea within 24 hours prior to immunization, younger age, or weight less than 2000 g at the time of immunization and 12-hour Score for Neonatal Acute Physiology II less than 10 have been associated with development of postimmunization apnea, and it may be prudent to observe such infants for 48 hours after immunization. However, these postimmunization cardiorespiratory events generally do not have a detrimental effect on the clinical course of immunized infants.

Medically stable preterm infants who remain in the hospital at 2 months of chronologic age should be given all inactivated vaccines recommended at that age (see Recommended Immunization Schedule For Persons Aged 0 Through 6 Years, Fig 1.1, p 27–28). A medically stable infant is defined as one who does not require ongoing management for serious infection; metabolic disease; or acute renal, cardiovascular, neurologic, or respiratory tract illness and who demonstrates a clinical course of sustained recovery and pattern of steady growth. All immunizations required at 2 months of age can be administered simultaneously to preterm or low birth weight infants, except for rotavirus vaccine, which should be deferred unless the infant is being discharged from the hospital (see Rotavirus, p 626) to prevent potential spread of this live vaccine virus. The same volume of vaccine used for term infants is appropriate for medically stable preterm infants. The number of injections at 2 months of age can be minimized by using combination vaccines. When it is difficult to administer 3 or 4 injections simultaneously to hospitalized preterm infants because of limited injection sites, the vaccines recommended at 2 months of age can be administered at different times. Because recommended parenteral vaccines are inactivated, any interval between doses of individual vaccines is acceptable. However, to avoid superimposing local reactions, 2-week intervals may be reasonable. The choice of needle lengths used for intramuscular vaccine administration is determined by available muscle mass of the preterm or low birth weight infant (see Table 1.6, p 22).

Hepatitis B vaccine given to preterm or low birth weight infants weighing more than 2000 g at birth produces an immune response comparable to that in term infants. Medically stable and thriving infants weighing less than 2000 g demonstrate predictable, consistent, and sufficient hepatitis B antibody responses. Hepatitis B vaccine schedules for infants weighing <2000 g and infants weighing ≥2000 g born to mothers with positive, negative, and unknown hepatitis B surface antigen (HBsAg) status are given in Hepatitis B, Special Considerations, including Tables 3.20 (p 384) and 3.21 (p 386).

Only monovalent hepatitis B vaccine should be used for infants younger than 6 weeks of age. Giving a birth dose of monovalent hepatitis B vaccine when a combination vaccine containing hepatitis B vaccine subsequently is used means that 4 total doses will be administered.

Because all preterm infants are considered at increased risk of complications of influenza, 2 doses of inactivated influenza vaccine given 1 month apart should be offered for preterm infants beginning at 6 months of chronologic age as soon as influenza vaccine is available (see Influenza, p 439). Because preterm infants younger than 6 months of age and infants of any age with chronic complications of preterm birth are extremely vulnerable to influenza virus infection, household contacts, child care providers, and hospital nursery personnel caring for preterm infants should receive influenza vaccine annually (see Influenza, p 439).

Preterm infants younger than 6 months of age, who are too young to have completed the primary immunization series, are at increased risk of pertussis infection and pertussis-related complications. For people who previously have not received tetanus toxoid, reduced diphtheria toxoid, and acellular pertussis (Tdap) vaccine, Tdap should be administered to hospital personnel caring for pregnant women and infants, to pregnant women during pregnancy (after 20 weeks' gestation), to postpartum women as soon as possible after the infant's birth if not administered during pregnancy, and to household contacts and child-care providers of all infants younger than 1 year of age (see Pertussis, p 553).

Appropriately selected preterm infants born at less than 32 weeks of gestational age, infants with chronic lung disease and prematurity, and infants with specified cardiovascular conditions up to 2 years of age may benefit from monthly immunoprophylaxis with palivizumab (respiratory syncytial virus monoclonal antibody) during respiratory syncytial virus season (see Respiratory Syncytial Virus, p 609). Palivizumab use does not interfere with immune response to routine childhood immunizations in preterm or low birth weight infants.

Preterm infants can receive rotavirus vaccine under the following circumstances: the infant is at least 6 weeks and less than 15 weeks, 0 days of chronologic age, the infant is medically stable, and the first dose is given at the time of hospital discharge or after hospital discharge.

Pregnancy[1]

Immunization during pregnancy poses theoretical risks to the developing fetus. Although no evidence indicates that vaccines currently in use have detrimental effects on the fetus, pregnant women should receive a vaccine only when the vaccine is unlikely to cause harm, the risk of disease exposure is high, and the infection would pose a significant risk to the pregnant woman or fetus. When a vaccine is to be given during pregnancy, delaying administration until the second or third trimester, when possible, is a reasonable precaution to minimize theoretical concern about possible teratogenicity.

The only vaccines recommended for routine administration during pregnancy in the United States, provided they are indicated (either for primary or booster immunization), are tetanus toxoid, reduced diphtheria, and acellular pertussis (Tdap) or adult-type tetanus and diphtheria toxoids (Td) and inactivated influenza vaccines.[1] The Centers for Disease Control and Prevention (CDC) recommends administration of Tdap during pregnancy, preferably during the third or late-second trimester (after 20 weeks' gestation) if the woman previously had not received Tdap.[2] If not administered during pregnancy, Tdap should be administered immediately postpartum. Women who are unimmunized or only partially immunized against tetanus should complete the primary series. For complete recommendations regarding use of Td and Tdap vaccines in pregnancy, see Pertussis (p 553). In resource-limited countries with a high incidence of neonatal tetanus, Td vaccine routinely is administered during pregnancy without evidence of adverse effects and with striking decreases in the occurrence of neonatal tetanus.

---

[1] See adult immunization schedule available at **www.cdc.gov/vaccines.**

[2] Centers for Disease Control and Prevention. Updated recommendations for use of tetanus toxoid, reduced diphtheria toxoid and acellular pertussis vaccine (Tdap) in pregnant women and persons who have or anticipate having close contact with an infant aged <12 months—Advisory Committee on Immunization Practices (ACIP), 2011. *MMWR Morb Mortal Wkly Rep.* 2011;60(41):1424–1426

Studies indicate that women who are pregnant and have no other underlying medical conditions are at increased risk of complications and hospitalization from influenza. Therefore, inactivated influenza vaccine should be administered to all women who will be pregnant during the influenza season, regardless of trimester (see Influenza, p 439). Influenza immunization of pregnant women also protects infants younger than 6 months of age who cannot be immunized actively and in whom antiviral prophylaxis and treatment options are limited. Influenza vaccines are not approved for use in infants younger than 6 months of age. Live-attenuated influenza vaccine should not be given to pregnant women.

Pneumococcal and meningococcal vaccines can be given to a pregnant woman at high risk of serious or complicated illness from infection with *Streptococcus pneumoniae* or *Neisseria meningitidis*. Meningococcal conjugate vaccine can be given to a pregnant woman when there is increased risk of disease, such as during epidemics or before travel to an area with hyperendemic infection. Infection with hepatitis A or hepatitis B can result in severe disease in a pregnant woman and, in the case of hepatitis B, chronic infection in the newborn infant. Hepatitis A or hepatitis B immunizations, if indicated, can be given to pregnant women. Although data on safety of these vaccines for a pregnant woman or developing fetus are not available, no risk would be expected. Inactivated poliovirus (IPV) vaccine can be given to pregnant women who never have received poliovirus vaccine, are immunized partially, or are immunized completely but require a booster dose (see Poliovirus Infections, p 588). Oral poliovirus (OPV) vaccine should not be administered to pregnant women.

Pregnancy is a contraindication to administration of all live-virus vaccines, except when susceptibility and exposure are highly probable and the disease to be prevented poses a greater threat to the pregnant woman or fetus than does the vaccine. Although only a theoretical risk to the fetus exists with a live-virus vaccine, the background rate of anomalies in uncomplicated pregnancies may result in a defect that could be attributed inappropriately to a vaccine. Therefore, live-virus vaccines should be avoided during pregnancy.

Because measles, mumps, rubella, and varicella vaccines are contraindicated for pregnant women, efforts should be made to immunize susceptible women against these illnesses before they become pregnant or after pregnancy. Although of theoretical concern, no case of embryopathy caused by the attenuated rubella vaccine strain has been reported. However, a rare theoretical risk of embryopathy from inadvertent rubella vaccine administration cannot be excluded. The effect of varicella vaccine on the fetus, if any, is unknown. The manufacturer, in collaboration with the Centers for Disease Control and Prevention (CDC), established the VARIVAX Pregnancy Registry to monitor the maternal and fetal outcomes of women who inadvertently are given varicella vaccine during the 3 months before or at any time during pregnancy. From March 1995 through March 2010, there were 827 prospectively reported women with known pregnancy outcomes exposed to VARIVAX enrolled in the Pregnancy Registry. Of the 827, 54 chose elective termination for unknown reasons, 168 were seronegative, and 605 were unknown or seropositive. Seven hundred twelve of these women were known to have received varicella vaccine inadvertently within 3 months before or during pregnancy and had known pregnancy outcomes available for analysis and considered complete. No offspring had clinical features consistent with congenital varicella, and there were no birth defects consistent with congenital varicella syndrome in reports of pregnancies that ended in spontaneous abortion or elective termination. The prevalence estimates of birth defects were compatible with the background number of congenital anomalies expected in the general population. Reporting of instances of inadvertent immunization with a varicella/zoster virus-containing vaccine during pregnancy by telephone is encouraged (1-800-986-8999).

A pregnant mother or other household member is not a contraindication for varicella immunization of a child in that household. Transmission of vaccine virus from an immunocompetent vaccine recipient to a susceptible person has been reported only rarely, and only when a vaccine-associated rash develops in the vaccinee (see Varicella-Zoster Infections, p 774). Breastfeeding is not a contraindication for immunization of varicella-susceptible women after pregnancy. Varicella has not been detected by polymerase chain reaction assay in human milk specimens after immunization, and infants breastfed by mothers immunized with varicella vaccine do not seroconvert to varicella. Varicella-Zoster Immune Globulin should be considered strongly for susceptible, pregnant women who have been exposed to natural varicella infection. If Varicella-Zoster Immune Globulin is not available, some experts suggest use of Immune Globulin Intravenous; use of acyclovir in this circumstance has not been evaluated.

Pregnant women at risk of exposure to unusual pathogens should be considered for immunization when the potential benefits outweigh the potential risks to the mother and fetus.

- Zoster vaccine is a live-attenuated vaccine. It should not be administered to pregnant women, and pregnancy should be avoided for 3 months following a dose.
- Human papillomavirus (HPV) vaccine contains no live virus, but data on immunization during pregnancy are limited. Initiation of the vaccine series should be delayed until after completion of the pregnancy. If a woman is found to be pregnant after initiating the immunization series, the remainder of the 3-dose regimen should be delayed until after completion of the pregnancy. If a vaccine dose has been administered during pregnancy, no intervention is needed. Two vaccine registries have been established for reporting of inadvertent exposure to HPV vaccine during pregnancy (quadrivalent HPV vaccine, Merck and Co Inc, telephone: 800-986-8999; bivalent HPV vaccine, GlaxoSmithKline, telephone: 888-452-9622).
- Rabies vaccine should be given to pregnant women after exposure to rabies under the same circumstances as nonpregnant women. There has been no reported association between rabies immunization and adverse fetal outcomes. If the risk of exposure to rabies is substantial, preexposure prophylaxis also may be indicated.
- Yellow fever vaccine is a live-attenuated virus vaccine, which is a precaution for pregnant women, but if travel of a pregnant woman cannot be postponed and mosquito exposure cannot be avoided, immunization should be considered.[1,2]
- No specific information is available on the safety of Japanese encephalitis virus vaccine for pregnant women. Women should be immunized before conception, if possible, but Japanese encephalitis virus vaccine should be considered if travel to regions with endemic infection and mosquito exposure is unavoidable and the risk of disease

---

[1] See **wwwn.cdc.gov/travel/contentDiseases.aspx.**

[2] Centers for Disease Control and Prevention. Yellow fever vaccine—recommendations of the Advisory Committee on Immunization Practices (ACIP). *MMWR Recomm Rep.* 2010;59(RR-07):1–27

outweighs the theoretical risk of adverse events in pregnant woman and fetus (see Arboviruses, p 232).[1]

- The parenteral typhoid vaccine should be considered on a case-by-case basis; oral typhoid vaccine is a live-attenuated vaccine and should not be administered to pregnant women.[2]

- Anthrax vaccine is inactivated, so there is no theoretical risk to the fetus, but the vaccine has not been evaluated for safety in pregnant women (see Anthrax, p 228).

- Vaccinia virus vaccine should be given only when there is a definite and significant exposure to smallpox. Because smallpox causes more severe disease in pregnant than nonpregnant women, the potential risks of immunization may be outweighed by the risk of disease. Immunized household contacts should avoid contact with pregnant women until the vaccination site is healed.

Immunocompromised Children

PRIMARY AND SECONDARY IMMUNE DEFICIENCIES

The safety and effectiveness of vaccines in people with immune deficiency are determined by the nature and degree of immunosuppression. Immunocompromised people vary in their degree of immunosuppression and susceptibility to infection and represent a heterogeneous population with regard to immunization. Immunodeficiency conditions can be grouped into primary and secondary (acquired) disorders. Primary disorders of the immune system generally are inherited, usually as single-gene disorders; may involve any part of the immune defenses, including B-lymphocyte (humoral) immunity, T-lymphocyte (cell)-mediated immunity, complement and phagocytic function, and abnormalities of innate immunity; and share the common feature of susceptibility to infection.[3] Secondary disorders of the immune system are acquired and occur in people with human immunodeficiency virus (HIV) infection/acquired immunodeficiency syndrome (AIDS) or malignant neoplasms; people who have undergone stem cell or solid organ transplantation, people without a functioning spleen; people receiving immunosuppressive, antimetabolic, or radiation therapy; and people with a variety of other illnesses, such as severe malnutrition, protein loss, and uremia (see Table 1.16, p 75). Published studies of experience with vaccine administration to immunocompromised children are limited. In many situations, theoretical considerations are the primary guide to vaccine administration, because experience with individual vaccines in people with a specific disorder is lacking. However, experience in HIV-infected children provides reassurance that the risk of adverse events in these children following immunization is low. The Infectious Diseases Society of America, in conjunction with the AAP, CDC, and other professional societies and organizations, is developing immunization guidelines for children and adults with primary and secondary immune deficiencies.

---

[1] Centers for Disease Control and Prevention. Japanese encephalitis virus vaccines—recommendations of the Advisory Committee on Immunization Practices (ACIP). *MMWR Recomm Rep.* 2010;59(RR-01):1–27

[2] See **wwww.cdc.gov/travel/contentDiseases.aspx.**

[3] Centers for Disease Control and Prevention. Applying public health strategies to primary immunodeficiency diseases: a potential approach to genetic disorders. *MMWR Recomm Rep.* 2004;53(RR-1):1–29

Table 1.16. Immunization of Children and Adolescents With Primary and Secondary Immune Deficiencies

Category	Example of Specific Immunodeficiency	Vaccine Contraindications	Effectiveness and Comments, Including Risk-Specific Vaccines[a]
Primary[b]			
B lymphocyte (humoral)	Severe antibody deficiencies (eg, X-linked agammaglobulinemia and common variable immuno-deficiency)	OPV,[c] smallpox, LAIV, yellow fever (YF), and live-bacteria vaccines[d], consider measles vaccine; no data for varicella or rotavirus vaccines	Effectiveness of any vaccine is uncertain if it depends only on humoral response (eg, PPSV23 or MPSV4); IGIV therapy interferes with measles and possibly varicella immune response. Pneumococcal vaccine recommended. Consider measles and varicella vaccines.
	Less severe antibody deficiencies (eg, selective IgA deficiency and IgG subclass deficiencies)	OPV,[c] BCG, YF vaccines; other live vaccines[e] appear to be safe, but caution is urged	All vaccines probably effective; immune response may be attenuated. Pneumococcal vaccine recommended.
T lymphocyte (cell-mediated and humoral)	Complete defects (eg, severe combined immunodeficiency; complete DiGeorge syndrome)	All live vaccines[d,e,f]	All vaccines probably ineffective. Pneumococcal vaccine recommended.
	Partial defects (eg, most patients with DiGeorge syndrome, Wiskott-Aldrich syndrome, ataxia telangiectasia)	All live vaccines[d,e]	Effectiveness of any vaccine depends on degree of immune suppression. Pneumococcal and meningococcal vaccines recommended. Consider Hib vaccine if not administered during infancy.
Complement	Persistent complement component, properdin, or factor B deficiency	None	All routine vaccines probably effective. Pneumococcal and meningococcal vaccines recommended.
Phagocytic function	Chronic granulomatous disease, leukocyte adhesion defects, myeloperoxidase deficiency	Live-bacterial vaccines[d]	All inactivated vaccines safe and probably effective. Live-virus vaccines probably safe and effective.

Table 1.16. Immunization of Children and Adolescents With Primary and Secondary Immune Deficiencies, continued

Category	Example of Specific Immunodeficiency	Vaccine Contraindications	Effectiveness and Comments, Including Risk-Specific Vaccines[a]
Secondary[a]			
	HIV/AIDS	OPV,[c] smallpox, BCG, MMRV, LAIV[e]; withhold MMR and varicella in severely immunocompromised children; YF vaccine may have a contraindication or precaution depending on indicators of immune function[g]	MMR, varicella, rotavirus, and all inactivated vaccines, including inactivated influenza, may be effective.[h] Pneumococcal vaccine recommended. Consider Hib vaccine (if not administered during infancy) and meningococcal vaccine.
	Malignant neoplasm, transplantation, autoimmune disease, immunosuppressive or radiation therapy	Live-virus and -bacteria vaccines, depending on immune status[d,e]	Effectiveness of any vaccine depends on degree of immune suppression. Pneumococcal vaccine recommended.
	Asplenia	None	All routine vaccines likely effective. Pneumococcal and meningococcal vaccines recommended. Consider Hib vaccine (if not administered during infancy).
	Chronic renal disease	LAIV	Pneumococcal vaccine and hepatitis B vaccine (because of risk of dialysis-based bloodborne transmission) recommended.

Table 1.16. Immunization of Children and Adolescents With Primary and Secondary Immune Deficiencies, continued

Category	Example of Specific Immunodeficiency	Vaccine Contraindications	Effectiveness and Comments, Including Risk-Specific Vaccines[a]

OPV indicates oral poliovirus; LAIV, live-attenuated influenza vaccine; IGIV, Immune Globulin Intravenous; Ig, immunoglobulin; HIV, human immunodeficiency virus; AIDS, acquired immunodeficiency syndrome; BCG, bacille Calmette-Guérin; Hib, *Haemophilus influenzae* type b; MMR, measles-mumps-rubella.

[a] Other vaccines that are recommended universally or routinely should be given if not contraindicated.

[b] All children and adolescents should receive an annual age-appropriate inactivated influenza vaccine. LAIV is indicated only for healthy people 2 through 49 years of age.

[c] OPV vaccine no longer is available in the United States.

[d] Live-bacteria vaccines: BCG and Ty21a *Salmonella typhi* vaccine.

[e] Live-virus vaccines: LAIV, MMR, measles-mumps-rubella-varicella (MMRV), herpes zoster (ZOS), OPV, varicella, YF, vaccinia (smallpox), and rotavirus.

[f] Regarding T-lymphocyte immunodeficiency as a contraindication to rotavirus vaccine, data only exist for severe combined immunodeficiency syndrome.

[g] Symptomatic HIV-infection or CD4+ T-lymphocyte values less than 200/mm³ or less than 15% of total lymphocytes for children younger than 6 years is a contraindication to YF vaccine. Aysmptomatic HIV-infected people 6 years of age and older with CD4+ T-lymphocyte values of 200 to 499/mm³, or 15% to 24% of total lymphocytes for children younger than 6 years, is a precaution for YF vaccine (Centers for Disease Control and Prevention. Yellow fever vaccine: recommendations of the Advisory Committee on Immunization Practices [ACIP]. *MMWR Recomm Rep.* 2010;59[RR-07];1–27).

[h] HIV-infected children should receive Immune Globulin after exposure to measles (see Measles, p 489) and may receive varicella vaccine if CD4+ lymphocyte count ≥15% of expected for age (see Varicella-Zoster Infections, p 774).

LIVE VACCINES. In general, people who are severely immunocompromised or in whom immune function is uncertain should not receive live vaccines, either viral or bacterial, because of the risk of disease caused by the vaccine strains. There are particular immune deficiency disorders with which some live vaccines are safe, and for certain immunocompromised children and adolescents, the benefits may outweigh risks for use of particular live vaccines.

INACTIVATED VACCINES AND PASSIVE IMMUNIZATION. Inactivated vaccines and Immune Globulin (IG) preparations should be used when appropriate. All children 6 months of age and older and adolescents with primary and secondary immunodeficiencies should receive an annual age-appropriate inactivated influenza vaccine to prevent influenza and secondary bacterial infections associated with influenza disease. However, immune responses of immunocompromised children to inactivated vaccines, including trivalent inactivated influenza vaccine, may be inadequate. In children with secondary immunodeficiency, the ability to develop an adequate immunologic response depends on the presence of immunosuppression during or within 2 weeks of immunization. In children with malignant neoplasms, if possible, inactivated influenza immunization should be given no sooner than 3 to 4 weeks after a course of chemotherapy is discontinued and when peripheral granulocyte and lymphocyte counts >1000 cells/μL $(1.0 \times 10^9/L)$ are achieved. In children, an adequate response to vaccines usually occurs between 3 months and 1 year after discontinuation of immunosuppressive therapy.

PRIMARY IMMUNODEFICIENCIES. In general, live vaccines should not be given to children with major B-lymphocyte disorders, because the safety is unknown, and optimal antibody response may not occur because of the underlying disease and because the patient may be receiving Immune Globulin Intravenous (IGIV) periodically. Oral poliovirus (OPV) vaccine, which no longer is available in the United States, is contraindicated, because it has been associated with an increased incidence of paralytic disease in people with B-lymphocyte or combined immunodeficiency disorders. Live vaccines can be given to children with isolated immunoglobulin A deficiency. All live vaccines are contraindicated for all patients with severe T-lymphocyte–mediated disorders of immune function, such as severe combined immunodeficiency syndrome (SCID) and complete DiGeorge syndrome (thymic aplasia) (see Table 1.16, p 75). Fatal or chronic poliomyelitis, measles, and vaccinia have occurred in children with severe disorders of T-lymphocyte function after administration of the respective live-virus vaccines. Inactivated vaccines, including poliovirus and trivalent influenza vaccines, should be administered. Immunization of children with less severe T-lymphocyte associated immunodeficiencies, such as partial DiGeorge syndrome (thymic hypoplasia), should be decided on an individual basis with expert advice. Children with deficiency in antibody-synthesizing capacity may be incapable of developing an antibody response to vaccines and may benefit from regular doses of IG (usually IGIV) to provide passive protection against many infectious diseases. Specific immune globulins are available for postexposure prophylaxis for some infections (see Specific Immune Globulins, p 59). Children with milder B-lymphocyte and antibody deficiencies have an intermediate degree of vaccine responsiveness and may require monitoring of postimmunization antibody concentrations to confirm responses to vaccination.

The live-attenuated vaccines for rotavirus are not safe in children with severe combined immunodeficiency and are of unproven safety in infants with other immunodeficiencies, including other primary and acquired immunodeficiency conditions, infants on immunosuppressive therapy, or infants who are HIV exposed or infected. SCID is a contraindication to rotavirus vaccines.[1] Because these vaccines are recommended for infants beginning at 6 weeks of age, some recipients will have these as-yet undiagnosed diseases and have the potential for prolonged shedding and illness. Many experts would administer rotavirus vaccine to HIV-infected or -exposed infants. The potential risks should be weighed against the benefits of administering rotavirus vaccine to infants with known or suspected altered immunocompetence (see Rotavirus, p 626).[2,3]

Most experts believe that attenuated live-virus vaccines are safe to administer to children with complement deficiencies and disorders of phagocyte function. Children with early or late complement deficiencies should receive all routinely recommended immunizations, including live-virus vaccines. In addition, children with early complement deficiencies should receive pneumococcal vaccine (including pneumococcal polysaccharide vaccine) and meningococcal conjugate vaccine (see Pneumococcal Infections, p 571, and Meningococcal Infections, p 500, for specific details). Children with late complement deficiencies should receive meningococcal conjugate vaccine starting at 9 months of age. Children with phagocytic function disorders, including chronic granulomatous disease and leukocyte adhesion defects, should receive all recommended childhood vaccines. Live-bacterial vaccines (bacille Calmette Guérin and *Salmonella typhi*) should not be administered to children with phagocytic disorders.

SECONDARY (ACQUIRED) IMMUNODEFICIENCIES. Several factors should be considered in immunization of children with secondary immunodeficiencies, including the underlying disease, the specific immunosuppressive regimen (dose and schedule), and the infectious disease and immunization history of the person. Live-viral vaccines generally are contraindicated because of a proven or theoretical increased risk of prolonged shedding and disease. Exceptions include children 1 through 8 years of age with HIV infection who are in Centers for Disease Control and Prevention (CDC) clinical categories N, A, and B, in whom measles-mumps-rubella (MMR) vaccine is recommended (see Human Immunodeficiency Virus Infection, p 418) and in whom varicella vaccine is recommended if CD4+ T-lymphocyte percentage is 15% or greater (see Varicella-Zoster Infections, p 774).[4] Immunization with MMR (2 doses administered at least 4 weeks apart) and varicella (2 doses administered 3 months apart) vaccines of people 9 years of age and older who have CD4+ T-lymphocyte counts 200 cells/mm^3 or greater or a CD4+ T-lymphocyte

[1] Centers for Disease Control and Prevention. Addition of severe combined immunodeficiency as a contraindication for administration of rotavirus vaccine. *MMWR Morb Mortal Wkly Rep.* 2010;59(22):687–688

[2] Centers for Disease Control and Prevention. Prevention of rotavirus gastroenteritis among infants and children: recommendations of the Advisory Committee on Immunization Practices (ACIP). *MMWR Recomm Rep.* 2009;58(RR-2):1–25

[3] American Academy of Pediatrics, Committee on Infectious Diseases. Prevention of rotavirus disease: updated guidelines for use of rotavirus vaccine. *Pediatrics.* 2009;123(5):1412–1420

[4] Centers for Disease Control and Prevention. Guidelines for prevention and treatment of opportunistic infections among HIV-exposed and HIV-infected children: recommendations from CDC, the National Institutes of Health, the HIV Medical Association of the Infectious Diseases Society of America, the Pediatric Infectious Diseases Society, and the American Academy of Pediatrics. *MMWR Recomm.* 2009;58(RR-11):1–166

percentage of 15% or greater also can be considered.[1] Although varicella vaccine has been studied in children with acute lymphoblastic leukemia in remission, varicella vaccine generally should not be given to children with acute lymphocytic leukemia or another malignancy, because (a) many children will have received varicella vaccine prior to immune suppression and may retain protective immunity; (b) the risk of acquiring varicella has diminished in some countries with universal immunization programs; (c) antiviral agents are available for treatment; and (d) chemotherapy regimens change frequently and often are more immunosuppressive than regimens under which the safety and efficacy of varicella vaccine was studied (see Varicella-Zoster Infections, p 774). Measles-mumps-rubella-varicella (MMRV) vaccine has not been studied in immunocompromised people. When appropriate, MMR and varicella vaccines should be administered as separate immunizations at separate sites.

Live-virus vaccines usually are withheld for an interval of at least 3 months after immunosuppressive cancer chemotherapy has been discontinued. For corticosteroid therapy (see Corticosteroids, p 81), the interval is based on the assumption that immune response will have been restored in 3 months and that the underlying disease for which immunosuppressive therapy was given is in remission or under control. Immunodeficiency that follows use of recombinant human proteins with antiinflammatory properties, including tumor necrosis factor-alpha antagonists (eg, adalimumab, certolizumab, infliximab, etanercept, and golimumab) or anti–B-lymphocyte monoclonal antibodies (eg, rituximab), appears to be prolonged. The interval until immune reconstitution varies with the intensity and type of immunosuppressive therapy, radiation therapy, underlying disease, and other factors. Therefore, often it is not possible to make a definitive recommendation for an interval after cessation of immunosuppressive therapy when live-virus vaccines can be administered safely and effectively.

MONITORING SEROLOGIC RESPONSE. Because patients with congenital or acquired immunodeficiencies may not have an adequate response to vaccines, they may remain susceptible despite having been immunized. If there is an available test for a known antibody correlate of protection, specific postimmunization serum antibody titers can be determined 4 to 6 weeks after immunization to assess immune response and guide further immunization and management of future exposures.

HOUSEHOLD CONTACTS. Immunocompetent siblings and other household contacts of people with an immunologic deficiency should not receive smallpox vaccine or OPV vaccines, because vaccine virus may be transmitted to immunocompromised people. However, siblings and household contacts should receive MMR and rotavirus vaccines if indicated. The viruses in MMR vaccine are not transmitted, and transmission of rotavirus vaccine virus is rare. Varicella vaccine is recommended for susceptible contacts of immunocompromised children, because transmission of varicella vaccine virus from healthy people is rare, and vaccine-associated illness, if it develops, is mild. Either MMRV or separate MMR and varicella vaccine can be given to contacts. No precautions need to be taken after immunization unless the vaccine recipient develops a rash, particularly a vesicular rash. In such instances, the vaccine recipient should avoid direct contact with

---

[1] Centers for Disease Control and Prevention. Guidelines for prevention and treatment of opportunistic infections in HIV-infected adults and adolescents: recommendations from CDC, the National Institutes of Health, and the HIV Medicine Association of the Infectious Diseases Society of America. *MMWR Recomm.* 2009;58(RR-4):1–207

immunocompromised, susceptible hosts for the duration of the rash. If contact occurs inadvertently, risk of transmission is low. Therefore, administration of Varicella-Zoster Immune Globulin (VariZIG) or IGIV is not indicated. Also, when transmission has occurred, the virus has maintained its attenuated characteristics. In most instances, antiviral therapy is not necessary but can be initiated if illness occurs (see Varicella-Zoster Infections, p 774). Household contacts 6 months of age and older should receive influenza vaccine annually to prevent infection and subsequent transmission to the immunocompromised person. Limited data assessing risk of transmission of live attenuated influenza vaccine (LAIV) from healthy vaccine recipients to contacts indicate that this is a rare event. Trivalent inactivated influenza vaccine (TIV) or LAIV (for healthy people 2 through 49 years of age) is recommended for household members of immunosuppressed people. TIV should be used preferentially if the immunosuppressed person is a hematopoietic stem cell transplant (HSCT) recipient in a protected environment.

CORTICOSTEROIDS

Children who receive systemic corticosteroid therapy can become immunocompromised. The minimal amount of systemic corticosteroids and duration of administration sufficient to cause immunosuppression in an otherwise healthy child are not well defined. The frequency and route of administration of corticosteroids, the underlying disease, and concurrent therapies are additional factors affecting immunosuppression. Despite these uncertainties, sufficient experience exists to recommend empiric guidelines for administration of attenuated live-virus vaccines to previously healthy children receiving corticosteroid therapy. A dosage equivalent to ≥2 mg/kg per day of prednisone or equivalent to a total of ≥20 mg/day for children who weigh more than 10 kg, particularly when given for more than 14 days, is considered sufficient to raise concern about the safety of immunization with attenuated live-virus vaccines. Accordingly, guidelines for administration of attenuated live-virus vaccines to recipients of corticosteroids are as follows:

- **Topical therapy, local injections, or aerosol use of corticosteroids.** Application of low-potency topical corticosteroids to focal areas on the skin; administration by aerosolization in the respiratory tract; application on conjunctiva; or intraarticular, bursal, or tendon injections of corticosteroids usually do not result in immunosuppression that would contraindicate administration of attenuated live-virus vaccines. However, attenuated live-virus vaccines should not be administered if there is clinical or laboratory evidence of systemic immunosuppression until corticosteroid therapy has been discontinued for at least 1 month.
- **Physiologic maintenance doses of corticosteroids.** Children who are receiving only maintenance physiologic doses of corticosteroids can receive attenuated live-virus vaccines.
- **Low or moderate doses of systemic corticosteroids given daily or on alternate days.** Children receiving <2 mg/kg per day of prednisone or its equivalent, or <20 mg/day if they weigh more than 10 kg, can receive attenuated live-virus vaccines during corticosteroid treatment.
- **High doses of systemic corticosteroids given daily or on alternate days for fewer than 14 days.** Children receiving ≥2 mg/kg per day of prednisone or its equivalent, or ≥20 mg/day if they weigh more than 10 kg, can receive attenuated live-virus vaccines immediately after discontinuation of treatment. Some experts, however, would

delay immunization with attenuated live-virus vaccines until 2 weeks after corticosteroid therapy has been discontinued.

- **High doses of systemic corticosteroids given daily or on alternate days for 14 days or more.** Children receiving ≥2 mg/kg per day of prednisone or its equivalent, or ≥20 mg/day if they weigh more than 10 kg for 14 days or more, should not receive attenuated live-virus vaccines until corticosteroid therapy has been discontinued for at least 1 month.[1]
- **Children who have a disease (eg, systemic lupus erythematosus) that, in itself, is considered to suppress the immune response and/or are receiving immunosuppressant medication other than corticosteroids and who are receiving systemic or locally administered corticosteroids.** These children should not be given attenuated live-virus vaccines, except in special circumstances.

These guidelines are based on concerns about vaccine safety in recipients of high doses of corticosteroids. When deciding whether to administer attenuated live-virus vaccines, the potential benefits and risks of immunization for an individual patient and the specific circumstances should be considered.

The guidelines also are based on considerations of safety concerning attenuated live-virus vaccines and do not correlate necessarily with those for optimal protection. For example, some children receiving moderate doses of prednisone, such as 1.5 mg/kg per day for several weeks or longer, may have a less than optimal immune response to some vaccine antigens. In contrast, some children receiving relatively high doses of corticosteroids (eg, 30 mg/day of prednisone) may respond adequately to immunization. Immunization can be deferred temporarily until corticosteroids are discontinued if timely return for immunization is ensured. Otherwise, children should be immunized despite corticosteroid use to enhance the likelihood of protection in the case of exposure to disease.

BIOLOGIC RESPONSE MODIFIERS USED TO DECREASE INFLAMMATION

Biologic response modifiers, also known as cytokine inhibitors, are a novel class of drugs used to treat immune-mediated conditions, including juvenile idiopathic arthritis, rheumatoid arthritis, and inflammatory bowel disease. These drugs are antibodies to proinflammatory cytokines or proteins that target cytokine receptors. Their purpose is to block the action of cytokines involved in inflammation, resulting in inhibition of the normal inflammatory processes involved in the immune response. The immune-modulating effects can last for weeks after discontinuation. Tumor necrosis factor-alpha (TNF-α) inhibitors (adalimumab, certolizumab, etanercept, golimumab, infliximab) are the prototype agents, but newer biologic response modifiers in this class target other cytokines, such as interleukin-1 (anakinra), -6 (tocilizumab), -12, and -23, or the proteins that target cytokine receptors on lymphocytes. These agents often are used in combination with other immunosuppressive drugs, such as methotrexate or steroids.

Patients treated with biologic response modifiers are at risk of infections caused by *Mycobacterium tuberculosis*, molds and endemic fungi, *Legionella* species, *Listeria* species, and other intracellular pathogens as well as lymphomas and other cancers. Inhibition of this

---

[1] Centers for Disease Control and Prevention. General recommendations on immunization: recommendations of the Advisory Committee on Immunization Practices (ACIP). *MMWR Recomm Rep.* 2011;60(RR-2):1–64

inflammatory immune response potentially permits reactivation of infections that have been controlled previously and/or leads to an inadequate immune response to new pathogens requiring cell-mediated immunity. The Canadian Paediatric Society has developed guidelines on preventive strategies that should be considered in patients who will be or who are taking these immune-modifying agents (Table 1.17, p 84).[1] Adverse events related to use of these products should be reported to the FDA MedWatch Program (**www.fda. gov/Safety/MedWatch/default.htm**).

HEMATOPOIETIC STEM CELL TRANSPLANT RECIPIENTS

Patients for whom hematopoietic stem cell transplantation is planned should receive all routinely recommended vaccines that are not contraindicated because of immunosuppression. This recommendation includes varicella vaccine if the time interval to start of conditioning regimen is no less than 4 weeks. Many factors can affect immunity to vaccine-preventable diseases for a child recovering from successful hematopoietic stem cell transplantation.[2] These include the donor's immunity, type of transplantation (ie, autologous or allogeneic, blood or hematopoietic stem cell), interval since the transplantation, receipt of immunosuppressive medications, and presence of graft-versus-host disease (GVHD). Although many children who are hematopoietic stem cell transplant (HSCT) recipients acquire the immunity of the donor, some will lose serologic evidence of immunity. Retention of donor immune memory can be facilitated if recalled by antigenic stimulation soon after transplantation. Clinical studies of HSCT recipients indicate that administration of diphtheria and tetanus toxoids to the donor before harvest and immediate administration to the recipient after transplantation can facilitate response to these antigens; serum antibody titers did not increase when immunization of the recipient was delayed until 5 weeks after transplantation. In theory, these results could be expected with other inactivated vaccine antigens. However, immunization of the donor is often impractical and may be difficult ethically to justify immunization of a donor if given solely for the benefit of the HSCT recipient.

Three doses of diphtheria, tetanus toxoids, and acellular pertussis (DTaP) vaccine or 3 doses of tetanus and diphtheria toxoid-containing vaccine, including 2 doses of tetanus and diphtheria (TD) vaccine and 1 dose of adolescent tetanus toxoid, reduced diphtheria toxoid, and acellular pertussis (Tdap), should be administered starting at 6 months after hematopoietic stem cell transplantation for patients younger than 7 years and 7 years or older, respectively. People with tetanus-prone wounds sustained during the first year after transplantation should be given Tetanus Immune Globulin, regardless of their tetanus immunization status.

---

[1] Le Saux N; Canadian Paediatric Society, Infectious Diseases and Immunization Committee. *Paediatrics & Child Health.* Ottawa, Ontario: Canadian Paediatric Society; 2012:17(3):147–150

[2] Tomblyn M, Chiller T, Einsele H, et al; Center for International Blood and Marrow Transplant Research, National Marrow Donor Program, European Blood and Marrow Transplant Group, American Society of Blood and Marrow Transplantation, Canadian Blood and Marrow Transplant Group, Infectious Disease Society of America, Society for Healthcare Epidemiology of America, Association of Medical Microbiology and Infectious Diseases Canada, Centers for Disease Control and Prevention. Guidelines for preventing infectious complications among hematopoietic cell transplantation recipients: a global perspective. *Biol Blood Marrow Transplant.* 2009;15(10):1143–1238

Table 1.17. Recommendations for Patient Evaluation Prior to Initiation of Biologic Response Modifiers

- Tuberculin skin test and/or blood-based assay for tuberculosis (the latter if 5 years of age or older)

- Chest radiograph

- Document vaccination status and verify that all recommended inactivated vaccines for age are up-to-date, including yearly injectable influenza vaccine

- Document vaccination status and, if required, administer all live-virus vaccines a minimum 4 weeks before initiation of biologic response modifier therapy, unless contraindicated

- Counsel household members regarding risk of disease and ensure vaccination for prevention of exposure to varicella and influenza and other transmissible infections

- Depending on risk of past exposure, consider serologic testing for *Histoplasma* species, *Toxoplasma* species, and other intracellular pathogens

- Consider serologic testing for hepatitis B virus, varicella-zoster virus, and Epstein-Barr virus

- Counseling with respect to:
  - food safety (**www.cdc.gov/foodsafety**)
  - maintenance of dental hygiene
  - exposure to heavy concentrations of garden soil, pets, and other animals
  - high-risk activities (eg, excavation sites or spelunking and *Histoplasma capsulatum*)
  - travel to areas with endemic pathogenic fungi (eg, southwestern United States and *Coccidioides* species) or to areas where tuberculosis is endemic

Reprinted with permission from Le Saux N; Canadian Paediatric Society, Infectious Diseases and Immunization Committee. *Paediatrics & Child Health.* Ottawa, Ontario: Canadian Paediatric Society; 2012:17(3):147–150

HSCT recipients are at high risk of invasive pneumococcal disease. Studies have shown good immunogenicity after 3 doses of 13-valent pneumococcal conjugate vaccine (PCV13) starting 3 to 6 months after transplantation. At 12 months after hematopoietic stem cell transplantation in children 2 years of age or older, a dose of pneumococcal polysaccharide vaccine should be given to broaden the serotype coverage provided the patient does not have chronic GVHD. For patients with chronic GVHD, a fourth dose of PCV13 can be given at 12 months after transplantation (see Pneumococcal Infections, p 571). Three doses of conjugated *Haemophilus influenzae* type b (Hib) vaccine, 3 doses of hepatitis B vaccine, 3 doses of inactivated poliovirus vaccine, and 1 dose of conjugated meningococcal vaccine should be administered, starting 6 to 12 months after hematopoietic stem cell transplantation. Postimmunization serologic testing for antibody to hepatitis B surface antigen (HBsAg) may be considered following completion of the 3-dose hepatitis B series. Additional doses of vaccine (maximum of 3) may be given to vaccine nonresponders. For HSCT recipients who are seronegative to measles and without chronic GVHD or ongoing immunosuppression, 1 dose of MMR vaccine can be administered to adolescents and adults and 2 doses can be administered to children, at least 24 months after transplantation. Administration of varicella vaccine can be considered at least 24 months after hematopoietic stem cell transplantation in patients who are seronegative and without chronic GVHD or ongoing immunosuppression. Susceptible people who are exposed to measles should receive passive immunoprophylaxis (see Measles, p 489). Varicella vaccine is contraindicated for HSCT recipients less than 24 months after transplantation. Passive immunization with VariZIG or IGIV is recommended for susceptible people with known exposure to varicella (see Varicella-Zoster Infections, p 774).

Administration of inactivated influenza vaccine annually is recommended starting at 4 to 6 months after hematopoietic stem cell transplantation using an age-appropriate schedule. Even in patients in whom there is no serologic response, T-lymphocyte responses may be elicited that may prevent serious disease. If the vaccine is given during the 6 months after hematopoietic stem cell transplantation, a second dose can be administered 4 or more weeks later. During community outbreaks, HSCT recipients should be vaccinated against influenza immediately using inactivated vaccine if it has been more than 4 months since they underwent HSCT. Because the risk of influenza disease and its complications are substantial, inactivated influenza vaccine should be administered annually during early autumn (see Influenza, p 439) to people who underwent hematopoietic stem cell transplantation more than 6 months previously, even if the interval is less than 12 months. For children and adolescents for whom less than 6 months has elapsed after undergoing HSCT, influenza chemoprophylaxis should be considered (see Influenza, p 439). Live-attenuated influenza vaccine should not be administered to children and adolescents who have undergone HSCT.

Administration of a 2-dose hepatitis A vaccine series may be considered 12 months or longer after HSCT for people who have chronic liver disease or chronic GVHD, people traveling to areas with endemic disease, or people for whom immunity against hepatitis A is desired (see Hepatitis A, p 361). Household and health care contacts of HSCT recipients should have proven immunity to or be immunized against poliovirus, measles, mumps, rubella, varicella, influenza, and hepatitis A.

SOLID ORGAN TRANSPLANT RECIPIENTS

Children and adolescents being considered for solid organ transplantation should receive immunizations recommended for their age at least 2 weeks before the transplantation is performed. In general, vaccines will be more immunogenic before transplantation, because the medications given after transplantation to prevent and treat organ rejection adversely affect numbers and/or function of T and B lymphocytes. Live-virus vaccines should be given at least 1 month before transplantation and, in general, should not be given to patients receiving immunosuppressive medications after transplantation. MMR vaccine may be given before transplantation to patients as young as 6 months of age if transplantation is anticipated before 12 through 15 months of age. For transplantation candidates who are older than 12 months of age, if previously immunized, serum concentrations of antibody to measles, mumps, rubella, and varicella should be measured. Children who are susceptible should be immunized before transplantation.

Information about use of live-virus vaccines in patients after solid organ transplantation is limited. Some transplant centers have reported administration of live-virus vaccines (eg, MMR and varicella vaccines) in patients who are stable at least 6 months after transplantation, who are receiving minimal immunosuppressive agents, and who have not had recent episodes of organ rejection. No serious adverse reactions have been reported among these children, but too few children have been studied to recommend general use of live-virus vaccines in this population. MMR vaccine may be considered for susceptible solid organ transplant recipients in the event of an outbreak of measles, mumps, or rubella in the local community. Serum antibody concentrations for measles, mumps, rubella, and varicella should be measured in all patients 1 year or more after transplantation. Susceptible household and close contacts of a solid organ transplant recipient should receive MMR and varicella vaccines to reduce the risk of transmission of wild-type virus to the immunosuppressed child. OPV, which is not available in the United States, is contraindicated for transplant recipients and their household contacts. Inactivated poliovirus should be used for protection against poliovirus. Live-bacterial vaccines (eg, bacille Calmette-Guérin [BCG] and Ty21a *Salmonella typhi vaccines*) are contraindicated in patients receiving immunosuppressive medications after solid organ transplantation.

After solid organ transplantation, DTaP, Hib, hepatitis B, hepatitis A, inactivated influenza, and pneumococcal and meningococcal conjugate and polysaccharide vaccines can be administered, if indicated. Safety and immunogenicity data for these vaccines in children after transplantation are limited. Most experts recommend waiting at least 6 months after transplantation, when immune suppression is less intense, for resumption of immunization schedules. However, immunization schedules vary among transplant centers. Hepatitis A vaccine should be administered to patients undergoing liver transplantation because of increased disease severity associated with hepatitis A infection in patients with chronic liver disease. Annual influenza immunization with inactivated vaccine is indicated before and after solid organ transplantation. Live-attenuated influenza vaccine is contraindicated for solid organ transplant recipients because of immunosuppressive therapy. Solid organ transplant recipients at highest risk of infection with *S pneumoniae* appear to be those who have undergone cardiac transplantation or splenectomy. Pneumococcal conjugate and polysaccharide vaccine should be considered in all transplant recipients (see Pneumococcal Infections, p 571).

The decision to use passive immunization with an IG preparation (see Passive Immunization, p 56) should be made on the basis of serologic evidence of susceptibility and exposure to disease. Household and health care contacts of HSCT and solid organ transplant recipients should have immunity to or be immunized against poliovirus, measles, mumps, rubella, varicella, influenza, and hepatitis A.

HIV INFECTION (SEE ALSO HUMAN IMMUNODEFICIENCY VIRUS INFECTION, P 418)

Although data on use of currently available live-virus vaccines in HIV-infected children are limited, studies are available on safety and immunogenicity for many childhood vaccines. A vaccine schedule approved by the Advisory Committee on Immunization Practices (ACIP) of the CDC for HIV-exposed and infected children and adolescents is available and is similar to recommendations in the recommended immunization schedules for people 0 through 18 years of age.[1] Complications have been reported after BCG, measles, and varicella immunizations in severely immunocompromised HIV-infected children, including vaccine-related measles pneumonitis in a severely immunocompromised child 1 year after measles immunization. Because there have been reports of severe wild-type measles in symptomatic HIV-infected children, with fatalities in as many as 40% of cases, measles immunization (given as MMR vaccine) is recommended for HIV-infected

[1] Centers for Disease Control and Prevention. Guidelines for prevention and treatment of opportunistic infections among HIV-exposed and HIV-infected children. Recommendations from CDC, the National Institutes of Health, the HIV Medical Association of the Infectious Diseases Society of America, the Pediatric Infectious Diseases Society, and the American Academy of Pediatrics. *MMWR Recomm Rep.* 2009;58(RR-11):1–166

children with CD4+ T-lymphocyte percentages of 15% or greater. MMR vaccine should be given at 12 months of age to enhance the likelihood of an appropriate immune response. The second dose after the 12-month immunization can be administered as soon as 28 days later to induce seroconversion as early as possible. In a measles epidemic, MMR vaccine may be given to infants 6 months of age and older. Children immunized before their first birthday should be immunized with 2 additional doses of MMR vaccine (see Measles, Immunization During an Outbreak, p 495). Severely immunocompromised patients with HIV infection, as defined by age-specific low CD4+ T-lymphocyte counts or low percentage of total circulating lymphocytes, should not receive measles vaccine (see Human Immunodeficiency Virus Infection, p 418, and Table 3.27, p 427).

No safety or efficacy data are available to support administration of rotavirus vaccine to infants who potentially are immunocompromised, including infants who are HIV exposed or HIV infected. However, the following considerations support immunization of HIV-exposed or HIV-infected infants: (1) the HIV diagnosis may not be established in infants born to HIV-infected mothers before the age when the first rotavirus vaccine dose is due, and only 1.5% to 3% of HIV-exposed infants in the United States will acquire HIV infection; and (2) rotavirus vaccines are attenuated considerably and, therefore, are unlikely to pose the risk of increased shedding or serious disease.

Because children infected with HIV are at increased risk of morbidity from varicella and zoster compared with children not infected with HIV, after the potential risks and benefits are weighed, monovalent varicella vaccine (2 doses, 3 months apart) should be considered for HIV-infected children and adolescents with CD4+ T-lymphocyte percentages of 15% or more of the expected for age or 200 cells/mm^3 (see Varicella-Zoster Infections, p 774). Data are not available regarding safety, immunogenicity, or efficacy of MMRV vaccine in HIV-infected children; therefore, monovalent varicella vaccine should be used.

Children and adolescents with asymptomatic or symptomatic HIV infection should receive all inactivated vaccines, including DTaP, Tdap, IPV, hepatitis B, hepatitis A, Hib, and pneumococcal and meningococcal conjugate and/or polysaccharide vaccines, according to the recommended childhood and adolescent immunization schedule (see Fig 1.1–1.3, p 27–31). Annual inactivated influenza immunization of HIV-infected children 6 months of age or older and adolescents is recommended; LAIV is not licensed for use in this population (see Influenza, p 439). Household contacts of any child infected with HIV should receive LAIV or inactivated influenza vaccine annually. Immunization with pneumococcal conjugate and/or polysaccharide vaccine is indicated on the basis of age- and vaccine-specific recommendations (see Pneumococcal Infections, p 571).

In the United States, BCG vaccine is contraindicated for HIV-infected patients. In areas of the world with a high incidence of tuberculosis, the World Health Organization (WHO) recommends giving BCG vaccine to HIV-infected children who are asymptomatic.

Routine or widespread screening to detect HIV infection in asymptomatic children before routine immunizations is not recommended. Children without clinical manifestations of or known risk factors for HIV infection should be immunized in accordance with the recommended childhood and adolescent immunization schedule. For screening of newborn infants for HIV infection, see Human Immunodeficiency Virus Infection (p 418).

Because the ability of HIV-infected children to respond to vaccine antigens likely is related to the degree of immunosuppression at the time of immunization and may be inadequate, these children should be considered potentially susceptible to vaccine-preventable diseases, even after appropriate immunization, unless a recent serologic test demonstrates adequate antibody concentrations. Hence, passive immunoprophylaxis or chemoprophylaxis after exposure to these diseases should be considered, even if the child previously has received the recommended vaccines. Children with HIV infection given recommended vaccines when they had high HIV RNA concentrations and/or low CD4+ T-lymphocyte percentages (eg, before the diagnosis of HIV infection was made or before institution of therapy) may benefit from reimmunization after improvement of their immune status that may occur after institution of antiretroviral therapy.

Vaccine-strain varicella-zoster virus rarely has been transmitted from healthy people. Therefore, household contacts of HIV-infected people can be immunized with live-virus varicella vaccine (see Varicella-Zoster Infections, p 774). No precautions are needed after immunization of healthy children who do not develop a rash. Vaccine recipients who develop a rash should avoid direct contact with susceptible immunocompromised hosts for the duration of the rash. If the immunocompromised contact develops varicella caused by the vaccine strain, disease likely will be mild, and use of VariZIG, if available, or IGIV to prevent transmission is not indicated.

CHILDREN WITH ASPLENIA OR FUNCTIONAL ASPLENIA

The asplenic state results from the following: (1) surgical removal of the spleen (eg, after trauma, for treatment of hemolytic conditions); (2) certain diseases, such as sickle cell disease (functional asplenia); or (3) congenital asplenia or polysplenia. All infants, children, adolescents, and adults with asplenia, regardless of the reason for the asplenic state, have an increased risk of fulminant bacteremia, especially associated with encapsulated bacteria, which is associated with a high mortality rate. In comparison with immunocompetent children who have not undergone splenectomy, the incidence of and mortality rate from septicemia are increased in children who have had splenectomy after trauma and in children with sickle cell disease by as much as 350-fold, and the rate may be even higher in children who have had splenectomy for thalassemia. The risk of bacteremia is higher in younger children than in older children, and risk may be greater during the years immediately after splenectomy. Fulminant septicemia, however, has been reported in adults as long as 25 years after splenectomy.

Streptococcus pneumoniae is the most common pathogen that causes bacteremia in children with asplenia. Less common causes of bacteremia include *H influenzae* type b, *N meningitidis*, other streptococci, *Escherichia coli*, *Staphylococcus aureus*, and gram-negative bacilli, such as *Salmonella* species, *Klebsiella* species, and *Pseudomonas aeruginosa*. People with functional or anatomic asplenia also are at increased risk of fatal malaria and severe babesiosis.

Pneumococcal conjugate and polysaccharide vaccines are indicated for all children with asplenia at the recommended age (see Pneumococcal Infections, p 571). Following administration of appropriate number of doses of PCV13, pneumococcal polysaccharide vaccine (PPSV23) should be administered starting at 24 months of age. A second dose should be administered 5 years later (see Pneumococcal Infections, p 571). For children 2 through 5 years of age with a complete PCV7 series who have not received PCV13, a supplemental dose of PCV13 should be administered. For asplenic people

6 through 18 years of age who have not received a dose of PCV13, a supplemental dose of PCV13 should be considered. Hib immunization should be initiated at 2 months of age, as recommended for otherwise healthy young children (see Fig 1.1–1.3, p 27–31) and for all previously unimmunized children with asplenia.

Two primary doses of quadrivalent meningococcal conjugate vaccine should be administered 2 months apart to children with asplenia from 2 years of age through adolescence, and a booster dose should be administered every 5 years[1] (see Meningococcal Infections, p 500), although the efficacy of meningococcal vaccines in children with asplenia has not been established. No known contraindication exists to giving these vaccines at the same time as other required vaccines in separate syringes at different sites.

Daily antimicrobial prophylaxis against pneumococcal infections is recommended for many children with asplenia, regardless of immunization status. For infants with sickle cell anemia, oral penicillin prophylaxis against invasive pneumococcal disease should be initiated as soon as the diagnosis is established and preferably by 2 months of age. Although the efficacy of antimicrobial prophylaxis has been proven only in patients with sickle cell anemia, other children with asplenia at particularly high risk, such as children with malignant neoplasms or thalassemia, also should receive daily chemoprophylaxis. Less agreement exists about the need for prophylaxis for children who have had splenectomy after trauma. In general, antimicrobial prophylaxis (in addition to immunization) should be considered for all children with asplenia younger than 5 years of age and for at least 1 year after splenectomy.

The age at which chemoprophylaxis is discontinued often is an empiric decision. On the basis of a multicenter study, prophylactic penicillin can be discontinued at 5 years of age in children with sickle cell disease who are receiving regular medical attention and who have not had a severe pneumococcal infection or surgical splenectomy. The appropriate duration of prophylaxis for children with asplenia attributable to other causes is unknown. Some experts continue prophylaxis throughout childhood and into adulthood for particularly high-risk patients with asplenia.

For antimicrobial prophylaxis, oral penicillin V (125 mg, twice a day, for children younger than 5 years of age; and 250 mg, twice a day, for children 5 years of age and older) is recommended. Some experts recommend amoxicillin (20 mg/kg per day). For children with anaphylactic allergy to penicillin, erythromycin can be given (250 mg, twice daily). A substantial percentage of pneumococcal isolates have intermediate or high-level resistance to penicillin, resistance to macrolides and azalides, or both. Administration of pneumococcal conjugate vaccine reduces carriage of penicillin-nonsusceptible vaccine strains of pneumococci. Ongoing surveillance for resistant pneumococci is needed to determine whether changes to the recommended chemoprophylaxis will be required.

When antimicrobial prophylaxis is used, the limitations must be stressed to parents and patients, who should recognize that some bacteria capable of causing fulminant septicemia are not susceptible to the antimicrobial agents given for prophylaxis. Parents should be aware that all febrile illnesses potentially are serious in children with asplenia and that immediate medical attention should be sought, because the initial signs and symptoms of fulminant septicemia can be subtle. When bacteremia or septicemia is a

---

[1] Centers for Disease Control and Prevention. Recommendation of the Advisory Committee on Immunization Practices (ACIP) for use of quadrivalent meningococcal conjugate vaccine (MenACWY-D) among children aged 9 through 23 months at increased risk for invasive meningococcal disease. *MMWR Morb Mortal Wkly Rep.* 2011;60(40):1391–1392

possibility, health care professionals should obtain specimens for blood and other cultures as indicated; begin treatment immediately with an antimicrobial regimen effective against *S pneumoniae, H influenzae* type b, and *N meningitidis;* and consider hospitalizing the child. In some clinical situations, other antimicrobial agents, such as aminoglycosides, may be indicated. If a child with asplenia travels to or resides in an area where medical care is not accessible, an appropriate antimicrobial agent should be readily available, and the child's caregiver should be instructed in appropriate use.

Whenever possible, alternatives to splenectomy should be considered. Management options include postponement of splenectomy for as long as possible in people with congenital hemolytic anemia, preservation of accessory spleens, performance of partial splenectomy for benign tumors of the spleen, conservative (nonoperative) management of splenic trauma, or when feasible, repair rather than removal, and if possible, avoidance of splenectomy when immunodeficiency is present (eg, Wiskott-Aldrich syndrome). When surgical splenectomy is planned, immunization status for Hib, pneumococcus, and meningococcus should be ascertained, and needed vaccines should be administered at least 2 weeks before surgery, if possible. If splenectomy is emergent, administration of indicated vaccines is recommended 2 weeks after surgery.

Children With a Personal or Family History of Seizures

Infants and children with a personal or family history of seizures are at increased risk of having a seizure after receipt of diphtheria and tetanus toxoids and whole-cell pertussis (DTP) or combination measles-mumps-rubella-varicella (MMRV) vaccine or simultaneously administered influenza and 13-valent pneumococcal conjugate (PCV13) vaccines. Seizures following immunizations are brief, self-limited, and generalized and occur in conjunction with fever, indicating that such vaccine-associated seizures usually are febrile seizures. No evidence indicates that febrile seizures cause permanent brain damage or epilepsy, aggravate neurologic disorders, or affect the prognosis for children with underlying disorders. Universal use of diphtheria and tetanus toxoids and acellular pertussis (DTaP) has reduced greatly the incidence of febrile seizures associated with DTP immunization.

In the case of pertussis immunization during infancy, administration of DTaP could coincide with or hasten the recognition of a disorder associated with seizures, such as infantile spasms or severe myoclonic epilepsy of infancy, and cause confusion about the role of pertussis immunization. Hence, pertussis immunization in infants with a history of recent seizures should be deferred until a progressive neurologic disorder is excluded or the cause of the earlier seizure has been determined. In contrast, measles and varicella immunization is given at an age when the cause and nature of any seizures and related neurologic status are more likely to have been established. This difference provides the basis for the recommendation that measles immunization should not be deferred for children with a history of recent seizures.

A family history of a seizure disorder is not a contraindication to pertussis, measles, or varicella immunization or a reason to defer immunization. Children with a personal or family history of seizures generally should be given measles-mumps-rubella (MMR) and varicella vaccine as separate immunizations rather than MMRV for the first dose at 12 through 47 months of age[1] (see Measles, p 489). Postimmunization seizures in these children are uncommon, and if they occur, usually are febrile in origin, have a benign outcome, and are not likely to be confused with manifestations of a previously unrecognized neurologic disorder.

Children With Chronic Diseases

Chronic diseases may make children more susceptible to the severe manifestations and complications of common infections. Unless specifically contraindicated, immunizations recommended for healthy children should be given to children with chronic diseases. However, live-virus vaccines are contraindicated in children with severe immunologic disorders (see Immunocompromised Children, p 74). Children with human immunodeficiency virus (HIV) infection who are not severely immunocompromised may receive measles-mumps-rubella (MMR), varicella, and rotavirus vaccines. For children with conditions that may require organ transplantation or immunosuppression, administering recommended immunizations before the start of immunosuppressive therapy is important. Children with certain chronic diseases (eg, cardiorespiratory, allergic, hematologic, metabolic, and renal disorders; cystic fibrosis; and diabetes mellitus) are at increased risk of complications of influenza, varicella, and pneumococcal infection and should receive inactivated influenza vaccine, live-varicella vaccine, and pneumococcal conjugate or polysaccharide vaccine as recommended for age and immunization status and condition (see Influenza, p 439, Varicella-Zoster Infections, p 774, and Pneumococcal Infections, p 571). People with chronic liver disease are at risk of severe clinical manifestations of acute infection with hepatitis viruses and should receive hepatitis A and hepatitis B vaccines on a catch-up schedule if they have not received vaccines routinely (see Hepatitis A, p 361, and Hepatitis B, p 369). Siblings of children with chronic diseases and children in households of adults with chronic diseases should receive recommended vaccines (see Fig 1.1–1.3, p 27–31, and Immunocompromised Children, p 74).

Active Immunization After Exposure to Disease

Because not all susceptible people receive vaccines before exposure, active immunization may be considered for a person who has been exposed to a specific disease. The following situations are the most commonly encountered (see the disease-specific chapters in Section 3 for detailed recommendations).

- **Measles.** Live-virus measles vaccine given to susceptible (ie, lack of antibody or receipt of fewer than 2 doses of measles virus-containing vaccine after 12 months of age) immunocompetent children 12 months of age and older, adolescents, and adults within 72 hours of exposure will provide protection against measles in some cases (see Measles, p 489). Determining the time of exposure may be difficult, because measles can be spread from 4 days before to 4 days after onset of the rash.

Immune Globulin (IG), administered intramuscularly within 6 days of exposure, also can prevent or attenuate measles in an immunocompetent or immunocompromised susceptible person (see Measles, p 489). Because measles morbidity rate is high in children younger than 1 year of age, administration of IG is recommended for

---

[1] Centers for Disease Control and Prevention. Use of combination measles, mumps, rubella, and varicella vaccine: recommendations of the Advisory Committee on Immunization Practices (ACIP). *MMWR Recomm Rep.* 2010;59(RR-03):1–12

infants, immunocompromised people at any age, and pregnant women exposed to measles. Immunocompromised children who receive Immune Globulin Intravenous (IGIV) regularly are considered to be protected against measles.

- **Varicella.** Susceptible (ie, lack of antibody, lack of a reliable history of varicella, or receipt of fewer than 2 doses of varicella-virus containing vaccine after 12 months of age) immunocompetent children 12 months of age or older and household contacts exposed to a person with varicella disease should be given varicella vaccine within 72 hours of the appearance of the rash in the index case (see Varicella-Zoster Infections, p 774). Immunization is safe even in the event that the exposure results in clinical varicella disease. Susceptible immunocompromised children should receive passive immunoprophylaxis as soon as possible but within 10 days after contact with an infected person or acyclovir preemptively starting 7 days after exposure (see Varicella-Zoster Infections, p 774). Immunocompromised children who receive IGIV regularly are considered to be protected against varicella.

- **Hepatitis B.** Postexposure immunization is highly effective if combined with administration of Hepatitis B Immune Globulin (HBIG). Administration of HBIG does not inhibit active immunization from hepatitis B vaccine. For postexposure prophylaxis in a newborn infant whose mother is a carrier of hepatitis B surface antigen (HBsAg), administration of HBIG and hepatitis B immunization is essential. For percutaneous or mucosal exposure to hepatitis B virus, combined active and passive immunization is recommended for susceptible people (see Hepatitis B, p 369). People with continuing household or sexual contact with an HBsAg carrier also should be immunized.

- **Hepatitis A.** Availability of highly effective inactivated hepatitis A vaccines and results from a randomized, double-blind noninferiority clinical trial comparing the efficacy of hepatitis A vaccine and IG after exposure to hepatitis A virus led to a change in recommendations of postexposure prophylaxis (see Hepatitis A, p 361).[1]

  People who recently have been exposed to hepatitis A virus and who previously have not received hepatitis A vaccine (HAV) should receive a single dose of single-antigen HAV (or IG, 0.02 mL/kg, if not a vaccine candidate and exposure was within 2 weeks [see Hepatitis A, p 361]).

  - For healthy people 12 months through 40 years of age, single-antigen HAV at the age-appropriate dose is preferred.
  - For people older than 40 years of age, IG is preferred; vaccine can be used if IG cannot be obtained.
  - For infants younger than 12 months of age, immunocompromised people, people who have chronic liver disease, and people for whom vaccine is contraindicated, IG should be used.

- **Tetanus.** In wound management, cleaning and débriding all dirty wounds as soon as possible is essential. Unimmunized and incompletely immunized people or people who have not received a booster dose in the past 5 years should be given a tetanus toxoid-containing vaccine immediately. Some people may require Tetanus Immune Globulin in addition to immunization (see Table 3.73, p 709).

---

[1] Centers for Disease Control and Prevention. Update: prevention of hepatitis A after exposure to hepatitis A virus and in international travelers: updated recommendations of the Advisory Committee on Immunization Practices (ACIP). *MMWR Morb Mortal Wkly Rep.* 2007;56(41):1080–1084

- **Rabies.** Thorough local cleansing and débridement of the wound and postexposure active and passive immunization are essential aspects of immunoprophylaxis for rabies after proven or suspected exposure to rabid animals (see Rabies, p 600).
- **Mumps and Rubella.** Exposed susceptible people are not necessarily protected by postexposure administration of live-virus vaccine. However, a common practice for people exposed to mumps or rubella is to administer vaccine to presumed susceptible people so that permanent immunity will be afforded by immunization if mumps or rubella does not result from the current exposure. Administration of live-virus vaccine is recommended for adults born in the United States in 1957 or after who previously have not been immunized against or had mumps or rubella.

American Indian/Alaska Native Children

Compared with children from other racial groups, American Indian/Alaska Native (AI/AN) children historically have been at greater risk of acquiring certain vaccine-preventable diseases, such as hepatitis A, hepatitis B, *Haemophilus influenzae* type b, and *Streptococcus pneumoniae* infections, and for being hospitalized for respiratory syncytial virus infection and other lower respiratory tract infections. Mortality from pneumonia and influenza among AI/AN infants is 4 times higher than the rate reported for white people in the United States. The rate of diarrhea-associated hospitalizations is significantly higher in AI/AN infants than in other US infants. In addition, cervical cancer (now largely a vaccine-preventable disease) rates among AI/AN women are higher than rates among non-Hispanic white women.

High incidences of hepatitis A and hepatitis B infections also have been demonstrated among urban AI/AN children. During the past decade, childhood immunization for hepatitis B and targeted immunization for hepatitis A in the United States have eliminated disease disparities for these pathogens in most populations of AI/AN children, and significant decreases in disease have been demonstrated for *H influenzae* type b and *S pneumoniae*. Continued immunization is critical to maintaining this success. Disparities for some vaccine-preventable diseases, however, persist, likely related in part to adverse living conditions such as poverty, household crowding, poor indoor air quality, and absence of indoor plumbing. The historically high rates of infection and ongoing disparities highlight the importance of ensuring that recommendations for universal childhood immunization for hepatitis A and hepatitis B, *S pneumoniae*, human papillomaviruses (HPV), rotavirus, influenza, and *H influenzae* type b be implemented optimally in AI/AN children. Children in AI/AN communities should be targeted specifically to receive immunizations on time and to receive the full schedule of immunizations even in times of vaccine shortages. Specific vulnerabilities are noted here.

- **Respiratory Syncytial Virus.** The rates of hospitalization for respiratory syncytial virus (RSV) are much higher for AI/AN children in the Alaska and southwestern Indian Health Service regions (71 and 48 RSV hospitalizations per 1000 births, respectively) than for other US children (27 per 1000 births); data for other areas are lacking. AI/AN infants born before 35 weeks' gestation often have several risk factors for severe RSV disease. Additionally, one quarter of rural Alaska Native communities lack in-home running water and flush toilets, and this lack of availability of water service is associated with increased risk of hospitalization for lower respiratory tract infections. Use of RSV-specific monoclonal antibody prophylaxis (palivizumab), as recommended by the American Academy of Pediatrics (AAP), should be optimized among high-risk

AI/AN infants (see Respiratory Syncytial Virus, p 609). RSV season length may be prolonged in northern latitudes, including Alaska, and RSV prophylaxis should reflect local seasonality and risk factors in this population.

- **Haemophilus influenzae *type B*.** There are important differences in the currently available *H influenzae* type b (Hib) vaccine products that should be considered by physicians caring for AI/AN children. Before availability and public use of conjugated Hib vaccines, the incidence of invasive *H influenzae* type b disease was approximately 10 times higher for young AI/AN children than for non-AI/AN children. Because of the high risk of invasive *H influenzae* type b disease within the first 6 months of life in many AI/AN infant populations, the Indian Health Service and AAP recommend that the first dose of Hib conjugate vaccine contain polyribosylribitol phosphate-meningococcal outer membrane protein (PRP-OMP) as a single-antigen vaccine or in a combination vaccine with other antigens. The administration of a PRP-OMP–containing vaccine leads to more rapid seroconversion to protective concentrations of antibody compared with other Hib vaccines, and failure to use vaccine containing PRP-OMP has been associated with excess cases of Hib disease in Alaska Native infants. For subsequent doses, PRP-OMP or any of the other Hib conjugate vaccines can be used with apparently equal efficacy (see *Haemophilus influenzae* Infections, p 345), but if the second dose is a vaccine other than PRP-OMP, a third dose of Hib vaccine should be given approximately 2 months later. Availability of more than 1 Hib vaccine in a clinic has been shown to lead to errors in the vaccine administration. To avoid confusion for health care professionals who serve AI/AN children predominantly, it may be prudent to use only a PRP-OMP–containing Hib vaccine.
- **Streptococcus pneumoniae.** Recommendations for 13-valent pneumococcal conjugate vaccine (PCV13) for AI/AN children are the same as for other US children. However, in special situations, public health authorities may recommend use of pneumococcal polysaccharide vaccine (PPSV23) after PCV13 for AI/AN children 24 through 59 months of age who are living in areas where the risk of invasive pneumococcal disease (IPD) is increased. Prior to introduction of heptavalent pneumococcal conjugate vaccine (PCV7), the incidence of IPD in certain AI/AN children was 5 to 24 times higher than the incidence among other US children. Use of PCV7 in AI/AN infants resulted in decreased incidence of IPD. PCV13 was tested in AI/AN children, among others, in Phase III trials, and gives promise of further reducing IPD. However, AI/AN children continue to have a twofold increased risk of acquiring IPD compared with non-AI/AN children.
- **Hepatitis viruses.** Before the advent of immunization initiatives, rates of hepatitis A and hepatitis B in the AI/AN population greatly exceeded those of the general US population. Universal immunization reduced incidence of hepatitis A and hepatitis B to that of the general US population. Special efforts should be made to ensure catch-up hepatitis B immunization of previously unimmunized adolescents.
- **Influenza virus.** The disparity in influenza-related mortality rates in the AI/AN population compared with the general US population was confirmed during the 2009 H1N1 epidemic; the H1N1 death rate among AI/AN in 12 states (representing 50% of the AI/AN population in the United States) was 4 times higher than the H1N1 death rate of all other racial and ethnic populations combined. For this reason, the AI/AN population is listed among the groups at risk of medical complications from influenza; therefore, when vaccine supplies are limited, AI/AN people should be considered a

high-risk priority group. Maternal immunization can provide protection of young infants who are at high risk of influenza and complications.

Children in Residential Institutions

Children housed in institutions pose special problems for control of certain infectious diseases. Ensuring appropriate immunization is important because of the risk of transmission within the facility and because conditions that led to institutionalization can increase the risk of complications from the disease. All children entering a residential institution should have received recommended immunizations for their age (see Fig 1.1–1.3, p 27–31). If children have not been immunized appropriately, arrangements should be made to administer these immunizations as soon as possible. Staff members should be familiar with standard precautions and procedures for handling blood and body fluids that might be contaminated by blood. For residents who acquire potentially transmissible infectious agents while living in an institution, isolation precautions similar to those recommended for hospitalized patients should be followed (see Infection Control for Hospitalized Children, p 160). Specific diseases of concern include the following (see the disease-specific chapters in Section 3 for detailed recommendations).

- **Measles.** Epidemics can occur among susceptible children in institutional settings. Recommendations for managing children in an institutional setting when a case of measles is recognized are as follows: (1) within 72 hours of exposure, administer live-virus measles vaccine (as measles-mumps-rubella [MMR] vaccine) to all susceptible children 12 months of age or older for whom immunization is not contraindicated; (2) administer Immune Globulin (IG) to immunocompromised children (see Measles, p 489) as soon as possible; and (3) administer IG within 6 days of exposure to all exposed susceptible children younger than 1 year of age. Immunocompetent IG recipients also will require live-virus vaccine (as MMR vaccine) at 12 months of age or thereafter, depending on the age and dose of IG administration (see Table 1.9, p 38, for the appropriate interval between IG administration and MMR immunization).
- **Mumps.** Epidemics can occur among susceptible children in institutions. Hazards are disruption of activities, the need for acute nursing care in difficult settings, and occasional serious complications (eg, in susceptible adult staff).

  If mumps is introduced, prophylaxis is not available to limit the spread or to attenuate the disease in a susceptible person. IG is not effective, and Mumps Immune Globulin is not available. Although mumps virus vaccine may not be effective after exposure, MMR should be administered to people 12 months of age and older who lack documentation of immunity to protect against infection from future exposures.
- **Influenza.** Influenza can be unusually severe in a residential or custodial institutional setting. Rapid spread, intensive exposure, and underlying disease can result in a high risk of severe illness that may affect many residents simultaneously or in close sequence. Current measures for control of influenza in institutions include: (1) a program of annual influenza immunization of residents and staff; (2) appropriate use of chemo-prophylaxis during influenza epidemics; and (3) initiation of an appropriate infection-control policy (see Influenza, p 439).
- **Pertussis.** Because progressive neurologic disorders may have resulted in a deferral of pertussis immunization, many children in an institutional setting may not be immunized appropriately against pertussis. Children who are not immunized fully and who are younger than 7 years of age should be immunized with diphtheria and tetanus

toxoids and acellular pertussis (DTaP), and those 7 through 10 years of age should receive 1 dose of reduced diphtheria toxoid, and acellular pertussis (Tdap) vaccine. If pertussis is recognized, infected people and their close contacts should receive chemoprophylaxis (see Pertussis, p 553).

- **Hepatitis A.** Outbreaks of hepatitis A affecting residents and staff can occur in institutions for custodial care by fecal-oral transmission. Infection usually is mild or asymptomatic in young children but can be severe in adults. Hepatitis A vaccine may be indicated for postexposure prophylaxis (PEP) for staff and people 12 months through 40 years of age in institutions in which a hepatitis A outbreak is occurring. Hepatitis A vaccine is preferable to IG for PEP of contacts in this age range. Contacts under 12 months of age and people older than 40 years of age should receive IG if PEP is indicated (see Hepatitis A, p 361).

- **Hepatitis B.** Children with developmental disabilities living in residential institutions and their caregivers are assumed to be at increased risk of acquiring HBV infection. The high prevalence of markers of HBV infection among children living in these facilities indicates that HBV infections have the propensity for spread in an institutional setting, presumably by exposure to blood and body fluids containing HBV. Factors associated with high prevalence of HBV markers include crowding, high resident-to-staff ratios, and lack of in-service educational programs for staff. In the presence of such factors, the prevalence of HBV infection increases with the duration of time spent at the institution. Thus, susceptible residents entering or already residing and staff in institutions for children with developmental disabilities should be immunized against HBV; preimmunization serologic screening for HBV may not be cost-effective.

  After parenteral or sexual exposure to an institutionalized patient recognized to be an HBsAg carrier, contacts who are unimmunized and susceptible should receive active and passive immunoprophylaxis (see also Hepatitis B, p 369, for recommendations for previously immunized people).

- **Pneumococcal Infections.** Children 6 years of age or older with severe physical or mental disabilities, particularly children who are bedridden, who suffer from a compromised respiratory status, or who are capable of only limited physical activity, may benefit from pneumococcal conjugate or polysaccharide vaccine (see Pneumococcal Infections, p 571).

- **Varicella.** Because varicella is highly contagious, disease can occur in a large proportion of susceptible people in an institutional setting. All healthy people 12 months of age or older who lack a reliable history of varicella disease or immunization should be immunized (see Varicella-Zoster Infections, p 774). In addition, during a varicella outbreak, a dose of varicella vaccine is recommended for people who have not received 2 doses of varicella vaccine, provided that the appropriate interval has elapsed since the first dose (3 months for people 12 months through 12 years of age and at least 4 weeks for people 13 years of age and older). If varicella vaccine is administered to a child from 12 months through 12 years of age 28 days or more after the first dose, the second dose does not need to be repeated. Passive immunization during outbreaks currently is recommended only for immunocompromised, susceptible children at risk of serious complications or death from varicella (see Varicella-Zoster Infections, p 774).

- **Other Infections.** Other organisms causing diseases that spread in institutions and for which no immunizations are available include *Shigella* species, *Escherichia coli* O157:H7 and other Shiga toxin-producing *E coli, Clostridium difficile,* other enteric pathogens, *Streptococcus pyogenes, Staphylococcus aureus, Mycobacterium tuberculosis,* respiratory tract viruses other than influenza, cytomegalovirus, scabies, and lice.

US Children Living Outside the United States

In general, US children living outside the United States require the same immunizations as children living in the United States and may require additional vaccines related to regional pathogens. If delay in any immunization occurs for any reason, parents should be warned that the risk of contracting diseases in countries where immunization is not administered routinely is substantial. For children and adolescents living or traveling internationally, the risk of exposure to hepatitis A virus, hepatitis B virus, measles, pertussis, diphtheria, *Neisseria meningitidis,* poliovirus, yellow fever, Japanese encephalitis, and other organisms or infections may be increased and may necessitate additional immunizations (see International Travel, p 103). In these instances, the choice of immunizations will be dictated by the country of proposed residence, duration of residence abroad, expected itinerary, and age and health of the child. For information on the risk of specific diseases in different countries and preventive measures, see International Travel (p 103) or consult the CDC Web site (**wwwn.cdc.gov/travel/default.aspx**) or the WHO Web site (**www.who.int/ith/en/**). For children (especially children younger than 5 years of age) who will reside for a year or longer in countries with high rates of endemic tuberculosis, some experts recommend bacille Calmette Guérin (BCG) immunization. Other methods of preventing tuberculosis exposure and disease often are not practical or available. In many cases, it may be desirable for the child to receive the BCG vaccine as soon as possible after entering the foreign country.

Adolescent and College Populations

Adolescents and young adults may not be protected against all vaccine-preventable diseases. Lack of protection may occur in people who have escaped natural infection and who (1) were not immunized with all recommended vaccines and doses; (2) received appropriate vaccines but at too young an age (eg, measles vaccine before 12 months of age); (3) failed to respond to vaccines administered at appropriate ages; or (4) have waned immunity despite appropriate immunization.

The adolescent population presents many challenges with regard to immunization, including infrequent visits that adolescents have with health care professionals and lack of payer coverage of annual visits. As a result, many adolescents do not receive routine preventive care that provides an opportunity for immunization.

For many years, the adolescent immunization schedule was relatively simple, consisting of only routine administration of the tetanus-diphtheria booster. However, new vaccines have been added to the adolescent immunization schedule, and recommendations for other vaccines have been expanded. In January 2007, the childhood and adolescent immunization schedule was divided into 2 separate tables; 1 of the tables provides recommendations for people from 7 through 18 years of age (see Childhood and Adolescent Immunization Schedules, Fig 1.2, p 29–30). The adult immunization schedule includes people 19 years of age and older (**www.cdc.gov/vaccines/recs/schedules/adult-schedule.htm**). Recommended vaccines for adolescents can be grouped into 3 categories:

- Vaccines for routine administration:
  - ◆ Human papillomavirus (HPV; 3-dose primary series for females and males)
  - ◆ Meningococcal conjugate vaccine (1 primary dose and 1 booster dose)
  - ◆ Tetanus, diphtheria, and acellular pertussis (1 booster dose of Tdap)
  - ◆ Influenza (annual dose)
- Catch-up vaccines:
  - ◆ Hepatitis B
  - ◆ Inactivated poliovirus
  - ◆ Measles-mumps-rubella (MMR)
  - ◆ Varicella
- Vaccines based on individual activities or risk (see Recommended Immunization Schedules):
  - ◆ Hepatitis A
  - ◆ Pneumococcal vaccine

To ensure age-appropriate immunization, all children should have a routine appointment at 11 through 12 years of age for administration of appropriate vaccines and to provide other preventive health care services that are indicated.[1] During all adolescent visits, immunization status should be reviewed and deficiencies should be corrected. Specific indications for each of these vaccines are given in the respective disease-specific chapters in Section 3.

School immunization laws encourage "catch-up" programs for older adolescents. Accordingly, school and college health services should establish a system to ensure that all students are protected against vaccine-preventable diseases. Because outbreaks of vaccine-preventable diseases, including measles, mumps, and meningococcal disease, have occurred at colleges and universities, many colleges and universities are implementing the American College Health Association recommendations for prematriculation immunization requirements, mandating protection against measles, mumps, rubella, tetanus, diphtheria, poliovirus, varicella, and hepatitis B virus (**www.acha.org/topics/vaccine.cfm**). In addition, *Neisseria meningitidis* vaccine is required by some colleges and universities for people who have not been immunized previously. Information regarding state laws requiring prematriculation immunization is available at **www.immunize.org/laws.**

Because adolescents and young adults commonly travel internationally, their immunization status and travel plans should be reviewed 2 or more months before departure to allow time to administer any needed vaccines (see International Travel, p 103). Pediatricians should assist in providing information on benefits and risks of immunization to ensure that adolescents are immunized appropriately. Vaccine refusal should be documented after emphasis of the importance of immunization.

The possible occurrence of illness attributable to a vaccine-preventable disease in a school or college should be reported promptly to local health officials according to individual state guidelines (see Appendix VI, p 902).

---

[1] American Academy of Pediatrics, Committee on Practice and Ambulatory Medicine and Bright Futures Steering Committee. Recommendations for preventive pediatric health care. *Pediatrics.* 2007;120(6):1376 (Reaffirmed January 2011)

Health Care Personnel[1]

Adults whose occupations place them in contact with patients with contagious diseases are at increased risk of contracting vaccine-preventable diseases and, if infected, transmitting them to their patients. All health care personnel should protect themselves and susceptible patients by receiving appropriate immunizations. Physicians, health care facilities, and schools for health care professionals should play an active role in implementing policies to maximize immunization of health care personnel. Vaccine-preventable diseases of special concern to people involved in the health care of children are as follows (see the disease-specific chapters in Section 3 for further recommendations).

- *Rubella.* Transmission of rubella from health care personnel to pregnant women has been reported. Although the disease is mild in adults, the risk to a fetus necessitates documentation of rubella immunity in health care personnel of both sexes. People should be considered immune on the basis of a positive serologic test result for rubella antibody or documented proof of rubella immunization on or after the first birthday. A history of rubella disease is unreliable and should not be used in determining immune status. All people without evidence of immunity should be immunized with measles-mumps-rubella (MMR) vaccine before initial or continuing contact with patients.

- *Measles.* Because measles in health care personnel has contributed to spread of this disease during outbreaks, evidence of immunity to measles should be required for health care personnel. Proof of immunity is established by a positive serologic test result for measles antibody or documented receipt of 2 appropriately spaced doses of live virus-containing measles vaccine, the first of which is given on or after the first birthday. Health care personnel born before 1957 generally have been considered immune to measles. However, because measles cases have occurred in health care personnel in this age group, health care facilities should consider offering at least 1 dose of measles-containing vaccine to health care personnel who lack proof of immunity to measles. In communities with documented measles outbreaks, unless evidence of serologic immunity is demonstrated, 2 doses of MMR vaccine are recommended for unvaccinated health care professionals born before 1957.

- *Mumps.* Transmission of mumps in health care facilities can be disruptive and costly. All people who work in health care facilities should be immune to mumps. Proof of immunity is established by a positive serologic test result for mumps antibody or documented receipt of 2 appropriately spaced doses of live virus-containing mumps vaccine, the first of which is given on or after the first birthday. Adequate mumps immunization for health care professionals born during or after 1957 consists of 2 doses of MMR vaccine. Health care personnel with no history of mumps immunization and no other evidence of immunity should receive 2 doses (at a minimum interval of 28 days between doses) of MMR vaccine. Health care personnel who have received only 1 dose previously should receive a second dose. Because birth before 1957 is only presumptive evidence of immunity, health care facilities should consider recommending 1 dose of MMR vaccine for unimmunized health care personnel born before 1957

---

[1] Centers for Disease Control and Prevention. Immunization of health-care providers: recommendations of the Advisory Committee on Immunization Practices (ACIP) and the Hospital Infection Control Practices Advisory Committee (HICPAC). *MMWR Recomm Rep.* 2011;60(RR-7):1–45

who do not have a history of physician-diagnosed mumps or laboratory evidence of mumps immunity and should recommend 2 doses during an outbreak.[1]

- **Hepatitis B.** Vaccine is recommended for all health care personnel who are likely to be exposed to blood or blood-containing body fluids. The Occupational Safety and Health Administration of the US Department of Labor issued a regulation requiring employers of personnel at risk of occupational exposure to HBV to offer hepatitis B immunization to personnel at the employer's expense. Personnel who refuse recommended immunizations should sign a declination form.

  In some cases, susceptible health care personnel immunized appropriately with hepatitis B vaccines fail to develop serologic evidence of immunity—antibody to hepatitis B surface antigen (HBsAg [anti-HBs]). Serologic evidence of immunity is defined as serum anti-HBs concentration $\geq$10 mIU/mL. People who do not respond to the primary immunization series should complete a second 3-dose vaccine series with reevaluation of anti-HBs titers 1 to 2 months after the series is completed. People who do not respond to the second series and are HBsAg negative should be considered susceptible to HBV infection and will need to receive Hepatitis B Immune Globulin (HBIG) prophylaxis after any known or probable exposure to blood or body fluids infected with hepatitis B virus.[2]

- **Influenza.** Because health care professionals can transmit influenza to patients and because health care-associated outbreaks do occur, annual influenza immunization should be considered a patient safety responsibility and a mandatory requirement for employment in a health care facility unless an individual has a contraindication to immunization.[3] Health care professionals should be educated about the benefits of influenza immunization and the potential health consequences of influenza illness for themselves and their patients. Influenza vaccine should be offered at no cost annually to all eligible people and should be available to personnel on all shifts in a convenient manner and location, such as through use of mobile immunization carts. A signed declination form should be obtained from personnel who decline for reasons other than medical contraindications in any facility that does not have a formal mandatory vaccine policy. The utility of mandatory masking for unimmunized health care professionals is not clear.[4] Either inactivated vaccine or live-attenuated vaccine (according to age and health status limitations) is appropriate. Live-attenuated vaccine should not be used for personnel who will have direct contact with hematopoietic stem cell transplant recipients in the 7 days following vaccine administration.

- **Varicella.** Proof of varicella immunity is recommended for all health care professionals. In health care institutions, serologic screening of personnel who have an uncorroborated, negative, or uncertain history of varicella before immunization is likely to be cost-effective but need not be performed. All health care personnel without

---

[1] Centers for Disease Control and Prevention. Notice to readers: updated recommendations of the Advisory Committee on Immunization Practices (ACIP) for the control and elimination of mumps. *MMWR Morb Mortal Wkly Rep.* 2006;55(22):629–630

[2] Centers for Disease Control and Prevention. A comprehensive immunization strategy to eliminate transmission of hepatitis B virus infection in the US. Recommendations of the Advisory Committee on Immunization Practices (ACIP). Part II: immunization of adults. *MMWR Recomm Rep.* 2006;55(RR-16):1–25

[3] American Academy of Pediatrics, Committee on Infectious Diseases. Recommendation for mandatory influenza immunization of all health care personnel. *Pediatrics.* 2011;128(4):813–825

[4] See **www.cdc.gov/flu/professionals/vaccination/index.htm#ACIP.**

evidence of immunity to varicella should receive 2 doses of varicella vaccine. Evidence of immunity to varicella in health care professionals includes any of the following: (1) documentation of 2 doses of varicella vaccine at least 4 weeks apart; (2) history of varicella diagnosed or verified by a health care professionals (for a patient reporting a history of or presenting with an atypical case, a mild case, or both, health care professionals should seek either an epidemiologic link with a typical varicella case or evidence of laboratory confirmation, if it was performed at the time of acute disease); (3) history of herpes zoster diagnosed by a health care professional; or (4) laboratory evidence of immunity or laboratory confirmation of disease.

- **Pertussis.** Pertussis outbreaks involving adults occur in the community and the workplace. Health care professionals frequently are exposed to *Bordetella pertussis* and have substantial risk of illness and can be sources for spread of infection to patients, colleagues, their families, and the community. Health care professionals in hospitals or ambulatory-care settings of all ages should receive a single dose of tetanus toxoid, reduced diphtheria toxoid, and acellular pertussis (Tdap) vaccine as soon as is feasible if they previously have not received Tdap. Hospitals and ambulatory-care facilities should provide Tdap for health care personnel using approaches that maximize immunization rates.[1]

Refugees and Immigrants

Prevention of infectious diseases in refugee and immigrant children presents special challenges because of the diseases to which these children may have been exposed and the different immunization practices in their native countries. In addition, other aspects of providing care (including testing for exposure to environmental toxins, such as lead) to immigrant, refugee, and immigrant children should be considered.[2] In 1996, Congress amended the Immigration and Nationality Act (INA), requiring immigrant visa applicants to provide "proof of vaccination" with at least the first dose of vaccines recommended by the Advisory Committee on Immunization Practices (ACIP) of the Centers for Disease Control and Prevention (CDC) before entry into the United States. Although these regulations apply to most immigrant children entering the United States, internationally adopted children who are 10 years of age or younger from countries that are parties to the Hague Convention may obtain an exemption from these requirements. Adoptive parents are required to sign an affidavit indicating their intention to comply with the ACIP immunization requirements within 30 days or at the earliest medically appropriate time after the child's arrival in the United States.

Refugees are not required to meet immunization requirements of the INA at the time of initial entry into the United States but must show proof of immunization when they apply for permanent residency, typically 1 year after arrival. However, in outbreak settings, selected refugees bound for the United States are immunized in their country of origin before arrival in the United States. Clinicians should review the CDC Refugee Health Web site (**www.cdc.gov/ncidod/dq/refugee/index.htm**) for information about which refugee populations currently are receiving immunization outside the United

---

[1] Centers for Disease Control and Prevention. Immunization of health-care personnel: recommendations of the Advisory Committee on Immunization Practices (ACIP). *MMWR Recomm Rep.* 2011;60(RR-7):1–42

[2] American Academy of Pediatrics, Committee on Community Health Services. Providing care for immigrant, homeless, and migrant children. *Pediatrics.* 2005;115(4):1095–1100 (Reaffirmed January 2010)

States. Information about immunization requirements for immigrants is available at **www.cdc.gov/immigrantrefugeehealth/**.

Children who have resided in refugee processing camps for a few months often have had access to medical and treatment services, which may have included some immunizations. However, these children almost universally are immunized incompletely and often have no immunization records. For refugee children whose immunizations are not up-to-date, as documented by a written immunization record (see Immunizations Received Outside the United States, p 36), vaccines as recommended for their age should be administered (see Fig 1.1–1.3, p 27–31). For children without documentation of immunizations, a new vaccine schedule may be initiated. Alternatively, measurement of antibody concentrations to diphtheria, tetanus, hepatitis A, measles, mumps, rubella, varicella, and poliovirus (each serotype) as well as anti-HBs, HBsAg, and antibody to hepatitis B core antigen (anti-HBc), may be considered to determine whether the child needs additional immunizations or initiation of the immunization schedule appropriate for that child's age (see Table 2.17, p 199). Although many children will have received diphtheria and tetanus toxoids and whole-cell pertussis (DTP), poliovirus, measles, and hepatitis B vaccines, most will not have received *Haemophilus influenzae* type b (Hib), pneumococcal, hepatitis A, rubella, mumps, and varicella vaccines. Measles antibody may be measured to determine whether the child is immune; however, many children may need mumps and rubella vaccines, because these vaccines are not given routinely in developing countries. A clinical diagnosis of measles, mumps, rubella, or hepatitis A without serologic testing should not be accepted as evidence of immunity. Varicella vaccine is not administered in most countries, and history of varicella infection may be unavailable or unreliable in these populations; therefore, children should be immunized for varicella or have antibody testing performed.

All refugees and immigrants from areas with endemic hepatitis B infection, particularly Asia and Africa, should be screened for hepatitis B with serologic tests for HBsAg, anti-HBs, and anti-HBc. A child who has positive test results for HBsAg has active infection and may be defined as a chronic carrier if HBsAg persists for longer than 6 months. Most children who are HBsAg carriers are asymptomatic. Therefore, screening is important to identify children who need follow-up and management and to limit transmission of disease. Transmission risks should be minimal among children in the United States because of universal infant HBV immunization programs. However, unimmunized adult care providers should be given hepatitis B vaccine if they are susceptible and HBIG if they have had a significant exposure to blood of a carrier (see Hepatitis B, p 369). Serologic screening of all pregnant refugees and immigrants for HBsAg is imperative to identify women whose infants need passive as well as active immunoprophylaxis.

Tuberculosis and human immunodeficiency virus (HIV) infection are important public health concerns, because many refugees and immigrants come from countries with high prevalences of tuberculosis and HIV infection. Tuberculosis cases in foreign-born people now account for more than 50% of all tuberculosis cases in the United States. Although tuberculosis rates have decreased among children born in the United States in the last decade, rates remain high among children from developing countries. The overseas screening requirements for tuberculosis for immigrants and refugees bound for the United States underwent a major revision in 2007 and included tuberculosis screening for all people. Information about the screening and implementation is available at **www.cdc.gov/immigrantrefugeehealth/pdf/tuberculosis-ti-2009.pdf.** The risk of HIV infection among refugees and immigrants depends on the country of origin and on individual risk factors, especially among vulnerable refugee populations. As part of the required overseas medical assessment, HIV testing previously was performed on all immigrants and refugees 15 years of age and older. Children younger than 15 years of age were tested for HIV if history or examination raised concern about possible HIV infection (eg, maternal history of HIV infection, history of rape or sexual assault). As of January 2010, HIV testing no longer is required for immigration medical assessment. HIV testing still is recommended for people who are diagnosed with active tuberculosis as part of the overseas medical assessment. HIV testing after arrival in the United States is recommended for refugees 13 through 64 years of age and encouraged for refugees 12 years of age or younger and older than 64 years of age (**http://www.cdc.gov/ immigrantrefugeehealth/guidelines/domestic/screening-hiv-infection- domestic.html**). The decision to screen immigrant children for HIV after arrival in the United States should depend on history and risk factors (eg, receipt of blood products, maternal drug use), physical examination findings, and prevalence of HIV infection in the child's country of origin. If there is a suspicion of HIV infection, testing should be performed before administration of live vaccines.

International Travel

Up to 60% of children will become ill during international travel and up to 19% will require medical care. At particular risk are children of immigrants visiting friends and relatives abroad. Medical planning for travel requires 6 to 8 weeks at minimum. Yellow fever vaccine is only available at select clinics. Japanese encephalitis immunization requires 30 days to complete, and catch-up immunization for routine pediatric vaccines may take longer. Routinely recommended immunizations should be up-to-date before international travel; some routinely recommended immunizations should be given early or on an accelerated schedule. Parents should be made aware that there is increased risk for their children of exposure to vaccine-preventable diseases overseas, even in many countries in Europe. Additional vaccines to prevent yellow fever, meningococcal disease, typhoid fever, rabies, and Japanese encephalitis may be indicated depending on the destination and type of international travel (see Table 1.18, p 104). Travelers to tropical and subtropical areas often risk exposure to malaria, dengue, diarrhea, and skin diseases for which vaccines are not available. For travelers to areas with endemic malaria, antimalarial chemoprophylaxis and insect precautions vitally are important (see Malaria, p 483). Attention to hand hygiene, safer foods, insect vectors, and contaminated sand, soil, and water reduce travelers' risk of acquiring other communicable diseases.

Up-to-date information, including alerts about current disease outbreaks that may affect international travelers, is available on the Centers for Disease Control and Prevention (CDC) Travelers' Health Web site at **http://wwwnc.cdc.gov/travel/** or the World Health Organization (WHO) Web site at **www.who.int/ith/.** *Health Information for International Travel* (the "Yellow Book") is revised every 2 years by the CDC and is an excellent reference for travelers and for practitioners who advise international travelers of health risks. Travel information and recommendations can be obtained from the CDC (800-CDC-INFO). Local and state health departments and travel clinics also can provide updated information. Information about cruise ship sanitation inspection scores and reports can be found at **www.cdc.gov/nceh/vsp/default.htm.** In June 2007, federal agencies developed a public health Do Not Board (DNB) list, enabling

Table 1.18. Recommended Immunizations for Travelers to Developing Countries[a]

| | Length of Travel | | |
| | Brief, <2 wk | Intermediate, 2 wk through 3 mo | Long-term Residential, >3 mo |
Immunizations			
Review and complete age-appropriate childhood schedule (see text for details)	+	+	+
• DTaP, poliovirus, pneumococcal, meningococcal, *Haemophilus influenzae* type b, and hepatitis vaccines may be given at 4-wk intervals if necessary to complete the recommended schedule before departure			
• Measles: 2 additional doses given if younger than 12 mo of age at first dose			
• Varicella			
• Hepatitis A[b]			
• Hepatitis B[c]			
Yellow fever[d]	+	+	+
Typhoid fever[e]	±	+	+
Meningococcal disease[f]	±	±	±
Rabies[g]	±	+	+
Japanese encephalitis[h]	±	±	+

DTaP indicates diphtheria and tetanus toxoids and acellular pertussis; +, recommended; ±, consider.

[a] See disease-specific chapters in Section 3 for details. For further sources of information, see text.

[b] Indicated for travelers to areas with intermediate or high endemic rates of HAV infection.

[c] If insufficient time to complete 6-month primary series, accelerated series can be given (see text for details).

[d] For regions with endemic infection (see *Health Information for International Travel*, p 4, and Centers for Disease Control and Prevention. Yellow fever vaccine: recommendations of the Advisory Committee on Immunization Practices [ACIP]. *MMWR Recomm Rep.* 2010;59[RR-7]:1–27).

[e] Indicated for travelers to areas of poor sanitation.

[f] Recommended for regions of Africa with endemic infection and during local epidemics and required for travel to Saudi Arabia for the Hajj.

[g] Indicated for people with high risk of animal exposure (especially to dogs) and for travelers to countries with endemic infection.

[h] For regions with endemic infection (see *Health Information for International Travel*, p 4), and Centers for Disease Control and Prevention. Japanese encephalitis vaccines: recommendations of the Advisory Committee on Immunization Practices [ACIP]. *MMWR Recomm Rep.* 2010;59[RR-1]:1–26). For high-risk activities in areas experiencing outbreaks, vaccine is recommended, even for brief travel.

domestic and international public health officials to request that people with communicable diseases who meet specific criteria and pose a serious threat to the public be restricted from boarding commercial aircraft from or arriving in the United States.[1]

RECOMMENDED IMMUNIZATIONS

Transmission of pathogens prevented by the US schedule of childhood and adolescent immunization is more intense in other areas of the world, including some industrialized nations. Infants and children embarking on international travel should be up-to-date on receipt of immunizations recommended for their age. For travel to any developing

[1] Centers for Disease Control and Prevention. Federal air travel restrictions for public health purposes—United States, June 2007–May 2008. *MMWR Morb Mortal Wkly Rep.* 2008;57(37):1009–1012

country, immunization with hepatitis A virus (HAV) vaccine is recommended for any child or adolescent not immunized previously (see Hepatitis A, p 361). To optimize immunity before departure, vaccines may need to be given on an accelerated schedule (see Table 1.18, p 104).

POLIOVIRUS. Polio remains endemic in a few countries in Africa and Asia (an up-to-date listing of polio cases can be found at **www.polioeradication.org**). The Western Hemisphere was declared free of wild-type poliovirus in 1994, and the Western Pacific Region was declared free in 2000. The finding of vaccine-derived poliovirus in stool samples from several asymptomatic unimmunized people in a United States community raises concerns about the risk of transmission of polio within other communities with a low level of immunization.[1] To ensure protection, all children should be immunized fully against poliovirus. The Advisory Committee on Immunization Practices recommends the following[2] (see Poliovirus Infections, p 588):

• The 4-dose IPV series should be administered at 2 months, 4 months, 6 through 18 months, and 4 through 6 years of age.
• The final dose in the IPV series should be administered at 4 through 6 years of age, regardless of the number of previous doses.
• The minimum interval from dose 3 to dose 4 is 6 months.
• The minimum interval from dose 1 to dose 2, and from dose 2 to dose 3, is 4 weeks.
• The minimum age for dose 1 remains 6 weeks of age.

MEASLES. People traveling abroad should be immune to measles to provide personal protection and minimize importation of the infection. Importation of measles remains an important source for measles cases in the United States.[3] People should be considered susceptible to measles unless they have documentation of appropriate immunization, physician-diagnosed measles, laboratory evidence of immunity to measles, or were born in the United States before 1957. For people born in the United States in 1957 or after, 2 doses of measles vaccine, the first administered at or after 12 months of age, are required to ensure immunity (see Measles, p 489). Children who travel or live abroad should be vaccinated at an earlier age than recommended for children remaining in the United States. Before their departure from the United States, children 12 months of age and older should have received 2 doses of measles-mumps-rubella (MMR) vaccine separated by at least 28 days, with the first dose administered on or after the first birthday. Children 6 through 11 months of age should receive 1 dose of MMR vaccine before departure; 2 doses of MMR vaccine separated by at least 28 days will be required at 12 months or older to complete the required schedule.

HEPATITIS A. HAV vaccine is recommended routinely for all children at 12 through 23 months of age in the United States and should be considered for all ages traveling to areas with intermediate or high rates of HAV infection. These include all areas of the world except Australia, Canada, Japan, New Zealand, and Western Europe. Inactivated

---

[1] Centers for Disease Control and Prevention. Poliovirus infections in four unvaccinated children—Minnesota, August–October 2005. *MMWR Morb Mortal Wkly Rep.* 2005;54(41):1053–1055

[2] Centers for Disease Control and Prevention. Updated recommendations of the Advisory Committee on Immunization Practices (ACIP) regarding routine poliovirus vaccination. *MMWR Morb Mortal Wkly Rep.* 2009;58(30):829–830

[3] Centers for Disease Control and Prevention. Measles—United States, January–May 20, 2011. *MMWR Morb Mortal Wkly Rep.* 2011;60(20):666–668

vaccine is used for immunoprophylaxis for people 1 year of age and older. A combination HAV-hepatitis B virus (HBV) vaccine is available for people 18 years of age and older. For children younger than 1 year of age, Immune Globulin is indicated, because HAV vaccine is not licensed in the United States for use in this age group. Administration of IG may interfere with the immune response to varicella and MMR vaccines for up to 6 months (Table 1.9, p 38).

HEPATITIS B. HBV vaccine is recommended routinely for all children in the United States and should be considered for susceptible travelers of all ages visiting areas where hepatitis B infection is endemic, such as countries in Asia, Africa, and some parts of South America (see Hepatitis B, p 369). An accelerated dosing schedule is licensed for 1 hepatitis B vaccine (Engerix-B), during which the first 3 doses are given at 0, 1, and 2 months. In another accelerated schedule, doses are given on days 0, 7, and 14. This schedule may benefit travelers who have insufficient time to complete a standard schedule before departure. If the accelerated schedule is used, a fourth dose should be given at least 6 months after the third dose (see Hepatitis B, p 369). A combination HAV-HBV vaccine is available for people 18 years of age and older.

REQUIRED OR RECOMMENDED TRAVEL-RELATED IMMUNIZATIONS

Depending on the destination, planned activity, and length of stay, other immunizations may be required or recommended (see Table 1.18, p 104, **http://wwwnc.cdc.gov/ travel/** and disease-specific chapters in Section 3).

YELLOW FEVER. Yellow fever vaccine, a live-attenuated virus vaccine, is required by some countries as a condition of entry, including travelers arriving from regions with endemic infection.[1] The vaccine is available in the United States only in centers designated by state health departments. Current requirements and recommendations for yellow fever immunization on the basis of travel destination can be obtained from the CDC Travelers' Health Web site (**http://wwwnc.cdc.gov/travel/**). Yellow fever occurs year-round predominantly in rural areas of sub-Saharan Africa and South America; in recent years, outbreaks have been reported, including in some urban areas. Although rare, yellow fever continues to be reported among unimmunized travelers and may be fatal. Prevention measures against yellow fever should include protection against mosquito bites (see Prevention of Mosquitoborne Infections, p 209) and immunization. Yellow fever vaccine rarely has been found to be associated with a risk of viscerotropic disease (multiple-organ system failure) and neurotropic disease (postvaccinal encephalitis). There is increased risk of adverse events in people of any age with thymic dysfunction and people older than 60 years of age. Administration of YF vaccine is recommended for people 9 months of age and older who are traveling to or living in areas of South America and Africa in which risk exists for YF transmission. Because serious adverse events can follow YF vaccine administration, only people at risk of exposure to YF or who require proof of vaccination for country entry should be immunized. The contraindications and precautions should be followed (Table 1.19). Consultation with a travel medicine expert or the CDC Division of Vector-Borne Infectious Diseases (970-221-6400) or the Division of Global Migration and Quarantine (404-498-1600) to weigh risks and benefits is advised.

---

[1] Centers for Disease Control and Prevention. Yellow fever vaccine. Recommendations of the Advisory Committee on Immunization Practices. *MMWR Recomm Rep.* 2010;59(RR-07):1–27

Table 1.19. Contraindications and Precautions to Yellow Fever Vaccine Administration

Contraindications	Precautions
Allergy to vaccine component	Age 6 through 8 mo
Age less than 6 months	Age ≥60 y
Symptomatic HIV infection or CD4+ T-lymphocytes <200/mm^3 (or <15% of total in children <6 years of age)[a]	Asymptomatic HIV infection and CD4+ T-lymphocytes 200–499/mm^3 (or 15%–24% of total in children aged <6 y)
Thymus disorder associated with abnormal immune function	Pregnancy
	Breastfeeding
Primary immunodeficiencies	
Malignant neoplasms	
Transplantation	
Immunosuppressive and immunomodulatory therapies	

[a]Symptoms of HIV have been classified (Panel on Antiretroviral Guidelines for Adults and Adolescents. Guidelines for the use of antiretroviral agents in HIV-1-infected adults and adolescents; US Department of Health and Human Services; 2008. Available at: **http://aidsinfo.nih.gov/Guidelines/html/1/adult-and-adolescent-treatment-guidelines/0/** and Working Group on Antiretroviral Therapy and Medical Management of HIV-Infected Children. Guidelines for the Use of Antiretroviral Agents in Pediatric HIV Infection; 2009. Available at: **http://aidsinfo.nih.gov/ContentFiles/PediatricGuidelines.pdf**).

Whenever possible, immunization should be delayed until 9 months of age to minimize the risk of vaccine-associated encephalitis. People who cannot receive yellow fever vaccine because of contraindications should consider alternative itineraries or destinations.

CHOLERA. The whole-cell inactivated cholera vaccine no longer is produced in the United States. According to WHO regulations, no country may require cholera immunization as a condition for entry. However, despite WHO recommendations, some local authorities may require documentation of immunization. In such cases, a notation of vaccine contraindication should be sufficient to satisfy local requirements.

TYPHOID. Typhoid vaccine is recommended for travelers who may be exposed to contaminated food or water. Two typhoid vaccines are available for civilian use in the United States: an oral vaccine containing live-attenuated *Salmonella typhi* (Ty21a strain) and a parenteral Vi capsular polysaccharide (ViCPS) vaccine. Travelers should be reminded that typhoid immunization is not 100% effective, and typhoid fever still can occur; both vaccines protect 50% to 80% of recipients. For specific recommendations, see *Salmonella* Infections (p 635). Mefloquine or chloroquine may be administered simultaneously with oral Ty21a vaccine. The oral vaccine capsules should be refrigerated. Because the vaccine is not completely efficacious, typhoid immunization is not a substitute for careful selection of food and drink.

MENINGOCOCCUS. Quadrivalent meningococcal conjugate vaccines (MCV4) are licensed for use among people 9 months through 55 years of age traveling to areas where meningococcal disease is hyperendemic, such as sub-Saharan Africa, and countries with current meningococcal epidemics. Saudi Arabia requires a certificate of immunization for pilgrims to Mecca or Medina during the Hajj. Quadrivalent meningococcal polysaccharide vaccine (MPSV4) is recommended for travelers 56 years of age and older traveling to the same destinations. Revaccination with a conjugate vaccine is recommended after 3 years in children vaccinated with MPSV4 at ages 2 through 6 years and after 5 years if vaccinated at 7 years of age or older.

RABIES.[1] Rabies immunization should be considered for children who will be traveling to areas with endemic rabies where they may encounter wild or domestic animals (particularly dogs). The 3-dose preexposure series is given by intramuscular injection (see Rabies, p 600). In the event of a bite by a potentially rabid animal, all travelers (whether they have received preexposure rabies vaccine or not) should be counseled to clean the wound thoroughly with soap and water and then promptly receive postexposure prophylaxis (PEP). Prior receipt of preexposure vaccination avoids the need for Rabies Immune Globulin, which is critical to the success of PEP but often is not available or of equine origin in developing countries. Travelers who have completed a 3-dose preexposure series or have received the full postexposure prophylaxis series do not require routine boosters, except after a likely rabies exposure. Periodic serum testing for rabies virus neutralizing antibody is not necessary for routine international travelers.

JAPANESE ENCEPHALITIS.[2] Japanese encephalitis (JE) virus, a mosquitoborne flavivirus, is the most common cause of encephalitis in Asia. The overall incidence of JE reported among people from countries without endemic infection traveling to Asia is less than 1 case per million travelers. Short-term travelers whose visits are restricted to major urban areas are at minimal risk of JE, but risk varies on the basis of season, destination, duration, and activities. JE virus transmission occurs principally in rural agricultural areas, often associated with rice production. In temperate areas of Asia, JE cases usually peak in summer and fall. In the tropics, transmission varies with monsoon rains and irrigation practices, and cases may occur year-round. Short-term travelers should be encouraged to avoid high-risk areas or not to take their children to these high-risk areas. Expatriates and travelers staying for prolonged periods in rural areas with active JE virus transmission likely are at similar risk as the susceptible resident population (0.1 to 2 cases per 100 000 people per week). Two JE vaccines are licensed for use in the United States. An inactivated mouse brain-derived JE vaccine (JE-VAX [JE-MB]) was licensed since 1992 to prevent JE in people 1 year of age or older traveling to countries with endemic JE, but this vaccine no longer is available in the United States. In March 2009, an inactivated Vero cell culture-derived vaccine (IXIARO [JE-VC]) was licensed for use in people 17 years of age or older. For information on JE immunization of people younger than 18 years of age and prevention of arboviral diseases, see Arboviruses (p 232).

INFLUENZA. In addition to recommended annual influenza immunization, vaccine may be warranted at other times for international travelers, depending on the destination, duration of travel, risk of acquisition of disease (in part on the basis of the season of the year), and the travelers' underlying health status. Because the influenza season is different in the northern and southern hemispheres and epidemic strains may differ, the antigenic composition of influenza vaccines used in North America may be different from those used in the southern hemisphere, and timing of administration may vary (see Influenza, p 439).

[1] Centers for Disease Control and Prevention. Human rabies prevention—United States, 2008: recommendations of the Advisory Committee on Immunization Practices. *MMWR Recomm Rep.* 2008;57(RR-3):1–28

[2] Centers for Disease Control and Prevention. Japanese encephalitis vaccines: recommendations of the Advisory Committee on Immunization Practices (ACIP). *MMWR Recomm Rep.* 2010;59(RR-01):1–26

TUBERCULOSIS. The risk of acquiring latent tuberculosis infection (LTBI) during international travel depends on the activities of the traveler and the epidemiology of tuberculosis in the areas in which travel occurs. In general, the risk of acquiring LTBI during usual tourism activities appears to be low, and no pre- or post-travel testing is recommended routinely. When travelers live or work among the general population of a country with a high prevalence of tuberculosis, the risk may be appreciably higher. In most high-prevalence countries, contact investigation of tuberculosis cases is not performed, and treatment of LTBI is not available. Children returning to the United States who have signs or symptoms compatible with tuberculosis should be evaluated appropriately for tuberculosis disease. It may be prudent to perform a tuberculin skin test 8 to 12 weeks after return for children who spent 3 months or longer in a high-prevalence country. Pretravel administration of bacille Calmette-Guérin (BCG) vaccine generally is not recommended. However, some countries may require BCG vaccine for issuance of work and residency permits for expatriate workers and their families.

OTHER CONSIDERATIONS. In addition to vaccine-preventable diseases, travelers to the tropics will be exposed to other diseases, such as malaria, which can be life threatening. Prevention strategies for malaria are twofold: prevention of mosquito bites and use of antimalarial chemoprophylaxis. For recommendations on appropriate use of chemoprophylaxis, including recommendations for pregnant women, infants, and breastfeeding mothers, see Malaria (p 483). Prevention of mosquito bites will decrease the risk of malaria, dengue, chikungunya, and other mosquito-transmitted diseases (see Prevention of Mosquitoborne Infections, p 209).

Traveler's diarrhea affects up to 60% of travelers but may be mitigated by attention to foods and beverages ingested (including ice). Chemoprophylaxis generally is not recommended. Educating families about self-treatment, particularly oral rehydration, is critical. Packets of oral rehydration salts can be obtained before travel and are available in most pharmacies throughout the world, especially in developing countries where diarrheal diseases are most common. During international travel, families may want to carry an antimicrobial agent (eg, fluoroquinolone for people 16 years of age and older and azithromycin for younger children) for treatment of significant diarrheal symptoms. Antimotility agents may be considered for older children and adolescents (see *Escherichia coli* Diarrhea, p 324) but should not be used if diarrhea is bloody or for patients with diarrhea attributable to Shiga toxin-producing *Escherichia coli*, *Clostridium difficile*, or *Shigella* species.

Travelers should be aware of potential acquisition of respiratory tract viruses, including novel strains of influenza. They should be counseled on hand hygiene and avoidance of close contact with animals (dead or live). Swimming, water sports, and ecotourism around freshwater carry risks of acquisition of infections from environmental contamination. Pyogenic skin infections and cutaneous larva migrans are common. Travelers should avoid direct skin contact with sand, soil, and animals.

Recommendations for Care of Children in Special Circumstances

BIOLOGICAL TERRORISM

Some infectious agents have the potential to be used in acts of bioterrorism. The Centers for Disease Control and Prevention (CDC) previously designated 3 categories (Table 2.1, p 112) of biological agents to stratify the potential impact and risk to civilians and guide national public health bioterrorism preparedness and response.[1] The highest-priority agents for preparedness were designated **category A**, because they have a moderate to high potential for large-scale dissemination, cause high rates of mortality with potential for major public health effects, could cause public panic and social disruption, and require special action for public health preparedness. Organisms in category A cause anthrax, smallpox, plague, tularemia, botulism, and viral hemorrhagic fevers, including Ebola, Marburg, Lassa, Junin, and other related viruses. **Category B** agents are moderately easy to disseminate, cause moderate morbidity and low mortality rates, but still require enhanced diagnostic capacity and disease surveillance. Some examples of these agents include *Coxiella burnetii* (Q fever), *Brucella* species (brucellosis), *Burkholderia mallei* (glanders), *Burkholderia pseudomallei* (melioidosis), alphaviruses (Venezuelan equine, eastern equine, and western equine encephalitis), *Rickettsia prowazekii* (typhus), and toxins such as ricin toxin from *Ricinus communis* (castor beans) and *Staphylococcus* enterotoxin B. Additional category B agents that are foodborne or waterborne safety threats include, but are not limited to, *Salmonella* species, *Shigella dysenteriae*, *Escherichia coli* O157:H7, and *Vibrio cholerae*. **Category C** agents include emerging pathogens that could present a potential bioterrorism threat as scientific information about these organisms increases. Examples include Nipah virus, hantavirus, tickborne hemorrhagic fever viruses, and tickborne encephalitis viruses. The US Department of Homeland Security (DHS) now conducts biennial bioterrorism risk assessments for evaluation and prioritization of potential bioterrorism threats, as mandated by the Homeland Security Presidential Directive 10 (**http://www.fas.org/irp/offdocs/nspd/hspd-10.html**).

Children particularly may be vulnerable to a bioterrorist attack, because children have a more rapid respiratory rate, frequent hand-to-mouth behavior, increased skin permeability, higher ratio of skin surface area to mass, and less fluid reserve, compared with adults. Accurate and rapid diagnosis may be more difficult in children because of their inability to describe symptoms. In addition, adults on whom children depend for their health and safety may become ill or require quarantine during a bioterrorism event. Many preventive and therapeutic agents recommended for adults exposed or potentially exposed to agents of bioterrorism have not been studied in infants and children, and pediatric doses have not been established or approved by the US Food and Drug

---

[1] Rotz LD, Khan AS, Ostroff S, Hughes J, Lillibridge SR. Public health assessment and prioritization of potential biological terrorism agents. *Emerg Infect Dis.* 2002;8(2):225–230

Table 2.1. Bioterrorism Agents and Categories

Category A

Category A agents are high-priority agents that include organisms that pose a risk to national security because they:
1. Can be easily disseminated or transmitted from person to person;
2. Result in high mortality rates and have the potential for major public health impact;
3. Might cause public panic and social disruption; and
4. Require special action for public health preparedness.

Category A agents include:
1. Anthrax (*Bacillus anthracis*)
2. Botulism (*Clostridium botulinum* toxin)
3. Plague (*Yersinia pestis*)
4. Smallpox (variola major)
5. Tularemia (*Francisella tularensis*)
6. Viral hemorrhagic fever (filoviruses [eg, Ebola, Marburg] and arenaviruses [eg, Lassa, Machupo])

Category B

Category B agents are second highest priority agents and include agents that:
1. Are moderately easy to disseminate;
2. Result in moderate morbidity rates and low mortality rates; and
3. Require specific enhancements of the Centers for Disease Control and Prevention's diagnostic capacity and enhanced disease surveillance.

Category B agents include:
1. Brucellosis (*Brucella* species)
2. Epsilon toxin of *Clostridium perfringens*
3. Food safety threats (eg, *Salmonella* species, *Escherichia coli* O157:H7, *Shigella* species)
4. Glanders (*Burkholderia mallei*)
5. Melioidosis (*Burkholderia pseudomallei*)
6. Psittacosis (*Chlamydophila psittaci)*
7. Q fever (*Coxiella burnetii*)
8. Ricin toxin from *Ricinus communis* (castor beans)
9. Staphylococcal enterotoxin B
10. Typhus fever (*Rickettsia prowazekii*)
11. Viral encephalitis (alphavirus [eg, Venezuelan equine encephalitis, eastern equine encephalitis, western equine encephalitis])
12. Water safety threats (eg, *Vibrio cholerae, Cryptosporidium parvum*)

Category C

Category C agents are third highest priority agents, which include emerging pathogens that could be engineered for mass dissemination because of:
1. Their availability;
2. Their ease of production and dissemination; and
3. Their potential for high morbidity and mortality rates and major health impact.

Category C agents include emerging infectious diseases, such as Nipah virus and hantavirus.

Administration for use in children.[1] Children also may be at risk of unique adverse effects from preventive and therapeutic agents that are recommended for treating exposure to agents of bioterrorism. Further, availability of appropriate pediatric formulations of medical countermeasures may be limited. Parents, pediatricians, and other adults should be cognizant of the psychological responses of children to a disaster or terrorist incident to reduce the possibility of long-term psychological morbidity.[2]

Fever, malaise, headache, vomiting, and diarrhea are common early manifestations of illness caused by many bioterrorism agents and other infectious diseases. Some bioterrorism agents can cause typical distinctive signs and symptoms and incubation periods and require unique diagnostic tests, isolation, and recommended treatment and prophylaxis. Agents are discussed in Section 3 under specific pathogens, and extensive information and advice are available elsewhere. Table 2.2 (below) lists resources, including telephone numbers and Internet sites, where updated information concerning clinical recognition, prevention, diagnosis, and treatment of illness caused by potential agents of bioterrorism can be found.

Table 2.2. Emergency Contacts and Educational Resources

Health Department Information
- State Health Department Web sites: **www.cdc.gov/mmwr/international/relres.html**

Emergency Contacts
- Centers for Disease Control and Prevention (CDC) 24-Hour Emergency Operations Center: **770-488-7100**
- US Army Medical Research Institute of Infectious Disease (USAMRIID) Emergency Response Line: **888-872-7443**

Selected Web Information Resources
- American Academy of Pediatrics bioterrorism information: **www.aap.org/disasters/terrorism-biological.cfm and www.aap.org/disasters/index.cfm**
- CDC Emergency Preparedness and Response: **http://emergency.cdc.gov**
- Infectious Diseases Society of America: **www.idsociety.org/Bioterrorism_Agents/**
- American Society for Microbiology: **www.asm.org/asm/index.php/policy/biodefense-resources-center.html**
- US Department of Health and Human Services Public Health Emergency: **www.phe.gov/emergency/pages/default.aspx**
- University of Pittsburgh Medical Center, Center for Biosecurity: **www.upmc-biosecurity.org**
- USAMRIID: **www.usamriid.army.mil/**
- US Food and Drug Administration (FDA) Drug Preparedness: **www.fda.gov/Drugs/EmergencyPreparedness/BioterrorismandDrugPreparedness/default.htm**

---

[1] American Academy of Pediatrics, Committee on Environmental Health and Committee on Infectious Diseases. Chemical-biological terrorism and its impact on children. *Pediatrics.* 2006;118(3):1267–1278 (Reaffirmed January 2011)

[2] Hagan JF Jr; American Academy of Pediatrics, Committee on Psychosocial Aspects of Child and Family Health. Psychosocial implications of disaster or terrorism on children: a guide for the pediatrician. *Pediatrics.* 2005;116(3):787–795

Clinicians should be familiar with reporting requirements within their public health jurisdiction for these conditions. When clinicians suspect that illness is caused by an act of bioterrorism, they should contact their local public health authority immediately so that appropriate infection-control measures and outbreak investigations can begin. In the event of a bioterrorist attack, clinicians should review the CDC Emergency Preparedness and Response Web site (**http://emergency.cdc.gov**) for current information and specific prophylaxis and treatment guidelines. Public health authorities should be contacted before obtaining and submitting patient specimens for identification of suspected agents of bioterrorism.

Blood Safety: Reducing the Risk of Transfusion-Transmitted Infections

In the United States, risk of transmission of screened infectious agents through transfusion of blood components (Red Blood Cells, Platelets, and Plasma) and plasma derivatives (clotting factor concentrates, immune globulins, and protein-containing plasma volume expanders) is extremely low. Continued vigilance is crucial, however, because of risk from newly identified or emerging infections as well as lack of a uniform nationwide system for transfusion reaction surveillance. This chapter reviews blood and plasma collection procedures in the United States, factors that have contributed to enhancing the safety of the blood supply, some of the known and emerging infectious agents and related blood safety concerns, and approaches to decreasing the risk of transfusion-transmitted infections.

Blood Components and Plasma Derivatives

Blood collection, preparation, and testing are regulated by the US Food and Drug Administration (FDA). In the United States, Whole Blood is collected from volunteer donors and separated into **components,** including Red Blood Cells, Platelets, Plasma, and (rarely) Leukocytes, for further manufacturing; granulocytes and other white blood cells, although sometimes transfused, are not FDA-licensed products (although they generally are prepared in FDA-registered facilities). Platelets and, less commonly, Red Blood Cells and Plasma can be collected through apheresis, in which blood passes through a machine that separates blood components and returns uncollected components to the donor. Plasma for transfusion or further manufacturing into plasma derivatives can be prepared from Whole Blood or collected by apheresis. Most Plasma in the United States is obtained from paid donors at specialized collection centers. **Plasma derivatives** are prepared by pooling plasma from many donors and subjecting the plasma to a fractionation process that separates the desired proteins, including immune globulin and clotting factors.

From an infectious disease standpoint, plasma derivatives differ from blood components in several ways. For economic and therapeutic reasons, plasma from thousands of donors is pooled, and therefore, recipients of plasma derivatives have vastly greater donor exposure than do blood component recipients. However, plasma derivatives are able to withstand vigorous viral inactivation processes that would destroy Red Blood Cells and Platelets. Most recognized infectious organisms, with the notable exception of non–lipid-enveloped viruses and prions, have been shown to be inactivated easily by plasma processing methods. Development and evaluation of various novel strategies for inactivation of infectious agents are ongoing for cellular components.

Current Blood Safety Measures

The safety of the blood supply relies on multiple steps, including donor interview and selection, donor screening by serologic testing and use of nucleic acid amplification tests (NAATs) for markers of infection, deferral registries to avoid collection and use of unsuitable units, inventory quarantines and controls to prevent release of unsuitable or untested blood, investigation of errors and accidents followed by corrective action, inactivation procedures for plasma-derived products, and leukodepletion of certain blood components (see Tables 2.3, below, and 2.4, p 116). Blood donors are interviewed

Table 2.3. Blood Donor Screening Measures[a]

Measure	Targeted Infectious Agents
General interview and screening	Bloodborne phase of multiple agents
• Previous donor history (ie, no deferral in effect)	
• General health, current illness, temperature at time of donation	
• Donor confidential unit exclusion option[b]	
• Remember to notify blood collector of illness (eg, fever, diarrhea after donation, or any other pertinent information recalled)	
Specific risk factor history	
• High-risk sexual behaviors or injection drug use in donor or donor's partner(s)	HIV, HCV, HBV, HTLV
• Geographic risks (travel and residence)	Malaria, vCJD, leishmaniasis, Chagas disease, babesiosis (within the United States)
• History of specific infections	HIV, HBV, HCV, other hepatitis agents, parasites (those causing malaria, Chagas disease, babesiosis, and leishmaniasis)
• Previous parenteral exposure to blood via transfusion or occupational exposure; not lifetime deferral	HIV, HCV, HBV
Laboratory screening	HIV-1 (antibody and NAAT); HIV-2 (antibody); HCV (antibody and NAAT); HBV (HBsAg and anti-HBc; ALT sometimes is performed but not recommended by the FDA); HTLV-I and HTLV-II (antibodies); syphilis (antibodies); WNV (NAAT); screens for bacteria; *Trypanosoma cruzi* (antibody)

HIV indicates human immunodeficiency virus; HCV, hepatitis C virus; HBV, hepatitis B virus; HTLV, human T-lymphotropic virus; vCJD, variant Creutzfeldt-Jakob disease; NAAT, nucleic acid amplification test; HBsAg, hepatitis B surface antigen; anti-HBc, antibody to hepatitis B core antigen; ALT alanine transaminase; FDA, US Food and Drug Administration; WNV, West Nile virus.

[a] Screening of Source Plasma (paid) donors is similar but not identical. For example, because HTLV-I and HTLV-II are cell-associated agents, Plasma donations are not tested for anti-HTLV-I and anti-HTLV-II. Donors are tested for syphilis at least every 4 months.

[b] Donor is given the opportunity during the screening process to exclude himself or herself without disclosing the reason.

Table 2.4. Selected Known and Potential Transfusion-Transmitted Agents

Agents and Products	Transfusion-Transmitted	Pathogenic	Estimated per-Unit Risk of Contamination (US Studies, Except as Noted)[a]
Viruses for which all blood donors tested			
HIV	Yes	Yes	1 in 1 467 000
HCV	Yes	Yes	1 in 1 149 000
HBV	Yes	Yes	1 in 357 000 to 280 000
HTLV-I and HTLV-II	Yes	Yes	1 in 641 000
Other viruses			
CMV	Yes	Yes	Most donors harbor virus
Parvovirus B19	Yes	Yes	1 in 10 000
HAV	Yes	Yes	Less than 1 in 1 million contaminated per units transfused
TT virus	Yes	Unknown	1 in 10 (Japan), 1 in 50 (Scotland)
SEN virus	Yes	Unknown	Unknown
HHV-8	Probable	Yes	Unknown
Bacteria			
Red Blood Cells: *Yersinia enterocolitica* and other gram-negative bacteria	Yes	Yes	1 in 5 million units
Platelets: *Staphylococcus epidermidis,* *Bacillus* species, *Staphylococcus aureus,* *Salmonella* species, *Serratia* species	Yes	Yes	1 in 100 000 units
Parasites[b]			
Malaria *(Plasmodium falciparum)*	Yes	Yes	Varies widely depending on location
Chagas disease *(Trypanosoma cruzi)*	Yes	Yes	Unknown
Prion diseases (TSEs)			
CJD/vCJD	Yes	Yes	Unknown
Tickborne (in nature)			
Babesia species	Yes	Yes	Unknown
Rickettsia rickettsii	Yes	Yes	Unknown
Colorado tick fever virus	Yes	Yes	Unknown
Borrelia burgdorferi	Unknown	Yes	Unknown
Ehrlichia species	Unknown	Yes	Unknown
Mosquitoborne (in nature)			
West Nile virus	Yes	Yes	Variable (depends on epidemic year)

HIV indicates human immunodeficiency virus; HCV, hepatitis C virus; HBV, hepatitis B virus; HTLV, human T-lymphotropic virus; CMV, cytomegalovirus; HAV, hepatitis A virus; HHV, human herpesvirus; CJD, Creutzfeldt-Jakob disease; and vCJD, variant CJD. (TT and SEN viruses were named for the initials of patients from whom the viruses first were isolated.)

[a]Not all studies are performed by all blood centers.

[b]Other parasites that can be transmitted by transfusion include *Toxoplasma gondii* and leishmanial species.

to exclude people with a history of exposures or behaviors that increase the risk that their blood contains an infectious agent. All blood donations are tested routinely for syphilis, hepatitis B virus (HBV), hepatitis C virus (HCV), human T-lymphotropic virus (HTLV) types I and II, and human immunodeficiency virus (HIV) types 1 and 2; selected donations are tested for cytomegalovirus (CMV). Since July 2003, most donations are tested for West Nile virus. Since January 2007, most donations also have been tested for antibodies to *Trypanosoma cruzi*, the etiologic agent of Chagas disease, on an investigational basis. In December 2010, the FDA recommended steps to reduce the risk of transfusion-transmitted Chagas disease, including one-time testing of all donors of allogeneic units of blood using a licensed test for antibodies to *T cruzi*.

Transfusion-Transmitted Agents: Known Threats and Potential Pathogens

Any infectious agent that has an infectious blood phase potentially can be transmitted by blood transfusion. Factors that influence the risk of transmission by transfusion of an infectious agent and development of clinical disease in the recipient include the prevalence and incidence of the agent in donors, the duration of its hematogenous phase (particularly when asymptomatic), tolerance of the agent to processing and storage, the infectivity and pathogenicity of the agent, and the recipient's health status. Table 2.4 (p 116) lists major known transfusion-transmitted infections and some of the emerging agents under investigation.

VIRUSES

HIV (P 418), HCV (P 391), HBV (P 369). The probability of infection in recipients who are exposed to HIV, HCV, or HBV in transfused blood products is approximately 90%. Although blood donations are screened for these viruses, there is a very small residual risk of infection resulting almost exclusively from donations collected during the "window period" of infection—the period soon after infection during which a blood donor is infectious but screening results are negative.

To decrease the time period when donor HIV and HCV infection may be undetected, routine use of NAATs for blood and plasma donations was implemented beginning in 1999 in the United States and is performed on blood and plasma donations. At present, the NAAT for HBV is an optional donor screening test. Various estimates suggest that performing NAATs on pooled units can decrease the preantibody seroconversion window period from 22 days to 13 to 15 days for HIV and from 70 days to 10 to 29 days for HCV. Mathematical models have been developed to estimate the current very low risks of transfusion transmission of HIV, HCV, and HBV using currently accepted screening policies (Table 2.4, p 116).

HTLV-I AND HTLV-II. Infections with HTLV are relatively common in certain geographic areas of the world and in specific populations. For example, HTLV-I is more common in Japan, the Caribbean, and the southern United States, and HTLV-II is more common in indigenous people of North America, Central America, and South America and among injection drug users in the United States and Europe. HTLV-I and HTLV-II are transmitted by transfusion of cellular components of blood but not by plasma or plasma derivatives. The risk of HTLV transmission from screened blood donated during the window period has been estimated at 1 per 641 000 units screened. However, transmission of HTLV from an infected transfusion is less likely to lead to infection than is transmission of HIV, HBV, or HCV, with an approximate 27% seroconversion rate in people in the United States who receive nonleukocyte-reduced cellular blood components from infected donors.

CYTOMEGALOVIRUS (P 300). Immunocompromised people, including preterm infants and stem cell and solid organ transplant recipients, are at risk of severe, life-threatening illness from transfusion-transmitted CMV. Consequently, in many centers, only blood from donors who lack CMV antibodies is given to people in these categories. Leukoreduction decreases the risk of CMV transmission, because CMV resides in a latent phase within white blood cells.

PARVOVIRUS B19 (P 539). Blood donations generally are not screened for parvovirus B19, because previous infection with this virus is common in adults. Seroprevalence rates in adult blood donors range from 29% to 79%. Estimates of parvovirus B19 viremia in blood donors have ranged from 0 to 2.6 per 10 000 donors. Parvovirus, like CMV, usually does not cause severe disease in immunocompetent hosts but may be a threat to certain groups (eg, fetuses of nonimmune pregnant women; people with hemoglobinopathies, such as sickle cell disease and thalassemia; and immunocompromised patients). The risk of transmission of parvovirus B19 from Whole Blood donations is unknown but thought to be rare. However, pooled plasma derivatives commonly test positive for parvovirus B19 DNA, because parvovirus B19 lacks a lipid envelope and, therefore, is resistant to solvent/detergent treatment. To increase safety, manufacturers of plasma derivatives test plasma minipools for parvovirus DNA and exclude those containing parvovirus above a threshold concentration.

HEPATITIS A VIRUS (P 361). As with parvovirus, hepatitis A virus (HAV) lacks a lipid envelope and may survive solvent/detergent treatment. Infection with HAV leads to a relatively short period of viremia, and a chronic carrier state does not occur. Cases of transfusion-transmitted HAV infection have been reported but are rare. Clusters of HAV infections transmitted from clotting factor concentrates have occurred among people with hemophilia in Europe, South Africa, and the United States.

NON-A THROUGH -E HEPATITIS VIRUSES. A small proportion of people with post-transfusion hepatitis as well as community-acquired hepatitis will have negative test results for all known hepatitis agents. Several other viruses have been evaluated as possible etiologic agents. Although 3 of these viruses—hepatitis G virus/GB virus type C (strain variants of a member of the *Flaviviridae* family), TT virus, and SEN virus (the latter 2 of which were named for the patients from whom the viruses first were isolated in Japan)—can be found in blood donors and can be transmitted by transfusion, none of these viruses have been associated with post-transfusion hepatitis; hence, technically, they are not "hepatitis" viruses. No test has been licensed to screen donors for any of these viruses, and no data suggest that such tests would be beneficial.

HUMAN HERPESVIRUS 8 (P 416). Human herpesvirus 8 (HHV-8) is associated with Kaposi sarcoma, particularly in the setting of HIV infection and certain rare malignant neoplasms. The predominant modes of transmission are male-to-male sexual contact in the United States and close, nonsexual contact in Africa and Mediterranean Europe. Because HHV-8 DNA has been detected in peripheral blood mononuclear cells and serum specimens, there is concern that HHV-8 could be transmitted through blood and blood products. Serologic evidence from several US-based studies suggests that HHV-8 infection may have resulted from receipt of nonleukoreduced blood components as well as with injection drug use. More direct evidence for HHV-8 transmission by blood transfusion was provided by a case-controlled transfusion study in Uganda, where HHV-8 is endemic. However, HHV-8 seroprevalence rates are far lower in the United States than in areas with endemic infection (2%–5% versus 40%–60%, respectively), and transmission has not been shown in US studies with small numbers of recipients of blood from known HHV-8–seropositive donors. Among people with exposure to blood and blood products (eg, people with hemophilia), HHV-8 seroprevalence generally is comparable with that among healthy, HIV-seronegative people. Research on larger populations of recipients of blood or blood products from HHV-8–positive people will be needed to evaluate this risk.

WEST NILE VIRUS (P 792). West Nile virus (WNV) can be transmitted through blood transfusions. To reduce transfusion-associated transmission, blood collection agencies have implemented use of NAATs for WNV. Blood collection agencies primarily use an algorithm starting with minipools of donation samples. Donations constituting a reactive minipool are retested individually and, if results are positive, the reactive units are removed from the blood supply. If there is evidence of local epidemic WNV transmission, local blood collection agencies switch to individual donation testing to improve the sensitivity of finding blood donations containing WNV. Along with an overall decline in WNV incidence in recent years, these steps have reduced substantially but not eliminated the risk of WNV transmission via blood products. Cases of WNV disease in patients who have received blood transfusions within 28 days before illness onset should be reported promptly to the supplying blood center and the Centers for Disease Control and Prevention (CDC) through state and local public health authorities. Serum and tissue samples should be retained for later studies. In addition, cases of WNV disease diagnosed in people who have donated blood within 2 weeks before onset of illness should be reported promptly.

DENGUE VIRUSES (P 305). A case of transfusion-transmitted dengue hemorrhagic fever was recognized during a recent outbreak of dengue fever in Puerto Rico (and other transfusion-transmitted dengue cases in East Asia). Small outbreaks of dengue fever in Florida, Texas, and Hawaii resulted in no recognized transfusion transmissions. In 2009, an AABB Transfusion Transmitted Diseases Committee identified dengue viruses (4 types) as among the emerging pathogens that pose a major potential risk of transmission by transfusion. Currently, healthy blood donors recently returning to the continental United States from areas with endemic or epidemic dengue are not deferred, and no licensed tests to screen donors for dengue infection are available, although some blood establishments have implemented investigational donor screening and deferral programs; similar programs are under consideration nationally.

VIRUSES RELATED TO MURINE LEUKEMIA VIRUS. Several reports have suggested a possible causal relationship between viruses related to murine leukemia virus—particularly the exotropic murine retrovirus (XMRV)—and 2 common diseases: prostate cancer and chronic fatigue syndrome. Although the association is disputed and controversial, several national authorities outside the United States and some US blood organizations have recommended precautionary deferral of donors who report diagnoses of chronic fatigue syndrome.

BACTERIA

Although major advances in blood safety have been made, bacterial contamination of blood products remains an important cause of transfusion reaction. Bacterial contamination can occur during collection, processing, and transfusion of blood components.

Platelets are stored at room temperature, which can facilitate growth of contaminating bacteria. Bacterial contamination of blood products historically has been underestimated. The predominant bacterium that contaminates Platelets is *Staphylococcus epidermidis. Bacillus* species; more virulent organisms, such as *Staphylococcus aureus;* and various gram-negative bacteria, including *Salmonella* and *Serratia* species, also have been reported. Transfusion reactions attributable to contaminated Platelets potentially are underrecognized, because episodes of bacteremia with skin organisms are common in patients requiring Platelets, and the link to the transfusion may not be suspected.

On March 1, 2004, the AABB (formerly known as the American Association of Blood Banks) adopted a new standard that requires member blood banks and transfusion services to implement measures to detect and limit bacterial contamination of all Platelet components. As a result, most apheresis platelets are screened using liquid culture methods, whereas pooled platelets generally are screened using nonculture-based, less-sensitive methods. However, all widely used detection methods have been associated with failures. The American Red Cross has estimated that current culture methods may detect only 50% of bacterial contamination. Hospitals should ensure that protocols are in place to communicate results of bacterial contamination, both for quarantine of components from individual donors and for prompt treatment of any transfused recipients. Post-transfusion notification of appropriate personnel is required if cultures identify bacteria after product release or transfusion. If bacterial contamination of a component is suspected, the transfusion should be stopped immediately, the unit should be saved for further testing, and blood cultures should be obtained from the recipient. Bacterial isolates from cultures of the recipient and unit should be saved for further investigation. The AABB should be consulted for management algorithms (**www.aabb.org/**), and suspected bacterial transmission should be reported to public health authorities. In 2007, the FDA cleared for marketing a rapid test to screen for bacterial contamination of Platelets before transfusion (**www.fda.gov/NewsEvents/Newsroom/PressAnnouncements/2007/ucm108986.htm**).

Red Blood Cell units are much less likely than are Platelets to contain bacteria at the time of transfusion, because refrigeration kills or inhibits growth of many bacteria. However, certain bacteria, most notably gram-negative organisms such as *Yersinia enterocolitica,* may contaminate Red Blood Cells, because they survive cold storage. Cases of septic shock and death attributable to transfusion-transmitted *Y enterocolitica* and other gram-negative organisms have been documented.

Reported rates of transfusion-associated bacterial sepsis have varied widely depending on study methodology and microbial detection methods used. A prospective, voluntary multisite study (the Assessment of the Frequency of Blood Component Bacterial Contamination Associated with Transfusion Reaction [BaCon] Study) estimated the rate of transfusion-transmitted sepsis to be 1 in 100 000 units for single-donor and pooled Platelets and 1 in 5 million units for Red Blood Cells. Other studies that did not require matching bacterial cultures and/or molecular typing of both the component and the recipient's blood, as in the BaCon Study, or that included less severe recipient reactions in addition to sepsis have found higher rates of bacterial transmission.

PARASITES

Several parasitic agents have been reported to cause transfusion-transmitted infections, including malaria, Chagas disease, babesiosis, toxoplasmosis, and leishmaniasis. Increasing travel to and immigration from areas with endemic infection have led to a need for increased vigilance in the United States. Babesiosis and toxoplasmosis are endemic in the United States.

MALARIA (SEE P 483). The incidence of transfusion-associated malaria has decreased over the last 30 years in the United States. During the last decade, the rate has ranged from 0 to 0.18 cases per million units transfused—that is, no more than 1 to 2 cases per year. Most cases are attributed to infected donors who have immigrated to the United States rather than people born in the United States who traveled to areas with endemic infection. *Plasmodium falciparum* is the species most commonly transmitted. Prevention of transfusion-transmitted malaria relies on interviewing donors for risk factors related to residence in or travel to areas with endemic infection or previous treatment for malaria. Donation should be delayed until 3 years after either completing treatment of malaria or living in a country where malaria is found and 12 months after returning from a trip to an area where malaria is found. There is no licensed laboratory test to screen donated blood for malaria.

CHAGAS DISEASE (SEE AMERICAN TRYPANOSOMIASIS, P 734). The immigration of millions of people from areas with endemic *T cruzi* infection (parts of Central America, South America, and Mexico) and increased international travel have raised concern about the potential for transfusion-transmitted Chagas disease. To date, fewer than 10 cases of transfusion-transmitted Chagas disease have been reported in North America. However, studies of blood donors likely to have been born in or to have traveled to areas with endemic infection have found antibodies to *T cruzi* in as many as 0.5% of people tested. Although recognized transfusion transmissions of *T cruzi* in the United States have been rare, in some areas of the United States, the prevalence of Chagas disease estimated by detection of antibodies appears to have increased in recent years. In the absence of treatment, seropositive people can remain potential sources of infection by blood transfusion for decades after immigration from a region of the world with endemic disease. Screening for Chagas disease by donor history is not adequately sensitive or specific to identify infected donors. In December 2006, the FDA approved the first test to screen for antibodies to *T cruzi* (**www.fda.gov/NewsEvents/Newsroom/PressAnnouncements/2006/ucm108802.htm**); a second manufacturer's test was approved in 2010 (**www.fda.gov/NewsEvents/Newsroom/PressAnnouncements/2010/ucm210429.htm**). The American Red Cross and Blood Systems Inc began screening all blood donations in January 2008, and currently, most of the US blood supply is screened. In the first 16 months of screening, more than 14 million donations were tested, yielding a seroprevalence of 1:27 500; the highest rates were in Florida (1:3800) and California (1:8300). The AABB offered recommendations to member facilities regarding appropriate use of the Chagas disease screening test, and in March 2009, the FDA issued draft guidance for appropriate use of the test for all blood donations (**www.fda.gov/BiologicsBloodVaccines/GuidanceComplianceRegulatoryInformation/Guidances/Tissue/ucm125678.htm**). However, more recent discussions have suggested that donors only be screened a limited number of times, depending on their risk of continued exposure.

BABESIOSIS (P 244). Babesiosis is the most commonly reported transfusion-associated tickborne infection in the United States. More than 70 transfusion-associated cases have been documented; most were attributed to *Babesia microti,* but *Babesia duncani* (formerly the WA1-type *Babesia* parasite) also has been implicated. *Babesia* organisms are intracellular parasites that infect red blood cells. However, at least 4 cases have been associated with receipt of whole blood-derived Platelets, which often contain a small number of red blood cells. Although most infections are asymptomatic, *Babesia* infection can cause severe, life-threatening disease, particularly in the elderly and people without spleens. Severe infection can result in hemolytic anemia, thrombocytopenia, and renal failure. Surveys using indirect immunofluorescent antibody assays in areas of Connecticut and New York with highly endemic infection have revealed seropositivity rates for *B microti of* approximately 1% and 4%, respectively. In a study of blood donors in Connecticut, 19 (56%) of 34 seropositive donors had positive results for nucleic acid, as determined by PCR assay.

No licensed test is available to screen donors for evidence of *Babesia* infection. Donors with a history of babesiosis are deferred indefinitely from donating blood. Although people with acute illness or fever are not suitable to donate blood, people infected with *Babesia* species commonly are asymptomatic or experience only mild and nonspecific symptoms. In addition, *Babesia* species can cause asymptomatic infection for months and even years in untreated, otherwise healthy people. Questioning donors about recent tick bites has been shown to be ineffective, in part because donors who are seropositive for antibody to tickborne agents are no more likely than seronegative donors to recall tick bites. In 2009, an AABB Transfusion Transmitted Diseases Committee identified *Babesia* species as emerging pathogens posing a major potential risk of transmission by transfusion.

TRANSMISSIBLE SPONGIFORM ENCEPHALOPATHIES: PRION DISEASE

CREUTZFELDT-JAKOB DISEASE, AND VARIANT CREUTZFELDT-JAKOB DISEASE (P 595).

Creutzfeldt-Jakob disease (CJD) and variant CJD (vCJD) are fatal neurologic illnesses caused by unique infectious agents known as prions (see Transmissible Spongiform Encephalopathies, p 595).

SPORADIC CJD. The risk of transmitting most forms of CJD through blood has been considered theoretical. No cases of CJD resulting from receipt of blood transfusion from donors who later developed sporadic, familial, or iatrogenic forms of CJD have been documented, and case-control studies have not found an association between receipt of blood and development of CJD.

Nevertheless, because blood of animals with a number of naturally acquired and experimental transmissible spongiform encephalopathies (TSEs) may be infective, concerns have remained about the theoretical risk of transmitting CJD by blood transfusion. Since 1987, the FDA has recommended that certain people at increased risk of having CJD be deferred as blood donors. Concern increased after 4 reports of transfusion-transmitted vCJD (see below) infection and one infection attributed to injections of plasma-derived coagulation factor VIII. People with signs of sporadic CJD or who are at increased risk of iatrogenic or inherited forms of CJD (eg, receipt of pituitary-derived growth hormone or dura mater transplant or family history of CJD unless TSE-associated mutation is ruled out) should be deferred as donors. In addition, if postdonation information reveals that a donor should have been rejected because of increased CJD risk, in-date Whole Blood and components, including unpooled Plasma remaining from previous donations, should be retrieved and discarded; if those units already have been distributed, a biological product deviation report should be submitted to the FDA by the blood establishment. However, since 1998, withdrawal of plasma derivatives no longer has been recommended in such a situation, because epidemiologic and laboratory data suggest that most plasma derivatives are much less likely to transmit TSE agents than are blood components, because Plasma undergoes extensive processing during fractionation. The FDA continues to recommend retrieval of derivatives from any Plasma pool to which a person subsequently diagnosed with vCJD donated—something that has not occurred in the United States—and case-by-case decision, in consultation with CDC, when a person younger than 55 years of age with a diagnosis of any other form of CJD is subsequently reported to have donated to a Plasma pool.

VARIANT CJD. In 1996, cases of a new clinically and histopathologically distinct variant form of CJD (vCJD) first were reported in the United Kingdom. There is now scientific evidence that the agent responsible for the outbreak of prion disease in cows, bovine spongiform encephalopathy (BSE), is the same agent responsible for the outbreak of vCJD in humans. BSE in cattle first was recognized in the United Kingdom in 1986 and later in 24 other countries.

Transmission of vCJD infections to 4 elderly people in the United Kingdom has been attributed presumptively to transfusions received years earlier with nonleukoreduced Red Blood Cells from healthy donors who became ill with vCJD 16 months to 3.5 years after the donations. Three of the recipients had typical vCJD, and a fourth had evidence of preclinical or subclinical infection. The asymptomatic incubation periods in the clinically ill recipients lasted from 6.3 to 8.5 years; the patient with evidence of preclinical infection died of an unrelated illness approximately 5 years after receiving the implicated transfusion. Recipients of blood components from other donors later diagnosed with vCJD remain under surveillance in the United Kingdom and France. The magnitude of the risk of acquiring vCJD from transfusion is uncertain. To date, one case of vCJD presumptively has been attributed to treatment with a plasma derivative. However, one 73-year-old United Kingdom resident with hemophilia who died without neurologic symptoms had evidence of a vCJD infection in his spleen at autopsy; his infection was attributed to receipt of plasma products from the United Kingdom.

In the United States, the following categories of potential blood and plasma donors are deferred as donors: people who received a blood or blood component transfusion in the United Kingdom or in France after January 1, 1980, when the BSE epidemic is believed to have begun; people who have lived in the United Kingdom for any combined period of 3 months or more from the beginning of 1980 until the end of 1996 (after which rigorous food-protection measures were implemented fully throughout the United Kingdom); people who spent a total of 5 years or more in most other European countries (excluding countries of the former Soviet Union) from 1980 to the present; people injected with bovine insulin, unless it is confirmed that the insulin was not manufactured from cattle in the United Kingdom; and military personnel, civilian employees, and dependents who resided or worked on US military bases from 1980 through the end of 1990 in northern Europe or the end of 1996 in southern Europe (as defined by the US Department of Defense). Policies regarding CJD donor deferral may change, and blood and Plasma programs are expected to remain informed about such changes, which are announced promptly by trade organizations and the FDA. In 2009, an AABB Transfusion Transmitted Diseases Committee identified the vCJD agent as emerging pathogen posing a major potential risk of transmission by transfusion.

Improving Blood Safety

A number of strategies have been proposed or implemented to further decrease the risk of transmission of infectious agents through blood and blood products. Various safety strategies are as follows.

ELIMINATION OF INFECTIOUS AGENTS

AGENT INACTIVATION. Virtually all Plasma derivatives, including Immune Globulin Intravenous (IGIV) and clotting factors, are treated to eliminate infectious agents that may be present despite screening measures. Methods used for this include wet and dry heat and treatment with a solvent/detergent. Solvent/detergent-treated pooled Plasma for transfusion no longer is marketed in the United States, but methods of treating single-donor Plasma are under study. Solvent/detergent treatment dissolves the lipid envelope of HIV, HBV, and HCV but is not effective against non–lipid-enveloped viruses, such as HAV and parvovirus B19. Transmission of HIV through administration of IGIV never has been documented.

Because of the fragility of Red Blood Cells and Platelets, pathogen inactivation is more difficult. However, several methods have been developed, such as addition of psoralens followed by exposure to ultraviolet A, which binds nucleic acids and blocks replication of bacteria and viruses. Clinical trials of these treated components are underway.

AGENT REMOVAL. Leukoreduction, in which filters are used to remove donor white blood cells, is performed increasingly in the United States. Benefits of this process include decreasing febrile transfusion reactions related to white blood cells and their products and decreasing the immune modulation associated with transfusion. Leukoreduction also decreases cell-associated agents (eg, intracellular viruses, such as CMV, Epstein-Barr virus, HHV-8, and HTLV). Several countries have adopted this practice.

DECREASING EXPOSURE TO BLOOD PRODUCTS

Current screening policies have decreased the risk of transfusion associated infections dramatically, but blood products remain a source of known and potentially unknown infectious agents.

ALTERNATIVES TO HUMAN BLOOD PRODUCTS. Many alternatives to human blood products have been developed. Established alternatives include recombinant clotting factors for patients with hemophilia and factors such as erythropoietin used to stimulate red blood cell production. Physicians should use the lowest erythropoiesis-stimulating agent (ESA) dose that will increase the hemoglobin level gradually to a concentration not exceeding 12 g/dL. Increased risks of death and serious cardiovascular and thrombotic events have been described when ESAs were administered to achieve a target hemoglobin concentration greater than 12 g/dL in people with chronic kidney failure and surgical candidates. These adverse safety outcomes and shortened time to tumor progression have been observed in certain patients with cancer who have chemotherapy-related anemia, such as people with advanced head and neck cancer receiving radiation therapy and metastatic breast cancer.

Other agents currently in clinical trials include hemoglobin-based oxygen carriers, Red Blood Cell substitutes, such as human hemoglobin extracted from Red Blood Cells, recombinant human hemoglobin, animal hemoglobin, and various oxygen-carrying chemicals.

AUTOLOGOUS TRANSFUSION. Another means of decreasing recipient exposure is autologous transfusion. Blood may be donated by the patient several weeks before a surgical procedure (preoperative autologous donation) or, alternatively, donated immediately before surgery and replaced with a volume expander (acute normovolemic hemodilution). In either case, the patient's blood can be reinfused if needed. Autologous blood is not completely risk free, because bacterial contamination may occur.

Blood-recycling techniques (autotransfusion) also are in this category. During surgery, blood lost by the patient may be collected, processed, and reinfused into the patient.

SURVEILLANCE FOR TRANSFUSION-TRANSMITTED INFECTION

Transfusion-transmitted infection surveillance is crucial and must be coupled with the capacity to investigate reported cases rapidly and to implement measures needed to prevent additional infections. The CDC has developed a Hemovigilance Module in the National Healthcare Safety Network for transfusion-related adverse events, including patient transfusion reactions and quality-control incidents (eg, errors and accidents). The National Healthcare Safety Network is a secure Internet-based surveillance system that collects data from voluntary participating health care facilities in the United States. The CDC also has had a blood safety monitoring system since 1998, the Universal Data Collection Program, for recipients of processed plasma factors. The program provides annual testing for hepatitis and HIV and stores blood specimens in a serum bank for use in blood safety investigations. A similar system has been established in several centers in the United States that treat patients with thalassemia who depend on frequent blood transfusions. For regulatory purposes, serious adverse reactions and product problems should be reported to the manufacturer (or, alternatively, to the supplier for transmission to the manufacturer). Health care professionals also may report such information directly to the FDA through MedWatch. Reports can be made by telephone (1-800-FDA-1088), fax (1-800-FDA-0178), Internet (**www.fda.gov/medwatch/report/hcp.htm**), or mail (see MedWatch, p 869). Voluntary reporting is considered vital for monitoring product safety.

ORGAN AND TISSUE TRANSPLANTATION

Each year, more than 25 000 organs and 2 000 000 tissues are distributed for transplantations (eg, musculoskeletal allografts, cornea, and skin), and numerous cell therapy infusions (eg, bone marrow and peripheral stem cell transplants) occur each year in the United States. The proliferation of these products also has increased the opportunities for transmission of infectious pathogens, including bacteria, viruses, and parasites. Transmission of Chagas disease, *Strongyloides* species, *Mycobacterium tuberculosis*, lymphocytic choriomeningitis virus, rabies, WNV, HIV, and HCV have been reported through organ transplantation. CJD transmission has occurred through corneal transplantation.

In 2005, the FDA final rule, Current Good Tissue Practice for Human Cells, Tissues, and Cellular and Tissue-Based Products (HCT/Ps), became effective. The purpose of this rule is to improve the safety of HCT/Ps by preventing introduction, transmission, and spread of communicable disease through transplantation of HCT/Ps.[1] The Joint Commission adopted some of these standards, which will apply to accredited organizations that store or use tissue. Solid organs are overseen by the Health Resources and Services Administration through the Organ Procurement and Transplant Network, which also compiles donor-derived disease reports. All suspected disease-transmission cases, notifiable diseases, and clusters should be reported to public health agencies. A Transplantation Transmission Sentinel Network has been piloted by the CDC to facilitate recognition of adverse events associated with transplanted allografts (organs, tissues, and eyes), but standard tissue nomenclature and tracking is needed for national implementation. Along with receiving mandatory reports of adverse events from HCT/P establishments that manufacture tissue, the FDA encourages direct voluntary reporting through its MedWatch program by using MedWatch Form FDA-3500 (available at **www.fda. gov/medwatch**). Additional information about the FDA and HCT/Ps is available at **www.fda.gov/cber/tiss.htm**.

·······················
HUMAN MILK

Breastfeeding provides numerous health benefits to infants, including protection against morbidity and mortality from infectious diseases of bacterial, viral, and parasitic origin. In addition to providing an ideal source of infant nutrition, human milk contains immune-modulating factors, including secretory antibodies, glycoconjugates, anti-inflammatory components, and other factors. Breastfed infants have high concentrations of protective bifidobacteria and lactobacilli in their gastrointestinal tracts, which diminish the risk of colonization and infection with pathogenic organisms. Protection by human milk is established most clearly for pathogens causing gastrointestinal tract infection. In addition, human milk seems to provide protection against otitis media, invasive *Haemophilus influenzae* type b infection, and other causes of upper and lower respiratory tract infections. Evidence also indicates that human milk may modulate development of the immune system of infants.

The American Academy of Pediatrics (AAP) publishes policy statements and a manual on infant feeding[2] that provide further information about the benefits of breastfeeding, recommended feeding practices, and potential contaminants of human milk. In the *Pediatric Nutrition Handbook*[3] and in the AAP policy statement on human milk,[4] issues regarding immunization of lactating mothers and breastfeeding infants, transmission of infectious agents via human milk, and potential effects on breastfed infants of antimicrobial agents administered to lactating mothers are addressed.

---

[1] Centers for Disease Control and Prevention. Notice to readers: FDA rule for current good tissue practice for human cells, tissues, and cellular and tissue-based products. *MMWR Morb Mortal Wkly Rep.* 2005;54(19):490

[2] American Academy of Pediatrics. *Breastfeeding Handbook for Physicians.* Schanler RJ, Gartner LM, Krebs NF, Dooley S, Mass SB, eds. Elk Grove Village, IL: American Academy of Pediatrics; 2006

[3] American Academy of Pediatrics, Committee on Nutrition. *Pediatric Nutrition Handbook.* 6th ed. Elk Grove Village, IL: American Academy of Pediatrics; 2009

[4] American Academy of Pediatrics, Section on Breastfeeding. Breastfeeding and the use of human milk. *Pediatrics.* 2012;129(3):e827–e841

Immunization of Mothers and Infants

EFFECT OF MATERNAL IMMUNIZATION

Women who have not received recommended immunizations before or during pregnancy may be immunized during the postpartum period regardless of lactation status. No evidence exists to validate concern about the potential presence of live viruses from vaccines in maternal milk if the mother is immunized during lactation. Lactating women may be immunized as recommended for adults and adolescents to protect against many infectious diseases (**www.cdc.gov/vaccines** [see adult immunization schedule]). If previously unimmunized or if traveling to an area with endemic infection, a lactating mother may be given inactivated poliovirus vaccine. Attenuated rubella can be detected in human milk and transmitted to breastfed infants with seroconversion; infections usually are asymptomatic or mild. Rubella-seronegative mothers who could not be immunized during pregnancy should be immunized with measles-mumps-rubella (MMR) vaccine during the early postpartum period. In women who receive live-attenuated varicella vaccine while breastfeeding, neither varicella DNA in human milk (by polymerase chain reaction assay) nor varicella antibody in the infant can be detected. Women who previously have not received tetanus toxoid, reduced diphtheria toxoid, and acellular pertussis (Tdap) should receive a dose of Tdap vaccine during pregnancy, preferably during the third or late-second trimester (after 20 weeks' gestation). If not administered during pregnancy, Tdap should be administered immediately postpartum.[1,2] Pregnant women should receive their annual, seasonal inactivated influenza immunization for the current season during pregnancy if not previously received. Breastfeeding women should receive a seasonal influenza immunization for the current season when available, if not received while pregnant. Either inactivated or live-attenuated influenza immunizations may be administered during the postpartum period.[3,4] Yellow fever vaccine is a live-attenuated viral vaccine. Transmission of yellow fever vaccine virus via breastfeeding has resulted in meningoencephalitis in the nursing infant. Yellow fever vaccine is contraindicated in the breastfeeding mother in nonemergency situations.[5]

---

[1] American Academy of Pediatrics, Committee on Infectious Diseases. Additional recommendations for use of tetanus toxoid, reduced-content diphtheria toxoid, and acellular pertussis vaccine (Tdap). *Pediatrics.* 2011;128(4):809–812

[2] Centers for Disease Control and Prevention. Updated recommendations for use of tetanus toxoid, reduced diphtheria toxoid and acellular pertussis vaccine (Tdap) in pregnant women and persons who have or anticipate having close contact with an infant aged <12 months—Advisory Committee on Immunization Practices (ACIP), 2011. *MMWR Morb Mortal Wkly Rep* 2011;60(41):1424–1426

[3] Centers for Disease Control and Prevention. Prevention and control of influenza with vaccines. Recommendations of the Advisory Committee on Immunization Practices (ACIP), 2011. *MMWR Morb Mortal Wkly Rep.* 2011;60(33):1128–1132. For annual updates, see **www.cdc.gov/vaccines**.

[4] American Academy of Pediatrics, Committee on Infectious Diseases. Recommendations for prevention and control of influenza, 2011–2012. *Pediatrics.* 2011;128(4):813–825. For updates, see **www.aapredbook. aappublications.org/flu/**

[5] Centers for Disease Control and Prevention. Yellow fever vaccine. Recommendations of the Advisory Committee on Immunization Practices (ACIP). *MMWR Recomm Rep.* 2010;59(RR-7):1–26

EFFICACY OF IMMUNIZATION IN BREASTFED INFANTS

Infants should be immunized according to the childhood and adolescent immunization schedule regardless of the mode of infant feeding. The immunogenicity of some recommended vaccines is enhanced by breastfeeding, but data are lacking as to whether the efficacy of these vaccines is enhanced. Although high concentrations of antipoliovirus antibody in human milk of some mothers theoretically could interfere with the immunogenicity of oral poliovirus vaccine, this is not a concern with inactivated poliovirus vaccine. The effectiveness of rotavirus vaccine in breastfed infants is comparable to that in nonbreastfed infants.

Transmission of Infectious Agents via Human Milk

BACTERIA

Postpartum mastitis occurs in one third of breastfeeding women in the United States and leads to breast abscesses in up to 10% of cases. Mastitis and breast abscesses have been associated with the presence of bacterial pathogens in human milk. Breast abscesses have the potential to rupture into the ductal system, releasing large numbers of organisms, such as *Staphylococcus aureus*, into milk. Although an increase in mastitis attributable to community-associated methicillin-resistant *S aureus* (MRSA) corresponding to an increase in overall prevalence of community-associated MRSA has been noted, cases of infant infection were not increased in a single-center cohort study from 1998–2005. Temporary discontinuation of breastfeeding on the affected breast for 24 to 48 hours after surgical drainage and appropriate antimicrobial therapy may be necessary. In general, infectious mastitis resolves with continued lactation during appropriate antimicrobial therapy and does not pose a significant risk for the healthy term infant. Even when breastfeeding is interrupted on the affected breast, breastfeeding may continue on the unaffected breast.

Women with tuberculosis who have been treated appropriately for 2 or more weeks and who are not considered contagious may breastfeed. Women with tuberculosis disease suspected of being contagious should refrain from breastfeeding and other close contact with the infant because of potential spread through respiratory tract droplet or airborne transmission (see Tuberculosis, p 736). *Mycobacterium tuberculosis* rarely causes mastitis or a breast abscess, but if a breast abscess caused by *M tuberculosis* is present, breastfeeding should be discontinued until the mother has received treatment and no longer is considered to be contagious.

Expressed human milk can become contaminated with a variety of bacterial pathogens, including *Staphylococcus* species and gram-negative bacilli. Outbreaks of gram-negative bacterial infections in neonatal intensive care units occasionally have been attributed to contaminated human milk specimens that have been collected or stored improperly. Expressed human milk may be a reservoir for multiresistant *S aureus* and other pathogens. Human milk from women other than the biologic mother should be treated according to the guidelines of the Human Milk Banking Association of North America (**www.hmbana.org**) before being fed to the infant. Routine culturing or heat treatment of a mother's milk fed to her infant has not been demonstrated to be necessary or cost-effective (see Human Milk Banks, p 131).

VIRUSES

CYTOMEGALOVIRUS. Cytomegalovirus (CMV) may be shed intermittently in human milk. Although CMV has been found in human milk of women who delivered preterm infants, none of the case reviews have demonstrated sequelae in follow-up over several years after infants were discharge from the neonatal intensive care unit (NICU). Very low birth weight preterm infants, however, are at greater potential risk of symptomatic disease. Decisions about breastfeeding of preterm infants by mothers known to be CMV seropositive should include consideration of the potential benefits of human milk and the risk of CMV transmission. Holder pasteurization (62.5°C [144.5°F] for 30 minutes) and short-term pasteurization (72°C [161.6°F] for 5 seconds) of milk seems to inactivate CMV; short-term pasteurization may be less harmful to the beneficial constituents of human milk. Freezing milk at −20°C (−4°F) will decrease viral titers but does not eliminate CMV reliably.

HEPATITIS B VIRUS. Hepatitis B surface antigen (HBsAg) has been detected in milk from HBsAg-positive women. However, studies from Taiwan and England have indicated that breastfeeding by HBsAg-positive women does not increase significantly the risk of infection among their infants. In the United States, infants born to known HBsAg-positive women should receive the initial dose of hepatitis B vaccine within 12 hours of birth and Hepatitis B Immune Globulin should be administered concurrently but at a different anatomic site. This effectively will eliminate any theoretical risk of transmission through breastfeeding (see Hepatitis B, p 369). There is no need to delay initiation of breastfeeding until after the infant is immunized.

HEPATITIS C VIRUS. Hepatitis C virus (HCV) RNA and antibody to HCV have been detected in milk from mothers infected with HCV. Transmission of HCV via breastfeeding has not been documented in mothers who have positive test results for anti-HCV but negative test results for human immunodeficiency virus (HIV) antibody. Mothers infected with HCV should be counseled that transmission of HCV by breastfeeding theoretically is possible but has not been documented. Mothers infected with HCV should consider abstaining from breastfeeding from a breast with cracked or bleeding nipples. According to current guidelines of the US Public Health Service, maternal HCV infection is not a contraindication to breastfeeding. The decision to breastfeed should be based on an informed discussion between a mother and her health care professional.

HUMAN IMMUNODEFICIENCY VIRUS. HIV has been isolated from human milk and can be transmitted through breastfeeding. The risk of transmission is higher for women who acquire HIV infection during lactation (ie, postpartum) than for women with preexisting infection. In populations such as the United States, in which the risk of infant mortality from infectious diseases and malnutrition is low and in which safe and effective alternative sources of feeding are available readily, HIV-infected women, including women receiving antiretroviral therapy, should be counseled not to breastfeed their infants or donate their milk. Randomized clinical trials have demonstrated that infant prophylaxis with daily nevirapine or nevirapine/zidovudine during breastfeeding significantly decreases the risk of postnatal transmission via human milk. Observational data suggest that maternal antiretroviral therapy (ART) during breastfeeding may decrease postnatal infection. However, neither maternal nor infant postpartum antiretroviral therapy is sufficient to eliminate the risk of HIV transmission through breastfeeeding.[1] Available data indicate that various antiretroviral drugs have differential penetration into human milk; some antiretroviral drugs have concentrations in human milk that are much higher than concentrations in maternal plasma, and other drugs have concentrations in human milk that are much lower than concentrations in plasma or are not detectable. This raises potential concerns regarding infant toxicity as well as the potential for selection of antiretroviral-resistant virus within human milk. Therefore, breastfeeding is not recommended for HIV-infected women in the United States (including women receiving ART), where safe and affordable alternatives are available.

All pregnant women in the United States should be screened for HIV infection to allow implementation of effective interventions to prevent mother-to-child HIV transmission (eg, antiretroviral prophylaxis and elective cesarean delivery) should the woman be found to have HIV infection and to permit appropriate counseling of the woman regarding breastfeeding.[2] HIV screening should occur as part of a panel of prenatal testing unless evaluation is declined (see Human Immunodeficiency Virus Infection, p 418).

In areas where infectious diseases and malnutrition are important causes of infant mortality and where safe, affordable, and sustainable replacement feeding may not be available, infant feeding decisions are more complex. In resource-poor locations, women whose HIV status is unknown are encouraged to continue breastfeeding, because the morbidity associated with artificial feeding is unacceptably high. For HIV-infected mothers, studies in Africa revealed that exclusive breastfeeding for the first 3 to 6 months after birth appeared to lower the risk of HIV transmission through human milk compared with infants who received mixed feedings (breastfeeding and other foods or milks). Exclusive breastfeeding by HIV-infected women does not eliminate postnatal transmission, and HIV transmission is higher than in infants who receive only replacement feeding from birth. Current World Health Organization, UNICEF, and UNAIDS infant feeding guidelines state that if replacement feeding is affordable, feasible, acceptable, sustainable, and safe, replacement of human milk from HIV-infected women with nutritional substitutes is recommended to decrease the risk of HIV transmission. If these criteria are not met, HIV-infected women are recommended to breastfeed exclusively for the first 6 months of life, with weaning after that time when replacement feeding meets the affordable, feasible, acceptable, sustainable, and safe criteria. Thus, in resource-poor countries, the most appropriate feeding option for an HIV-infected mother needs to be based on her individual circumstances and should weigh the benefits of breastfeeding against the risk of breastfeeding associated transmission of HIV (see Human Immunodeficiency Virus Infection, p 418).

HUMAN T-LYMPHOTROPIC VIRUS TYPE 1. Human T-lymphotropic virus type 1 (HTLV-1), endemic in Japan, the Caribbean, and parts of South America, is associated with development of malignant neoplasms and neurologic disorders among adults. Epidemiologic and laboratory studies suggest that mother-to-infant transmission of human HTLV-1 occurs primarily through breastfeeding, although freezing/thawing of

---

[1] Perinatal HIV Guidelines Working Group. Public Health Service Task Force Recommendations for use of Antiretroviral Drugs in Pregnant HIV-Infected Women for Maternal Health and Interventions to Reduce Perinatal HIV Transmission in the United States. September 14, 2011:1–207. Available at: **http://aidsinfo. nih.gov/ContentFiles/PerinatalGL.pdf**

[2] Centers for Disease Control and Prevention. Revised recommendations for HIV testing of adults, adolescents, and pregnant women in health-care settings. *MMWR Recomm Rep.* 2006;55(RR-14):1–17

expressed human milk may decrease infectivity of human milk. Women in the United States who are HTLV-1 seropositive should be advised not to breastfeed. Routine screening for HTLV-1 or HTLV type 2 (HTLV-2) during pregnancy is not recommended.

HUMAN T-LYMPHOTROPIC VIRUS TYPE 2. HTLV-2 is a retrovirus that has been detected among American and European injection drug users and some American Indian/Alaska Native groups. Although apparent maternal-infant transmission has been reported, the rate and timing of transmission have not been established. Until additional data about possible transmission through breastfeeding become available, women in the United States who are HTLV-2 seropositive should be advised not to breastfeed.

HERPES SIMPLEX VIRUS TYPE 1. Women with herpetic lesions may transmit herpes simplex virus (HSV) to their infants by direct contact with the lesions. Transmission may be reduced with hand hygiene and covering of lesions with which the infant might come into contact. Women with herpetic lesions on a breast or nipple should refrain from breastfeeding an infant from the affected breast until lesions have resolved but may breastfeed from the unaffected breast when lesions on the affected breast are covered completely to avoid transmission.

RUBELLA. Wild and vaccine strains of rubella virus have been isolated from human milk. However, the presence of rubella virus in human milk has not been associated with significant disease in infants, and transmission is more likely to occur via other routes. Women with rubella or women who have been immunized recently with live-attenuated rubella virus vaccine may continue to breastfeed.

VARICELLA. Secretion of varicella vaccine virus and infection of a breastfeeding infant of a mother who received varicella vaccine has not been noted in the few instances where it has been studied. Varicella vaccine may be considered for a susceptible breastfeeding mother if the risk of exposure to natural varicella-zoster virus is high. Recommendations for use of passive immunization and varicella vaccine for breastfeeding mothers who have had contact with people in whom varicella has developed or for contacts of a breastfeeding mother in whom varicella has developed are available (see Varicella-Zoster Infections, p 774).

WEST NILE VIRUS. West Nile virus RNA has been detected in human milk collected from a woman with disease attributable to West Nile virus; her breastfed infant developed West Nile virus immunoglobulin M antibodies but remained asymptomatic. Animal experiments have shown that West Nile virus can be transmitted in animal milk, and other related flaviviruses can be transmitted to humans via unpasteurized milk from ruminants. The degree to which West Nile virus is transmitted in human milk and the extent to which breastfeeding infants become infected are unknown. Because the health benefits of breastfeeding have been established and the risk of West Nile virus transmission through breastfeeding is unknown, women who reside in an area with endemic West Nile virus infection should continue to breastfeed.

HUMAN MILK BANKS

Some circumstances, such as preterm delivery, may preclude breastfeeding, but infants in these circumstances still may be fed milk collected from their own mothers or from individual donors. The potential for transmission of infectious agents through donor human milk requires appropriate selection and screening of donors and careful collection, processing, and storage of milk. Currently, US donor milk banks that belong to the

Human Milk Banking Association of North America (**www.hmbana.org/**) voluntarily follow guidelines drafted in consultation with the US Food and Drug Administration and the Centers for Disease Control and Prevention. These guidelines include screening of all donors for HBsAg and antibodies to HIV-1, HIV-2, HTLV-1, HTLV-2, hepatitis C virus, and syphilis. Donor milk is dispensed only by prescription after it is heat treated at 62.5°C (144.5°F) for 30 minutes and prepasteurization bacterial cultures reveal no growth of pathogenic organisms (*Staphylococcus aureus*, group B streptococcus, and lactose-fermenting coliform) and no more than 100 000 colony-forming units/mL of normal skin bacteria and no viable bacteria after pasteurization.

INADVERTENT HUMAN MILK EXPOSURE

Policies to deal with occasions when an infant inadvertently is fed expressed human milk not obtained from his or her mother have been developed. These policies require documentation, counseling, and observation of the affected infant for signs of infection and potential testing of the source mother for infections that could be transmitted via human milk. Recommendations for management of a situation involving an accidental exposure may be found at **www.cdc.gov/breastfeeding/recommendations/other_mothers_milk.htm.** A summary of the recommendations include the following:

1. Inform the donor mother about the inadvertent exposure, and ask:
   - Whether she has had a recent HIV test and, if so, would she agree to have the results shared anonymously with the parent(s) of the infant given her milk?
   - If the donor mother does not know her HIV status, would she be willing to be tested and have the results shared anonymously with parent(s) of the recipient infant?
2. Discuss inadvertent administration of the donor milk with the parent(s) of the recipient infant.
   - Inform the parent(s) of the recipient infant that the risk of transmission of HIV infection via this exposure is low. Explain that factors present in human milk act, together with time and cold temperatures, to destroy HIV, if present in expressed human milk. Furthermore, explain that transmission of HIV from single human milk exposure has never been documented.
   - Recommend that a baseline HIV antibody test be performed from blood of the recipient infant.

Collection of milk from the birth mother of a preterm infant does not require processing if fed to her infant, but proper collection and storage procedures should be followed. Heat treatment at 56°C or greater (133°F or greater) for 30 minutes reliably eliminates bacteria, inactivates HIV, and decreases titers of other viruses but may not eliminate CMV completely. Holder pasteurization (62.5°C [144.5°F] for 30 minutes) reliably inactivates HIV and CMV and eliminates or decreases significantly titers of most other viruses. Short-term pasteurization (72°C [161.6°F] for 5 seconds) also appears to inactivate CMV.

Freezing at −20°C (−4°F) eliminates HTLV-1 and decreases the concentration of CMV but does not destroy most other viruses or bacteria. Microbiologic quality standards for fresh, unpasteurized, expressed milk are not available. The presence of gram-negative bacteria, *S aureus*, or alpha- or beta-hemolytic streptococci may preclude use of expressed human milk. Routine culture of milk that a birth mother provides to her own infant is not warranted.

Antimicrobial Agents in Human Milk

Antimicrobial agents often are prescribed for lactating women. Although these drugs may appear in milk, the potential risk to an infant must be weighed against the known benefits of continued breastfeeding. As a general guideline, an antimicrobial agent is safe to administer to a lactating woman if it is safe to administer to an infant. Only in rare cases will interruption of breastfeeding be necessary because of maternal medications.

The amount of drug an infant receives from a lactating mother depends on a number of factors, including maternal dose, frequency and duration of administration, absorption, timing of medication administration and breastfeeding, and distribution characteristics of the drug. When a lactating woman receives appropriate doses of an antimicrobial agent, the concentration of the compound in her milk usually is less than the equivalent of a therapeutic dose for the infant. A breastfed infant who requires antimicrobial therapy should receive the recommended doses, independent of administration of the agent to the mother.

Current information about drugs and lactation can be found at the Toxicology Data Network Web site (**www.toxnet.nlm.nih.gov/help/LactMedRecordFormat. htm**). Data for drugs, including antimicrobial agents, administered to lactating women are provided in several categories, including maternal and infant drug levels, effects in breastfed infants, possible effects on lactation, the category into which the drug has been placed by the American Academy of Pediatrics, alternative drugs to consider, and references.

CHILDREN IN OUT-OF-HOME CHILD CARE[1]

Infants and young children who are cared for in group settings have an increased rate of communicable infectious diseases and an increased risk of acquiring antimicrobial-resistant organisms. Prevention and control of infection in out-of-home child care settings is influenced by several factors, including the following: (1) health status, practice of personal hygiene, and immunization status of care providers; (2) environmental sanitation; (3) food-handling procedures; (4) age and immunization status of children; (5) ratio of children to care providers; (6) physical space and quality of facilities; (7) frequency of use of antimicrobial agents in children in child care; and (8) adherence to standard precautions for infection control. Adequately addressing problems of infection control in child care settings requires collaborative efforts of public health officials, licensing agencies, child care providers, physicians, nurses, parents, employers, and other members of the community.

Child care programs should require that all enrollees and staff members receive age-appropriate immunizations and routine health care. In addition, these programs have the opportunity to provide parents with ongoing instruction in child development, hygiene, appropriate nutrition, and management of minor illnesses. Many early education and child care programs have access to health consultants who can assist providers and parents with these issues (**www.healthychildcare.org/contacts.html**). People involved

---

[1] American Academy of Pediatrics. *Managing Infectious Diseases in Child Care and Schools: A Quick Reference Guide.* Aronson SS, Shope TR, eds. 2nd ed. Elk Grove Village, IL: American Academy of Pediatrics; 2009

with early education and child care can use the published national standards[1] related to these topics to provide specific education and implementation measures.

Classification of Care Service

Child care services commonly are classified by the type of setting, number of children in care, and age and health status of the children. **Small family child care homes** provide care and education for up to 6 children simultaneously, including any preschool-aged relatives of the care provider, in a residence that usually is the home of the care provider. **Large family child care homes** provide care and education for between 7 and 12 children at a time, including any preschool-aged relatives of the care provider, in a residence that usually is the home of one of the care providers. A **child care center** is a facility that provides care and education to any number of children in a nonresidential setting or to 13 or more children in any setting if the facility is open on a regular basis. A **facility for ill children** provides care for 1 or more children who are excluded temporarily from their regular child care setting for health reasons. A facility for children with special needs provides specialized care and education for 1 child or more who cannot be accommodated in a setting with typically developing children. All 50 states regulate out-of-home child care; however, regulation enforcement is directed toward center-based child care; few states or municipalities license or enforce regulations as carefully for small or large child care homes. Regulatory requirements for every state can be accessed through the Web site of the National Resource Center for Health and Safety in Child Care and Early Education (**www.nrckids.org**).

Grouping of children by age varies, but in child care centers, common groups consist of **infants** (birth through 12 months of age), **toddlers** (13 through 35 months of age), **preschoolers** (36 through 59 months of age), and **school-aged children** (5 through 12 years of age). Age grouping reflects developmental status. Infants and toddlers who require diapering or assistance in using a toilet have significant hands-on contact with care providers. Furthermore, they have oral contact with the environment, have poor control over their secretions and excretions, and have immunity to fewer common pathogens. Toddlers also have frequent direct contact with each other and with secretions of other toddlers. Therefore, child care programs that provide infant and toddler care should be vigilant about practice of infection-control measures.

Management and Prevention of Illness

Modes of transmission of bacteria, viruses, parasites, and fungi within child care settings are listed in Table 2.5 (p 135). In most instances, the risk of introducing an infectious agent into a child care group is related directly to prevalence of the agent in the population and to the number of susceptible children in that group. Transmission of an agent within the group depends on the following: (1) characteristics of the organism, such as mode of spread, infective dose, and survival in the environment; (2) frequency of asymptomatic infection or carrier state; and (3) immunity to the respective pathogen. Transmission also can be affected by behaviors of the child care providers, particularly hygienic

---

[1] American Academy of Pediatrics, American Public Health Association, National Resource Center for Health and Safety in Child Care and Early Education. *Caring for Our Children: National Health and Safety Performance Standards: Guidelines for Out-of-Home Child Care.* 3rd ed. Elk Grove Village, IL: American Academy of Pediatrics; and Washington, DC: American Public Health Association; 2011

Table 2.5. Modes of Transmission of Organisms in Child Care Settings

Usual Route of Transmission[a]	Bacteria	Viruses	Other[b]
Fecal-oral	*Campylobacter* organisms, *Clostridium difficile*, *Escherichia coli* O157:H7, *Salmonella* organisms, *Shigella* organisms	Astrovirus, norovirus, enteric adenovirus, enteroviruses, hepatitis A virus, rotaviruses	*Cryptosporidium species*, *Enterobius vermicularis*, *Giardia intestinalis*
Respiratory	*Bordetella pertussis*, *Haemophilus influenzae* type b, *Mycobacterium tuberculosis*, *Neisseria meningitidis*, *Streptococcus pneumoniae*, group A streptococcus, *Kingella kingae*	Adenovirus, influenza virus, human metapneumovirus, measles virus, mumps virus, parainfluenza virus, parvovirus B19, respiratory syncytial virus, rhinovirus, coronavirus, rubella virus, varicella-zoster virus	...
Person-to-person contact	Group A streptococcus, *Staphylococcus aureus*	Herpes simplex virus, varicella-zoster virus	Agents causing pediculosis, scabies, and ringworm[e]
Contact with blood, urine, and/or saliva	...	Cytomegalovirus, herpes simplex virus	...
Bloodborne	...	Hepatitis B virus	...

[a]The potential for transmission of microorganisms in the child care setting by food and animals also exists (see Appendix X, Clinical Syndromes Associated With Foodborne Diseases, p 921, and Appendix XI, Diseases Transmitted by Animals, p 926, and Diseases Transmitted by Animals [Zoonoses]: Household Pets, Including Nontraditional Pets, and Exposure to Animals in Public Settings, p 215).

[b]Parasites, fungi, mites, and lice.

[e]Transmission also may occur from contact with objects in the environment.

aspects of child handling; by environmental sanitation practices; and by age and immunization status of children enrolled. Children infected in a child care group can transmit organisms not only within the group but also within their households and the community. Appropriate hand hygiene and adherence to immunization recommendations are the most important factors for decreasing transmission of disease in child care settings.

Options for management of ill or infected children in child care and for reducing transmission of pathogens include the following: (1) antimicrobial treatment or prophylaxis when appropriate; (2) immunization when appropriate; (3) exclusion of ill or infected children from the facility when appropriate; (4) provision of alternative care at a separate site; (5) cohorting to provide care (eg, segregation of infected children in a group with separate staff and facilities); (6) limiting new admissions; (7) hand hygiene; and (8) closing the facility (a rarely exercised option). Recommendations for controlling spread of specific infectious agents differ according to the epidemiology of the pathogen (see disease-specific chapters in Section 3) and characteristics of the setting.

Infection-control procedures in child care programs that decrease acquisition and transmission of communicable diseases include: (1) periodic (at least annual) review of facility-maintained child and employee illness records, including current immunization status; (2) hygienic and sanitary procedures for toilet use, toilet training, and diaper changing; (3) review and enforcement of hand-hygiene procedures; (4) environmental sanitation; (5) personal hygiene for children and staff; (6) sanitary preparation and handling of food; (7) communicable disease surveillance and reporting; and (8) appropriate handling of animals in the facility. Policies that include education and implementation of procedures for full- and part-time employees and volunteers as well as exclusion policies aid in control of infectious diseases. Health departments should have plans for responding to reportable and nonreportable communicable diseases in child care programs and should provide training, written information, and technical consultation to child care programs when requested or alerted. Evaluation of the well-being of each child should be performed by a trained staff member each day as the child enters the site and throughout the day as needed. Parents should be required to report their child's immunization status on an ongoing basis and should be encouraged to share information with child care staff about their child's acute and chronic illnesses and medication use.

Recommendations for Inclusion or Exclusion

Mild illness is common among children. Most children will not need to be excluded from their usual source of care for mild respiratory tract illnesses, because transmission is likely to have occurred before symptoms developed in the child. Disease may occur as a result of contact with children with asymptomatic infection. The risk of illness can be decreased by following standard hygienic practices.

Exclusion of sick children and adults from out-of-home child care settings has been recommended when such exclusion could decrease the likelihood of secondary cases. In many situations, the expertise of the program's health consultant and that of the responsible local and state public health authorities are helpful for determining the benefits and risks of excluding children from their usual care program. Most states have laws about isolation of people with specific communicable diseases. Local or state health departments should be contacted for information about these laws, and public health authorities in these areas should be notified about cases of nationally notifiable infectious diseases and unusual outbreaks of other illnesses involving children or adults in the child care environment (see Appendix VI, Nationally Notifiable Infectious Diseases in the United States, p 902).

General recommendations for exclusion of children in out-of-home care are shown in Table 2.6. Disease- or condition-specific recommendations for exclusion from out-of-home care and management of contacts are shown in Table 2.7 (p 138).

Most minor illnesses do not constitute a reason for excluding a child from child care unless the illness prevents the child from participating in normal activities, as determined by the child care staff, or the illness requires a need for care that is greater than staff can

Table 2.6. General Recommendations for Exclusion of Children in Out-Of-Home Child Care

Symptom(s)	Management
Illness preventing participation in activities, as determined by child care staff	Exclusion until illness resolves and able to participate in activities
Illness that requires a need for care that is greater than staff can provide without compromising health and safety of others	Exclusion or placement in care environment where appropriate care can be provided, without compromising care of others
Severe illness suggested by fever with behavior changes, lethargy, irritability, persistent crying, difficulty breathing, progressive rash with above symptoms	Medical evaluation and exclusion until symptoms have resolved
Rash with fever or behavioral change	Medical evaluation and exclusion until illness is determined not to be communicable
Persistent abdominal pain (2 hours or more) or intermittent abdominal pain associated with fever, dehydration, or other systemic signs and symptoms	Medical evaluation and exclusion until symptoms have resolved
Vomiting 2 or more times in preceding 24 hours	Exclusion until symptoms have resolved, unless vomiting is determined to be caused by a non-communicable condition and child is able to remain hydrated and participate in activities
Diarrhea if stool not contained in diaper. If stool frequency exceeds 2 or more stools above normal for that child or stools containing blood or mucus	Medical evaluation for stools with blood or mucus; exclusion until stools are contained in the diaper or when toilet-trained children no longer have accidents using the toilet and when stool frequency becomes less than 2 stools above that child's normal frequency
Oral lesions	Exclusion if unable to contain drool or if unable to participate because of other symptoms or until child or staff member is considered to be noninfectious (lesions smaller or resolved).
Skin lesions	Keep lesions on exposed skin surfaces covered with a waterproof dressing

Table 2.7. Disease- or Condition-Specific Recommendations for Exclusion of Children in Out-Of-Home Child Care

Condition	Management of Case	Management of Contacts
Hepatitis A virus (HAV) infection	Serologic testing to confirm HAV infection in suspected cases. Exclusion until 1 week after onset of jaundice.	If 1 or more cases confirmed in child or staff attendees or 2 or more cases in households of staff or attendees, HAV vaccine or Immune Globulin (IG) should be administered within 14 days of exposure to unimmunized staff and attendees. In centers without diapered children, HAV vaccine or IG should be given to unimmunized classroom contacts of index case. Asymptomatic IG recipients may return after receipt of IG (see Hepatitis A, p 361).
Impetigo	Exclusion until 24 hours after treatment has been initiated. Lesions on exposed skin should be covered with watertight dressing.	No intervention unless additional lesions develop.
Measles	Exclusion until 4 days after beginning of rash and when the child is able to participate.	Immunize exposed children without evidence of immunity within 72 hours of exposure. Children who do not receive vaccine within 72 hours or who remain unimmunized after exposure should be excluded until at least 2 weeks after onset of rash in the last case of measles. For use of IG, see Measles (p 489).
Mumps	Exclusion until 5 days after onset of parotid gland swelling.	In outbreak setting, people without documentation of immunity should be immunized or excluded. Immediate readmission may occur following immunization. Unimmunized people should be excluded for 26 or more days following onset of parotitis in last case.
Pediculosis capitis (head lice)	Treatment at end of program day and readmission on completion of first treatment.	Household and close contacts should be examined and treated if infested. No exclusion necessary.

Table 2.7. Disease- or Condition-Specific Recommendations for Exclusion of Children in Out-Of-Home Child Care, continued

Condition	Management of Case	Management of Contacts
Pertussis	Exclusion until 5 days of appropriate antimicrobial therapy course completed (see Pertussis, p 553).	Immunization and chemoprophylaxis should be administered as recommended for household contacts. Symptomatic children and staff should be excluded until completion of 5 days of antimicrobial therapy course. Untreated adults should be excluded until 21 days after onset of cough (see Pertussis Infections, p 553).
Rubella	Exclusion until 6 days after onset of rash for postnatal infection.	Pregnant contacts should be evaluated (see Rubella, p 629).
Salmonella serotype Typhi infection	Exclusion until diarrhea resolves. Three negative stool culture results required before readmission.	Stool cultures should be performed for attendees and staff; infected people should be excluded on the basis of age (see *Salmonella* Infections, p 635).
Non-serotype Typhi *Salmonella* infection or unknown *Salmonella* serotype	Exclusion until diarrhea resolves. Negative stool culture results not required for non-serotype Typhi *Salmonella* species.	Symptomatic contacts should be excluded until symptoms resolve. Stool cultures are not required for asymptomatic contacts. Antimicrobial therapy is not recommended for asymptomatic infection or uncomplicated diarrhea or for contacts.
Scabies	Exclusion until after treatment given.	Close contacts with prolonged skin-to-skin contact should have prophylactic therapy. Bedding and clothing in contact with skin of infected people should be laundered (see Scabies, p 641).
Shiga toxin-producing *Escherichia coli* (*STEC*), including *E coli* O157:H7, or *Shigella* infection	Exclusion until diarrhea resolves and results of 2 stool cultures are negative for these organisms, depending on state regulations.	Meticulous hand hygiene; stool cultures should be performed for any contacts. Center(s) with cases should be closed to new admissions during *STEC* outbreak (see *Escherichia coli* diarrhea, p 324, and *Shigella* infections, p 645).

Table 2.7. Disease- or Condition-Specific Recommendations for Exclusion of Children in Out-Of-Home Child Care, continued

Condition	Management of Case	Management of Contacts
Staphylococcus aureus skin infections	Exclusion only if skin lesions are draining and cannot be covered with a watertight dressing.	Meticulous hand hygiene; cultures of contacts are not recommended.
Streptococcal pharyngitis	Exclusion until 24 hours after treatment has been initiated and the child is able to participate in activities.	Symptomatic contacts of documented cases of group A streptococcal infection should be tested and treated if test results are positive.
Tuberculosis	For active disease, exclusion until determined to be noninfectious by physician or health department authority. May return to activities after therapy is instituted, symptoms have diminished, and adherence to therapy is documented. No exclusion for latent tuberculosis infection (LTBI).	Local health department personnel should be informed for contact investigation (see Tuberculosis, p 736).
Varicella (see Varicella-Zoster Infections, p 774)	Exclusion until all lesions have dried and crusted (usually 6 days after onset of rash in immuno-competent people; may be longer in immuno-compromised people). Breakthrough cases are modified and may be maculopapular only and may not crust. In these cases, isolate for 24 hours following appearance of last lesions.	For people without evidence of immunity, varicella vaccine should be administered within 3 days but up to 5 days after exposure, or when indicated, Varicella-Zoster Immune Globulin should be administered up to 10 days after exposure.

provide. Examples of illnesses and conditions that do not necessitate exclusion include the following:

- Common cold.
- Diarrhea, as long as stools are contained in the diaper (for infants), there are no accidents using the toilet (for older children), and stool frequency is less than 2 stools above normal for that child.
- Rash without fever and without behavioral change.
- Parvovirus B19 infection in an immunocompetent host.
- Cytomegalovirus (CMV) infection.
- Chronic hepatitis B virus (HBV) infection (see p 145 for possible exceptions).
- Conjunctivitis without fever and without behavioral change; if 2 or more children in a group care setting develop conjunctivitis in the same period, seek advice from the program's health consultant or public health authority.
- Human immunodeficiency virus (HIV) infection (see p 147 for possible exceptions).
- Known methicillin-resistant *Staphylococcus aureus* (MRSA) carriers or children with colonization of MRSA but without an illness that would otherwise require exclusion.

Asymptomatic children who excrete an enteropathogen usually do not need to be excluded, except when an infection with Shiga toxin-producing *Escherichia coli (STEC)*, *Shigella* species, or *Salmonella* serotype Typhi has occurred in the child care program. Because these infections are transmitted easily and can be severe, exclusion is warranted until results of 2 stool cultures are negative for STEC or *Shigella* species (see *Escherichia coli* Diarrhea, p 324, *Shigella* Infections, p 645) and results of 3 stool cultures are negative for *Salmonella* serotype Typhi *(see Salmonella* Infections, p 635). Other *Salmonella* serotypes do not require negative test results from stool cultures. Local health ordinances may differ with respect to number and timing of specimens. Child care staff and families of enrolled children need to be fully informed about inclusion and exclusion criteria.

During the course of an identified outbreak of a nonreportable or reportable communicable illness in a child care setting (see Nationally Notifiable Infectious Diseases, Appendix VI, p 902), a child determined to be contributing to transmission of organisms causing the illness at the program may be excluded. The child may be readmitted when the risk of transmission no longer is present. For most outbreaks of vaccine-preventable illnesses, unvaccinated children should be excluded until they are vaccinated.

Infectious Diseases—Epidemiology and Control

(Also see disease-specific chapters in Section 3.)

ENTERIC DISEASES

The close personal contact and suboptimal hygiene of young children provide ready opportunities for spread of enteric bacteria, viruses, and parasites in child care settings. Enteropathogens transmitted by the person-to-person route, such as rotaviruses, enteric adenoviruses, astroviruses, noroviruses, *Shigella* species, *E coli* O157:H7, *Giardia intestinalis,* *Cryptosporidium* species, and hepatitis A virus (HAV), have been the principal organisms implicated in outbreaks. Since administration of rotavirus vaccine was recommended routinely, disease and hospitalization for diarrhea attributable to rotavirus have decreased dramatically. *Salmonella* species, *Clostridium difficile,* and *Campylobacter* species infrequently have been associated with outbreaks of disease in children in child care.

Human-animal contact involving family and classroom pets, animal displays, and petting zoos expose children to pathogens harbored by these animals. Most reptiles and many rodents (eg, hamsters, mice, rats) are colonized with *Salmonella* organisms, lymphocytic choriomeningitis virus, and other viruses that may be transmitted to children via contact (see Diseases Transmitted by Animals [Zoonoses]: Household Pets, Including Nontraditional Pets, and Exposure to Animals in Public Settings, p 215). Management of contact between young children and animals known to transmit disease to children is difficult in group child care settings. Children should not have contact with these animals or their habitats. Optimal hand hygiene, especially after contact with animals and before eating or drinking, is essential to prevent transmission of zoonoses in the child care setting.

Young children who are not toilet trained have an increased frequency of diarrhea and of fecal contamination of the environment. Enteropathogen spread is common in child care programs and is highest in infant and toddler areas, especially among attendees who are not toilet trained completely. Enteropathogens are spread by the fecal-oral route, either directly by person-to-person transmission or indirectly via fomites, environmental surfaces, and food, resulting in transmission of disease. The risk of food contamination can be increased when staff members who assist with toilet use and diaper-changing activities also prepare or serve food. Several enteropathogens, including rotaviruses, norovirus, HAV, *G intestinalis* cysts, *Cryptosporidium* oocysts, and *C difficile* spores survive on environmental surfaces for periods ranging from hours to weeks.

Before universal hepatitis A immunization of children 12 through 23 months of age was recommended in 2006, child care programs were a source of HAV spread within the community. HAV infection differs from most other diseases in child care facilities, because symptomatic illness occurs primarily among adult contacts of infected asymptomatic children. To recognize outbreaks and initiate appropriate control measures, health care professionals and child care providers should be aware of this epidemiologic characteristic (see Hepatitis A, p 361). Hepatitis A vaccine should be considered for staff of child care centers with ongoing or recurrent outbreaks, in communities where cases in a child care center are a major source of HAV infection, and routinely for all children 12 months of age and older, including children older than 23 months of age who have not been immunized previously with hepatitis A vaccine for whom immunity against hepatitis A is desired (see Hepatitis A, p 361).

The single most important procedure to minimize fecal-oral transmission is frequent hand hygiene measures combined with staff training and monitoring of staff implementation. A child in whom jaundice develops should not have contact with other children or staff until 7 days after symptom onset. Exclusion criteria are provided in Table 2.6 (p 137) and Table 2.7 (p 138).

RESPIRATORY TRACT DISEASES

Organisms spread by the respiratory route include viruses causing acute upper respiratory tract infections or bacterial organisms associated with invasive infections, such as *Haemophilus influenzae* type b, *Streptococcus pneumoniae*, *Neisseria meningitidis*, *Bordetella pertussis*, *Mycobacterium tuberculosis*, and *Kingella kingae*. Possible modes of spread of respiratory tract viruses include aerosols, respiratory droplets, and direct hand contact with contaminated secretions and fomites. The viral pathogens responsible for respiratory tract disease in child care settings are those that cause disease in the community, including respiratory syncytial virus, parainfluenza virus, influenza virus, human metapneumovirus, adenovirus, and rhinovirus. The incidence of viral infections of the respiratory tract is increased in child care settings. Hand hygiene measures can decrease the incidence of acute respiratory tract disease among children in child care (see Recommendations for Inclusion and Exclusion, p 136). Influenza virus and rhinovirus have been detected on samples from toys, indicating that environmental sanitation may be important in decreasing the incidence of acute respiratory tract disease in children in child care.

The occurrence of invasive disease attributable to *H influenzae* type b (Hib) is rare since immunization of infants and children with Hib conjugate vaccine was recommended routinely (see *Haemophilus influenzae* infections, p 345). Infections caused by *N meningitidis* occur in all age groups. The age group experiencing the highest incidence is children younger than 1 year of age. Extended close contact between children and staff exposed to an index case of meningococcal disease predisposes to secondary transmission. Because outbreaks may occur in child care settings, chemoprophylaxis is indicated for exposed child care contacts (see Meningococcal Infections, p 500).

In the prevaccine era, the risk of primary invasive disease attributable to *S pneumoniae* among children in child care settings was increased compared with children not in child care settings. Secondary spread of *S pneumoniae* in child care centers has been reported, but the degree of risk of secondary spread in child care facilities is unknown. Prophylaxis for contacts after an occurrence of one or more cases of invasive *S pneumoniae* disease is not recommended. Use of *S pneumoniae* conjugate vaccine has decreased dramatically the incidence of both invasive disease and pneumonia among children and other age groups not targeted for vaccination and has decreased carriage of serotypes of *S pneumoniae* contained in the pneumococcal conjugate vaccine. In 2010, the US Food and Drug Administration (FDA) licensed 13-valent pneumococcal conjugate vaccine (PCV13), which replaced PCV7. The PCV13 vaccine will add coverage for 6 additional serotypes, potentially providing protection for two thirds of the most common pneumococcal serotypes in children younger than 5 years of age (see Pneumococcal Infections, p 571).

Group A streptococcal infection among children in child care has been reported, including an association with varicella outbreaks. A child with proven group A streptococcal infection should be excluded from classroom contact until 24 hours after initiation of antimicrobial therapy. Although outbreaks of streptococcal pharyngitis in these settings have occurred, the risk of secondary transmission after a single case of mild or even severe invasive group A streptococcal infection remains low. Chemoprophylaxis for contacts after group A streptococcal infection in child care facilities generally is not recommended (see Group A Streptococcal Infections, p 668).

Infants and young children with tuberculosis disease are not as contagious as adults, because children are less likely to have cavitary pulmonary lesions and are unable to expel large numbers of organisms into the air forcefully. If approved by health care officials, children with tuberculosis disease may attend group child care if the following criteria are met: (1) chemotherapy has begun; (2) ongoing adherence to therapy is documented; (3) clinical symptoms have resolved; (4) children are considered noninfectious to others; and (5) children are able to participate in activities. Because an adult with tuberculosis disease poses a hazard to children in group child care, tuberculin screening with a tuberculin skin test (TST) or an interferon-gamma release blood assay of all adults who have contact with children in a child care setting is recommended before caregiving activities are initiated. This includes noncare providers present in family child care homes. However, adults with tuberculosis, especially adults with diminished or altered immunologic function, may not have a reaction to a TST, and further evaluation may be required (see Tuberculosis, p 736). The need for periodic subsequent tuberculin screening for people without clinically important reactions should be determined on the basis of their risk of acquiring a new infection and local or state health department recommendations. Adults with symptoms compatible with tuberculosis should be evaluated for the disease as soon as possible. Child care providers with suspected or confirmed tuberculosis disease should be excluded from the child care facility and should not be allowed to care for children until their evaluation is negative or chemotherapy has rendered them noninfectious (see Tuberculosis, p 736).

OTHER CONDITIONS

PARVOVIRUS B19. Isolation or exclusion of immunocompetent people with parvovirus B19 infection in child care settings is unwarranted, because little or no virus is present in respiratory tract secretions at the time of occurrence of the rash of erythema infectiosum. In addition, because fewer than 1% of pregnant teachers during erythema infectiosum outbreaks would be expected to experience an adverse fetal outcome, exclusion of pregnant women from employment in child care or teaching is not recommended (see Parvovirus B19, p 539). This is based on the equivalent risk of acquisition of parvovirus B19 from a community source not affiliated with the child care facility.

VARICELLA-ZOSTER VIRUS. The epidemiology of varicella has changed dramatically since licensure of the varicella vaccine in 1995. In the prevaccine era, attendance in child care was a described risk factor for children acquiring varicella at earlier ages. However, varicella is now an uncommon disease in child care settings. Children with varicella who have been excluded from child care may return after all lesions have dried and crusted, which usually occurs on the sixth day after onset of rash. Varicella in vaccinated people usually is less severe clinically. Immunized children with breakthrough varicella with only maculopapular lesions can return to child care or school if no new lesions have appeared within a 24-hour period. All staff members and parents should be notified when a case of varicella occurs; they should be informed about the greater likelihood of serious infection in susceptible adults and adolescents and in susceptible immunocompromised people in addition to the potential for fetal sequelae if infection occurs during the pregnancy of a susceptible woman. Less than 5% of adults may be susceptible to varicella-zoster virus. Adults without evidence of immunity should be offered 2 doses of varicella vaccine unless contraindicated. Susceptible child care staff members who are pregnant and exposed to children with varicella should be referred promptly to a qualified physician or other health care professional for counseling and management. The American Academy of Pediatrics and Centers for Disease Control and Prevention (CDC) recommend use of varicella vaccine in nonpregnant immunocompetent people 12 months of age or older without evidence of immunity within 72 and possibly up to 120 hours after exposure to varicella (see Varicella-Zoster Infections, p 774). During a varicella outbreak, people who have received 1 dose of varicella vaccine should, resources permitting, receive a second dose of vaccine, provided the appropriate interval has elapsed since the first dose (3 months for children 12 months through 12 years of age and at least 4 weeks for people 13 years of age and older).

The decision to exclude staff members or children with herpes zoster infection (shingles) whose lesions cannot be covered should be made on the basis of criteria similar to criteria for varicella. In immunocompetent people, herpes zoster lesions that can be covered pose a minimal risk, because transmission usually occurs as a result of direct contact with fluid from lesions (see Varicella-Zoster Infections, p 774).

HERPES SIMPLEX VIRUS. Children with herpes simplex virus (HSV) gingivostomatitis who do not have control of oral secretions (drooling) should be excluded from child care when active lesions are present. Although HSV can be transmitted from a mother to her fetus or newborn infant, maternal HSV infections that are a threat to offspring usually are acquired by the infant during birth from genital tract infection of the mother. Exposure of a pregnant woman to HSV in a child care setting carries little risk for her fetus. Child care providers should be educated on the importance of hand hygiene and other measures for limiting transfer of infected material from children with varicella-zoster virus or HSV infection (eg, saliva, tissue fluid, or fluid from a skin lesion).

CMV INFECTION. Spread of CMV from an asymptomatic infected child in child care to his or her mother or to child care providers is the most important consequence of child care-related CMV infection (see Cytomegalovirus Infection, p 300). Children enrolled in child care programs are more likely to acquire CMV than are children primarily cared for at home. The highest rates (eg, 70%) of viral shedding in oral secretions and urine occur in children between 1 and 3 years of age, and excretion commonly continues (sometimes intermittently) for years. Studies of CMV seroconversion among female child care providers have found annualized seroconversion rates of 8% to 20%. Women who are or who may become pregnant and who are CMV naive are at risk of being infected during pregnancy and transmitting CMV to their infant.

In view of the risk of CMV infection in child care staff and the potential consequences of gestational CMV infection, child care staff members should be counseled about risks. This counseling may include testing for serum antibody to CMV to determine the child care provider's protection against primary CMV infection, but routine serologic testing is not recommended. CMV excretion is so prevalent that attempts at isolation or segregation of children who excrete CMV are impractical and inappropriate. Similarly, testing of children to detect CMV excretion is inappropriate, because excretion often is intermittent, and results of testing can be misleading. Therefore, use of standard precautions and hand hygiene are the optimal methods of prevention of transmission of infection.

BLOODBORNE VIRUS INFECTIONS

HBV, HIV, and hepatitis C virus (HCV) are bloodborne pathogens. Although risk of contact with blood containing one of these viruses is low in the child care setting, appropriate infection-control practices will prevent transmission of bloodborne pathogens if exposure occurs. All child care providers should receive regular training on how to prevent transmission of bloodborne infections and how to respond should an exposure occur (**www.osha.gov/SLTC/bloodbornepathogens/index.html**).

HEPATITIS B VIRUS. Transmission of HBV in the child care setting has been described but occurs rarely. Because of the low risk of transmission, high immunization rates against HBV in children, and implementation of infection-control measures, children known to have chronic HBV infection (hepatitis B surface antigen [HBsAg] positive) may attend child care in most circumstances.

Transmission of HBV in a child care setting is most likely to occur through direct exposure to blood after an injury or from bites or scratches that break the skin and introduce blood or body secretions from an HBV carrier into a susceptible person. Indirect transmission through environmental contamination with blood or saliva is possible. This occurrence has not been documented in a child care setting in the United States. Because saliva contains much less virus than does blood, the potential infectivity of saliva is low. Infectivity of saliva has been demonstrated only when inoculated through the skin of gibbons and chimpanzees.

On the basis of limited data, the risk of disease transmission from a child or staff member who has chronic HBV infection but who does not exhibit behavioral risk factors and is without injury, generalized dermatitis, or bleeding problems is minimal. This slight risk usually does not justify exclusion of a child who has chronic HBV infection from child care or the necessity of HBV immunization of the child's contacts at the care program, most of whom already should be protected by previous HBV immunization as part of their recommended immunization schedule.

Routine screening of children for HBsAg before admission to child care is not justified. Admission of a child previously identified to have chronic HBV infection with one or more risk factors for transmission of bloodborne pathogens (eg, biting, frequent scratching, generalized dermatitis, or bleeding problems) should be determined by the child's physician, in conjunction with the child care provider and program director. The responsible public health authority or child care health consultant should be consulted when appropriate. Regular assessment of behavioral risk factors and medical conditions of enrolled children with chronic HBV infection is necessary.

Children who bite pose an additional concern. Existing data in humans suggest a small risk of HBV transmission from the bite of a child with chronic HBV infection. For a susceptible child (not fully immunized with HBV vaccine) who is bitten by a child with chronic HBV infection, prophylaxis with Hepatitis B Immune Globulin (HBIG) and hepatitis B immunization is recommended (see Hepatitis B, p 369).

The risk of HBV acquisition when a susceptible child bites a child who has chronic HBV infection is unknown. A theoretical risk exists if HBsAg-positive blood enters the oral cavity of the biter, but transmission by this route has not been reported. Most experts would initiate or complete the hepatitis B vaccine series but not give HBIG to a susceptible biting child (not fully immunized with HBV vaccine) who does not have oral mucosal disease when the amount of blood transferred from a child with chronic HBV infection is small.

In the common circumstance in which the HBsAg status of both the biting child and the victim is unknown, the risk of HBV transmission is extremely low because of the expected low seroprevalence of HBsAg in most groups of preschool-aged children, the low efficiency of disease transmission from bites, and routine hepatitis B immunization of preschool children. Serologic testing generally is not warranted for the biting child or the recipient of the bite, but each situation should be evaluated individually.

Efforts to decrease the risk of HBV transmission in child care through hygienic and environmental standards generally should focus on precautions for blood exposures and limiting potential saliva contamination of the environment. Toothbrushes and pacifiers should be labeled individually and should not be shared among children. Accidents that lead to bleeding or contamination with blood-containing body fluids by any child should be handled as follows: (1) disposable gloves should be used when cleaning or removing any blood or blood-containing body fluid spills; (2) the material should be absorbed using disposable towels or tissues; (3) the area should be disinfected with a freshly prepared solution of a 1:10 dilution of household bleach, applied for at least 2 minutes and wiped after the minimum contact time; (4) people involved in cleaning contaminated surfaces should avoid exposure of open skin lesions or mucous membranes to blood or blood-containing body fluids and to wound or tissue exudates; (5) hands should be washed thoroughly after exposure to blood or blood-containing body fluids after gloves are removed and discarded properly; (6) disposable towels or tissues should be used and discarded properly, and mops should be rinsed in disinfectant; (7) blood-contaminated paper towels, diapers, gloves, and other materials should be placed in a leak-proof plastic bag with a secure tie for disposal; and (8) staff members should be educated about standard precautions for handling blood or blood-containing material.

HIV INFECTION (ALSO SEE HUMAN IMMUNODEFICIENCY VIRUS INFECTION, P 418).
Children who enter child care should not be required to be tested for HIV or to disclose their HIV status. There is no need to restrict placement of HIV-infected children without risk factors for transmission of bloodborne pathogens in child care facilities to protect other children or staff members in these settings. Because HIV-infected children whose status is unknown may attend child care, standard precautions should be adopted for handling all spills of blood and blood-containing body fluids and wound exudates of all children, as described in the preceding HBV section.

The decision to admit known HIV-infected children to child care is best made on an individual basis by qualified people, including the child's physician, who are able to evaluate whether the child will receive optimal care in the program and whether an HIV-infected child poses a significant risk to others. Specifically, admission of each HIV-infected child with one or more potential risk factors for transmission of bloodborne pathogens (eg, frequent scratching, generalized dermatitis, or bleeding problems) should be assessed by the child's physician and the program director. Local or state public health authorities should be consulted as appropriate. If a bite results in blood exposure to either person involved, the US Public Health Service recommends evaluation, including consideration of postexposure prophylaxis (see Human Immunodeficiency Virus Infection, p 418). Information about a child who has immunodeficiency, regardless of cause, should be available to care providers who need to know how to help protect the child against other infections. For example, immunodeficient children exposed to measles or varicella should receive postexposure immunoprophylaxis as soon as possible (see Measles, p 489, and Varicella-Zoster Infections, p 774).

HIV-infected adults who do not have open and uncoverable skin lesions, other conditions that would allow contact with their body fluids, or a transmissible infectious disease may care for children in child care programs. However, immunosuppressed adults with HIV infection may be at increased risk of acquiring infectious agents from children and should consult their physician about the safety of continuing to work in child care. All child care providers, especially providers known to be HIV infected, should be notified immediately if they have been exposed to varicella, parvovirus B19, tuberculosis, diarrheal disease, or measles through children or other adults in the facility.

HEPATITIS C VIRUS. Transmission risks of HCV infection in child care settings are unknown. The general risk of HCV infection from percutaneous exposure to infected blood is estimated to be 10 times greater than that of HIV but lower than that of HBV. The risk of transmission of HCV via contamination of mucous membranes or broken skin probably is between the risk of transmission of HIV and the risk of transmission of HBV via contaminated blood. Standard precautions (see Hepatitis C, p 391) should be followed to prevent infection with HCV.

IMMUNIZATIONS

Routine immunization at appropriate ages is important for children in child care, because preschool-aged children can have high age-specific incidence rates of measles, rubella, *H influenzae* type b disease, hepatitis A, varicella, pertussis, rotavirus, influenza, and invasive *S pneumoniae* disease attributable to serotypes contained in respective vaccines.

Written documentation of immunizations appropriate for age should be provided by parents or guardians of all children in out-of-home child care. Unless contraindications exist or children have received medical, religious, or philosophic exemptions, immunization records should demonstrate complete immunization for age as shown in the recommended childhood and adolescent immunization schedules (see Fig 1.1–1.3, p 27–31). Immunization mandates by state for children in child care can be found online (**www.immunize.org/laws**).

Children who have not received recommended age-appropriate immunizations before enrollment should be immunized as soon as possible, and the series should be completed according to Fig 1.1–1.3 (p 27–31). In the interim, permitting unimmunized or inadequately immunized children to attend child care should depend on medical and legal counsel regarding how to handle the risk and whether to inform parents of enrolled infants and children about potential exposure to this risk. These children place other children at risk of contracting a vaccine-preventable disease. If a vaccine-preventable disease to which children may be susceptible occurs in the child care program, all underimmunized children should be excluded for the duration of possible exposure or until they have completed their immunizations.

All adults who work in a child care facility should have received all immunizations routinely recommended for adults (**www.cdc.gov/vaccines** [see adult immunization schedule]) according to guidelines for adult immunization of the Advisory Committee on Immunization Practices of the CDC, the American College of Physicians, the American College of Obstetricians and Gynecologists, and the American Academy of Family Physicians. Child care providers should be immunized against influenza annually and should be immunized appropriately against measles as shown in the adult immunization schedule. Requirements of the Occupational Safety and Health Administration (OSHA) state that employers must offer employees hepatitis B vaccine if they are, as a part of their duties, likely to come in contact with blood. Child care providers are expected to render first aid, which may expose them to blood. All child care providers should receive written information about hepatitis B disease and its complications as well as means of prevention with immunization.

Child care providers should be asked to document evidence of varicella immunity. Child care providers born after 1980 with a negative or uncertain history of varicella and no history of immunization should be immunized with 2 doses of varicella vaccine or undergo serologic testing for susceptibility; providers who are not immune should be offered 2 doses of varicella vaccine unless it is contraindicated medically. All child care providers should receive written information about varicella, particularly disease manifestations in adults, complications, and means of prevention.

Because HAV can cause symptomatic illness in adult contacts and because child care programs have been a source of infection in the community, hepatitis A vaccine in some circumstances may be justified (see Hepatitis A, p 361). However, because the prevalence of HAV infection does not seem to be significantly increased in staff members of child care centers in comparison with the prevalence in the general population and because routine HAV immunization of children 12 through 23 months of age and beyond is indicated, routine immunization of staff members is not recommended. During HAV outbreaks, immunization should be considered (see Hepatitis A, p 361).

All adults who work in child care facilities should receive a one-time dose of Tdap (tetanus toxoid, reduced diphtheria toxoid, and acellular pertussis) vaccine regardless of how recently they received their last dose of Td for booster immunization against tetanus, diphtheria, and pertussis. Pregnant women not immunized previously with Tdap should be immunized at more than 20 weeks' gestation, or if not immunized during pregnancy, they should receive Tdap immediately postpartum. For other recommendations for Tdap vaccine use in adults, including unimmunized or partially immunized adults, see Pertussis (p 553) and the adult immunization schedule.

General Practices

The following practices are recommended to decrease transmission of infectious agents in a child care setting:

- Each child care facility should have **written policies** for managing child and provider illness in child care.
- **Toilet areas and toilet-training equipment** should be maintained in sanitary condition.
- **Diaper-changing surfaces** should be nonporous and disinfected between uses. The changing surface should be covered with nonabsorbent paper liners large enough to cover the surface from the child's shoulders to beyond the child's feet. The liner is discarded after each use. If the surface becomes wet or soiled, it should be cleaned. The changing surface should be cleaned and disinfected after each use.
- **Diaper-changing procedures** should be posted at the changing area. Soiled disposable diapers, training pants, and soiled disposable wiping cloths should be discarded in a secure, hands-free, plastic-lined container with a lid. Diapers should contain all urine and stool and minimize fecal contamination of children, child care providers, environmental surfaces, and objects in the child care environment. Disposable diapers with absorbent gelling material or carboxymethylcellulose or single-unit reusable systems with an inner cotton lining attached to an outer waterproof covering that are changed as a unit should be used. Clothes should be worn over diapers while the child is in the child care facility. This clothing, including shoes, should be removed and placed where it will not have contact with diaper contents during the diaper change. Soiled clothing should be bagged and sent home for laundering. Both the child's and caregiver's hands should be washed after the diaper change is complete.

- **Diaper-changing areas** never should be located in or in proximity to food preparation areas and never should be used for temporary placement of food, drinks, or eating utensils.
- The use of **child-sized toilets** or access to steps and modified toilet seats that provide for easier maintenance should be encouraged. The use of potty chairs should be discouraged, but if used, potty chairs should be emptied into a toilet, cleaned in a utility sink, and disinfected after each use. Staff members should disinfect potty chairs, toilets, and diaper-changing areas with a freshly prepared solution of a 1:64 dilution of household bleach (one quarter cup of bleach diluted in 1 gallon of water) applied for at least 2 minutes and allowed to dry.
- **Written procedures for hand hygiene** should be established and enforced.[1] Handwashing sinks should be adjacent to all diaper-changing and toilet areas. These sinks should be washed and disinfected at least daily and should not be used for food preparation. Food and drinking utensils should not be washed in sinks in diaper-changing areas. Handwashing sinks should not be used for rinsing soiled clothing or for cleaning potty chairs. Children should have access to height-appropriate sinks, soap dispensers, and disposable paper towels. Children should not have independent access to alcohol-based hand sanitizing gels or use them without adult supervision, because they are flammable and toxic if ingested because of their high alcohol content. Alcohol-based sanitizing gels should be limited to areas where there are no sinks.
- Written **personal hygiene policies** for staff and children are necessary.
- Written **environmental sanitation policies and procedures** should include daily cleaning of floors, covering sandboxes, cleaning and sanitizing play tables, and cleaning and disinfecting spills of blood or body fluids and wound or tissue exudates. In general, routine housekeeping procedures using a freshly prepared solution of commercially available cleaner (eg, detergents, disinfectant detergents, or chemical germicides) compatible with most surfaces are satisfactory for cleaning spills of vomitus, urine, and feces. For spills of blood or blood-containing body fluids and of wound and tissue exudates, the material should be removed using gloves to avoid contamination of hands, and the area then should be disinfected using a freshly prepared solution of a 1:10 dilution of household bleach applied for at least 2 minutes and wiped with a disposable cloth after the minimum contact time.
- Each item of **sleep equipment** should be used only by a single child and should be cleaned weekly and before being used by another child. Crib mattresses should have a nonporous easy-to-wipe surface and should be cleaned and sanitized when soiled or wet. Sleeping cots should be stored so that contact with the sleeping surface of another mat does not occur. Bedding (sheets and blankets) should be assigned to each child and cleaned and sanitized when soiled or wet.
- Optimally, **toys** that are placed in children's mouths or otherwise contaminated by body secretions should be cleaned with water and detergent, sanitized, rinsed if the manufacturer's label on the product used requires it, and air-dried before handling by another child. All frequently touched toys in rooms that house infants and toddlers should be cleaned and sanitized daily. Toys in rooms for older continent children

---

[1] Centers for Disease Control and Prevention. Guideline for hand hygiene in health-care settings. Recommendations of the Healthcare Infection Control Practices Advisory Committee and the HICPAC/SHEA/APIC/IDSA Hand Hygiene Task Force. *MMWR Recomm Rep.* 2002;51(RR-16):1–45

should be cleaned at least weekly and when soiled. Soft, nonwashable toys should not be used in infant and toddler areas of child care programs.

- **Food** should be handled safely and appropriately to prevent growth of bacteria and to prevent contamination by enteropathogens, insects, or rodents.[1] Tables and countertops used for food preparation, food service, and eating should be cleaned and sanitized between uses and between preparation of raw and cooked food. People with signs or symptoms of illness, including vomiting, diarrhea, jaundice, or infectious skin lesions that cannot be covered or with potential foodborne pathogen infections should not be responsible for food handling. Hands should be washed using soap and water before handling food. Because of their frequent exposure to feces and children with enteric diseases, staff members whose primary function is the preparation of food should not change diapers. Except in home-based care, staff members who work with diapered children should not prepare food for, or serve food to, older groups of children. Staff members involved in changing diapers should not be involved in food preparation or serving on the same day. If doing both is necessary, staff members should prepare food before doing diaper changing, do both tasks for as few children as possible, and handle food only for infants and toddlers in their own group and only after thoroughly washing their hands. Caregivers who prepare food for infants should be aware of the importance of careful hand hygiene. Pasteurized milk and juice products should be served (see Appendix IX, Potentially Contaminated Food Products, p 917).

- The living quarters of **pets** should be enclosed and kept clean of waste to decrease the risk of human contact with the waste. Hands should be washed after handling all animals or animal wastes. Dogs and cats should be in good health, immunized appropriately for age, and kept away from child play areas and handled only with staff supervision. Such animals should be given flea-, tick-, and worm-control programs. Reptiles, rodents, amphibians, and baby poultry and their habitats should not be handled by children (see Diseases Transmitted by Animals [Zoonoses]: Household Pets, Including Nontraditional Pets, and Exposure to Animals in Public Settings, p 215).[2]

- Written policies that comply with local and state regulations for filing and regularly updating **immunization records** of each child and child care provider should be maintained. Children in group child care settings should receive all recommended immunizations, including annual influenza vaccine.

- Each child care program should use the services of a **health consultant** to assist in development and implementation of written policies for prevention and control of communicable diseases and provision of related health education to children, staff, and parents. The health consultant should conduct program observations to correct hazards and risky practices.

- The child care provider should, when registering each child, **inform parents of inclusion and exclusion policies and the need to share information about nationally notifiable infectious diseases** that could be communicable in the child or in any member of the immediate household to facilitate prompt reporting of disease and institution of any measures necessary to prevent transmission. The child care

---

[1] Centers for Disease Control and Prevention. Surveillance for foodborne disease outbreaks—United States, 2011. *MMWR Morb Mortal Wkly Rep.* 2011;60(35):1197–1202

[2] Centers for Disease Control and Prevention. Compendium of measures to prevent disease associated with animals in public settings, 2011: National Association of State Public Health Veterinarians, Inc. *MMWR Recomm Rep.* 2011;60(RR-4):1–24

provider or program director, after consulting with the program's health consultant or the responsible public health official, should follow recommendations of the consultant or public health official for **notification of parents** of children who attend the program about exposure of their child to a communicable disease.

- Local and/or state **public health authorities should be contacted** about cases of reportable diseases involving children or care providers in the child care setting.

- In settings where human milk is stored and delivered to infants, there should be a written policy and a quality-improvement program (as is done routinely for blood products) to ensure administration of human milk to the designated infant. Monitoring of the program results and developing protocols to deal with incidents when human milk inadvertently is fed to an infant other than the designated infant also are necessary (see Human Milk Banks, p 131). Health care facilities have developed policies that could be adapted to the child care setting to address such incidents. These policies require documentation, counseling, observation of the affected infant for signs of infection, and verification of the donor mother's infectious disease status. Meticulous labeling, storage, and verification of recipient identity before providing human milk should be practiced by child care providers.

····································

SCHOOL HEALTH

Clustering of children together in a school setting provides opportunities for transmission of infectious diseases. Determining the likelihood that infection in one or more children will pose a risk for schoolmates depends on an understanding of several factors: (1) the mechanism by which the organism causing infection is spread; (2) the ease with which the organism is spread (contagion); and (3) the likelihood that classmates are immune because of immunization or previous infection. Decisions to intervene to prevent spread of infection within a school should be made through collaboration among school officials, local public health officials, and health care professionals, considering the availability and effectiveness of specific methods of prevention and risk of serious complications from infection.

Generic methods for control and prevention of spread of infection in the school setting include the following:

- For vaccine-preventable diseases, documentation of the immunization status of enrolled children should be reviewed. Schools have a legal responsibility to ensure that students have been immunized against vaccine-preventable diseases at the time of enrollment, in accordance with state requirements (see Appendix XII, State Immunization Requirements for School Attendance, p 934). Although specific laws vary by state, most states require proof of protection against poliomyelitis, tetanus, pertussis, diphtheria, measles, mumps, rubella, and varicella. Immunizations against hepatitis B (HBV), varicella, and meningococcal disease are mandatory in many states (**www. immunize.org/laws** or **www.cdc.gov/other.htm#states**). Hepatitis A virus (HAV) immunization is required for school entry in some states. In 2007, the Centers for Disease Control and Prevention recommended that all states require that children entering elementary school have received 2 doses of varicella vaccine or have other evidence of immunity to varicella. Policies established by state health departments concerning exclusion of unimmunized children and exemptions for children with certain underlying medical conditions and families with religious or philosophic objection to immunization should be followed. Exemption rates by state can be found at **www2. cdc.gov/nip/schoolsurv/rptgmenu.asp.**

* Infected children should be excluded from school until they no longer are considered contagious (for recommendations on specific diseases, see relevant disease-specific chapters in Section 3).
* In some instances, administration of appropriate antimicrobial therapy will limit further spread of infection (eg, streptococcal pharyngitis and pertussis).
* Antimicrobial prophylaxis administered to close contacts of children with infections caused by specific pathogens may be warranted in some circumstances (eg, meningococcal infection and pertussis).
* Temporary school closing can be used in limited circumstances: (1) to prevent spread of infection; (2) when an infection is expected to affect a large number of susceptible students and available control measures are considered inadequate (eg, outbreak of influenza); or (3) when an infection is expected to have a high rate of morbidity or mortality.

Physicians involved with school health should be aware of current public health guidelines to prevent and control infectious diseases. In all circumstances requiring intervention to prevent spread of infection within the school setting, the privacy of children who are infected should be protected.

Diseases Preventable by Routine Childhood Immunization

Children and adolescents immunized according to the recommended childhood and adolescent immunization schedule (see Fig 1.1–1.3, p 27–31) should be considered to be protected against diseases for which they were immunized. Disease-specific chapters should be consulted for details.

Measles and varicella vaccines have been demonstrated to provide protection in some susceptible people if administered within 72 hours after exposure. Measles or varicella immunization should be recommended immediately for all nonimmune people during a measles or varicella outbreak, respectively, except for people with a contraindication to immunization. Many people without evidence of immunity may not yet have been exposed; therefore, vaccinating at any stage of an outbreak can prevent disease. Students immunized for measles or varicella for the first time under these circumstances should be allowed to return to school after immunization. Susceptible children and adolescents 12 months of age or older exposed to HAV should receive single-antigen HAV vaccine (or Immune Globulin) within 14 days after exposure. People who are immunocompromised, are older than 40 years of age, or have liver disease should receive Immune Globulin (see Hepatitis A, p 361).[1]

Mumps and rubella vaccines given after exposure have not been demonstrated to prevent infection among susceptible contacts, but immunization should be administered to unimmunized students to protect them from infection from subsequent exposure.

---

[1] Advisory Committee on Immunization Practices (ACIP) Centers for Disease Control and Prevention (CDC). Update: Prevention of hepatitis A after exposure to hepatitis A virus and in international travelers. Updated recommendations of the Advisory Committee on Immunization Practices (ACIP). *MMWR Morb Mortal Wkly Rep.* 2007;56(41):1080–1084

Infections Spread by the Respiratory Route

Some pathogens that cause severe lower respiratory tract disease in infants and toddlers, such as respiratory syncytial virus and metapneumovirus, are of less concern in healthy school-aged children. Respiratory tract viruses, however, are associated with exacerbations of reactive airway disease and an increase in the incidence of otitis media and can cause significant complications for children with chronic respiratory tract disease, such as cystic fibrosis, or for children who are immunocompromised. Infection control principles of respiratory etiquette—hand hygiene and covering mouth and nose with tissue when coughing or sneezing (if no tissue is available, use the upper shoulder or elbow area rather than hands)—should be taught and implemented in schools.

Influenza virus infection is a common cause of febrile respiratory tract disease and school absenteeism. Annual influenza immunization should be administered to children and adults 6 months of age and older (see Influenza Vaccine, p 445).

Mycoplasma pneumoniae causes upper and lower respiratory tract infection in school-aged children, and outbreaks of *M pneumoniae* infection occur in communities and schools. The nonspecific symptoms and signs associated with this organism make distinguishing *M pneumoniae* infection from other causes of respiratory tract illness difficult. Antimicrobial therapy does not necessarily eradicate the organism or prevent spread. Thus, intervention to prevent secondary infection in the school setting is difficult. Mass prophylaxis may be considered in certain limited outbreak situations. *Mycoplasma* outbreaks in schools should be reported to the local health department.

Symptomatic contacts of students with pharyngitis attributable to group A streptococcal infection should be evaluated and treated if streptococcal infection is demonstrated. Infected students may return to school 24 hours after initiation of antimicrobial therapy. Students awaiting results of culture or antigen-detection tests who are not receiving antimicrobial therapy may attend school during the culture incubation period unless there is an associated fever or the infection involves a child with poor hygiene and poor control of secretions. Asymptomatic contacts usually require neither evaluation nor therapy.

Bacterial meningitis in school-aged children may be caused by *Neisseria meningitidis*. Infected people are not considered contagious after 24 hours of appropriate antimicrobial therapy. After discharge from the hospital, they pose no risk to classmates and may return to school. Prophylactic antimicrobial therapy is not recommended for school contacts in most circumstances. Close observation of contacts is recommended, and they should be evaluated promptly if a febrile illness develops. Students who have been exposed to oral secretions of an infected student, such as through kissing or sharing of food and drink, should receive chemoprophylaxis (see Meningococcal Infections, p 500). Immunization of school contacts with meningococcal conjugate vaccine (MCV4), which in the United States contains antigens for serogroups A, C, Y, and W-135, should be considered in consultation with local public health authorities if evidence suggests an outbreak within a school attributable to one of the meningococcal serogroups contained in the vaccine. Immunization recommendations for administration of MCV4 for all adolescents 11 through 18 years of age and for certain high-risk groups 2 through 10 years of age and 19 through 55 years of age should be followed (see Meningococcal Infections, p 500.

Students and staff members with documented pertussis should be excluded until they have received at least 5 days of the recommended course of azithromycin, clarithromycin, or erythromycin therapy and are able to participate in school-related activities. In some circumstances, chemoprophylaxis is recommended for their school contacts (see Pertussis, p 553). Tetanus toxoid, reduced diphtheria toxoid, and acellular pertussis (Tdap) vaccine should be substituted for a single dose of tetanus and diphtheria toxoids (Td) vaccine for children 7 years of age or older and adults in the primary catch-up series or as a booster dose if age appropriate (see Fig 1.1–1.3, p 27–31).

Before adolescence, children with tuberculosis generally are not contagious, but students who are in close contact with a child, teacher, or other adult with tuberculosis should be evaluated for infection, including tuberculin skin testing or interferon-gamma release assay (see Tuberculosis, p 736). An adolescent or adult with tuberculosis almost always is the source of infection for young children. If an adult source outside the school is identified (eg, parent or grandparent of a student), efforts should be made to determine whether other students have been exposed to the same source and whether they warrant evaluation for infection.

Children with erythema infectiosum should be allowed to attend school, because the period of contagion occurs before a rash is evident. Parvovirus B19 infection poses no risk of significant illness for healthy classmates, although aplastic crisis can develop in infected children and adults with sickle cell disease or other hemoglobinopathies. The relatively low risk of fetal damage should be explained to pregnant students and teachers exposed to children in the early stages of parvovirus B19 infection, 5 to 10 days before appearance of the rash. Exposed pregnant women should be referred to their physician for counseling and possible serologic testing.

Infections Spread by Direct Contact

Infection and infestation of skin, eyes, and hair can spread through direct contact with the infected area or through contact with contaminated hands or fomites, such as hair brushes, hats, and clothing. *Staphylococcus aureus* (including methicillin-resistant *S aureus* [MRSA]) and group A streptococcal organisms may colonize skin, oropharynx, or nasal mucosa of asymptomatic people. Lesions may develop when these organisms are passed from a person with infected skin to another person. Organisms also can be transmitted to open skin lesions in the same child or to other children. Although most skin infections attributable to *S aureus* and group A streptococcal organisms are minor and require only topical or oral antimicrobial therapy, person-to-person spread should be interrupted by appropriate treatment whenever lesions are recognized. Local and systemic infections associated with MRSA pose a diagnostic and therapeutic challenge (see Staphylococcal Infections, p 653). Exclusion of any infected child with an open or draining lesion that cannot be covered is recommended.

Herpes simplex virus (HSV) infection of the mouth and skin is common among school-aged children. Infection is spread through direct contact with herpetic lesions or asymptomatic shedding of virus from oral or genital secretions. "Cold sore" lesions of herpes labialis represent active infection, but no evidence suggests that these students pose any greater risk to their classmates than do unidentified asymptomatic shedders. For immuno-compromised children and for children with open skin lesions (eg, severe eczema), exposure to another child with HSV infection may pose an increased risk of HSV acquisition and of severe or disseminated infection. Because of the frequency of symptomatic and asymptomatic shedding of HSV among classmates and staff members, careful hygienic practices are the best means of preventing infection (see Herpes Simplex, p 398).

Infectious conjunctivitis can be caused by bacterial (eg, nontypable *Haemophilus influenzae* and *Streptococcus pneumoniae*) or viral (eg, adenoviruses, enteroviruses, and HSV) pathogens. Bacterial conjunctivitis is less common in children older than 5 years of age. Infection occurs through direct contact or through contamination of hands followed by autoinoculation. Respiratory tract spread from large droplets also may occur. Topical antimicrobial therapy is indicated for bacterial conjunctivitis, which usually is distinguished by a purulent exudate. HSV conjunctivitis usually is unilateral and may be accompanied by vesicles on adjacent skin and preauricular adenopathy. Evaluation of HSV conjunctivitis by an ophthalmologist and administration of specific antiviral therapy are indicated. Conjunctivitis attributable to adenoviruses or enteroviruses is self-limited and requires no specific antiviral therapy. Spread of infection is minimized by careful hand hygiene, and infected people should be presumed contagious until symptoms have resolved. Except when viral or bacterial conjunctivitis is accompanied by systemic signs of illness, infected children should be allowed to remain in school once any indicated therapy is implemented, unless their behavior is such that close contact with other students cannot be avoided. The local health department should be notified of an outbreak of conjunctivitis.

Fungal infections of the skin and hair are spread by direct person-to-person contact and through contact with contaminated surfaces or objects. *Trichophyton tonsurans,* the predominant cause of tinea capitis, remains viable for long periods on combs, hair brushes, furniture, and fabric. The fungi that cause tinea corporis (ringworm) are transmissible by direct contact. Tinea cruris (jock itch) and tinea pedis (athlete's foot) occur in adolescents and young adults. The fungi that cause these infections have a predilection for moist areas and are spread through direct contact and contact with contaminated surfaces.

Students with fungal infections of the skin or scalp should be encouraged to receive treatment both for their benefit and to prevent spread of infection. However, lack of treatment does not necessitate exclusion from school unless the nature of their contact with other students could potentiate spread. Students with tinea capitis should be instructed not to share combs, hair brushes, hats, or hair ornaments with classmates until they have been treated. Students with tinea pedis should be excluded from swimming pools and from walking barefoot on locker room and shower floors until treatment has been initiated. Spread of infection by students with tinea capitis may be decreased by use of selenium sulfide shampoos, but treatment requires systemic antifungal therapy (see Tinea Capitis, p 712). Sharing of towels and shower shoes during sports activities should be discouraged.

Sarcoptes scabiei (scabies) and *Pediculus capitis* (head lice) are transmitted primarily through person-to-person contact. The scabies parasite survives on clothing for only 3 to 4 days without skin contact. Combs, hair brushes, hats, and hair ornaments can transmit head lice, but away from the scalp, lice do not remain viable.

Children identified as having scabies or head lice should be referred for treatment at the end of the school day and subsequently excluded from school only until treatment recommended by the child's health care professional has been started. School contacts generally should not be treated prophylactically. Caregivers who have prolonged skin-to-skin contact with students infested with scabies may benefit from prophylactic treatment (see Scabies, p 641).

Shampooing with an appropriate pediculicide and manually removing nits by combing usually are effective in eradicating viable lice. Manual removal of nits after treatment with a pediculicide is not necessary to prevent reinfestation (see Pediculosis Capitis, p 543).

Infections Spread by the Fecal-Oral Route

For developmentally typical school-aged children, pathogens spread via the fecal-oral route constitute a risk only if the infected person fails to maintain good hygiene, including hand hygiene after toilet use, or if contaminated food is shared between or among schoolmates.

Outbreaks attributable to HAV can occur in schools, but these outbreaks usually are associated with community outbreaks. Schoolroom exposure generally does not pose an appreciable risk of infection, and administration of HAV vaccine or Immune Globulin to susceptible people for postexposure prophylaxis is not indicated. However, if transmission within a school is documented, HAV vaccine should be considered as a means of prophylaxis and prolonged protection for immunocompetent people 12 months through 40 years of age (see Hepatitis A, p 361). If an outbreak occurs, consultation with local public health authorities is indicated before initiating interventions. Ultimately, implementation of the recommended immunization of preschool-aged children with HAV vaccine should help reduce school outbreaks of disease.

Enteroviral infections probably are spread via the oral-oral route as well as by the fecal-oral route. The incidence is so high when outbreaks occur during summer and fall epidemics that control measures specifically aimed at the school classroom likely would be futile. Person-to-person spread of bacterial, viral, and parasitic enteropathogens within school settings occurs infrequently, but foodborne outbreaks attributable to enteric pathogens can occur. Symptomatic people with gastroenteritis attributable to an enteric pathogen should be excluded until symptoms resolve.

Children in diapers at any age and in any setting constitute a far greater risk of spread of gastrointestinal tract infection attributable to enteric pathogens. Guidelines for control of these infections in child care settings should be applied for school-aged students with developmental disabilities who are diapered (see Children in Out-of-Home Child Care, p 133).

Infections Spread by Blood and Body Fluids

Contact with blood and other body fluids of another person requires more intimate exposure than usually occurs in the school setting. However, care required for children with developmental disabilities may result in exposure of caregivers to urine, saliva, and in some cases, blood. The application of Standard Precautions for prevention of transmission of bloodborne pathogens, as recommended for children in out-of-home child care, prevents spread of infection from these exposures (see Children in Out-of-Home Child Care, p 133). School staff members who routinely provide acute care for children with epistaxis or bleeding from injury should wear disposable gloves and use appropriate hand hygiene measures immediately after glove removal for protection from bloodborne pathogens. Staff members at the scene of an injury or bleeding incident who do not have access to gloves need to use some type of barrier to avoid exposure to blood or blood-containing materials, use appropriate hand hygiene measures, and adhere to proper protocols for handling contaminated material. Routine use of these precautions helps avoid the necessity of identifying children known to be infected with human immunodeficiency virus (HIV), hepatitis B virus (HBV), or hepatitis C virus (HCV) and acknowledges that an unknown exposure poses at least as much risk as does exposure from an identified infected child.

Students infected with HIV, HBV, or HCV do not need to be identified to school personnel. Because HIV-, HBV-, and HCV-infected children and adolescents will not be identified, policies and procedures to manage all potential exposures to blood or blood-containing materials should be established and implemented. Parents and students should be educated about the types of exposure that present a risk for school contacts. Although a student's right to privacy should be maintained, decisions about activities at school should be made by parents or guardians together with a physician on a case-by-case basis, keeping the health needs of the infected student and the student's classmates in mind.

Prospective studies to aid in determining the risk of transmission of HIV, HBV, or HCV during contact sports among high school students have not been performed, but the available evidence indicates that risk is low. Guidelines for management of bleeding injuries have been developed for college and professional athletes in recognition of the possibility of unidentified HIV, HBV, or HCV infection in any competitor. The American Academy of Pediatrics (AAP) has published recommendations for prevention of transmission of HIV and other bloodborne pathogens in the athletic setting.[1,2]

- Athletes infected with HIV, HBV, or HCV should be allowed to participate in competitive sports.
- Physicians should respect the rights of infected athletes to confidentiality. The infection status of patients should not be disclosed to other participants or the staff of athletic programs.
- Testing for bloodborne pathogens should not be mandatory for athletes or sports participants.
- Pediatricians are encouraged to counsel athletes who are infected with HIV, HBV, or HCV and assure them that they have a low risk of infecting other competitors. Infected athletes should consider choosing a sport in which this risk is minimal. This may be protective for other participants and for infected athletes themselves, decreasing their possible exposure to bloodborne pathogens other than the one(s) with which they are infected. Wrestling and boxing probably have the greatest potential for contamination of injured skin by blood. The AAP opposes boxing as a sport for youth for other reasons.[3]
- Athletic programs should inform athletes and their parents that the program is operating under the policies of the aforementioned recommendations and that the athletes have a low risk of becoming infected with a bloodborne pathogen.

[1] American Academy of Pediatrics, Committee on Sports Medicine and Fitness. Human immunodeficiency virus and other blood-borne viral pathogens in the athletic setting. *Pediatrics.* 1999;104(6):1400–1403 (Reaffirmed October 2008)

[2] Rice SG; American Academy of Pediatrics, Council on Sports Medicine and Fitness. Medical conditions affecting sports participation. *Pediatrics.* 2008;121(4):841–848 (Reaffirmed May 2011)

[3] American Academy of Pediatrics, Council on Sports Medicine and Fitness; Canadian Paediatric Society, Healthy Active Living and Sports Medicine Committee. Boxing participation by children and adolescents. *Pediatrics.* 2011;128(3):617–623

- Clinicians and staff of athletic programs should promote HBV immunization among all athletes and among coaches, athletic trainers, equipment handlers, laundry personnel, and any other people at risk of exposure to blood of athletes as an occupational hazard.
- Each coach and athletic trainer must receive training in first aid and emergency care and in prevention of transmission of bloodborne pathogens in the athletic setting. These staff members then can help implement these recommendations.
- Coaches and members of the health care team should educate athletes about precautions described in these recommendations. Such education should include the greater risks of transmission of HIV and other bloodborne pathogens through sexual activity and needle sharing during the use of injection drugs, including anabolic steroids. Athletes should be told not to share personal items, such as razors, toothbrushes, and nail clippers, that might be contaminated with blood.
- Depending on law in some states, schools may need to comply with Occupational Safety and Health Administration (OSHA) regulations[1] for prevention of bloodborne pathogens. The athletic program must determine what rules apply. Compliance with OSHA regulations is a reasonable and recommended precaution even if this is not required specifically by the state.
- The following precautions should be adopted in sports with direct body contact and other sports in which an athlete's blood or other body fluids visibly tinged with blood may contaminate the skin or mucous membranes of other participants or staff members of the athletic program. Even if these precautions are adopted, the risk that a participant or staff member may become infected with a bloodborne pathogen in the athletic setting will not be eliminated entirely.
  - Athletes must cover existing cuts, abrasions, wounds, or other areas of broken skin with an occlusive dressing before and during participation. Caregivers should cover their own damaged skin to prevent transmission of infection to or from an injured athlete.
  - Disposable, water-impervious vinyl or latex gloves should be worn to avoid contact with blood or other body fluids visibly tinged with blood and any objects, such as equipment, bandages, or uniforms, contaminated with these fluids. Hands should be cleaned with soap and water or an alcohol-based antiseptic agent as soon as possible after gloves are removed.
  - Athletes with active bleeding should be removed from competition as soon as possible until bleeding is stopped. Wounds should be cleaned with soap and water. Skin antiseptic agents may be used if soap and water are not available. Wounds must be covered with an occlusive dressing that will remain intact and not become soaked through during further play before athletes return to competition.
  - Athletes should be advised to report injuries and wounds in a timely fashion before or during competition.
  - Minor cuts or abrasions that are not bleeding do not require interruption of play but can be cleaned and covered during scheduled breaks. During these breaks, if an athlete's equipment or uniform fabric is wet with blood, the equipment should be cleaned and disinfected (see next bullet), or the uniform should be replaced.

---

[1] Occupational Safety and Health Administration (**www.osha.gov**)

- Equipment and playing areas contaminated with blood must be cleaned using gloves and disposable absorbent material until all visible blood is gone and then disinfected with an appropriate germicide, such as a freshly made bleach solution containing 1 part bleach in 10 parts of water.[1] The decontaminated equipment or area should be in contact with the bleach solution for at least 30 seconds. The area then may be wiped with a disposable cloth after the minimum contact time or allowed to air dry.
- Emergency care must not be delayed because gloves or other protective equipment are not available. If the caregiver does not have appropriate protective equipment, a towel may be used to cover the wound until an off-the-field location is reached where gloves can be used during more definitive treatment.
- Breathing bags (eg, Ambu manual resuscitators) and oropharyngeal airways should be available for use during resuscitation.
- Equipment handlers, laundry personnel, and janitorial staff must be educated in proper procedures for handling washable or disposable materials contaminated with blood.
- For guidelines on control and prevention of MRSA in athletes and other school settings, see Staphylococcal Infections (p 653).

··

INFECTION CONTROL AND PREVENTION FOR HOSPITALIZED CHILDREN

Health care-associated infections are a major cause of morbidity and mortality in hospitalized children, particularly children in intensive care units. Hand hygiene before and after each patient contact remains the single most important practice in prevention and control of health care-associated infections. A comprehensive set of guidelines for preventing and controlling health care-associated infections, including isolation precautions, personnel health recommendations, and guidelines for prevention of postoperative and device-related infections, can be found on the Centers for Disease Control and Prevention (CDC) Web site (**www.cdc.gov/hicpac/pubs.html**). Guidelines for prevention of intravascular catheter-related infections are available.[2] Additional guidelines are available from the principal infection control societies in the United States, the Society for Healthcare Epidemiology of America and the Association for Professionals in Infection Control and Epidemiology, as well as subspecialty societies and regulatory agencies, such as the Occupational Safety and Health Administration (OSHA). The Cystic Fibrosis Foundation published an evidence-based guideline for prevention of transmission of infectious agents among cystic fibrosis patients in 2003. The Joint Commission also has established infection control standards. Physicians and infection control professionals should be familiar with this increasingly complex array of guidelines, regulations, and standards. Ongoing infection prevention and control programs should educate, implement, reinforce, document, and evaluate recommendations on a regular basis.

---

[1] Centers for Disease Control and Prevention. Guidelines for environmental infection control in health-care facilities. Recommendations of CDC and the Healthcare Infection Control Practices Advisory Committee (HICPAC). *MMWR Recomm Rep.* 2003;52(RR-10):1–42

[2] O'Grady NP, Alexander M, Burns LA, et al; Healthcare Infection Control Practices Advisory Committee. Guidelines for the prevention of intravascular catheter-related infections. *Am J Infect Control.* 2011;39 (4 Suppl 1):S1–S34

Isolation Precautions

Isolation precautions are designed to protect hospitalized children, health care personnel, and visitors from health care-associated infections. The Healthcare Infection Control Practices Advisory Committee in 2007 updated evidence-based isolation guidelines for preventing transmission of infectious agents in health care settings.[1] Adherence to these isolation policies, supplemented by health care facility policies and procedures for other aspects of infection and environmental control and occupational health, should result in reduced transmission and safe patient care. Adaptations should be made according to the conditions and population served by each facility.

Routine and optimal performance of **Standard Precautions** is appropriate for care of all patients regardless of diagnosis or suspected or confirmed infection status. In addition to Standard Precautions, pathogen- and syndrome-based **Transmission-Based Precautions** are used when caring for patients who are infected or colonized with pathogens transmitted by airborne, droplet, or contact routes.

STANDARD PRECAUTIONS

Standard Precautions are used to prevent transmission of all infectious agents through contact with any body fluid except sweat (regardless of whether these fluids contain visible blood), nonintact skin, or mucous membranes. Barrier techniques are recommended to decrease exposure of health care personnel to body fluids. Precautions are used with all patients when exposure to blood and body fluids is anticipated, because medical history and examination cannot reliably identify all patients infected with human immunodeficiency virus or other bloodborne infectious agents. Standard Precautions decrease transmission of microorganisms from patients who are not recognized as harboring potential pathogens, such as antimicrobial-resistant bacteria. See Table 2.8, p 162, for new elements added to Standard Precautions (respiratory hygiene/cough etiquette). Standard Precautions include the following practices:

- **Hand hygiene**[2] is necessary before and after all patient contact and after touching blood, body fluids, secretions, excretions, and contaminated items, whether gloves are worn or not. Hand hygiene should be performed either with alcohol-based agents or soap and water before wearing and immediately after removing gloves, between patient contacts, and when otherwise indicated to avoid transfer of microorganisms to other patients and to items in the environment. When hands are visibly dirty or contaminated with proteinaceous material, such as blood or other body fluids, hands should be washed with soap and water for at least 20 seconds. When exposure to spores (eg, *Clostridium difficile*) or norovirus is likely, handwashing with soap and water is preferred.

---

[1] Centers for Disease Control and Prevention. Guideline for isolation precautions: preventing transmission of infectious agents in healthcare settings 2007. Recommendations of the Healthcare Infection Control Practices Advisory Committee. Atlanta, GA: Centers for Disease Control and Prevention; 2007. Available at: **www.cdc. gov/ncidod/dhqp/pdf/guidelines/isolation2007.pdf**

[2] Centers for Disease Control and Prevention. Guideline for hand hygiene in health-care settings. Recommendations of the Healthcare Infection Control Practices Advisory Committee and the HICPAC/SHEA/APIC/IDSA Hand Hygiene Task Force. *MMWR Recomm Rep.* 2002;51(RR-16):1–45

Table 2.8. Recommendations for Application of Standard Precautions for Care of All Patients in All Health Care Settings

Component	Recommendations
Hand hygiene	Before and after each patient contact, regardless of whether gloves are used. After touching blood, body fluids, secretions, excretions, or contaminated items; immediately after removing gloves. Alcohol-containing antiseptic hand rubs preferred except when hands are soiled visibly with blood or other proteinaceous materials or if exposure to spores (eg, *Clostridium difficile, Bacillus anthracis*) is likely to have occurred.
Personal protective equipment (PPE)	
Gloves	For touching blood, body fluids, secretions, excretions, or contaminated items; for touching mucous membranes and nonintact skin.
Gown	During procedures and patient-care activities when contact of clothing/exposed skin with blood/body fluids, secretions, and excretions is anticipated.
Mask, eye protection (goggles), face shield	During procedures and patient-care activities likely to generate splashes or sprays of blood, body fluids, or secretions, especially suctioning and endotracheal intubation, to protect health care personnel. For patient protection, use of a mask by the person inserting an epidural anesthesia needle or performing myelograms when prolonged exposure of the puncture site is likely to occur.
Soiled patient-care equipment	Handle in a manner that prevents transfer of microorganisms to others and to the environment; wear gloves if visibly contaminated; perform hand hygiene.
Environmental control	Develop procedures for routine care, cleaning, and disinfection of environmental surfaces, especially frequently touched surfaces in patient care areas.
Textiles (linens) and laundry	Handle in a manner that prevents transfer of microorganisms to others and the environment.

Table 2.8. Recommendations for Application of Standard Precautions for Care of All Patients in All Health Care Settings, continued

Component	Recommendations
Injection practices (use of needles and other sharps)	Do not recap, bend, break, or hand manipulate used needles; if recapping is required, use a one-handed scoop technique only; use needle-free safety devices when available; place used sharps in conveniently placed, puncture-resistant container. Use a sterile, single-use, disposable needle and syringe for each injection given. Single-dose medication vials are preferred when medications are administered to more than one patient.
Patient resuscitation	Use mouthpiece, resuscitation bag, or other ventilation devices to prevent contact with mouth and oral secretions.
Patient placement	Prioritize for single-patient room if patient is at increased risk of transmission, is likely to contaminate the environment, does not maintain appropriate hygiene, or is at increased risk of acquiring infection or developing adverse outcome following infection.
Respiratory hygiene/cough etiquette (source containment of infectious respiratory tract secretions in symptomatic patients) beginning at the initial point of encounter (eg, triage and reception areas in emergency departments and physician offices)	Instruct symptomatic people to cover mouth/nose when sneezing/coughing; use tissues and dispose in no-touch receptacle; observe hand hygiene after soiling of hands with respiratory tract secretions; wear surgical mask if tolerated or maintain spatial separation more than 3 feet, if possible.

- **Gloves** (clean, nonsterile) should be worn when touching blood, body fluids, secretions, excretions, and items contaminated with these fluids except for wiping a child's tears or nose or for routine wet diaper changing. Clean gloves should be used before touching mucous membranes and nonintact skin. Gloves should be changed between tasks and procedures on the same patient after contact with material that may contain a high concentration of microorganisms (eg, purulent drainage).
- **Masks, eye protection, and face shields** should be worn to protect mucous membranes of the eyes, nose, and mouth during procedures and patient care activities likely to generate splashes or sprays of blood, body fluids, secretions, or excretions.

  Masks should be worn when placing a catheter or injecting material into the spinal canal or subdural space (eg, during myelograms and spinal or epidural anesthesia).
- **Nonsterile gowns** that are fluid-resistant will protect skin and prevent soiling of clothing during procedures and patient care activities likely to generate splashes or sprays of blood, body fluids, secretions, or excretions. Soiled gowns should be removed promptly and carefully to avoid contamination of clothing.
- **Patient care equipment** that has been used should be handled in a manner that prevents skin or mucous membrane exposures and contamination of clothing or the environment.
- **All used textiles (linens)** are considered to be contaminated and should be handled, transported, and processed in a manner that prevents aerosolization of microorganisms, skin and mucous membrane exposure, and contamination of clothing.
- **Safe injection practices:** Bloodborne pathogen exposure of health care personnel should be avoided by taking precautions to prevent injuries caused by needles, scalpels, and other sharp instruments or devices during procedures; when handling sharp instruments after procedures; when cleaning used instruments; and during disposal of used needles. To prevent needlestick injuries, needles should not be recapped, purposely bent or broken by hand, removed from disposable syringes, or otherwise manipulated by hand. After use, disposable syringes and needles, scalpel blades, and other sharp items should be placed in puncture-resistant containers for disposal; puncture-resistant containers should be located as close as practical to the use area. Large–bore reusable needles should be placed in a puncture-resistant container located close to the site of use for transport to the reprocessing area to ensure maximal patient safety. Sharp devices with safety features are preferred whenever such devices have function equivalent to conventional sharp devices and should be evaluated and implemented by users. Single-dose vials of medication are preferred.
- **Mouthpieces, resuscitation bags, and other ventilation devices** should be available in all patient care areas and used instead of mouth-to-mouth resuscitation.

TRANSMISSION-BASED PRECAUTIONS

Transmission-Based Precautions are designed for patients documented or suspected to have colonization or infection with pathogens for which additional precautions beyond **Standard Precautions** are recommended to prevent transmission. The 3 types of transmission routes on which these precautions are based are: airborne, droplet, and contact.

- **Airborne transmission** occurs by dissemination of airborne droplet nuclei (small-particle residue [≤5 μm in size] of evaporated droplets containing microorganisms that remain suspended in the air for long periods) or small respirable particles containing the infectious agent or spores. Microorganisms transmitted by the airborne route can be dispersed widely by air currents and can be inhaled by a susceptible host within the same room or a long distance from the source patient, depending on environmental factors. Special air handling and ventilation are required to prevent airborne transmission. Examples of microorganisms transmitted by airborne droplet nuclei are *Mycobacterium tuberculosis*, rubeola (measles) virus, and varicella-zoster virus. Specific recommendations for **Airborne Precautions** are as follows:

- Provide infected or colonized patients with a single-patient room (if unavailable, consult an infection control professional).
- Use special ventilation, including 6 to 12 air changes per hour, air flow direction from surrounding area to the room, and room air exhausted directly to the outside or recirculated through a high-efficiency particulate air (HEPA) filter.
- If infectious pulmonary tuberculosis is suspected or proven, respiratory protective devices (ie, National Institute for Occupational Safety and Health-certified personally "fitted" and "sealing" respirator, such as N95 or N100 respirators, powered air-purifying respirators) should be worn while inside the patient's room.
- Susceptible health care personnel should not enter rooms of patients with measles or varicella-zoster virus infections. If susceptible people must enter the room of a patient with measles or varicella infection or an immunocompromised patient with local or disseminated zoster infection, a mask or a respiratory protective device (eg, N95 respirator) that has been fit-tested should be worn. People with proven immunity to these viruses need not wear a mask.

- **Droplet transmission** occurs when droplets containing microorganisms generated from an infected person, primarily during coughing, sneezing, or talking and during the performance of certain procedures, such as suctioning and bronchoscopy, are propelled a short distance (3 feet or less) and deposited into conjunctivae, nasal mucosa, or the mouth. Because these relatively large droplets do not remain suspended in air, special air handling and ventilation are not required to prevent droplet transmission. Droplet transmission should not be confused with airborne transmission via droplet nuclei, which are much smaller. Specific recommendations for **Droplet Precautions** are as follows:
  - Provide the patient with a single-patient room if possible. If unavailable, consider cohorting patients infected with the same organism. Spatial separation of more than 3 feet should be maintained between the bed of the infected patient and the beds of the other patients in multiple bed rooms. Standard precautions plus a mask should be used.
  - Wear a mask on entry into the room or into the cubical space.
  Specific illnesses and infections requiring **Droplet Precautions** include the following:
- Adenovirus pneumonia
- Diphtheria (pharyngeal)
- *Haemophilus influenzae* type b (invasive)
- Influenza
- Mumps
- *Mycoplasma pneumoniae*
- *Neisseria meningitidis* (invasive)
- Parvovirus B19 during the phase of illness before onset of rash in immunocompetent patients (see Parvovirus B19, p 539)
- Pertussis
- Plague (pneumonic)

- Rhinovirus
- Rubella
- Severe acute respiratory syndrome (SARS): airborne preferred; droplet if unavailable
- Group A streptococcal pharyngitis, pneumonia, or scarlet fever
- Viral hemorrhagic fevers

- **Contact Transmission** is the most common route of transmission of health care–associated infections. *Direct contact* transmission involves a direct body surface-to-body surface contact and physical transfer of microorganisms between a person with infection or colonization and a susceptible host, such as occurs when a health care professional turns a patient, gives a patient a bath, or performs other patient care activities that require direct personal contact. Direct contact transmission also can occur between 2 patients when one serves as the source of the infectious microorganisms and the other serves as a susceptible host. *Indirect contact* transmission involves contact of a susceptible host with a contaminated intermediate object, usually inanimate, such as contaminated instruments, needles, dressings, toys, or contaminated hands that are not cleansed or gloves that are not changed between patients.

  Specific recommendations for **Contact Precautions** are as follows:
  - Provide the patient with a single-patient room if possible. If unavailable, cohorting patients likely to be infected with the same organism and use of standard and contact precautions are permissible.
  - Gloves (clean, nonsterile) should be used at all times.
  - Hand hygiene should be performed after glove removal.
  - Gowns should be used during direct contact with a patient, environmental surfaces, or items in the patient room. Gowns should be worn on entry into the room and should be removed before leaving the patient's room or area.
  - Specific illnesses and infections with organisms requiring **Contact Precautions** include the following:
    - Colonization or infection with multidrug-resistant bacteria judged by the infection control practitioner on the basis of current state, regional, or national recommendations to be of special clinical and epidemiologic significance (eg, vancomycin-resistant enterococci; methicillin-resistant *Staphylococcus aureus;* multidrug-resistant, gram-negative bacilli) or other epidemiologically important susceptible bacteria
    - *C difficile*
    - Conjunctivitis, viral and hemorrhagic
    - Diphtheria (cutaneous)
    - Enteroviruses
    - *Escherichia coli* O157:H7 and other Shiga toxin-producing *E coli*
    - Hepatitis A virus
    - Herpes simplex virus (neonatal, mucocutaneous, or cutaneous)
    - Herpes zoster (localized with no evidence of dissemination)
    - Human metapneumovirus
    - Impetigo
    - Major (noncontained) abscess, decubitus ulcer
    - Parainfluenza virus
    - Pediculosis (lice)
    - Respiratory syncytial virus
    - Rotavirus

— *Salmonella* species
— Scabies
— *Shigella* species
— *S aureus* (cutaneous or draining wounds)
— Viral hemorrhagic fevers (Ebola, Lassa, or Marburg)

Airborne, Droplet, and **Contact Precautions** should be combined for diseases caused by organisms that have multiple routes of transmission. When used alone or in combination, these transmission-based precautions always are to be used in addition to **Standard Precautions,** which are recommended for all patients. The specifications for these categories of isolation precautions are summarized in Table 2.9, and Table 2.10 (p 168) lists syndromes and conditions that are suggestive of contagious infection and require empiric isolation precautions pending identification of a specific pathogen. When the specific pathogen is known, isolation recommendations and duration of isolation are given in the pathogen- or disease-specific chapters in Section 3.

PEDIATRIC CONSIDERATIONS

Unique differences in pediatric care necessitate modifications of these guidelines, including the following: (1) diaper changing and wiping a child's tears or nose; (2) use of single-patient room isolation; and (3) use of common areas, such as hospital waiting rooms, playrooms, and schoolrooms.

Because diapering or wiping a child's nose or tears does not soil hands routinely, wearing gloves is not mandatory except when gloves are required as part of Transmission-Based Precautions. However, it may be prudent for women who are pregnant or likely to be pregnant to use gloves when changing diapers.

Single-patient rooms are recommended for all patients for **Transmission-Based Precautions** (ie, **Airborne, Droplet,** and **Contact**). Patients placed on Transmission-Based Precautions should not leave their rooms to use common areas, such as child life

Table 2.9. Transmission-Based Precautions for Hospitalized Patients[a]

Category of Precautions	Single-Patient Room	Respiratory Tract/ Mucous Membrane Protection	Gowns	Gloves
Airborne	Yes, with negative air-pressure ventilation, 6–12 air exchanges per hour, ± HEPA filtration	Respirators: N95 or higher level	No[b]	No[b]
Droplet	Yes[c]	Surgical masks[d]	No[b]	No[b]
Contact	Yes[c]	No	Yes	Yes

HEPA indicates high-efficiency particulate air.

[a] These recommendations are in addition to those for **Standard Precautions** for all patients.

[b] Gowns and gloves may be required as a component of **Standard Precautions** (eg, for blood collection or during procedures likely to cause blood splashes or if there are skin lesions containing transmissible infectious agents).

[c] Preferred. Cohorting of children infected with the same pathogen is acceptable if a single-patient room is not available, a distance of more than 3 feet between patients can be maintained, and precautions are observed between all contacts with different patients in the room.

[d] Masks should be donned on entry into the room.

Table 2.10. Clinical Syndromes or Conditions Warranting Precautions in Addition to Standard Precautions to Prevent Transmission of Epidemiologically Important Pathogens Pending Confirmation of Diagnosis[a]

Clinical Syndrome or Condition[b]	Potential Pathogens[c]	Empiric Precautions[d]
Diarrhea		
Acute diarrhea with a likely infectious cause	Enteric pathogens[e]	Contact
Diarrhea in patient with a history of recent antimicrobial use	*Clostridium difficile*	Contact; use soap and water for handwashing
Meningitis	*Neisseria meningitidis*	Droplet
	Enteroviruses	Contact
Rash or exanthems, generalized, cause unknown		
Petechial or ecchymotic with fever	*N meningitidis*	Droplet
	Hemorrhagic fever viruses	Add Contact plus face/eye protection
Vesicular	Varicella-zoster virus	Airborne and Contact
Maculopapular with coryza and fever	Measles virus	Airborne
Respiratory tract infections		
Pulmonary cavitary disease	*Mycobacterium tuberculosis*	Airborne
Paroxysmal or severe persistent cough during periods of pertussis activity in the community	*Bordetella pertussis*	Droplet
Viral infections, particularly bronchiolitis and croup, in infants and young children	Respiratory viral pathogens	Contact and Droplet until adenovirus, rhinovirus, and influenza virus excluded

Table 2.10. Clinical Syndromes or Conditions Warranting Precautions in Addition to Standard Precautions to Prevent Transmission of Epidemiologically Important Pathogens Pending Confirmation of Diagnosis,[a] continued

Clinical Syndrome or Condition[b]	Potential Pathogens[c]	Empiric Precautions[d]
Risk of multidrug-resistant microorganisms[f]		
History of infection or colonization with multidrug-resistant organisms	Resistant bacteria	Contact
Skin, wound, or urinary tract infection in a patient with a recent stay in a hospital or chronic care facility	Resistant bacteria	Contact until resistant organism is excluded by cultures
Skin or wound infection		
Abscess or draining wound that cannot be covered	*Staphylococcus aureus*, group A *Streptococcus* species	Contact

[a] Infection-control professionals are encouraged to modify or adapt this table according to local conditions. To ensure that appropriate empiric precautions are implemented, hospitals must have systems in place to evaluate patients routinely according to these criteria as part of their preadmission and admission care.

[b] Patients with the syndromes or conditions listed may have atypical signs or symptoms (eg, pertussis in neonates may present with apnea, paroxysmal or severe cough may be absent in pertussis in adults). The clinician's index of suspicion should be guided by the prevalence of specific conditions in the community and clinical judgment.

[c] The organisms listed in this column are not intended to represent the complete or even most likely diagnoses but, rather, possible causative agents that require additional precautions beyond **Standard Precautions** until a causative agent can be excluded.

[d] Duration of isolation varies by agent and the antimicrobial treatment administered.

[e] These pathogens include Shiga toxin–producing *Escherichia coli* including *E coli* O157:H7, *Shigella* organisms, *Salmonella* organisms, *Campylobacter* organisms, hepatitis A virus, enteric viruses including rotavirus, *Cryptosporidium* organisms, and *Giardia* organisms. Use masks when cleaning vomitus or stool during norovirus outbreak.

[f] Resistant bacteria judged by the infection control program on the basis of current state, regional, or national recommendations to be of special clinical or epidemiologic significance.

playrooms, schoolrooms, or waiting areas, except under special circumstances as defined by the facility infection control personnel. The guidelines for **Standard Precautions** state that patients who cannot control body excretions should be in single-patient rooms. Because most young children are incontinent, this recommendation does not apply to routine care of uninfected children.

CDC isolation guidelines were developed for preventing transmission of infection in hospitals and other settings in which health care is delivered. These recommendations do not apply to schools, out-of-home child care centers, and other settings in which healthy children congregate in shared space.

Strategies to Prevent Health Care-Associated Infections

Health care-associated infections in patients in acute care hospitals are associated with substantial morbidity and some mortality. Important infections include central line-associated bloodstream infections, central nervous system shunt infections, surgical site infections, bladder catheter-associated urinary tract infections, ventilator-associated pneumonias, infections caused by viruses (eg, respiratory syncytial virus and rotavirus), and colitis attributable to *Clostridium difficile*. Infection-prevention strategies exist for each of these infections. Occurrence of these preventable infections is viewed as a patient safety issue, and there has been an increased emphasis on prevention. Reports[1] have suggested that rates of some of these infections can be further reduced by implementing evidence-based "best practices." Successful strategies typically have included several practice improvements, often referred to as a "bundle," that are implemented simultaneously and with multidisciplinary participation and collaboration with members of the health care team, including administrators, physicians, nurses, therapists, and housekeeping services. Most studies documenting a favorable effect of implementation of infection-prevention "bundles" have been performed in adults, and studies of infection prevention in pediatric patients are limited.

Prevention of central line-associated bloodstream infection has been studied in pediatric patients in a multicenter investigation.[2] "Bundles" to prevent such infections include a bundle directed at catheter insertion and a bundle directed at catheter maintenance. Such bundles may include the following elements:

- Education of health care personnel in central venous catheter insertion and maintenance relevant to infection prevention, typically with a course or video
- Insertion practices:
  - ◆ Use maximal sterile barrier precautions, including a large sterile drape for the patient and a mask and cap and sterile gown and gloves for the person inserting the catheter
  - ◆ Use a chlorhexidine-based antiseptic for skin preparation in neonates weighing more than 1500 g at birth and children and an iodine-based antiseptic for smaller infants
  - ◆ Use a catheter insertion checklist and a trained observer who is empowered to halt the procedure if there is a break in the sterile technique protocol

[1] A compendium of strategies to prevent healthcare-associated infections in acute care hospitals. *Infect Control Hosp Epidemiol*. 2008;29(Suppl 1):S1–S92

[2] Miller MR, Griswold M, Harris JM II, et al. Decreasing PICU catheter-associated bloodstream infections: NACHRI's quality transformation efforts. *Pediatrics*. 2010;125(2):206–213

- Maintenance practices:
  - Catheter site care:
    - Use a chlorhexidine gluconate scrub to sites for dressing changes (scrub for 30 seconds, air dry for 30 seconds)
    - Change gauze dressings every 2 days and when they are soiled, dampened, or loosened
    - Change clear dressings every 7 days and when they are soiled, dampened, or loosened
    - Use a prepackaged dressing-change kit or supply area
  - Disinfect catheter hubs, injection ports, and needleless connectors by vigorous rubbing with an alcohol- or chlorhexidine-soaked swab or pad for at least 10 seconds prior to catheter accessing, a procedure sometimes called "scrub the hub"
- Evaluate patients daily to determine whether there is a continued need for the central venous catheter and remove catheter if not needed
- Monitor infection rates and adherence to infection-prevention measures

Occupational Health

Transmission of infectious agents within health care settings is facilitated by close contact between patients and health care personnel and lack of hygienic practices by infants and young children. Standard Precautions and Transmission-Based Precautions are designed to prevent transmission of infectious agents in health care settings to limit transmission among patients and health care personnel. To further limit risks of transmission of organisms between children and health care personnel, health care facilities should have established personnel health policies and services. Specifically, personnel should be protected against vaccine-preventable diseases by establishing appropriate screening and immunization policies (see adult immunization schedule at **www.cdc.gov/vaccines/ recs/schedules/adult-schedule.htm**). Guidelines for immunization of health care personnel have been published.[1]

For infections that are not vaccine preventable, personnel should be counseled about exposures and the possible need for leave if they are exposed to, ill with, or a carrier of a specific pathogen, whether the exposure occurs in the home, community, or health care setting.

The frequency and need for screening of health care personnel for tuberculosis should be determined by local epidemiologic data, as described in the CDC guideline for prevention of transmission of tuberculosis in health care settings.[2] People with commonly occurring infections, such as gastroenteritis, dermatitis, herpes simplex virus lesions on exposed skin, or upper respiratory tract infections, should be evaluated to determine the resulting risk of transmission to patients or to other health care personnel.

Health care personnel education, including understanding of hospital policies, is of paramount importance in infection control. Pediatric health care professionals should be knowledgeable about the modes of transmission of infectious agents, proper hand hygiene techniques, and serious risks to children from certain mild infections in adults.

---

[1] Centers for Disease Control and Prevention. Immunization of health-care personnel: recommendations of the Advisory Committee on Immunization Practices (ACIP). *MMWR Recomm Rep.* 2011;60(RR-7):1–44

[2] Centers for Disease Control and Prevention. Guidelines for preventing the transmission of *Mycobacterium tuberculosis* in health-care settings, 2005. *MMWR Recomm Rep.* 2005;54(RR-17):1–141

Frequent educational sessions will reinforce safe techniques and the importance of infection-control policies. Written policies and procedures relating to needlestick or sharp injuries are mandated by OSHA.[1] Recommendations for postinjury prophylaxis are available (see Human Immunodeficiency Virus Infection, p 418, and Table 3.27, p 427).[2,3]

Pregnant health care personnel who follow recommended precautions should not be at increased risk of infections that have possible adverse effects on the fetus (eg, parvovirus B19, cytomegalovirus, rubella, and varicella). The risk of severe influenza infection for pregnant health care personnel can be reduced by influenza immunization. Personnel who are immunocompromised and at increased risk of severe infection (eg, *M tuberculosis,* measles virus, herpes simplex virus, and varicella-zoster virus) should seek advice from their primary health care professional.

The consequences to pediatric patients of acquiring infections from adults can be significant. Mild illness in adults, such as viral gastroenteritis, upper respiratory tract viral infection, pertussis, or herpes simplex virus infection, can cause life-threatening disease in infants and children. People at greatest risk are preterm infants, children who have heart disease or chronic pulmonary disease, and people who are immunocompromised.

Sibling Visitation

Sibling visits to birthing centers, postpartum rooms, pediatric wards, and intensive care units are encouraged. Neonatal intensive care, with its increasing sophistication, often results in long hospital stays for the preterm or sick newborn, making family visits important. If guidelines are followed, subsequent infection is not increased in the sick or preterm newborn infant visited by siblings.

Guidelines for sibling visits should be established to maximize opportunities for visiting and to minimize the risks of transmission of pathogens brought into the hospital by young visitors. Guidelines may need to be modified by local nursing, pediatric, obstetric, and infectious diseases staff members to address specific issues in their hospital settings. Basic guidelines for sibling visits to pediatric patients are as follows:

- Sibling visits may benefit hospitalized children.
- Before the visit, a trained health care professional should interview the parents at a site outside the unit to assess the health of each sibling visitor. These interviews should be documented, and approval for each sibling visit should be noted. No child with fever or symptoms of an acute infection, including upper respiratory tract infection, gastroenteritis, or cellulitis, should be allowed to visit. Siblings who recently have been exposed to a person with a known communicable disease and are susceptible should not be allowed to visit.
- Siblings who are visiting should have received all recommended immunizations for age. Before and during influenza season, siblings who visit should have received influenza vaccine.

---

[1] Occupational Safety and Health Administration (**www.osha.gov**)

[2] American Academy of Pediatrics, Committee on Pediatric AIDS. Postexposure prophylaxis in children and adolescents for nonoccupational exposure to human immunodeficiency virus. *Pediatrics.* 2003;111(5):1475–1489 (Reaffirmed January 2007)

[3] Centers for Disease Control and Prevention. Updated US Public Health Service guidelines for the management of occupational exposures to HIV and recommendations for postexposure prophylaxis. *MMWR Recomm Rep.* 2005;54(RR-9):1–17

- Asymptomatic siblings who recently have been exposed to varicella but have been immunized previously can be assumed to be immune.
- The visiting sibling should visit only his or her sibling and not be allowed in playrooms with groups of patients.
- Children should perform recommended hand hygiene before any patient contact.
- Throughout the visit, sibling activity should be supervised by parents or a responsible adult and limited to the mother's or patient's patient room or other designated areas where other patients are not present.

Adult Visitation

Guidelines should be established for visits by other relatives and close friends. Anyone with fever or contagious illnesses ideally should not visit. Medical and nursing staff members should be vigilant about potential communicable diseases in parents and other adult visitors (eg, a relative with a cough who may have pertussis or tuberculosis; a parent with a cold visiting a highly immunosuppressed child). Before and during influenza season, it is prudent to encourage all visitors to receive influenza vaccine. Adherence to these guidelines especially is important for oncology, hematopoietic stem cell transplant units, and neonatal intensive care units.

Pet Visitation

Pet visitation in the health care setting includes visits by a child's personal pet and pet visitation as a part of child life therapeutic programs. Guidelines for pet visitation should be established to minimize risks of transmission of pathogens from pets to humans or injury from animals. The specific health care setting and the level of concern for zoonotic disease will influence establishment of pet visitation policies. The pet visitation policy should be developed in consultation with pediatricians, infection-control professionals, nursing staff, the hospital epidemiologist, and veterinarians. Basic principles for pet visitation policies in health care settings are as follows[1]:

- Personal pets other than cats and dogs should be excluded from the hospital. No reptiles (eg, iguanas, turtles, snakes), amphibians, birds, primates, ferrets, or rodents should be allowed to visit. Exceptions may be made for end-of-life patients who are in single-patient rooms.
- Visiting pets should have a certificate of immunization from a licensed veterinarian and verification that the pet is healthy.
- The pet should be bathed and groomed for the visit.
- Pet visitation should be discouraged in an intensive care unit, but individual circumstances can be considered.
- The visit of a pet should be approved by an appropriate personnel member (eg, the director of the child life therapy program), who should observe the pet for temperament and general health at the time of visit. The pet should be free of obvious bacterial skin infections, infections caused by superficial dermatophytes, and ectoparasitic infections (fleas and ticks).

---

[1] Writing Panel of Working Group; Lefebvre SL, Golab GC, Christensen E, et al. Guidelines for animal-assisted interventions in health care facilities. *Am J Infect Control.* 2008;36(2):78–85

- Pet visitation should be confined to designated areas. Contact should be confined to the petting and holding of animals, as appropriate. All contact should be supervised throughout the visit by appropriate personnel and should be followed by hand hygiene performed by the patient and all who had contact with the pet. Supervisors should be familiar with institutional policies for managing animal bites and cleaning pet urine, feces, or vomitus.
- Patients having contact with pets must have approval from a physician or physician representative before animal contact. Documented allergy to dogs or cats should be considered before approving contact. For patients who are immunodeficient or for people receiving immunosuppressive therapy, the risks of exposure to the microflora of pets may outweigh the benefits of contact. Contact of children with pets should be approved on a case-by-case basis.
- Care should be taken to protect indwelling catheter sites (eg, central venous catheters, peritoneal dialysis catheters). These sites should have dressings that provide an effective barrier to pet contact, including licking, and be covered with clothing or gown. Concern for contamination of other body sites should be considered on a case-by-case basis.

The pet policy should not apply to professionally trained service animals. These animals are not pets, and separate policies should govern their uses and presence in the hospital according to the American Disabilities Act recommendations.

INFECTION CONTROL AND PREVENTION IN AMBULATORY SETTINGS

Infection control and prevention is an integral part of pediatric practice in ambulatory care settings as well as in hospitals. All health care personnel should be aware of the routes of transmission and techniques to prevent transmission of infectious agents. Written policies and procedures for infection prevention and control should be developed, implemented, and reviewed at least every 2 years. Standard Precautions, as outlined for the hospitalized child (see Infection Control for Hospitalized Children, p 160) and by the Centers for Disease Control and Prevention,[1] with a modification by the American Academy of Pediatrics exempting the use of gloves for routine diaper changes and wiping a child's nose or tears,[2] are appropriate for most patient encounters. In addition, to help curb ambulatory health care-associated infections, the CDC has created a guideline (**www.cdc.gov/HAI/settings/outpatient/outpatient-care-guidelines.html**) and checklist (**www.cdc.gov/HAI/settings/outpatient/checklist/outpatient-care-checklist.html**) that clinicians working in outpatient settings can use to help ensure that appropriate infection control practices are being followed. Key principles of infection prevention and control in an outpatient setting are as follows:

---

[1] Centers for Disease Control and Prevention. Guideline for isolation precautions: preventing transmission of infectious agents in health care settings 2007. Recommendations of the Healthcare Infection Control Practices Advisory Committee. Atlanta, GA: Centers for Disease Control and Prevention; 2007. Available at: **www.cdc.gov/ncidod/dhqp/pdf/guidelines/isolation2007.pdf**

[2] American Academy of Pediatrics, Committee on Infectious Diseases. Infection prevention and control in pediatric ambulatory settings. *Pediatrics.* 2007;120(3):650–665 (Reaffirmed August 2010)

- Infection control and prevention should begin when the child's appointment is scheduled and initiated when the child enters the office or clinic.
- Standard Precautions should be used when caring for all patients.
- Contact between contagious children and uninfected children should be minimized. Policies for children who are suspected of having contagious infections, such as varicella or measles, should be implemented. Immunocompromised children and neonates should be kept away from people with potentially contagious infections.
- In waiting rooms of ambulatory care facilities, use of some or all components of respiratory hygiene/cough etiquette should be implemented for patients and accompanying people with suspected respiratory tract infection.[1]
- All health care personnel should perform hand hygiene before and after each patient contact. In health care settings, alcohol-based products are preferred for decontaminating hands routinely. Soap and water are preferred when hands are visibly dirty or contaminated with proteinaceous material, such as blood or other body fluids. Parents and children should be taught the importance of hand hygiene.
- Health care personnel should receive influenza immunization annually as well as immunizations against other vaccine-preventable infections that can be transmitted in an ambulatory setting to patients or to other health care personnel. Other recommended vaccines include tetanus and diphtheria toxoids and acellular pertussis (Tdap), measles-mumps-rubella (MMR), varicella, and hepatitis B.[2]
- Health care personnel should be familiar with aseptic technique, particularly regarding insertion or manipulation of intravascular catheters, performance of other invasive procedures, and preparation and administration of parenteral medications. This includes selection and use of appropriate skin antiseptics. Alcohol is preferred for skin preparation before immunization or routine venipuncture. Skin preparation for incision, suture, or collection of blood for culture requires 70% alcohol, alcohol tinctures of iodine (10%), or alcoholic chlorhexidine (>0.5%) preparations that may be superior to povidone iodine.
- Needles and sharps should be handled with great care. The use of safer medical devices designed to reduce the risk of needle sticks should be implemented. Sharps disposal containers that are impermeable and puncture resistant should be available adjacent to the areas where sharps are used (eg, areas where injections or venipunctures are performed). Sharps containers should be replaced before they become overfilled and kept out of reach of young children. Policies should be established for removal and the disposal of sharps containers consistent with state and local regulations.
- A written bloodborne pathogen exposure control plan that includes policies for management of exposures to blood and body fluids, such as through needle sticks and exposures of nonintact skin and mucous membranes, should be developed, readily available to all staff, and reviewed regularly (see Hepatitis B, p 369; Hepatitis C, p 391; and Human Immunodeficiency Virus Infection, p 418).
- Standard guidelines for decontamination, disinfection, and sterilization should be followed.

---

[1] Centers for Disease Control and Prevention. Respiratory Hygiene/Cough Etiquette in Healthcare Settings. Available at: **www.cdc.gov/flu/professionals/infectioncontrol/resphygiene.htm**

[2] Centers for Disease Control and Prevention. Immunization of healthcare personnel. Recommendations of the Advisory Committee on Immunization Practices (ACIP). *MMWR Recomm Rep*. 2011;60(RR-7):1–45

- Appropriate use of antimicrobial agents is essential to limit the emergence and spread of drug-resistant bacteria (see Appropriate Use of Antimicrobial Agents, p 802).
- Policies and procedures should be developed for communication with local and state health authorities about reportable diseases and suspected outbreaks.
- Ongoing educational programs that encompass appropriate aspects of infection control should be implemented, reinforced, documented, and evaluated on a regular basis.
- Physicians should be aware of requirements of government agencies, such as the Occupational Safety and Health Administration, as they relate to the operation of physicians' offices.

··

SEXUALLY TRANSMITTED INFECTIONS IN ADOLESCENTS AND CHILDREN

Physicians and other health care professionals perform a critical role in preventing and treating sexually transmitted infections (STIs) in the pediatric population. STIs are a major problem for adolescents; an estimated 25% of adolescents will acquire an STI before 18 years of age. Although an STI in an infant or child early in life can be the result of vertical transmission or autoinoculation, certain STIs (eg, gonorrhea, syphilis, chlamydia, herpes simplex virus [HSV] type 2]) are pathognomonic of sexual abuse if acquired after the neonatal period. For infants and children, detection of an STI is a highly concerning probability of sexual abuse. Whenever sexual abuse is suspected, appropriate social service and law enforcement agencies must be involved to ensure the child's or adolescent's protection and to provide appropriate counseling.

STIs in Adolescents

EPIDEMIOLOGY

Adolescents and young adults continue to have higher rates of STIs when compared with any other age group. Adolescents are at greater risk of STIs, because they frequently have unprotected intercourse, may be more susceptible biologically to infection, often are engaged in multiple sequential monogamous partnerships of varying durations, and face multiple obstacles in accessing confidential health care services.[1] The rate of diagnosed STIs is higher in women than in men by a factor of 3:1, but far fewer sexually active male than female adolescents are screened for STIs. Data underestimate the incidence of STIs among sexually experienced adolescents, because *all* adolescents, including those who never have had sexual intercourse, are included in the denominators used to calculate age-specific STI rates, and because many cases are not diagnosed or reported.

MANAGEMENT

At each annual checkup and at visits for acute illness, the physician should meet with the teen apart from the parent(s) or guardian(s) during the evaluation. Physicians can prepare patients and families about the need for private time by educating both parents and pre-adolescents about the need for confidentiality as adolescence approaches. Pediatricians

---

[1] Centers for Disease Control and Prevention. Youth risk behavior surveillance—United States, 2009. *MMWR Surveill Summ.* 2010;59(SS-5):1–142

should screen for risk of STIs by asking all adolescent patients—apart from their parents—whether they ever have had sexual intercourse, currently are sexually active, or are planning to be sexually active in the near future. It is important that adolescents recognize that oral and anal intercourse, as well as vaginal intercourse, put them at risk of STIs. Although some groups of adolescents are at increased risk of STIs, all teenagers should be screened for risk and appropriately tested and treated (see Table 2.11, p 178). More detailed recommendations for preventive health care for adolescents are available in the American Academy of Pediatrics' *Bright Futures: Guidelines for Health Supervision of Infants, Children, and Adolescents,* Third Edition[1] and the Centers for Disease Control and Prevention (CDC) 2010 "Sexually Transmitted Diseases Treatment Guidelines."[2] All 50 states allow minors to give their own consent for confidential STI screening, diagnosis, and treatment. Despite the high prevalence of STIs among adolescents, health care professionals frequently fail to provide the time to confidentially inquire about sexual behaviors, assess for STI risks, counsel about risk reduction, and screen for STIs.

Recommendations have been published suggesting that annual Papanicolaou smears to screen for cervical dysplasia associated with human papillomavirus (HPV) infection should be delayed until a young woman's 21st birthday, regardless of sexual history. For adolescent females who are immunosuppressed or immunocompromised, yearly Papanicolaou smears should begin with the initiation of consensual sexual intercourse or with a history of nonconsensual sexual intercourse. Sexually active adolescent females should be screened at least annually for chlamydia and gonorrhea. The 2010 "Sexually Transmitted Infections Treatment Guidelines" from the CDC (**www.cdc.gov/std/ treatment**) suggest that screening of asymptomatic sexually active adolescent males should be considered in clinical settings with a high prevalence of chlamydia (eg, adolescent clinics, correctional facilities, and STI clinics). Sexually active adolescents should receive human immunodeficiency virus (HIV) and syphilis prevention counseling at least annually, and the CDC recommends HIV screening once for everyone 13 years of age and older, with additional testing based on risk. All adolescents should receive hepatitis B virus immunization if they were not immunized earlier in childhood. The HPV immunization series should be started for females and males, at the 11- through 12-year visit (or at 13 through 18 years of age if they were not immunized previously). Hepatitis A vaccine should be offered to adolescent males who have sex with males (see Recommended Childhood and Adolescent Immunization Schedules, Fig 1.1–1.3, p 27–31) and others at high risk of hepatitis A virus infection (see Hepatitis A, p 361).

For treatment recommendations for specific STIs, see the disease-specific chapters in Section 3 and Table 4.3, Guidelines for Treatment of Sexually Transmitted Infections in Children and Adolescents According to Syndrome (p 821). Patients and their partners treated for gonorrhea, *Chlamydia trachomatis* infection, and trichomoniasis should be advised to refrain from sexual intercourse for 1 week after completion of appropriate treatment. Retesting to detect therapeutic failure (tests of cure) for patients who receive recommended treatment regimens for *Neisseria gonorrhoeae* or *C trachomatis* infection is not recommended unless therapeutic adherence is in question or symptoms persist. If a

[1] American Academy of Pediatrics, Bright Futures Steering Committee. *Bright Futures: Guidelines for Health Supervision of Infants, Children, and Adolescents.* Hagan JF Jr, Shaw JS, Duncan P, eds. 3rd ed. Elk Grove Village, IL: American Academy of Pediatrics; 2008

[2] Centers for Disease Control and Prevention. Sexually transmitted diseases treatment guidelines, 2010. *MMWR Morb Mortal Wkly Rep.* 2010;59(RR-12):1–110

Table 2.11. Approaches to Clinical Sexually Transmitted Disease (STD) Prevention[a]

1. Partners
   - "Do you have sex with men, women, or both?"
   - "In the past 2 months, how many partners have you had sex with?"
   - "In the past 12 months, how many partners have you had sex with?"
   - "Is it possible that any of your sex partners in the past 12 months had sex with someone else while they were still in a sexual relationship with you?"

2. Prevention of Pregnancy
   - "What are you doing to prevent pregnancy?"

3. Protection From STDs
   - "What do you do to protect yourself from STDs and HIV?"

4. Practices
   - "To understand your risks for STDs, I need to understand the kind of sex you have had recently."
   - "Have you had vaginal sex, meaning 'penis in vagina sex'?" If yes, "Do you use condoms: never, sometimes, or always?"
   - "Have you had anal sex, meaning 'penis in rectum/anus sex'?" If yes, "Do you use condoms: never, sometimes, or always?"
   - "Have you had oral sex, meaning 'mouth on penis/vagina'?"

   For Condom Answers:
   - If "never:" "Why don't you use condoms?"
   - If "sometimes:" "In what situations (or with whom) do you not use condoms?"

5. Past history of STDs
   - "Have you ever had an STD?"
   - "Have any of your partners had an STD?"

   Additional Questions to Identify HIV and Viral Hepatitis Risk Include:
   - "Have you or any of your partners ever injected drugs?"
   - "Have any of your partners exchanged money or drugs for sex?"
   - "Is there anything else about your sexual practices that I need to know about?"

[a]From Centers for Disease Control and Prevention. Sexually transmitted diseases treatment guidelines, 2010. *MMWR Morb Mortal Wkly Rep.* 2010;59(RR-12):1–110. Available at: **www.cdc.gov/std/treatment.**

multiple-dose regimen is used, nonadherence is possible. Retesting for chlamydia infection using nonculture techniques such as nucleic acid amplification tests (NAATs) less than 3 weeks after treatment may yield false-positive results attributable to residual nonviable organisms. Repeat testing is recommended for these infections within 3 months because of the likelihood of reinfection as a result of nontreatment of a current sexual partner and/or new infection from a new sexual partner.

PREVENTION

Pediatricians can contribute to primary prevention of STIs by supporting a teenager's decision to postpone initiating sexual intercourse. For teenagers who become sexually active, physicians should discuss methods of protecting against STIs and unwanted pregnancies, including the correct and consistent use of condoms. Teenagers need to be made aware and to be reminded of the strong association between alcohol or drug use and failure to appropriately use barrier methods correctly when either person is "under the influence." Adolescents should be reminded that barrier methods should be used with all forms of sexual intercourse (vaginal, oral, and anal). Pediatricians also should discuss other ways to decrease risk of acquiring STIs, including limiting number of partners and deciding to abstain even if initiation of sexual intercourse already has occurred.

The US Food and Drug Administration has licensed a quadrivalent vaccine against HPV types 6, 11, 16, and 18 for females and males 9 through 26 years of age and a bivalent HPV vaccine against HPV types 16 and 18 for females 9 through 26 years of age.[1,2]

Diagnosis and Treatment of STIs in Children[3]

Because of social and legal implications, STIs in children must be diagnosed using tests with high specificity, because the low prevalence of STIs in children increases the probability that rapid detection tests for STIs will give false-positive results. Therefore, tests that allow for isolation of the organism and have the highest specificities must be used.

Because of the serious implications of the diagnosis of an STI in a child, antimicrobial therapy for children with suspected STIs may need to be withheld until the final outcome of the diagnostic test is known. Specimens for culture to screen for *N gonorrhoeae* and *C trachomatis* should be obtained from the rectum and vagina of girls and from the rectum and urethra of boys. Specimens for culture to screen for *N gonorrhoeae* also should be obtained from the pharynx, even in the absence of symptoms. An NAAT should be performed for diagnosing *C trachomatis* and *N gonorrhoeae* in females with cervicitis; this testing can be performed on either vaginal, cervical, or urine samples. Culture and nucleic acid hybridization tests require female endocervical or male urethral swab specimens. Endocervical specimens for culture are not required for prepubertal girls but are required for culture of *C trachomatis* and *N gonorrhoeae* if the female is pubertal or postmenarcheal. If vaginal discharge is present, specimens for wet mount for *Trichomonas vaginalis* and wet mount or Gram stain for bacterial vaginosis may be obtained as well. Serum specimens for testing for syphilis and HIV should be obtained. Completion of the hepatitis B immunization series should be documented, or the patient should be screened for hepatitis B surface antibody. For more detailed diagnosis and treatment recommendations for specific STIs, see the disease-specific chapters in Section 3 and Table 4.3, Guidelines for Treatment of Sexually Transmitted Infections in Children and Adolescents According to Syndrome (p 821).

Social Implications of STIs in Children

Children can acquire STIs through vertical transmission, by autoinoculation, or by sexual contact. Each of these mechanisms should be given appropriate consideration in evaluation of a preadolescent child with an STI. Evaluation solely on the basis of suspicion of an STI should not proceed until the STI diagnosis has been confirmed. Factors to be considered in assessing the likelihood of sexual abuse in a child with an STI include the

---

[1] Centers for Disease Control and Prevention. FDA licensure of bivalent human papillomavirus vaccine (HPV2, Cervarix) for use in females and updated HPV vaccination recommendations from the Advisory Committee on Immunization Practices (ACIP). *MMWR Morb Mortal Wkly Rep.* 2010;59(20):626–629

[2] Centers for Disease Control and Prevention. Use of quadrivalent human papillomavirus vaccine in males: recommendations of the Advisory Committee on Immunization Practices (ACIP). *MMWR.* 2011; in press

[3] Centers for Disease Control and Prevention. Sexually transmitted diseases treatment guidelines, 2010. *MMWR Morb Mortal Wkly Rep.* 2010;59(RR-12):1–110

biological characteristics of the STI in question, the age of the child, and whether the child reports a history of sexual victimization (see Table 2.12, below).

Anogenital gonorrhea in a prepubertal child indicates sexual abuse in virtually every case. All confirmed cases of gonorrhea in prepubertal children beyond the neonatal period should be reported to the local child protective services agency for investigation.

First-episode symptomatic HSV infection has a short incubation period but can be transmitted by sexual or nonsexual contact with another person or by self-inoculation. In an infant or toddler in diapers, genital herpes may arise from any of these mechanisms. In a prepubertal child whose toilet-use activities are independent, the new occurrence of genital herpes should prompt a careful investigation, including a child protective services investigation, for suspected sexual abuse. Viral typing for HSV-1 and HSV-2 may yield additional helpful information, but a significant percentage of genital herpes acquired sexually now is caused by HSV-1 in adolescent and adult populations.

Trichomoniasis is transmitted perinatally or by sexual contact. In a perinatally infected infant, vaginal discharge can persist for several weeks; accordingly, intense social investigation may not be warranted. However, a new diagnosis of trichomoniasis in an older infant or child should prompt a careful investigation, including a child protective services investigation, for suspected sexual abuse.

Infections that have long incubation periods (eg, HPV infection) and that can be asymptomatic for a period of time after vertical transmission (eg, syphilis, HIV infection, and *C trachomatis* infection) are more problematic. The possibility of vertical transmission

Table 2.12. Implications of Commonly Encountered Sexually Transmitted Infections (STIs) for Diagnosis and Reporting of Suspected or Diagnosed Sexual Abuse of Infants and Prepubertal Children[a]

STI Confirmed	Sexual Abuse	Suggested Action
Gonorrhea[b]	Diagnostic[c]	Report[d]
Syphilis[b]	Diagnostic	Report
Human immunodeficiency virus infection[e]	Diagnostic	Report
Chlamydia trachomatis infection[b]	Diagnostic[c]	Report
Trichomonas vaginalis infection	Highly suspicious	Report
Condylomata acuminata infection[b] (anogenital warts)	Suspicious	Report
Herpes (genital location)	Suspicious	Report[f]
Bacterial vaginosis	Inconclusive	Medical follow-up

[a] Adapted from Kellogg N; American Academy of Pediatrics, Committee on Child Abuse and Neglect. The evaluation of sexual abuse in children. *Pediatrics*. 2005;116(2):506–512.

[b] If not likely to be perinatally acquired and if rare nonsexual, vertical transmission is excluded.

[c] Although the culture technique is the "gold standard," studies are investigating the use of nucleic acid amplification testing as an alternative diagnostic method in children.

[d] Report to the agency mandated in the community to receive reports of suspected sexual abuse.

[e] If not likely to be acquired perinatally or through transfusion.

[f] Unless there is a clear history of herpes simplex virus type 1 autoinoculation.

should be considered in these cases, but an evaluation of the patient's circumstances by the local child protective services agency usually is warranted.

Although hepatitis B virus, scabies, and pediculosis pubis may be transmitted sexually, other modes of transmission can occur. The discovery of any of these conditions in a prepubertal child does not warrant child protective services involvement unless the clinician finds other information that suggests abuse. The presence of *T vaginalis* and bacterial vaginosis in a pubertal and postpubertal female suggests sexual contact and should be investigated appropriately (see Bacterial Vaginosis, p 247).

Sexual Victimization and STIs

GENERAL CONSIDERATIONS

Child sexual abuse has been defined as the exploitation of a child, either by physical contact or by other interactions, for the sexual stimulation of an adult or a minor who is in a position of power over the child. Physicians are required by law to report abuse to their state child protective services agency. Approximately 5% of sexually abused children acquire an STI as a result of the victimization.

SCREENING ASYMPTOMATIC SEXUALLY VICTIMIZED CHILDREN FOR STIs

Factors that influence the likelihood that a sexually victimized child will acquire an STI include the regional prevalence of STIs in the adult population, the number of assailants, the type and frequency of physical contact between the perpetrator(s) and the child, the infectivity of various microorganisms, the child's susceptibility to infection, and whether the child has received intercurrent antimicrobial treatment. The time interval between a child's physical contact with an assailant and the medical evaluation influences the likelihood that an exposed child will demonstrate signs or symptoms of an STI.

The decision to obtain specimens from genital or other areas from a child who has been victimized sexually to conduct an STI evaluation must be made on an individual basis. The following situations involve a high risk of STIs and constitute a strong indication for testing:

- The child has or has had signs or symptoms of an STI or an infection that can be transmitted sexually, even in the absence of suspicion of sexual abuse.
- A sibling, another child, or an adult in the household or child's immediate environment has an STI.
- A suspected assailant is known to have an STI or to be at high risk of STIs (eg, has had multiple sexual partners or a history of STIs) or has an unknown history.
- The patient or family requests testing.
- Evidence of genital, oral, or anal penetration or ejaculation is present.
  See Table 2.13 (p 182) if STI testing of a child is to be performed.

Most experts recommend universal screening of postpubertal patients who have been victims of sexual abuse or assault because of the possibility of a preexisting asymptomatic infection. When STI screening is performed, it should focus on likely anatomic sites of infection (as determined by the patient's history and physical examination or by epidemiologic considerations) and should include assessment for HIV infection if the patient, family, or both consent to serologic screening; assessment for bacterial vaginosis

Table 2.13. Sexually Transmitted Infection (STI) Testing in a Child[a] When Sexual Abuse Is Suspected

Organism/Syndrome	Specimens
Neisseria gonorrhoeae[b]	Rectal, throat, urethral (male), and/or vaginal cultures[c]
Chlamydia trachomatis[b]	Rectal, urethral (male), and vaginal cultures[c]
Syphilis	Darkfield examination of chancre fluid, if present; blood for serologic tests at time of abuse and 6, 12, and 24 wk later
Human immunodeficiency virus	Serologic testing of abuser (if possible); serologic testing of child at time of abuse and 6, 12, and 24 wk later
Hepatitis B virus	Serum hepatitis B surface antigen testing of abuser or hepatitis B surface antibody testing of child, unless the child has received 3 doses of hepatitis B vaccine
Herpes simplex virus (HSV)	Culture of lesion specimen; in addition, polymerase chain reaction assay of lesion specimen if lesion crusted; all virologic specimens should be typed (HSV-1 vs HSV-2)
Bacterial vaginosis	Wet mount, pH, and potassium hydroxide testing of vaginal discharge or Gram stain in pubertal and post-menarcheal girls
Human papillomavirus	Clinical examination, with biopsy of lesion specimen if diagnosis unclear
Trichomonas vaginalis	Wet mount and culture of vaginal discharge
Pediculosis pubis	Identification of eggs, nymphs, and lice with naked eye or using hand lens

[a] See text for indications for testing for STIs (Screening Asymptomatic Sexually Victimized Children for STIs, p 181).
[b] Nucleic acid amplification tests can be used as an alternative to culture with vaginal specimens or urine from girls.
[c] Cervical specimens are not recommended or necessary for prepubertal girls, but cervical specimens must be obtained in pubertal premenarchal and pubertal postmenarcheal girls.

and trichomoniasis for female patients; and testing for *N gonorrhoeae* infection, *C trachomatis* infection, and syphilis. To preserve the "chain of custody" for information that may later constitute legal evidence, specimens for laboratory analysis obtained from sexually victimized patients should be labeled carefully, and standard hospital procedures for transferring specimens from site to site should be followed carefully. Only tests with high specificities should be used, and whenever possible, specimens should be obtained by health care professionals with experience in the evaluation of children who have been sexually abused or assaulted. Data on the utility of NAATs are limited for *N gonorrhoeae*, and performance is test dependent. Consultation with an expert is necessary before using NAATs in this context to minimize the possibility of cross-reaction with nongonococcal *Neisseria* species. NAATs may be an alternative for *C trachomatis* if confirmation with another test is available and culture systems are unavailable. Confirmation tests should consist of a second US Food and Drug Administration-cleared NAAT that targets a different sequence from the initial test. A follow-up visit approximately 2 to 6 weeks after the most recent sexual exposure may include a repeat physical examination and collection of additional specimens. Another follow-up visit at 3 and 6 months after the most recent sexual exposure may be necessary to obtain convalescent sera to test for hepatitis B (if indicated), syphilis, and HIV infection.

PROPHYLAXIS AFTER SEXUAL VICTIMIZATION

Most experts do not recommend antimicrobial prophylaxis for asymptomatic **prepubertal** children who have been sexually abused, because their incidence of STIs is low, the risk of spread to the upper genital tract in prepubertal girls is low, and follow-up usually can be ensured. If a test result for an STI is positive, treatment then can be given. Factors that may increase the likelihood of infection or that constitute an indication for prophylaxis are the same as those listed under Screening Asymptomatic Sexually Victimized Children for STIs (p 181).

Many experts believe that prophylaxis is warranted for **postpubertal** female patients who seek care within 72 hours after an episode of sexual victimization because of the possibility of a preexisting asymptomatic infection, the potential risk for acquisition of new infections with the assault, and the substantial risk of pelvic inflammatory disease in this age group.[1] All patients who receive prophylaxis should be offered screening for relevant STIs (see Table 2.13, p 182) before treatment is given. Postmenarcheal patients should be tested for pregnancy before antimicrobial treatment or emergency contraception is given. Regimens for prophylaxis are presented in Tables 2.14 (children [p 184]) and 2.15 (adolescents [p 185]).

Because of the demonstrated effectiveness of prophylaxis to prevent HIV infection after perinatal and occupational exposures, the question arises whether HIV prophylaxis is warranted for children and adolescents after sexual assault (also see Human Immunodeficiency Virus Infection, Control Measures, p 434, and Table 3.28, p 435). The risk of HIV transmission from a single sexual assault that involves transfer of secretions and/or blood is low. Prophylaxis may be considered for patients who seek care within 72 hours after an assault if the assault involved mucosal exposure to secretions; repeated abuse; multiple assailants; oral, vaginal, and/or anal trauma; and particularly if the alleged perpetrator(s) is known to have or is at high risk of having HIV infection (see Human Immunodeficiency Virus Infection, p 418).[2]

The following are recommendations for postexposure assessment of children within 72 hours of sexual assault:

- Review HIV/acquired immunodeficiency syndrome (AIDS) local epidemiology and assess risk of HIV infection in the assailant.
- Evaluate circumstances of assault that may affect risk of HIV transmission.
- Consult with a specialist in treating HIV-infected children if postexposure prophylaxis is considered.
- If the child appears to be at risk of HIV transmission from the assault, discuss postexposure prophylaxis with the caregiver(s), including toxicity and unknown efficacy.
- If caregivers choose for the child to receive antiretroviral postexposure prophylaxis, provide enough medication until the return visit at 3 to 7 days after initial assessment to reevaluate the child and to assess tolerance of medication; dosages should not exceed those for adults.
- Perform HIV antibody test at original assessment and 6, 12, and 24 weeks later.

---

[1] Kaufmann M; American Academy of Pediatrics, Committee on Adolescence. Care of the adolescent sexual assault victim. *Pediatrics*. 2008;122(2):462–470. Available at: **http://aappolicy.aappublications.org/cgi/reprint/pediatrics;122/2/462.pdf**

[2] Centers for Disease Control and Prevention. Antiretroviral postexposure prophylaxis after sexual, injection-drug use, or other nonoccupational exposure to HIV in the United States: recommendations from the US Department of Health and Human Services. *MMWR Recomm Rep.* 2005;54(RR-2):1–20

Table 2.14. Prophylaxis After Sexual Victimization of Preadolescent Children

Weight <100 lb (<45 kg)		Weight ≥100 lb (≥45 kg)
	For prevention of gonorrhea	
1. Ceftriaxone, 125 mg, intra-muscularly, in a single dose		1A. Ceftriaxone, 250 mg, intra-muscularly, in a single dose **OR** 1B. Cefixime, 400 mg, orally, in a single dose
PLUS	**For prevention of Chlamydia trachomatis infection**	**PLUS**
2A. Azithromycin, 20 mg/kg (maximum 1 g), orally, in a single dose **OR** 2B. Erythromycin base or ethylsuccinate, 50 mg/kg per day, divided into 4 doses for 14 days		2A. Azithromycin, 1 g, orally, in a single dose **OR** 2B. Doxycycline, 100 mg, twice daily, for 7 days (if at least 8 years of age)
PLUS	**For prevention of hepatitis B virus infection**	**PLUS**
3. Begin or complete hepatitis B virus immunization series if not fully immunized		3. Begin or complete hepatitis B virus immunization series if not fully immunized
PLUS	**For prevention of trichomoniasis and bacterial vaginosis**	**PLUS**
4. Consider adding prophy-laxis for trichomoniasis and bacterial vaginosis (metro-nidazole, 15 mg/kg per day, orally, in 3 divided doses for 7 days; maximum 2 g)		4. Consider adding prophylaxis against trichomoniasis and bacterial vaginosis (metro-nidazole, 2 g, orally, in a single dose)

See text for human immunodeficiency virus infection prophylaxis in children following sexual abuse or assault.

Table 2.15. Prophylaxis After Sexual Victimization of Adolescents[a]

Antimicrobial prophylaxis[b] is recommended to include an empiric regimen to prevent *Chlamydia trachomatis* infection, gonorrhea, trichomoniasis, and bacterial vaginosis	
For gonorrhea[c]	Ceftriaxone, 250 mg, intramuscularly, in a single dose **OR** Cefixime, 400 mg orally, in a single dose **PLUS**
For *C trachomatis* infection	Azithromycin, 1 g, orally, in a single dose **OR** Doxycycline, 100 mg, orally, twice a day for 7 days (for those ≥8 years of age and not pregnant) **PLUS**
For trichomoniasis and bacterial vaginosis	Metronidazole, 2 g, orally, in a single dose **PLUS**
For hepatitis B virus infection	Hepatitis B virus immunization at time of initial examination, if not fully immunized. Follow-up doses of vaccine should be administered 1–2 and 4–6 mo after the first dose **PLUS**
For human immunodeficiency virus (HIV) infection[b]	Consider offering prophylaxis for HIV, depending on circumstances (see Table 3.28, p 435)

Emergency contraception[d]

Plan B, 2 tablets (levonorgestrel, 0.75 mg) at the same time; or 1 tablet (levonorgestrel, 1.5 mg) once

OR

Oral contraceptive pills, each containing 20 or 30 µg of ethinyl estradiol plus 0.1 mg or 0.15 mg of levonorgestrel or 0.3 mg of norgestrel: each of 2 doses must be given 12 h apart. Each dose must contain at least 100 to 120 µg of ethinyl estradiol and 0.5 to 0.6 mg of levonorgestrel or 1 mg of norgestrel.

[a] Source: Centers for Disease Control and Prevention. Sexually transmitted diseases treatment guidelines, 2010. *MMWR Morb Mortal Wkly Rep.* 2010;59(RR-12):1–110 (**www.cdc.gov/std/treatment**).
[b] See text for discussion of prophylaxis for human immunodeficiency virus (HIV) infection after sexual abuse or assault.
[c] Fluoroquinolones no longer are recommended for treatment of gonococcal infections because of increasing prevalence of resistant organisms (Centers for Disease Control and Prevention. Update to CDC's sexually transmitted diseases treatment guidelines, 2006: fluoroquinolones no longer recommended for treatment of gonococcal infections). *MMWR Recomm Rep.* 2007;56[RR-14]:332–336).
[d] The patient should have a negative pregnancy test result before emergency contraception is given. Although emergency contraception is most effective if taken within 72 hours of event, data suggest it is effective up to 120 hours.

HEPATITIS AND YOUTH IN CORRECTIONAL SETTINGS[1]

Pediatricians should work with state and local public health agencies and administrators of correctional facilities to address the health needs of youth in detention and to protect the community. The number of arrests of juveniles (younger than 18 years of age) in the United States was 2.11 million in 2008, 3% fewer than the number of arrests in 2007 and 16% fewer than in 1999.[2] Juveniles accounted for 16% of all violent crime arrests and 26% of all property crime arrests in 2008. On any given day, approximately 120 000 adolescents are held in juvenile correctional facilities or adult prisons or jails. Incarceration periods of at least 90 days await 60% of juvenile inmates, and 15% can expect to be confined for a year or more behind bars. Males account for approximately 85% of juvenile offenders in residential placement, and 61% of juveniles in correctional facilities are members of ethnic or racial minority groups. Female juveniles in custody represent a much larger proportion of "status" offenders, with offenses including ungovernability, running away, truancy, curfew violation, and underage drinking, than "delinquent" offenders who have committed offenses against other people or property (40% vs 14%, respectively).

Juvenile offenders commonly lack regular access to preventive health care in their communities and suffer significantly greater health deficiencies, including psychosocial disorders, chronic illness, exposure to illicit drugs, and physical trauma when compared with adolescents who are not in the juvenile justice system. Detained youth are more likely to have contracted sexually transmitted infections (STIs) early in adolescence, and delayed or incomplete treatment places them at increased risk of chronic complications of chlamydia, gonorrhea, syphilis, and human papillomavirus infections. Tuberculosis (TB) is more common in correctional populations, and although current juvenile detainees continue to have a low prevalence of human immunodeficiency virus (HIV) infection, their high-risk behaviors place them at significant risk. Hepatitis A virus (HAV), hepatitis B virus (HBV), and hepatitis C virus (HCV) infections are of particular concern because of the increased frequency of alcohol and injection drug use and the increased rate of unprotected sex with multiple partners early in life. The rate of juvenile arrests for drug abuse violations increased 47% between 1990 and 2005, and a history of injection drug use has played a major role in explaining the increased incidence of HCV infections in adolescent offenders. Infected juveniles place their communities at risk after their release from detention. Personal knowledge of an infection and its transmissibility may allow youth to take preventive measure to reduce their risk to others.

Up to 15% of all chronic HBV infections and more than 30% of all HCV infections known to exist in the United States are found among people with a history of incarceration. High-risk behaviors make adolescents particularly vulnerable to HAV, HBV, and HCV infections well before their first incarceration. Fewer than 3% of new hepatitis virus infections of all types are acquired once incarceration has occurred. Most juvenile offenders ultimately are returned to their community and, without intervention, resume

---

[1] Centers for Disease Control and Prevention. Prevention and control of infections with hepatitis viruses in correctional settings. *MMWR Recomm Rep.* 2003;52(RR-1):1–33

[2] Puzzanchera C. Juvenile arrests 2008. *Juvenile Justice Bulletin.* December 2009. Available at: **www.ncjrs.gov/ pdffiles1/ojjdp/228479.pdf**

a high-risk lifestyle. High recidivism rates lead many juvenile offenders to adult prisons, where the prevalence of HBV and HCV infections may be significantly higher than those found in juvenile correctional facilities. Viral hepatitis also can be a comorbid condition with other diseases, including TB and HIV infection. Correctional facilities, in partnership with public health departments and other community resources, have the opportunity to assess, contain, control, and prevent liver infection in a highly vulnerable segment of the population. HCV presents the greatest challenge to correctional facilities overall because of the lack of a vaccine to protect prisoners and the public. The extremely high rate of chronic carriage after infection increases the risk of transmission when youth are released into their communities. The controlled nature of the correctional system facilitates initiation of many hepatitis-prevention and -treatment strategies for an adolescent population that otherwise is difficult to reach.

Hepatitis A

Correctional facilities in the United States rarely report cases of hepatitis A, and national prevalence data for incarcerated populations are not available. States that have assessed prevalence of past infection in incarcerated populations younger than 20 years of age show a similar ethnic distribution of predominance in American Indian/Alaska Native and Hispanic inmates and documented and undocumented people from Mexico, as is reflected in the population as a whole. Some estimates suggest an overall seroprevalence of antibody to HAV between 22% and 39% in the adult prison population, with up to a 43% prevalence found in older prisoners between 40 and 49 years of age. Risk factors that could contribute to outbreaks of hepatitis A among adolescents include using injection and noninjection street drugs, having multiple sexual partners, and participating in male-with-male sexual activity.

RECOMMENDATIONS FOR CONTROL OF HAV INFECTIONS IN INCARCERATED YOUTH. Routine screening of incarcerated youth for HAV serologic markers is not recommended. However, adolescents who have signs or symptoms of hepatitis should be tested for seromarkers of acute hepatitis A, acute hepatitis B, and hepatitis C. HAV vaccine (see Hepatitis A Vaccine, p 362) should be given to all adolescents who have acknowledged identified risk behaviors (eg, use of injection and noninjection street drugs, having multiple sexual partners, and participating in male-with-male sexual activity) or who are incarcerated in residential facilities located in states with existing programs for routine HAV immunization of adolescents, generally in states that historically had the highest HAV infection rates. Correctional facilities in all states should consider routine HAV immunization of all adolescents under their care because of the likelihood that most adolescents in the juvenile correctional system have indications for HAV immunization. If this is not possible, HAV vaccine should be provided to juveniles with high-risk profiles, including illicit drug users and male adolescents who may engage in sex with males. Routine postimmunization serologic testing is not recommended. There is no contraindication to giving HAV vaccine to a person who may be immune as the result of a previous HAV infection or immunization. Incarcerated juveniles found to have acute hepatitis A disease should be reported to the local health department, and appropriate postexposure prophylaxis with HAV vaccine should be given to other susceptible residents who may have been exposed (see Hepatitis A, p 361).

Hepatitis B

HBV in the United States is transmitted mainly through exposure to blood, saliva, semen, and vaginal fluid; chronic infection with HBV mainly is found among people born in countries with prevalence higher than 2%, where most infections are transmitted in the perinatal period or during early childhood (see Hepatitis B, p 369). Adolescents in correctional facilities may include foreign-born (eg, Asia, Africa) residents who can have chronic infection and can transmit infection to susceptible residents. Resident adolescents also can include people with high-risk behaviors, including adolescents engaged in injection drug use with needle sharing; inmates who have had early initiation of sexual intercourse, unprotected sexual activity, multiple sexual partners, or history of STIs; and male adolescents who engage in sex with males. Although no published national studies have determined HBV infection prevalence rates for incarcerated juveniles, rates of HBV seroprevalence in homeless and high-risk street youth are higher when compared with peers lacking risk factors. Studies investigating hepatitis B outbreaks in prison settings also suggest that horizontal transmission may occur when people with chronic HBV infection are present. Adolescent female inmates present additional challenges for hepatitis B assessment and management if they are pregnant during incarceration, in which case coordination of care for mother and infant become paramount.

RECOMMENDATIONS FOR CONTROL OF HBV INFECTIONS IN INCARCERATED YOUTH.
Routine screening of juvenile inmates for HBV markers generally is not recommended, although testing for chronic infection is recommended in certain populations (see Hepatitis B, p 369). However, in states with school entry laws (**www.immunize.org/laws**) where high levels of adolescent HBV immunization have been achieved, adolescents who entered school when a law was in effect may be considered immunized. In other states, in the absence of proof of immunization, initial testing for HBV immunity may save vaccine costs, provided the timing of testing does not delay HBV immunization should the patient lack immunity. Correctional facilities may wish to survey juvenile inmates periodically for HBV immunity as they enter the institution to approximate HBV infection prevalence and determine the desirability of preimmunization testing. Adolescent detainees with signs and symptoms of hepatitis disease should be tested for serologic markers for acute hepatitis A, acute hepatitis B, and hepatitis C to determine the presence of acute or chronic infection and coinfection.

All adolescents receiving medical evaluation in a correctional facility should begin the HBV vaccine series or complete a previously begun series unless they have proof of completion of a previous HBV immunization series. Beginning an HBV vaccine series is critical, because a single dose of vaccine may confer protection from infection and subsequent complications of chronic carriage in a high-risk adolescent who may be lost to follow-up. Routine preimmunization and postimmunization serologic screening is not recommended. In states where HBV vaccine school entry requirements are in place, correctional facilities may use a combination of immunization history, immunization registry data, school entry immunization laws, and serologic testing to develop institutional policies regarding the need for HBV immunization in specific age groups of adolescents. Correctional facilities should have mechanisms in place for completion of the HBV vaccine series in the community after release of the juvenile. Immunization information should be made available to the inmate, the parents or legal guardian, the state immunization registry, and the patient's future medical home in the community.

Postexposure hepatitis B prophylaxis regimens for unimmunized incarcerated adolescents after potential percutaneous or sexual exposures to HBV are available (see Hepatitis B, Care of Exposed People, p 386). Should the source of the exposure be found to be hepatitis B surface antigen (HBsAg) positive, the unimmunized inmate exposed percutaneously should receive Hepatitis B Immune Globulin (HBIG) as soon as possible after exposure (preferably within 24 hours, and not more than 14 days after exposure). Exposed juveniles who have begun but not completed their HBV vaccine series should receive an appropriate dose of HBIG and complete the remainder of the series as scheduled (see Hepatitis B, p 369). If the source of exposure is unknown and not available for HBsAg testing, the exposed person should receive HBV vaccine or complete a vaccine series already initiated.

All pregnant adolescents should be tested for HBsAg at the time a pregnancy is discovered, regardless of HBV immunization history and previous results of tests for HBsAg and antibody to HBsAg. Unimmunized pregnant adolescents who are HBsAg negative should begin the HBV vaccine series as soon as possible during the course of pregnancy. Pregnancy is not a contraindication to receiving HBV vaccine in any trimester. The HBsAg status of a pregnant adolescent should be reported to the patient's prenatal care facility, the hospital where she will deliver her infant, and the state health department where case-management assistance will occur. Infants born to HBsAg-positive mothers must receive a dose of HBV vaccine and HBIG within 12 hours of birth (see Hepatitis B, Care of Exposed People, p 386).

Incarcerated adolescents who are found to have evidence of chronic HBV infection should be evaluated by a specialist to determine the extent of their liver disease and their eligibility for antiviral therapy. Detainees who are HBsAg positive should be reported to the local health department to facilitate long-term follow-up after release.

All adolescents with chronic liver disease should be immunized with HAV vaccine to prevent fulminant liver disease should infection with HAV occur. Adolescents who chronically are infected with HBV should be counseled against the use and abuse of alcohol and street drugs, both of which can degrade liver function in patients with HBV-induced cirrhosis. Chronically infected people may remain infectious to sexual and household contacts for life and must be counseled accordingly to protect sexual partners and household contacts.

Hepatitis C

Of the nearly 4 million people chronically infected with HCV in the United States, approximately 30% have been incarcerated in one or more of the nation's correctional institutions. The most common mode of acquisition of HCV is injection drug use; exposure to multiple sexual partners is a distant second. Up to 80% of inmates who use illicit injection drugs will be infected with HCV within 5 years after onset of their drug use. Tattooing and body piercing in regulated settings are not thought to be significant sources of transmission of HCV, but tattoos received in a correctional facility can be associated with hepatitis C. Prevalence studies of HCV infection in incarcerated youth are limited but show an approximate two- to fourfold increase over youth who are not in the juvenile justice system. Injection drug use is the predominant HCV infection risk factor for detained juveniles.

Testing inmates for HCV infection has created conflicts for administrators of correctional facilities. Many do not view the diagnosis and potential treatment of their residents with HCV infection as part of the correctional mission. Inmates commonly refuse testing, even when at high risk of hepatitis, to avoid persecution from fellow prisoners. The lack of a vaccine for hepatitis C places a substantial burden on prevention counseling to elicit changes in high-risk behaviors and health maintenance counseling to decrease health risks in people already infected. This includes lifestyle alterations and avoidance of street drug and alcohol abuse, which increase morbidity and mortality from hepatitis C.

RECOMMENDATIONS FOR CONTROL OF HCV INFECTIONS IN INCARCERATED YOUTH.
Routine screening of incarcerated adolescents for HCV infection is not recommended. Focused screening of adult inmates on the basis of risk criteria has proven reliable and cost-effective for correctional facilities that use it consistently. Risk factor assessments of newly admitted juvenile inmates being considered for HCV testing might include (1) self-reported history of injection drug use; (2) history of liver disease; (3) presence of antibody to hepatitis B core antigen; (4) increased alanine transaminase concentration; or (5) history of hemodialysis or receipt of clotting factors made before 1987, or blood transfusions before 1992, or organ transplants. Testing of detainees with one or more of these factors for antibody to hepatitis C virus can detect more than 90% of HCV infections in correctional facilities. Some juvenile offenders may withhold reporting risk behaviors and yet express interest in HCV testing when offered. These requests, in most instances, should be accommodated. Adolescents with signs or symptoms of hepatitis should undergo diagnostic testing for acute hepatitis A, acute hepatitis B, and HCV infection.

Adolescents who test positive for antibody to HCV should receive ongoing medical attention to determine the likelihood of chronic infection, and cases should be reported to the local health department. The presence of HCV antibody and the absence of HCV RNA do not preclude the possibility of active liver disease. HCV antigenemia is variable from day to day and occurs in the presence of circulating HCV antibody. Juveniles found to be chronically infected with HCV should receive ongoing medical evaluation (in consultation with an expert in caring for chronic live disease) to monitor the course of their liver disease and to determine their suitability for therapeutic interventions (see Hepatitis C, p 391). Incarcerated adolescents with HCV infection should be enrolled in a risk-reduction program for drug and alcohol avoidance as indicated and should receive counseling for safe sex practices for the safety of their sexual partners and the protection of the community at large (**www.cdc.gov/ncidod/diseases/hepatitis/resource/index.htm#training**). Incarcerated adolescents with hepatitis C-related chronic liver disease or with ongoing risk behaviors should receive HAV and HBV vaccines if not already immunized.

MEDICAL EVALUATION OF INTERNATIONALLY ADOPTED CHILDREN FOR INFECTIOUS DISEASES[1,2]

Annually, thousands of children from other countries are adopted by families in the United States. In recent years, more than 90% of international adoptees are from Asian (China, South Korea, Vietnam, India, Kazakhstan, and Philippines), Latin American and Caribbean (Guatemala, Colombia, and Haiti), Eastern European (Russia and the Ukraine), and African (Ethiopia, Nigeria, Liberia, and Ghana) countries. The Middle East is a less common origin for international adoptees. The diverse birth countries of these children, their unknown medical histories before adoption, their previous living circumstances (eg, orphanages and/or foster care), and the limited availability of reliable health care in some resource-limited countries make the medical evaluation of internationally adopted children a challenging but important task.

Internationally adopted children typically differ from refugee children in terms of their access to medical care and treatment before arrival in the United States and in the frequency of certain infectious diseases. Many refugee children may have resided in refugee camps for months before resettlement in the United States and will have had access to limited medical care and treatment services. The history of access to and quality of medical care for international adoptees can be variable. Before admission to the United States, all internationally adopted children are required to have a medical examination performed by a physician designated by the US Department of State in their country of origin. However, this examination is limited to completing legal requirements for screening for certain communicable diseases and examination for serious physical or mental defects that would prevent the issue of an immigrant visa. Information about this required health assessment is available at **www.cdc.gov/immigrantrefugeehealth/**. This evaluation is not a comprehensive assessment of the child's health. During preadoption visits, pediatricians can stress to prospective parents the importance of acquiring immunization and other health records. The Immigration and Nationality Act of 1996 requires immigrant visa applicants to provide "proof of vaccination" with vaccines recommended by the Advisory Committee on Immunization Practices (ACIP) before entry into the United States. Internationally adopted children who are 10 years of age and younger may obtain a waiver of exemption from the Immigration and Nationality Act regulations pertaining to immunization of immigrants before arrival in the United States (see Refugees and Immigrants, p 101). Children adopted from countries that are not part of the Hague Convention can receive waivers to have their immunizations delayed until arrival in the United States (**www.adoption.state.gov**). When an exemption is granted, adoptive parents are required to sign a waiver indicating their intention to comply with ACIP-recommended immunizations within 30 days after the child arrives in the United States. However, the child should be seen by his or her pediatrician or a physician

---

[1] For additional information, see Canadian Paediatric Society. *Children and Youth New to Canada: Health Care Guide.* Ottawa, Ontario: Canadian Paediatric Society; 2000; and the CDC (**www.cdc.gov/travel/default.aspx**) and World Health Organization (**www.who.int**) Web sites.

[2] Information for parents can be found at **www.cdc.gov/immigrantrefugeehealth/adoption/index. html/**.

who specializes in adoption medicine as soon as possible after arrival in the United States to begin all preventive health services, including immunizations.

Infectious diseases are among the most common medical diagnoses identified in international adoptees after arrival in the United States. Children may be asymptomatic, and therefore, the diagnoses must be made by screening tests in addition to history and physical examination. Because of inconsistent use of the birth dose of hepatitis B vaccine; inconsistent perinatal screening for hepatitis B, syphilis, and human immunodeficiency virus (HIV); and the high prevalence of certain intestinal parasites and tuberculosis, all international adoptees should be screened for these infections on arrival in the United States. Recommended screening tests for infectious diseases are listed in Table 2.16 (also see disease-specific chapters in Section 3). In addition to these infectious disease screening tests, other medical and developmental issues, including hearing and vision assessment, evaluation of growth and development, nutritional assessment, blood lead concentration, complete blood cell count with red blood cell indices and differential of white blood cells

Table 2.16. Screening Tests for Infectious Diseases in International Adoptees[a]

Hepatitis B virus serologic testing:
  Hepatitis B surface antigen (HBsAg)

Hepatitis C virus serologic testing

Syphilis serologic testing:
  Nontreponemal test (RPR, VDRL, or ART)
  Treponemal test (MHA-TP, FTA-ABS, or TPPA)

Human immunodeficiency virus 1 and 2 serologic testing

Complete blood cell count with red blood cell indices and differential

Stool examination for ova and parasites (3 specimens)[b] with specific request for *Giardia intestinalis* and *Cryptosporidium* species testing

Tuberculin skin test[b]

In children from countries with endemic infection[b]:
  Trypanosoma cruzi serologic testing

In children with eosinophilia (absolute eosinophil count exceeding 450 cells/mm³) and negative stool ova and parasite examinations[c]:
  Strongyloides species serologic testing
  Schistosoma species serologic testing (for sub-Saharan African, Southeast Asian, and certain Latin American adoptees)

Serologic testing for lymphatic filariasis(for children >2 years of age from endemic countries)[b]

RPR indicates rapid plasma reagin; VDRL, Venereal Disease Research Laboratories; ART, automated reagin test; MHA-TP, microhemagglutination test for *Treponema pallidum;* FTA-ABS, fluorescent treponemal antibody absorption; TPPA, *T pallidum* particle agglutination.
[a] For evaluation of noninfectious disease conditions, see text.
[b] See text.
[c] Some experts would perform serologic tests for schistosomiasis in children from areas with high endemicity regardless of eosinophil count because of its poor positive- and negative-predictive values.

to evaluate for eosinophilia, glucose-6-phosphate dehydrogenase screening, hemoglobin electrophoresis, measurement of thyroid-stimulating hormone concentration, and examination for congenital anomalies (including fetal alcohol syndrome), should be part of the initial evaluation of any internationally adopted child.

Parents generally will have limited information about a child before adoption. Optimally, parents should obtain all information available for that child and meet with the child's physician before their child arrives home to review available information and to discuss common medical issues regarding internationally adopted children. Parents who have not met with a physician before adoption should notify their physician when their child arrives so that a timely medical evaluation can be arranged. Internationally adopted children should be examined as soon as possible after arrival in the United States, preferably within the first 2 weeks after arrival. A list of pediatricians with special interest in adoption and foster care medicine is available on the American Academy of Pediatrics Web site at **www2.aap.org/sections/adoption/directory/map-adoption.cfm.**

Viral Hepatitis

In studies conducted primarily during the 1990s, the prevalence of hepatitis B surface antigen (HBsAg) in internationally adopted children ranged from 1% to 5%, depending on the country of origin and the year studied. Hepatitis B virus (HBV) infection was prevalent in adoptees from Asia and Africa, regions of high endemicity, and in some countries of central and Eastern Europe (eg, Romania and Bulgaria) and states of the former Soviet Union (eg, Russia and the Ukraine). Over the past 5 to 10 years, the number of countries with routine infant hepatitis B immunization programs has increased markedly. By 2006, 163 countries, encompassing 84% of the world's population, had implemented routine infant hepatitis B immunization nationwide. However, administration of a birth dose of hepatitis B vaccine, needed to prevent perinatal transmission from an infected mother, is not routine in many countries, and coverage among infants can be suboptimal. Therefore, all children should be tested for HBsAg to identify cases of chronic infection, regardless of immunization status (see Hepatitis B, p 369). Although hepatitis B serologic tests are performed routinely in the country of origin, testing may be incomplete and children may become infected after testing. Unimmunized children with a negative HBsAg laboratory result should be immunized according to the recommended childhood and adolescent immunization schedules (Fig 1.1–1.3, p 27–31).

Children with a positive HBsAg laboratory result should be reported to the local or state health department. To verify the presence of chronic HBV infection, HBsAg-positive children should be retested. The absence of immunoglobulin M antibody to hepatitis B core antigen (IgM anti-HBc) or the persistence of HBsAg for at least 6 months indicates chronic HBV infection (see Hepatitis B, p 369). Children with chronic HBV infection should be tested for biochemical evidence of liver disease and followed by a specialist who cares for patients with chronic hepatitis B (see Hepatitis B, p 369). All unimmunized household contacts of children with chronic HBV infection should be immunized (see Hepatitis B, p 369).

Hepatitis D virus (HDV), which occurs only in conjunction with the presence of HBsAg, can infect adoptees, particularly from North Africa, parts of South America, and the Mediterranean Basin. Serologic tests for diagnosis of HDV infection are not available widely (see Hepatitis D, p 396). Routine testing is recommended as part of further clinical evaluation of children found to have chronic HBV infection.

Because hepatitis A virus (HAV) is endemic in the countries of origin of internationally adopted children, many international adoptees may have acquired hepatitis A virus (HAV) infection early in life in their country of origin and may be immune. However, because HAV is endemic in many of these countries, internationally adopted children are at ongoing risk of HAV infection while in their countries of origin. Serologic testing for acute infection (hepatitis A IgM) and immunity (total hepatitis A antibody) can be performed at the initial visit to determine whether the child has a current hepatitis A infection or immunity. Children incubating HAV infection at the time of adoption could transmit the virus to their adoptive families and others on arrival in the United States. Adoptive parents and any accompanying family members should ensure they are immunized or otherwise immune to HAV infection before international travel to pick up their child. In addition, hepatitis A vaccine should be administered to all susceptible nontraveling people who anticipate having close personal contact with a child adopted internationally from a country with high or intermediate hepatitis A endemicity before arrival of the adoptee. Adopted children or their household or other close contacts with symptoms consistent with acute viral hepatitis should be evaluated promptly. Children without hepatitis A immunity who are 12 months of age and older should receive hepatitis A vaccine as recommended according to the routine immunization schedule (Fig 1.1, p 27–31).

Routine testing for hepatitis C virus (HCV) infection is recommended for all children, given that most international adoptees in recent years have been adopted from countries with higher prevalence rates (China, Russia, southeast Asia) and because risk factors for infection are rarely known. An enzyme immunoassay (EIA) should be used as the initial screening test. Passively transferred maternal antibody may remain detectable by EIA for up to 18 months (see Hepatitis C, p 391); therefore, in young children, positive EIA results may be from maternal antibody. A positive EIA result needs to be confirmed with a more specific assay, such as a recombinant immunoblot assay or polymerase chain reaction testing, and those with positive results should be seen by a liver specialist (see Hepatitis C, p 391).

Intestinal Pathogens

Fecal examinations for ova and parasites by an experienced laboratory will identify a pathogen in 15% to 35% of internationally adopted children. The prevalence of intestinal parasites varies by age of the child and country of origin. The most common pathogens identified are *Giardia intestinalis, Dientamoeba fragilis, Hymenolepis* species, *Ascaris lumbricoides,* and *Trichuris trichiura. Strongyloides stercoralis, Entamoeba histolytica,* and hookworm are recovered less commonly. If gastrointestinal tract signs or symptoms are present, 3 stool specimens, collected daily, should be examined for ova and parasites, with direct fluorescent antibody or EIA testing for *Giardia* species and *Cryptosporidium* species. Therapy for intestinal parasites generally will be successful, but complete eradication may not occur. Therefore, repeat ova and parasite testing after treatment is important to ensure successful elimination of parasites if symptoms persist. Children who fail to demonstrate adequate catch-up growth, who have unexplained anemia, or who have gastrointestinal tract symptoms or signs that occur or recur months or even years after arrival in the United States should be reevaluated for intestinal parasites. In addition, when newly arrived adoptees have diarrhea, stool specimens should be tested for *Salmonella* species,

Shigella species, *Campylobacter* species, and Shiga toxin-producing *Escherichia coli*, including *E coli* O157:H7, and antimicrobial susceptibility testing should be performed if bacterial pathogens are isolated and if treatment is planned.

Tuberculosis

Latent tuberculosis infection commonly is encountered in international adoptees from all countries, although incidence rates of tuberculosis vary by country. Reported rates of latent *Mycobacterium tuberculosis* infection range from 0.6% to 30%. All immigrants, including international adoptees, are required to have screening for tuberculosis before arriving in the United States. The screening requirements for tuberculosis underwent a major revision in 2007. Information about the screening and implementation requirements is available at **www.cdc.gov/ncidod/dq/panel_2007.htm.**

Because tuberculosis may be more severe in young children and may reactivate in later years, screening with the tuberculin skin test (TST) in all children or an interferon-gamma release assay in children 5 years of age or older is important in this high-risk population (see Tuberculosis, p 736). Routine chest radiography is not indicated in asymptomatic children in whom the TST result is negative. However, some international adoptees may be anergic because of malnutrition, which is common in malnourished children. If malnutrition is suspected, the TST should be repeated once the child is nourished appropriately. Presence or absence of a bacille Calmette-Guérin (BCG) vaccine scar should be noted. Receipt of BCG vaccine is not a contraindication to a TST, and a positive TST result should not be attributed to BCG vaccine. In these children, further investigation is necessary to determine whether latent tuberculosis infection or active disease is present and therapy is needed (see Tuberculosis, p 736). Some children will have had recent exposure to a person with tuberculosis disease. Preventive therapy should be considered if such a history is available. Some experts repeat the TST 3 to 6 months after the initial TST in children with an initial TST <10 mm of induration, because the initial test may have been falsely negative because of anergy or recent infection. However, a boosting phenomenon attributable to a previous TST also can occur, which confounds interpretation. In children 5 years of age and older, interferon-gamma release assay (IGRA) could be performed to help determine whether a "positive" TST result in a child who previously received BCG vaccine is attributable to latent tuberculosis infection. When active tuberculosis is suspected in an international adoptee, efforts to isolate and test the organism for drug susceptibilities are imperative because of the high prevalence of drug resistance in many countries.

Syphilis

Congenital syphilis, especially with involvement of the central nervous system, may not have been diagnosed or may have been treated inadequately in adoptees from some resource-limited countries. Children 15 years of age and older should have had serologic testing for syphilis as part of the required overseas medical assessment. Children who had positive test results are required to complete treatment before arrival in the United States. After arrival in the United States, clinicians should screen each international adoptee for syphilis by reliable nontreponemal and treponemal serologic tests, regardless of history or a report of treatment (see Syphilis, p 690). Children with positive treponemal serologic test results should be evaluated by a health care professional with special expertise to assess the differential diagnosis of pinta, yaws, and syphilis and to determine extent of infection so appropriate treatment can be administered (see Syphilis, p 690).

HIV Infection

The risk of HIV infection in internationally adopted children depends on the country of origin and individual risk factors. Because of the rapidly changing epidemiology of HIV infection and because adoptees may come from populations at high risk of infection, screening for HIV should be performed for all internationally adopted children. Although many children will have HIV test results documented in their referral information, test results from the child's country of origin may not be reliable. Transplacentally acquired maternal antibody in the absence of infection can be detected in a child younger than 18 months of age. Hence, positive HIV antibody test results in asymptomatic children of this age require clinical evaluation, further testing, and counseling (see Human Immunodeficiency Virus Infection, p 418).

Chagas Disease (American Trypanosomiasis)

Chagas disease is endemic throughout much of Mexico and Central and South America (see American Trypanosomiasis, p 734). Risk of Chagas disease varies by region within countries with endemic infection. Although the risk of Chagas disease is low in internationally adopted children from countries with endemic infection, treatment of infected children is highly effective. Countries with endemic Chagas disease include Argentina, Belize, Bolivia, Brazil, Chile, Colombia, Costa Rica, Ecuador, El Salvador, French Guiana, Guatemala, Guyana, Honduras, Mexico, Nicaragua, Panama, Paraguay, Peru, Suriname, Uruguay, and Venezuela. Transmission within countries with endemic infection is focal, but if a child comes from a country with endemic Chagas disease, testing for *Trypanosoma cruzi* should be considered. Serologic testing should be performed only in children 12 months of age or older because of the potential presence of maternal antibody.

Other Infectious Diseases

Skin infections that occur commonly in international adoptees include bacterial (eg, impetigo) and fungal (eg, candidiasis) infections and ectoparasitic infestations (eg, scabies and pediculosis). Adoptive parents should be instructed on how to examine their child for signs of scabies, pediculosis, and tinea so treatment can be initiated and transmission to others can be prevented (see Scabies, p 641, and Pediculosis, p 543–547).

Diseases such as typhoid fever, malaria, leprosy, or melioidosis are encountered infrequently in internationally adopted children. Although routine screening for these diseases is not recommended, findings of fever, splenomegaly, respiratory tract infection, anemia, or eosinophilia should prompt an appropriate evaluation on the basis of the epidemiology of infectious diseases that occur in the child's country of origin. If the child came from a country where malaria is present, malaria should be considered in the differential diagnosis (see Malaria, p 483).

In the United States, multiple outbreaks of measles have been reported in children adopted from China and in their United States contacts. Measles outbreaks among children in orphanages in China also were reported. In 2002 and 2004, adoptions from affected orphanages were suspended temporarily while Chinese authorities implemented measures to control and prevent further transmission of measles among the children. Measles elimination has been achieved only in the Americas; transmission continues in other parts of the world. In 2011, measles importation into the United States occurred from more than 22 countries, but because of high immunization rates, secondary cases were minimal. Prospective parents who are traveling internationally to adopt children, as well as their household contacts, should ensure that they have a history of natural disease or have been immunized adequately for measles according to US guidelines. All people born after 1957 should receive 2 doses of measles-containing vaccine in the absence of documented measles infection or contraindication to the vaccine (see Measles, p 489).

Clinicians should be aware of potential diseases in internationally adopted children and their clinical manifestations. Some diseases, such as central nervous system cysticercosis, may have incubation periods as long as several years and, thus, may not be detected during initial screening. On the basis of findings at the initial evaluation, consideration should be given to a repeat evaluation 6 months after adoption. In most cases, the longer the interval from adoption to development of a clinical syndrome, the less likely the syndrome can be attributed to a pathogen acquired in the country of origin.

In international adoptees who have negative stool ova and parasite test results and in whom eosinophilia (absolute eosinophil count exceeding 450 cells/mm^3) is found on review of complete blood cell count, serologic testing for strongyloidiasis, schistosomiasis, and lymphatic filariasis should be considered. Serologic testing for *Strongyloides stercoralis* should be performed on all international adoptees with eosinophilia and no identified pathogen commonly associated with an increased eosinophil count, regardless of country of origin. Serologic testing for *Schistosoma* species should be performed on international adoptees with eosinophilia and no identified pathogen commonly associated with eosinophilia who are from Sub-Saharan Africa, South East Asia, or areas of Latin America where schistosomiasis is endemic. Serologic testing for lymphatic filariasis should be considered in international adoptees older than 2 years of age with eosinophilia who are from countries with endemic lymphatic filariasis (**www.cdc.gov/parasites/lymphaticfilariasis/index.html**).

Immunizations

Only written documentation of immunizations received by an adoptee should be accepted. Immunizations such as BCG, diphtheria and tetanus toxoids and pertussis (DTP or DTaP), poliovirus, measles, and hepatitis B vaccines are given routinely in many parts of the world and may be documented in an immunization record. However, because other immunizations such as *Haemophilus influenzae* type b, *Streptococcus pneumoniae*, mumps, rubella, hepatitis A, and varicella vaccines are given less frequently or are not part of the routine immunization schedule in other countries, written documentation may be available less often. Internationally adopted children and adolescents should receive immunizations according to the recommended schedule in the United States for healthy children and adolescents (see Fig 1.1–1.3, p 27–31). Although some vaccines with inadequate potency are used in other countries, most vaccines available worldwide are produced with adequate quality-control standards and are reliable. However, information about storage, handling, site of administration, vaccine potency, and provider generally is not available. In general, written documentation of immunizations can be accepted as evidence of adequacy of previous immunization if the vaccines, dates of administration, number of doses, intervals between doses, and age of the child at the time of immunization are consistent internally and comparable to current US or World Health Organization schedules (see Immunizations Received Outside the United States, p 36). Given the limited data available regarding verification of immunization records from other countries, evaluation of concentrations of antibody to the antigens given repeatedly is an option to ensure that vaccines were given and were immunogenic. Serologic testing may be performed to determine whether protective antibody concentrations are present. An acceptable alternative when doubt exists is to reimmunize the child. Table 2.17 (p 199) lists the vaccines for which antibody testing can be performed, specifies the types of tests to be ordered, and provides recommended and alternative approaches. In children older than 6 months of age with or without written documentation of immunization, serologic testing for antibodies to diphtheria and tetanus toxoids and poliovirus may be considered to determine whether the child has protective antibody concentrations. If the child has protective antibody concentrations, then the immunization series should be completed as appropriate for that child's age. In children older than 12 months of age, hepatitis A, measles, mumps, rubella, and varicella antibody concentrations may be measured to determine whether the child is immune; these antibody tests should not be performed in children younger than 12 months of age because of the potential presence of maternal antibody. Many children will need mumps and rubella vaccines, administered as MMR vaccine, because mumps and rubella vaccines are administered infrequently in resource-limited countries. Two doses of measles-mumps-rubella (MMR) vaccine could be administered for mumps coverage, even if measles antibodies are present. Rubella coverage is achieved following 1 dose of a rubella-containing vaccine. At this time, no antibody testing is reliable or available routinely to assess immunity to pertussis. Serologic testing for HBsAg should be performed for all children to identify chronic infection. If serologic testing is not available and receipt of immunogenic vaccines cannot be ensured, the prudent course is to provide the immunization series.

Table 2.17. Approaches to the Evaluation and Immunization of Children Adopted From Outside the United States[a]

Vaccine	Recommended Approach	Alternative Approach
Hepatitis B	Complete serologic testing for hepatitis B; if HBsAg positive or HBsAb and HBcAb positive, no immunization is needed. If only HBsAb positive, review record to determine whether hepatitis B vaccine doses were age and interval appropriate. If they were, no additional immunization is needed; if not, administer 1 dose of HBV vaccine.	—
Diphtheria, pertussis and tetanus toxoids (DTaP, Tdap, DT, Td)	Immunize with diphtheria, pertussis, and tetanus-containing vaccine as appropriate for age (see Diphtheria, p 307, Pertussis, p 553, and Tetanus, p 707). Serologic testing for antitoxoid antibodies 4 wk after dose 1 if severe local reaction occurs.	Serologic testing for diphtheria and tetanus IgG antibodies; if protective, continue immunizations appropriate for age; if nonprotective, reimmunize.
Haemophilus influenzae type b (Hib)	Age-appropriate immunization.	—
Pertussis (DTaP, Tdap)	No serologic test routinely available. May use antibodies to diphtheria or tetanus toxoids as a marker of receipt of diphtheria, tetanus, and pertussis-containing vaccine.	—
Poliovirus	Immunize with inactivated poliovirus (IPV) vaccine.	Serologic testing for neutralizing antibody to poliovirus types 1, 2, and 3 or administration of a single dose of IPV, followed by serologic testing for neutralizing antibody to poliovirus types 1, 2, and 3.
Hepatitis A	Serologic testing with immunization if nonimmune.	Age-appropriate immunization.
Measles-mumps-rubella (MMR)	Immunize with MMR vaccine or obtain measles and mumps antibody and if positive, administer 1 dose of MMR vaccine for rubella protection.	Serologic testing for IgG antibody to vaccine viruses.
Varicella	Serologic testing and immunization if nonimmune.	Age-appropriate immunization.
Pneumococcal	Age-appropriate immunization.	—

HBsAg indicates hepatitis B surface antigen; HBsAb, hepatitis B surface antibody; HBcAb, hepatitis B core antibody; HBV, hepatitis B virus; DTaP, diphtheria and tetanus toxoids and acellular pertussis; Tdap, tetanus and diphtheria toxoids and reduced acellular pertussis; DT, diphtheria and tetanus toxoids; Td, tetanus and diphtheria toxoids; IgG, immunoglobulin G.

[a]Centers for Disease Control and Prevention. General recommendations on immunization. Recommendations of the Advisory Committee on Immunization Practices. *MMWR Recomm Rep.* 2011;60(2):1–64. Also see Fig 1.1–1.3 (p 27–31)

INJURIES FROM DISCARDED NEEDLES IN THE COMMUNITY

Contact with and injuries from hypodermic needles and syringes discarded in public places, presumably by injection drug users, may pose a risk of transmission of bloodborne pathogens, including human immunodeficiency virus (HIV), hepatitis B virus (HBV), and hepatitis C virus (HCV). An epidemiologic study of 274 pediatric-aged children (mean age, 7.4 years) identified with a community-acquired needlestick injury over a 19-year period observed no seroconversions, confirming that the risk of transmission of bloodborne viruses in these events is low.[1] Infection risks and options for postexposure prophylaxis (PEP) vary depending on the virus and type of injury and exposure. Although nonoccupational needlestick injuries may pose a lower risk of infection transmission than do occupational needlestick injuries, a person injured by a needle in a nonoccupational setting needs evaluation, counseling, and in some cases, PEP. Even if the potential for the discarded syringe to contain a specific bloodborne pathogen can be estimated from the background prevalence rates of these infections in the local community, the need to test the injured or exposed person usually is not influenced significantly by this assessment.

Wound Care and Tetanus Prophylaxis

Management of people with needlestick injuries includes acute wound care and consideration of the need for antimicrobial prophylaxis. Standard wound cleansing and care is indicated; such wounds rarely require closure. Tetanus toxoid vaccine, with or without Tetanus Immune Globulin, should be considered as appropriate for the age, the severity of the injury, the immunization status of the exposed person, and the potential for dirt or soil contamination of the needle (see Tetanus, p 707). The preferred tetanus toxoid vaccine is tetanus and diphtheria toxoids and reduced acellular pertussis (Tdap; see Pertussis, p 553), but tetanus and diphtheria toxoids (Td) vaccine should be used if the patient has already received Tdap at some point in the past, because current recommendations are for only a single administration of Tdap.

Bloodborne Pathogens

Consideration of the need for prophylaxis for HBV and HIV is the next step in exposure management; currently, there is no recommended PEP for HCV. Risk of acquisition of various pathogens depends on the nature of the wound, the ability of the pathogens to survive on environmental surfaces, the volume of source material, the concentration of virus in the source material, prevalence rates among local injection drug users, the probability that the syringe and needle were used by a local injection drug user, and the immunization status of the exposed person. Unlike an occupational blood or body fluid exposure, in which the status of the exposure source for HBV, HCV, and HIV often is

---

[1] Papenburg J, Blais D, Moore D, et al. Pediatric injuries from needles discarded in the community: epidemiology and risk of seroconversion. *Pediatrics.* 2008;122(2):e487–e487

known, these data usually are not available to help in the decision-making process in a nonoccupational exposure.[1,2]

Hepatitis B Virus

HBV is the hardiest of the major bloodborne pathogens and can survive on environmental surfaces at room temperature for at least 7 days. It has been shown to be transmitted at a rate of 23% to 62% during needlestick injury between health care personnel and HBV-positive sources. Prompt and appropriate PEP intervention reduces this risk. The effectiveness of PEP diminishes the longer after exposure it is initiated. Children who have needlestick injuries and who have not completed the 3-dose hepatitis B vaccine series should receive a dose of HBV vaccine and, if indicated, should be scheduled to receive the remaining doses to complete the schedule. Administration of Hepatitis B Immune Globulin usually is not indicated if the child has received the 3-dose regimen of hepatitis B vaccine. If the child has received 2 doses of hepatitis B vaccine 4 or more months previously, the immediate administration of the third dose of vaccine alone should be sufficient in most cases. Experts differ in opinion about the need for Hepatitis B Immune Globulin at the time of an injury of an incompletely immunized child. If the needle is from a person known to be hepatitis B surface antigen (HBsAg) positive, consideration could be given to testing the child for hepatitis B surface antibody and providing Hepatitis B Immune Globulin, in addition to continuing with the vaccination series.

Human Immunodeficiency Virus

Infection with HIV usually is the greatest concern of the victim and family. The risk of HIV transmission from a needle discarded in public is low. To date, no cases in which HIV was transmitted by needlestick injury outside a health care setting have been reported to the Centers for Disease Control and Prevention. Risk of HIV transmission from a puncture wound caused by a needle found in the community is lower than the 0.3% risk of HIV transmission to a health care professional from a needlestick injury from a person with known HIV infection. In most reports of occupational HIV transmission by percutaneous injury, needlestick injury occurred shortly after needle withdrawal from the vein or artery of the source patient with HIV infection. HIV RNA was detected in only 3 (3.8%) of 80 discarded disposable syringes that had been used by health care professionals for intramuscular or subcutaneous injection of patients with HIV infection, indicating that most syringes will not contain transmissible HIV even after being used to draw blood from a person with HIV infection. HIV is susceptible to drying, and when HIV is placed on a surface exposed to air, the 50% tissue culture infective dose decreases by approximately 1 log every 9 hours.

Despite the low risk, there may be situations in which HIV testing in the child who suffered the needlestick is appropriate. In this situation, HIV antibody testing should be performed at baseline, and follow-up testing should be performed at 6 weeks, 12 weeks,

---

[1] Centers for Disease Control and Prevention. Updated US Public Health Service guidelines for the management of occupational exposures to HBV, HCV, and HIV and recommendations for postexposure prophylaxis. *MMWR Recomm Rep.* 2001;50(RR-11):1–52

[2] US Department of Health and Human Services. Antiretroviral postexposure prophylaxis after sexual, injection-drug use, or other nonoccupational exposure to HIV in the United States: recommendations from the US Department of Health and Human Services. *MMWR Recomm Rep.* 2005;54(RR-2):1–20

and 6 months after injury. Testing also is indicated if an illness consistent with acute HIV-related syndrome develops before the 6-week testing. Negative results from these initial tests support the conclusion that any subsequent positive test result likely reflects infection acquired from the needlestick. A positive initial test result in a pediatric patient requires further investigation of the cause, such as perinatal transmission, sexual abuse or activity, or drug use. An alternative option is to obtain and save a baseline serum specimen for later testing for HIV antibody in the unlikely event that a subsequent test result is positive. Counseling is necessary before and after testing (see Human Immunodeficiency Virus Infection, p 418).

A specialist in HIV infection should be consulted before deciding whether to initiate PEP. Antiretroviral therapy is not without risk and often is associated with significant adverse effects (see Human Immunodeficiency Virus Infection, p 418). In the rare event that the needle owner is known to be HIV positive, PEP should be started immediately. If the needle owner is known and has a low risk of being HIV-infected, most experts agree that PEP does not need to be administered pending test results of the owner. In most situations, the needle owner is not known. Data are not available on the efficacy of PEP with antiretroviral drugs in these circumstances for adults or children, and as a result, the US Public Health Service is unable to recommend for or against prophylaxis in this circumstance.[1,2] PEP should be considered on a case–by-case basis, taking into consideration type of exposure and prevalence in the setting concerned. Some experts recommend that antiretroviral chemoprophylaxis be considered if the needle and/or syringe are available and found to contain visible blood; testing the syringe for HIV is not practical or reliable and is not recommended. If the decision to begin prophylaxis is made, any delay before starting the medications should be minimized (see Human Immunodeficiency Virus Infection, p 418). Medication should begin within 72 hours and should continue for 28 days in combination of 2 or 3 antiretroviral drugs. The suggested medication options are the same for the HIV occupational exposure (see Human Immunodeficiency Virus Infection, p 418).

Hepatitis C Virus

The third bloodborne pathogen of concern is HCV, which can last in the environment for at least 16 to 23 hours. The prevalence of chronic HCV infection in the United States varies by race/ethnicity, age group, geographic location, and individual history of risk behaviors. Although transmission by sharing syringes among injection drug users is efficient, the risk of transmission from a discarded syringe is likely to be low. Testing for HCV is not recommended routinely in the absence of a risk factor for infection or a known exposure to a HCV-positive source. If performed, antibody to HCV (anti-HCV) can be detected in 80% of newly infected patients within 15 weeks after exposure and in 97% of newly infected patients by 6 months after exposure. If earlier diagnosis is desired, testing for HCV RNA may be performed at 4 to 6 weeks after exposure. Positive test results should be confirmed by supplemental confirmatory laboratory tests (see Hepatitis

---

[1] Centers for Disease Control and Prevention. Antiretroviral postexposure prophylaxis after sexual injection-drug-use, or other nonoccupational exposure to HIV in the United States: recommendations from the US Department of Health and Human Services. *MMWR Recomm Rep.* 2005;54(RR-2):1–20

[2] Havens PL; American Academy of Pediatrics, Committee on Pediatric AIDS. Postexposure prophylaxis in children and adolescents for nonoccupational exposure to human immunodeficiency virus. *Pediatrics.* 2003;111(6):1475–1489 (Reaffirmed October 2008)

C, p 391). There is no recommended PEP for HCV using antiviral drugs or Immune Globulin preparations, because any HCV antibody-positive donor is excluded from the pool from which Immune Globulin products are prepared.

Preventing Needlestick Injuries

Needlestick injuries of both children and adults can be minimized by implementing public health programs on safe needle disposal and programs for exchange of used syringes and needles from injection drug users for sterile needles. Syringe and needle exchanges decrease improper disposal and spread of bloodborne pathogens without increasing the rate of injection drug use. The American Academy of Pediatrics supports needle-exchange programs in conjunction with drug treatment and within the context of continuing research to assess their effectiveness.

BITE WOUNDS

As many as 1% of all pediatric visits to emergency departments during summer months are for treatment of human or animal bite wounds. An estimated 5 million bites occur annually in the United States; dog bites account for approximately 90% of those wounds. The rate of infection after cat bites is as high as 50%; rates of infection after dog or human bites are 10% to 15%. The bites of humans, wild animals, or nontraditional pets potentially are sources of serious infection. Parents should be informed to teach children to avoid contact with wild animals and should secure garbage containers so that raccoons and other animals will not be attracted to the home and places where children play. Most nontraditional pets, including ferrets, iguanas, and other reptiles, and wild animals pose an infection as well as an injury risk for children, and their ownership should be discouraged in households with children younger than 8 years of age. Potential transmission of rabies is increased when a bite, particularly unprovoked, is from a wild animal (especially a bat or a carnivore) or from a domestic animal that cannot be observed for 10 days after the bite (see Rabies, p 600). Dead animals should be avoided, because they can harbor rabies virus in their nervous system tissues and saliva and can be infested with arthropods (fleas or ticks) infected with a variety of bacterial, rickettsial, protozoan, or viral agents.

Recommendations for bite wound management are given in Table 2.18 (p 204). Sufficient prospective, controlled studies on which to base recommendations about the closure of bite wounds are lacking. In general, recent, apparently uninfected, low-risk lesions can be sutured after thorough wound cleansing, irrigation, and débridement. Use of local anesthesia can facilitate these procedures. Because suturing enhances risk of wound infection, some clinicians prefer to manage small wounds by approximation of the wound edges with adhesive strips or tissue adhesive. Bite wounds on the face seldom become infected, but if a wound has important cosmetic considerations, it should be closed whenever possible. Hand wounds have a higher risk of infection, and serious hand wounds should be managed in consultation with an appropriate surgical specialist. Specimens for aerobic and anaerobic culture should be obtained from wounds that appear infected. Approximation of margins and closure by delayed primary or secondary intent is prudent for infected nonfacial wounds, but sealing an infected wound with a tissue adhesive should be avoided. Elevation of injured areas to minimize swelling is important.

Table 2.18. Prophylactic Management of Human or Animal Bite Wounds to Prevent Infection

Category of Management	Management
Cleansing	Remove visible dirt
	Cleanse the wound surface with soap and water, saline, 1% povidone–iodine, or 1% benzalkonium chloride
	Irrigate with a copious volume of sterile saline solution by high-pressure syringe irrigation[a]
	Do not irrigate puncture wounds; Standard Precautions should be used
Wound culture	No for fresh wounds, unless signs of infection exist
	Yes for wounds that appear infected[b]
Diagnostic imaging	Indicated for penetrating injuries overlying bones or joints, for suspected fracture, or to assess foreign body inoculation
Débridement	Remove superficial devitalized tissue
Operative débridement and exploration	Yes if any of the following:
	• Extensive wounds (devitalized tissue)
	• Involvement of the metacarpophalangeal joint (clenched fist injury)
	• Cranial bites by large animal
Wound closure	Yes for selected fresh, nonpuncture bite wounds (see text)
Assess tetanus immunization status[c]	Yes
Assess risk of rabies from animal bites[d]	Yes
Assess risk of hepatitis B virus infection from human bites[e]	Yes
Assess risk of human immunodeficiency virus from human bites[f]	Yes
Initiate antimicrobial therapy[g]	Yes for:
	• Moderate or severe bite wounds, especially if edema or crush injury is present
	• Puncture wounds, especially if penetration of bone, tendon sheath, or joint has occurred
	• Facial bite wounds
	• Hand and foot bite wounds
	• Genital area bite wounds
	• Wounds in immunocompromised and asplenic people
	• Wounds with signs of infection
Follow-up	Inspect wound for signs of infection within 48 h

[a] Use of an 18-gauge needle with a large-volume syringe is effective. Antimicrobial or anti-infective solutions offer no advantage and may increase tissue irritation.
[b] Both aerobic and anaerobic bacterial culture should be performed.
[c] See Tetanus, p 707.
[d] See Rabies, p 600.
[e] See Hepatitis B, p 369.
[f] See Human Immunodeficiency Virus Infection, p 418.
[g] See Table 2.19 (p 206) for suggested drug choices.

Limited data exist to guide antimicrobial prophylaxis or therapy for patients with wounds that are not overtly infected. Patients with mild injuries in which the skin is abraded do not need to be treated with antimicrobial agents. The use of an antimicrobial agent within 8 to 12 hours of injury for a 3- to 5-day course of therapy may decrease the rate of infection. Children at high risk of infection (eg, children who are immunocompromised or who have joint penetration) should receive preemptive antimicrobial therapy. Guidelines for initial choice of antimicrobial prophylaxis and therapy for human and animal bites are provided in Table 2.19 (p 206). In the child with an overt bite wound-associated infection, initial therapy should be modified when culture results become available. Methicillin-resistant *Staphylococcus aureus* (MRSA) is a potential bite wound pathogen; empiric therapy may require modification if MRSA is isolated from an infected wound (see Staphylococcal Infections, p 653). Coverage for MRSA should be considered in severe bite wound infections while cultures are pending.

Prophylaxis or treatment of the child with a serious allergy to penicillin and a human or animal bite wound is problematic. Oral or parenteral treatment with trimethoprim-sulfamethoxazole, which is effective against *S aureus* including MRSA, *Pasteurella multocida*, and *Eikenella corrodens*, in conjunction with clindamycin, which is active in vitro against anaerobic bacteria, streptococci, and many strains of *S aureus*, may be effective for preventing or treating bite wound infections. Extended-spectrum cephalosporins, such as cefotaxime or ceftriaxone parenterally or cefpodoxime orally, do not have good anaerobic spectra of activity but can be used in conjunction with clindamycin as alternative therapy for penicillin-allergic patients who can tolerate cephalosporins. Doxycycline is an alternative agent that has activity against *P multocida*; use of doxycycline in children younger than 8 years of age must be weighed against the risk of dental staining. Azithromycin and fluoroquinolones display good in vitro activity against organisms that commonly cause bite wound infections, but clinical trial data are lacking and fluoroquinolones are not approved for this indication in children. Meropenem is an option for children with penicillin allergy, but cross-reactions with penicillins can occur infrequently. If meropenem is used as monotherapy, it should be noted that meropenem does not have activity against MRSA. A 7- to 10-day course usually is sufficient for soft tissue infections. Longer courses of treatment may be indicated, depending on severity of infection, feasibility of draining abscesses if these occur, and patient's clinical responses. The duration of treatment for bite wound-associated bone infections is based on location, severity, and pathogens isolated.

Table 2.19. Antimicrobial Agents for Human or Animal Bite Wounds

Source of Bite	Organism(s) Likely to Cause Infection	Antimicrobial Agent			
		Oral Route	Oral Alternatives for Penicillin-Allergic Patients[a]	Intravenous Route[b,c]	Intravenous Alternatives for Penicillin-Allergic Patients[a,b,c]
Dog, cat, or mammal[d]	*Pasteurella* species, *Staphylococcus aureus*, streptococci, anaerobes, *Capnocytophaga* species, *Moraxella* species, *Corynebacterium* species, *Neisseria* species	Amoxicillin-clavulanate	Extended-spectrum cephalosporin or trimethoprim-sulfamethoxazole[e] PLUS Clindamycin	Ampicillin-sulbactam[f]	Extended-spectrum cephalosporin or trimethoprim-sulfamethoxazole PLUS Clindamycin OR Meropenem
Reptile[g]	Enteric gram-negative bacteria, anaerobes	Amoxicillin-clavulanate	Extended-spectrum cephalosporin or trimethoprim-sulfamethoxazole[e] PLUS Clindamycin	Ampicillin-sulbactam[f] PLUS Gentamicin	Clindamycin PLUS Gentamicin OR Meropenem
Human	Streptococci, *S aureus*, *Eikenella corrodens*, *Haemophilus* species, anaerobes	Amoxicillin-clavulanate	Extended-spectrum cephalosporin or trimethoprim-sulfamethoxazole[e] PLUS Clindamycin	Ampicillin-sulbactam[f]	Extended spectrum cephalosporin or trimethoprim-sulfamethoxazole PLUS Clindamycin OR Meropenem

[a] For patients with history of allergy to penicillin or one of its congeners, alternative drugs are recommended. In patients without a history of anaphylaxis, wheezing, angioedema, or urticaria, an extended-spectrum cephalosporin or other beta-lactam–class drug may be acceptable. For example, ceftriaxone, rather than trimethoprim-sulfamethoxazole, could be used intravenously. These drugs should not be used for patients with an immediate hypersensitivity (anaphylaxis) to penicillin, because approximately 5% to 10% of penicillin-allergic patients also will be allergic to cephalosporins.

[b] Coverage for methicillin-resistant *S aureus* with vancomycin should be considered for severe bite wounds.

[c] Note that use of ampicillin-sulbactam or meropenem monotherapy will not include activity against methicillin-resistant *S aureus* isolates.

[d] Data are lacking to guide antimicrobial use for bites that are not overtly infected from small mammals, such as guinea pigs and hamsters.

[e] Doxycycline is an alternative for children 8 years of age and older.

[f] Piperacillin-tazobactam or ticarcillin-clavulanate can be used as alternatives.

[g] The role of empirical antimicrobial use for noninfected snake bite wounds is not well-defined. Therapy should be chosen on the basis of results of cultures from infected wounds.

PREVENTION OF TICKBORNE INFECTIONS

Tickborne infectious diseases in the United States include diseases caused by bacteria (eg, tularemia), spirochetes (Lyme disease and relapsing fever), rickettsiae (eg, Rocky Mountain spotted fever, ehrlichiosis, anaplasmosis), viruses (eg, Colorado tick fever, Powassan virus), and protozoa (eg, babesiosis) (see Table 2.20, and disease-specific chapters in Section 3). Different species of ticks transmit different infectious agents (eg, brown dog ticks are 1 vector of the agent that causes Rocky Mountain spotted fever; black-legged ticks transmit the agent of Lyme disease), and some species of ticks (eg, the

Table 2.20. Some Tick-Transmitted Pathogens (Domestic and Imported)

Human Disease Type	Pathogens in the United States	Pathogens in Other Countries
Bacteria		
Human anaplasmosis	*Anaplasma phagocytophilum*	*Anaplasma phagocytophilum*
Human ehrlichiosis	*Ehrlichia chaffeensis, Ehrlichia ewingii, Ehrlichia muris-like species*	*Ehrlichia muris,* possibly *Ehrlichia canis,* other species
Lyme disease, Lyme borreliosis	*Borrelia burgdorferi sensu stricto*	*Borrelia burgdorferi sensu lato,* including *Borrelia afzelii, Borrelia garinii, Borrelia burgdorferi sensu stricto,* and other genomospecies in Europe
Q fever (uncommon tick transmission)	*Coxiella burnetii*	*Coxiella burnetii*
Spotted fever group of rickettsioses	*Rickettsia rickettsii, Rickettsia parkeri, Rickettsia* species serotype 364D, perhaps other species	*Rickettsia rickettsii, Rickettsia conorii, Rickettsia africae, Rickettsia honei, Rickettsia japonica, Rickettsia sibirica, Rickettsia slovaca,* other species
Tickborne relapsing fever	*Borrelia hermsii, Borrelia turicatae, Borrelia parkeri,* and other species	*Borrelia duttonii,* other species
Tularemia	*Francisella tularensis*	*Francisella tularensis*
Protozoa		
Human babesiosis	*Babesia microti, Babesia* species (MO1), *Babesia duncani* (WA1, CA2)	*Babesia microti, Babesia divergens,* other species
Viruses		
Coltivirus infection	Colorado tick fever virus	European Eyach virus
Flavivirus infection	Powassan virus, Deer tick virus	Powassan virus, tickborne encephalitis virus, Kyasanur Forest disease virus, Russian spring-summer encephalitis virus, Omsk hemorrhagic fever virus

black-legged tick) may transmit more than 1 agent. Physicians should be aware of the epidemiology of tickborne infections in their local areas. Prevention of tickborne diseases is accomplished by avoiding tick-infested habitats, decreasing tick populations in the environment, using personal protection against tick bites, and limiting the length of time ticks remain attached to the human host. Control of tick populations in the field often is not practical but can be effective in more defined areas around places where children reside and play. Using consumer-applied acaricides (pesticides targeting ticks) or contracting with a licensed pest-control operator can be efficient approaches to reducing tick populations and, therefore, the risk of tickborne disease in highly tick-infested areas. Specific measures for prevention are as follows:

- Physicians, parents, and children should be made aware that ticks can transmit pathogens that cause human and animal diseases.
- Tick-infested areas should be avoided whenever possible. Most ticks prefer dense woods with thick growth of shrubs and small trees as well as along the edges of the woods, where the woods abut lawns. Ticks require humidity to survive, and drier areas usually are less infested. For homes located in tick-prone areas, risk of exposure can be reduced by locating play equipment in sunny, dry areas away from forest edges, by creating a barrier of wood chips or gravel between recreation areas and forest, and keeping leaves raked and underbrush cleared. The brown dog tick is able to survive in more arid environments and can be introduced indoors. This species may be found in cracks and crevices of housing or in animal housing or bedding.
- If a tick-infested area is entered, light-colored clothing that covers the arms, legs, and other exposed areas should be worn. Pants should be tucked into boots or socks, and long-sleeved shirts should be buttoned at the cuff. Permethrin (a synthetic pyrethroid) can be sprayed onto clothes to decrease tick attachment. Permethrin should not be sprayed onto skin, and treated clothing should be dried before wearing. In 2003, the US Environmental Protection Agency approved commercial sale of outdoor clothing treated with permethrin for children of all ages and for pregnant women. Permethrin-treated clothing remains effective for approximately 20 washings.
- Tick and insect repellents that contain diethyltoluamide (DEET) applied to the skin provide additional protection but may require reapplication every 1 to 2 hours for maximum effectiveness. Some newer formulations are microencapsulated to increase the time before reapplication to 8 to 12 hours. Although there have been rare reports of serious neurologic complications in children possibly associated with exposure to DEET-containing insect repellents, the risk is extremely low when these products are used properly. Products containing DEET should be applied as recommended (see Prevention of Mosquitoborne Infections, p 209). For children 2 months of age and older, products with 10% to 30% DEET can be used. Products containing DEET should not be used on infants younger than 2 months of age. Repellents should not be used on clothing or mosquito nets on which young children may chew or suck.
- Picaridin (KBR 3023), the plant-based oil of eucalyptus, IR3535 (3-[N-Butyl-N-acetyl]-aminopropionic acid, ethyl ester), and other active ingredients have been registered for use as tick repellents by the US Environmental Protection Agency. These products are readily available and may be more acceptable to some families, because they do not damage certain synthetic fabrics and plastics as DEET-containing products can.

- People should inspect themselves and their children's bodies and clothing daily after possible tick exposure. Special attention should be given to the exposed hairy regions of the body where ticks often attach, including the head, neck, and behind the ears in children (*Dermacentor* ticks). Ticks (especially *Ixodes* ticks) also may attach at areas of tight clothing (eg, belt line, axillae, groin).
- Ticks should be removed as soon as possible, because risk of transmission of pathogens increases with time of tick attachment. For removal, a tick should be grasped with a fine tweezers close to the skin and gently pulled straight out without twisting motions. Although not recommended, if fingers are used to remove ticks, they should be protected with a barrier such as tissue and washed after removal of the tick. The bite site should be washed with soap and water to reduce the risk of secondary skin infections.
- Maintaining tick-free pets also will decrease tick exposure. Daily inspection of pets and removal of ticks are indicated, as is the routine use of appropriate veterinary products to prevent ticks on pets. Consult a veterinarian for information on suitable products.
- Chemoprophylaxis to prevent Lyme disease may be considered under certain circumstances in areas with highly endemic Lyme disease (see Lyme Disease, p 474).

PREVENTION OF MOSQUITOBORNE INFECTIONS

Mosquitoborne infectious diseases in the United States are caused by arboviruses (eg, West Nile, La Crosse, St. Louis encephalitis, eastern equine encephalitis, and western equine encephalitis viruses [see Arboviruses, p 232]). International travelers may encounter other arboviral (eg, Yellow fever, dengue, Japanese encephalitis) or other mosquitoborne infections (eg, malaria) during travel (also see disease-specific chapters in Section 3). Physicians should be aware of the epidemiology of arbovirus infections in their local areas. Prevention involves protection from the bite of an infected mosquito. In areas with arbovirus transmission, protection of children is recommended during outdoor activities, including activities related to school, child care, or camping. Education of families and other caregivers is an important component of prevention. Specific measures include:

- **Eliminate local mosquito breeding sites.** Mosquitoes develop in standing water. Often, large numbers of mosquitoes are produced from sources at or very near the home. Measures to limit mosquito breeding sites around the home include drainage or removal of receptacles for standing water (old tires, toys, flower pots, cans, buckets, barrels, other containers that collect rain water); keeping swimming pools, decorative pools, children's wading pools, and bird-baths clean; and cleaning clogged rain gutters. Under certain circumstances, large-scale mosquito control measures may be conducted by community mosquito-control programs or public health officials. These efforts include drainage of standing water, use of larvicides in waters that are sources of mosquitoes, and use of pesticides to control biting adult mosquitoes.
- **Reduce exposure to mosquitoes.** Avoiding mosquito bites by limiting outdoor activities at times of high mosquito activity, which primarily occur at dusk and dawn, and screening of windows and doors can help reduce exposure to mosquitoes. Many parts of the United States also have mosquitoes that bite during the day, and some of these have been found to transmit La Crosse, dengue, and West Nile virus. Mosquito

traps, electrocutors (bug zappers), ultrasonic repellers, and other devices marketed to prevent mosquitoes from biting people are not effective and should not be relied on to reduce mosquito bites.

- **Use barriers to protect skin.** Barriers include mosquito nets and screens for baby strollers or other areas where immobile children are placed. Additional protection can be gained, when practical, by using clothing to cover exposed skin (ie, long sleeves, long pants, socks, shoes, and hats).
- **Discourage mosquitoes from biting.** Mosquitoes are attracted to people by odors on the skin and by carbon dioxide from the breath. The active ingredients in repellents make the user unattractive for feeding, but they do not kill the mosquitoes. Repellents should be used during outdoor activities when mosquitoes are present, especially in regions with arbovirus transmission, and should always be used according to the label instructions. Repellents are synthetic compounds or derivatives of plant oils. The most effective repellents for use on skin are products that contain either diethyltoluamide (DEET), picaridin (KBR 3023), IR3535 (3-[N-Butyl-N-acetyl]-aminopropionic acid, ethyl ester), or the plant-based oil of lemon eucalyptus (OLE) and its synthetic equivalent p-menthane-3,8-diol. Products containing these active ingredients have been shown to have good repellent activity. Products with a higher concentration of active ingredients protect longer and are appropriate for people who will be exposed to mosquitoes during outdoor activities lasting many hours. Products with lower concentrations of active ingredients may be used when more transient protection is required, but they may require repeated applications to provide a longer duration of protection. Studies in human volunteers document the association of active ingredient concentration with duration of repellent activity. For example, results of one study demonstrated an average duration of protection of 5 hours, 4 hours, 2 hours, and 1.5 hours for products with DEET concentrations of 23.8%, 20%, 6.7%, and 4.5%, respectively. Picaridin is available in 7%, 15%, and 20% formulations in the United States and has been shown to be as effective as lower concentrations of DEET, with higher concentrations offering longer protection, but frequent reapplication is necessary for lasting protection. IR3535 is available in formulations ranging from 7.5% to 20%, with estimated protection times ranging from 2 hours for the lower concentrations to up to 8 hours with the higher concentrations. OLE appears to have similar duration of action as products containing lower concentrations of DEET, with a product containing 30% OLE providing protection roughly equivalent to a product containing 15% DEET. All other plant products studied, including those based on citronella, protected for less than 20 minutes. Ingestion of garlic or vitamin B_1, wearing devices that emit sounds, and impregnated wristbands are ineffective measures.

DEET has been used worldwide since 1957, has been studied more extensively than any other repellent, and has a good safety profile. Concerns about potential toxicity, especially in children, are unfounded. Adverse effects are rare; are most often associated with ingestions, chronic use, or excessive use; and do not appear to be related to DEET concentration used. Urticaria and contact dermatitis have been reported in a small number of people. Reports of encephalopathy have been rare, with 13 cases reported after skin application in children. Encephalopathy also has been reported after unintentional ingestion. DEET is irritating to eyes and mucous membranes. Concentrated formulations can damage plastic and certain fabrics. If used appropriately, DEET does not present a health problem.

Although concentrations of 10% to 15% DEET or lower have been recommended for children, there is no evidence that these concentrations are safer than 30% DEET. Products with DEET concentrations of 10% or less should not be used for exposures lasting more than 1 to 2 hours. There is no evidence that repellents that do not contain DEET are safer, and there are no safety data for other products in children. In 2001, the US Environmental Protection Agency (EPA) concluded that appropriate use of DEET at concentrations of up to 30% posed no significant risk to children or adults but that DEET should not be used in children younger than 2 months of age because of increased skin permeability. The American Academy of Pediatrics has supported this recommendation.[1] The Centers for Disease Control and Prevention currently recommends DEET at concentrations up to 50% for both adults and children older than 2 months of age.

Picaridin-containing compounds have been used as an insect repellent for years in Europe and Australia as a 20% formulation with no serious toxicity reported. Except for eye irritation, products containing oil of eucalyptus appear safe, although the EPA specifies that they should not be used on children younger than 3 years of age.

Permethrin-containing repellents are registered by the EPA for use on clothing, shoes, bed nets, and camping gear. Permethrin is a synthetic pyrethroid that is highly effective both as an insecticide and as a repellent for ticks, mosquitoes, and other arthropods. Permethrin can be sprayed onto clothes but should not be sprayed onto skin. Some manufacturers now offer permethrin-treated clothing, and beginning in 2003, the EPA approved commercial sale of outdoor clothing treated with permethrin for children of all ages and for pregnant women. Repellents should not be used on clothing or mosquito nets on which young children may chew or suck.

The EPA recommends the following precautions when using insect repellents. Recommendations for use of any of these insect repellents should be followed for children:
- Do not apply over cuts, wounds, or irritated or sunburned skin. Avoid areas around eyes and mouth.
- Do not spray onto the face; apply with hands.
- Use just enough to cover exposed skin.
- Do not apply to young children's hands, because they may rub it into their eyes or mouth.
- Do not allow young children to apply a product themselves.
- Do not apply under clothing.
- Do not use sprays in enclosed areas or near food.
- Repellents containing DEET, applied according to label instructions, can be used along with a separate sunscreen. No data are available regarding the use of other active repellent ingredients in combination with a sunscreen.
- Reapply if washed off by sweating or by getting wet.
- After returning indoors, wash treated skin with soap and water or bathe. Also, wash treated clothing before wearing again.
- If a child develops a rash or other reaction from any insect repellent, wash the repellent off with soap and water and contact the child's physician or the US poison control center (800-222-1222) for guidance.

---

[1] American Academy of Pediatrics, Committee on Environmental Health. Pesticides. In: Etzel RA, Balk SJ, eds. *Pediatric Environmental Health. 3rd* ed. Elk Grove Village, IL: American Academy of Pediatrics; 2012:515–548

···

PREVENTION OF ILLNESSES ASSOCIATED WITH RECREATIONAL WATER USE

Pathogen transmission through ingestion or use of recreational water (eg, swimming pools, interactive fountains, lakes, oceans) is a growing source of illness in the United States. Since the mid-1980s, the number of outbreaks related to recreational water activities has increased substantially, particularly outbreaks associated with treated recreational venues (eg, swimming pools).[1] Therefore, preventing recreational water-related illness is becoming increasingly important for the health of children and adults. Recreational water illnesses (RWIs) are caused by pathogens transmitted by ingesting, inhaling mists or aerosols, or having contact with contaminated water from swimming pools, interactive fountains, water parks, spas, lakes, rivers, or oceans. RWIs also can be caused by chemicals in the water or chemicals that volatilize from the water and cause indoor air quality problems. Illnesses caused by recreational water exposure can involve the gastrointestinal tract, respiratory tract, central nervous system, skin, ears, and eyes. During 2007–2008, 134 waterborne disease outbreaks associated with recreational water were reported.[1] This represents the largest number of outbreaks reported in a 2-year period and a more than 300% increase compared with 1997–1998. Of the 134 outbreaks, 60% involved the gastrointestinal tract, 18% involved the skin, and 18% involved the respiratory tract. The most common organism associated with treated recreational water venues was *Cryptosporidium* species (see Cryptosporidiosis, p 296).

Swimming is a communal bathing activity by which the same water is shared by dozens to thousands of people each day, depending on venue size (eg, small wading pools, municipal pools, water parks). Fecal contamination of recreational water venues is a common occurrence because of the high prevalence of diarrhea and fecal incontinence (particularly in young children) and the presence of residual fecal material on bodies of swimmers (up to 10 g on young children). The largest outbreaks of waterborne disease tend to affect children less than 5 years of age disproportionately, tend to occur during the summer months, and result in gastroenteritis.

To protect swimmers from pathogens, water at public swimming venues is chlorinated to oxidize fecal matter and pathogens. Although many pathogens are inactivated rapidly by chlorination, some pathogens are moderately to highly tolerant to chlorination and can survive for extended periods of time in chlorinated water. *Cryptosporidium* oocysts can remain infectious for days in chlorine concentrations typically mandated in swimming pools, thus contributing to the role of *Cryptosporidium* species as the leading cause of treated recreational water-associated outbreaks of gastroenteritis. *Giardia* species have been shown to survive for up to 45 minutes in water chlorinated at concentrations typically used in swimming pools and are well documented as causes of recreational water-associated disease outbreaks.

Recreational water use is an ideal means of amplifying pathogen transmission within a community because of chlorine-tolerant pathogens, coupled with low infectious doses, a high prevalence of diarrhea in the general population, high pathogen-excretion concentrations, and heavy use of swimming venues. As a result, one or more swimmers ill with

---

[1] Centers for Disease Control and Prevention. Surveillance for waterborne disease outbreaks and other health events associated with recreational water—United States, 2007–2008. *MMWR Surveill Summ*. 2011;60(SS-12):1–32

diarrhea can contaminate large volumes of water and expose large numbers of coswimmers to pathogens, particularly if pool disinfection is inadequate or the pathogen is chlorine tolerant. However, RWI outbreaks generally are preventable and can be decreased substantially through a combination of proper pool maintenance, water disinfection, and improved swimmer hygiene and behavior.

CONTROL MEASURES

Swimming continues to be a safe and effective means of exercise. Transmission of pathogens that cause RWIs can be prevented by reducing contamination of swimming venues and exposure to contaminated water through adoption of the following practices:

- Do not participate in recreational water activities such as swimming while ill with diarrhea.
  - After cessation of symptoms, people who had diarrhea attributable to *Cryptosporidium* also should avoid recreational water activities for an additional 2 weeks. This is because of prolonged excretion of infectious *Cryptosporidium* oocysts after cessation of symptoms, the potential for intermittent diarrhea that might cause infected people to think symptoms have resolved, and the increased transmission potential in treated venues (eg, swimming pools) because of the parasite's high chlorine tolerance.
  - After cessation of symptoms, children who had diarrhea attributable to other potentially waterborne pathogens (eg, *Shigella* species, *Giardia* species, and norovirus) and who have not been toilet trained should avoid recreational water activities for 1 additional week.
- Do not participate in recreational water activities if you have open wounds or sores until the wounds or sores heal. Open wounds can serve as portals of entry for pathogens.
- Avoid ingestion of recreational water.
- Practice good swimming hygiene by:
  - Taking a cleansing shower, using soap and water, before entering recreational water.
  - Washing children thoroughly, especially the perianal area, with soap and water before allowing them to participate in recreational water activities.
  - Taking young children for regular bathroom breaks often or checking diapers every 30 to 60 minutes.
  - Washing hands with soap and water after toilet use and diaper-changing activities. Toilet use and diaper changing should occur away from the recreational water source.
  - Washing hands with soap and water before and after consumption of food and drink.
    Recommendations for responding to fecal incidents in treated recreational water venues have been published.[1]

"SWIMMER'S EAR"/ACUTE OTITIS EXTERNA

Participation in recreational water activities can predispose children to infections of the external auditory canal. Acute otitis externa (AOE) or "swimmer's ear" is diffuse inflammation of the external auditory canal and usually is attributed to bacterial infection. Recreational water activities, showering, and bathing can introduce water into the ear canal, wash away protective ear wax, and cause maceration of the thin skin of the ear

---

[1] Centers for Disease Control and Prevention. Notice to readers: revised recommendations for responding to fecal accidents in disinfected swimming venues. *MMWR Morb Mortal Wkly Rep.* 2008;57(6):151–152. Available at: **www.cdc.gov/mmwr/preview/mmwrhtml/mm5706a5.htm**

canal, predisposing the ear canal to bacterial infection. AOE is most common among children 5 to 14 years of age but can occur in all age groups, including adults. A marked seasonality is observed, with cases peaking during the summer months. Warm, humid environments and frequent submersion of the head while swimming are risk factors for AOE.

The 2 bacteria most commonly associated with AOE are *Pseudomonas aeruginosa* and *Staphylococcus aureus*. Many cases are polymicrobial. *Aspergillus* species and *Candida* species have been identified rarely in AOE. Cultures of swab specimens taken from the external ear canal in AOE may reflect normal ear canal flora or pathogenic organisms.

AOE readily responds to treatment with topical antimicrobial agents with or without a topical steroid. Unless the infection has spread to surrounding tissues or the patient has complicating factors (eg, diabetes or immunosuppression), topical treatment alone should be sufficient and no additional oral antimicrobial agent is required. Polymyxin B sulfate/neomycin sulfate, gentamicin sulfate, and ciprofloxacin for 7 to 10 days are topical antibiotic agents used commonly. If clinical improvement is not noted by 48 to 72 hours, foreign body obstruction of the canal, noncompliance with therapy, or alternate diagnoses such as contact dermatitis or traumatic cellulitis following piercing should be considered. Some topical agents have the potential for ototoxicity (eg, gentamicin, neomycin, agents with a low pH, hydrocortisone-neomycin-polymyxin). These ototoxic agents should not be used in children with tympanostomy tubes or a perforated tympanic membrane. Patients with AOE should avoid submerging their head in water for 7 to 10 days, but competitive swimmers might be able to return to the pool if pain has resolved and they use well-fitting ear plugs.

Swimmers should be instructed to keep their ear canals as dry as possible. This can be accomplished by covering the opening of the external auditory canal with a bathing cap or by using ear plugs or swim molds. Following swimming or showering, the ears should be dried thoroughly.

If a patient experiences recurring episodes of AOE, consideration can be given to use of ear drops after recreational water exposure as an additional preventive measure. Commercial ear-drying agents are available for use as directed, or patients may drop a 1:1 mixture of acetic acid (white vinegar) and isopropanol (rubbing alcohol) in the external ear canal after swimming or showering to restore the proper acidic pH to the ear canal and to dry residual water. Note that these drops should not be used in the presence of ear tubes, tympanic membrane perforation, or acute external ear infection.

DISEASES TRANSMITTED BY ANIMALS (ZOONOSES): HOUSEHOLD PETS, INCLUDING NONTRADITIONAL PETS, AND EXPOSURE TO ANIMALS IN PUBLIC SETTINGS[1,2]

Disease transmission from animals to humans is possible for children who interact with pets or other domestic or wild animals. Important zoonoses that may be encountered in North America, the common animal source or vector, and major modes of transmission are reviewed in disease-specific chapters in Section 3 and are listed in Appendix XI (p 926). Most households in the United States contain 1 or more pets. The number of families with nontraditional pets, defined as (1) imported, nonnative species or species that originally were nonnative but now are bred in the United States; (2) indigenous wildlife; or (3) wildlife hybrids (offspring of wildlife crossbred with domestic animals), has increased in recent years. Infants and children also come in contact with animals at many venues outside the home, including zoos, farms, shopping malls, schools, hospitals, animal swap meets, agricultural fairs, and petting zoos. Examples of nontraditional pets and animals commonly encountered in public settings are listed in Table 2.21, p 216.

Exposure to animals can pose significant infection risks to all people, but children younger than 5 years of age, pregnant women, the elderly, and people of all ages with immunodeficiencies are at higher risk of serious infections. The increased infection risk for children younger than 5 years of age is attributable, in part, to children's less-than-optimal hygiene practices and developing immune systems. Children younger than 5 years of age also are at increased risk of injury from animals because of their size and behavior. Bites, scratches, kicks, falls, and crush injuries to hands or feet or from being pinned between an animal and a fixed object can occur.

Nontraditional pets pose a potential risk of infection and injury. Most imported nonnative animal species are caught in the wild rather than bred in captivity. These animals are held and transported in close contact with multiple other species, thus increasing the transmission risk of potential pathogens for humans and domestic animals. Some nonnative animals are brought into the United States illegally, thus bypassing rules established to reduce introduction of disease and potentially dangerous animals. In addition, as an animal matures, its physical and behavioral characteristics can result in an increased risk of injuries to children. The behavior of captive indigenous wildlife and wildlife hybrids cannot be predicted. These potential risks are enhanced when there is an inadequate understanding of disease transmission and methods to prevent transmission; animal behavior; or how to maintain appropriate facilities, environment, or nutrition for captive animals. Among nontraditional pets, reptiles pose a particular risk because of high carriage rates of *Salmonella* species, the intermittent shedding of *Salmonella* organisms in their feces, and persistence of *Salmonella* organisms in the environment. The US Food and Drug Administration's ban on

[1] Pickering LK; Marano N; Bocchini JA; Angulo FJ; American Academy of Pediatrics, Committee on Infectious Diseases. Exposure to nontraditional pets at home and to animals in public settings: risks to children. *Pediatrics*. 2008;122(4):876–886 (Reaffirmed December 2011)

[2] National Association of State Public Health Veterinarians. Compendium of measures to prevent disease associated with animals in public settings, 2011. *MMWR Recomm Rep*. 2011;60(RR-04):1–24

Table 2.21. Nontraditional Pets and/or Animals That May Be Encountered in Public Settings[a]

Category	Examples
Amphibians	Frogs, toads, newts, salamanders
Fish	Many types
Mammals	
Wildlife	Raccoons, skunks, foxes, coyotes, civet cats, tigers, lions, bobcats, bears, nonhuman primates
Domesticated livestock	Cattle, pigs, goats, sheep
Poultry	Chickens, ducks, geese, and turkeys
Equines	Horses, mules, donkeys, zebras
Weasels	Ferrets, minks, sables, skunks
Lagomorphs	Rabbits, hares, pikas
Rodents	Mice, rats, hamsters, gerbils, guinea pigs, chinchillas, gophers, lemmings, squirrels, chipmunks, prairie dogs, hedgehogs
Feral animals	Cats, dogs, horses, swine
Reptiles	Turtles, lizards, iguanas, snakes, alligators

[a] Pickering LK; Marano N; Bocchini JA; Angulo FJ; American Academy of Pediatrics, Committee on Infectious Diseases. Exposure to nontraditional pets at home and to animals in public settings: risks to children. *Pediatrics.* 2008;122(4):876–886 (Reaffirmed December 2011)

commercial distribution of turtles with shells less than 4 inches long in 1975 resulted in a sustained reduction of human *Salmonella* infections. *Salmonella* infections also have been described as a result of contact with aquatic frogs, hedgehogs, hamsters, and other rodents and with baby chicks and other poultry, including ducks, ducklings, geese, goslings, and turkeys. Additionally, pet products, such as dry dog and cat food, and pet treats, such as pig ears, have been sources of *Salmonella* infections, especially among young children.

Infectious diseases, injuries, and other health problems can occur after contact with animals in public settings. Enteric bacteria and parasites pose the highest infection risk. Individual cases and outbreaks associated with *Salmonella* species, *Escherichia coli* O157:H7, *Campylobacter* species, and *Cryptosporidium* species have been reported. Ruminant livestock (cattle, sheep, and goats) are the major source of infection, but poultry, rodents, and other domestic and wild animals also are potential sources and often are asymptomatic carriers of potential human pathogens. Direct contact with animals (especially young animals), contamination of the environment or food or water sources, and inadequate hand hygiene facilities at animal exhibits all have been implicated as reasons for infection in these public settings. Unusual infection or exposure has been reported occasionally; rabies has occurred in animals in a petting zoo, pet store, animal shelter, and county fair, necessitating prophylaxis of adults and children.

Contact with animals has numerous positive benefits, including opportunities for education and entertainment. However, many pet owners and people in the process of choosing a pet are unaware of the potential risks posed by pets. Pediatricians, veterinarians, and other health care professionals are in a unique position to offer advice on proper pet selection, provide information about safe pet ownership and responsibility, and minimize risks to infants and children. Pet size and temperament should be matched to the age and behavior of an infant or child. Acquisition and ownership of nontraditional pets should be discouraged in households with young children. Information brochures and posters are available for display in physician and veterinarian offices so parents can be educated about the guidelines available for safe pet selection and appropriate handling (**www.cdc.gov/healthypets/index.htm, www.cdc.gov/Features/ HealthyPets/** and **https://ebusiness.avma.org/ebusiness50/product catalog/ProductCategory.aspx?ID=132**). The Black Pines Animal Park (**www.blackpineanimalpark.com**) offers the following guidance on pet selection:

G How much will this animal **G**row?

O How **O**ld can this animal live to be?

O Will this animal create **O**dors I won't like?

D What kind of **D**iet does this animal require?

L Can this animal be **L**ethal to me and others?

I Is it **I**llegal for me to own this animal?

F Just how much **F**un will it really be to own this animal?

E What are the **E**nvironmental requirements for this animal?

Young children should be supervised closely when in contact with animals at home or in public settings, and children should be educated about appropriate human-animal interactions. Parents should be made aware of recommendations for prevention of human diseases and injuries from exposure to pets, including nontraditional pets and animals in the home, animals in public settings, and pet products including food and pet treats (Table 2.22).

Questions regarding pet and animal contact should be part of well-child evaluations and the evaluation of a suspected infectious disease.

Table 2.22. Guidelines for Prevention of Human Diseases From Exposure to Pets, Nontraditional Pets, and Animals in Public Settings[a,b]

General

- Always supervise children, especially children younger than 5 years of age, during interaction with animals
- Wash hands immediately after contact with animals, animal products, feed or treats, or animal environments
- Supervise hand washing for children younger than 5 years of age
- Do not allow children to kiss pets or to eat, drink, or put objects or hands into their mouths after handling animals or while in animal areas
- Do not permit nontraditional pets to roam or fly freely in the house or allow nontraditional or domestic pets to have contact with wild animals
- Do not permit animals in areas where food or drink are stored, prepared, or consumed
- Never bring wild animals home, and never adopt wild animals as pets
- Teach children never to handle unfamiliar, wild, or domestic animals, even if animals appear friendly
- Avoid rough play with animals to prevent scratches or bites
- Administer rabies vaccine to all dogs, cats, and ferrets; livestock animals with frequent human contact also should be up to date with all immunizations
- Keep animals clean and free of intestinal parasites, fleas, ticks, mites, and lice
- People at increased risk of infection or serious complications of salmonellosis and other enteric infections (eg, children younger than 5 years of age, older adults, and immunocompromised hosts) should avoid contact with high-risk animals (turtles, baby chicks, ducklings, aquatic frogs, farm animals) and animal-derived pet treats and pet foods

Table 2.22. Guidelines for Prevention of Human Diseases From Exposure to Pets, Nontraditional Pets, and Animals in Public Settings,[a,b] continued

Animals Visiting Schools and Child-Care Facilities

- Designate specific areas for animal contact
- Display animals in enclosed cages or under appropriate restraint
- Do not allow food in animal-contact areas
- Always supervise children, especially those younger than 5 y, during interaction with animals
- Obtain a certificate of veterinary inspection for visiting animals and/or proof of rabies immunization according to local or state requirements
- Properly clean and disinfect all areas where animals have been present
- Consult with parents or guardians to determine special considerations needed for children who are immunocompromised or who have allergies or asthma
- Animals not recommended in schools, child-care settings, and hospitals include nonhuman primates, inherently dangerous animals (lions, tigers, cougars, bears, wolf/dog hybrids), mammals at high risk of transmitting rabies (bats, raccoons, skunks, foxes, coyotes, and mongooses), aggressive animals or animals with unpredictable behavior, stray animals with unknown health history, reptiles, amphibians, or baby chicks or other live poultry
- Ensure that people who provide animals for educational purposes are knowledgeable regarding animal handling and zoonotic disease issues

Public Settings

- Venue operators must know about risks of disease and injury
- Venue operators and staff must maintain a safe environment
- Venue operators and staff must educate visitors about the risk of disease and injury and provide appropriate preventive measures

Animal Specific

- Children younger than 5 years of age and immunocompromised people should avoid contact in public settings with reptiles, amphibians, rodents, ferrets, baby poultry (chicks, ducklings), and any items that have been in contact with these animals or their environments
- Reptiles, amphibians, rodents, ferrets, and baby poultry (chicks, ducklings) should be kept out of households that contain children younger than 5 years of age, immunocompromised people, or people with sickle cell disease and should not be allowed in child-care centers
- Reptiles, amphibians, rodents, and baby poultry should not be permitted to roam freely throughout a home or living area and should not be permitted in kitchens or other areas where food and drink is prepared, served or consumed
- Disposable gloves should be used when cleaning fish aquariums, and aquarium water should not be disposed in sinks used for food preparation or for obtaining drinking water
- Mammals at high risk of transmitting rabies (bats, raccoons, skunks, foxes, and coyotes) should not be touched by children

[a]Pickering LK, Marano N, Bocchini JA, Angulo FJ; American Academy of Pediatrics, Committee on Infectious Diseases. Exposure to nontraditional pets at home and to animals in public settings: risks to children. *Pediatrics.* 2008;122(4):876–886 (Reaffirmed December 2011)

[b]National Association of State Public Health Veterinarians, Centers for Disease Control and Prevention. Compendium of measures to prevent disease associated with animals in public settings, 2011: National Association of State Public Health Veterinarians, Inc. *MMWR Recomm Rep.* 2011;60(RR-4):1–24

Summaries of Infectious Diseases

Actinomycosis

CLINICAL MANIFESTATIONS: Actinomycosis classically results from pathogen introduction following a breakdown in mucocutaneous protective barriers. Spread within the host is by direct invasion of adjacent tissues, typically forming sinus tracts that cross tissue planes. The most common species causing human disease is *Actinomyces israelii*.

There are 3 common anatomic sites. **Cervicofacial** is most common, often occurring after tooth extraction, oral surgery, other oral/facial trauma, or even from carious teeth. Localized pain and induration may progress to cervical abscess and "woody hard" nodular lesions ("lumpy jaw"), which can develop draining sinus tracts, usually at the angle of the jaw or in the submandibular region. Infection also may contribute to chronic tonsillar airway obstruction. **Thoracic** disease may be an extension of cervicofacial infection but most commonly is secondary to aspiration of oropharyngeal secretions. It occurs rarely after esophageal disruption secondary to surgery or nonpenetrating trauma. Presentations include pneumonia, which can be complicated by abscesses, empyema, and rarely, pleurodermal sinuses. Focal or multifocal mediastinal and pulmonary masses may be mistaken for tumors. **Abdominal** actinomycosis usually is attributable to penetrating trauma or intestinal perforation. The appendix and cecum are the most common sites; symptoms are similar to appendicitis. Slowly developing masses may simulate abdominal or retroperitoneal neoplasms. Intra-abdominal abscesses and peritoneal-dermal draining sinuses occur eventually. Chronic localized disease often forms draining sinus tracts with purulent discharge. **Other sites** of infection include liver, pelvis (which, in some cases, has been linked to use of intrauterine devices), heart, testicles, and brain (which usually is associated with a primary pulmonary focus). Noninvasive primary cutaneous actinomycosis has occurred.

ETIOLOGY: *A israelii* and at least 5 other *Actinomyces* species cause human disease. All are slow-growing, microaerophilic or facultative anaerobic, gram-positive, filamentous branching bacilli. They can be part of normal oral, gastrointestinal tract, or vaginal flora. *Actinomyces* species frequently are copathogens in tissues harboring multiple other anaerobic and/or aerobic species. Isolation of *Aggregatibacter (Actinobacillus) actinomycetemcomitans*, frequently detected with *Actinomyces species*, may predict the presence of actinomycosis.

EPIDEMIOLOGY: *Actinomyces* species occur worldwide, being components of endogenous oral and gastrointestinal tract flora. *Actinomyces* species are opportunistic pathogens (reported in patients with HIV and chronic granulomatous disease), with disease usually following penetrating (including human bite wounds) and nonpenetrating trauma. Infection is uncommon in infants and children, with 80% of cases occurring in adults. The male-to-female ratio in children is 1.5:1. Overt, microbiologically confirmed, monomicrobial disease caused by *Actinomyces* species has become rare in the era of antimicrobial agents.

The **incubation period** varies from several days to several years.

DIAGNOSTIC TESTS: Microscopic demonstration of beaded, branched, gram-positive bacilli in purulent material or tissue specimens suggests the diagnosis. Only normally sterile site specimens should be submitted for culture. Acid-fast staining can distinguish *Actinomyces* species, which are acid-fast negative, from *Nocardia* species, which are variably acid-fast positive. Yellow "sulfur granules" visualized microscopically or macroscopically in drainage or loculations of purulent material suggest the diagnosis. A Gram stain of "sulfur granules" discloses a dense aggregate of bacterial filaments mixed with inflammatory debris. Immunofluorescent stains for *Actinomyces* species are available. *Actinomyces israelii* forms "spiderlike" microcolonies on culture medium after 48 hours. *Actinomyces* species can be identified in tissue specimens using the 16s rRNA sequencing and polymerase chain reaction assay. Although most *Actinomyces* species are microaerophilic or facultative anaerobic, specimens must be obtained, transported, and cultured anaerobically on semiselective (kanamycin/vancomycin) media.

TREATMENT: Initial therapy should include intravenous penicillin G or ampicillin for 4 to 6 weeks followed by high doses of oral penicillin (up to 2 g/day for adults), usually for a total of 6 to 12 months. Amoxicillin, erythromycin, clindamycin, doxycycline, and tetracycline are alternative antimicrobial choices. Amoxicillin/clavulanate, piperacillin/tazobactam, ceftriaxone, clarithromycin, linezolid, and meropenem also show high activity in vitro, and all *Actinomyces* appear resistant to ciprofloxacin and metronidazole.

Tetracyclines are not recommended for pregnant women or children younger than 8 years of age (see Tetracyclines, p 801). Surgical drainage often is a necessary adjunct to medical management and may allow for a shorter duration of antimicrobial treatment.

ISOLATION OF THE HOSPITALIZED PATIENT: Standard precautions are recommended. There is no person-to-person spread.

CONTROL MEASURES: Appropriate oral hygiene, regular dental care, and careful cleansing of wounds, including human bite wounds, can prevent infection.

Adenovirus Infections

CLINICAL MANIFESTATIONS: Adenovirus infections of the upper respiratory tract are common and, although often subclinical, can result in symptoms of the common cold, pharyngitis, tonsillitis, otitis media, and pharyngoconjunctival fever. Life-threatening disseminated infection, severe pneumonia, hepatitis, meningitis, and encephalitis occur occasionally, especially among young infants and immunocompromised hosts. Adenoviruses occasionally cause a pertussis-like syndrome, croup, bronchiolitis, exudative tonsillitis, pneumonia, hemorrhagic cystitis, and gastroenteritis. Ocular adenovirus infections may present as a follicular conjunctivitis or as epidemic keratoconjunctivitis. In epidemic keratoconjunctivitis, there is an autoimmune infiltration of the cornea in addition to the follicular conjunctivitis. In both cases, ophthalmologic illness frequently presents acutely in one eye followed by involvement of the other eye. In epidemic keratoconjunctivitis, corneal inflammation produces symptoms including light sensitivity and vision loss.

ETIOLOGY: Adenoviruses are double-stranded, nonenveloped DNA viruses; at least 51 distinct serotypes divided into 6 species (A through F) cause human infections. Some adenovirus types are associated primarily with respiratory tract disease, and others are associated primarily with gastroenteritis (types 40 and 41).

Adenovirus type 14 is emerging as a type that can cause severe and sometimes fatal respiratory tract illness in patients of all ages, including healthy young adults, such as military recruits. During 2007, 140 cases of confirmed adenovirus type 14 respiratory tract illness were identified in clusters in several states. Of these patients, 38% were hospitalized, including 17% who were admitted to intensive care units; 5% of the patients died. The isolates were distinct from the type 14 reference strain isolated in 1955, suggesting the emergence and spread of a new and possibly more virulent type 14 variant in the United States.[1] Occasional outbreaks involving smaller numbers of people have occurred since that time.

EPIDEMIOLOGY: Infection in infants and children can occur at any age. Adenoviruses causing respiratory tract infections usually are transmitted by respiratory tract secretions through person-to-person contact, airborne droplets, and fomites, the latter because adenoviruses are stable in the environment. The conjunctiva can provide a portal of entry. Outbreaks of febrile respiratory tract illness can be a common, significant problem in military trainees. Community outbreaks of adenovirus-associated pharyngoconjunctival fever have been attributed to water exposure from contaminated swimming pools and fomites, such as shared towels. Health care-associated transmission of adenoviral respiratory tract, conjunctival, and gastrointestinal tract infections can occur in hospitals, residential institutions, and nursing homes from exposures between infected health care personnel, patients, or contaminated equipment. Adenovirus infections in transplant recipients can occur from donor tissues. Epidemic keratoconjunctivitis commonly occurs by direct contact, has been associated with equipment used during eye examinations, and is caused principally serotypes 8 and 19. Enteric strains of adenoviruses are transmitted by the fecal-oral route. Adenoviruses do not demonstrate the marked seasonality of other respiratory tract viruses and circulate throughout the year. Enteric disease occurs throughout the year and primarily affects children younger than 4 years of age. Adenovirus infections are most communicable during the first few days of an acute illness, but persistent and intermittent shedding for longer periods, even months, is common. Asymptomatic infections are common. Reinfection can occur.

The **incubation period** for respiratory tract infection varies from 2 to 14 days; for gastroenteritis, the incubation period is 3 to 10 days.

DIAGNOSTIC TESTS: The preferred methods for diagnosis of adenovirus infection include cell culture, antigen detection, and DNA detection. Adenoviruses associated with respiratory tract disease can be isolated from pharyngeal and eye secretions and feces by inoculation of specimens into susceptible cell cultures. A pharyngeal or ocular isolate is more suggestive of recent infection than is a fecal isolate, which may indicate either recent infection or prolonged carriage. Rapid detection of adenovirus antigens is possible in a variety of body fluids by commercial immunoassay techniques, including direct fluorescent assay. These rapid assays can be useful for diagnosis of respiratory tract infections, ocular disease, and diarrheal disease. Enteric adenovirus types 40 and 41 usually cannot

---

[1] Centers for Disease Control and Prevention. Outbreak of adenovirus 14 respiratory illness—Prince of Wales Island, Alaska, 2008. *MMWR Morb Mortal Wkly Rep.* 2010;59(1):6–10

be isolated in standard cell cultures. Adenoviruses also can be identified by electron microscopic examination of respiratory tract or stool specimens, but this modality lacks sensitivity. Polymerase chain reaction assays for adenovirus DNA rapidly are replacing other detection methods because of improved sensitivity and increasing commercial availability. Adenovirus typing is available from some reference and research laboratories, although its clinical utility is limited. Serotyping can be determined by hemagglutination inhibition or serum neutralization tests with selected antisera or by molecular methods. Serodiagnosis is used primarily for epidemiologic studies.

TREATMENT: Treatment of adenovirus infection is supportive. Randomized clinical trials evaluating specific antiviral therapy have not been performed. However, case reports of the successful use of intravenous cidofovir in immunocompromised patients with severe adenoviral disease have been published, albeit without a uniform dose or dosing strategy.

ISOLATION OF THE HOSPITALIZED PATIENT: In addition to standard precautions for young children with respiratory tract infections, contact and droplet precautions are indicated for the duration of hospitalization. For patients with conjunctivitis and for diapered and incontinent children with adenoviral gastroenteritis, contact precautions in addition to standard precautions are indicated for the duration of illness.

CONTROL MEASURES: Children who are in group child care, particularly children from 6 months through 2 years of age, are at increased risk of adenoviral respiratory tract infections and gastroenteritis. Effective measures for preventing spread of adenovirus infection in this setting have not been determined, but frequent hand hygiene is recommended. If 2 or more children in a group child care setting develop conjunctivitis in the same period, advice should be sought from the health consultant of the program or the state health department.

Adequate chlorination of swimming pools is recommended to prevent pharyngoconjunctival fever. Epidemic keratoconjunctivitis associated with ophthalmologic practice can be difficult to control and requires use of single-dose medication dispensing and strict attention to hand hygiene and instrument sterilization procedures.

Health care professionals with known or suspected adenoviral conjunctivitis should avoid direct patient contact for 14 days after onset of disease in the most recently involved eye. Because adenoviruses are difficult to inactivate, they can remain viable on skin, fomites, and environmental surfaces. Thus, assiduous adherence to hand hygiene and use of disposable gloves when caring for infected patients are recommended.

A live, oral adenovirus vaccine for types 4 and 7 (2 oral tablets) has been licensed by the US Food and Drug Administration for prevention of febrile, acute respiratory tract disease and is being used in military personnel 17 through 50 years of age.

Amebiasis

CLINICAL MANIFESTATIONS: Clinical syndromes associated with *Entamoeba histolytica* infection include noninvasive intestinal tract infection, intestinal amebiasis (amebic colitis), ameboma, and liver abscess. Disease is more severe in very young people, elderly people, malnourished people, and pregnant women. Patients with noninvasive intestinal tract infection may be asymptomatic or may have nonspecific intestinal tract complaints. People with intestinal amebiasis generally have a gradual onset of symptoms over 1 to 3 weeks. The mildest form of intestinal tract disease is nondysenteric colitis. However, amebic dysentery is the most common manifestation of amebiasis and generally includes diarrhea with either gross or microscopic blood in the stool, lower abdominal pain, and tenesmus. Weight loss is common because of the gradual onset, but fever occurs only in a minority of patients (8%–38%). Symptoms may be chronic and may mimic those of inflammatory bowel disease. Progressive involvement of the colon may produce toxic megacolon, fulminant colitis, ulceration of the colon and perianal area, and rarely, perforation. Colonic progression may occur at multiples sites and carries a high fatality rate. Progression may occur in patients inappropriately treated with corticosteroids or antimotility drugs. An ameboma may occur as an annular lesion of the colon and may present as a palpable mass on physical examination. Amebomas can occur in any area of the colon but are more common in the cecum. They may be mistaken for colonic carcinoma. Amebomas usually resolve with antiamebic therapy and do not require surgery.

In a small proportion of patients, extraintestinal disease may occur. The liver is the most common extraintestinal site, and infection may spread from there to the pleural space, lungs, and pericardium. Liver abscess may be acute, with fever, abdominal pain, tachypnea, liver tenderness, and hepatomegaly, or may be chronic, with weight loss, vague abdominal symptoms, and irritability. Rupture of abscesses into the abdomen or chest may lead to death. Evidence of recent intestinal tract infection usually is absent. Infection also may spread from the colon to the genitourinary tract and the skin. The organism may spread hematogenously to the brain and other areas of the body.

ETIOLOGY: The genus *Entamoeba* includes 6 species that live in the human intestine. Three of these species are identical morphologically: *E histolytica*, *Entamoeba dispar*, and *Entamoeba moshkovskii*. The pathogenic *E histolytica* and the nonpathogenic *E dispar* and *E moshkovskii* are excreted as cysts or trophozoites in stools of infected people.

EPIDEMIOLOGY: *E histolytica* can be found worldwide but is more prevalent in people of lower socioeconomic status who live in resource-limited countries, where the prevalence of amebic infection may be as high as 50% in some communities. Groups at increased risk of infection in industrialized countries include immigrants from or long-term visitors to areas with endemic infection, institutionalized people, and men who have sex with men. *E histolytica* is transmitted via amebic cysts by the fecal-oral route. Ingested cysts, which are unaffected by gastric acid, undergo excystation in the alkaline small intestine and produce trophozoites that infect the colon. Cysts that develop subsequently are the source of transmission, especially from asymptomatic cyst excreters. Infected patients excrete cysts intermittently, sometimes for years if untreated. Transmission has been associated with contaminated food or water. Fecal-oral transmission also can occur in the setting of anal sexual practices or direct rectal inoculation through colonic irrigation devices.

The **incubation period** is variable, ranging from a few days to months or years but commonly is 2 to 4 weeks.

DIAGNOSTIC TESTS: A presumptive diagnosis of intestinal tract infection depends on identifying trophozoites or cysts in stool specimens. Examination of serial specimens may be necessary. Specimens of stool may be examined microscopically by wet mount within 30 minutes of collection or may be fixed in formalin or polyvinyl alcohol (available in kits) for concentration, permanent staining, and subsequent microscopic examination. Biopsy specimens and endoscopy scrapings (not swabs) may be examined using similar methods. *E histolytica* is not distinguished easily from the noninvasive and more prevalent but nonpathogenic *E dispar* and *E moshkovskii*, although trophozoites containing ingested red blood cells are more likely to be *E histolytica*. Polymerase chain reaction, isoenzyme analysis, and monoclonal antibody-based antigen detection assays can differentiate *E histolytica* from *E dispar* and *E moshkovskii*.

The indirect hemagglutination (IHA) test has been replaced by commercially available enzyme immunoassay (EIA) kits for routine serodiagnosis of amebiasis. The EIA detects antibody specific for *E histolytica* in approximately 95% of patients with extraintestinal amebiasis, 70% of patients with active intestinal tract infection, and 10% of asymptomatic people who are passing cysts of *E histolytica*. Patients may continue to have positive serologic test results even after adequate therapy. Diagnosis of an *E histolytica* liver abscess is aided by serologic testing, because stool tests and abscess aspirate frequently are not revealing.

Ultrasonography, computed tomography, and magnetic resonance imaging can identify liver abscesses and other extraintestinal sites of infection. Aspirates from a liver abscess usually show neither trophozoites nor leukocytes.

TREATMENT[1]: Treatment involves elimination of the tissue-invading trophozoites as well as organisms in the intestinal lumen. *E dispar* and *E moshkovskii* infections are considered to be nonpathogenic and do not require treatment. Corticosteroids and antimotility drugs administered to people with amebiasis can worsen symptoms and the disease process. In settings where tests to distinguish species are not available, treatment should be given to symptomatic people on the basis of positive results of microscopic examination. The following regimens are recommended:

- **Asymptomatic cyst excreters (intraluminal infections):** treat with a luminal amebicide, such as iodoquinol, paromomycin, or diloxanide. Metronidazole is not effective against cysts.
- **Patients with mild to moderate or severe intestinal tract symptoms or extraintestinal disease (including liver abscess):** treat with metronidazole or tinidazole, followed by a therapeutic course of a luminal amebicide (iodoquinol or paromomycin). Nitazoxanide also may be effective for mild to moderate intestinal amebiasis, although it is only approved by the US Food and Drug Administration for treatment of diarrhea caused by *Giardia lamblia* or *Cryptosporidium parvum*. An alternate treatment for liver abscess is chloroquine phosphate administered concomitantly with metronidazole or tinidazole, followed by a therapeutic course of a luminal amebicide.

Dehydroemetine followed by a therapeutic course of a luminal amebicide may be considered for patients for whom treatment of invasive disease has failed or cannot be tolerated. However, dehydroemetine has significant toxicity and should be used with caution. Chloroquine or dehydroemetine have been added to metronidazole for rare cases of amebic liver abscesses not responding to metronidazole alone.

Percutaneous or surgical aspiration of large liver abscesses occasionally may be required when response of the abscess to medical therapy is unsatisfactory. In most cases of liver abscess, though, drainage is not required and does not speed recovery.

Follow-up stool examination is recommended after completion of therapy, because no pharmacologic regimen is effective in eradicating intestinal tract infection completely. Household members and other suspected contacts also should have adequate stool examinations performed and be treated if results are positive for *E histolytica*.

---

[1] For further information, see Drugs for Parasitic Infections, p 848.

ISOLATION OF THE HOSPITALIZED PATIENT: In addition to standard precautions, contact precautions are recommended for the duration of illness.

CONTROL MEASURES: Careful hand hygiene after defecation, sanitary disposal of fecal material, and treatment of drinking water will control spread of infection. Sexual transmission may be controlled by use of condoms and avoidance of sexual practices that may permit fecal-oral transmission. Because of the risk of shedding infectious cysts, people diagnosed with amebiasis should refrain from using recreational water venues (eg, swimming pools, water parks) until after their course of luminal chemotherapy has completed and any diarrhea they might have been experiencing has stopped.

Amebic Meningoencephalitis and Keratitis
(*Naegleria fowleri, Acanthamoeba species,* and *Balamuthia mandrillaris*)

CLINICAL MANIFESTATIONS: *Naegleria fowleri* can cause a rapidly progressive, almost always fatal, primary amebic meningoencephalitis. Early symptoms include fever, headache, vomiting, and sometimes disturbances of smell and taste. The illness progresses rapidly to signs of meningoencephalitis, including nuchal rigidity, lethargy, confusion, personality changes, and altered level of consciousness. Seizures are common, and death generally occurs within a week of onset of symptoms. No distinct clinical features differentiate this disease from fulminant bacterial meningitis.

Granulomatous amebic encephalitis (GAE) caused by *Acanthamoeba* species and *Balamuthia mandrillaris* has a more insidious onset and progression of manifestations occurring weeks to months after exposure. Signs and symptoms may include personality changes, seizures, headaches, nuchal rigidity, ataxia, cranial nerve palsies, hemiparesis, and other focal deficits. Fever often is low grade and intermittent. The course may resemble that of a bacterial brain abscess or a brain tumor. Chronic granulomatous skin lesions (pustules, nodules, ulcers) may be present without central nervous system (CNS) involvement, particularly in patients with acquired immunodeficiency syndrome, and lesions may present for months before brain involvement in immunocompetent hosts.

The most common symptoms of amebic keratitis, usually attributable to *Acanthamoeba* species, are pain (often out of proportion to clinical signs), photophobia, tearing, and foreign body sensation. Characteristic clinical findings include radial keratoneuritis and stromal ring infiltrate. Acanthamoeba keratitis generally follows an indolent course and initially may resemble herpes simplex or bacterial keratitis; delay in diagnosis is associated with worse outcomes.

ETIOLOGY: *N fowleri, Acanthamoeba* species, and *B mandrillaris* are free-living amebae that exist as motile, infectious trophozoites and environmentally hardy cysts.

EPIDEMIOLOGY: *N fowleri* is found in warm fresh water and moist soil. Most infections with *N fowleri* have been associated with swimming in natural bodies of warm fresh water, such as ponds, lakes, and hot springs, but other sources have included tap water from geothermal sources and contaminated and poorly chlorinated swimming pools. Disease has been reported worldwide but is uncommon. In the United States, infection occurs primarily in the summer and usually affects children and young adults. The trophozoites of the parasite invade the brain directly from the nose along the olfactory nerves via the cribriform plate. In infections with *N fowleri*, trophozoites but not cysts can be visualized in sections of brain or in cerebrospinal fluid (CSF).

The **incubation period** for *N fowleri* infection typically is 3 to 7 days.

Acanthamoeba species are distributed worldwide and are found in soil; dust; cooling towers of electric and nuclear power plants; heating, ventilating, and air conditioning units; fresh and brackish water; whirlpool baths; and physiotherapy pools. The environmental niche of *B mandrillaris* is not delineated clearly, although it has been isolated from soil. CNS infection attributable to *Acanthamoeba* occurs primarily in debilitated and immunocompromised people. However, some patients infected with *B mandrillaris* have had no demonstrable underlying disease or defect. Central nervous system infection by both amebae probably occurs by inhalation or direct contact with contaminated soil or water. The primary foci of these infections most likely are skin or respiratory tract, followed by hematogenous spread to the brain. *Acanthamoeba* keratitis occurs primarily in people who wear contact lenses, although it also has been associated with corneal trauma. Poor contact lens hygiene and/or disinfection practices as well as swimming with contact lenses are risk factors.

The **incubation periods** for *Acanthamoeba* and *Balamuthia* GAE are unknown. It is thought to take several weeks or months to develop the first symptoms of CNS disease following exposure to the amebae. However, patients exposed to *Balamuthia* through solid organ transplantation can develop symptoms of *Balamuthia* GAE more quickly—within a few weeks. The incubation period for *Acanthamoeba* keratitis also is unknown but thought to range from several days to several weeks.

DIAGNOSTIC TESTS: In *N fowleri* infection, computed tomography scans of the head without contrast are unremarkable or show only cerebral edema but with contrast might show meningeal enhancement of the basilar cisterns and sulci. However, these changes are not specific for amebic infection. CSF pressure usually is elevated (300 to >600 mm water), and CSF indices may show a polymorphonuclear pleocytosis, an increased protein concentration, and a normal to very low glucose concentration; Gram stains are negative for bacteria. *N fowleri* infection can be documented by microscopic demonstration of the motile trophozoites on a wet mount of centrifuged CSF. Smears of CSF should be stained with Giemsa, Trichome, or Wright stains to identify the trophozoites, if present; Gram stain is not useful. The organism also can be cultured on nonnutrient agar plates layered with *Escherichia coli* or on monolayers of E6 and human lung fibroblast cells. Trophozoites can be visualized in sections of the brain. Immunofluorescence and polymerase chain reaction (PCR) assays performed on CSF and biopsy material to identify the organism are available through the Centers for Disease Control and Prevention.

In infection with *Acanthamoeba* species and *B mandrillaris*, trophozoites and cysts can be visualized in sections of brain, lungs, and skin; in cases of *Acanthamoeba* keratitis, they also can be visualized in corneal scrapings and by confocal microscopy in vivo in the cornea. In GAE infections, CSF indices typically reveal a lymphocytic pleocytosis and an increased protein concentration, with normal or low glucose but no organisms. Computed tomography and magnetic resonance imaging scans of the head show single or multiple space-occupying, ring-enhancing lesions that can mimic brain abscesses, tumors, cerebrovascular accidents, or other diseases. *Acanthamoeba* species, but not *Balamuthia* species, can be cultured by the same method used for *N fowleri*. *B mandrillaris* can be grown using mammalian cell culture. Like *N fowleri*, immunofluorescence and PCR assays can be performed on clinical specimens to identify *Acanthamoeba* species and *Balamuthia* species; these tests are available through the Centers for Disease Control and Prevention.

TREATMENT: If meningoencephalitis caused by *N fowleri* is suspected because of the presence of amebic organisms in CSF, therapy should not be withheld while waiting for results of confirmatory diagnostic tests. Although an effective treatment regimen for primary amebic meningoencephalitis has not been identified, amphotericin B is the drug of choice, although treatment usually is unsuccessful, with only a few cases of complete recovery having been documented. Two survivors recovered after treatment with amphotericin B in combination with an azole drug (either miconazole or fluconazole) plus rifampin, although rifampin probably had no additional effect; these patients also received dexamethasone to control cerebral edema. Although these 2 patients did not receive azithromycin, this drug has both in vitro and in vivo efficacy against *Naegleria* species and also may be tried as an adjunct to amphotericin B. Early diagnosis and institution of high-dose drug therapy is thought to be important for optimizing outcome.

Effective treatment for infections caused by *Acanthamoeba* species and *B mandrillaris* has not been established. Several patients with *Acanthamoeba* GAE and *Acanthamoeba* cutaneous infections without CNS involvement have been treated successfully with a multidrug regimen consisting of various combinations of pentamidine, sulfadiazine, flucytosine, either fluconazole or itraconazole, trimethoprim-sulfamethoxazole, and topical application of chlorhexidine gluconate and ketoconazole for skin lesions. Voriconazole, miltefosine, and azithromycin also might be of some value in treating *Acanthamoeba* infections. Three patients survived *B mandrillaris* infection following treatment with pentamidine, sulfadiazine, fluconazole, and either azithromycin or clarithromycin, in addition to surgical resection of the CNS lesions; in 2 of these cases, flucytosine was used as well. Of these 3 survivors, all had GAE and 1 had an accompanying cutaneous lesion. Miltefosine also has been used to successfully treat other patients with *B mandrillaris* GAE and cutaneous lesions. Unlike with *Acanthamoeba*, voriconazole has virtually no effect on *Balamuthia* species in vitro. Patients with *Acanthamoeba* keratitis should be evaluated by an ophthalmologist. Early diagnosis and therapy are important for a good outcome (see Drugs for Parasitic Infections, p 848).

ISOLATION OF THE HOSPITALIZED PATIENT: Standard precautions are recommended.

CONTROL MEASURES: People should assume that there is always a slight risk of developing primary amebic meningoencephalitis caused by *N fowleri* when entering warm fresh water. Only avoidance of such water-related activities can prevent *Naegleria* infection, although the risk might be reduced by taking measures to limit water exposure through known routes of entry, such as getting water up the nose. Presently, no clearly defined recommendations are available to prevent GAE attributable to *Acanthamoeba* species or *B mandrillaris*. To prevent *Acanthamoeba* keratitis, steps should be taken to avoid corneal trauma, such as the use of protective eyewear during high-risk activities, and contact lens users should maintain good contact lens hygiene and disinfection practices, use only sterile solutions as applicable, change lens cases frequently, and avoid swimming and showering while wearing contact lenses. Advice for people who wear contact lenses can be found at **www.cdc.gov/parasites/acanthamoeba/contact_wearers.html.**

Anthrax[1]

CLINICAL MANIFESTATIONS: Depending on the route of infection, anthrax can occur in 3 forms: cutaneous, inhalation, and gastrointestinal. **Cutaneous** anthrax begins as a pruritic papule or vesicle that enlarges and ulcerates in 1 to 2 days, with subsequent formation of a central black eschar. The lesion itself characteristically is painless, with surrounding edema, hyperemia, and painful regional lymphadenopathy. Patients may have associated fever, lymphangitis, and extensive edema. **Inhalation** anthrax is a frequently lethal form of the disease and is a medical emergency. A nonspecific prodrome of fever, sweats, nonproductive cough, chest pain, headache, myalgia, malaise, and nausea and vomiting may occur initially, but illness progresses to the fulminant phase 2 to 5 days later. In some cases, the illness is biphasic with a period of improvement between prodromal symptoms and overwhelming illness. Fulminant manifestations include hypotension, dyspnea, hypoxia, cyanosis, and shock occurring as a result of hemorrhagic mediastinal lymphadenitis, hemorrhagic pneumonia, and hemorrhagic pleural effusions, bacteremia, and toxemia. In addition, the liver and central nervous system (CNS) may be involved. A widened mediastinum is the classic finding on imaging of the chest. Chest radiography also may show pleural effusions and/or infiltrates, both of which may be hemorrhagic in nature. **Gastrointestinal tract** disease can present as 2 clinical syndromes—intestinal or oropharyngeal. Patients with the intestinal form have symptoms of nausea, anorexia, vomiting, and fever progressing to severe abdominal pain, massive ascites, hematemesis, bloody diarrhea, and submucosal intestinal hemorrhage. Oropharyngeal anthrax also may have dysphagia with posterior oropharyngeal necrotic ulcers, which may be associated with marked, often unilateral neck swelling, regional adenopathy, fever, and sepsis. Hemorrhagic meningitis can result from hematogenous spread of the organism after acquiring any form of disease and may develop without any other apparent clinical presentation. The case-fatality rate for patients with appropriately treated cutaneous anthrax usually is less than 1%, but for inhalation or gastrointestinal tract disease, mortality often exceeds 50% and approaches 100% for meningitis in the absence of antimicrobial therapy.

ETIOLOGY: *Bacillus anthracis* is an aerobic, gram-positive, encapsulated, spore-forming, nonhemolytic, nonmotile rod. *B anthracis* has 3 major virulence factors: an antiphagocytic capsule and 2 exotoxins, called lethal and edema toxins. The toxins are responsible for the significant morbidity and clinical manifestations of hemorrhage, edema, and necrosis.

EPIDEMIOLOGY: Anthrax is a zoonotic disease most commonly affecting domestic and wild herbivores that occurs in many rural regions of the world. *B anthracis* spores can remain viable in the soil for decades, representing a potential source of infection for livestock or wildlife through ingestion. In susceptible hosts, the spores germinate to become viable bacteria. Natural infection of humans occurs through contact with infected animals or contaminated animal products, including carcasses, hides, hair, wool, meat, and bone meal. Outbreaks of gastrointestinal tract anthrax have occurred after ingestion of undercooked or raw meat from infected animals. Historically, the vast majority (more

---

[1] Center for Infectious Disease Research and Policy, University of Minnesota. Anthrax: Current, comprehensive information on pathogenesis, microbiology, epidemiology, diagnosis, treatment, and prophylaxis. Available at: **www.cidrap.umn.edu/cidrap/content/bt/anthrax/index.html**; and Stern EJ, Uhde KB, Shadomy SV, Messonnier N. Conference report on public health and clinical guidelines for anthrax. *Emerg Infect Dis.* 2008;14(4). Available at: **www.cdc.gov/eid/content/14/4/e1.htm**

than 95%) of cases of anthrax in the United States were cutaneous infections among animal handlers or mill workers. Severe disseminated anthrax following soft tissue infection among heroin users has been reported. The incidence of naturally occurring human anthrax decreased in the United States from an estimated 130 cases annually in the early 1900s to 0 to 2 cases per year by the end of the first decade of the 21st century. Recent cases of inhalation, cutaneous, and gastrointestinal tract anthrax have occurred in drum makers working with animal hides contaminated with *B anthracis* spores or people exposed to drumming events where spore-contaminated drums were used.[1]

B anthracis is one of the most likely agents to be used as a biological weapon, because (1) its spores are highly stabile; (2) spores can infect via the respiratory route; and (3) the resulting inhalation anthrax has a high mortality rate. In 1979, an accidental release of *B anthracis* spores from a military microbiology facility in the former Soviet Union resulted in at least 69 deaths. In 2001, 22 cases of anthrax (11 inhalation, 11 cutaneous) were identified in the United States after intentional contamination of the mail; 5 (45%) of the inhalation anthrax cases were fatal. In addition to aerosolization, there is a theoretical health risk associated with *B anthracis* spores being introduced into food products or water supplies. Use of *B anthracis* in a biological attack would require immediate response and mobilization of public health resources. Anthrax meets the definition of a nationally and immediately notifiable condition as specified by the US Council of State and Territorial Epidemiologists; therefore, every suspected case should be reported immediately to the local or state health department (see Biological Terrorism, p 111).

The **incubation period** typically is 1 week or less for cutaneous or gastrointestinal tract anthrax. However, because of spore dormancy and slow clearance from lungs, the incubation period for inhalation anthrax may be prolonged and has been reported to range from 1 to 43 days in humans and up to 2 months in experimental nonhuman primates. Discharge from cutaneous lesions potentially is infectious, but person-to-person transmission rarely has been reported. Both inhalation and cutaneous anthrax have occurred in laboratory workers.

DIAGNOSTIC TESTS: Depending on the clinical presentation, Gram stain, culture, and PCR for anthrax should be performed on specimens of blood, pleural fluid, cerebrospinal fluid, and tissue biopsy specimens or on swabs of vesicular fluid or eschar material from cutaneous or oropharyngeal lesions, rectal swabs, or stool. These tests should be obtained before initiating antimicrobial therapy, because previous treatment with antimicrobial agents makes isolation by culture unlikely. Gram-positive bacilli seen on unspun peripheral blood smears or in vesicular fluid or cerebrospinal fluid can be an important initial finding. Definitive identification of suspect *B anthracis* isolates can be performed through the Laboratory Response Network (LRN) in each state. Additional diagnostic tests for anthrax can be accessed through state health departments, including tissue immunohistochemistry, an enzyme immunoassay that measures immunoglobulin G antibodies against *B anthracis* protective antigen in paired sera, or a MALDI-TOF mass spectrometry assay measuring lethal factor activity in serum samples. The commercially available QuickELISA Anthrax-PA Kit can be used as a screening test. Clinical evaluation of patients with suspected inhalation anthrax should include a chest radiograph and/or

---

[1] Centers for Disease Control and Prevention. Gastrointestinal anthrax after an animal-hide drumming event— New Hampshire and Massachusetts, 2009. *MMWR Morb Mortal Wkly Rep.* 2010;59(28):872–877

computed tomography scan to evaluate for widened mediastinum, pleural effusion, and/ or pulmonary infiltrates.

TREATMENT: A high index of suspicion and rapid administration of appropriate antimicrobial therapy to people suspected of being infected, along with access to critical care support, are essential for effective treatment of anthrax. No controlled trials in humans have been performed to validate current treatment recommendations for anthrax, and there is limited clinical experience. Case reports suggest that naturally occurring cutaneous disease can be treated effectively with a variety of antimicrobial agents, including penicillins and tetracyclines, for 7 to 10 days. For bioterrorism-associated cutaneous disease in adults or children, ciprofloxacin (30 mg/kg per day, orally, divided 2 times/day for children, not to exceed 1000 mg every 24 hours) or doxycycline (100 mg, orally, 2 times/ day for children 8 years of age or older; or 4.4 mg/kg per day, orally, divided 2 times/ day for children younger than 8 years of age [see Tetracyclines, p 801]) are recommended for initial treatment until antimicrobial susceptibility data are available. Because of the risk of spore dormancy in mediastinal lymph nodes, the antimicrobial regimen should be continued for a total of 60 days to provide postexposure prophylaxis, in conjunction with administration of vaccine (see Control Measures). A multidrug approach is recommended if there also are signs of systemic disease, extensive edema, or lesions of the head and neck.

On the basis of in vitro data and animal studies, ciprofloxacin (400 mg, intravenously, every 8–12 hours) is recommended as the primary antimicrobial agent as part of an initial multidrug regimen for treating inhalation anthrax, anthrax meningitis, cutaneous anthrax with systemic signs or extensive edema, and gastrointestinal tract/oropharyngeal anthrax until results of antimicrobial susceptibility testing are known.[1] Meningitis treatment requires agents with known CNS penetration; meningeal involvement should be suspected in cases of inhalation anthrax or other systemic anthrax infections. The addition of 1 or 2 other agents with adequate CNS penetration is recommended for use in conjunction with ciprofloxacin; the list of additional antimicrobial agents to consider includes clindamycin (which also may decrease toxin production via its inhibition of protein synthesis), rifampin, penicillin, ampicillin, vancomycin, meropenem, chloramphenicol, and clarithromycin. Other fluoroquinolones, including levofloxacin and ofloxacin, have excellent in vitro activity against *B anthracis*, as do other agents, such as quinupristin/dalfopristin and the ketolide telithromycin. Because of intrinsic resistance, cephalosporins and trimethoprim-sulfamethoxazole should not be used. Treatment should continue for at least 60 days, but a switch from intravenous to oral therapy may occur when clinically appropriate. Neither ciprofloxacin nor tetracyclines are used routinely in children or pregnant women because of safety concerns. However, ciprofloxacin or doxycycline should be used for treatment of life-threatening anthrax infections in children until antimicrobial susceptibility patterns are known (see Tetracyclines, p 801). For severe anthrax, Anthrax-Specific Hyperimmune Globulin 5% should be considered in consultation with the Centers for Disease Control and Prevention (CDC) under the CDC-sponsored Investigational New

---

[1] Centers for Disease Control and Prevention. Update: investigation of bioterrorism-related anthrax and interim guidelines for exposure management and antimicrobial therapy, October 2001. *MMWR Morb Mortal Wkly Rep.* 2001;50(42):909–919; and Centers for Disease Control and Prevention. Notice to readers: update: interim recommendations for antimicrobial prophylaxis for children and breastfeeding mothers and treatment of children with anthrax. *MMWR Morb Mortal Wkly Rep.* 2001;50(45):1014–1016

Drug (IND) use protocol. In addition, aggressive pleural fluid drainage is recommended if effusions exist and is recommended for treatment of all patients with inhalation anthrax.

ISOLATION OF THE HOSPITALIZED PATIENT: Standard precautions are recommended. In addition, contact precautions should be implemented when draining cutaneous lesions are present. Contaminated dressings and bedclothes should be incinerated or steam sterilized (121°C for 30 minutes) to destroy spores. Autopsies performed on patients with systemic anthrax require special precautions.

CONTROL MEASURES: BioThrax (AVA [formerly known as Anthrax Vaccine Adsorbed]), the only vaccine for prevention of anthrax licensed in the United States for use in humans, is prepared from a cell-free culture filtrate. The vaccine efficacy of AVA is based on animal studies, a single controlled trial of the alum-precipitated precursor to AVA, observational data from humans, and immunogenicity data from humans and other mammals. In the controlled trial in adult mill workers, AVA had a demonstrated 93% efficacy for preventing cutaneous and inhalation anthrax. Multiple reviews and publications evaluating AVA safety have found adverse events usually are local injection site reactions with rare systemic symptoms, including fever, chills, muscle aches, and hypersensitivity. The CDC updated its recommendations on preexposure and postexposure use of anthrax vaccine in 2010 (**http://www.cdc.gov/mmwr/preview/mmwrhtml/rr5906a1. htm?s_cid=rr5906a1_w**).[1]

In a preevent or preexposure setting, AVA is administered in a schedule consisting of five 0.5-mL intramuscular injections (at 0, 1, 6, 12, and 18 months) and 0.5-mL booster injections at 1- year intervals after the 18-month dose. People with medical contraindications to intramuscular administration (eg, people with coagulation disorders) may continue to receive the vaccine by subcutaneous administration.

Postexposure management for previously unvaccinated people older than 18 years of age who have been exposed to aerosolized *B anthracis* spores consists of 60 days of appropriate antimicrobial prophylaxis combined with 3 subcutaneous doses of AVA (administered at 0, 2, and 4 weeks postexposure). AVA is not licensed for use in pregnant women; in a postevent setting that poses a high risk of exposure to aerosolized *B anthracis* spores, pregnancy is neither a precaution nor a contraindication to postexposure prophylaxis (PEP). AVA is not licensed for use in pediatric populations and has not been studied in children; however, there is no reason to suggest an increased risk of adverse events associated with the use of anthrax vaccine in pediatric populations. The extraordinary morbidity of inhalation anthrax should affect decision making. During an event, the US Food and Drug Administration and appropriate public health authorities will determine whether to offer vaccine to children and the mechanism under which it should be offered.

When no information is available about antimicrobial susceptibility of the implicated strain of *B anthracis*, ciprofloxacin and doxycycline are equivalent first-line antimicrobial agents for initial PEP for adults or children (see Tetracyclines, p 801). Levofloxacin is a second-line antimicrobial agent for PEP for people 6 months of age or older. Safety data on extended use of levofloxacin in any population for longer than 28 days are limited; therefore, levofloxacin should only be used when the benefit outweighs the risk. Although fluoroquinolones and tetracyclines are not recommended as first-choice drugs in children

---

[1] Centers for Disease Control and Prevention. Use of anthrax vaccine in the United States. Recommendations of the Advisory Committee on Immunization Practices (ACIP), 2009. *MMWR Recomm Rep.* 2010;59 (RR-06):1–30

because of adverse effects, these concerns may be outweighed by the need for prophylaxis to prevent disease in pregnant women and children exposed to *B anthracis* after a biological terrorism event. As soon as susceptibility of the organism to penicillin has been confirmed, PEP antimicrobial therapy for children should be changed to oral amoxicillin. Because of the lack of data on amoxicillin dosages for treating anthrax (and the associated high mortality rate), the American Academy of Pediatrics recommends a higher dosage of oral amoxicillin, 80 mg/kg per day, divided into 3 daily doses administered every 8 hours (each dose not to exceed 500 mg). Because of intrinsic resistance, cephalosporins and trimethoprim-sulfamethoxazole should not be used for prophylaxis.

Arboviruses (also see Dengue, p 305, and West Nile Virus, p 792)

(Including California Serogroup, Chikungunya, Colorado Tick Fever, Eastern Equine Encephalitis, Japanese Encephalitis, Powassan, St. Louis Encephalitis, Tickborne Encephalitis, Venezuelan Equine Encephalitis, Western Equine Encephalitis, and Yellow Fever Viruses)

CLINICAL MANIFESTATIONS: More than 150 arthropodborne viruses (arboviruses) are known to cause human disease. Although most infections are subclinical, symptomatic illness usually manifests as 1 of 3 primary clinical syndromes: systemic febrile illness, neuroinvasive disease, or hemorrhagic fever (Table 3.1, p 233).

- *Systemic febrile illness.* Most arboviruses are capable of causing a systemic febrile illness that often includes headache, arthralgia, myalgia, and rash. Some viruses also can cause more characteristic clinical manifestations, including severe joint pain (eg, chikungunya) or jaundice (yellow fever). With some arboviruses, fatigue, malaise, and weakness can linger for weeks following the initial infection.
- *Neuroinvasive disease.* Many arboviruses cause neuroinvasive diseases, including aseptic meningitis, encephalitis, or acute flaccid paralysis. Illness usually presents with a prodrome similar to the systemic febrile illness followed by neurologic symptoms. The specific symptoms vary by virus and clinical syndrome but can include vomiting, stiff neck, mental status changes, seizures, or focal neurologic deficits. The severity and long-term outcome of the illness vary by etiologic agent and the underlying characteristics of the host, such as age, immune status, and preexisting medical condition.
- *Hemorrhagic fever.* Hemorrhagic fevers can be caused by dengue or yellow fever viruses. After several days of nonspecific febrile illness, the patient may develop overt signs of hemorrhage (eg, petechiae, ecchymoses, bleeding from the nose and gums, hematemesis, and melena) and septic shock (eg, decreased peripheral circulation, azotemia, tachycardia, and hypotension). Hemorrhagic fever caused by dengue and yellow fever viruses may be confused with hemorrhagic fevers transmitted by rodents (eg, Argentine hemorrhagic fever, Bolivian hemorrhagic fever, and Lassa fever) or those caused by Ebola or Marburg viruses. For information on other potential infections causing hemorrhagic manifestations, see Hemorrhagic Fevers Caused by Arenaviruses (p 356) and Hemorrhagic Fevers and Related Syndromes Caused by Viruses of the Family Bunyaviridae (p 358).

Table 3.1. Clinical Manifestations for Select Domestic and International Arboviral Diseases

Virus	Systemic Febrile Illness	Neuroinvasive Disease[a]	Hemorrhagic Fever
Domestic			
Colorado tick fever	Yes	Rare	No
Dengue	Yes	Rare	Yes
Eastern equine encephalitis	Yes	Yes	No
California serogroup[b]	Yes	Yes	No
Powassan	Yes	Yes	No
St. Louis encephalitis	Yes	Yes	No
Western equine encephalitis	Yes	Yes	No
West Nile	Yes	Yes	No
International			
Chikungunya	Yes[c]	Rare	No
Japanese encephalitis	Yes	Yes	No
Tickborne encephalitis	Yes	Yes	No
Venezuelan equine encephalitis	Yes	Yes	No
Yellow fever	Yes	No	Yes

[a] Aseptic meningitis, encephalitis, or acute flaccid paralysis.
[b] In this group, most human cases are caused by La Crosse virus. Other known or suspected human pathogens in the group include California encephalitis, Jamestown Canyon, snowshoe hare, and trivittatus viruses.
[c] Most often characterized by sudden onset of high fever and severe joint pain.

ETIOLOGY: Arboviruses are RNA viruses that are transmitted to humans primarily through bites of infected arthropods (mosquitoes, ticks, sand flies, and biting midges). The viral families responsible for most arboviral infections in humans are Flaviviridae (genus *Flavivirus*), Togaviridae (genus *Alphavirus*), and Bunyaviridae (genus *Bunyavirus*). Reoviridae (genus *Coltivirus*) also are responsible for a smaller number of human arboviral infections (eg, Colorado tick fever) (Table 3.2, p 234).

EPIDEMIOLOGY: Most arboviruses maintain cycles of transmission between birds or small mammals and arthropod vectors. Humans and domestic animals usually are infected incidentally as "dead-end" hosts (Table 3.2, p 234). Important exceptions are dengue, yellow fever, and chikungunya viruses, which can be spread from person-to-arthropod-to-person (anthroponotic transmission). For other arboviruses, humans usually do not develop a sustained or high enough level of viremia to infect arthropod vectors. Direct person-to-person spread of arboviruses can occur through blood transfusion, organ transplantation, intrauterine transmission, and possibly human milk (see Blood Safety, p 114, and Human Milk, p 126). Percutaneous and aerosol transmission of arboviruses can occur in the laboratory setting.

In the northern United States, arboviral infections occur during summer and autumn, when mosquitoes and ticks are most active. In the southern United States, cases occur throughout the year because of warmer temperatures, which are conducive to year-round

Table 3.2. Genus, Geographic Location, Vectors, and Average Number of Annual Cases for Selected Domestic and International Arboviral Diseases

Virus	Genus	Geographic Location		Vectors	Number of US Cases/Year (Range)[a]
		United States	Non-United States		
Domestic					
Colorado tick fever	*Coltivirus*	West	Canada	Ticks	8 (2–12)
Dengue	*Flavivirus*	Puerto Rico, Florida, Texas, and Hawaii	Worldwide in tropical areas	Mosquitoes	45 (20–71)[b]
Eastern equine encephalitis	*Alphavirus*	Eastern and gulf states	Canada, Central and South America	Mosquitoes	8 (3–21)
California serogroup	*Bunyavirus*	Widespread, most prevalent in Midwest and East	Canada	Mosquitoes	93 (46–167)
Powassan	*Flavivirus*	Northeast and north central	Canada, Russia	Ticks	2 (0–7)
St. Louis encephalitis	*Flavivirus*	Widespread	Canada, Caribbean, Mexico, Central and South America	Mosquitoes	21 (2–79)
Western equine encephalitis	*Alphavirus*	Central and West	Central and South America	Mosquitoes	Less than 1
West Nile	*Flavivirus*	Widespread	Canada, Europe, Africa, Asia	Mosquitoes	1215 (19–2946)[c]
International					
Chikungunya	*Alphavirus*	Imported only	Asia, Africa	Mosquitoes	27 (12–42)[d]
Japanese encephalitis	*Flavivirus*	Imported only	Asia	Mosquitoes	Less than 1
Tickborne encephalitis	*Flavivirus*	Imported only	Europe, northern Asia	Ticks	Less than 1
Venezuelan equine encephalitis	*Alphavirus*	Imported only	Mexico, Central and South America	Mosquitoes	Less than 1
Yellow fever	*Flavivirus*	Imported only	South America, Africa	Mosquitoes	Less than 1

[a]Average annual number of domestic and/or imported cases from 2000 to 2009 unless otherwise noted.
[b]Domestic and imported cases from 1997–2006; excludes indigenous transmission in Puerto Rico.
[c]Neuroinvasive disease only.
[d]Cases imported to the United States from 2006 to 2009 only.

arthropod activity. The number of domestic or imported arboviral disease cases reported in the United States varies greatly by specific etiology and year (Table 3.2, p 234).

Overall, the risk of severe clinical disease for most arboviral infections in the United States is higher among adults than among children. One notable exception is La Crosse virus infections, for which children are at highest risk of severe neurologic disease and possible long-term sequelae. Eastern equine encephalitis virus causes a low incidence of disease but high case-fatality rate (40%) across all age groups.

The **incubation periods** for arboviral diseases typically range between 2 and 15 days. Longer incubation periods can occur in immunocompromised people and for tickborne viruses, such as tickborne encephalitis and Powassan viruses.

DIAGNOSTIC TESTS: Arboviral infections are confirmed most frequently by measurement of virus-specific antibody in serum or cerebrospinal fluid (CSF). Acute-phase serum specimens should be tested for virus-specific immunoglobulin (Ig) M antibody using an enzyme immunoassay (EIA) or microsphere immunoassay (MIA). With clinical and epidemiologic correlation, a positive IgM test has good diagnostic predictive value, but cross-reaction with related arboviruses from the same family can occur. For most arboviral infections, IgM is detectable 3 to 8 days after onset of illness and persists for 30 to 90 days, but longer persistence has been documented. Therefore, a positive IgM test result occasionally may reflect a past infection. Serum collected within 10 days of illness onset may not have detectable IgM, and the test should be repeated on a convalescent sample. IgG antibody generally is detectable shortly after IgM and persists for years. A plaque-reduction neutralization test (PRNT) can be performed to measure virus-specific neutralizing antibodies. A fourfold or greater increase in virus-specific neutralizing antibodies between acute- and convalescent-phase serum specimens collected 2 to 3 weeks apart may be used to confirm recent infection or discriminate between cross-reacting antibodies in primary arboviral infections. In patients who have been immunized against or infected with another arbovirus from the same virus family in the past, cross-reactive antibodies in both the EIA and neutralization assays may make it difficult to identify which arbovirus is causing the patient's illness. For some arboviral infections (eg, Colorado tick fever), the immune response may be delayed, with IgM antibodies not appearing until 2 to 3 weeks after onset of illness and neutralizing antibodies taking up to a month to develop. Immunization history, date of symptom onset, and information regarding other arboviruses known to circulate in the geographic area that may cross-react in serologic assays should be considered when interpreting results.

Viral culture and nucleic acid amplification tests (NAATs) for RNA can be performed on acute-phase serum, CSF, or tissue specimens. Arboviruses that are more likely to be detected using culture or NAATs early in the illness include chikungunya, dengue, and yellow fever viruses. Immunohistochemical staining (IHC) can detect specific viral antigen in fixed tissue.

Antibody testing for common domestic arboviral diseases is performed in most state public health laboratories and many commercial laboratories. Confirmatory PRNTs, viral culture, NAATs, IHC, and testing for less common domestic and international arboviruses are performed only at the Centers for Disease Control and Prevention (CDC; telephone: 970-221-6400) and selected other reference laboratories.

TREATMENT: The primary treatment for all arboviral disease is supportive. Although various therapies have been evaluated for several arboviral diseases, none have shown specific benefit.

ISOLATION OF THE HOSPITALIZED PATIENT: Standard precautions are recommended.

CONTROL MEASURES: Reduction of vectors in areas with endemic transmission is important to reduce risk of infection. Use of certain personal protective strategies can help decrease the risk of human infection. These strategies include using insect repellent, wearing long pants and long-sleeved shirts while outdoors, staying in screened or air-conditioned dwellings, and limiting outdoor activities during peak vector feeding times (see Prevention of Mosquitoborne Infections, p 209). Select arboviral infections also can be prevented through screening of blood and organ donations and through immunization. The blood supply in the United States has been screened for West Nile virus since 2003. Blood donations from areas with endemic transmission also are screened for dengue virus. Although some arboviruses can be transmitted through human milk, transmission appears rare. Because the benefits of breastfeeding seem to outweigh the risk of illness in breastfeeding infants, mothers should be encouraged to breastfeed even in areas of ongoing arboviral transmission.

Vaccines are available in the United States to protect against travel-related yellow fever and Japanese encephalitis:

Yellow Fever Vaccine.[1] Live-attenuated (17D strain) vaccine is available at state-approved immunization centers. A single dose provides protection for 10 years or longer. Unless contraindicated, yellow fever immunization is recommended for all people 9 months of age or older living in or traveling to areas with endemic disease and is required by international regulations for travel to and from certain countries (**wwwn.cdc.gov/travel/**). Infants younger than 6 months of age should not be immunized, because they have an increased risk of vaccine-associated encephalitis. The decision to immunize infants between 6 and 9 months of age must balance the infant's risk of exposure with the theoretical risks of vaccine-associated encephalitis.

Yellow fever vaccine is a live-virus vaccine produced in embryonic chicken eggs and, thus, is contraindicated in people who have an allergic reaction to eggs or chicken proteins and people who are immunocompromised. Pregnancy and breastfeeding are precautions to yellow fever vaccine administration, because rare cases of in utero or breastfeeding transmission of the vaccine virus have been documented. Pregnant or breastfeeding women should be excused from immunization and issued a medical waiver letter to fulfill health regulations unless travel to an area with endemic infection is unavoidable and the risk of exposure outweighs the risks of immunization. Procedures for immunizing people with egg allergy are described in the vaccine package insert. For more detailed information on the yellow fever vaccine, including adverse events, precautions, and contraindications, visit **wwwn.cdc.gov/travel/** or see Required or Recommended Travel-Related Immunizations (p 106).

---

[1] Centers for Disease Control and Prevention. Yellow fever vaccine: recommendations of the Advisory Committee on Immunization Practices (ACIP). *MMWR Recomm Rep.* 2010;59(RR-7):1–27

Japanese Encephalitis (JE) Vaccine.[1] The risk of JE for most travelers to Asia is low but varies on the basis of destination, duration, season, and activities. All travelers to countries with endemic JE should be informed of the risks of JE and use personal protective measures to reduce the risk of mosquito bites. For some travelers who will be in high-risk settings, JE vaccine can further reduce the risk for infection. The US Centers for Disease Control and Prevention recommends JE vaccine for travelers who plan to spend a month or longer in areas with endemic infection during the JE virus transmission season. JE vaccine also should be considered for shorter-term travelers if they plan to travel outside of an urban area and have an itinerary or activities that will increase their risk of JE virus exposure. Information on the location of JE virus transmission and detailed information on vaccine recommendations and adverse events can be obtained from CDC (**wwwnc.cdc.gov/travel/**).

In 2009, an inactivated Vero cell culture-derived JE vaccine (IXIARO [JE-VC]) was licensed in the United States for use in people 17 years of age and older. The primary vaccination series is 2 doses administered 28 days apart. A booster dose may be given at 1 year or longer after the primary series and prior to potential JE virus exposure. Data on the response to a booster dose administered more than 2 years after the primary series are not available. Data on the need for and timing of additional booster doses also are not available.

No efficacy data exist for JE-VC. The vaccine was licensed on the basis of its ability to induce JE virus-neutralizing antibodies as a surrogate for protection and safety evaluations in fewer than 5000 adults. Pain (33%), tenderness (36%), and erythema (10%) are the most common local reactions, but severe reactions occur in fewer than 1% of recipients. Reported systemic adverse events in the 7 days following vaccination usually are mild but include headache (26%), myalgia (21%), influenza-like illness (13%), and fatigue (13%). No serious hypersensitivity reactions or neurologic adverse events were identified among JE-VC recipients enrolled in the clinical trials. Postlicensure studies and monitoring of surveillance data are ongoing to evaluate the safety of JE-VC in a larger population.

There currently is no JE vaccine that is licensed and available for use in children in the United States. An inactivated mouse brain-derived JE vaccine (JE-VAX) that had been licensed in the United States since 1992 for use in people 1 year of age and older no longer is being produced, and all remaining doses expired in 2011. Pediatric clinical trials with JE-VC are ongoing in the Philippines, Australia, Europe, and the United States. More information regarding the clinical trial is available at **http://clinicaltrials.gov/ct2/show/NCT01047839?term=Japanese+encephalitis&rank=26**. Other JE vaccines are manufactured and routinely used for children in Asia but are not licensed in the United States. Information regarding options for obtaining JE vaccine for US children is available.[2] A partial list of international travelers' health clinics in Asia that administer JE vaccines to children is available online from the CDC at **www.cdc.gov/ncidod/dvbid/jencephalitis/children.htm**.

Other Arboviral Vaccines. An inactivated vaccine for tickborne encephalitis virus is licensed in Canada and some countries in Europe where the disease is endemic, but this vaccine is not available in the United States. Experimental vaccines also exist against

---

[1] Centers for Disease Control and Prevention. Inactivated Japanese encephalitis vaccines: recommendations of the Advisory Committee on Immunization Practices (ACIP). *MMWR Recomm Rep.* 2010;59(RR-1):1–27

[2] Centers for Disease Control and Prevention. Update on Japanese encephalitis vaccine for children— United States, May 2011. *MMWR Morb Mortal Wkly Rep.* 2011;60(20):664–665

chikungunya, eastern equine encephalitis, Venezuelan equine encephalitis, and western equine encephalitis viruses but are used primarily to protect laboratory workers and other people with occupational exposure to these viruses and are not available for public use. Dengue and West Nile virus vaccines are under development.

REPORTING: Arboviral diseases are nationally notifiable conditions and should be reported to the appropriate local and state health authorities. For select arboviruses (eg, chikungunya, dengue, and yellow fever viruses), patients may remain viremic during their acute illness. Such patients pose a risk for further person-to-mosquito-to-person transmission, increasing the importance of timely reporting.

Arcanobacterium haemolyticum Infections

CLINICAL MANIFESTATIONS: Acute pharyngitis attributable to *Arcanobacterium haemolyticum* often is indistinguishable from that caused by group A streptococci. Fever, pharyngeal exudate, lymphadenopathy, rash, and pruritus are common, but palatal petechiae and strawberry tongue are absent. In almost half of all reported cases, a maculopapular or scarlatiniform exanthem is present, beginning on the extensor surfaces of the distal extremities, spreading centripetally to the chest and back, and sparing the face, palms, and soles. Rash is associated primarily with cases presenting with pharyngitis and typically develops 1 to 4 days after onset of sore throat, although cases have been reported with rash preceding pharyngitis. Respiratory tract infections that mimic diphtheria, including membranous pharyngitis, sinusitis, and pneumonia; and skin and soft tissue infections, including chronic ulceration, cellulitis, paronychia, and wound infection, have been attributed to *A haemolyticum.* Invasive infections, including septicemia, peritonsillar abscess, Lemierre syndrome, brain abscess, orbital cellulitis, meningitis, endocarditis, pyogenic arthritis, osteomyelitis, urinary tract infection, pneumonia, spontaneous bacterial peritonitis, and pyothorax have been reported. No nonsuppurative sequelae have been reported.

ETIOLOGY: *A haemolyticum* is a catalase-negative, weakly acid-fast, facultative, hemolytic, anaerobic, gram-positive, slender, sometimes club shaped bacillus formerly classified as *Corynebacterium haemolyticum.*

EPIDEMIOLOGY: Humans are the primary reservoir of *A haemolyticum,* and spread is person to person, presumably via droplet respiratory tract secretions. Severe disease occurs almost exclusively among immunocompromised people. Pharyngitis occurs primarily in adolescents and young adults. Although long-term pharyngeal carriage with *A haemolyticum* has been described after an episode of acute pharyngitis, isolation of the bacterium from the nasopharynx of asymptomatic people is rare. An estimated 0.5% to 3% of acute pharyngitis is attributable to *A haemolyticum.* Case reports also document isolation in combination with other pathogens. Person-to-person spread is inferred from studies of families and epidemiologic reports.

The **incubation period** is unknown.

DIAGNOSTIC TESTS: *A haemolyticum* grows on blood-enriched agar, but colonies are small, have narrow bands of hemolysis, and may not be visible for 48 to 72 hours. The organism will not be detected on routine evaluation of pharyngitis by the antigen test for group A streptococci. Detection is enhanced by culture on rabbit or human blood agar rather than on more commonly used sheep blood agar because of larger colony size and wider zones of hemolysis. Growth also is enhanced by addition of 5% carbon dioxide. Routine throat cultures are inoculated onto sheep blood agar, and *A haemolyticum* may be missed if laboratory personnel are not trained to look for the organism. Pits characteristically form under the colonies on blood agar plates. Two biotypes of *A haemolyticum* have been identified: a rough biotype predominates in respiratory tract infections and a smooth biotype is most commonly associated with skin and soft-tissue infections.

TREATMENT: Erythromycin is the drug of choice for treating tonsillopharyngitis attributable to *A haemolyticum*, but no prospective therapeutic trials have been performed. *A haemolyticum* is susceptible in vitro to azithromycin, erythromycin, clindamycin, cefuroxime, vancomycin, and tetracycline. Failures in treatment of pharyngitis with penicillin have been reported, perhaps because of penicillin tolerance or intracellular residing pathogens. Resistance to trimethoprim-sulfamethoxazole is common. In rare cases of disseminated infection, susceptibility tests should be performed. In disseminated infection, parenteral penicillin plus an aminoglycoside may be used initially as empiric treatment.

ISOLATION OF THE HOSPITALIZED PATIENT: Standard precautions are recommended.

CONTROL MEASURES: None.

Ascaris lumbricoides Infections

CLINICAL MANIFESTATIONS: Most infections with *Ascaris lumbricoides* are asymptomatic, although moderate to heavy infections may lead to malnutrition and nonspecific gastrointestinal tract symptoms. During the larval migratory phase, an acute transient pneumonitis (Löffler syndrome) associated with fever and marked eosinophilia may occur. Acute intestinal obstruction has been associated with heavy infections. Children are prone to this complication because of the small diameter of the intestinal lumen and their propensity to acquire large worm burdens. Worm migration can cause peritonitis secondary to intestinal wall perforation and common bile duct obstruction resulting in biliary colic, cholangitis, or pancreatitis. Adult worms can be stimulated to migrate by stressful conditions (eg, fever, illness, or anesthesia) and by some anthelmintic drugs. *A lumbricoides* has been found in the appendiceal lumen in patients with acute appendicitis.

ETIOLOGY: *A lumbricoides* is the most prevalent of all human intestinal nematodes (roundworms), with more than 1 billion people infected worldwide.

EPIDEMIOLOGY: Adult worms live in the lumen of the small intestine. Female worms produce approximately 200 000 eggs per day, which are excreted in stool and must incubate in soil for 2 to 3 weeks for an embryo to become infectious. Following ingestion of embryonated eggs, usually from contaminated soil, larvae hatch in the small intestine, penetrate the mucosa, and are transported passively by portal blood to the liver and lungs. After migrating into the airways, larvae ascend through the tracheobronchial tree to the pharynx, are swallowed, and mature into adults in the small intestine. Infection with *A lumbricoides* is most common in resource-limited countries, including rural and urban communities characterized by poor sanitation. Adult worms can live for 12 to 18 months, resulting in daily fecal excretion of large numbers of ova. Female worms are longer than male worms and can measure 40 cm in length and 6 mm in diameter.

The **incubation period** (interval between ingestion of eggs and development of egg-laying adults) is approximately 8 weeks.

DIAGNOSTIC TESTS: Ova routinely are detected by examination of a fresh stool specimen using light microscopy. Infected people also may pass adult worms from the rectum, from the nose after migration through the nares, and from the mouth, usually in vomitus. Adult worms may be detected by computed tomographic scan of the abdomen or by ultrasonographic examination of the biliary tree.

TREATMENT: Albendazole (taken with food in a single dose), mebendazole for 3 days, or ivermectin (taken on an empty stomach in a single dose) are recommended for treatment of ascariasis (see Drugs for Parasitic Infections, p 848). Nitazoxanide taken twice a day for 3 days also is effective against *A lumbricoides*. Although widely accepted for treatment of ascariasis, albendazole is not labeled for this indication. Likewise, ivermectin and nitazoxanide are not labeled for use for treatment of ascariasis. The safety of ivermectin in children weighing less than 15 kg and in pregnant women has not been established. In 1-year-old children, the World Health Organization recommends reducing the albendazole dose to half of that given to older children and adults. Reexamination of stool specimens 2 weeks after therapy to determine whether the worms have been eliminated is helpful for assessing therapy.

Conservative management of small bowel obstruction, including nasogastric suction and intravenous fluids, may result in resolution of major symptoms before administration of anthelmintic therapy. Piperazine, which is not available in the United States, causes worms to be paralyzed, allows them to be eliminated in stool, and may relieve intestinal obstruction caused by heavy worm burden. Surgical intervention occasionally is necessary to relieve intestinal or biliary tract obstruction or for volvulus or peritonitis secondary to perforation. Endoscopic retrograde cholangiopancreatography has been used successfully for extraction of worms from the biliary tree.

ISOLATION OF THE HOSPITALIZED PATIENT: Standard precautions are recommended, because there is no direct person-to-person transmission.

CONTROL MEASURES: Sanitary disposal of human feces prevents transmission. Vegetables cultivated in areas where uncomposted human feces are used as fertilizer must be thoroughly cooked before eating. Periodic mass treatment of preschool- and school-aged children in areas where ascariasis is endemic can reduce the prevalence and intensity of infection of *Ascaris lumbricoides* as well as of other soil-transmitted helminths.

Aspergillosis

CLINICAL MANIFESTATIONS: Aspergillosis manifests as invasive, noninvasive, chronic, or allergic disease depending on the immune status of the host.

- Invasive aspergillosis occurs almost exclusively in immunocompromised patients with prolonged neutropenia (eg, cytotoxic chemotherapy), graft-versus-host disease, or impaired phagocyte function (eg, chronic granulomatous disease, immunosuppressive therapy, corticosteroids). Children at highest risk include children with new-onset or a relapse of hematologic malignancy and allogeneic hematopoietic stem cell transplant recipients. Invasive infection usually involves pulmonary, sinus, cerebral, or cutaneous sites. Rarely, endocarditis, osteomyelitis, meningitis, infection of the eye or orbit, and esophagitis occur. The hallmark of invasive aspergillosis is angioinvasion with resulting thrombosis, dissemination to other organs, and occasionally, erosion of the blood vessel wall with catastrophic hemorrhage. Aspergillosis in patients with chronic granulomatous disease rarely displays angioinvasion.

- Aspergillomas and otomycosis are 2 syndromes of nonallergic colonization by *Aspergillus* species in immunocompetent children. Aspergillomas ("fungal balls") grow in preexisting pulmonary cavities or bronchogenic cysts without invading pulmonary tissue; almost all patients have underlying lung disease, such as cystic fibrosis or tuberculosis. Patients with otomycosis have chronic otitis media with colonization of the external auditory canal by a fungal mat that produces a dark discharge.
- Allergic bronchopulmonary aspergillosis is a hypersensitivity lung disease that manifests as episodic wheezing, expectoration of brown mucus plugs, low-grade fever, eosinophilia, and transient pulmonary infiltrates. This form of aspergillosis occurs most commonly in immunocompetent children with asthma or cystic fibrosis and can be a trigger for asthmatic flares.
- Allergic sinusitis is a far less common allergic response to colonization by *Aspergillus* species than is allergic bronchopulmonary aspergillosis. Allergic sinusitis occurs in children with nasal polyps or previous episodes of sinusitis or children who have undergone sinus surgery. Allergic sinusitis is characterized by symptoms of chronic sinusitis with dark plugs of nasal discharge.

ETIOLOGY: *Aspergillus* species are ubiquitous molds that grow on decaying vegetation and in soil. *Aspergillus fumigatus* is the most common cause of invasive aspergillosis, with *Aspergillus flavus* being the next most common. Several other species, including *Aspergillus terreus, Aspergillus nidulans,* and *Aspergillus niger,* also cause invasive human infections.

EPIDEMIOLOGY: The principal route of transmission is inhalation of conidia (spores) originating from multiple environmental sources (plants, vegetables, dust from construction or demolition), soil, and water supplies (eg, shower heads). Incidence of disease in transplant recipients is highest during periods of neutropenia or during treatment for graft-versus-host disease. Health care-associated outbreaks of invasive pulmonary aspergillosis in susceptible hosts have occurred in which the probable source of the fungus was a nearby construction site or faulty ventilation system. Transmission by direct inoculation of skin abrasions or wounds is less likely. Person-to-person spread does not occur.

The **incubation period** is unknown.

DIAGNOSTIC TESTS: Dichotomously branched and septate hyphae, identified by microscopic examination of 10% potassium hydroxide wet preparations or of Gomori methenamine-silver nitrate stain of tissue or bronchoalveolar lavage specimens, are suggestive of the diagnosis. Isolation of *Aspergillus* species is required for definitive diagnosis. The organism usually is not recoverable from blood (except *A terreus*) but is isolated readily from lung, sinus, and skin biopsy specimens when cultured on Sabouraud dextrose agar or brain-heart infusion media (without cycloheximide). *Aspergillus* species can be a laboratory contaminant, but when evaluating results from ill, immunocompromised patients, recovery of this organism frequently indicates infection. Biopsy of a lesion usually is required to confirm the diagnosis, and care should be taken to distinguish aspergillosis from zygomycosis, which appears similar by diagnostic imaging studies. An enzyme immunosorbent assay serologic test for detection of galactomannan, a molecule found in the cell wall of *Aspergillus* species, is available commercially and has been found to be useful in children and adults. A test result of ≥ 0.5 supports a diagnosis of invasive aspergillosis, and monitoring of serum antigen concentrations twice weekly in periods of highest risk (eg, neutropenia and active graft-versus-host disease) may be useful for early detection of invasive aspergillosis in at-risk patients. False-positive test results have been reported and can be related to consumption of food products containing galactomannan (eg, rice and pasta) or from cross-reactivity with antimicrobial agents derived from fungi (eg, penicillins). A negative galactomannan test result does not exclude diagnosis of invasive aspergillosis. False-negative galactomannan test results consistently occur in patients with chronic granulomatous disease, so the test should not be used in these patients. Limited data suggest that other biomarkers, including 1,3-β-D glucan testing may be useful in the diagnosis of aspergillosis. Unlike adults, children frequently do not manifest cavitation or the air crescent or halo signs on chest radiography, and lack of these characteristic signs does not exclude the diagnosis of invasive aspergillosis. In allergic aspergillosis, diagnosis is suggested by a typical clinical syndrome with elevated total concentrations of immunoglobulin (Ig) E (≥1000 ng/mL) and *Aspergillus*-specific serum IgE, eosinophilia, and a positive result from a skin test for *Aspergillus* antigens. In people with cystic fibrosis, the diagnosis is more difficult, because wheezing, eosinophilia, and a positive skin test result not associated with allergic bronchopulmonary aspergillosis often are present.

TREATMENT[1]: Voriconazole is the drug of choice for invasive aspergillosis, except in neonates, for whom amphotericin B deoxycholate in high doses is recommended (see Drugs for Invasive and Other Serious Fungal Infections, p 835). Voriconazole has been shown to be superior to amphotericin B in a large, randomized trial in adults. Therapy is continued for at least 12 weeks, but treatment duration should be individualized. Monitoring of serum galactomannan serum concentrations twice weekly may be useful to assess response to therapy concomitant with clinical and radiologic evaluation. Voriconazole is metabolized in a linear fashion in children (nonlinear in adults), so the recommended adult dosing is too low for children. The optimal pediatric dose is 7 to 8 mg/kg, intravenously, every 12 hours. Posaconazole has been used as salvage therapy in adults with invasive aspergillosis. Posaconazole may be used in children 13 years of age and older. Pharmacokinetics and safety of posaconazole have not been evaluated in younger children.

Caspofungin has been studied in pediatric patients older than 3 months of age as salvage therapy for invasive aspergillosis. The pharmacokinetics of caspofungin in adults differ from those in children, in whom a body-surface area dosing scheme is preferred to a weight-based dosing regimen. Itraconazole alone is an alternative for mild to moderate cases of aspergillosis, although extensive drug interactions and poor absorption (capsular form) limit the utility of itraconazole. Lipid formulations of amphotericin B can be considered, but *A terreus* is resistant to all amphotericin B products. Data are limited on the safety and efficacy of voriconazole, itraconazole, posaconazole, and caspofungin in children. The efficacy and safety of combination antifungal therapy for invasive aspergillosis in children have not been evaluated adequately. Immune reconstitution can occur during treatment in some patients. Decreasing immunosuppression, if possible, specifically decreasing corticosteroid dose, is important to disease control.

Surgical excision of a localized invasive lesion (eg, cutaneous eschars, a single pulmonary lesion, sinus debris, accessible cerebral lesions) usually is warranted. In pulmonary disease, surgery is indicated only when a mass is impinging on a great vessel. Allergic bronchopulmonary aspergillosis is treated with corticosteroids and adjunctive antifungal therapy is recommended. Allergic sinus aspergillosis also is treated with corticosteroids,

[1] Walsh TJ, Anaissie EJ, Denning DW, et al. Treatment of aspergillosis: clinical practice guidelines of the Infectious Diseases Society of America. *Clin Infect Dis.* 2008;46(3):327–360

and surgery has been reported to be beneficial in many cases. Antifungal therapy has not been found to be useful.

ISOLATION OF THE HOSPITALIZED PATIENT: Standard precautions are recommended.

CONTROL MEASURES: Outbreaks of invasive aspergillosis have occurred among hospitalized immunosuppressed patients during construction in hospitals or at nearby sites. Environmental measures reported to be effective include erecting suitable barriers between patient care areas and construction sites, routine cleaning of air-handling systems, repair of faulty air flow, and replacement of contaminated air filters. High-efficiency particulate air filters and laminar flow rooms markedly decrease the risk of exposure to conidia in patient care areas. These latter measures may be expensive and difficult for patients to tolerate.

Posaconazole has been shown to be effective in 2 randomized controlled trials as prophylaxis against invasive aspergillosis for patients 13 years of age and older who have undergone hematopoietic stem cell transplantation and have graft-versus-host disease and in patients with hematologic malignancies with prolonged neutropenia. Low-dose amphotericin B, itraconazole, voriconazole, or posaconazole prophylaxis has been reported for other high-risk patients, but controlled trials have not been completed in pediatric patients.

Patients at risk of invasive infection should have their home conditions evaluated before discharge from hospital and avoid environmental exposure (eg, gardening). People with allergic aspergillosis should take measures to reduce exposure to *Aspergillus* species in the home.

Astrovirus Infections

CLINICAL MANIFESTATIONS: Illness is characterized by diarrhea of short duration accompanied by vomiting, fever, and occasionally, abdominal pain and mild dehydration. Illness in an immunocompetent host is self-limited, lasting a median of 5 to 6 days. Asymptomatic infections are common.

ETIOLOGY: Astroviruses are nonenveloped, single-stranded RNA viruses with a characteristic starlike appearance when visualized by electron microscopy. Eight human antigenic types originally were described, and several novel species have been identified since 2008.

EPIDEMIOLOGY: Human astroviruses have a worldwide distribution. Multiple antigenic types cocirculate in the same region. Astroviruses have been detected in as many as 10% to 34% of sporadic cases of nonbacterial gastroenteritis among young children in the community but appear to cause a lower proportion of cases of more severe childhood gastroenteritis requiring hospitalization. Astrovirus infections occur predominantly in children younger than 4 years of age and have a seasonal peak during the late winter and spring in the United States. Transmission is person to person via the fecal-oral route. Outbreaks tend to occur in closed populations of the young and the elderly, and incidence is high among hospitalized children and children in child care centers. Excretion lasts a median of 5 days after onset of symptoms, but asymptomatic excretion after illness can last for several weeks in healthy children. Persistent excretion may occur in immunocompromised hosts.

The **incubation period** is 1 to 4 days.

DIAGNOSTIC TESTS: Commercial tests for diagnosis are not available in the United States, although enzyme immunoassays are available in many other countries. The following tests are available in some research and reference laboratories: electron microscopy for detection of viral particles in stool, enzyme immunoassay for detection of viral antigen in stool or antibody in serum, latex agglutination in stool, and reverse transcriptase polymerase chain reaction (RT-PCR) assay for detection of viral RNA in stool. Of these tests, RT-PCR assay is the most sensitive.

TREATMENT: No specific antiviral therapy is available. Oral or parenteral fluids and electrolytes are given to prevent and correct dehydration.

ISOLATION OF THE HOSPITALIZED PATIENT: In addition to standard precautions, contact precautions are recommended for diapered or incontinent children with possible or proven astrovirus infection for the duration of illness.

CONTROL MEASURES: No specific control measures are available. The spread of infection in child care settings can be decreased by using general measures for control of diarrhea, such as training care providers about infection-control procedures, maintaining cleanliness of surfaces, keeping food preparation duties and areas separate from child care activities, exercising adequate hand hygiene, cohorting ill children, and excluding ill child care providers, food handlers, and children (see Children in Out-of-Home Child Care, p 133).

Babesiosis

CLINICAL MANIFESTATIONS: *Babesia* infection often is asymptomatic or associated with mild, nonspecific symptoms. The infection also can be severe and life threatening, particularly in people who are asplenic, immunocompromised, or elderly. In general, babesiosis, like malaria, is characterized by the presence of fever and hemolytic anemia; however, some infected people who are immunocompromised or at the extremes of age (eg, preterm infants) are afebrile. Infected people may have a prodromal illness, with gradual onset of symptoms, such as malaise, anorexia, and fatigue, followed by development of fever and other influenza-like symptoms (eg, chills, sweats, myalgia, arthralgia, headache, anorexia, nausea, vomiting). Less common findings include hyperesthesia, sore throat, abdominal pain, conjunctival injection, photophobia, weight loss, and nonproductive cough. Clinical signs generally are minimal, often consisting only of fever and tachycardia, although hypotension, respiratory distress, mild hepatosplenomegaly, jaundice, and dark urine may be noted. Thrombocytopenia is common; disseminated intravascular coagulation can be a complication of severe babesiosis. If untreated, illness can last for several weeks or months; even asymptomatic people can have persistent low-level parasitemia, sometimes for longer than 1 year.

ETIOLOGY: *Babesia* species are intraerythrocytic protozoa. The etiologic agents of babesiosis in the United States include *Babesia microti*, which has caused most of the reported cases, and several other genetically and antigenically distinct organisms, such as *Babesia duncani* (formerly the WA1-type parasite).

EPIDEMIOLOGY: Babesiosis predominantly is a tickborne zoonosis. *Babesia* parasites also can be transmitted by blood transfusion and through congenital/perinatal routes. In the United States, the primary reservoir host for *B microti* is the white-footed mouse *(Peromyscus leucopus)*, and the primary vector is the tick *Ixodes scapularis*, which also can transmit *Borrelia* *burgdorferi*, the causative agent of Lyme disease, and *Anaplasma phagocytophilum*, the causative agent of human granulocytic anaplasmosis. Humans become infected through tick bites, which typically are not noticed. The white-tailed deer *(Odocoileus virginianus)* is an important host for blood meals for the tick but is not a reservoir host of *B microti*. An increase in the deer population in some geographic areas, including some suburban areas, during the past few decades is thought to be a major factor in the spread of *I scapularis* and the increase in numbers of reported cases of babesiosis. The reported vectorborne cases of *B microti* infection have been acquired in the Northeast (particularly, but not exclusively, in Connecticut, Massachusetts, New Jersey, New York, and Rhode Island) and in the upper Midwest (Wisconsin and Minnesota). Occasional human cases of babesiosis caused by other species have been described in various regions of the United States; tick vectors and reservoir hosts for these agents typically have not yet been identified. Whereas most US vectorborne cases of babesiosis occur during late spring, summer, or autumn, transfusion-associated cases can occur year round.

The **incubation period** ranges from approximately 1 week to several months.

DIAGNOSTIC TESTS: Babesiosis is diagnosed by microscopic identification of the organism on Giemsa- or Wright-stained thick or thin blood smears. If seen, the tetrad (Maltese-cross) form is pathognomonic. *B microti* and other *Babesia* species can be difficult to distinguish from *Plasmodium falciparum;* examination of blood smears by a reference laboratory should be considered for confirmation of the diagnosis. Serologic and molecular testing are performed at the Centers for Disease Control and Prevention and at some other reference laboratories and are important adjunctive tests. If indicated, the possibility of concurrent *B burgdorferi* or *Anaplasma* infection should be considered.

TREATMENT: Clindamycin plus oral quinine for 7 to 10 days or atovaquone plus azithromycin for 7 to 10 days had comparable efficacy in a controlled clinical trial conducted among adult patients who did not have life-threatening babesiosis (see Drugs for Parasitic Infections, p 848). Therapy with atovaquone plus azithromycin is associated with fewer adverse effects. However, the combination of clindamycin and quinine remains the standard of care for severely ill patients. In addition, exchange blood transfusions should be considered for patients who are critically ill (eg, hemodynamically unstable), especially but not exclusively for patients with parasitemia concentrations 10% or greater.

ISOLATION OF THE HOSPITALIZED PATIENT: Standard precautions are recommended.

CONTROL MEASURES: Specific recommendations concern prevention of tick bites and are similar to those for prevention of Lyme disease and other tickborne infections (see Prevention of Tickborne Infections, p 207).

Bacillus cereus Infections

CLINICAL MANIFESTATIONS: Two clinical syndromes are associated with *Bacillus cereus* foodborne illness. The first is the emetic syndrome, which, like staphylococcal foodborne illness, develops after a short incubation period and is characterized by nausea, vomiting, abdominal cramps, and in approximately 30% of patients, diarrhea. The second is the diarrhea syndrome, which, like *Clostridium perfringens* foodborne illness, has a slightly longer incubation period and is characterized predominantly by moderate to severe abdominal cramps and watery diarrhea, with vomiting in approximately 25% of patients. Both syndromes are mild, usually are not associated with fever, and abate within 24 hours.

B cereus also can cause local skin and wound infections (some can be severe, resembling gas-gangrene), periodontitis, ocular infections, and invasive disease, including bacteremia, central line-associated bloodstream infection, endocarditis, osteomyelitis, pneumonia, brain abscess, and meningitis. Ocular involvement includes panophthalmitis, endophthalmitis, and keratitis.

ETIOLOGY: *B cereus* is an aerobic and facultatively anaerobic, spore-forming, gram-positive bacillus. The emetic syndrome is caused by a preformed heat-stable enterotoxin. The emetic toxin is cytotoxic, can cause rhabdomyolysis, and has been associated with fulminant liver failure. The diarrhea syndrome is caused by in vivo production of 1 or 2 heat-labile enterotoxins.

EPIDEMIOLOGY: *B cereus* is ubiquitous in the environment and commonly is present in small numbers in raw, dried, and processed foods. The organism is thought to be a fairly common cause of foodborne illness in the United States but rarely is diagnosed, because clinical laboratories do not test for it. Spores of *B cereus* are heat resistant and can survive pasteurization, brief cooking, or boiling. Vegetative forms can grow and produce enterotoxins over a wide range of temperatures, from 25°C to 42°C (77°F–108°F). The emetic syndrome occurs after eating food containing preformed toxin, most commonly fried rice. Disease can result from eating food contaminated with *B cereus* spores, which produce enterotoxin in the gastrointestinal tract. Spore-associated disease most commonly is caused by contaminated meat or vegetables and manifests as the diarrhea syndrome. Foodborne illness caused by *B cereus* is not transmissible from person to person.

Risk factors for invasive disease attributable to *B cereus* include history of injection drug use, presence of indwelling intravascular catheters or implanted devices, neutropenia or immunosuppression, and preterm birth. *B cereus* endophthalmitis has occurred after penetrating ocular trauma and injection drug use. *Bacillus*-contaminated 70% alcohol pads not labeled as sterile can lead to outbreaks.

The **incubation period** for the emetic syndrome is 0.5 to 6 hours; for the diarrhea syndrome, the incubation period is 6 to 24 hours.

DIAGNOSTIC TESTS: For foodborne illness, isolation of *B cereus* in a concentration of 10^5 colony-forming units/g or greater of epidemiologically incriminated food establishes the diagnosis. Because the organism can be recovered from stool specimens from some well people, the presence of *B cereus* in feces or vomitus of ill people is not definitive evidence of infection. Food can be tested for the diarrhea syndrome toxins using commercially available tests. Phage typing, DNA hybridization, plasmid analysis, enzyme electrophoresis, and multilocus sequence typing have been used as epidemiologic tools in outbreaks of foodborne illness.

In patients with risk factors for invasive disease, isolation of *B cereus* from wounds, blood, or other usually sterile body fluids is significant.

TREATMENT: People with *B cereus* food poisoning require only supportive treatment. Oral rehydration or, occasionally, intravenous fluid and electrolyte replacement for patients with severe dehydration is indicated. Antimicrobial agents are not indicated.

Patients with invasive disease require antimicrobial therapy. Prompt removal of any potentially infected foreign bodies, such as central lines or implants, is essential. *B cereus* usually is susceptible to vancomycin, which is the drug of choice, and also to alternative drugs, including clindamycin, meropenem, imipenem, and ciprofloxacin. *B cereus* is resistant to beta-lactam antimicrobial agents.

ISOLATION OF THE HOSPITALIZED PATIENT: Standard precautions are recommended.

CONTROL MEASURES: Proper cooking and appropriate storage of foods, particularly rice cooked for later use, will help prevent foodborne outbreaks. Food should be kept at temperatures higher than 60°C (140°F) or rapidly cooled to less than 10°C (50°F) after cooking.

Hand hygiene and strict aseptic technique in caring for immunocompromised patients or patients with indwelling intravascular catheters are important to minimize the risk of invasive disease.

Bacterial Vaginosis

CLINICAL MANIFESTATIONS: Bacterial vaginosis (BV), a polymicrobial clinical syndrome diagnosed primarily in sexually active postpubertal females, is characterized by changes in vaginal flora. Classic signs, when present, include a thin white or grey, homogenous, adherent vaginal discharge with a fishy odor often noted to increase after intercourse. Although 84% of females with BV have no symptoms, the remainder of affected females have vaginal discharge that rarely can be accompanied by abdominal pain, pruritus or dysuria. In pregnant women, BV has been associated with adverse outcomes including chorioamnionitis, preterm delivery, and postpartum endometritis.

Vaginitis and vulvitis in prepubertal girls rarely, if ever, are manifestations of BV. Causes of vaginitis in prepubertal girls frequently are nonspecific but include foreign bodies or infections attributable to group A streptococci, *Escherichia coli*, herpes simplex virus, *Neisseria gonorrhoeae, Chlamydia trachomatis, Trichomonas vaginalis,* or enteric bacteria, including *Shigella* species.

ETIOLOGY: The microbiologic cause of BV has not been delineated fully. Typical microbiologic findings of vaginal specimens show an increase in concentrations of *Gardnerella vaginalis*, genital mycoplasmas, anaerobic bacteria (eg, *Prevotella* species and *Mobiluncus* species), *Ureaplasma* species, *Mycoplasma* species, and a marked decrease in concentration of hydrogen peroxide-producing *Lactobacillus* species.

EPIDEMIOLOGY: BV is the most prevalent cause of vaginal discharge in sexually active adolescents and adult women. In this population, BV can accompany other conditions associated with vaginal discharge, such as trichomoniasis or cervicitis secondary to other infections, such as *Neisseria gonorrhoeae* and *Chlamydia trachomatis*. Although evidence of sexual transmission of BV is inconclusive, the correct and consistent use of condoms reduces the risk of acquisition. An increased prevalence of BV is associated significantly with increasing number of sexual partners, a new sex partner, lack of condom use, and douching. Women who never have been sexually active also can be affected. Preexisting symptomatic or asymptomatic BV may be a risk factor for pelvic inflammatory disease. BV increases the risk of complications after gynecologic surgery, complications during pregnancy, and acquisition of many other sexually transmitted infections, including human immunodeficiency virus, *N gonorrhoeae*, herpes simplex virus-2, and *C trachomatis*.

The **incubation period** for BV is unknown.

DIAGNOSTIC TESTS: The clinical diagnosis of BV requires the presence of 3 or more of the following symptoms or signs (Amsel criteria):
- Homogenous, thin grey or white, noninflammatory vaginal discharge that smoothly coats the vaginal walls

- Vaginal fluid pH greater than 4.5
- A fishy odor (amine test) of vaginal discharge before or after addition of 10% potassium hydroxide (ie, the "whiff test")
- Presence of "clue cells" (squamous vaginal epithelial cells covered with bacteria, which cause a stippled or granular appearance and ragged "moth-eaten" borders) on microscopic examination of at least 20% of vaginal epithelial cells.

A Gram stain of vaginal secretions is an alternative means of establishing a diagnosis and is considered by some experts the gold standard for making the diagnosis. A paucity of large gram-positive bacilli consistent with decreased lactobacilli and a predominance of gram-negative and gram-variable rods and cocci (eg, *G vaginalis*, *Prevotella* species, *Porphyromonas* species, and *Peptostreptococcus* species) with or without the presence of curved gram-negative rods (*Mobiluncus* species) are characteristic. Douching, recent intercourse, menstruation, and coexisting infection can alter findings on Gram stain. Culture for *G vaginalis* is not recommended, because the organism is found in females without BV, including females who are not sexually active. Sexually active females with BV should be evaluated for coinfection with other sexually transmitted infections, including syphilis, gonorrhea, chlamydia, trichomoniasis, and human immunodeficiency virus (HIV) infection. Completion of hepatitis B immunization series and HPV immunization series both should be documented.

TREATMENT: The principal goal of treatment is to relieve vaginal symptoms and signs of infection and decrease the risk of infectious complications and acquisition of other sexually transmitted infections. All nonpregnant patients who are symptomatic should be treated after discussion of patient preference for oral versus intravaginal treatment, possible adverse effects, and need to evaluate for other coinfections. Nonpregnant patients with symptoms should be treated with metronidazole for 7 days, tinidazole for 2 days, metronidazole gel intravaginally for 5 days, or clindamycin cream intravaginally, at bedtime, for 7 days (see Table 4.3, p 821). Use of these agents for young children generally has not been evaluated; doses should be based on age of the child. Clindamycin cream can weaken latex condoms and diaphragms for up to 5 days after completion of therapy. Alternative regimens that have a lower efficacy for BV include clindamycin, 300 mg, orally, twice daily for 7 days, or clindamycin ovales, 100 mg, intravaginally, once at bed time for 3 days. Approximately 30% of appropriately treated females have a recurrence within 3 months. Early relapse can occur. Retreatment with the same topical regimen is reasonable. For patients with multiple recurrences, metronidazole gel, twice weekly for 4 to 6 months, may be considered. Monthly metronidazole plus fluconazole also has been used. Probiotic therapies have not been studied sufficiently to recommend their use.

Pregnant or breastfeeding women with symptoms of BV should be treated, regardless of history of prior risk factors for adverse pregnancy outcomes. Asymptomatic pregnant women with a history of adverse pregnancy outcomes (eg, previous preterm birth, premature rupture of membranes, chorioamnionitis) may be considered for treatment. Metronidazole (500 mg, twice daily for 7 days; or 250 mg, orally, 3 times a day for 7 days) is the preferred treatment during pregnancy. Current data suggest that oral treatment regimens are preferred, although intravaginal clindamycin may be an option but only during the first half of pregnancy. Because treatment of BV in high-risk pregnant women who are asymptomatic might prevent adverse pregnancy outcomes, a follow-up evaluation 1 month after completion of treatment is advised.

For nonpregnant women, routine follow-up visits on completion of therapy for BV are unnecessary if symptoms resolve. Recurrences are common and can be treated with the same regimen that was given initially. The presence of a foreign body in the vagina should be excluded. Routine treatment of male sexual partners is not recommended.

ISOLATION OF THE HOSPITALIZED PATIENT: Standard precautions are recommended.

CONTROL MEASURES: None.

Bacteroides and *Prevotella* Infections

CLINICAL MANIFESTATIONS: *Bacteroides* and *Prevotella* organisms from the oral cavity can cause chronic sinusitis, chronic otitis media, dental infection, peritonsillar abscess, cervical adenitis, retropharyngeal space infection, aspiration pneumonia, lung abscess, pleural empyema, or necrotizing pneumonia. Species from the gastrointestinal tract are recovered in patients with peritonitis, intra-abdominal abscess, pelvic inflammatory disease, postoperative wound infection, or vulvovaginal and perianal infections. Soft tissue infections include synergistic bacterial gangrene and necrotizing fasciitis. Invasion of the bloodstream from the oral cavity or intestinal tract can lead to brain abscess, meningitis, endocarditis, arthritis, or osteomyelitis. Skin involvement includes omphalitis in newborn infants; cellulitis at the site of fetal monitors, human bite wounds, or burns; infections adjacent to the mouth or rectum; and decubitus ulcers. Neonatal infections, including conjunctivitis, pneumonia, bacteremia, or meningitis, rarely occur. Most *Bacteroides* and *Prevotella* infections are polymicrobial.

ETIOLOGY: Most *Bacteroides* and *Prevotella* organisms associated with human disease are pleomorphic, non-spore–forming, facultatively anaerobic, gram-negative bacilli.

EPIDEMIOLOGY: *Bacteroides* species and *Prevotella* species are part of the normal flora of the mouth, gastrointestinal tract, and female genital tract. Members of the *Bacteroides fragilis* group predominate in the gastrointestinal tract flora; members of the *Prevotella melaninogenica* (formerly *Bacteroides melaninogenicus*) and *Prevotella oralis* (formerly *Bacteroides oralis*) groups are more common in the oral cavity. These species cause infection as opportunists, usually after an alteration of the body's physical barrier and in conjunction with other endogenous species. Endogenous infection results from aspiration, spillage from the bowel, or damage to mucosal surfaces from trauma, surgery, or chemotherapy. Mucosal injury or granulocytopenia predispose to infection. Except in infections resulting from human bites, no evidence of person-to-person transmission exists.

The **incubation period** is variable and depends on the inoculum and the site of involvement but usually is 1 to 5 days.

DIAGNOSTIC TESTS: Anaerobic culture media are necessary for recovery of *Bacteroides* or *Prevotella* species. Because infections usually are polymicrobial, aerobic cultures also should be obtained. A putrid odor suggests anaerobic infection. Use of an anaerobic transport tube or a sealed syringe is recommended for collection of clinical specimens. Rapid diagnostic tests, including polymerase chain reaction and fluorescent in situ hybridization, are available in research laboratories.

TREATMENT: Abscesses should be drained when feasible; abscesses involving the brain, liver, and lungs may resolve with effective antimicrobial therapy. Necrotizing soft tissue lesions should be débrided surgically.

The choice of antimicrobial agent(s) is based on anticipated or known in vitro susceptibility testing. *Bacteroides* infections of the mouth and respiratory tract generally are susceptible to penicillin G, ampicillin, and extended-spectrum penicillins, such as ticarcillin or piperacillin. Clindamycin is active against virtually all mouth and respiratory tract *Bacteroides* and *Prevotella* isolates and is recommended by some experts as the drug of choice for anaerobic infections of the oral cavity and lungs. Some species of *Bacteroides* and almost 50% of *Prevotella* species produce beta-lactamase. A beta-lactam penicillin active against *Bacteroides* species combined with a beta-lactamase inhibitor (ampicillin-sulbactam, amoxicillin-clavulanate, ticarcillin-clavulanate, or piperacillin-tazobactam) can be useful to treat these infections. *Bacteroides* species of the gastrointestinal tract usually are resistant to penicillin G but are susceptible predictably to metronidazole, beta-lactam plus beta-lactamase inhibitors, chloramphenicol, and sometimes, clindamycin. Tigecycline has demonstrated in vitro activity against *Prevotella* species and *Bacteroides* species but is not approved by the US Food and Drug Administration for use in people younger than 18 years of age. More than 80% of isolates are susceptible to cefoxitin, ceftizoxime, linezolid, imipenem, and meropenem. Cefuroxime, cefotaxime, and ceftriaxone are not reliably effective.

ISOLATION OF THE HOSPITALIZED PATIENT: Standard precautions are recommended.

CONTROL MEASURES: None.

Balantidium coli Infections
(Balantidiasis)

CLINICAL MANIFESTATIONS: Most human infections are asymptomatic. Acute symptomatic infection is characterized by rapid onset of nausea, vomiting, abdominal discomfort or pain, and bloody or watery mucoid diarrhea. In many patients, the course is chronic with intermittent episodes of diarrhea, anorexia, and weight loss. Rarely, organisms spread to mesenteric nodes, pleura, or liver. Inflammation of the gastrointestinal tract and local lymphatic vessels can result in bowel dilation, ulceration, and secondary bacterial invasion. Colitis produced by *Balantidium coli* often is indistinguishable from colitis produced by *Entamoeba histolytica*. Fulminant disease can occur in malnourished or otherwise debilitated or immunocompromised patients.

ETIOLOGY: *B coli*, a ciliated protozoan, is the largest pathogenic protozoan known to infect humans.

EPIDEMIOLOGY: Pigs are the primary host reservoir of *B coli*, but other sources of infection have been reported. Infections have been reported in most areas of the world but are rare in industrialized countries. Cysts excreted in feces can be transmitted directly from hand to mouth or indirectly through fecally contaminated water or food. Excysted trophozoites infect the colon. A person is infectious as long as cysts are excreted in stool. Cysts may remain viable in the environment for months.

The **incubation period** is not established, but may be several days.

DIAGNOSTIC TESTS: Diagnosis of infection is established by scraping lesions via sigmoidoscopy, histologic examination of intestinal biopsy specimens, or ova and parasite examination of stool. The diagnosis usually is established by demonstrating trophozoites (or less frequently, cysts) in stool or tissue specimens. Stool examination is less sensitive, and repeated stool examination may be necessary to diagnose infection, because shedding of organisms can be intermittent. Microscopic examination of fresh diarrheal stools must be performed promptly, because trophozoites degenerate rapidly.

TREATMENT: The drug of choice is a tetracycline, which should not be given to children younger than 8 years of age or during pregnancy unless the benefits of therapy are greater than the risks of dental staining (see Tetracyclines, p 801). Alternative drugs are metronidazole and iodoquinol (see Drugs for Parasitic Infections, p 848). Successful use of nitazoxanide also has been reported.

ISOLATION OF THE HOSPITALIZED PATIENT: In addition to standard precautions, contact precautions are recommended, because human-to-human transmission can occur rarely.

CONTROL MEASURES: Control measures include sanitary disposal of human feces and avoidance of contamination of food and water with porcine feces. Despite chlorination of water, waterborne outbreaks of disease have occurred.

Baylisascaris Infections

CLINICAL MANIFESTATIONS: *Baylisascaris procyonis,* a raccoon roundworm, is a rare cause of acute eosinophilic meningoencephalitis. In a young child, acute central nervous system (CNS) disease (eg, altered mental status and seizures) accompanied by peripheral and/or cerebrospinal fluid (CSF) eosinophilia occurs 2 to 4 weeks after infection. Severe neurologic sequelae or death are usual outcomes. *B procyonis* also is a rare cause of extraneural disease in older children and adults. Ocular larva migrans can result in diffuse unilateral subacute neuroretinitis; direct visualization of worms in the retina sometimes is possible. Visceral larval migrans can present with nonspecific signs, such as macular rash, pneumonitis, and hepatomegaly. Similar to visceral larva migrans caused by *Toxocara,* subclinical or asymptomatic infection is thought to be the most common infection.

ETIOLOGY: *B procyonis* is a 10- to 25-cm roundworm (nematode) with a life cycle usually limited to its definitive host, the raccoon, and to soil. Domestic dogs and some exotic pets, such as kinkajous and ringtails, can serve as definitive hosts and a potential source of human disease.[1]

EPIDEMIOLOGY: *B procyonis* is distributed focally throughout the United States; in endemic foci, an estimated 22% to 80% of raccoons can harbor the parasite in their intestines. Reports of infections in dogs raise concern regarding potential for the infection to be moved into closer contact with people. Embryonated eggs containing infective larvae are ingested from the soil by raccoons, rodents, and birds. When infective eggs or an infected host is eaten by a raccoon, the larvae grow to maturity in the small intestine, where adult female worms shed millions of eggs per day. The eggs are 60 to 80 μm in size and have an outer shell that permits long-term viability in soil. Cases of raccoon infection have been reported in the Midwest, Northeast, West Coast, and more recently, in the South in areas where significant raccoon populations live near humans.

Risk factors for *Baylisascaris* infection include contact with raccoon latrines and uncovered sand boxes, geophagia/pica, age younger than 4 years, and in older children, developmental delay and exposure to kinkajous and other related pets that may harbor this organism. Nearly all reported cases have been in males.

[1] Centers for Disease Control and Prevention. Raccoon roundworms in pet kinkajous—three states, 1999 and 2010. *MMWR Morb Mortal Wkly Rep.* 2011;60(10):302–305

DIAGNOSTIC TESTS: *Baylisascaris* infection is confirmed by identification of larvae in biopsy specimens. Serologic assays (serum, CSF) are available only in research laboratories. A presumptive diagnosis can be made on the basis of clinical (meningoencephalitis, diffuse unilateral subacute neuroretinitis, pseudotumor), epidemiologic (raccoon exposure), and laboratory (blood and CSF eosinophilia) findings. Neuroimaging results can be normal initially, but as larvae grow and migrate through CNS tissue, focal abnormalities are found in periventricular white matter and elsewhere. In ocular disease, ophthalmologic examination can reveal characteristic chorioretinal lesions or rarely larvae. Because eggs are not shed in human feces, stool examination is not helpful. The disease is not transmitted from person to person.

TREATMENT: No drug has been demonstrated to be effective. On the basis of CNS and CSF penetration and in vitro activity, albendazole, in conjunction with high-dose corticosteroids, has been advocated most widely. Treatment with anthelmintic agents and corticosteroids may not affect clinical outcome once severe CNS disease manifestations are evident. Some experts advocate use of additional anthelmintic agents. Limited data are available regarding safety and efficacy of these therapies in children. Preventive therapy with albendazole should be considered for children with a history of ingestion of soil potentially contaminated with raccoon feces; however, no definitive preventive dosing regimen has been established. Worms localized to the retina may be killed by direct photocoagulation (see Drugs for Parasitic Infections, p 848).

ISOLATION OF THE HOSPITALIZED PATIENT: Standard precautions are recommended.

CONTROL MEASURES: *Baylisascaris* infections are prevented by avoiding ingestion of soil contaminated with stool of infective animal reservoirs, primarily raccoons; avoiding raccoon defecation sites, such as flat tree stumps and rocks; washing hands after contact with soil or with pets or other animals; discouraging raccoon presence by limiting access to human or pet food sources; and decontaminating raccoon latrines (especially if located near homes) by treating the area with boiling water or a propane torch, in keeping with local fire safety regulations.

Blastocystis hominis Infections

CLINICAL MANIFESTATIONS: The importance of *Blastocystis hominis* as a cause of gastrointestinal tract disease is controversial. The asymptomatic carrier state is well documented. *B hominis* has been associated with symptoms of bloating, flatulence, mild to moderate diarrhea without fecal leukocytes or blood, abdominal pain, nausea, and poor growth. When *B hominis* is identified in stool from symptomatic patients, other causes of this symptom complex, particularly *Giardia intestinalis* and *Cryptosporidium parvum*, should be investigated before assuming that *B hominis* is the cause of the signs and symptoms. Polymerase chain reaction fingerprinting suggests that some *B hominis* organisms are disease associated but others are not.

ETIOLOGY: *B hominis* previously has been classified as a protozoan, but molecular studies have characterized it as a stramenopile (a eukaryote). Multiple forms have been described: vacuolar, which is observed most commonly in clinical specimens; granular; which is seen rarely in fresh stools; ameboid; and cystic.

EPIDEMIOLOGY: *B hominis* is recovered from 1% to 20% of stool specimens examined for ova and parasites. Because transmission is believed to be via the fecal-oral route, presence of the organism may be a marker for presence of other pathogens spread by fecal contamination. Transmission from animals occurs.

The **incubation period** has not been established.

DIAGNOSTIC TESTS: Stool specimens should be preserved in polyvinyl alcohol and stained with trichrome or iron-hematoxylin before microscopic examination. The parasite may be present in varying numbers, and infections may be reported as light to heavy. The presence of 5 or more organisms per high-power ($\times$400 magnification) field can indicate heavy infection with many organisms, which, to some experts suggests causation when other enteropathogens are absent. Other experts consider the presence of 10 or more organisms per 10 oil immersion fields ($\times$1000 magnification) to represent many organisms.

TREATMENT: Indications for treatment are not established. Some experts recommend that treatment should be reserved for patients who have persistent symptoms and in whom no other pathogen or process is found to explain the gastrointestinal tract symptoms; randomized controlled treatment trials for both nitazoxanide and metronidazole have demonstrated benefit in symptomatic patients. Trimethoprim-sulfamethoxazole and iodoquinol have been used with limited success (see Drugs for Parasitic Infections, p 848). Other experts believe that *B hominis* does not cause symptomatic disease and recommend only a careful search for other causes of symptoms.

ISOLATION OF THE HOSPITALIZED PATIENT: In addition to standard precautions, contact precautions are recommended for diapered or incontinent children.

CONTROL MEASURES: Personal hygiene measures, including hand washing with soap and warm water, both after using the toilet and changing diapers and before preparing food, should be practiced.

Blastomycosis

CLINICAL MANIFESTATIONS: Infections can be acute, chronic, or fulminant but are asymptomatic in up to 50% of infected people. The most common clinical manifestation of blastomycosis in children is pulmonary disease, with fever, chest pain and nonspecific symptoms, such as fatigue and myalgia. Rarely, patients may develop acute respiratory distress syndrome (ARDS). Typical radiographic patterns include patchy pneumonitis, a mass-like infiltrate, or nodules. Blastomycosis can be misdiagnosed as bacterial pneumonia, tuberculosis, sarcoidosis, or malignant neoplasm. Disseminated blastomycosis, which can occur in up to 25% of cases, most commonly involves the skin, osteoarticular structures, and the genitourinary tract. Cutaneous manifestations can be verrucous, nodular, ulcerative, or pustular. Abscesses usually are subcutaneous but can involve any organ. Central nervous system infection is rare as is intrauterine or congenital infection.

ETIOLOGY: Blastomycosis is caused by *Blastomyces dermatitidis*, a dimorphic fungus existing in the yeast form at 37°C (98°F) , in infected tissues, and in a mycelial form at room temperature and in soil. Conidia, produced from hyphae of the mycelial form, are infectious.

EPIDEMIOLOGY: Infection is acquired through inhalation of conidia from soil. Person-to-person transmission does not occur. Blastomycosis is endemic in certain areas of the United States, with most cases occurring in the Ohio and Mississippi river valleys, the southeastern states, and states that border the Great Lakes. Sporadic cases also have been reported in Hawaii, Israel, India, Africa, and Central and South America. Blastomycosis can occur in immunocompetent and immunocompromised hosts.

The **incubation period** ranges from 2 weeks to 3 months.

DIAGNOSTIC TESTS: Definitive diagnosis of blastomycosis is based on identification of characteristic thick-walled, broad-based, single budding yeast cells either by culture or histopathologic testing. The organism may be seen in sputum, tracheal aspirates, cerebrospinal fluid, urine, or material from lesions processed with 10% potassium hydroxide or a silver stain. Children with pneumonia who are unable to produce sputum may require bronchoalveolar lavage or open biopsy to establish the diagnosis. Organisms can be cultured on brain-heart infusion media and Sabouraud dextrose agar at room temperature. Chemiluminescent DNA probes are available for identification of *B dermatitidis.* Because serologic tests (immunodiffusion and complement fixation) lack adequate sensitivity, every effort should be made to obtain appropriate specimens for culture. An assay that detects *Blastomyces* antigen in urine is available commercially, but cross-reactivity occurs in patients with other endemic mycoses. Clinical and epidemiologic findings often aid with interpretation.

TREATMENT[1]: Amphotericin B is the treatment of choice for severe infection. Liposomal amphotericin B is recommended for central nervous system infection (see Drugs for Invasive and Other Serious Fungal Infections, p 835). Oral itraconazole or fluconazole can be used for mild or moderate infections, either alone or after a short course of amphotericin B. Data regarding the efficacy of fluconazole therapy in children are limited. Although itraconazole is indicated for treatment of nonmeningeal, non–life-threatening infections in adults, the safety and efficacy of this agent in children with blastomycosis has not been established; however, its use in children in this setting has been recommended.[1]

Therapy usually is continued for at least 6 months for pulmonary and extrapulmonary disease. Some experts suggest 1 year of therapy for patients with osteomyelitis.

ISOLATION OF THE HOSPITALIZED PATIENT: Standard precautions are recommended.

CONTROL MEASURES: None.

Borrelia Infections
(Relapsing Fever)

CLINICAL MANIFESTATIONS: Two types of relapsing fever occur in humans: tickborne and louseborne. Both are characterized by sudden onset of high fever, shaking chills, sweats, headache, muscle and joint pain, and nausea. A fleeting macular rash of the trunk and petechiae of the skin and mucous membranes sometimes occur. Findings and complications can differ between types of relapsing fever and include hepatosplenomegaly, jaundice, thrombocytopenia, iridocyclitis, cough with pleuritic pain, pneumonitis, meningitis, and myocarditis. Mortality rates are 10% to 70% in untreated louseborne relapsing fever (possibly related to comorbidities in refugee-type settings where this disease typically is found) and 4% to 10% in untreated tickborne relapsing fever. Death occurs predominantly in people with underlying illnesses, infants, and elderly people. Early treatment

---

[1] Chapman SW, Dismukes WE, Proia LA, et al. Clinical guidelines for the management of blastomycosis: 2008 update by the Infectious Diseases Society of America. *Clin Infect Dis.* 2008;46(12):1801–1812

reduces mortality to less than 5%. Untreated, an initial febrile period of 2 to 7 days terminates spontaneously by crisis. The initial febrile episode is followed by an afebrile period of several days to weeks, then by one relapse or more (0–13 for tickborne, 1–5 for louseborne). Relapses typically become shorter and milder progressively as afebrile periods lengthen. Relapse is associated with expression of new borrelial antigens, and resolution of symptoms is associated with production of antibody specific to those new antigenic determinants. Infection during pregnancy often is severe and can result in preterm birth, abortion, stillbirth, or neonatal infection.

ETIOLOGY: Relapsing fever is caused by certain spirochetes of the genus *Borrelia*. *Borrelia recurrentis* is the only species that causes louseborne (epidemic) relapsing fever, and there is no animal reservoir of *B recurrentis*. Worldwide, at least 14 *Borrelia* species cause tickborne (endemic) relapsing fever, including *Borrelia hermsii, Borrelia turicatae,* and *Borrelia parkeri* in North America.

EPIDEMIOLOGY: Louseborne epidemic relapsing fever has been reported in Ethiopia, Eritrea, Somalia, and the Sudan, especially in refugee and displaced populations. Epidemic transmission occurs when body lice *(Pediculus humanus)* become infected by feeding on humans with spirochetemia; infection is transmitted when infected lice are crushed and their body fluids contaminate a bite wound or skin abraded by scratching.

Endemic tickborne relapsing fever is distributed widely throughout the world, is transmitted by soft-bodied ticks *(Ornithodoros* species), and occurs sporadically and in small clusters, often within families. Ticks become infected by feeding on rodents or other small mammals and transmit infection via their saliva and other fluids when they take subsequent blood meals. Ticks may serve as reservoirs of infection as a result of transovarial and trans-stadial transmission. Soft-bodied ticks inflict painless bites and feed briefly (10–30 minutes), usually at night, so people often are unaware of bites.

Most tickborne relapsing fever in the United States is caused by *B hermsii*. Infection typically results from tick exposures in rodent-infested cabins in western mountainous areas, including state and national parks. *B turicatae* infections occur less frequently; most cases have been reported from Texas and often are associated with tick exposures in rodent-infested caves. A single human infection has been reported with *B parkeri*; however, the tick infected with this *Borrelia* species is associated with burrows, rodent nests, and caves in arid areas or grasslands in the western United States.

Infected body lice and ticks remain alive and infectious for several years without feeding. Relapsing fever is not transmitted between individual humans, but perinatal transmission from an infected mother to her infant does occur and can result in preterm birth, stillbirth, and neonatal death.

The **incubation period** is 2 to 18 days, with a mean of 7 days.

DIAGNOSTIC TESTS: Spirochetes can be observed by dark-field microscopy and in Wright-, Giemsa- , or acridine orange-stained preparations of thin or dehemoglobinized thick smears of peripheral blood or in stained buffy-coat preparations. Organisms often can be detected in blood obtained while the person is febrile. Spirochetes can be cultured from blood in Barbour-Stoenner-Kelly medium or by intraperitoneal inoculation of immature laboratory mice. Serum antibodies to *Borrelia* species can be detected by enzyme immunoassay and Western immunoblot analysis at some reference and commercial specialty laboratories; these tests are not standardized and are affected by antigenic variations among and within *Borrelia* species and strains. Serologic cross-reactions occur with other spirochetes, including *Borrelia burgdorferi*, *Treponema pallidum*, and *Leptospira* species. Biological specimens for laboratory testing can be sent to the Division of Vector-Borne Diseases, Centers for Disease Control and Prevention, Fort Collins, CO 80521 (telephone: 970-221-6400).

TREATMENT: Treatment of tickborne relapsing fever with a 5- to 10-day course of one of the tetracyclines, usually doxycycline, produces prompt clearance of spirochetes and remission of symptoms. For children younger than 8 years of age and for pregnant women, penicillin and erythromycin are the preferred drugs (see Tetracyclines, p 801). Penicillin G procaine or intravenous penicillin G is recommended as initial therapy for people who are unable to take oral therapy, although low-dose penicillin G has been associated with a higher frequency of relapse. A Jarisch-Herxheimer reaction (an acute febrile reaction accompanied by headache, myalgia, and an aggravated clinical picture lasting less than 24 hours) commonly is observed during the first few hours after initiating antimicrobial therapy. Because this reaction sometimes is associated with transient hypotension attributable to decreased effective circulating blood volume (especially in louseborne relapsing fever), patients should be hospitalized and monitored closely, particularly during the first 4 hours of treatment. However, the Jarisch-Herxheimer reaction in children typically is mild and usually can be managed with antipyretic agents alone.

Single-dose treatment using a tetracycline, penicillin, erythromycin, or chloramphenicol is effective for curing louseborne relapsing fever.

ISOLATION OF THE HOSPITALIZED PATIENT: Standard precautions are recommended. If louse infestation is present, contact precautions also are indicated (see Pediculosis, p 543–547).

CONTROL MEASURES: Soft ticks often frequent rodent nests; exposure is reduced most effectively by preventing rodent infestations of homes or cabins by blocking rodent access to foundations and attics and other forms of rodent control. Dwellings infested with soft ticks should be rodent proofed and treated professionally with chemical agents. When in a louse-infested environment, body lice can be controlled by bathing, washing clothing at frequent intervals, and use of pediculicides (see Pediculosis, p 543–547). Reporting of suspected cases of relapsing fever to health authorities is required in most western states and is important for initiation of prompt investigation and institution of control measures.

Brucellosis

CLINICAL MANIFESTATIONS: Onset of brucellosis in children can be acute or insidious. Manifestations are nonspecific and include fever, night sweats, weakness, malaise, anorexia, weight loss, arthralgia, myalgia, abdominal pain, and headache. Physical findings may include lymphadenopathy, hepatosplenomegaly, and arthritis. Abdominal pain and peripheral arthritis are reported more frequently in children than in adults. Neurologic deficits, ocular involvement, epididymo-orchitis, liver or spleen abscesses, anemia, thrombocytopenia, and pancytopenia also are reported. Serious complications include meningitis, endocarditis, and osteomyelitis. Chronic disease is less common among children than among adults, although rate of relapse has been found to be similar.

ETIOLOGY: *Brucella* bacteria are small, nonmotile, gram-negative coccobacilli. The species that are known to infect humans are *Brucella abortus, Brucella melitensis, Brucella suis,* and rarely, *Brucella canis.* Three recently identified species, *Brucella ceti, Brucella pinnipedialis,* and *Brucella inopinata,* are potential human pathogens.

EPIDEMIOLOGY: Brucellosis is a zoonotic disease of wild and domestic animals. It is transmissible to humans by direct or indirect exposure to aborted fetuses or tissues or fluids of infected animals. Transmission occurs by inoculation through mucous membranes or cuts and abrasions in the skin, inhalation of contaminated aerosols, or ingestion of undercooked meat or unpasteurized dairy products. People in occupations such as farming, ranching, and veterinary medicine as well as abattoir workers, meat inspectors, and laboratory personnel are at increased risk. Clinicians should alert the laboratory if they anticipate *Brucella* may grow from microbiologic specimens so that appropriate laboratory precautions can be taken. In the United States, 100 to 200 cases of brucellosis are reported annually, and 3% to 10% of cases occur in people younger than 19 years of age. The majority of pediatric cases reported in the United States result from ingestion of unpasteurized dairy products. Although human-to-human transmission is rare, in utero transmission has been reported, and infected mothers can transmit *Brucella* to their infants through breastfeeding.

The **incubation period** varies from less than 1 week to several months, but most people become ill within 3 to 4 weeks of exposure.

DIAGNOSTIC TESTS: A definitive diagnosis is established by recovery of *Brucella* species from blood, bone marrow, or other tissue specimens. A variety of media will support growth of *Brucella* species, but the physician should contact laboratory personnel and ask them to incubate cultures for a minimum of 4 weeks. Newer BACTEC systems have greater reliability and can detect *Brucella* species within 5 to 7 days. In patients with a clinically compatible illness, serologic testing using the serum agglutination test can confirm the diagnosis with a fourfold or greater increase in antibody titers between acute and convalescent serum specimens collected at least 2 weeks apart. The serum agglutination test, the gold standard test for diagnosis, will detect antibodies against *B abortus, B suis,* and *B melitensis* but not *B canis,* which requires use of *B canis*-specific antigen. Although a single titer is not diagnostic, most patients with active infection in an area without endemic infection will have a titer of 1:160 or greater within 2 to 4 weeks of clinical disease onset. Lower titers may be found early in the course of infection. Immunoglobulin (Ig) M antibodies are produced within the first week, followed by a gradual increase in IgG synthesis. Low IgM titers may persist for months or years after initial infection. Increased concentrations of IgG agglutinins are found in acute infection, chronic infection, and relapse. When interpreting serum agglutination test results, the possibility of cross-reactions of *Brucella* antibodies with antibodies against other gram-negative bacteria, such as *Yersinia enterocolitica* serotype 09, *Francisella tularensis,* and *Vibrio cholerae,* should be considered. Enzyme immunoassay is a sensitive method for determining IgG, IgA, and IgM anti-*Brucella* antibody titers. Until better standardization is established, enzyme immunoassay should be used only for suspected cases with negative serum agglutination test results or for evaluation of patients with suspected chronic brucellosis, reinfection, or complicated cases. Polymerase chain reaction tests have been developed but are not available in most clinical laboratories.

TREATMENT: Prolonged antimicrobial therapy is imperative for achieving a cure. Relapses generally are not associated with development of *Brucella* resistance but rather with premature discontinuation of therapy. Monotherapy is associated with a high rate of relapse; combination therapy is recommended.

Oral doxycycline (2–4 mg/kg per day, maximum 200 mg/day, in 2 divided doses) or oral tetracycline (30–40 mg/kg per day, maximum 2 g/day, in 4 divided doses) is the drug of choice and should be administered for a minimum of 6 weeks. However, tetracyclines including doxycycline should be avoided, if possible, in children younger than 8 years of age (see Tetracyclines, p 801). Oral trimethoprim-sulfamethoxazole (trimethoprim, 10 mg/kg per day, maximum 480 mg/day; and sulfamethoxazole, 50 mg/kg per day, maximum 2.4 g/day) divided in 2 doses for at least 4 to 6 weeks is appropriate therapy for younger children.

To decrease the rate of relapse, combination therapy with a tetracycline (or trimethoprim-sulfamethoxazole if tetracyclines are contraindicated) and rifampin (15–20 mg/kg per day, maximum 600–900 mg/day, in 1 or 2 divided doses) is recommended. Because of the potential emergence of rifampin resistance, rifampin monotherapy is not recommended.

For treatment of serious infections or complications, including endocarditis, meningitis, spondylitis and osteomyelitis, gentamicin for the first 7 to 14 days of therapy, in addition to a tetracycline and rifampin for a minimum of 6 weeks (or trimethoprim-sulfamethoxazole, if tetracyclines are not used), are recommended. For life-threatening complications of brucellosis, such as meningitis or endocarditis, the duration of therapy often is extended for 4 to 6 months. Surgical intervention should be considered in patients with complications, such as deep tissue abscesses, endocarditis, mycotic aneurysm, and foreign body infections.

The benefit of corticosteroids for people with neurobrucellosis is unproven. Occasionally, a Jarisch-Herxheimer-like reaction (an acute febrile reaction accompanied by headache, myalgia, and an aggravated clinical picture lasting less than 24 hours) occurs shortly after initiation of antimicrobial therapy, but this reaction rarely is severe enough to require corticosteroids.

ISOLATION OF THE HOSPITALIZED PATIENT: In addition to standard precautions, contact precautions are indicated for patients with draining wounds.

CONTROL MEASURES: The control of human brucellosis depends on eradication of *Brucella* species from cattle, goats, swine, and other animals. Pasteurization of dairy products for human consumption is important to prevent disease, especially in children. The certification of raw milk does not eliminate the risk of transmission of *Brucella* organisms.

Burkholderia Infections

CLINICAL MANIFESTATIONS: *Burkholderia cepacia* complex has been associated with severe pulmonary infections in patients with cystic fibrosis, with significant bacteremia in preterm infants after prolonged hospitalization, and with infection in children with chronic granulomatous disease, hemoglobinopathies, or malignant neoplasms. Health care-associated infections include wound and urinary tract infections and pneumonia. Pulmonary infections in people with cystic fibrosis occur late in the course of disease, usually after respiratory epithelial damage caused by infection with *Pseudomonas aeruginosa*. Patients with positive culture results can become chronically infected and experience no change in the rate of pulmonary decompensation or exhibit a more rapid decline in pulmonary function or experience an unexpectedly rapid deterioration in clinical status that results in death. In patients with chronic granulomatous disease, pneumonia is the most common manifestation of *B cepacia* complex infection; lymphadenitis also occurs. Disease onset is insidious, with low-grade fever early in the course and systemic effects occurring 3 to 4 weeks later. Pleural effusion is common, and lung abscess can occur.

Burkholderia pseudomallei is the cause of **melioidosis**, which is endemic in Southeast Asia and northern Australia but also is found in other tropical and subtropical areas, including the Indian Subcontinent and South and Central America. Melioidosis can occur in the United States, usually among travelers returning from areas with endemic disease. Melioidosis can be asymptomatic or can manifest as a localized infection or as fulminant septicemia. Pericarditis, septic arthritis, prostatic abscess, and brain abscess associated with nonsepticemic melioidosis also have been reported. Acute suppurative parotitis is a frequent manifestation that occurs in children in Thailand. Localized infection usually is nonfatal and most commonly manifests as pneumonia, but skin, soft tissue, and skeletal infections also occur. In severe cutaneous infection, necrotizing fasciitis has been reported. In disseminated infection, hepatic and splenic abscesses can occur, and relapses are common without prolonged therapy.

ETIOLOGY: *Burkholderia* organisms are nutritionally diverse, oxidase- and catalase-producing, non–lactose-fermenting, gram-negative bacilli. *B cepacia* complex comprises at least 10 species (*B cepacia, Burkholderia multivorans, Burkholderia cenocepacia, Burkholderia stabilis, Burkholderia vietnamiensis, Burkholderia dolosa, Burkholderia ambifaria, Burkholderia anthina, Burkholderia pyrrocinia,* and *Burkholderia ubonensis*) Additional members of the complex continue to be identified but are rare human pathogens. Other species of *Burkholderia* include *Burkholderia gladioli, Burkholderia mallei* (the agent responsible for glanders), *Burkholderia thailandensis, Burkholderia oklahomensis,* and *B pseudomallei*.

EPIDEMIOLOGY: *Burkholderia* species are waterborne and soilborne organisms that can survive for prolonged periods in a moist environment. Epidemiologic studies of recreational camps and social events attended by people with cystic fibrosis from different geographic areas have demonstrated person-to-person spread of *B cepacia* complex. The source for acquisition of *B cepacia* complex by patients with chronic granulomatous disease has not been identified. Health care-associated spread of *B cepacia* complex most often is associated with contamination of disinfectant solutions used to clean reusable patient equipment, such as bronchoscopes and pressure transducers, or to disinfect skin. Contaminated medical products, including mouthwash and inhaled medications, have been identified as a cause of multistate outbreaks of colonization and infection. *B gladioli* also has been isolated from sputum from people with cystic fibrosis and may be mistaken for *B cepacia*. The clinical significance of *B gladioli* is not known.

In areas with highly endemic infection, *B pseudomallei* is acquired early in life, with the highest seroconversion rates between 6 and 42 months of age. Disease can be acquired by direct inhalation of aerosolized organisms or dust particles containing organisms, by percutaneous or wound inoculation with contaminated soil or water, or by ingestion of contaminated soil or water. Symptomatic infection can occur in people as young as 1 year of age. Risk factors for disease include frequent contact with soil and water as well as underlying chronic disease, such as diabetes mellitus and renal insufficiency, with most people presenting with melioidosis in areas with endemic disease. *B pseudomallei* also has been reported to cause pulmonary infection in people with cystic fibrosis and people traveling to areas with endemic infection as well as septicemia in children with chronic granulomatous disease.

The **incubation period** is 1 to 21 days, with a median of 9 days, but can be prolonged (years) for melioidosis.

DIAGNOSTIC TESTS: Culture is the appropriate method to diagnose *B cepacia* complex infection. In cystic fibrosis lung infection, culture of sputum on selective agar is recommended to decrease the potential for overgrowth by mucoid *Pseudomonas aeruginosa*. *B cepacia* and *B gladioli* can be identified by polymerase chain reaction assay, but this assay is not available routinely. Definitive diagnosis of melioidosis is made by isolation of *B pseudomallei* from blood or other infected sites. The likelihood of successfully isolating the organism is increased by culture of sputum, throat, rectum, and ulcer or skin lesion specimens. A positive result by the indirect hemagglutination assay for a traveler who has returned from an area with endemic infection may support the diagnosis of melioidosis, but definitive diagnosis still requires isolation of *B pseudomallei* from an infected site. Other rapid assays are being developed for diagnosis of melioidosis, but none are available commercially.

TREATMENT: Meropenem is the agent most active against the majority of *B cepacia* complex isolates, although other drugs that may be effective include imipenem, trimethoprim-sulfamethoxazole, ceftazidime, doxycycline, and chloramphenicol. Most experts recommend combinations of antimicrobial agents that provide synergistic activity against *B cepacia* complex. The majority of *B cepacia* complex isolates are resistant intrinsically to aminoglycosides and polymyxin B.

The drugs of choice for initial treatment of melioidosis include ceftazidime and meropenem or imipenem for a minimum of 10 to 14 days. After acute therapy is completed, eradication therapy with trimethoprim-sulfamethoxazole and doxycycline for 12 to 24 weeks is recommended to reduce recurrence. Further studies to determine the optimal duration and regimen are ongoing.

ISOLATION OF THE HOSPITALIZED PATIENT: Contact and droplet precautions are recommended for patients infected with multidrug-resistant strains of *B cepacia* complex. Standard precautions are recommended for people with *B pseudomallei* infection.

CONTROL MEASURES: Because some strains of *B cepacia* complex are highly transmissible and virulence is not well understood, many centers limit contact between *B cepacia* complex-infected and -uninfected patients with cystic fibrosis. This includes inpatient, outpatient, and social settings. For example, patients with cystic fibrosis who are infected with *B cepacia* complex are cared for in single rooms and have unique clinic hours. Education of patients and families about hand hygiene and appropriate personal hygiene is recommended.

Prevention of infection with *B pseudomallei* in areas with endemic disease can be difficult, because contact with contaminated water and soil is common. People with diabetes mellitus, renal insufficiency, or skin lesions should avoid contact with soil and standing water in these areas. Wearing boots and gloves during agricultural work in areas with endemic disease is recommended.

Human Calicivirus Infections (Norovirus and Sapovirus)

CLINICAL MANIFESTATIONS: Abrupt onset of vomiting accompanied by watery diarrhea, abdominal cramps, and nausea are characteristic but not pathognomonic of human calicivirus (HuCV) infections. Mild to moderate diarrhea without vomiting is common in children. Symptoms last from 24 to 60 hours. Systemic manifestations, including myalgia, malaise, and headache, may accompany gastrointestinal tract symptoms.

ETIOLOGY: Caliciviruses are 20- to 40-nm, nonenveloped, single-stranded RNA viruses of the family *Caliciviridae*. This family is divided into 5 genera (*Lagovirus, Nebovirus, Vesivirus, Sapovirus,* and *Norovirus*), with the noroviruses and sapoviruses associated with disease in humans and hence referred to as HuCVs. HuCVs are diverse genetically and antigenically, but for epidemiologic purposes, they are classified into genogroups and genotypes.

EPIDEMIOLOGY: Although noroviruses and sapoviruses include some viruses found in animals, humans are considered the primary reservoir for HuCVs that cause human disease. HuCVs have a worldwide distribution, with multiple antigenic types circulating simultaneously in the same region. The most commonly detected HuCVs are noroviruses, which are a major cause of both sporadic cases and outbreaks of gastroenteritis. The norovirus genogroup 2 type 4 (GII.4) has been predominant during the past decade in the United States, Europe, and Oceania. Sapovirus infections are reported mainly among children with sporadic acute diarrhea, although sapoviruses increasingly have been recognized as a cause of outbreaks. Asymptomatic norovirus excretion is common across all age groups, with the highest prevalence in children. In the United States, noroviruses are the most common cause of outbreaks of gastroenteritis. Outbreaks with high incidences tend to occur in closed populations, such as nursing homes, child care centers, and cruise ships. Transmission is by person-to-person spread via the fecal-oral route or through contaminated food or water. Norovirus is recognized as the most common cause of foodborne illness and foodborne disease outbreaks in the United States.[1] Common-source outbreaks have been described after ingestion of ice, shellfish, and a variety of ready-to-eat foods, including salads and bakery products, usually contaminated by infected food handlers. Transmission via vomitus has been documented, and exposure to contaminated surfaces and aerosolized vomitus has been implicated in some outbreaks. Viral excretion peaks 4 days after exposure and may persist for as long as 3 weeks. Prolonged excretion can occur in immunocompromised hosts. Infection occurs year round but is more common during the colder months of the year.

The **incubation period** is 12 to 48 hours.

DIAGNOSTIC TESTS: Commercial assays for diagnosis of individual cases are not available in the United States. The following tests are available in some research and reference laboratories: electron microscopy for detection of viral particles in stool, enzyme immunoassay for detection of viral antigen in stool or antibody in serum, and reverse transcriptase-polymerase chain reaction (RT-PCR) assay for detection of viral RNA in stool. The most sensitive assay available is a quantitative real-time RT-PCR assay (RT-qPCR) that includes multiple primers in a single reaction to detect the broad range of norovirus genotypes. Laboratory and epidemiologic support for investigation of suspected calicivirus outbreaks is available at the Centers for Disease Control and Prevention (CDC) by

---

[1] Centers for Disease Control and Prevention. Surveillance for foodborne disease outbreaks—United States, 2008. *MMWR Morb Mortal Wkly Rep.* 2011;60(35):1197–1202

request, and the RT-qPCR assay for viral detection in stool is available at all state and public health laboratories.

TREATMENT: Supportive therapy includes oral or intravenous rehydration solutions to replace and maintain fluid and electrolyte balance.

ISOLATION OF THE HOSPITALIZED PATIENT: Contact precautions are recommended for suspected cases of acute gastroenteritis attributable to HuCV infection until 48 hours after symptom resolution.

CONTROL MEASURES: Several factors favor transmission. HuCVs are extremely contagious, large numbers of virus particles can be excreted, and shedding can last for several weeks after symptoms have subsided. The spread of infection can be decreased by standard measures for control of diarrhea, such as educating child care providers and all food handlers about infection control, maintaining cleanliness of surfaces and food preparation areas, using appropriate disinfectants approved by the US Environmental Protection Agency, excluding caregivers or food handlers who are ill and for a period after recovery (eg, 24–72 hours), exercising appropriate hand hygiene, and excluding children from group child care (see Children in Out-of-Home Child Care, p 133). If a source of transmission can be identified (eg, contaminated food or water) during an outbreak, then specific interventions to interrupt transmission can be effective. Candidate vaccines are at an early stage of development. Producing a highly effective vaccine may be challenging, because protective immunity elicited by natural HuCV infection is short-lived, with limited cross-protection to different antigenic types. Sporadic cases of HuCV are not nationally notifiable, but outbreaks of HuCV should be reported to local and state public health authorities as required and to the CDC via the National Outbreak Reporting System (NORS). Updated guidance on norovirus is available at **www.cdc.gov/mmwr/pdf/ rr/rr6003.pdf**.[1] A toolkit designed to help health care professionals control and prevent norovirus gastroenteritis in health care settings is available **(http://www.cdc.gov/hai/ pdfs/norovirus/229110-ANorovirusIntroLetter508.pdf)**.

Campylobacter Infections

CLINICAL MANIFESTATIONS: Predominant symptoms of *Campylobacter* infections include diarrhea, abdominal pain, malaise, and fever. Stools can contain visible or occult blood. In neonates and young infants, bloody diarrhea without fever can be the only manifestation of infection. Fever can be pronounced in children and results in febrile seizures that can have onset before gastrointestinal tract symptoms. Abdominal pain can mimic that produced by appendicitis or intussusception. Mild infection lasts 1 or 2 days and resembles viral gastroenteritis. Most patients recover in less than 1 week, but 10% to 20% have a relapse or a prolonged or severe illness. Severe or persistent infection can mimic acute inflammatory bowel disease. Bacteremia is uncommon but can occur in children, including neonates. Immunocompromised hosts can have prolonged, relapsing, or extraintestinal infections, especially with *Campylobacter fetus* and other *Campylobacter* species. Immunoreactive complications, such as acute idiopathic polyneuritis (Guillain-Barré syndrome), Miller Fisher syndrome (ophthalmoplegia, areflexia, ataxia), reactive arthritis,

---

[1] Centers for Disease Control and Prevention. Updated norovirus outbreak management and disease prevention guidelines. *MMWR Recomm Rep.* 2011;60(3):1–15

Reiter syndrome (arthritis, urethritis, and bilateral conjunctivitis), myocarditis, pericarditis, and erythema nodosum, can occur during convalescence.

ETIOLOGY: *Campylobacter* species are motile, comma-shaped, gram-negative bacilli that cause gastroenteritis. There are 21 species within the genus *Campylobacter*, but *Campylobacter jejuni* and *Campylobacter coli* are the species isolated most commonly from patients with diarrhea. *C fetus* predominantly causes systemic illness in neonates and debilitated hosts. Other *Campylobacter* species, including *Campylobacter upsaliensis*, *Campylobacter lari*, and *Campylobacter hyointestinalis*, can cause similar diarrheal or systemic illnesses in children.

EPIDEMIOLOGY: Data from the Foodborne Diseases Active Surveillance Network[1] (**www.cdc.gov/foodnet**) indicate a 30% decrease in the incidence of infections since 1996 but little change in incidence since 2004. In 2009, the incidence of culture-confirmed cases was 13 per 100 000 population. The highest rates of infection occur in children younger than 4 years of age (28.7 per 100 000 in 2009). In susceptible people, as few as 500 *Campylobacter* organisms can cause infection.

The gastrointestinal tracts of domestic and wild birds and animals are reservoirs of infection. *C jejuni* and *C coli* have been isolated from feces of 30% to 100% of healthy chickens, turkeys, and water fowl. Poultry carcasses usually are contaminated. Many farm animals and meat sources can harbor the organism, and pets (especially young animals), including dogs, cats, hamsters, and birds, are potential sources of infection. Transmission of *C jejuni* and *C coli* occurs by ingestion of contaminated food or by direct contact with fecal material from infected animals or people. Improperly cooked poultry, untreated water, and unpasteurized milk have been the main vehicles of transmission. *Campylobacter* infections usually are sporadic; outbreaks are rare but have occurred among school children who drank unpasteurized milk, including children who participated in field trips to dairy farms. Person-to-person spread occurs occasionally, particularly among very young children, and outbreaks of diarrhea in child care centers have been reported uncommonly. Person-to-person transmission also has occurred in neonates of infected mothers and has resulted in health care-associated outbreaks in nurseries. In perinatal infection, *C jejuni* and *C coli* usually cause neonatal gastroenteritis, whereas *C fetus* often causes neonatal septicemia or meningitis. Enteritis occurs in people of all ages. Person-to-person transmission is uncommon but is greatest during the acute phase of illness. Excretion of *Campylobacter* organisms typically lasts 2 to 3 weeks without treatment.

The **incubation period** usually is 2 to 5 days but can be longer.

DIAGNOSTIC TESTS: *C jejuni* and *C coli* can be cultured from feces, and *Campylobacter* species, including *C fetus*, can be cultured from blood. Laboratory identification of *C jejuni* and *C coli* in stool specimens requires selective media, microaerophilic conditions, and an incubation temperature of 42° to 43°C. Unless the laboratory uses a nonselective isolation technique, many *Campylobacter* species other than *C jejuni and C coli* will not be detected. *C upsaliensis*, *C hyointestinalis*, and *C fetus* may not be isolated because of susceptibility to antimicrobial agents present in routinely used *Campylobacter* selective media. The presence of motile curved, spiral, or S-shaped rods resembling *Vibrio cholerae* by stool phase contrast or darkfield microscopy can provide rapid, presumptive evidence for *Campylobacter* species infection. This is less sensitive than culture and is not performed

---

[1] Centers for Disease Control and Prevention. Vital signs: incidence and trends of infections with pathogens transmitted commonly through food—Foodborne Diseases Active Surveillance Network, 10 US sites, 1996–2010. *MMWR Morb Mortal Wkly Rep.* 2011;60(22):749–755

routinely. *C jejuni* and *C coli* can be detected directly in stool specimens by commercially available enzyme immunoassays, which provide rapid and reliable methods for laboratory diagnosis of enteric infections with *C jejuni* and *C coli*. *Campylobacter* genus- and species-specific polymerase chain reaction (PCR) assay can detect *Campylobacter* organisms directly in stool, but PCR assay is not available commercially.

TREATMENT: Rehydration is the mainstay for all children with diarrhea. Azithromycin and erythromycin shorten the duration of illness and excretion of organisms and prevent relapse when given early in gastrointestinal tract infection. Treatment with azithromycin (10 mg/kg/day for 3 days) or erythromycin (40 mg/kg/day in 4 divided doses for 5 days) usually eradicates the organism from stool within 2 or 3 days. A fluoroquinolone, such as ciprofloxacin, may be effective, but resistance to ciprofloxacin is common (22% of *C coli* isolates and 23% of *C jejuni* isolates in the United States in 2009 [**www.cdc.gov/NARMS**]), and fluoroquinolones are not approved for this indication by the US Food and Drug Administration for people younger than 18 years of age (see Fluoroquinolones, p 800). If antimicrobial therapy is given for treatment of gastroenteritis, the recommended duration is 3 to 5 days. Antimicrobial agents for bacteremia should be selected on the basis of antimicrobial susceptibility tests. *C fetus* generally is susceptible to aminoglycosides, extended-spectrum cephalosporins, meropenem, imipenem, ampicillin, and erythromycin.

ISOLATION OF THE HOSPITALIZED PATIENT: In addition to standard precautions, contact precautions are recommended for diapered and incontinent children for the duration of illness.

CONTROL MEASURES:
- Exercise hand hygiene after handling raw poultry, wash cutting boards and utensils with soap and water after contact with raw poultry, avoid contact of fruits and vegetables with juices of raw poultry, and cook poultry thoroughly.
- Exercise hand hygiene after contact with feces of dogs and cats, particularly stool of puppies and kittens with diarrhea.
- Pasteurization of milk and chlorination of water supplies are important.
- People with diarrhea should be excluded from food handling, care of patients in hospitals, and care of people in custodial care and child care centers.
- Infected food handlers and hospital employees who are asymptomatic need not be excluded from work if proper personal hygiene measures, including hand hygiene, are maintained.
- Outbreaks are uncommon in child care centers. General measures for interrupting enteric transmission in child care centers are recommended (see Children in Out-of-Home Child Care, p 133). Infants and children in diapers who have symptomatic infection should be excluded from child care or cared for in a separate area until diarrhea has subsided. Azithromycin or erythromycin treatment may further limit the potential for transmission.
- Stool cultures of asymptomatic exposed children are not recommended.

Candidiasis
(Moniliasis, Thrush)

CLINICAL MANIFESTATIONS: Mucocutaneous infection results in oral-pharyngeal (thrush) or vaginal or cervical candidiasis; intertriginous lesions of the gluteal folds, buttocks, neck, groin, and axilla; paronychia; and onychia. Dysfunction of T lymphocytes, other immunologic disorders, and endocrinologic diseases are associated with chronic mucocutaneous candidiasis. Chronic or recurrent oral candidiasis can be the presenting sign of human immunodeficiency virus (HIV) infection or primary immunodeficiency. Esophageal and laryngeal candidiasis can occur in immunocompromised patients. Disseminated or invasive candidiasis occurs in very low birth weight newborn infants and in immunocompromised or debilitated hosts, can involve virtually any organ or anatomic site, and rapidly can be fatal. Candidemia can occur with or without systemic disease in patients with indwelling central vascular catheters, especially patients receiving prolonged intravenous infusions with parenteral alimentation or lipids. Peritonitis can occur in patients undergoing peritoneal dialysis, especially in patients receiving prolonged broad-spectrum antimicrobial therapy. Candiduria can occur in patients with indwelling urinary catheters, focal renal infection, or disseminated disease.

ETIOLOGY: *Candida* species are yeasts that reproduce by budding. *Candida albicans* and several other species form long chains of elongated yeast forms called pseudohyphae. *C albicans* causes most infections, but in some regions and patient populations, the non-*albicans Candida* species now account for more than half of invasive infections. Other species, including *Candida tropicalis, Candida parapsilosis, Candida glabrata, Candida krusei, Candida guilliermondii, Candida lusitaniae,* and *Candida dubliniensis,* also can cause serious infections, especially in immunocompromised and debilitated hosts. *C parapsilosis* is second only to *C albicans* as a cause of systemic candidiasis in very low birth weight neonates.

EPIDEMIOLOGY: Like other *Candida* species, *C albicans* is present on skin and in the mouth, intestinal tract, and vagina of immunocompetent people. Vulvovaginal candidiasis is associated with pregnancy, and newborn infants can acquire the organism in utero, during passage through the vagina, or postnatally. Mild mucocutaneous infection is common in healthy infants. Person-to-person transmission occurs rarely. Invasive disease typically occurs in people with impaired immunity, with infection usually arising endogenously from colonized sites. Factors such as extreme prematurity, neutropenia, or treatment with corticosteroids or cytotoxic chemotherapy increases the risk of invasive infection. People with diabetes mellitus generally have localized mucocutaneous lesions. An estimated 5% to 20% of newborn infants weighing less than 1000 g at birth develop invasive candidiasis. Patients with neutrophil defects, such as chronic granulomatous disease or myeloperoxidase deficiency, also are at increased risk. Patients undergoing intravenous alimentation or receiving broad-spectrum antimicrobial agents, especially extended-spectrum cephalosporins, carbapenems, and vancomycin, or requiring long-term indwelling central venous or peritoneal dialysis catheters have increased susceptibility to infection. Postsurgical patients can be at risk, particularly after cardiothoracic or abdominal procedures.

The **incubation period** is unknown.

DIAGNOSTIC TESTS: The presumptive diagnosis of mucocutaneous candidiasis or thrush usually can be made clinically, but other organisms or trauma also can cause clinically similar lesions. Yeast cells and pseudohyphae can be found in *C albicans*-infected tissue and are identifiable by microscopic examination of scrapings prepared with Gram, calcofluor white, or fluorescent antibody stains or suspended in 10% to 20% potassium hydroxide. Endoscopy is useful for diagnosis of esophagitis. Ophthalmologic examination can reveal typical retinal lesions that can result from candidemia. Lesions in the brain, kidney, liver, or spleen can be detected by ultrasonography, computed tomography, or magnetic resonance imaging; however, these lesions typically do not appear by imaging until late in the course of disease or after neutropenia has resolved.

A definitive diagnosis of invasive candidiasis requires isolation of the organism from a normally sterile body site (eg, blood, cerebrospinal fluid, bone marrow) or demonstration of organisms in a tissue biopsy specimen. Negative results of culture for *Candida* species do not exclude invasive infection in immunocompromised hosts; in some settings, blood culture is only 50% sensitive. Recovery of the organism is expedited using blood culture systems that are biphasic or that use a lysis-centrifugation method. Special fungal culture media are not needed to grow *Candida* species. A presumptive species identification of *C albicans* can be made by demonstrating germ tube formation, and molecular fluorescence *in situ* hybridization (FISH) testing rapidly can distinguish *C albicans* from non-*albicans Candida* species. Another method of detection is the assay for (1,3)-beta-D-glucan from fungal cell walls, which does not distinguish *Candida* species from other fungi. Data on use of this assay for children are limited.

TREATMENT[1]:

Mucous Membrane and Skin Infections. Oral candidiasis in immunocompetent hosts is treated with oral nystatin suspension or clotrimazole troches applied to lesions. Troches should not be used in infants. Fluconazole may be more effective than oral nystatin or clotrimazole troches and may be considered if other treatments fail. Fluconazole or itraconazole can be beneficial for immunocompromised patients with oropharyngeal candidiasis. Voriconazole or posaconazole are alternative drugs. Although cure rates with fluconazole are greater than with nystatin, relapse rates are comparable. Safety and efficacy of itraconazole in HIV-infected children with oropharyngeal candidiasis have been demonstrated.

Esophagitis caused by *Candida* species is treated with oral or intravenous fluconazole or oral itraconazole solutions for 14 to 21 days after clinical improvement. Alternatively, intravenous amphotericin B, voriconazole, caspofungin, micafungin, or anidulafungin (for people 18 years of age and older) can be used for refractory, azole-resistant, or severe esophageal candidiasis. Duration of treatment depends on severity of illness and patient factors, such as age and degree of immunocompromise.

Skin infections are treated with topical nystatin, miconazole, clotrimazole, naftifine, ketoconazole, econazole, or ciclopirox (see Topical Drugs for Superficial Fungal Infections, p 836). Nystatin usually is effective and is the least expensive of these drugs.

Vulvovaginal candidiasis is treated effectively with many topical formulations, including clotrimazole, miconazole, butoconazole, terconazole, and tioconazole. Such topically applied azole drugs are more effective than nystatin. Oral azole agents (fluconazole, itraconazole, and ketoconazole) also are effective and should be considered for recurrent or refractory cases (see Recommended Doses of Parenteral and Oral Antifungal Drugs, p 831).

---

[1] Infectious Diseases Society of America. Clinical practice guidelines for the management of candidiasis: 2009 update by the Infectious Diseases Society of America. *Clin Infect Dis.* 2009;48(5):503–535

For chronic mucocutaneous candidiasis, fluconazole, itraconazole, and voriconazole are effective drugs. Low-dose amphotericin B administered intravenously is effective in severe cases. Relapses are common with any of these agents once therapy is terminated, and treatment should be viewed as a lifelong process, hopefully using only intermittent pulses of antifungal agents. Invasive infections in patients with this condition are rare.

Keratomycosis is treated with corneal baths of amphotericin B (1 mg/mL of sterile water) in conjunction with systemic therapy. Patients with cystitis caused by *Candida*, especially patients with neutropenia, patients with renal allographs, and patients undergoing urologic manipulation, should be treated with fluconazole for 7 days because of the concentrating effect of fluconazole in the urinary tract. An alternative is a short course (7 days) of low-dose amphotericin B intravenously (0.3 mg/kg per day). Repeated bladder irrigations with amphotericin B (50 μg/mL of sterile water) have been used to treat patients with candidal cystitis, but this does not treat disease beyond the bladder and is not recommended routinely. A urinary catheter in a patient with candidiasis should be removed or replaced promptly.

Invasive Disease. Treatment of invasive candidiasis in neonates and nonneutropenic adults should include prompt removal of any infected vascular or peritoneal catheters and replacement, if necessary, when infection is controlled. Avoidance or reduction of systemic immunosuppression also is advised when feasible. Immediate replacement of a catheter over a wire in the same catheter site is not recommended.

Amphotericin B deoxycholate is the drug of choice for treating neonates with systemic candidiasis; if urinary tract involvement and meningitis are excluded, lipid formulations can be considered. Echinocandins should be used with caution in neonates, because dosing and safety have not been established. Treatment for neonates is at least 3 weeks. In nonneutropenic and clinically stable children and adults, fluconazole or an echinocandin (caspofungin, micafungin, anidulafungin) is the recommended treatment; amphotericin B deoxycholate or lipid formulations are alternative therapies (see Drugs for Invasive and Other Serious Fungal Infections, p 835). In nonneutropenic patients with candidemia and no metastatic complications, treatment is 2 weeks after documented clearance of *Candida* from the bloodstream and resolution of clinical manifestations associated with candidemia.

In critically ill neutropenic patients, an echinocandin or a lipid formulation of amphotericin B is recommended because of the fungicidal nature of these agents when compared with fluconazole, which is fungistatic. In less seriously ill neutropenic patients, fluconazole is the alternative treatment for patients who have not had recent azole exposure, but voriconazole can be considered. The duration of treatment for candidemia without metastatic complications is 2 weeks after documented clearance of *Candida* organisms from the bloodstream and resolution of neutropenia.

Most *Candida* species are susceptible to amphotericin B, although *C lusitaniae* and some strains of *C glabrata* and *C krusei* have decreased susceptibility or resistance. Among patients with persistent candidemia despite appropriate therapy, investigation for a deep focus of infection should be conducted. Short-course therapy (ie, 7–10 days) can be used for intravenous catheter-associated infections if the catheter is removed promptly, there is rapid resolution of candidemia once treatment is initiated, and there is no evidence of infection beyond the bloodstream. Lipid-associated preparations of amphotericin B can be used as an alternative to amphotericin B deoxycholate in patients who experience significant toxicity during therapy. Published reports in adults and anecdotal reports in preterm infants indicate that lipid-associated amphotericin B preparations have failed to eradicate renal candidiasis, because these large-molecule drugs may not penetrate well into the renal parenchyma. Flucytosine is not recommended routinely for use with amphotericin B deoxycholate for *C albicans* infection involving the central nervous system because of difficulty in maintaining appropriate serum concentrations and the risk of toxicity.

Fluconazole may be appropriate for patients with impaired renal function or for patients with meningitis. However, data on fluconazole use for *Candida* meningitis are limited. Fluconazole is not an appropriate choice for therapy before the infecting *Candida* species has been identified, because *C krusei* is resistant to fluconazole, and more than 50% of *C glabrata* isolates also can be resistant. Although voriconazole is effective against *C krusei*, it is often ineffective against *C glabrata*. The echinocandins (caspofungin, micafungin, and anidulafungin) all are active in vitro against most *Candida* species and are appropriate first-line drugs for *Candida* infections in severely ill or neutropenic patients (see Echinocandins, p 830). The echinocandins should be used with caution against *C parapsilosis* infection, because some decreased *in vitro* susceptibility has been reported. If an echinocandin is initiated empirically and *C parapsilosis* is isolated in a recovering patient, then the echinocandin can be continued. Echinocandins are not recommended for treatment of central nervous system infections.

Ophthalmologic evaluation is recommended for all patients with candidemia. Evaluation should occur once candidemia is controlled, and in patients with neutropenia, evaluation should be deferred until recovery of the neutrophil count.

Chemoprophylaxis. Invasive candidiasis in neonates is associated with prolonged hospitalization and neurodevelopmental impairment or death in almost 75% of affected infants with extremely low birth weight (ELBW [less than 1000 g]). The poor outcomes, despite prompt diagnosis and therapy, make prevention of invasive candidiasis in this population desirable. Four prospective randomized controlled trials and 10 retrospective cohort studies of fungal prophylaxis in neonates with birth weight less than 1000 g or less than 1500 g have demonstrated significant reduction of *Candida* colonization, rates of invasive candidiasis, and *Candida*-related mortality in nurseries with a moderate or high incidence of invasive candidiasis. Besides birth weight, other risk factors for invasive candidiasis in neonates include inadequate infection-prevention practices and injudicious use of antimicrobial agents. Adherence to optimal infection control practices, including "bundles" for intravascular catheter insertion and maintenance and antimicrobial stewardship, can diminish infection rates and should be optimized before implementation of chemoprophylaxis as standard practice in a neonatal intensive care unit. On the basis of current data, fluconazole is the preferred agent for prophylaxis, because it has been shown to be effective and safe. Fluconazole prophylaxis is recommended for ELBW infants cared for in neonatal intensive care units with moderate (5%–10%) or high (≥10%) rates of invasive candidiasis. The recommended regimen for ELBW neonates is fluconazole administered intravenously during the first 48 to 72 hours after birth at a dose of 3 mg/kg, twice a week, for 4 to 6 weeks, or until intravenous access no longer is required for care. This dosage and duration of chemoprophylaxis has not been associated with emergence of fluconazole-resistant *Candida* species.

Fluconazole can decrease the risk of mucosal (eg, oropharyngeal and esophageal) candidiasis in patients with advanced HIV disease. However, an increased incidence of infections attributable to *C krusei* (which intrinsically is resistant to fluconazole) has been reported in non–HIV-infected patients receiving prophylactic fluconazole. Adults undergoing allogenic hematopoietic stem cell transplantation had significantly fewer *Candida* infections when given fluconazole, but limited data are available for children. Prophylaxis should be considered for children undergoing allogenic hematopoietic stem cell transplantation during the period of neutropenia. Prophylaxis is not recommended routinely for other immunocompromised children, including children with HIV infection.

ISOLATION OF THE HOSPITALIZED PATIENT: Standard precautions are recommended.

CONTROL MEASURES: Prolonged broad-spectrum antimicrobial therapy and use of systemic corticosteroids in susceptible patients promote overgrowth of and predispose to invasive infection with *Candida* organisms. Meticulous care of central intravascular catheters is recommended for any patient requiring long-term intravenous alimentation.

Cat-Scratch Disease
(Bartonella henselae)

CLINICAL MANIFESTATIONS: The predominant manifestation of cat-scratch disease (CSD) in an immunocompetent person is regional lymphadenopathy. Fever and mild systemic symptoms occur in approximately 30% of patients. A skin papule or pustule often is found at the presumed site of inoculation and usually precedes development of lymphadenopathy by approximately 2 weeks (range, 7 to 60 days). Lymphadenopathy involves nodes that drain the site of inoculation, typically axillary, but cervical, submental, epitrochlear, or inguinal nodes can be involved. The skin overlying affected lymph nodes typically is tender, warm, erythematous, and indurated. Most CSD lymph nodes will resolve spontaneously within 4 to 6 weeks, but approximately 25% of affected nodes suppurate spontaneously. Most people with CSD are afebrile or have low grade fever with mild systemic symptoms such as malaise, anorexia, fatigue, and headache. Inoculation of the eyelid conjunctiva can result in Parinaud oculoglandular syndrome, which consists of conjunctivitis and ipsilateral preauricular lymphadenopathy. Less common manifestations of *Bartonella henselae* infection (approximately 25% of cases) most likely reflect bloodborne disseminated disease and include fever of unknown origin, conjunctivitis, uveitis, neuroretinitis, encephalopathy, aseptic meningitis, osteolytic lesions, hepatitis, granulomata in the liver and spleen, abdominal pain, glomerulonephritis, pneumonia, thrombocytopenic purpura, erythema nodosum, and endocarditis. Neuroretinitis is characterized by unilateral painless vision impairment, papillitis, macular edema, and lipid exudates (macular star).

ETIOLOGY: *B henselae*, the causative organism of CSD, is a fastidious, slow-growing, gram-negative bacillus that also is the causative agent of bacillary angiomatosis (vascular proliferative lesions of skin and subcutaneous tissue) and bacillary peliosis (reticuloendothelial lesions in visceral organs, primarily the liver). The latter 2 manifestations of infection are reported primarily in patients with human immunodeficiency virus infection. *B henselae* is related closely to *Bartonella quintana*, the agent of louseborne trench fever and a causative agent of bacillary angiomatosis and bacillary peliosis. *B quintana* also can cause endocarditis.

EPIDEMIOLOGY: CSD is a common infection, although its true incidence is unknown. *B henselae* is one of the most common causes of benign regional lymphadenopathy in children. Cats are the natural reservoir for *B henselae*, with a seroprevalence of in 13%

to 90% of domestic and stray cats in the United States. Other animals, including dogs, can be infected and occasionally are associated with human infection. Cat-to-cat transmission occurs via the cat flea *(Ctenocephalides felis)*, with infection resulting in bacteremia that usually is asymptomatic in infected cats and lasts weeks to months. Fleas acquire the organism when feeding on a bacteremic cat and then shed infectious organisms in their feces. The bacteria are transmitted to humans by inoculation through a scratch or bite or hands contaminated by flea feces touching an open wound or the eye. Kittens (more often than cats) and animals that are from shelters or adopted as strays are more likely to be bacteremic. Most reported cases occur in people younger than 20 years of age, with most patients having a history of recent contact with apparently healthy cats, typically kittens. No evidence of person-to-person transmission exists. Infection occurs more often during the autumn and winter.

The **incubation period** from the time of the scratch to appearance of the primary cutaneous lesion is 7 to 12 days; the period from the appearance of the primary lesion to the appearance of lymphadenopathy is 5 to 50 days (median, 12 days).

DIAGNOSTIC TESTS: *B henselae* is a fastidious organism; recovery by routine culture rarely is achieved. Specialized laboratories experienced in isolating *Bartonella* organisms are recommended for processing of cultures. The indirect immunofluorescent antibody (IFA) assay for detection of serum antibodies to antigens of *Bartonella* species is useful for diagnosis of CSD. The IFA test is available at many commercial laboratories and through the Centers for Disease Control and Prevention (CDC). Enzyme immunoassays for detection of antibodies to *B henselae* have been developed; however, they have not been demonstrated to be more sensitive or specific than the IFA test. Polymerase chain reaction assays are available in some commercial and research laboratories and at the CDC for testing of tissue or body fluids, such as pleural or cerebrospinal fluid. If tissue (eg, lymph node) specimens are available, bacilli occasionally may be visualized using Warthin-Starry silver stain; however, this test is not specific for *B henselae*. Early histologic changes in lymph node specimens consist of lymphocytic infiltration with epithelioid granuloma formation. Later changes consist of polymorphonuclear leukocyte infiltration with granulomas that become necrotic and resemble granulomas from patients with tularemia, brucellosis, and mycobacterial infections.

TREATMENT: Management of localized CSD primarily is aimed at relief of symptoms, because the disease usually is self-limited, resolving spontaneously in 2 to 4 months. However, some experts recommend a 5-day course of azithromycin orally to speed recovery. Painful suppurative nodes can be treated with needle aspiration for relief of symptoms; incision and drainage should be avoided, and surgical excision generally is unnecessary.

Antimicrobial therapy may hasten recovery in acutely or severely ill patients with systemic symptoms, particularly people with hepatic or splenic involvement or painful adenitis, and is recommended for all immunocompromised people. Reports suggest that several oral antimicrobial agents (azithromycin, ciprofloxacin, trimethoprim-sulfamethoxazole, and rifampin) and parenteral gentamicin are effective, but the role of antimicrobial therapy is not clear. The optimal duration of therapy is not known but may be several weeks for systemic disease.

Antimicrobial therapy for patients with bacillary angiomatosis and bacillary peliosis has been shown to be beneficial and is recommended. Azithromycin or doxycycline are effective for treatment of these conditions; therapy should be administered for several months to prevent relapse in immunocompromised people.

ISOLATION OF THE HOSPITALIZED PATIENT: Standard precautions are recommended.

CONTROL MEASURES: People, especially children, should avoid playing roughly with cats and kittens to minimize scratches and bites. Immunocompromised people should avoid contact with cats that scratch or bite and should avoid cats younger than 1 year of age or stray cats. Sites of cat scratches or bites should be washed immediately. Care of cats should include flea control. Testing of cats for *Bartonella* infection is not recommended, nor is removal of the cat from the household.

Chancroid

CLINICAL MANIFESTATIONS: Chancroid is an acute ulcerative disease of the genitalia. An ulcer begins as an erythematous papule that becomes pustular and erodes over several days, forming a sharply demarcated, somewhat superficial lesion with a serpiginous border. The base of the ulcer is friable and can be covered with a gray or yellow, purulent exudate. Single or multiple ulcers can be present. Unlike a syphilitic chancre, which is painless and indurated, the chancroid ulcer often is painful and nonindurated and can be associated with a painful, unilateral inguinal suppurative adenitis (bubo). Without treatment, ulcer(s) can resolve in several weeks.

In most males, chancroid manifests as a genital ulcer with or without inguinal tenderness; edema of the prepuce is common. In females, most lesions are at the vaginal introitus and symptoms include dysuria, dyspareunia, vaginal discharge, pain on defecation, or anal bleeding. Constitutional symptoms are unusual.

ETIOLOGY: Chancroid is caused by *Haemophilus ducreyi*, which is a gram-negative coccobacillus.

EPIDEMIOLOGY: Chancroid is a sexually transmitted infection associated with poverty, prostitution, and illicit drug use. Chancroid is rare in the United States, and when it does occur, it usually is associated with sporadic outbreaks. Coinfection with syphilis or herpes simplex virus (HSV) occurs in as many as 10% of patients. Chancroid is a well-established cofactor for transmission of human immunodeficiency virus (HIV). Because sexual contact is the only known route of transmission, the diagnosis of chancroid in infants and young children is strong evidence of sexual abuse.

The **incubation period** is 3 to 10 days.

DIAGNOSTIC TESTS: Chancroid usually is diagnosed on the basis of clinical findings (one or more painful genital ulcers with tender suppurative inguinal adenopathy) and by excluding other genital ulcerative diseases, such as syphilis, HSV infection, or lymphogranuloma venereum. Confirmation is made by isolation of *Haemophilus ducreyi* from a genital ulcer or lymph node aspirate, although sensitivity is less than 80%. Because special culture media and conditions are required for isolation, laboratory personnel should be informed of the suspicion of chancroid. Buboes almost always are sterile. Fluorescent monoclonal antibody stains and polymerase chain reaction assays can provide a specific diagnosis but are not available in most clinical laboratories.

TREATMENT: Recommended regimens include azithromycin or ceftriaxone. Alternatives include erythromycin or ciprofloxacin (see Table 4.3, p 821). Ciprofloxacin is not approved by the US Food and Drug Administration for people younger than 18 years of age for this indication and should not be administered to pregnant or lactating women (see Tetracyclines, p 801). Patients with HIV infection and uncircumcised males may need prolonged therapy. *H ducreyi* strains with intermediate resistance to ciprofloxacin or erythromycin have been reported worldwide.

Clinical improvement occurs 3 to 7 days after initiation of therapy, and healing is complete in approximately 2 weeks. Adenitis often is slow to resolve and can require needle aspiration or surgical incision. Patients should be reexamined 3 to 7 days after initiating therapy to verify healing. If healing has not occurred, the diagnosis can be incorrect or the patient may have an additional sexually transmitted infection, so further testing is required. Slow clinical improvement and relapses can occur after therapy, especially in HIV-infected people. Close clinical follow-up is recommended; retreatment with the original regimen usually is effective in patients who experience a relapse.

Patients should be evaluated for other sexually transmitted infections, including syphilis, hepatitis B virus infection, chlamydia, gonorrhea, and HIV infection at the time of diagnosis. Because chancroid is a risk factor for HIV infection and facilitates HIV transmission, if initial HIV or syphilis test results are negative, they should be repeated 3 months later. All people having sexual contact with patients with chancroid within 10 days before onset of the patient's symptoms need to be examined and treated, even if they are asymptomatic.

ISOLATION OF THE HOSPITALIZED PATIENT: Standard precautions are recommended.

CONTROL MEASURES: Identification, examination, and treatment of sexual partners of patients with chancroid are important control measures. Regular condom use may decrease transmission, and male circumcision is thought to be partially protective. Immunization status for hepatitis B and human papillomavirus should be reviewed and updated if necessary.

Chlamydial Infections

Chlamydophila (formerly Chlamydia) pneumoniae

CLINICAL MANIFESTATIONS: Patients may be asymptomatic or mildly to moderately ill with a variety of respiratory tract diseases caused by *Chlamydophila pneumoniae*, including pneumonia, acute bronchitis, prolonged cough, and less commonly, pharyngitis, laryngitis, otitis media, and sinusitis. In some patients, a sore throat precedes the onset of cough by a week or more. *C pneumoniae* can present as severe community-acquired pneumonia in immunocompromised hosts and has been associated with acute respiratory tract exacerbation in patients with cystic fibrosis and in acute chest syndrome in children with sickle cell disease. Physical examination may reveal nonexudative pharyngitis, pulmonary rales, and bronchospasm. Chest radiography may reveal an infiltrate(s) of a variety of patterns ranging from pleural effusion and bilateral infiltrates to a single patchy subsegmental infiltrate. Illness can be prolonged, with cough often persisting 2 to 6 weeks or longer. The clinical course can be biphasic, culminating in atypical pneumonia.

ETIOLOGY: *C pneumoniae* is an obligate intracellular bacterium. *C pneumoniae* is distinct antigenically, genetically, and morphologically from *Chlamydia* species and is grouped in the genus *Chlamydophila*. All isolates of *C pneumoniae* appear serologically to be closely related.

EPIDEMIOLOGY: *C pneumoniae* infection is presumed to be transmitted from person to person via infected respiratory tract secretions. It is unknown whether there is an animal reservoir. The disease occurs worldwide, but in tropical and less developed areas, disease occurs earlier in life than in industrialized countries in temperate climates. In the United States, approximately 50% of adults have *C pneumoniae*-specific serum antibody by 20 years of age, indicating prior infection by the organism. Initial infection peaks between 5 and 15 years of age. Recurrent infection is common, especially in adults. Clusters of infection have been reported in groups of children and young adults. There is no evidence of seasonality.

The mean **incubation period** is 21 days.

DIAGNOSTIC TESTS: No reliable diagnostic test to identify the organism is available commercially, and none has been approved by the US Food and Drug Administration for use in the United States. Serologic testing has been the primary laboratory means of diagnosis of *C pneumoniae* infection. Of the serologic tests, the microimmunofluorescent antibody test is the most sensitive and specific serologic test for acute infection and currently is the only endorsed approach. A fourfold increase in immunoglobulin (Ig) G titer between acute and convalescent sera or an IgM titer of 16 or greater is evidence of acute infection; use of acute and convalescent titers is preferable over an IgM titer. Use of a single IgG titer in diagnosis of acute infection is not recommended, because during primary infection, IgG antibody may not appear until 6 to 8 weeks after onset of illness and increases within 1 to 2 weeks with reinfection. In primary infection, IgM antibody appears approximately 2 to 3 weeks after onset of illness, but caution is advised when interpreting a single IgM antibody titer for diagnosis, because a single result can be either falsely positive because of cross-reactivity with other *Chlamydia* species or falsely negative in cases of reinfection, when IgM may not appear. Early antimicrobial therapy also may suppress antibody response. Past exposure is indicated by a stable IgG titer of 16 or greater. *C pneumoniae* can be isolated from swab specimens obtained from the nasopharynx or oropharynx or from sputum, bronchoalveolar lavage, or tissue biopsy specimens. Specimens should be placed into appropriate transport media and held at 4°C (39°F) until inoculated into cell culture; specimens that cannot be processed within 24 hours should be frozen and held at −70°C. Culturing *C pneumoniae* is difficult and often fails to detect presence of the organism. A positive culture is confirmed by propagation of the isolate or a positive polymerase chain reaction assay result. Nasopharyngeal shedding can occur for months after acute disease, even with treatment. Immunohistochemistry, used to detect *C pneumoniae* in tissue specimens, requires control antibodies and tissues in addition to skill in recognizing staining artifacts to avoid false-positive results. Because of difficulty of accurately detecting *C pneumoniae* via culture, serologic testing, or immunohistochemistry testing, several types of PCR, including multiplex, hybridization probe method, and fluorescent probe-based method, have been developed. Sensitivity and specificity of these different PCR techniques remains largely unknown, and reliability of results has been reported to vary widely between laboratories using the same PCR type. Currently, PCR testing for *C pneumoniae* is not available commercially, has not been validated for clinical use, and can be accessed only through reference laboratories.

TREATMENT: Most respiratory tract infections thought to be caused by *C pneumoniae* are treated empirically. For suspected *C pneumoniae* infections, treatment with macrolides (eg, erythromycin, azithromycin, or clarithromycin) is recommended. Tetracycline or doxycycline may be used but should not be given routinely to children younger than 8 years of age (see Tetracyclines, p 801). Newer fluoroquinolones (levofloxacin and moxifloxacin) are alternative drugs for patients who are unable to tolerate macrolide antibiotics but should not be used as first-line treatment. In vitro data suggest that *C pneumoniae* is not susceptible to sulfonamides. Duration of therapy typically is 10 to 14 days for erythromycin, clarithromycin, tetracycline, or doxycycline. With azithromycin, the treatment duration typically is 5 days. However, with all of these antimicrobial agents, the optimal duration of therapy is not clear.

ISOLATION OF THE HOSPITALIZED PATIENT: In addition to standard precautions, droplet precautions are recommended for the duration of symptomatic illness.

CONTROL MEASURES: Recommended prevention measures include minimizing crowding, maintaining personal hygiene, respiratory hygiene (or cough etiquette), and frequent hand hygiene.

Chlamydophila (formerly *Chlamydia*) *psittaci*
(Psittacosis, Ornithosis)

CLINICAL MANIFESTATIONS: Psittacosis (ornithosis) is an acute respiratory tract infection with systemic symptoms and signs that often include fever, nonproductive cough, headache, and malaise. Less common symptoms include pharyngitis, diarrhea, and altered mental status. Extensive interstitial pneumonia can occur, with radiographic changes characteristically more severe than would be expected from physical examination findings. Endocarditis, myocarditis, pericarditis, thrombophlebitis, nephritis, hepatitis, and encephalitis are rare complications.

ETIOLOGY: *Chlamydophila psittaci* is an obligate intracellular bacterial pathogen that is distinct antigenically, genetically, and morphologically from *Chlamydia* species and, following reclassification, is grouped in the genus *Chlamydophila*.

EPIDEMIOLOGY: Birds are the major reservoir of *C psittaci*. The term psittacosis commonly is used, although the term ornithosis more accurately describes the potential for nearly all domestic and wild birds to spread this infection, not just psittacine birds (eg, parakeets, parrots, and macaws). In the United States, psittacine birds, pigeons, and turkeys are important sources of human disease. Importation and illegal trafficking of exotic birds is associated with an increased incidence of disease in humans, because shipping, crowding, and other stress factors may increase shedding of the organism among birds with latent infection. Infected birds, whether asymptomatic or obviously ill, may transmit the organism. Infection usually is acquired by inhaling aerosolized excrement or secretions from the eyes or beaks of birds. Handling of plumage and mouth-to-beak contact are the modes of exposure described most frequently, although transmission has been reported through exposure to aviaries, bird exhibits, and lawn-mowing. Excretion of *C psittaci* from birds may be intermittent or continuous for weeks or months. Pet owners and workers at poultry slaughter plants, poultry farms, and pet shops are at increased risk of infection. Laboratory personnel working with *C psittaci* also are at risk. Psittacosis is worldwide in distribution and tends to occur sporadically in any season. Although rare, severe illness and abortion have been reported in pregnant women.

The **incubation period** usually is 5 to 14 days but may be longer.

DIAGNOSTIC TESTS: A confirmed case of psittacosis requires a clinically compatible illness with fever, chills, headache, cough, and myalgia and laboratory confirmation by one of the following: (1) isolation of *C psittaci* from respiratory tract specimens or blood, or (2) fourfold or greater increase in immunoglobulin G (IgG) by complement fixation (CF) or microimmunofluorescence (MIF) against *C psittaci* between paired acute- and convalescent-phase serum obtained at least 2 to 4 weeks apart. A probable case of psittacosis requires a clinically compatible illness and either: (1) supportive serologic test results (eg, *C psittaci* immunoglobulin M [IgM] ≥32 in at least 1 serum specimen obtained after onset of symptoms), or (2) detection of *C psittaci* DNA in a respiratory tract specimen by polymerase chain reaction (PCR) assay. For serologic testing, MIF is more sensitive and specific than CF for *C psittaci*; however, both CF and MIF can cross-react with other chlamydial species and should be interpreted cautiously. Additionally, a reverse-transcriptase polymerase chain reaction (RT-PCR) assay has been developed that can distinguish *C psittaci* from other chlamydial species. This assay has been validated in birds but has yet to be validated for use in humans. Treatment with antimicrobial agents may suppress the antibody response, and in such cases, a third serum sample obtained 4 to 6 weeks after the acute sample may be useful in confirming the diagnosis. Culturing the organism is difficult and should be attempted only by experienced personnel in laboratories where strict measures to prevent spread of the organism are used during collection and handling of all specimens because of occupational and laboratory safety concerns.

TREATMENT: Tetracycline or doxycycline is the drug of choice but should not be given routinely to children younger than 8 years of age or to pregnant women (see Tetracyclines, p 801). Therapy should be a minimum of 10 days and should continue for 10 to 14 days after fever abates. In patients with severe infection, intravenous doxycycline (4.4 mg/kg/day, divided into 2 infusions, maximum 100 mg/dose) may be considered. Erythromycin and azithromycin are alternative agents and are recommended for younger children and pregnant women.

ISOLATION OF THE HOSPITALIZED PATIENT: Standard precautions are recommended, because person-to-person transmission has been theorized but not proven.

CONTROL MEASURES: Human psittacosis is a nationally notifiable disease and should be reported to public health authorities. All birds suspected to be the source of human infection should be seen by a veterinarian for evaluation and management. Birds with *C psittaci* infection should be isolated and treated with appropriate antimicrobial agents for at least 30 to 45 days.[1] Birds suspected of dying from *C psittaci* infection should be sealed in an impermeable container and transported on dry ice to a veterinary laboratory for testing. All potentially contaminated caging and housing areas should be disinfected thoroughly before reuse to eliminate any infectious organisms. People cleaning cages or handling possibly infected birds should wear personal protective equipment including gloves, eyewear, a disposable hat, and a respirator with N95 or higher rating. *C psittaci* is susceptible to many but not all household disinfectants and detergents. Effective disinfectants include

---

[1] National Association of State Public Health Veterinarians. *Compendium of Measures to Control* Chlamydophila psittaci *Infection Among Humans (Psittacosis) and Pet Birds (Avian Chlamydiosis), 2008.* Available at: **www.nasphv. org/Documents/Psittacosis.pdf**

1:1000 dilutions of quaternary ammonium compounds, and freshly made 1:32 dilutions of household bleach (½ cup per gallon). People exposed to common sources of infection should be observed for development of fever or respiratory tract symptoms; early diagnostic tests should be performed, and therapy should be initiated if symptoms appear.

Chlamydia trachomatis

CLINICAL MANIFESTATIONS: *Chlamydia trachomatis* is associated with a range of clinical manifestations, including neonatal conjunctivitis, pneumonia in young infants, genital tract infection, lymphogranuloma venereum (LGV), and trachoma.

Neonatal chlamydial conjunctivitis is characterized by ocular congestion, edema, and discharge developing a few days to several weeks after birth and lasting for 1 to 2 weeks and sometimes longer. In contrast to trachoma, scars and pannus formation are rare.

Pneumonia in young infants usually is an afebrile illness of insidious onset occurring between 2 and 19 weeks after birth. A repetitive staccato cough, tachypnea, and rales in an afebrile 1-month-old infant are characteristic but not always present. Wheezing is uncommon. Hyperinflation usually accompanies infiltrates seen on chest radiographs. Nasal stuffiness and otitis media may occur. Untreated disease can linger or recur. Severe chlamydial pneumonia has occurred in infants and some immunocompromised adults.

Genitourinary tract manifestations, such as vaginitis in prepubertal girls; urethritis, cervicitis, endometritis, salpingitis, and perihepatitis (Fitz-Hugh-Curtis syndrome) in postpubertal females; urethritis and epididymitis in males; and Reiter syndrome (arthritis, urethritis, and bilateral conjunctivitis) also can occur. Infection can persist for months to years. Reinfection is common. In postpubertal females, chlamydial infection can progress to pelvic inflammatory disease and result in ectopic pregnancy or infertility.

LGV classically is an invasive lymphatic infection with an initial ulcerative lesion on the genitalia accompanied by tender, suppurative, inguinal, and/or femoral lymphadenopathy that typically is unilateral. However, anorectal infection is associated with anal intercourse and can cause hemorrhagic proctocolitis or stricture among women and men who engage in anal intercourse. The proctocolitis can be moderate to severe and can resemble inflammatory bowel disease.

Trachoma is a chronic follicular keratoconjunctivitis with neovascularization of the cornea that results from repeated and chronic infection. Blindness secondary to extensive local scarring and inflammation occurs in 1% to 15% of people with trachoma. Trachoma is rare in the United States.

ETIOLOGY: *C trachomatis* is an obligate intracellular bacterial agent with at least 18 serologic variants (serovars) divided between the following biologic variants (biovars): oculogenital (serovars A–K) and LGV (serovars L1, L2, and L3). Trachoma usually is caused by serovars A through C, and genital and perinatal infections are caused by B and D through K.

EPIDEMIOLOGY: *C trachomatis* is the most common reportable sexually transmitted infection (STI) in the United States, with high rates among sexually active adolescents and young adults. A significant proportion of patients are asymptomatic, thereby providing an ongoing reservoir for infection. Prevalence of the organism consistently is highest among adolescent females and was 5% among 14- to 19-year-old females in the recent National Health and Nutrition Examination Survey. Across 27 states, median prevalence among

15- to 24-year-old females screened in prenatal clinics was 7%, with a range of 2% to 20%. Oculogenital serovars of *C trachomatis* can be transmitted from the genital tract of infected mothers to their infants during birth. Acquisition occurs in approximately 50% of infants born vaginally to infected mothers and in some infants born by cesarean delivery with membranes intact. The risk of conjunctivitis is 25% to 50%, and the risk of pneumonia is 5% to 20% in infants who contract *C trachomatis.* The nasopharynx is the anatomic site most commonly infected.

Genital tract infection in adolescents and adults is transmitted sexually. The possibility of sexual abuse should be considered in prepubertal children beyond infancy who have vaginal, urethral, or rectal chlamydial infection. Asymptomatic infection of the nasopharynx, conjunctivae, vagina, and rectum can be acquired at birth. Nasopharyngeal cultures may remain positive for as long as 28 months, but spontaneous resolution of vaginal and rectal infection occurs by 16 to 18 months of age. Infection is not known to be communicable among infants and children. The degree of contagiousness of pulmonary disease is unknown but seems to be low.

LGV biovars are worldwide in distribution but particularly are prevalent in tropical and subtropical areas. Although disease occurs rarely in the United States, outbreaks of LGV have been reported in Europe, and cases have been reported in the United States in men who have sex with men. Infection often is asymptomatic in women. Perinatal transmission is rare. LGV is infectious during active disease. Little is known about the prevalence or duration of asymptomatic carriage.

The **incubation period** of chlamydial illness is variable, depending on the type of infection, but usually is at least 1 week.

DIAGNOSTIC TESTS: Nucleic acid amplification tests (NAATs) tests largely have replaced tissue culture isolation and nonamplified direct detection methods, such as DNA probe, direct fluorescent antibody (DFA) tests, or enzyme immunoassay (EIA), because of the generally better sensitivity and high specificity of NAATs. High sensitivity of NAATs enables testing of specimen types, such as urine and vaginal swabs, for which sensitivity is inadequate with the older methods. However, commercially available NAATs, such as polymerase chain reaction (PCR), transcription-mediated amplification (TMA), and strand-displacement amplification (SDA) tests, vary in specimen types and populations for which manufacturers have obtained approval from the US Food and Drug Administration (FDA). In addition, evaluation of NAATs still is limited for certain pediatric indications.

For **postpubescent individuals**, commercial NAATs have been approved by the FDA for testing of endocervical and male intraurethral swab and male or female urine specimens. Certain NAATs also have been approved by the FDA for testing of vaginal swab specimens collected by a clinician or by the patient in a clinical setting. NAATs have not been approved by the FDA for use with rectal specimens, but some laboratories have met Clinical Laboratory Improvement Amendments (CLIA) requirements and have validated NAATs of rectal swab specimens from males who engage in receptive rectal sexual exposure. Testing of pharyngeal specimens from postpubescent individuals for *C trachomatis* infection generally is not recommended.

NAATs have not been approved by the FDA for testing of conjunctival specimens from infants with suspected *C trachomatis* **conjunctivitis** or for testing of nasopharyngeal swab, tracheal aspirate, or lung biopsy specimens from infants with suspected *C trachomatis* **pneumonia**. Published evaluations of NAATs for these indications are limited, but sensitivity and specificity is expected to be at least as high as those for culture or the selected nonamplified direct detection methods that have been approved by the FDA but have become less available.

Tissue culture has been recommended for *C trachomatis* testing of specimens when **evaluating a child for possible sexual abuse**; culture of the organism may be the only acceptable diagnostic test in certain legal jurisdictions. NAATs are not approved by the FDA for this indication but are available more widely and are more sensitive than culture in limited published evaluations. Test specificity, which is of critical concern because of the potential legal consequences of positive test results, has been high in limited published evaluations of NAATs for this indication. Some experts and expert groups recommend that a positive NAAT result be followed by additional testing with a second NAAT that detects a different target and that specimens be saved according to forensic standards to permit additional evaluation.

Serum anti-*C trachomatis* antibody concentrations are difficult to determine, and only a few clinical laboratories perform this test. In **children with pneumonia**, an acute microimmunofluorescent serum titer of *C trachomatis*-specific immunoglobulin (Ig) M of 1:32 or greater is diagnostic. Diagnosis of **LGV** can be supported but not confirmed by a positive result (ie, titer >1:64) on a complement fixation test for chlamydia or a high titer (typically >1:128, but this can vary by laboratory) on a microimmunofluorescent serologic test for *C trachomatis*. However, most available serologic tests in the United States are based on EIAs and might not provide a quantitative "titer-based" result.

Diagnosis of genitourinary tract chlamydial disease in a child, adolescent, or adult should prompt investigation for **other STIs**, including syphilis, gonorrhea, and human immunodeficiency virus infection. In the case of an infant, evaluation of the mother also is advisable.

Diagnosis of **ocular trachoma** usually is made clinically in countries with endemic infection.

TREATMENT[1]:

- Infants with **chlamydial conjunctivitis** or **pneumonia** are treated with oral erythromycin base or ethylsuccinate (50 mg/kg/day in 4 divided daily doses) for 14 days. Limited data on azithromycin therapy for treatment of *C trachomatis* infections in infants suggest that dosing of 20 mg/kg as a single daily dose for 3 days may be effective. Oral sulfonamides may be used to treat chlamydial conjunctivitis after the immediate neonatal period for infants who do not tolerate erythromycin. Topical treatment of conjunctivitis is ineffective. Because the efficacy of erythromycin therapy is approximately 80%, a second course may be required, and follow-up of infants is recommended. A diagnosis of *C trachomatis* infection in an infant should prompt treatment of the mother and her sexual partner(s). The need for treatment of infants can be avoided by screening pregnant women to detect and treat *C trachomatis* infection before delivery.

An association between orally administered erythromycin and infantile hypertrophic pyloric stenosis (IHPS) has been reported in infants younger than 6 weeks of age. The risk of IHPS after treatment with other macrolides (eg, azithromycin and clarithromycin) is unknown, although IHPS has been reported after use of azithromycin. Because confirmation of erythromycin as a contributor to cases of IHPS will require additional

---

[1] Centers for Disease Control and Prevention. Sexually transmitted diseases treatment guidelines, 2010. *MMWR Recomm Rep.* 2010;59(RR-12):1–110

investigation and because alternative therapies are not as well studied, the American Academy of Pediatrics continues to recommend use of erythromycin for treatment of diseases caused by *C trachomatis*. Physicians who prescribe erythromycin to newborn infants should inform parents about the signs and potential risks of developing IHPS. Cases of pyloric stenosis after use of oral erythromycin or azithromycin should be reported to MedWatch (see MedWatch, p 869).

- Infants born to mothers known to have untreated chlamydial infection are at high risk of infection; however, prophylactic antimicrobial treatment is not indicated, because the efficacy of such treatment is unknown. Infants should be monitored clinically to ensure appropriate treatment if infection develops. If adequate follow-up cannot be ensured, some experts recommend that preemptive therapy be considered.

- For uncomplicated *C trachomatis* **anogenital tract infection in adolescents or adults**, oral doxycycline (200 mg/day in 2 divided daily doses) for 7 days or azithromycin in a single 1-g oral dose is recommended. Alternatives include oral erythromycin base (2.0 g/day in 4 divided daily doses) for 7 days, erythromycin ethylsuccinate (3.2 g/day in 4 divided daily doses) for 7 days, ofloxacin (600 mg/day in 2 divided daily doses) for 7 days, or levofloxacin (500 mg, orally, once per day) for 7 days. **For children who weigh <45 kg**, the recommended regimen is oral erythromycin base or ethylsuccinate 50 mg/kg/day divided into 4 doses daily for 14 days. **For children who weigh >45 kg but who are <8 years of age**, the recommended regimen is azithromycin, 1 g, orally, in a single dose. **For children >8 years of age**, the recommended regimen is azithromycin, 1 g, orally, in a single dose or doxycycline, 100 mg, orally, twice a day for 7 days. **For pregnant women**, the recommended treatment is azithromycin (1 g, orally, as a single dose) or amoxicillin (1.5 g/day in 3 divided daily doses) for 7 days. Erythromycin base (2 g/day in 4 divided daily doses) for 7 days is an alternative regimen. Doxycycline, ofloxacin, and levofloxacin are contraindicated during pregnancy.

    Follow-up Testing. Repeat testing (preferably by NAAT) is recommended 3 weeks after treatment of pregnant women. Because these regimens for pregnant women may not be highly efficacious, a second course of therapy may be required. Nonpregnant adult or adolescent patients treated for uncomplicated *Chlamydia* infection with azithromycin or doxycycline do not need to be retested unless compliance is in question, symptoms persist, or reinfection is suspected. A NAAT conducted less than 3 weeks after completion of therapy can yield false-positive results because of continued presence of dead organisms. Previously infected adolescents are a high priority for repeat testing for *C trachomatis*, usually 3 to 6 months after initial infection. Women recently treated for chlamydial infection have a high risk of reinfection. Thus, consideration should be given to retest all women treated for chlamydial infection whenever they next seek medical care within the following 3 to 12 months.

- For **LGV**, doxycycline (200 mg/day in 2 divided daily doses) for 21 days is the preferred treatment for children 8 years of age and older (see Tetracyclines, p 801). Erythromycin base (2 g/day in 4 divided daily doses) for 21 days is an alternative regimen; azithromycin (1 g, once weekly for 3 weeks) probably is effective.

- Treatment of **trachoma** is more difficult, and recommendations for therapy differ. The most widely used therapy is topical treatment with erythromycin, tetracycline, or sulfacetamide ointment twice a day for 2 months or twice a day for the first 5 days of the month for 6 consecutive months or oral erythromycin or doxycycline (for children

8 years of age and older [see Tetracyclines, p 801]) for 40 days if the infection is severe. However, because of improved adherence and greater efficacy, the World Health Organization encourages use of azithromycin (20 mg/kg, maximum 1 g) as a single dose or in 3 weekly doses as the first-line antimicrobial agent to treat trachoma.

ISOLATION OF THE HOSPITALIZED PATIENT: Standard precautions are recommended.

CONTROL MEASURES:

Pregnancy. Identification and treatment of women with *C trachomatis* genital tract infection during pregnancy can prevent disease in the infant. Pregnant women at high risk of *C trachomatis* infection, in particular women younger than 25 years of age and women with new or multiple sexual partners, should be targeted for screening. Some experts advocate routine testing of pregnant women at high risk during the first trimester and again during the third trimester.

Neonatal Chlamydial Conjunctivitis. Recommended topical prophylaxis with erythromycin or tetracycline for all newborn infants for prevention of gonococcal ophthalmia will not prevent neonatal chlamydial conjunctivitis or extraocular infection (see Prevention of Neonatal Ophthalmia, p 880).

Contacts of Infants With C trachomatis *Conjunctivitis or Pneumonia.* Mothers of infected infants (and mothers' sexual partners) should be treated for *C trachomatis.*

Gynecologic Examination. Sexually active adolescent and young adult females (younger than 26 years of age) should be tested at least annually for *Chlamydia* infection during preventive health care visits, even if no symptoms are present and even if barrier contraception is reported.

Management of Sexual Partners. All sexual contacts of patients with *C trachomatis* infection (whether symptomatic or asymptomatic), nongonococcal urethritis, mucopurulent cervicitis, epididymitis, or pelvic inflammatory disease should be evaluated and treated for *C trachomatis* infection if the last sexual contact occurred during the 60 days preceding onset of symptoms in the index case. Integrated recommendations for services provided to partners of people with STIs, including *C trachomatis,* are available.[1,2]

Lymphogranuloma Venereum. Nonspecific preventive measures for LGV are the same as measures for STIs in general and include education, case reporting, condom use, and avoidance of sexual contact with infected people. Partners exposed to an LGV-infected person within the 60 days before the patient's symptom onset should be tested and treated.

Trachoma. Although not observed in the United States for more than 2 decades, trachoma is the leading infectious cause of blindness worldwide. It generally is confined to poor populations in resource-limited nations of Africa, the Middle East, Asia, Latin America, the Pacific Islands, and remote aboriginal communities in Australia. Trachoma is transmitted by transfer of ocular discharge. Predictors of scarring and blindness for trachoma include increasing age and constant, severe trachoma. Prevention methods recommended by the World Health Organization for global elimination of blindness attributable to trachoma by 2020 include **s**urgery, **a**ntibiotics, **f**ace washing, and **e**nvironmental improvement (SAFE). Azithromycin (20 mg/kg, maximum 1 g) once a year as

---

[1] Centers for Disease Control and Prevention. Recommendations for partner services programs for HIV infection, syphilis, gonorrhea, and chlamydial infection. *MMWR Recomm Rep.* 2008;57(RR-9):1–63

[2] Centers for Disease Control and Prevention. Sexually transmitted diseases treatment guidelines, 2010. *MMWR Recomm Rep.* 2010;59(RR-12):1–110

a single oral dose is used in mass drug administration campaigns for trachoma control. Azithromycin typically is given to all the resident population older than 6 months of age, and a 6-week course of topical tetracycline eye ointment is given to infants younger than 6 months of age.

CLOSTRIDIAL INFECTIONS

Botulism and Infant Botulism
(Clostridium botulinum)

CLINICAL MANIFESTATIONS: Botulism is a neuroparalytic disorder characterized by an acute, afebrile, symmetric, descending, flaccid paralysis. Paralysis is caused by blockade of neurotransmitter release at the voluntary motor and autonomic neuromuscular junctions. Four distinct, naturally occurring forms of human botulism exist: foodborne, wound, adult intestinal colonization, and infant. Fatal cases of iatrogenic botulism, which result from injection of excess therapeutic botulinum toxin, have been reported. Onset of symptoms occurs abruptly within hours or evolves gradually over several days and includes diplopia, dysphagia, dysphonia, and dysarthria. Cranial nerve palsies are followed by symmetric, descending, flaccid paralysis of somatic musculature in patients who are fully alert. Classic infant botulism, which occurs predominantly in infants younger than 6 months of age (range, 1 day to 12 months), is preceded by or begins with constipation and manifests as decreased movement, loss of facial expression, poor feeding, weak cry, diminished gag reflex, ocular palsies, loss of head control, and progressive descending generalized weakness and hypotonia. Sudden infant death can be caused by rapidly progressing botulism.

ETIOLOGY: Botulism results from absorption of botulinum toxin into the circulation from a wound or mucosal surface. Seven antigenic toxin types of *Clostridium botulinum* have been identified. Human botulism is caused by neurotoxins A, B, E, and rarely, F. Non-*botulinum* species of *Clostridium* rarely may produce these neurotoxins and cause disease. Almost all cases of infant botulism are caused by toxin types A and B. A few cases of types E and F have been reported from *Clostridium butyricum* (type E), *C botulinum* (type E), and *Clostridium baratii* (type F) (especially in very young infants). *C botulinum* spores are ubiquitous in soils and dust worldwide.

EPIDEMIOLOGY: Foodborne botulism (annual average, 17 cases in 2006–2010; age range, 3–87 years) results when food contaminated with spores of *C botulinum* is preserved or stored improperly under anaerobic conditions that permit germination, multiplication, and toxin production. Illness follows ingestion of preformed botulinum toxin. Outbreaks have occurred after ingestion of restaurant-prepared foods, home-prepared foods, and commercially canned foods. Immunity to botulinum toxin does not develop in botulism. Botulism is not transmitted from person to person.

Infant botulism (annual average, 90 laboratory-confirmed cases in 2006–2010; age range, <1 to 60 weeks; median age, 15 weeks) results after ingested spores of *C botulinum* or related neurotoxigenic clostridial species germinate, multiply, and produce botulinum toxin in the intestine, probably through a mechanism of transient permissiveness of the intestinal microflora. Most cases occur in breastfed infants at the time of first introduction of nonhuman milk substances; the source of spores usually is not identified. Honey has been identified as an avoidable source. Manufacturers of light and dark corn syrups cannot ensure that any given product will be free of *C botulinum* spores, but no case of infant botulism has been proven to be attributable to consumption of contaminated corn syrup. Rarely, intestinal botulism can occur in older children and adults, usually after intestinal surgery and exposure to antimicrobial agents.

Wound botulism (annual average, 26 laboratory-confirmed cases in 2006–2010; age range, 23–66 years) results when *C botulinum* contaminates traumatized tissue, germinates, multiplies, and produces toxin. Gross trauma or crush injury can be a predisposing event. During the last decade, self-injection of contaminated black tar heroin has been associated with most cases.

The usual incubation period for foodborne botulism is 12 to 48 hours (range, 6 hours–8 days). In infant botulism, the incubation period is estimated at 3 to 30 days from the time of exposure to the spore-containing material. For wound botulism, the incubation period is 4 to 14 days from time of injury until onset of symptoms.

DIAGNOSTIC TESTS: A toxin neutralization bioassay in mice[1] is used to detect botulinum toxin in serum, stool, gastric aspirate, or suspect foods. Enriched selective media is required to isolate *C botulinum* from stool and foods. In infant and wound botulism, the diagnosis is made by demonstrating *C botulinum* toxin or organisms in feces, wound exudate, or tissue specimens. Toxin has been demonstrated in serum in only 1% of US infants with botulism. To increase the likelihood of diagnosis, suspect foods should be collected and serum and stool or enema specimens should be obtained from all people with suspected foodborne botulism. In foodborne cases, serum specimens may be positive for toxin as long as 16 days after admission. Stool or enema and gastric aspirates are the best diagnostic specimens for culture. In infant botulism cases, toxin assay and culture of a stool or enema specimen is the test of choice. Organisms and toxin may persist in stool for up to 5 months. If constipation makes obtaining a stool specimen difficult, a small enema of sterile, nonbacteriostatic water should be used promptly. Because results of laboratory bioassay testing may require several days, treatment with antitoxin should be initiated urgently on the basis of clinical suspicion. The most prominent electromyographic finding is an incremental increase of evoked muscle potentials at high-frequency nerve stimulation (20–50 Hz). In addition, a characteristic pattern of brief, small-amplitude, overly abundant motor action potentials (BSAPs) may be seen after stimulation of muscle. This pattern may not be seen in infants, and its absence does not exclude the diagnosis.

TREATMENT:

Meticulous Supportive Care. Neurologic recovery from botulism may take weeks to months. Therefore, an important aspect of therapy in all forms of botulism is meticulous supportive care, in particular respiratory and nutritional support.

Antitoxin for Infant Botulism. Human-derived antitoxin is given urgently. Botulism Immune Globulin for intravenous use (BabyBIG) is licensed by the US Food and Drug Administration (FDA) for treatment of infant botulism caused by *C botulinum* type A or type B. BabyBIG is made and distributed by the California Department of Public Health (24-hour telephone number: 510-231-7600; **www.infantbotulism.org/**). BabyBIG has been shown to decrease significantly days of mechanical ventilation, days of intensive care unit stay, and overall hospital stays. Equine-derived investigational

---

[1] For information, consult your state health department.

Heptavalent Botulinum Antitoxin (HBAT; see below) is available through the Centers for Disease Control and Prevention (CDC). HBAT is not recommended routinely for infant botulism but has been used to treat patients with type F infant botulism on a case-by-case basis.

Antitoxin for Non-Infant Forms of Botulism. Immediate administration of antitoxin is the key to successful therapy, because antitoxin arrests the progression of paralysis. However, because botulinum neurotoxin binds irreversibly, administration of antitoxin does not reverse paralysis. On suspicion of botulism, antitoxin should be procured immediately through the state health department; all states maintain a 24-hour telephone service for reporting suspected foodborne botulism. If contact cannot be made with the state health department, the CDC Emergency Operations Center should be contacted at 770-488-7100 for botulism case consultation and antitoxin. In 2010, investigational HBAT replaced the licensed type AB antitoxin and the investigational type E antitoxin. HBAT is the only botulinum antitoxin now available in the United States for treatment of noninfant forms of botulism.[1] HBAT contains antitoxin against all 7 (A-G) botulinum toxin types and has been "de-speciated" by enzymatic removal of the Fc immunoglobulin fragment, resulting in a product that is >90% Fab and F(ab')2 immunoglobulin fragments. HBAT is provided under a CDC-sponsored, FDA investigational new drug treatment protocol that includes specific, detailed instructions for intravenous administration of antitoxin and return of required paperwork to the CDC. Additional information may be found at **www.bt.cdc.gov/agent/botulism.**

Antimicrobial Agents. Antimicrobial therapy is not indicated in infant botulism. Aminoglycoside agents potentiate the paralytic effects of the toxin and should be avoided. Penicillin or metronidazole should be given to patients with wound botulism after antitoxin has been administered. The role of antimicrobial therapy in the adult intestinal colonization form of botulism is not established.

ISOLATION OF THE HOSPITALIZED PATIENT: Standard precautions are recommended.

CONTROL MEASURES:
- Any case of suspected botulism is a nationally notifiable disease and is required by law to be reported immediately (ie, by phone or fax) to local and state health departments. Immediate reporting of suspect cases is particularly important because of possible use of botulinum toxin as a bioterrorism weapon.
- Prophylactic equine antitoxin is not recommended for asymptomatic people who have ingested a food known to contain botulinum toxin. Physicians treating a patient who has been exposed to toxin or is suspected of having any type of botulism should contact their state health department immediately. People exposed to toxin who are asymptomatic should have close medical observation in nonsolitary settings.
- Honey should not be given to children younger than 12 months of age.

---

[1] Centers for Disease Control and Prevention. Investigational heptavalent botulinum antitoxin (HBAT) to replace licensed botulinum antitoxin AB and investigational botulinum antitoxin E. *MMWR Morb Mortal Wkly Rep*. 2010;59(10):299

- The investigational botulinum toxoid pentavalent vaccine (types A, B, C, D, and E) has been discontinued by the CDC for immunization of laboratory workers at high risk of exposure to botulinum toxin and no longer is available.[1]
- Education regarding safe practices in food preparation and home-canning methods should be promoted. Use of a pressure cooker (at 116°C [240.8°F]) is necessary to kill spores of *C botulinum*. Bringing the internal temperature of foods to 85°C (185°F) for 10 minutes will destroy the toxin. Time, temperature, and pressure requirements vary with altitude and the product being heated. Food containers that appear to bulge may contain gas produced by *C botulinum* and should be discarded. Other foods that appear to have spoiled should not be eaten or tasted (**www.cdc.gov/nczved/divisions/dfbmd/diseases/botulism/**).

Clostridial Myonecrosis
(Gas Gangrene)

CLINICAL MANIFESTATIONS: Onset is heralded by acute pain at the site of the wound, followed by edema, exquisite tenderness, exudate, and progression of pain. Systemic findings initially include tachycardia disproportionate to the degree of fever, pallor, diaphoresis, hypotension, renal failure, and later, alterations in mental status. Crepitus is suggestive but not pathognomonic of *Clostridium* infection and is not present always. Diagnosis is based on clinical manifestations, including the characteristic appearance of necrotic muscle at surgery. Untreated gas gangrene can lead to disseminated myonecrosis, suppurative visceral infection, septicemia, and death within hours.

ETIOLOGY: Clostridial myonecrosis is caused by *Clostridium* species, most often *Clostridium perfringens*, which are large, gram-positive, spore-forming, anaerobic bacilli with blunt ends. Other *Clostridium* species (eg, *Clostridium sordellii*, *Clostridium septicum*, *Clostridium novyi*) also can be associated with myonecrosis. Disease manifestations are caused by potent clostridial exotoxins (eg, *C sordellii* with medical abortion and *C septicum* with malignancy). Mixed infection with other gram-positive and gram-negative bacteria is common.

EPIDEMIOLOGY: Clostridial myonecrosis usually results from contamination of open wounds involving muscle. The sources of *Clostridium* species are soil, contaminated objects, and human and animal feces. Dirty surgical or traumatic wounds with significant devitalized tissue and foreign bodies predispose to disease. Nontraumatic gas gangrene occurs rarely in immunocompromised people.

The **incubation period** from the time of injury is 1 to 4 days.

DIAGNOSTIC TESTS: Anaerobic cultures of wound exudate, involved soft tissue and muscle, and blood specimens should be performed. Because *Clostridium* species are ubiquitous, their recovery from a wound is not diagnostic unless typical clinical manifestations are present. A Gram-stained smear of wound discharge demonstrating characteristic gram-positive bacilli and absent or sparse polymorphonuclear leukocytes suggests clostridial infection. Tissue specimens (not swab specimens) are appropriate for anaerobic culture. Because some pathogenic *Clostridium* species are exquisitely oxygen sensitive, care should be taken to optimize anaerobic growth conditions. A radiograph of the affected site can

---

[1] Centers for Disease Control and Prevention. Notice of CDC's discontinuation of investigational pentavalent (ABCDE) botulinum toxoid vaccine for workers at high risk for occupational exposure to botulinum toxins. *MMWR Morb Mortal Wkly Rep.* 2011;60(42):1454–1455

demonstrate gas in the tissue, but this is a nonspecific finding. Occasionally, blood cultures are positive and are considered diagnostic.

TREATMENT:
- Prompt and complete surgical excision of necrotic tissue and removal of foreign material is essential.
- Management of shock, fluid and electrolyte imbalance, hemolytic anemia, and other complications is crucial.
- High-dose penicillin G (250 000–400 000 U/kg per day) should be administered intravenously. Clindamycin, metronidazole, meropenem, ertapenem, and chloramphenicol can be considered as alternative drugs for patients with a serious penicillin allergy or for treatment of polymicrobial infections. The combination of penicillin G and clindamycin may be superior to penicillin alone because of the theoretical benefit of clindamycin inhibiting toxin synthesis.
- Hyperbaric oxygen may be beneficial, but data from adequately controlled studies on its efficacy are not available.

ISOLATION OF THE HOSPITALIZED PATIENT: Standard precautions are recommended.

CONTROL MEASURES: Prompt and careful débridement, flushing of contaminated wounds, and removal of foreign material should be performed.

Penicillin G (50 000 U/kg per day) or clindamycin (20–30 mg/kg per day) have been used for prophylaxis in patients with grossly contaminated wounds, but efficacy is unknown.

Clostridium difficile

CLINICAL MANIFESTATIONS: *Clostridium difficle* is associated with several syndromes as well as with asymptomatic carriage. Mild to moderate illness is characterized by watery diarrhea, low-grade fever, and mild abdominal pain. Pseudomembranous colitis generally is characterized by diarrhea with mucus in feces, abdominal cramps and pain, fever, and systemic toxicity. Occasionally, children have marked abdominal tenderness and distention with minimal diarrhea (toxic megacolon). The colonic mucosa often contains 2- to 5-mm, raised, yellowish plaques. Disease often begins while the child is hospitalized receiving antimicrobial therapy but can occur more than 2 weeks after cessation of therapy. Community-associated *C difficle* disease is less common but is occurring with increasing frequency. The illness typically is associated with antimicrobial therapy or prior hospitalization. Complications, which usually occur in older adults, can include toxic megacolon, intestinal perforation, systemic inflammatory response syndrome, and death. Severe or fatal disease is more likely to occur in neutropenic children with leukemia, in infants with Hirschsprung disease, and in patients with inflammatory bowel disease. Colonization by toxin-producing strains without symptoms occurs in children younger than 5 years of age and is common in infants younger than 1 year of age.

ETIOLOGY: *C difficile* is a spore-forming, obligate anaerobic, gram-positive bacillus. Disease is related to A and B toxins produced by these organisms.

EPIDEMIOLOGY: *C difficile* can be isolated from soil and is found commonly in the hospital environment. *C difficile* is acquired from the environment or from stool of other colonized or infected people by the fecal-oral route. Intestinal colonization rates in healthy infants can be as high as 50% but usually are less than 5% in children older than 5 years of age and adults. Hospitals, nursing homes, and child care facilities are major reservoirs for *C difficile*. Risk factors for acquisition include prolonged hospitalization and exposure to an infected person either in the hospital or the community. Risk factors for disease include antimicrobial therapy, repeated enemas, gastric acid suppression therapy, prolonged nasogastric tube intubation, gastrostomy and jejunostomy tubes, underlying bowel disease, gastrointestinal tract surgery, renal insufficiency, and humoral immunocompromise. *C difficile* colitis has been associated with almost every antimicrobial agent. A more virulent strain of *C difficile* with variations in toxin genes has emerged as a cause of outbreaks among adults and is associated with severe disease. Hospitalization of children for *C difficile* colitis is increasing.

The **incubation period** is unknown; colitis usually develops 5 to 10 days after initiation of antimicrobial therapy but can occur on the first day and up to 10 weeks after therapy cessation.

DIAGNOSTIC TESTS: The diagnosis of *C difficile* disease is based on the presence of diarrhea and of *C difficile* toxins in a diarrheal stool specimen. Isolation of the organism from stool is not a useful diagnostic test nor is testing of stool from an asymptomatic patient. Endoscopic findings of pseudomembranes and hyperemic, friable rectal mucosa suggest pseudomembranous colitis. The most common testing method for *C difficile* toxins is the commercially available enzyme immunoassay (EIA), which detects toxins A and B. Although EIAs are rapid and performed easily, their sensitivity is relatively low. The tissue cytotoxin assay, which also tests for toxin in stool, is more sensitive than the EIA but requires more labor and has a slow turnaround time, limiting its usefulness in the clinical setting. Two-step testing algorithms that use the sensitive but nonspecific glutamine dehydrogenase EIA combined with confirmatory toxin testing of positive results also can be used. Molecular assays using nucleic acid amplification tests (NAATs) have been developed, are FDA approved, and now are preferred. NAATs combine good sensitivity and specificity, provide results to clinicians in times comparable to EIAs, and are not required to be part of a 2- or 3-step algorithm. Many children's hospitals are converting to NAAT technology to diagnose *C difficile* infection, but more data are needed before this technology can be used routinely. The predictive value of a positive test result in a child younger than 5 years of age is unknown, because asymptomatic carriage of toxigenic strains often occurs in these children. *C difficile* toxin degrades at room temperate and can be undetectable within 2 hours after collection of a stool specimen. Stool specimens that are not tested promptly or maintained at 4°C can yield false-negative results. Because colonization with *C difficile* in infants is common, testing for other causes of diarrhea always is recommended in these patients. None of the assays are licensed or recommended for test of cure.

TREATMENT:
- Precipitating antimicrobial therapy should be discontinued as soon as possible.
- Antimicrobial therapy for *C difficile* infection is indicated for symptomatic patients.
- Strains of *C difficile* are susceptible to metronidazole and vancomycin. Metronidazole (30 mg/kg per day in 4 divided doses, maximum 2 g/day) is the drug of choice for the initial treatment of children and adolescents with mild to moderate diarrhea and for first relapse.

- Oral vancomycin (40 mg/kg per day, orally, in 4 divided doses, to a maximum daily dose not to exceed 2 grams) or vancomycin administered by enema plus intravenous metronidazole is indicated as initial therapy for patients with severe disease (hospitalized in an intensive care unit, pseudomembranous colitis by endoscopy, or underlying intestinal tract disease) and for patients who do not respond to oral metronidazole. Vancomycin for intravenous use can be prepared for oral use. Intravenously administered vancomycin is not effective for *C difficile* infection.
- Therapy with either metronidazole or vancomycin or the combination should be administered for at least 10 days.
- Up to 25% of patients experience a relapse after discontinuing therapy, but infection usually responds to a second course of the same treatment. Metronidazole should not be used for treatment of a second recurrence or for chronic therapy, because neurotoxicity is possible. Tapered or pulse regimens of vancomycin are recommended under this circumstance.
- Fidaxomicin has been approved for treatment of *C difficile*-associated diarrhea in adults.
- Drugs that decrease intestinal motility should not be administered.
- Follow-up testing for toxin is not recommended.
- Investigational therapies include other antimicrobial agents (nitazoxanide, rifaximin, tinidazole), Immune Globulin therapy, toxin binders, probiotics,[1] and restoring intestinal tract flora (intestinal microbiota transplantation).

ISOLATION OF THE HOSPITALIZED PATIENT: In addition to standard precautions, contact precautions and a private room (if feasible) are recommended for the duration of illness.

CONTROL MEASURES:
- Exercising meticulous hand hygiene, properly handling contaminated waste (including diapers), disinfecting fomites, and limiting use of antimicrobial agents are the best available methods for control of *C difficile* infection. Alcohol-based hand hygiene products do not inactivate *C difficile* spores. Washing hands with soap and water is more effective in removing *C difficile* spores from contaminated hands and should be performed after each contact with a *C difficile* infected patient. The most effective means of preventing hand contamination is the use of gloves when caring for infected patients or their environment, followed by hand hygiene after glove removal.
- Thorough cleaning of hospital rooms and bathrooms of patients with *C difficile* disease is essential. Because *C difficile* forms spores, which are difficult to kill, organisms can resist action of many common hospital disinfectants; many hospitals have instituted the use of disinfectants with sporicidal activity (eg, hypochlorite) when outbreaks of *C difficile* diarrhea are not controlled by other measures.
- Children with *C difficile* diarrhea should be excluded from child care settings for the duration of diarrhea, and infection-control measures should be enforced (see Children in Out-of-Home Child Care, p 133).

---

[1] Thomas DW; Greer FR; American Academy of Pediatrics, Committee on Nutrition. Probiotics and prebiotics in pediatrics. *Pediatrics.* 2010;126(6):1217–1231

Clostridium perfringens Food Poisoning

CLINICAL MANIFESTATIONS: *Clostridium perfringens* foodborne illness is characterized by a sudden onset of watery diarrhea and moderate to severe, crampy, midepigastric pain. Vomiting and fever are uncommon. Symptoms usually resolve within 24 hours. The short incubation period, short duration, and absence of fever in most patients differentiate *C perfringens* foodborne disease from shigellosis and salmonellosis, and the infrequency of vomiting and longer incubation period contrast with the clinical features of foodborne disease associated with heavy metals, *Staphylococcus aureus* enterotoxins, *Bacillus cereus* emetic toxin, and fish and shellfish toxins. Diarrheal illness caused by *B cereus* diarrheal enterotoxins can be indistinguishable from that caused by *C perfringens* (see Appendix X, Clinical Syndromes Associated With Foodborne Diseases, p 921). Enteritis necroticans (known locally as pigbel) results from necrosis of the midgut and is a cause of severe illness and death attributable to *C perfringens* food poisoning among children in Papua, New Guinea. Rare cases have been reported elsewhere associated with diabetes mellitus.

ETIOLOGY: Food poisoning is caused by a heat-labile enterotoxin produced in vivo by *C perfringens* type A; enteritis necroticans is caused by type C.

EPIDEMIOLOGY: *C perfringens* is a gram-positive, spore-forming bacillus that is ubiquitous in the environment and commonly is present in raw meat and poultry. At an optimum temperature, *C perfringens* has one of the fastest rates of growth of any bacterium. Spores of *C perfringens* can survive cooking. Spores germinate and multiply during slow cooling and storage at temperatures from 20°C to 60°C (68°C–140°F). Illness results from consumption of food containing high numbers of organisms ($>10^5$ colony forming units/g) followed by enterotoxin production in the intestine. Beef, poultry, gravies, and dried or precooked foods are common sources. Infection usually is acquired at banquets or institutions (eg, schools and camps) or from food provided by caterers or restaurants where food is prepared in large quantities and kept warm for prolonged periods. Illness is not transmissible from person-to-person.

The **incubation period** is 6 to 24 hours, usually 8 to 12 hours.

DIAGNOSTIC TESTS: Because the fecal flora of healthy people commonly includes *C perfringens*, counts of *C perfringens* spores of 10^6/g of feces or greater obtained within 48 hours of onset of illness are required to support the diagnosis in ill people. The diagnosis also can be supported by detection of *C perfringens* enterotoxin in stool by commercially available kits. *C perfringens* can be confirmed as the cause of an outbreak when the concentration of organisms is at least 10^5/g in the epidemiologically implicated food. Although *C perfringens* is an anaerobe, special transport conditions are unnecessary, because the spores are durable. Stool specimens, rather than rectal swab specimens, should be obtained.

TREATMENT: Oral rehydration or, occasionally, intravenous fluid and electrolyte replacement can be indicated to prevent or treat dehydration. Antimicrobial agents are not indicated.

ISOLATION OF THE HOSPITALIZED PATIENT: Standard precautions are recommended.

CONTROL MEASURES: Preventive measures depend on limiting proliferation of *C perfringens* in foods by cooking foods thoroughly and maintaining food at warmer than 60°C (140°F) or cooler than 7°C (45°F). Meat dishes should be served hot shortly after cooking. Foods never should be held at room temperature to cool; they should be refrigerated after removal from warming devices or serving tables. Foods should be reheated to at least 74°C (165.2°F) before serving. Roasts, stews, and similar dishes should be divided into small quantities for refrigeration.

Coccidioidomycosis

CLINICAL MANIFESTATIONS: Primary pulmonary infection is acquired by inhaling fungal spores and is asymptomatic or self-limited in 60% of children. Symptomatic disease can resemble influenza or community-acquired pneumonia, with malaise, fever, cough, myalgia, headache, and chest pain. Constitutional symptoms, including extreme fatigue and weight loss, are common and can persist for weeks or months. Acute infection can be associated only with cutaneous abnormalities, such as erythema multiforme, an erythematous maculopapular rash, and erythema nodosum. Chronic pulmonary lesions are rare, but up to 5% of infected people develop asymptomatic pulmonary radiographic residua (eg, cysts, nodules, or coin lesions). Nonpulmonary primary infection is rare and usually follows trauma associated with contamination of wounds by arthroconidia. Cutaneous lesions and soft tissue infections often are accompanied by regional lymphadenitis.

Disseminated infection occurs in less than 0.5% of infected people; common sites of dissemination include skin, bones and joints, central nervous system (CNS), and lungs. Dissemination is more common in infants than older children and adults. Meningitis almost invariably is fatal if untreated. Congenital infection is rare.

ETIOLOGY: *Coccidioides* species are dimorphic fungi. In soil, *Coccidioides* organisms exist in the mycelial phase as a mold growing in branching, septate hyphae. Infectious arthroconidia (ie, spores) produced from hyphae become airborne, infecting the host after inhalation or rarely, inoculation. In tissues, arthroconidia enlarge to form spherules; mature spherules release hundreds to thousands of endospores that develop into new spherules and continue the tissue cycle. Using molecular markers, the genus *Coccidioides* now is divided into 2 species: *Coccidioides immitis,* confined mainly to California, and *Coccidioides posadasii,* encompassing the remaining areas of distribution of the fungus within the southwestern United States, northern Mexico, and areas of Central and South America.

EPIDEMIOLOGY: *Coccidioides* species are found in soil in areas of the southwestern United States with endemic infection, including California, Arizona, New Mexico, west and south Texas, southern Nevada, and Utah; northern Mexico; and throughout certain parts of Central and South America. In areas with endemic coccidioidomycosis, clusters of cases can follow dust-generating events, such as storms, seismic events, archaeologic digging, or recreational activities. The majority of cases occur without a known preceding event. Infection is thought to provide lifelong immunity. Person-to-person transmission of coccidioidomycosis does not occur except in rare instances of cutaneous infection with actively draining lesions and congenital infection following in utero exposure. Preexisting impairment of T-lymphocyte mediated immunity is a major risk factor for severe primary coccidioidomycosis, disseminated disease, or relapse of past infection. Other people at risk of severe or disseminated disease include people of African or Filipino ancestry, women in the third trimester of pregnancy, people with diabetes, people with preexisting cardiopulmonary disease, and children younger than 1 year of age. Cases can occur in people who do not reside in regions with endemic infection but who previously have visited these areas. Donor organ-derived coccidioidomycosis has occurred, in which organs come from people who have been in an area with endemic infection or who have had active disease at time of organ donation. In regions without endemic infection, careful travel histories should be obtained from people with symptoms or findings compatible with coccidioidomycosis. *Coccidioides* species are listed by the Centers for Disease Control and Prevention as agents of bioterrorism.

The **incubation period** typically is 10 to 16 days and ranges from 7 to 28 days.

DIAGNOSTIC TESTS: Diagnosis of coccidioidomycosis is best established using serologic, histopathologic, and culture methods. Serologic tests are useful to confirm the diagnosis and provide prognostic information. The immunoglobulin (Ig) M response can be detected by enzyme immunoassay (EIA) or immunodiffusion methods. In approximately 50% and 90% of primary infections, IgM is detected in the first and third weeks, respectively. IgG response can be detected by immunodiffusion, EIA, or complement fixation (CF) tests. Immunodiffusion and CF tests are highly specific. CF antibodies in serum usually are of low titer and are transient if the disease is asymptomatic or mild. Persistent high titers ($\geq$1:16) occur with severe disease and almost always in disseminated infection. Cerebrospinal fluid (CSF) antibodies also are detectable by CF testing. Increasing serum and CSF titers indicate progressive disease, and decreasing titers usually suggest improvement. Complement fixation titers may not be reliable in immunocompromised patients; low or nondetectable titers in immunocompromised patients should be interpreted with caution. Because clinical laboratories use different diagnostic test kits, positive results should be confirmed in an experienced reference laboratory.

Spherules are as large as 80 μm in diameter and can be visualized with 100 to 400 × magnification in infected body fluid specimens (eg, pleural fluid, bronchoalveolar lavage) and biopsy specimens of skin lesions or organs. The presence of a mature spherule with endospores is pathognomonic of infection. Culture of organisms is possible but potentially hazardous to laboratory personnel, because spherules can convert to arthroconidia-bearing mycelia on culture plates. Clinicians should inform the laboratory if there is suspicion of coccidioidomycosis. Suspect cultures should be sealed and handled using appropriate safety equipment and procedures. A DNA probe can identify *Coccidioides* species in cultures, thereby decreasing risk of exposure to infectious fungi.

TREATMENT: Antifungal therapy for uncomplicated primary infection in people without risk factors for severe disease is controversial. Although most cases will resolve without therapy, some experts believe that treatment may reduce illness duration or risk for severe complications. Most experts would treat people at risk of severe disease or people with severe primary infection. Severe primary infection is manifested by complement fixation titers of 1:16 or greater, infiltrates involving more than half of one lung or portions of both lungs, weight loss of greater than 10%, marked chest pain, severe malaise, inability to work or attend school, intense night sweats, or symptoms that persist for more than 2 months. Fluconazole or itraconazole (200–400 mg daily) is recommended for 3 to 6 months. If itraconazole is administered, measurement of serum concentration is recommended to ensure that absorption is satisfactory. Repeated patient encounters every 1 to 3 months for up to 2 years, either to document radiographic resolution or to identify pulmonary or extrapulmonary complications, are recommended.

Oral itraconazole or fluconazole are the recommended initial therapy for disseminated infection not involving the CNS. Amphotericin B is recommended as alternative therapy if lesions are progressing or are in critical locations, such as the vertebral column. In patients experiencing failure of conventional amphotericin B deoxycholate therapy or experiencing drug-related toxicities, lipid formulation of amphotericin B can be substituted.

Oral fluconazole (400 mg/day, up to 800 or 1000 mg/day) is recommended for treatment of patients with CNS infections. Patients who respond to azole therapy should continue this treatment indefinitely. For CNS infections that are unresponsive to oral azoles or associated with severe basilar inflammation, intrathecal amphotericin B deoxycholate therapy (0.1–1.5 mg per dose) can be used to augment azole therapy. A subcutaneous reservoir can facilitate administration into the cisternal space or lateral ventricle. Consultation with a specialist for treatment of patients with CNS disease caused by *Coccidioides* species is recommended.

The role of newer azole antifungal agents, such as voriconazole, posaconazole, and echinocandins, in treatment of coccidiomycosis has not been established. These newer agents may be administered in certain clinical settings, such as therapeutic failure in severe coccidioidal disease (eg, meningitis). The newer azoles should be used in consultation with experts experienced with their use in treatment of coccidioidomycosis.

The duration of antifungal therapy is variable and depends on the site(s) of involvement, clinical response, and mycologic and immunologic test results. In general, therapy is continued until clinical and laboratory evidence indicates that active infection has resolved. Treatment for disseminated coccidioidomycosis is at least 6 months but for some patients maybe extended to 1 year. The required duration of treatment with azoles is uncertain, except for patients with CNS infection, osteomyelitis, underlying HIV infection, or solid organ transplant recipients, for whom suppressive therapy is lifelong. Women should be advised to avoid pregnancy while receiving fluconazole, which may be teratogenic.

Surgical débridement or excision of lesions in bone, pericardium, and lung has been advocated for localized, symptomatic, persistent, resistant, or progressive lesions. In some localized infections with sinuses, fistulae, or abscesses, amphotericin B has been instilled locally or used for irrigation of wounds.

ISOLATION OF THE HOSPITALIZED PATIENT: Standard precautions are recommended. Care should be taken in handling, changing, and discarding dressings, casts, and similar materials in which arthroconidial contamination could occur.

CONTROL MEASURES: Measures to control dust are recommended in areas with endemic infection, including construction sites, archaeologic project sites, or other locations where activities cause excessive soil disturbance. Immunocompromised people residing in or traveling to areas with endemic infection should be counseled to avoid exposure to activities that may aerosolize spores in contaminated soil.

Coronaviruses, Including SARS

CLINICAL MANIFESTATIONS: Human coronaviruses (HCoVs) 229E, OC43, NL63, and HKU1, are associated most frequently with the common cold, an upper respiratory tract infection characterized by rhinorrhea, nasal congestion, sore throat, sneezing, and cough that may be associated with fever. Symptoms are self-limiting and typically peak on day 3 or 4 of illness. HCoV infections also may be associated with acute otitis media or asthma exacerbations. Less frequently, HCoVs have been associated with lower respiratory tract infections, including bronchiolitis, croup (especially HCoV-NL63), and pneumonia, primarily in infants and immunocompromised children and adults.

SARS-CoV, the HCoV responsible for the 2002–2003 global outbreaks of severe acute respiratory syndrome (SARS), is associated with more severe symptoms. It disproportionately affects adults, who typically present with fever, myalgia, headache, malaise, and chills followed by a nonproductive cough and dyspnea generally 5 to 7 days later. Approximately 25% of infected adults develop watery diarrhea. Twenty percent develop worsening respiratory distress requiring intubation and ventilation. The overall associated mortality rate is approximately 10%, with most deaths occurring in the third week of illness. The case fatality rate in people older than 60 years of age approaches 50%. Typical laboratory abnormalities include lymphopenia and increased lactate dehydrogenase and creatinine kinase concentrations. Most have progressive unilateral or bilateral ill-defined airspace infiltrates on chest imaging. Pneumothoraces and other signs of barotrauma are common in critically ill patients receiving mechanical ventilation.

SARS-CoV infections in children are less severe than adults; notably, no infants or children died from SARS-CoV infection in the 2002–2003 outbreaks. Infants and children younger than 12 years of age who develop SARS typically present with fever, cough, and rhinorrhea. Associated lymphopenia is less severe, and radiographic changes are milder and generally resolve more quickly than in adolescents and adults. Adolescents who develop SARS have clinical courses more closely resembling those of adult disease, presenting with fever, myalgia, headache, and chills. They also are more likely to develop dyspnea, hypoxemia, and worsening chest radiographic findings. Laboratory abnormalities are comparable to those in adult disease.

ETIOLOGY: Coronaviruses are enveloped, nonsegmented, single-stranded, positive-sense RNA viruses named after their corona- or crown-like surface projections observed on electron microscopy that correspond to large surface spike proteins. Coronaviruses are classified in the Nidovirus family. Coronaviruses are host specific and can infect humans as well as a variety of different animals causing diverse clinical syndromes. Three serologically and genetically distinct groups of coronaviruses have been described. HCoVs 229E and NL63 belong to group I, and HCoVs OC43, -HKU1, and SARS-CoV belong to group II. Serogroups I and II have been isolated from mammals and serogroup III has been isolated from birds.

EPIDEMIOLOGY: Coronaviruses first were recognized as animal pathogens in the 1930s. Thirty years later, 229E and OC43 were identified as human pathogens, along with other coronavirus strains that were not investigated further and for which little is known regarding their prevalence and associated disease syndromes. In 2003, SARS-CoV was identified as a novel virus responsible for the 2002–2003 global outbreaks of SARS, which lasted for 9 months, infected 8096 people, and resulted in 774 deaths. Most experts believe SARS-CoV evolved from a natural reservoir of SARS-CoV-like viruses in bats through civet cats as intermediate hosts. Whether or not a large-scale reemergence of SARS will occur is debatable. Finding a novel HCoV sparked a renewed interest in HCoV research, and 2 years later, NL63 and HKU1 were identified as newly recognized HCoVs. One of the investigations has revealed that NL63 was present in archived human respiratory samples as early as 1981.

HCoVs other than SARS-CoV can be found worldwide. They cause most disease in the winter and spring months in temperate climates. Seroprevalence data suggest that exposure is common in early childhood, with approximately 90% of adults being seropositive for 229E, OC43, and NL63 and 60% being seropositive for HKU1. In contrast, SARS-CoV infection has not been detected in humans since early 2004, when 4 isolated cases of SARS with no associated transmission were identified in China and 2 isolated cases and a cluster of 11 cases (1 death) were identified in South East Asia related to breaches in biosafety practices in different laboratories culturing SARS-CoV.

The modes of transmission for HCoV other than SARS-CoV have not been well studied. However, on the basis of studies of other respiratory tract viruses, it is likely that transmission occurs primarily via a combination of droplet and direct and indirect contact spread. Which of these modes are most important remains to be determined, and the possible role of aerosol spread requires further study. For SARS-CoV, studies suggest that droplet and direct contact spread are likely the most common modes of transmission, although evidence of indirect contact spread and aerosol spread also exist. There is no evidence of vertical transmission of SARS-CoV.

HCoVs other than SARS-CoV are most likely to be transmitted during the first few days of illness, when symptoms and respiratory viral loads are at their highest. Further study is needed to confirm that this holds true for the NL63 and HKU1 viruses. SARS-CoV is most likely to be transmitted during the second week of illness, when both symptoms and respiratory viral loads peak.

The **incubation period** for HCoV infections, other than SARS-CoV, is estimated to be 2 to 5 days (median 3 days), primarily on the basis of studies with 229E. The **incubation period** for SARS-CoV is 2 to 10 days (median, 4 days).

DIAGNOSTIC TESTS: The 2002–2003 SARS outbreaks garnered renewed interest in better understanding the etiology of respiratory tract infections, and some clinical laboratories have since started offering comprehensive respiratory molecular diagnostic testing for non-SARS HCoVs using reverse transcriptase polymerase chain reaction assays. Diagnostic laboratory and clinical guidance for SARS is available on the Centers for Disease Control and Prevention Web site (**www.cdc.gov/sars/index.html**). Given the potential for false-positive test results and the associated public health implications, testing for SARS-CoV in the absence of known person-to-person transmission of SARS must be performed with caution and only in consultation with regional public health departments when there is a high degree of suspicion in a patient with no alternative diagnosis.

Specimens obtained from the upper and lower respiratory tract are the most appropriate samples for viral detection. Stool and serum samples also frequently are positive in patients with SARS-CoV. For 299E and OC43, specimens are most likely to be positive during the first few days of illness; whether this is also true for NL63 and HKU1 needs further study. For SARS-CoV, respiratory and stool specimens may not be positive until the second week of illness when symptoms and viral loads peak; serum samples are most likely positive in the first week of illness. Compared with adults, infants and children with SARS-CoV infections are less likely to have positive specimens consistent with the milder symptoms and presumed corresponding lower viral loads seen in this age group.

TREATMENT: Infections attributable to HCoVs generally are treated with supportive care. SARS-CoV infections are more serious. Steroids, type 1 interferons, convalescent plasma, ribavirin, and lopinavir/ritonavir all were used clinically to treat patients

with SARS, albeit without benefit of controlled data documenting efficacy. No definitive conclusions regarding efficacy of any treatment can be made. There are reports
of patients who were treated with supportive care only who recovered uneventfully. In
the event that SARS-CoV reemerges, clarification of the effectiveness of treatments
through controlled clinical trials is needed.

ISOLATION OF THE HOSPITALIZED PATIENT: Health care professionals should use
Droplet and Contact Precautions in addition to Standard Precautions when examining and caring for infants and young children with signs and symptoms of a respiratory
tract infection for the duration of their illness (**www.cdc.gov/hicpac/2007IP/
2007isolationPrecautions.html**). Droplet Precautions may be discontinued
when infectious agents that have been documented to be spread via the droplet route,
such as influenza virus, adenovirus, rhinovirus, and SARS-CoV, have been ruled out.
Airborne, Droplet, and Contact Precautions are recommended for patients with suspected
SARS-CoV infection for the duration of illness plus 10 days after resolution of fever,
provided respiratory symptoms are absent or improving.

CONTROL MEASURES: Practicing appropriate hand and respiratory hygiene likely is the
most useful and easily implemented control measure to curb spread of all respiratory tract
viruses, including HCoVs. For hospitalized patients, following additional infection control
practices as described previously is recommended. The control of the 2002–2003 SARS
outbreaks is credited to the rapid identification of cases and early implementation of
infection control and public health measures, such as contact tracing and quarantine.

Cryptococcus neoformans Infections
(Cryptococcosis)

CLINICAL MANIFESTATIONS: Primary infection is acquired by inhalation of aerosolized
fungal elements from contaminated soil and often is asymptomatic or mild. Pulmonary
disease, when symptomatic, is characterized by cough, chest pain, and constitutional
symptoms. Chest radiographs may reveal a solitary nodule or mass or focal or diffuse
infiltrates. Hematogenous dissemination to the central nervous system (CNS), bones,
skin, and other sites can occur, but dissemination is rare in children without defects in
T-lymphocyte mediated immunity (eg, children with leukemia, systemic lupus erythema-
tosis, chronic mucocutaneous candidiasis, other congenital immunodeficiency, or acquired
immunodeficiency syndrome [AIDS] or children who have undergone solid organ transplantation). Usually, several sites are infected, but manifestations of involvement at 1 site
predominate. Cryptococcal meningitis, the most common and serious form of cryptococcal disease, often follows an indolent course. Symptoms are characteristic of meningitis,
meningoencephalitis, or space-occupying lesions but can sometimes manifest only as
behavioral changes. Cryptococcal fungemia without apparent organ involvement occurs
in patients with human immunodeficiency virus (HIV) infection but is rare in children.

ETIOLOGY: *Cryptococcus neoformans* (var *neoformans* and var *grubii*) and *Cryptococcus
gattii* are, with rare exception, the only 2 species of the genus *Cryptococcus* that are
human pathogens.

EPIDEMIOLOGY: *C neoformans* var *neoformans* and *C neoformans* var *grubii* are isolated primarily from soil contaminated with pigeon or other bird guano and cause most human
infections, especially infections in immunocompromised hosts. *C neoformans* infects 5% to

10% of adults with AIDS, but infection is rare in HIV-infected children. *C gattii* (formerly *C neoformans* var *gattii*) is associated with trees and soil around trees and has emerged as an outbreak-associated pathogen in British Columbia, Canada, and the Pacific Northwest region of the United States. *C gattii* causes disease in immunocompetent and immuno-compromised people, but infection is rare in children. Person-to-person transmission does not occur.

The **incubation period** for *C neoformans* is unknown; for *C gattii*, it is 8 weeks to 13 months.

DIAGNOSTIC TESTS: Definitive diagnosis requires isolation of the organism from body fluid or tissue specimens. Blood should be cultured by lysis-centrifugation. Media containing cycloheximide, which inhibits growth of *C neoformans*, should not be used. Sabouraud dextrose agar is useful for isolation of *Cryptococcus* from sputum, bronchopulmonary lavage, tissue, or cerebrospinal fluid (CSF) specimens. Use of Niger seed (birdseed) can increase the rate of detection in sputum and urine specimens. *C gattii* will turn CGB agar blue, but *C neoformans* leaves CGB agar green. In refractory or relapse cases, susceptibility testing can be helpful, although antifungal resistance is uncommon. Few organisms may be present in CSF specimens, and a large quantity of CSF may be needed to recover the organism. In children with CNS disease, CSF cell count and protein and glucose concentrations can be normal. The latex agglutination test and enzyme immunoassay for detection of cryptococcal capsular polysaccharide antigen in serum or CSF specimens are excellent rapid diagnostic tests. Antigen is detected in CSF or serum specimens from more than 90% of patients with cryptococcal meningitis. In patients with cryptococcal meningitis, antigen test results can be negative when antigen concentrations are low or very high (prozone effect), if infection is caused by unencapsulated strains, or if the patient is less severely immunocompromised. Polymerase chain reaction assays are investigational. Encapsulated yeast cells can be visualized using India ink or other stains of CSF and bronchoalveolar lavage specimens. Focal pulmonary or skin lesions can be biopsied for fungal staining and culture.

TREATMENT: The Infectious Diseases Society of America has published practice management guidelines for cryptococcal disease.[1] Amphotericin B deoxycholate, 1 mg/kg/day (see Drugs for Invasive and Other Serious Fungal Infections, p 835), in combination with oral flucytosine, 25 mg/kg/dose, 4 times a day, is indicated as initial therapy for patients with meningeal and other serious cryptococcal infections. Serum flucytosine concentrations should be maintained between 40 and 60 µg/mL. Patients with meningitis should receive combination therapy for at least 2 weeks followed by consolidation therapy with fluconazole (12 mg/kg on day 1 and then 6–12 mg/kg [maximum dose, 800 mg] daily) for a minimum of 8 to 10 weeks or until CSF culture is sterile. Alternatively, the amphotericin B deoxycholate and flucytosine combination can be continued for 6 to 10 weeks. Lipid formulations of amphotericin B can be substituted for conventional amphotericin B in children with renal impairment. If flucytosine cannot be administered, amphotericin B alone is an acceptable alternative and is administered for 4 to 6 weeks. A lumbar puncture should be performed after 2 weeks of therapy to document microbiologic clearance. The 20% to 40% of patients in whom culture is positive after 2 weeks of therapy will require a more prolonged treatment course. When infection is refractory to systemic therapy,

---

[1] Perfect J, Dismukes WE, Dromer F, et al. Clinical practice guidelines for the management of cryptococcal disease: 2010 update by the Infectious Diseases Society of America. *Clin Infect Dis*. 2010;50(3):291–322

intraventricular amphotericin B can be administered. Monitoring of serum cryptococcal antigen is not useful to monitor response to therapy in patients with cryptococcal meningitis. Patients with less severe disease can be treated with fluconazole or itraconazole, but data on use of these drugs for children with *C neoformans* infection are limited. Another potential treatment option for HIV-infected patients with less severe disease is combination therapy with fluconazole and flucytosine. The combination of fluconazole and flucytosine has superior efficacy to fluconazole alone. The toxicity associated with this regimen often limits its usefulness. Increased intracranial pressure occurs frequently despite microbiologic response and often is associated with clinical deterioration. Significant elevation of intracranial pressure should be managed with frequent repeated lumbar punctures or placement of a lumbar drain.

Children with HIV infection who have completed initial therapy for cryptococcosis should receive lifelong suppressive therapy with fluconazole 6 mg/kg daily. Oral itraconazole daily or amphotericin B deoxycholate 1 to 3 times weekly are alternatives. Data regarding discontinuing this secondary prophylaxis after immune reconstitution as a consequence of antiretroviral therapy (ART) are available for adults but not for children. Discontinuing chronic suppressive therapy for cryptococcosis (after 6 months or longer of secondary prophylaxis) can be considered in asymptomatic children 6 years of age or older who are receiving ART and who have sustained ($\geq$6 months) increases in CD4+ T-lymphocyte counts to $\geq$200 cells/mm^3. Secondary prophylaxis should be reinstituted if the CD4+ T-lymphocyte count decreases to <200/mm^3.

ISOLATION OF THE HOSPITALIZED PATIENT: Standard precautions are recommended.

CONTROL MEASURES: None.

Cryptosporidiosis

CLINICAL MANIFESTATIONS: Frequent, nonbloody, watery diarrhea is the most common manifestation of cryptosporidiosis, although infection can be asymptomatic. Other symptoms include abdominal cramps, fatigue, fever, vomiting, anorexia, and weight loss. In infected immunocompetent adults and children, diarrheal illness is self-limited, usually lasting 6 to 14 days. Infected immunocompromised people, such as people with acquired immunodeficiency syndrome (AIDS), might experience chronic, severe diarrhea, which can lead to malnutrition and weight loss and, as such, could be a significant contributing factor leading to death. Pulmonary, biliary tract or disseminated infection occurs rarely in immunocompromised people.

ETIOLOGY: *Cryptosporidium* species are oocyst-forming coccidian protozoa. Oocysts are excreted in feces of an infected host and are transmitted via the fecal-oral route. *Cryptosporidium hominis*, which predominantly infects humans, and *Cryptosporidium parvum*, which infects humans, cattle, and other mammals, are the primary *Cryptosporidium* species that infect humans.

EPIDEMIOLOGY: Extensive waterborne disease outbreaks have been associated with contamination of drinking water and recreational water (eg, swimming pools, lakes, and interactive fountains). The incidence of cryptosporidiosis has been increasing since 2005 in the United States. In children, the incidence of cryptosporidiosis is greatest during summer and early fall, corresponding to the outdoor swimming season.[1] Because oocysts are chlorine tolerant, multistep treatment processes often are used to remove (eg, filter) and inactivate (eg, ultraviolet treatment) oocysts from contaminated water to protect public drinking water supplies. Typical filtration systems used for swimming pools are only partially effective in removing oocysts from contaminated water. As a result, *Cryptosporidium* species have become the leading cause of recreational water-associated outbreaks.[2]

In addition to waterborne transmission, humans can acquire infections from livestock and animals found in petting zoos, particularly preweaned calves, or pets. Person-to-person transmission occurs as well and can cause outbreaks in child care centers, in which 20% to 35% but as many as 70% of attendees reportedly have been infected. *Cryptosporidium* species also can cause traveler's diarrhea.

The **incubation period** usually is 3 to 14 days. In immunocompetent people, oocyst shedding usually ceases within 2 weeks of symptom resolution. In immunocompromised people, the period of oocyst shedding can continue for months.

DIAGNOSTIC TESTS: The detection of oocysts on microscopic examination of stool specimens is diagnostic. Routine laboratory examination of stool for ova and parasites might not include testing for *Cryptosporidium* species, so testing for the organism specifically should be requested. The direct immunofluorescent antibody (DFA) method for detection of oocysts in stool is the current test of choice for diagnosis of cryptosporidiosis. The formalin ethyl acetate stool concentration method is recommended before staining the stool specimen with a modified Kinyoun acid-fast stain. Oocysts generally are small (4–6 µm in diameter) and can be missed in a rapid scan of a slide.

Enzyme immunoassays (EIAs) and immune chromatography (point-of-care rapid tests) for detecting antigen in stool are available commercially. With EIAs and rapid tests, false-positive and false-negative results can occur, and confirmation by microscopy should be considered.

Because shedding can be intermittent, at least 3 stool specimens collected on separate days should be examined before considering test results to be negative. Organisms also can be identified in intestinal biopsy tissue or sampling of intestinal fluid.

TREATMENT: Generally, immunocompetent people need no specific therapy. A 3-day course of nitazoxanide oral suspension has been approved by the US Food and Drug Administration (FDA) for treatment of all people 1 year of age and older with diarrhea associated with cryptosporidiosis. The nitazoxanide dose for healthy and HIV-infected children is age based and can be found in Drugs for Parasitic Infections (p 848).

In HIV-infected patients, improvement in CD4+ T-lymphocyte count associated with antiretroviral therapy can lead to symptom resolution and cessation of oocyst shedding. For HIV-infected children 12 years of age and older, oral nitazoxanide, 500 mg, twice daily, can be considered. The duration of treatment in HIV-infected children can be up to 14 days. Nitazoxanide, paromomycin, or a combination of paromomycin and azithro-

---

[1] Yoder JS, Harral C, Beach MJ. Cryptosporidiosis surveillance—United States, 2006–2008. *MMWR Surveill Summ.* 2010;59(SS-6):1–14

[2] Centers for Disease Control and Prevention. Surveillance for waterborne disease outbreaks and other health events associated with recreational water—United States, 2007–2008 *MMWR Surveill Summ.* 2011;60(SS–12):1–32

mycin may be effective, but few data regarding efficacy are available. Mixed results have been reported for bovine immunotherapy in immunocompromised people.

ISOLATION OF THE HOSPITALIZED PATIENT: In addition to standard precautions, contact precautions are recommended for diapered or incontinent people for the duration of illness or to control institutional outbreaks.

CONTROL MEASURES: The following measures can help prevent and control cryptosporidiosis:

- Wash hands with soap and water for at least 20 seconds, rubbing hands together vigorously and scrubbing all surfaces:
  - before preparing or eating food,
  - after using the toilet or assisting someone with using the toilet,
  - after changing a diaper or having a diaper changed,
  - after caring for someone who is ill with diarrhea, and
  - after handling an animal or its waste.
- Do not participate in recreational water activities such as swimming while ill with diarrhea and for 2 weeks after symptoms have resolved.
- Avoid ingestion of recreational water. For additional information, see Prevention of Illnesses Associated with Recreational Water Use (p 212).
- Exclude children ill with diarrhea from child care settings until diarrhea has resolved.
- Do not drink inadequately treated water or ice. This includes water or ice from lakes, rivers, springs, ponds, streams, or shallow wells or when traveling in countries where the drinking water supply might be unsafe.
  - If the safety of drinking water is questionable:
    - Drink bottled water.
    - Disinfect water by heating it to a rolling boil for 1 minute. The time of boiling (1 minute at sea level) will depend on altitude.
    - Use a filter that has been tested and rated by NSF Standard 53 or NSF Standard 58 for cyst and oocyst reduction or has an absolute pore size of 1 µm or smaller; filtered water will need additional treatment to kill or inactivate bacteria and viruses.

For additional information on cryptosporidiosis, visit **www.cdc.gov/crypto.**

Cutaneous Larva Migrans

CLINICAL MANIFESTATIONS: Nematode larvae produce pruritic, reddish papules at the site of skin entry, a condition referred to as creeping eruption. As the larvae migrate through skin advancing several millimeters to a few centimeters a day, intensely pruritic, serpiginous tracks or bullae are formed. Larval activity can continue for several weeks or months but eventually is self-limiting. An advancing serpiginous tunnel in the skin with an associated intense pruritus virtually is pathognomonic. Rarely, in infections with a large burden of parasites, pneumonitis (Löeffler syndrome), which can be severe, and myositis may follow skin lesions. Occasionally, the larvae reach the intestine and may cause eosinophilic enteritis.

ETIOLOGY: Infective larvae of cat and dog hookworms (ie, *Ancylostoma braziliense* and *Ancylostoma caninum*) are the usual causes. Other skin-penetrating nematodes are occasional causes.

EPIDEMIOLOGY: Cutaneous larva migrans is a disease of children, utility workers, gardeners, sunbathers, and others who come in contact with soil contaminated with cat and dog feces. In the United States, the disease is most prevalent in the Southeast. Most cases in the United States are imported by travelers returning from tropical and subtropical areas.

DIAGNOSTIC TESTS: Because the diagnosis usually is made clinically, biopsies are not indicated. Biopsy specimens typically demonstrate an eosinophilic inflammatory infiltrate, but the migrating parasite is not visualized. Eosinophilia and increased immunoglobulin (Ig) E serum concentrations occur in some cases. Larvae have been detected in sputum and gastric washings in patients with the rare complication of pneumonitis. Enzyme immunoassay or Western blot analysis using antigens of *A caninum* have been developed in research laboratories, but these assays are not available for routine diagnostic use.

TREATMENT: The disease usually is self-limited, with spontaneous cure after several weeks or months. Orally administered albendazole or mebendazole is the recommended therapy (see Drugs for Parasitic Infection, p 848).

ISOLATION OF THE HOSPITALIZED PATIENT: Standard precautions are recommended.

CONTROL MEASURES: Skin contact with moist soil contaminated with animal feces should be avoided. In warm climates, beaches should be kept free of dog and cat feces. There is no licensed vaccine available for the agents of cutaneous larva migrans.

Cyclosporiasis

CLINICAL MANIFESTATIONS: Watery diarrhea is the most common symptom of cyclosporiasis and can be profuse and protracted. Anorexia, nausea, vomiting, substantial weight loss, flatulence, abdominal cramping, myalgia, and prolonged fatigue also can occur. Low-grade fever occurs in approximately 50% of patients. Biliary tract disease also has been reported. Infection usually is self-limited, but untreated people may have remitting, relapsing symptoms for weeks to months. Asymptomatic infection has been documented most commonly in settings where cyclosporiasis is endemic.

ETIOLOGY: *Cyclospora cayetanensis* is a coccidian protozoan; oocysts (rather than cysts) are passed in stools and become infectious days to weeks following excretion.

EPIDEMIOLOGY[1]: *C cayetanensis* is known to be endemic in many resource-limited countries. In the United States, 10% of cases occur in people younger than 20 years of age, and a history of travel has been reported in approximately one third of people in the United States with cyclosporiasis. Both foodborne and waterborne outbreaks have been reported, with most cases in the United States occurring in May through July. Most of the outbreaks in United States and Canada have been associated with consumption of imported fresh produce, including Guatemalan raspberries and Thai basil. Humans are the only known hosts for *C cayetanensis.* Direct person-to-person transmission is unlikely, because excreted oocysts take days to weeks under favorable environmental conditions to sporulate and become infective. The oocysts are resistant to most disinfectants used in food and water processing and can remain viable for prolonged periods in cool, moist environments.

---

[1] Centers for Disease Control and Prevention. Surveillance for laboratory-confirmed sporadic cases of cyclosporiasis—United States, 1997–2008. *MMWR Surveill Summ.* 2011;60(SS-2):1–11

The **incubation period** is approximately 7 days and ranges from 2 to 14 days.

DIAGNOSTIC TESTS: Diagnosis is made by identification of oocysts (8–10 μm in diameter) in stool, intestinal fluid/aspirate, or intestinal biopsy specimens. Oocysts may be shed at low levels, even by people with profuse diarrhea. This constraint underscores the utility of repeated stool examinations, sensitive recovery methods (eg, concentration procedures), and detection methods that highlight the organism. Oocysts are autofluorescent and variably acid-fast after modified acid-fast staining of stool specimens (ie, oocysts that either have retained or not retained the stain can be visualized). Investigational molecular diagnostic assays (eg, polymerase chain reaction) are available at the Centers for Disease Control and Prevention and some other reference laboratories.

TREATMENT: Trimethoprim-sulfamethoxazole, typically for 7 to 10 days, is the drug of choice. People infected with human immunodeficiency virus may need long-term maintenance therapy (see Drugs for Parasitic Infections, p 848).

ISOLATION OF THE HOSPITALIZED PATIENT: In addition to standard precautions, contact precautions are recommended for diapered or incontinent children.

CONTROL MEASURES: Fresh produce always should be washed thoroughly before it is eaten. This precaution, however, may not eliminate the risk of transmission.

Cytomegalovirus Infection

CLINICAL MANIFESTATIONS: Manifestations of acquired human cytomegalovirus (CMV) infection vary with the age and immunocompetence of the host. Asymptomatic infections are the most common, particularly in children. An infectious mononucleosis-like syndrome with prolonged fever and mild hepatitis, occurring in the absence of heterophile antibody production, may occur in adolescents and adults. Pneumonia, colitis, and retinitis may occur in immunocompromised hosts, including people receiving treatment for malignant neoplasms, people infected with human immunodeficiency virus (HIV), and people receiving immunosuppressive therapy for organ or hematopoietic stem cell transplantation.

Congenital infection has a spectrum of manifestations but usually is not evident at birth (asymptomatic congenital CMV infection). Approximately 10% of infants with congenital CMV infection have involvement that is evident at birth (symptomatic congenital CMV disease), with manifestations including intrauterine growth restriction, jaundice, purpura, hepatosplenomegaly, microcephaly, intracerebral calcifications, and retinitis; developmental delays are common among these infants as they grow. Sensorineural hearing loss (SNHL) is the most common sequela following congenital CMV infection, with the likelihood of SNHL being higher among infants with symptomatic infection noted at birth. Congenital CMV infection is the leading nongenetic cause of sensorineural hearing loss in children in the United States. Approximately 21% of all hearing loss at birth is attributable to congenital CMV infection (10% symptomatic at birth and 11% asymptomatic at birth), and 25% of all hearing loss at 4 years of age is attributable to congenital CMV infection. Late-onset and progressive hearing losses occur following congenital CMV infection. Hearing loss following congenital CMV infection may be present at birth or occur later in the first years of life. Approximately 33% to 50% of SNHL attributable to congenital CMV infection is late-onset loss. Approximately 50% of children with SNHL following congenital CMV infection will continue to have further deterioration or progression of their loss. As such, children with congenital CMV infection should be evaluated regularly for early detection and appropriate intervention of suspected hearing losses.

Infection acquired intrapartum from maternal cervical secretions or postpartum from human milk usually is not associated with clinical illness in term babies. In preterm infants, infection resulting from human milk or from transfusion from CMV-seropositive donors has been associated with systemic infections, including lower respiratory tract disease and interstitial pneumonia.

ETIOLOGY: Human CMV, also known as human herpesvirus 5, is a member of the herpesvirus family (*Herpesviridae*), the beta-herpesvirus sub-family (*Betaherpesvirinae*), and the cytomegalovirus genus (*Cytomegalovirus*). The viral genome contains double-stranded DNA.

EPIDEMIOLOGY: CMV is highly species specific, and only the human strains are known to produce human disease. The virus is ubiquitous and has numerous strains. Transmission occurs horizontally (by direct person-to-person contact with virus-containing secretions), vertically (from mother to infant before, during, or after birth), and via transfusions of blood, platelets, and white blood cells from infected donors (see Blood Safety, p 114). CMV also can be transmitted with organ or hematopoietic stem cell transplantation. Infections have no seasonal predilection. CMV persists in latent form after a primary infection or subclinical reactivation, and frequent and symptomatic reactivation can occur years later, particularly under conditions of immunosuppression. Reinfection with other strains of CMV can occur in seropositive hosts.

Horizontal transmission probably is the result of salivary exposure, but contact with infected urine also can have a role. Spread of CMV in households and child care centers is well documented. Excretion rates from urine or saliva in children 1 to 3 years of age who attend child care centers usually range from 30% to 40% but can be as high as 70%. Young children can transmit CMV to their parents, including mothers who may be pregnant, and other caregivers, including child care staff (also see Children in Out-of-Home Child Care, p 133). In adolescents and adults, sexual transmission also occurs, as evidenced by detection of virus in seminal and cervical fluids.

Seropositive healthy people have latent CMV in their leukocytes and tissues; hence, blood transfusions and organ transplantation can result in viral transmission. Severe CMV disease following transfusion or organ transplantation is more likely to occur if the recipient is immunosuppressed and seronegative or is a preterm infant. In contrast, among nonautologous hematopoietic stem cell transplant recipients, it is seropositive recipients who receive transplants from seronegative donors (which do not provide preexisting immunity to CMV) who are at greatest risk of disease when exposed after transplant. Latent CMV commonly will reactivate in immunosuppressed people and can result in disease if immunosuppression is severe (eg, in patients with acquired immunodeficiency syndrome [AIDS] or solid organ or hematopoietic stem cell transplant recipients).

Vertical transmission of CMV to an infant occurs in one of the following time periods: (1) in utero by transplacental passage of maternal bloodborne virus; (2) at birth by passage through an infected maternal genital tract; or (3) postnatally by ingestion of CMV-positive human milk. Approximately 1% of all live-born infants are infected in utero and excrete CMV at birth, making this the most common congenital viral infection. Congenital infection and associated disabilities can occur no matter in what trimester the mother is infected, but severe sequelae are associated most commonly with primary maternal infection acquired during the first half of gestation. In utero fetal infection can occur in women with no preexisting CMV immunity (maternal primary infection) or in women with preexisting antibody to CMV (maternal nonprimary infection) by either acquisition of a different viral strain during pregnancy or reactivation of latent virus. Damaging fetal infections following nonprimary maternal infection have been reported, and the role of acquisition of a different viral strain in women with preexisting CMV antibody as a cause of symptomatic infection with sequelae is an area of current research.

Cervical excretion is common among seropositive women, resulting in exposure of many infants to CMV at birth. Cervical excretion rates are highest among young mothers in lower socioeconomic groups. Similarly, although disease can occur in seronegative infants fed CMV-infected human milk, most infants who acquire CMV from ingestion of infected human milk do not develop clinical illness, most likely because of the presence of passively transferred maternal antibody. Among infants who acquire infection from maternal cervical secretions or human milk, preterm infants are at greater risk of CMV illness and possibly sequelae than are full-term infants.

The **incubation period** for horizontally transmitted CMV infections is unknown. Infection usually manifests 3 to 12 weeks after blood transfusions and between 1 and 4 months after organ transplantation.

DIAGNOSTIC TESTS: The diagnosis of CMV disease is confounded by the ubiquity of the virus, the high rate of asymptomatic excretion, the frequency of reactivated infections, development of serum immunoglobulin (Ig) M CMV-specific antibody in some episodes of reactivation, reinfection with different strains of CMV, and concurrent infection with other pathogens.

Virus can be isolated in cell culture from urine, pharynx, peripheral blood leukocytes, human milk, semen, cervical secretions, and other tissues and body fluids. Recovery of virus from a target organ provides strong evidence that the disease is caused by CMV infection. A presumptive diagnosis of CMV infection beyond the neonatal period can be made on the basis of a fourfold antibody titer increase in paired serum specimens or by demonstration of virus excretion. Techniques for detection of viral DNA in tissues and some fluids, such as cerebrospinal fluid, by polymerase chain reaction assay or hybridization are available. Detection of pp65 antigen or quantification of viral DNA (eg, by quantitative polymerase chain reaction [PCR] assay) in white blood cells also may be used to detect infection in immunocompromised hosts.

Various immunofluorescent assays, indirect hemagglutination assays, latex agglutination assays, and enzyme immunoassays are available for detecting CMV-specific antibodies.

Amniocentesis has been used in several small series of patients to establish the diagnosis of intrauterine infection. Proof of congenital infection requires isolation of CMV from urine, stool, respiratory tract secretions, or CSF obtained within 2 to 4 weeks of birth. The sensitivity of CMV DNA detection by PCR assay of dried blood spots is low, limiting use of this type of specimen for widespread screening for congenital CMV. A positive PCR assay result from a neonatal dried blood spot confirms congenital infection, but a negative result does not rule out congenital infection. Differentiation between intrauterine and perinatal infection is difficult at later than 2 to 4 weeks of age unless clinical manifestations of the former, such as chorioretinitis or intracranial calcifications, are present. A strongly positive CMV-specific IgM during early infancy is suggestive of congenital CMV infection, but IgM antibody assays vary in accuracy for identification of primary infection.

TREATMENT: Intravenous ganciclovir (see Antiviral Drugs, p 841) is approved for induction and maintenance treatment of retinitis caused by acquired or recurrent CMV infection in immunocompromised adult patients, including HIV-infected patients, and for prevention of CMV disease in adult transplant recipients. Valganciclovir, the oral prodrug of ganciclovir, also is approved for treatment (induction and maintenance) of CMV retinitis in immunocompromised adult patients, including HIV-infected patients, and for prevention of CMV disease in kidney, kidney-pancreas, or heart transplant recipients at high risk of CMV disease. Valganciclovir also is approved for prevention of CMV disease in kidney or heart transplant pediatric patients 4 months of age and older. Ganciclovir and valganciclovir also are used to treat CMV infections of other sites (esophagus, colon, lungs) and for preemptive treatment of immunosuppressed adults with CMV antigenemia or viremia. Oral ganciclovir no longer is available in the United States, but oral valganciclovir is available both in tablet and in powder for oral solution formulations.

Data in neonates with symptomatic congenital CMV disease involving the central nervous system (CNS) suggest possible benefit of 6 weeks of parenteral ganciclovir therapy (6 mg/kg/dose, administered intravenously every 12 hours) for protecting against hearing deterioration and potentially in decreasing developmental impairment at 1 to 2 years of age. Valganciclovir administered orally to young infants at 16 mg/kg/dose, twice daily, provides the same systemic ganciclovir exposure as does intravenous ganciclovir at 6 mg/kg/dose. Antiviral therapy is not recommended routinely in neonates and young infants because of possible toxicities, including neutropenia in a significant proportion of recipients. If parenteral ganciclovir or oral valganciclovir are used in management of neonates congenitally infected with CMV, their use should be limited to patients with symptomatic congenital CMV disease involving the CNS who are able to start treatment within the first month of life. Experts differ in opinion as to whether patients with isolated hearing loss should be classified as symptomatic with CNS involvement; however, patients with such limited involvement are not the group in which therapeutic benefit has been documented. Oral valganciclovir is being evaluated in a clinical trial conducted by the National Institute of Allergy and Infectious Diseases Collaborative Antiviral Study Group comparing 6 weeks to 6 months of treatment in infants with symptomatic congenital CMV disease.

Preterm infants with perinatally acquired CMV infection can have symptomatic, end-organ disease (eg, pneumonitis, hepatitis, thrombocytopenia). Antiviral treatment has not been studied in this population. If such patients are treated with parenteral ganciclovir, a reasonable approach is to treat for 2 weeks and then reassess responsiveness to therapy. If clinical data suggest benefit of treatment, an additional 1 to 2 weeks of parenteral ganciclovir can be considered if symptoms and signs have not been resolved.

In hematopoietic stem cell transplant recipients, the combination of Immune Globulin Intravenous (IGIV) or CMV Immune Globulin Intravenous (CMV-IGIV) and ganciclovir administered intravenously has been reported to be synergistic in treatment of CMV pneumonia. Unlike CMV-IGIV, IGIV products have varying anti-CMV antibody concentrations from lot to lot, are not tested routinely, and do not have a specified titer of antibodies to CMV. Valganciclovir and foscarnet also have been approved for treatment and maintenance of CMV retinitis in adults with acquired immunodeficiency syndrome (see Antiviral Drugs, p 841). Foscarnet is more toxic (with high rates of limiting nephrotoxicity) but may be advantageous for some patients with HIV infection, including people with disease caused by ganciclovir-resistant virus or people who are unable to tolerate ganciclovir. Cidofovir is efficacious for CMV retinitis in adults with AIDS, but cidofovir has not been studied in children and is nephrotoxic. Because all drugs used for CMV infections may have serious toxicities, it is important to appropriately monitor patients under treatment.

As in all human hosts, CMV establishes lifelong latency and, as such, is not eliminated from the body with antiviral treatment of CMV disease. Until immune reconstitution is achieved with antiretroviral therapy (ART), chronic suppressive therapy should be administered to HIV-infected patients with a history of CMV end-organ disease (eg, retinitis, colitis, pneumonitis) to prevent recurrence. Recognizing limitations of the pediatric data but drawing on the growing experience in adult patients, discontinuing prophylaxis may be considered for pediatric patients 1 through 5 years of age who are receiving ART and have a sustained (eg, >6 months) increase in CD4+ T-lymphocyte count to greater than 500 cells/mm^3 or an increase in CD4+ T-lymphocyte percentage to greater than 15% and for children 6 years of age and older who have an increase in CD4+ T-lymphocyte count to greater than 100 cells/mm^3 or an increase in CD4+ T-lymphocyte percentage to greater than 15%. For immunocompromised children with CMV retinitis, such decisions should be made in close consultation with an ophthalmologist and should take into account such factors as magnitude and duration of CD4+ T-lymphocyte increase, anatomic location of the retinal lesion, vision in the contralateral eye, and the feasibility of regular ophthalmologic monitoring. All patients who have had anti-CMV maintenance therapy discontinued should continue to undergo regular ophthalmologic monitoring at least 3 to 6 month intervals for early detection of CMV relapse as well as for immune reconstitution uveitis.[1]

ISOLATION OF THE HOSPITALIZED PATIENT: Standard precautions are recommended.

CONTROL MEASURES:

Care of Exposed People. When caring for children, hand hygiene, particularly after changing diapers, is advised to decrease transmission of CMV. Because asymptomatic excretion of CMV is common in people of all ages, a child with congenital CMV infection should not be treated differently from other children.

Although unrecognized exposure to people who are shedding CMV likely is common, concern may arise when immunocompromised patients or nonimmune pregnant women, including health care professionals, are exposed to patients with clinically recognizable CMV infection. Standard precautions should be sufficient to interrupt transmission of CMV (See Infection Control for Hospitalized Children, p 160).

Child Care. Awareness of CMV, its potential risks, and appropriate hand hygiene measures to minimize occupationally acquired infection should be available for female workers in child care centers (**www.cdc.gov/cmv/index.html**; see discussion of CMV in Children in Out-of-Home Child Care, p 133).

---

[1] Centers for Disease Control and Prevention. Guidelines for the prevention and treatment of opportunistic infections among HIV-exposed and HIV-infected children. Recommendations from the CDC, the National Institutes of Health, the HIV Medicine Association of the Infectious Diseases Society of America, the Pediatric Infectious Diseases Society, and the American Academy of Pediatrics. *MMWR Recomm Rep.* 2009;58(RR-11):1–166

Immunoprophylaxis. CMV-IGIV has been developed for prophylaxis of CMV disease in seronegative kidney, lung, liver, pancreas and heart transplant recipients. CMV-IGIV seems to be moderately effective in kidney and liver transplant recipients and has been used in combination with antiviral agents. Results of a study of its use in pregnant women to prevent CMV transmission to the fetus were compromised by methodologic difficulties in the conduct of the trial, and use of CMV-IGIV cannot be recommended for this purpose at the current time. Evaluation of investigational vaccines in healthy volunteers and renal transplant recipients is in progress, and recent data from a phase II trial in pregnant women appear promising.

Prevention of Transmission by Blood Transfusion. Transmission of CMV by blood transfusion to newborn infants or other immune-compromised hosts virtually has been eliminated by use of CMV antibody-negative donors, by freezing red blood cells in glycerol before administration, by removal of the buffy coat, or by filtration to remove white blood cells.

Prevention of Transmission by Human Milk. Pasteurization or freezing of donated human milk can decrease the likelihood of CMV transmission. Holder pasteurization (62.5°C [144.5°F] for 30 minutes) and short-term pasteurization (72°C [161.6°F] for 5 seconds) of milk appear to inactivate CMV; short-term pasteurization may be less harmful to the beneficial constituents of human milk. Freezing milk at −20°C (−4°F) will decrease viral titers but does not eliminate CMV reliably. If fresh donated milk is needed for infants born to CMV antibody-negative mothers, providing these infants with milk from only CMV antibody-negative women should be considered. For further information on human milk banks, see Human Milk (p 126).

Prevention of Transmission in Transplant Recipients. CMV antibody-negative recipients of tissue from CMV-seropositive donors are at high risk of CMV disease. If such circumstances cannot be avoided, administration of antiviral therapy or monitoring for viremia and administering preemptive antiviral therapy is beneficial for decreasing this risk.

Dengue

CLINICAL MANIFESTATIONS: Dengue has a wide range of clinical presentations, from a mild viral syndrome to classic dengue fever and severe dengue (ie, dengue hemorrhagic fever or dengue shock syndrome). Approximately 5% of patients develop severe dengue, which is more common with second or other subsequent infections. Less common clinical syndromes include myocarditis, pancreatitis, hepatitis, and neuroinvasive disease.

Dengue is a dynamic disease beginning with a nonspecific, acute febrile illness lasting 2 to 7 days (febrile phase), progressing to severe disease during fever defervescence (critical phase), and ending in a convalescent phase. Fever may be biphasic and usually is accompanied by muscle, joint, and/or bone pain, headache, retro-orbital pain, facial erythema, injected oropharynx, macular or maculopapular rash, leukopenia, and petechiae or other minor bleeding manifestations. Warning signs of progression to severe dengue occur in the late febrile phase and include persistent vomiting, abdominal pain, mucosal bleeding, difficulty breathing, early signs of shock, and a rapid decline in platelet count with an increase in hematocrit (hemoconcentration). Patients with nonsevere disease begin to improve during the critical phase, and people with clinically significant plasma leakage attributable to increased vascular permeability develop severe disease with pleural effusions and/or ascites, hypovolemic shock, and hemorrhage.

ETIOLOGY: Four related RNA viruses of the genus *Flavivirus*, dengue viruses (DENV)-1, -2, -3, and -4, cause symptomatic (~25%) and asymptomatic (~75%) infections. Infection with one DENV type produces lifelong immunity against that type and short-term (≤2 months) cross-protection against infection with the other 3 types of DENV. A person has a lifetime risk of up to 4 DENV infections.

EPIDEMIOLOGY: DENV primarily is transmitted to humans through the bite of infected *Aedes aegypti* (and less commonly *Ae. albopictus* or *Ae. polynesiensis*) mosquitoes. Humans are the main amplifying host of DENV and the main source of virus for *Aedes* mosquitoes. A sylvatic nonhuman primate DENV transmission cycle exists in parts of Africa and Southeast Asia but rarely crosses to humans. Because of the approximately 7 days of viremia, DENV can be transmitted following receipt of blood products, donor organs or tissue, percutaneous exposure to blood, and exposure in utero or at parturition.

Dengue is a major public health problem in the tropics and subtropics; an estimated 50 million cases occur annually, and 40% of the world's population lives in areas with DENV transmission. In the United States, dengue is endemic in Puerto Rico, the Virgin Islands, and American Samoa. In addition, millions of US travelers, including children, are at risk, because dengue is the leading cause of febrile illness among travelers returning from the Caribbean, Latin America, and South Asia. Outbreaks with local DENV transmission have occurred in Texas, Hawaii, and Florida in the last decade. However, although 16 states have *A aegypti* and 35 states have *A albopictus* mosquitoes, local dengue transmission is uncommon because of infrequent contact between people and infected mosquitoes. Dengue occurs in both children and adults and affects both sexes with no differences in infection rates or disease severity.

The **incubation period** for DENV replication in mosquitoes is 8 to 12 days (extrinsic incubation); mosquitoes remain infectious for life (approximately 1 month). In humans, the incubation period is 3 to 14 days before symptom onset (intrinsic incubation). Infected people, both symptomatic and asymptomatic, can transmit to mosquitoes 1 to 2 days before symptoms develop and throughout the approximately 7-day viremic period.

DIAGNOSTIC TESTS: Laboratory confirmation of a clinical diagnosis of dengue depends on when a serum sample is obtained during the course of illness and may require detection of anti-DENV immunoglobulin (Ig) M antibodies by enzyme immunosorbent assay (EIA), detection of DENV RNA by reverse-transcriptase polymerase chain reaction (RT-PCR) assay, or detection of DENV antigen by immunoassay. DENV RNA is detectable during the febrile phase, but anti-DENV IgM antibodies are not detectable until 4 to 5 days after illness onset. DENV nonstructural protein 1 (NS-1) antigen is detectable for the first 10 days of illness. Other approaches are fourfold or greater increase in reciprocal IgG anti-DENV titer or hemagglutination inhibition titer to DENV antigens in acute- and convalescent-phase sera or IgM anti-DENV in CSF. Diagnostic testing for DENV is available through commercial reference laboratories, some state public health laboratories, and the Dengue Branch of the Centers for Disease Control and Prevention. Anti-DENV IgM antibody testing is not useful, because it remains elevated for life after DENV infection and often is falsely positive in people with prior infection with or immunization against other flaviviruses (eg, West Nile, Japanese encephalitis, or yellow fever viruses).

TREATMENT: No specific antiviral therapy exists for dengue. During the febrile phase, patients should stay well hydrated and avoid use of aspirin (acetylsalicylic acid), aspirin-containing drugs, and other nonsteroidal anti-inflammatory drugs (eg, ibuprofen) to minimize the potential for bleeding. Additional supportive care is required if the patient becomes dehydrated or develops warning signs for severe disease at the time of fever defervescence.

Early recognition of shock and intensive supportive therapy can reduce risk of death from approximately 10% to less than 1% in severe dengue. During the critical phase, maintenance of fluid volume and hemodynamic status is central to management of severe cases. Patients should be monitored for early signs of shock, occult bleeding, and resolution of plasma leak to avoid prolonged shock, end organ damage, and fluid overload. Patients with refractory shock may require intravenous colloids and/or blood or blood products after an initial trial of intravenous crystalloids. Reabsorption of extravascular fluid occurs during the convalescent phase with stabilization of hemodynamic status and diuresis. It is important to watch for signs of fluid overload, which may manifest as a decrease in the patient's hematocrit as a result of the dilutional effect of reabsorbed fluid.

ISOLATION OF THE HOSPITALIZED PATIENT: Standard precautions are recommended, with attention to the potential for bloodborne transmission. When indicated, attention should be given to control of *Aedes* mosquitoes to prevent secondary transmission of DENV from patients to others.

CONTROL MEASURES: Vaccines are not available to prevent dengue. A number of candidates are in clinical trials to evaluate immunogenicity, safety, and efficacy. No chemoprophylaxis or antiviral medication is available to treat patients with dengue. People traveling to areas with endemic dengue (see DengueMap: **www.healthmap.org/dengue/**) are at risk of dengue and should take precautions to protect themselves from mosquito bites. Travelers should select accommodations that are air conditioned and/or have screened windows and doors. *Aedes* mosquitoes bite during the daytime, so bed nets are indicated for children sleeping during the day. Travelers should wear clothing that fully covers arms and legs, especially during early morning and late afternoon. Use of mosquito repellents containing up to 50% N,N-diethyl-meta-toluamide (DEET) for adults (including pregnant women) and up to 30% DEET for children older than 2 months of age is recommended when used accordingly to directions on product.

Dengue, acquired locally in the United States and during travel, became a nationally notifiable disease in 2010. Suspected cases should be reported to state health departments.

Diphtheria

CLINICAL MANIFESTATIONS: Respiratory tract diphtheria usually occurs as membranous nasopharyngitis or obstructive laryngotracheitis. Membranous pharyngitis associated with a bloody nasal discharge should suggest diphtheria. Local infections are associated with a low-grade fever and gradual onset of manifestations over 1 to 2 days. Less commonly, diphtheria presents as cutaneous, vaginal, conjunctival, or otic infection. Cutaneous diphtheria is more common in tropical areas and among the urban homeless. Extensive neck swelling with cervical lymphadenitis (bull neck) is a sign of severe disease. Life-threatening complications of respiratory diphtheria include upper airway obstruction caused by extensive membrane formation; myocarditis, which often is associated with heart block;

and cranial and peripheral neuropathies. Palatal palsy, characterized by nasal speech, frequently occurs in pharyngeal diphtheria.

ETIOLOGY: Diphtheria is caused by toxigenic strains of *Corynebacterium diphtheriae*. In industrialized countries, toxigenic strains of *Corynebacterium ulcerans* are emerging as an important cause of a diphtheria-like illness. *C diphtheriae* is an irregularly staining, gram-positive, nonspore-forming, nonmotile, pleomorphic bacillus with 4 biotypes (*mitis*, *intermedius*, *gravis*, and *belfanti*). All biotypes of *C diphtheriae* may be either toxigenic or nontoxigenic. Toxigenic strains express an exotoxin that consists of an enzymatically active A domain and a binding B domain, which promotes the entry of A into the cell. The toxin gene, *tox*, is carried by a family of related corynebacteria phages. The toxin, an ADP-ribosylase toxin, inhibits protein synthesis in all cells, including myocardial, renal, and peripheral nerve cells, resulting in myocarditis, acute tubular necrosis, and delayed peripheral nerve conduction. Nontoxigenic strains of *C diphtheriae* can cause sore throat and, rarely, other invasive infections, including endocarditis.

EPIDEMIOLOGY: Humans are the sole reservoir of *C diphtheriae*. Organisms are spread by respiratory tract droplets and by contact with discharges from skin lesions. In untreated people, organisms can be present in discharges from the nose and throat and from eye and skin lesions for 2 to 6 weeks after infection. Patients treated with an appropriate antimicrobial agent usually are communicable for less than 4 days. Transmission results from intimate contact with patients or carriers. People who travel to areas where diphtheria is endemic or people who come into contact with infected travelers from such areas are at increased risk of being infected with the organism; rarely, fomites and raw milk or milk products can serve as vehicles of transmission. Severe disease occurs more often in people who are unimmunized or inadequately immunized. Fully immunized people may be asymptomatic carriers or have mild sore throat. The incidence of respiratory diphtheria is greatest during autumn and winter, but summer epidemics can occur in warm climates in which skin infections are prevalent. During the 1990s, epidemic diphtheria occurred throughout the newly independent states of the former Soviet Union, with case-fatality rates ranging from 3% to 23%. Diphtheria remains endemic in these countries as well as in countries in Africa, Latin America, Asia, the Middle East, and parts of Europe, where childhood immunization coverage with diphtheria toxoid-containing vaccines is suboptimal (**www.cdc.gov/travel/yellowbook**). No case of respiratory tract diphtheria has been reported in the United States since 2003. Cases of cutaneous diphtheria likely still occur in the United States, but they are not reportable. Only respiratory tract cases are included for national notification.

The **incubation period** usually is 2 to 7 days but occasionally is longer.

DIAGNOSTIC TESTS: Specimens for culture should be obtained from the nose or throat or any mucosal or cutaneous lesion. Material should be obtained from beneath the membrane, or a portion of the membrane itself should be submitted for culture. Because special medium is required for isolation (cystine-tellurite blood agar or modified Tinsdale agar), laboratory personnel should be notified that *C diphtheriae* is suspected. Specimens collected for culture can be placed in any transport medium (eg, Amies, Stuart media) or in a sterile container and transported at 4°C or in silica gel packs to a reference laboratory for culture. When *C diphtheriae* is recovered from a patient with suspected diphtheria, the strain should be tested for toxigenicity at a laboratory recommended by state and local authorities. All *C diphtheriae* isolates should be sent through the state health department to the Centers for Disease Control and Prevention (CDC).

TREATMENT:

Antitoxin. Because the condition of patients with diphtheria may deteriorate rapidly, a single dose of equine antitoxin should be administered on the basis of clinical diagnosis, even before culture results are available. Antitoxin is available through the CDC (see Directory of Resources, p 883). To neutralize toxin from the organism as rapidly as possible, the preferred route of administration is intravenous. Before intravenous administration of antitoxin, tests for sensitivity to horse serum should be performed, initially with a scratch test of a 1:1000 dilution of antitoxin in saline solution followed by an intradermal test if the scratch test result is negative (see Sensitivity Tests for Reactions to Animal Sera, p 64). If the patient is sensitive to equine antitoxin, desensitization is necessary (see Desensitization to Animal Sera, p 64). Allergic reactions to horse serum can be expected in 5% to 20% of patients. The dose of antitoxin depends on the site and size of the diphtheria membrane, duration of illness, and degree of toxic effects; presence of soft, diffuse cervical lymphadenitis suggests moderate to severe toxin absorption. Suggested dose ranges are: pharyngeal or laryngeal disease of 2 days' duration or less, 20 000 to 40 000 U; nasopharyngeal lesions, 40 000 to 60 000 U; extensive disease of 3 or more days' duration or diffuse swelling of the neck, 80 000 to 120 000 U. Antitoxin probably is of no value for cutaneous disease, but some experts recommend 20 000 to 40 000 U of antitoxin, because toxic sequelae have been reported. Although Immune Globulin Intravenous (IGIV) preparations may contain variable amounts of antibodies to diphtheria toxin, use of IGIV for therapy of cutaneous or respiratory diphtheria has not been approved or evaluated for efficacy.

Antimicrobial Therapy. Erythromycin administered orally or parenterally for 14 days, penicillin G administered intramuscularly or intravenously for 14 days, or penicillin G procaine administered intramuscularly for 14 days constitute acceptable therapy. Antimicrobial therapy is required to stop toxin production, to eradicate *C diphtheriae,* and to prevent transmission but is not a substitute for antitoxin, which is the primary therapy. Elimination of the organism should be documented 24 hours after completion of treatment by 2 consecutive negative cultures from specimens taken 24 hours apart.

Immunization. Active immunization against diphtheria should be undertaken during convalescence from diphtheria; disease does not necessarily confer immunity.

Cutaneous Diphtheria. Thorough cleansing of the lesion with soap and water and administration of an appropriate antimicrobial agent for 10 days are recommended.

Carriers. If not immunized, carriers should receive active immunization promptly, and measures should be taken to ensure completion of the immunization schedule. If a carrier has been immunized previously but has not received a booster of diphtheria toxoid within 5 years, a booster dose of a vaccine containing diphtheria toxoid (DTaP, Tdap, DT, or Td, depending on age) should be given. Carriers should be given oral erythromycin or penicillin G for 10 to 14 days or a single intramuscular dose of penicillin G benzathine (600 000 U for children weighing less than 30 kg and 1.2 million U for children weighing 30 kg or more and adults). Two follow-up cultures should be obtained after completing antimicrobial treatment to ensure detection of relapse, which occurs in as many as 20% of patients treated with erythromycin. The first culture should be obtained 24 hours after completing treatment. If results of cultures are positive, an additional 10-day course of oral erythromycin should be given, and follow-up cultures should be performed again. Erythromycin-resistant strains have been identified, but their epidemiologic significance has not been determined. Fluoroquinolones (see Fluoroquinolones, p 800), rifampin, clarithromycin, and azithromycin have good in vitro activity and may be better tolerated than erythromycin, but they have not been evaluated in clinical infection or in carriers.

ISOLATION OF THE HOSPITALIZED PATIENT: In addition to standard precautions, droplet precautions are recommended for patients and carriers with pharyngeal diphtheria until 2 cultures from both the nose and throat collected 24 hours after completing antimicrobial treatment are negative for *C diphtheriae*. Contact precautions are recommended for patients with cutaneous diphtheria until 2 cultures of skin lesions taken at least 24 hours apart and 24 hours after cessation of antimicrobial therapy are negative.

CONTROL MEASURES:

Care of Exposed People. Whenever respiratory diphtheria is suspected or proven, local public health officials should be notified promptly. Cutaneous diphtheria is not included for national notification. All diphtheria isolates should be sent to the CDC through the state health department. Management of exposed people is based on individual circumstances, including immunization status and likelihood of adherence to follow-up and prophylaxis. The following are recommended:

- Close contacts of a person suspected to have diphtheria should be identified promptly. Contact tracing should begin in the household and usually can be limited to household members and other people with a history of direct, habitual close contact (including kissing or sexual contacts), health care personnel exposed to nasopharyngeal secretions, people sharing utensils or kitchen facilities, and people caring for infected children.
- For close contacts, *regardless of their immunization status,* the following measures should be taken: (1) surveillance for 7 days for evidence of disease; (2) culture for *C diphtheriae;* and (3) antimicrobial prophylaxis with oral erythromycin (40–50 mg/kg per day for 10 days, maximum 2 g/day) or a single intramuscular injection of penicillin G benzathine (600 000 U for children weighing less than 30 kg and 1.2 million U for children weighing 30 kg or more and adults). The efficacy of antimicrobial prophylaxis is presumed but not proven. Follow-up cultures of pharyngeal specimens should be performed after completion of therapy for contacts proven to be carriers after completion of therapy (see Carriers, p 309). If cultures are positive, an additional 10-day course of erythromycin should be given, and follow-up cultures of pharyngeal specimens should be performed.
- Asymptomatic, previously immunized close contacts should receive a booster dose of an age-appropriate diphtheria toxoid-containing vaccine (DTaP [or DT], Tdap, or Td) if they have not received a booster dose of a diphtheria toxoid-containing vaccine within 5 years (Tdap [10 years of age and older] is preferred over Td, if the person previously did not receive pertussis booster vaccine).
- Asymptomatic close contacts who have had fewer than 3 doses of a diphtheria toxoid-containing vaccine, children younger than 7 years of age in need of their fourth dose of DTaP (or DT), or people whose immunization status is not known should be immunized with an age-appropriate diphtheria toxoid-containing vaccine (DTaP [or DT], Tdap, or Td).

- Contacts who cannot be kept under surveillance should receive penicillin G benzathine but not erythromycin, because adherence to an oral regimen is less likely, and if not fully immunized or if immunization status is not known, they should be immunized with DTaP, Tdap, DT, or Td vaccine, as appropriate for age.

Use of equine diphtheria antitoxin in unimmunized close contacts is not recommended, because there is no evidence that antitoxin provides additional benefit for contacts who have received antimicrobial prophylaxis.

Immunization. Universal immunization with a diphtheria toxoid-containing vaccine is the only effective control measure. The schedules for immunization against diphtheria are presented in the childhood and adolescent (Fig 1.1–1.3, p 27–31) and adult (**www.cdc.gov/vaccines**) immunization schedules. The value of diphtheria toxoid immunization is proven by the rarity of disease in countries in which high rates of immunization with diphtheria toxoid-containing vaccines have been achieved. The decreased frequency of endogenous exposure to the organism in countries with high childhood coverage rates implies decreased boosting of immunity. Therefore, ensuring continuing immunity requires regular booster injections of diphtheria toxoid (as Tdap or as Td vaccine) every 10 years after completion of the initial immunization series.

Pneumococcal and meningococcal conjugate vaccines containing diphtheria toxoid or CRM_{197} protein, a nontoxic variant of diphtheria toxin, are not substitutes for diphtheria toxoid immunization.

Immunization of children from 2 months of age to the seventh birthday (see Fig 1.1–1.3, p 27–31) routinely consists of 5 doses of diphtheria and tetanus toxoid-containing and acellular pertussis vaccines (DTaP vaccine). Immunization against diphtheria and tetanus for children younger than 7 years of age in whom pertussis immunization is contraindicated (see Pertussis, p 553) should be accomplished with DT instead of DTaP vaccine (see Tetanus, p 707).

Other recommendations for diphtheria immunization, including recommendations for older children (7 through 18 years of age) and adults, can be found in the recommended childhood and adolescent (Fig 1.1–1.3, p 27–31) and adult (**www.cdc.gov/vaccines**) immunization schedules.

- When children and adults require tetanus toxoid for wound management (see Tetanus, p 707), the use of preparations containing diphtheria toxoid (DTaP, Tdap, DT, or Td vaccine, as appropriate for age or for a specific contraindication to pertussis immunization) is preferred to tetanus toxoid and will help to maintain diphtheria and, when appropriate, pertussis immunity.
- Travelers to countries with endemic or epidemic diphtheria should have their diphtheria immunization status reviewed and updated when necessary.

Precautions and Contraindications. See Pertussis (p 553) and Tetanus (p 707).

Ehrlichia and *Anaplasma* Infections
(Human Ehrlichiosis and Anaplasmosis)

CLINICAL MANIFESTATIONS: Previously collectively referred to as ehrlichiosis, 2 distinct names—ehrlichiosis and anaplasmosis—now commonly are used to describe infections caused by bacteria of the genus *Ehrlichia* and genus *Anaplasma*, respectively. In the United States, human ehrlichiosis is caused by 3 different *Ehrlichia* species: *Ehrlichia chaffeensis*, the etiologic agent of human monocytic ehrlichiosis (HME); *Ehrlichia ewingii*, and *Ehrlichia muris*-like agent. Infection with *Anaplasma phagocytophilum* causes human granulocytic anaplasmosis (HGA) (Table 3.3, p 313). These 4 infections have similar signs, symptoms, and clinical courses. All are acute, systemic, febrile illnesses that have some clinical similarities to Rocky Mountain spotted fever (RMSF), which often is considered in the differential diagnosis. However, *Ehrlichia* and *Anaplasma* species do not cause vasculitis or endothelial cell damage characteristic of other rickettsial diseases, such as RMSF.

Common systemic manifestations present in more than 50% of patients include fever, headache, chills, malaise, myalgia, and nausea. More variable symptoms include arthralgia, vomiting, diarrhea, cough, and confusion, usually present in 20% to 50% of patients. For *E chaffeensis*, rash is reported in approximately 60% of children, although it is reported less commonly in adults; rash is present in fewer than 10% of people with anaplasmosis. When present, rash is variable in appearance (usually involving the trunk and sparing the hands and feet) and location and typically develops approximately 1 week after onset of illness. More severe manifestations of these diseases include acute respiratory distress syndrome, encephalopathy, meningitis, disseminated intravascular coagulation, spontaneous hemorrhage, and renal failure. Significant laboratory findings in these diseases may include leukopenia, lymphopenia, thrombocytopenia, and elevated serum hepatic transaminase concentrations. Cerebrospinal fluid abnormalities (ie, pleocytosis with a predominance of lymphocytes and increased total protein concentration) are common. Symptoms typically last 1 to 2 weeks, and recovery generally occurs without sequelae; however, reports suggest the occurrence of neurologic complications in some children after severe disease. Fatal infections have been reported more commonly for *E chaffeensis* infections (approximately 1%–3% case fatality) than for HGA (less than 1% case fatality). Typically, *E chaffeensis* causes more severe disease than does *A phagocytophilum*. Secondary or opportunistic infections may occur in severe illness, resulting in a delay in recognition of ehrlichiosis and administration of appropriate antimicrobial treatment. People with underlying immunosuppression are at greater risk of severe disease. Fulminant disease has been reported in people who initially received trimethoprim-sulfamethoxazole before a correct diagnosis was confirmed.

ETIOLOGY: In the United States, human ehrlichiosis and anaplasmosis are caused by at least 4 different species of obligate intracellular bacteria with tropisms for different white blood cells. Ehrlichiosis results from infection with *E chaffeensis*, *E ewingii*, or *E muris*-like agent, and anaplasmosis is caused by *A phagocytophilum*. *Ehrlichia* and *Anaplasma* species are gram-negative cocci that measure 0.5 to 1.5 µm in diameter.

EPIDEMIOLOGY: Although the reported incidences of *E chaffeensis* and *A phagocytophilum* infections during 2007 each were only 3.0 cases per million population, the diseases are underrecognized, and selected active surveillance programs have shown the incidence to be substantially higher in some areas with endemic infection. Recent surveillance

Table 3.3. Human Ehrlichiosis and Anaplasmosis in the United States

Disease	Causal Agent	Major Target Cell	Tick Vector	Geographic Distribution
Ehrlichiosis caused by *Ehrlichia chaffeensis* (also known as human monocytic ehrlichiosis, or HME)	*E chaffeensis*	Usually monocytes	Lone star tick *(Amblyomma americanum)*	Predominately southeast, south central, and Midwest states
Anaplasmosis (also known as human granulocytic anaplasmosis, or HGA)	*Anaplasma phagocytophilum*	Usually granulocytes	Black-legged or deer tick *(Ixodes scapularis)* or Western black-legged tick *(Ixodes pacificus)*	Northeast and north central states and northern California
Ehrlichiosis caused by *Ehrlichia ewingii*	*E ewingii*	Usually granulocytes	Lone star tick *(A americanum)*	Southeast, south central, and Midwest states
Ehrlichiosis cause by the *Ehrlichia muris*-like agent	*E muris*-like agent	Not determined	*I scapularis* is identified as a possible vector	Minnesota, Wisconsin

data also show that the incidence of reported cases seems to be increasing. Most cases of *E chaffeensis* infection occur in people from the southeastern and south central United States, but a number of cases have been described from other areas. Cases attributable to the new *E muris*-like agent have been reported only from Minnesota and Wisconsin but possibly occur with the same distribution as Lyme disease. Ehrlichiosis caused by *E chaffeensis* and *E ewingii* are associated with the bite of the lone star tick *(Amblyomma americanum)*. However, the distribution of *A americanum* is expanding, and the geographic range of reported ehrlichiosis may be expected to expand in the future as well. Most cases of human anaplasmosis have been reported in the north central and northeastern United States, particularly Wisconsin, Minnesota, Connecticut, and New York, but cases in many other states, including California, have been identified. In most of the United States, *A phagocytophilum* is transmitted by the black-legged or deer tick *(Ixodes scapularis)*, which also is the vector for *Borrelia burgdorferi* (the agent of Lyme disease) and probably for the *E muris*-like agent. In the western United States, the western black-legged tick *(Ixodes pacificus)* is the main vector for *A phagocytophilum*. Various mammalian wildlife reservoirs for the agents of human ehrlichiosis have been identified, including white-tailed deer, white-footed mice, and *Neotoma* wood rats. Compared with patients with RMSF (see p 623), reported cases of symptomatic ehrlichiosis characteristically are in older people, with age-specific incidences greatest in people older than 40 years of age. However, recent seroprevalence data indicate that exposure to *Ehrlichia* is common in children. Most human infections occur between April and September, and the peak occurrence is from May through July. Coinfections of anaplasmosis with other tickborne diseases, including babesiosis and Lyme disease, have been described.

The **incubation period** of human ehrlichiosis and anaplasmosis typically is 5 to 10 days after a tick bite (median, 9 days).

DIAGNOSTIC TESTS: Differences between ehrlichiosis and anaplasmosis compared with RMSF are: (1) rash is present in more than 90% of patients with RMSF; (2) leukopenia and absolute lymphopenia and neutropenia are uncommon in RMSF; (3) morulae are not observed in RMSF; and (4) histopathologic vasculitis is a hallmark of RMSF but not ehrlichiosis and anaplasmosis. The Centers for Disease Control and Prevention (CDC) defines a confirmed case of human ehrlichiosis or anaplasmosis as:

- a clinically compatible illness (fever plus one or more of the following: headache, myalgia, anemia, leukopenia, thrombocytopenia, or any elevation of serum hepatic transaminase concentrations) plus serologic evidence of a fourfold change in IgG-specific antibody titer by indirect immunofluorescent antibody (IFA) assay between paired serum specimens (one taken in the first week of illness and a second 2–4 weeks later);
- detection of *Ehrlichia* or *Anaplasma* DNA in a clinical specimen via amplification of a specific target by polymerase chain reaction (PCR) assay;
- demonstration of *Ehrlichia* or *Anaplasma* antigen in a biopsy/autopsy sample by immunohistochemical methods; or
- isolation of *Ehrlichia* or *Anaplasma* bacteria from a clinical specimen in cell culture.

The CDC further defines a probable case as serologic evidence of elevated IgG or IgM antibody reactive with *Ehrlichia* or *Anaplasma* antigen by IFA, enzyme immunosorbent assay (EIA), dot-EIA, or serologic assays in other formats; or identification of morulae in the cytoplasm of monocytes or granulocytes by microscopic examination. Specific antigens are available for serologic testing of *E chaffeensis* and *A phagocytophilum* infections, although cross-reactivity between species can make it difficult to interpret the causative agent in areas where geographic distributions overlap. Similarly, because IgM and IgG rise concurrently and IgM-only assays may be more prone to false-positive reactions, concurrent examination of both classes of antibodies is recommended when assessing acutely infected patients. *E ewingii* and probably the *E muris*-like agent share some antigens with *E chaffeensis*, so most cases of *E ewingii* ehrlichiosis can be diagnosed serologically using *E chaffeensis* antigens. These tests are available in reference laboratories, in some commercial laboratories and state health departments, and at the CDC. The use of tests that are not approved by the US Food and Drug Administration should be discouraged. Testing should be limited to patients with clinical presentations consistent with the illness. Examination of peripheral blood smears to detect morulae in peripheral blood monocytes or granulocytes is insensitive. Use of PCR assay to amplify nucleic acid from peripheral blood of patients in the acute phase of ehrlichiosis appears to be sensitive, specific, and promising for early diagnosis. PCR assay for both anaplasmosis and ehrlichiosis is available increasingly at many commercial laboratories. Broth isolation can be conducted on appropriate clinical samples sent to specialty research laboratories or the CDC.

TREATMENT: Doxycycline is the drug of choice for treatment of human ehrlichiosis and anaplasmosis, regardless of patient age. The recommended dosage of doxycycline is 4.4 mg/kg per day, divided every 12 hours, intravenously or orally (maximum 100 mg/dose). Ehrlichiosis and anaplasmosis can be severe or fatal in untreated patients or patients with predisposing conditions, and initiation of therapy early in the course of disease helps minimize complications of illness. Failure to respond to doxycycline within the first 3 days suggests infection with an agent other than *Ehrlichia* or *Anaplasma* species.

Despite concerns regarding dental staining with older tetracycline-class antimicrobial agents in young children (see Tetracyclines, p 801), doxycycline has not been demonstrated to cause cosmetic staining of developing teeth when used in the dose and duration recommended to treat rickettsial diseases. Treatment should continue for at least 3 days after defervescence; the standard course of treatment is 7 to 14 days. Unequivocal evidence of clinical improvement generally is evident by 1 week, although some symptoms (eg, headache, weakness, malaise) can persist for weeks after adequate therapy. Severe or complicated disease may require longer treatment courses.

Clinical manifestations and geographic distributions of ehrlichiosis, anaplasmosis, and RMSF overlap. As with other rickettsial diseases, when a presumptive diagnosis of ehrlichiosis is made, doxycycline should be started immediately and should not be delayed pending laboratory confirmation of infection.

ISOLATION OF THE HOSPITALIZED PATIENT: Standard precautions are recommended. Human-to-human transmission of ehrlichiosis or anaplasmosis, except in rare cases associated with transfusion of blood products, has not been documented.

CONTROL MEASURES: Specific measures focus on limiting exposures to ticks and are similar to those for RMSF and other tickborne diseases (see Prevention of Tickborne Infections, p 207). A risk of blood transfusion infection should be considered in areas with endemic infection. Prophylactic administration of doxycycline after a tick bite is not indicated because of the low risk of infection. For additional information, see **www.cdc.gov/ehrlichiosis/.** In addition, a collaborative report providing recommendations for "Diagnosis and Management of Tickborne Rickettsial Diseases" is available at **www.cdc.gov/mmwr/preview/mmwrhtml/rr5504a1.htm.**

Enterovirus (Nonpoliovirus) and Parechovirus Infections
(Group A and B Coxsackieviruses, Echoviruses, Numbered Enteroviruses, and Human Parechoviruses)

CLINICAL MANIFESTATIONS: Nonpolio enteroviruses are responsible for significant and frequent illnesses in infants and children and result in protean clinical manifestations. The most common manifestation is nonspecific febrile illness, which in young infants may lead to evaluation for bacterial sepsis. Other manifestations can include the following: (1) respiratory: coryza, pharyngitis, herpangina, stomatitis, bronchiolitis, pneumonia, and pleurodynia; (2) skin: hand-foot-and-mouth disease, onychomadesis (periodic shedding of nails), and nonspecific exanthems; (3) neurologic: aseptic meningitis, encephalitis, and motor paralysis; (4) gastrointestinal/genitourinary: vomiting, diarrhea, abdominal pain, hepatitis, pancreatitis, and orchitis; (5) eye: acute hemorrhagic conjunctivitis and uveitis; (6) heart: myopericarditis; and (7) muscle: myositis. Neonates, especially those who acquire infection in the absence of serotype-specific maternal antibody, are at risk of severe disease, including sepsis, meningoencephalitis, myocarditis, hepatitis, coagulopathy, and pneumonitis. Infection with enterovirus 71 is associated with hand-foot-and-mouth disease, herpangina, and in a small proportion of cases, severe neurologic disease, including brainstem encephalomyelitis and paralytic disease, and secondary pulmonary edema/hemorrhage and cardiopulmonary collapse. Other noteworthy but not exclusive serotype associations include coxsackievirus A16 with hand-foot-and-mouth disease, coxsackievirus A24 variant and enterovirus 70 with acute hemorrhagic conjunctivitis, enterovirus 68 with respiratory illness, and coxsackieviruses B1 through B5 with pleurodynia and myopericarditis.

Patients with humoral and combined immune deficiencies can have persistent central nervous system infections, a dermatomyositis-like syndrome, and/or disseminated infection. Severe, multisystem disease is reported in hematopoietic stem cell transplant patients and children with malignancies.

As a group, human parechoviruses (formerly echoviruses 22 and 23, and others) appear to cause similar clinical diseases as enteroviruses, including febrile illnesses, exanthems, sepsis-like syndromes, and respiratory tract, gastrointestinal tract, and central nervous system infections. Neonates and young infants have presented with more severe clinical disease and long-term sequelae than have older children.

ETIOLOGY: The enteroviruses are RNA viruses. The nonpolio enteroviruses include more than 100 distinct serotypes formerly subclassified as group A coxsackieviruses, group B coxsackieviruses, echoviruses, and newer numbered enteroviruses. A new classification system groups these nonpolio enteroviruses into 4 species (human enterovirus [HEV] A, B, C, and D) on the basis of genetic similarity, although traditional serotype names are retained for individual serotypes.[1] Echoviruses 22 and 23 have been reclassified within a new genus (Parechovirus) and are termed human parechovirus (HPeV) 1 and 2, respectively. During 2006–2008, 21 HPeV 1 detections were reported.[1]

EPIDEMIOLOGY: Humans are the only known reservoir for human enteroviruses, although some primates can become infected. Enterovirus infections are common. They are spread by fecal-oral and respiratory routes and from mother to infant prenatally, in the peripartum period, and possibly via breastfeeding. Enteroviruses may survive on environmental surfaces for periods long enough to allow transmission from fomites. Hospital nursery and other institutional outbreaks may occur. Infection incidence, clinical attack rates, and disease severity typically are greatest in young children, and infections occur more frequently in tropical areas and where poor hygiene and overcrowding are present. Most enterovirus infections in temperate climates occur in the summer and fall (June through October), but seasonal patterns are less evident in the tropics. Epidemics of enterovirus meningitis, enterovirus 71-associated hand-foot-and-mouth disease with neurologic and cardiopulmonary complications, and enterovirus 70- and coxsackievirus A24-associated acute hemorrhagic conjunctivitis occur. Fecal viral shedding can continue for several weeks or months after onset of infection, but respiratory tract shedding usually is limited to 1 to 3 weeks or less. Viral shedding can occur without signs of clinical illness.

Seroepidemiologic studies of human parechoviruses suggest that infection occurs commonly during early childhood. Most school-aged children have serologic evidence of prior infection. HPeV 1 has been noted to circulate throughout the year, whereas other human parechoviruses occur more commonly during late spring and summer months.

The usual **incubation period** is 3 to 6 days, except for acute hemorrhagic conjunctivitis, in which the incubation period is 24 to 72 hours.

DIAGNOSTIC TESTS: Enteroviruses can be detected by reverse-transcriptase polymerase chain reaction (PCR) assay and culture from a variety of specimens, including stool, rectal swabs, throat swabs, conjunctival swabs, tracheal aspirates, urine, blood, and tissue biopsy specimens during acute illness and from cerebrospinal fluid (CSF) when meningitis

---

[1] Centers for Disease Control and Prevention. Nonpolio enterovirus and human parechovirus surveillance—United States, 2006–2008. *MMWR Morb Mortal Wkly Rep.* 2010;59(48):1577–1580

is present. Patients with enterovirus 71 neurologic disease often have negative results of culture and PCR of CSF even when they have CSF pleocytosis; in these patients, results of PCR assay and culture of throat or rectal swab and/or vesicle fluid specimens more frequently are positive. PCR assays for detection of enterovirus RNA are available at many reference and commercial laboratories for CSF and other specimens. PCR assay is more rapid and more sensitive than isolation of enteroviruses in cell culture and can detect all enteroviruses, including serotypes that are difficult to cultivate in viral culture. Sensitivity of culture ranges from 0% to 80% depending on serotype and cell lines used. Many group A coxsackieviruses grow poorly or not at all in vitro. Culture usually requires 3 to 8 days to detect growth. The serotype of enterovirus may be identified either by partial genomic sequencing of the VP1 capsid region from the original specimen or viral isolate or by neutralization assay of the viral isolate at select reference laboratories. Serotyping may be indicated in cases of special clinical interest or for epidemiologic purposes. Although used less frequently for diagnosis, acute infection with a known enterovirus serotype can be determined at reference laboratories by demonstration of a change in neutralizing or other serotype-specific antibody titer between acute and convalescent serum specimens or detection of serotype-specific IgM, but these methods are relatively insensitive, and commercially available serologic assays may lack specificity.

Commercially available enteroviral PCR assays will not detect any of the human parechoviruses. However, the Centers for Disease Control and Prevention has developed PCR primers that detect all known parechoviruses, and this represents the best diagnostic modality currently available. Similar tests are becoming available in clinical reference laboratories. Viral culture has been used for initial diagnosis of HPeV infections, but propagation in viral culture media has proven difficult. Serologic assays have been developed for research but are not available commercially for diagnostic purposes.

TREATMENT: No specific therapy is available for enteroviruses or parechoviruses. Immune Globulin Intravenous (IGIV) may be beneficial for chronic enteroviral meningoencephalitis in immunodeficient patients. IGIV also has been used in life-threatening neonatal infections, severe infections in people with malignancies, hematopoietic stem cell transplant recipients, people with suspected viral myocarditis, and people with enterovirus 71 neurologic disease, but proof of efficacy for these uses is lacking. Interferons occasionally have been used for treatment of enterovirus-associated myocarditis, again without definitive proof of efficacy. The antiviral drug pleconaril has activity against enteroviruses but is not available commercially. Pleconaril is being studied in neonatal enteroviral sepsis syndrome in a study conducted by the National Institute of Allergy and Infectious Disease Collaborative Antiviral Study Group.

ISOLATION OF THE HOSPITALIZED PATIENT: In addition to standard precautions, contact precautions are indicated for infants and young children for the duration of illness. Cohorting of infected neonates has been effective in controlling hospital nursery outbreaks.

CONTROL MEASURES: Hand hygiene, especially after diaper changing, is important in decreasing spread within families and institutions. Other measures include avoidance of contaminated utensils and fomites and disinfection of surfaces. Recommended chlorination treatment of drinking water and swimming pools may help prevent transmission.

Maintenance administration of IGIV in patients with severe deficits of B-lymphocyte function (eg, severe combined immunodeficiency syndrome, X-linked agammaglobulinemia) may prevent chronic enterovirus infection of the central nervous system. Prophylactic immune globulin has been used to help control hospital nursery outbreaks. Vaccines for virulent serotypes, such as enterovirus 71, are under investigation.

Epstein-Barr Virus Infections
(Infectious Mononucleosis)

CLINICAL MANIFESTATIONS: Infectious mononucleosis manifests typically as fever, pharyngitis with petechiae, exudative pharyngitis, lymphadenopathy, hepatosplenomegaly, and atypical lymphocytosis. The spectrum of diseases is wide, ranging from asymptomatic to fatal infection. Infections commonly are unrecognized in infants and young children. Rash can occur and is more common in patients treated with ampicillin or amoxicillin as well as with other penicillins. Central nervous system (CNS) complications include aseptic meningitis, encephalitis, myelitis, optic neuritis, cranial nerve palsies, transverse myelitis, and Guillain-Barré syndrome. Hematologic complications include splenic rupture, thrombocytopenia, agranulocytosis, hemolytic anemia, and hemophagocytic lymphohistiocytosis (HLH, or hemophagocytic syndrome). Pneumonia, orchitis, and myocarditis are observed infrequently. Replication of Epstein-Barr virus (EBV) in B lymphocytes results in T-lymphocyte proliferation, and inhibition of B-lymphocyte proliferation by T-lymphocyte cytotoxic responses. Fatal disseminated infection or B-lymphocyte or T-lymphocyte lymphomas can occur in children with no detectable immunologic abnormality as well as in children with congenital or acquired cellular immune deficiencies.

EBV is associated with several other distinct disorders, including X-linked lymphoproliferative syndrome, post-transplantation lymphoproliferative disorders, Burkitt lymphoma, nasopharyngeal carcinoma, and undifferentiated B- or T-lymphocyte lymphomas of the CNS. X-linked lymphoproliferative syndrome occurs in people with an inherited, maternally derived, recessive genetic defect in the SH2DIA gene, which is important in several lymphocyte signaling pathways. The syndrome is characterized by several phenotypic expressions, including occurrence of fatal infectious mononucleosis early in life among boys, nodular B-lymphocyte lymphomas often with CNS involvement, and profound hypogammaglobulinemia.

EBV-associated lymphoproliferative disorders result in a number of complex syndromes in patients who are immunocompromised, such as transplant recipients or people infected with human immunodeficiency virus (HIV). The highest incidence of these disorders occurs in liver and heart transplant recipients, in whom the proliferative states range from benign lymph node hypertrophy to monoclonal lymphomas. Other EBV syndromes are of greater importance outside the United States, including Burkitt lymphoma (a B-lymphocyte tumor), found primarily in Central Africa, and nasopharyngeal carcinoma, found in Southeast Asia and the Inuit population. EBV also has been associated with Hodgkin disease (B-lymphocyte tumor), non-Hodgkin lymphomas (B- and T-lymphocyte), gastric carcinoma "lymphoepitheliomas," and a variety of common epithelial malignancies.

Chronic fatigue syndrome is not related to EBV infection; however, fatigue lasting weeks to a few months may follow fewer than 10% of cases of classic infectious mononucleosis.

ETIOLOGY: EBV (also known as human herpesvirus 4) is a gammaherpesvirus of the *Lymphocryptovirus* genus and is the most common cause of infectious mononucleosis.

EPIDEMIOLOGY: Humans are the only known reservoir of EBV, and approximately 90% of US adults have been infected. Close personal contact usually is required for transmission. The virus is viable in saliva for several hours outside the body, but the role of fomites in transmission is unknown. EBV also may be transmitted by blood transfusion or transplantation. Infection commonly is contracted early in life, particularly among members of lower socioeconomic groups, in which intrafamilial spread is common. Endemic infectious mononucleosis is common in group settings of adolescents, such as in educational institutions. No seasonal pattern has been documented. Intermittent excretion in saliva may be lifelong after infection.

The **incubation period** of infectious mononucleosis is estimated to be 30 to 50 days.

DIAGNOSTIC TESTS: Routine diagnosis depends on serologic testing. Nonspecific tests for heterophile antibody, including the Paul-Bunnell test and slide agglutination reaction test, are available most commonly. The heterophile antibody response primarily is immunoglobulin (Ig) M, which appears during the first 2 weeks of illness and gradually disappears over a 6-month period. The results of heterophile antibody tests often are negative in children younger than 4 years of age with EBV infection, but heterophile antibody tests identify approximately 85% of cases of classic infectious mononucleosis in older children and adults during the second week of illness. An absolute increase in atypical lymphocytes during the second week of illness with infectious mononucleosis is a characteristic but nonspecific finding. However, the finding of greater than 10% atypical lymphocytes together with a positive heterophile antibody test result is considered diagnostic of acute infection.

Multiple specific serologic antibody tests for EBV infection are available in diagnostic virology laboratories (see Table 3.4). The most commonly performed test is for antibody against the viral capsid antigen (VCA). Because IgG antibodies against VCA occur in high titer early in infection and persist for life, testing of acute and convalescent serum specimens for anti-VCA may not be useful for establishing the presence of active infection. Testing for presence of IgM anti-VCA antibody and the absence of antibodies to Epstein-Barr nuclear antigen (EBNA) is useful for identifying active and recent infections. Because serum antibody against EBNA is not present until several weeks to months after onset of infection, a positive anti-EBNA antibody test excludes an active primary infection. Testing for antibodies against early antigen (EA) is not useful for interpretation of

Table 3.4. Serum Epstein-Barr Virus (EBV) Antibodies in EBV Infection

Infection	VCA IgG	VCA IgM	EA (D)	EBNA
No previous infection	−	−	−	−
Acute infection	+	+	+/−	−
Recent infection	+	+/−	+/−	+/−
Past infection	+	−	+/−	+

VCA IgG indicates immunoglobulin (Ig) G class antibody to viral capsid antigen; VCA IgM, IgM class antibody to VCA; EA (D), early antigen diffuse staining; and EBNA, EBV nuclear antigen.

serologic results because of unreliability of the assays that are used. Interpretations of EBV serologic testing are based on quantitative immunofluorescent antibody tests performed during various stages of mononucleosis and its resolution, although detection of antibodies by enzyme immunoassays usually is performed by clinical laboratories. Typical patterns of antibody responses to EBV infection are illustrated in Fig 3.1 (p 320).

Serologic tests for EBV are useful particularly for evaluating patients who have heterophile-negative infectious mononucleosis. Testing for other agents, especially cytomegalovirus, *Toxoplasma* species, human herpesvirus 6, and human immunodeficiency virus, also may be indicated for some of these patients. Diagnosis of the entire range of EBV-associated illness requires use of molecular and antibody techniques, particularly for patients with immune deficiencies.

Isolation of EBV from oropharyngeal secretions by culture in cord blood cells is possible, but techniques for performing this procedure usually are not available in routine diagnostic laboratories, and viral isolation does not necessarily indicate acute infection. Polymerase chain reaction (PCR) assay for detection of EBV DNA in serum, plasma, and tissue and reverse-transcriptase PCR assay for detection of EBV RNA in lymphoid cells or tissue are available commercially and may be useful in evaluation of immunocompromised patients and in complex clinical problems.

FIG 3.1. SCHEMATIC REPRESENTATION OF THE EVOLUTION OF ANTIBODIES TO VARIOUS EPSTEIN-BARR VIRUS ANTIGENS IN PATIENTS WITH INFECTIOUS MONONUCLEOSIS.

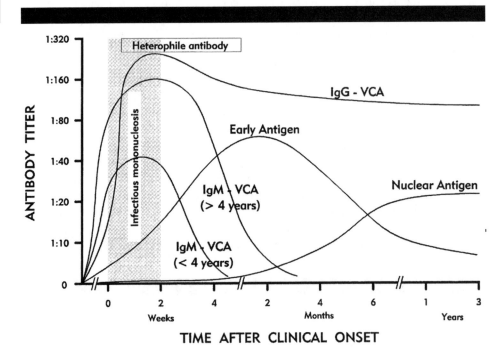

TREATMENT: Patients suspected to have infectious mononucleosis should not be given ampicillin or amoxicillin, which cause nonallergic morbilliform rashes in a high proportion of patients with active EBV infection. Although therapy with short-course corticosteroids may have a beneficial effect on acute symptoms, because of potential adverse effects, their use should be considered only for patients with marked tonsillar inflammation with impending airway obstruction, massive splenomegaly, myocarditis, hemolytic anemia, or HLH. The dosage of prednisone usually is 1 mg/kg per day, orally (maximum 20 mg/day), for 7 days with subsequent tapering. Life-threatening HLH has been treated with cytotoxic agents and immunomodulators, including cyclosporin and corticosteroids. Although acyclovir has in vitro antiviral activity against EBV, therapy is of no proven value in infectious mononucleosis or in EBV lymphoproliferative syndromes limited to cells with latent viral gene expression. Decreasing immunosuppressive therapy is beneficial for patients with EBV-induced post-transplant lymphoproliferative disorders, whereas an antiviral drug, such as acyclovir, valacyclovir, or ganciclovir, sometimes is used in patients with active replicating EBV infection with or without passive antibody therapy provided by IGIV.

Contact sports should be avoided until the patient is recovered fully from infectious mononucleosis and the spleen no longer is palpable. In the setting of acute infectious mononucleosis, sport participation in both strenuous and contact situations can result in splenic rupture. In the first 3 weeks following the onset of symptoms, the risk of rupture is related primarily to splenic fragility; thus, both strenuous and contact sports must be avoided regardless of the presence or absence of splenomegaly. Following the initial 3-week period, clearance for contact sport participation is determined primarily by the presence of splenomegaly and secondarily by the severity of clinical symptoms. Splenomegaly can be determined by palpation of an enlarged spleen, but clinical studies have shown historically that palpation has poor sensitivity. Imaging modalities, such as ultrasonography or computerized tomography, offer greater sensitivity and accuracy and may be useful in determining whether an athlete safely can be returned to competition in a contact sport.

ISOLATION OF THE HOSPITALIZED PATIENT: Standard precautions are recommended.

CONTROL MEASURES: None.

Escherichia coli and Other Gram-Negative Bacilli
(Septicemia and Meningitis in Neonates)

CLINICAL MANIFESTATIONS: Neonatal septicemia or meningitis caused by *Escherichia coli* and other gram-negative bacilli cannot be differentiated clinically from septicemia or meningitis caused by other organisms. The early signs of sepsis can be subtle and similar to signs observed in noninfectious processes. Signs of septicemia include fever, temperature instability, heart rate abnormalities, grunting respirations, apnea, cyanosis, lethargy, irritability, anorexia, vomiting, jaundice, abdominal distention, cellulitis, and diarrhea. Meningitis, especially early in the course, can occur without overt signs suggesting central nervous system involvement. Some gram-negative bacilli, such as *Citrobacter koseri*, *Chronobacter* (formerly *Enterobacter*) *sakazakii*, *Serratia marcescens*, and *Salmonella* species, are associated with brain abscesses in infants with meningitis caused by these organisms.

ETIOLOGY: *E coli* strains with the K1 capsular polysaccharide antigen cause approximately 40% of cases of *E coli* septicemia and 80% of cases of *E coli* meningitis. Other important gram-negative bacilli causing neonatal septicemia include non-K1 strains of *E coli* and *Klebsiella* species, *Enterobacter* species, *Proteus* species, *Citrobacter* species, *Salmonella* species, *Pseudomonas* species, *Acinetobacter* species, and *Serratia* species. Nonencapsulated strains of *Haemophilus influenzae* and anaerobic gram-negative bacilli are rare causes.

EPIDEMIOLOGY: The source of *E coli* and other gram-negative bacterial pathogens in neonatal infections during the first several days of life typically is the maternal genital tract. Reservoirs for gram-negative bacilli also can be present within the health care environment. Acquisition of gram-negative organisms can occur through person-to-person transmission from hospital nursery personnel and from nursery environmental sites, such as sinks, countertops, powdered infant formula, and respiratory therapy equipment, especially among very preterm infants who require prolonged neonatal intensive care management. Predisposing factors in neonatal gram-negative bacterial infections include maternal intrapartum infection, gestation less than 37 weeks, low birth weight, and prolonged rupture of membranes. Metabolic abnormalities (eg, galactosemia), fetal hypoxia, and acidosis have been implicated as predisposing factors. Neonates with defects in the integrity of skin or mucosa (eg, myelomeningocele) or abnormalities of gastrointestinal or genitourinary tracts are at increased risk of gram-negative bacterial infections. In neonatal intensive care units, systems for respiratory and metabolic support, invasive or surgical procedures, indwelling vascular lines, and frequent use of broad-spectrum antimicrobial agents enable selection and proliferation of strains of gram-negative bacilli that are resistant to multiple antimicrobial agents.

Multiple mechanisms of resistance in gram-negative bacilli can be present simultaneously. Resistance resulting from production of chromosomally encoded or plasmid-derived AmpC beta-lactamases or from plasmid-mediated extended-spectrum beta-lactamases (ESBLs), occurring primarily in *E coli* and *Klebsiella* species but reported in many other gram-negative species, has been associated with nursery outbreaks, especially in very low birth weight infants. Organisms that produce ESBLs typically are resistant to penicillins, cephalosporins, and monobactams and can be resistant to aminoglycosides. Carbapenem-resistant strains have emerged among *Enterobacteriaceae*, especially *Klebsiella pneumoniae*.

The **incubation period** is variable; time of onset of infection ranges from birth to several weeks after birth or longer in very low birth weight, preterm infants with prolonged hospitalizations.

DIAGNOSTIC TESTS: Diagnosis is established by growth of *E coli* or other gram-negative bacilli from blood, cerebrospinal fluid (CSF), or other usually sterile sites. Special screening and confirmatory laboratory procedures are required to detect some multiply drug-resistant gram-negative organisms.

TREATMENT:
- Initial empiric treatment for suspected early-onset gram-negative septicemia in neonates is ampicillin and an aminoglycoside. An alternative regimen of ampicillin and an extended-spectrum cephalosporin (such as cefotaxime) can be used, but rapid emergence of cephalosporin-resistant organisms, especially *Enterobacter* species, *Klebsiella* species, and *Serratia* species, and increased risk of colonization or infection with ESBL-producing *Enterobacteriaceae* can occur when use is routine. Hence, routine use of an

extended-spectrum cephalosporin is not recommended unless gram-negative bacterial meningitis is suspected.

- The proportion of *E coli* bloodstream infections with onset within 72 hours of life that are resistant to ampicillin is high among very low birth weight infants. These *E coli* infections almost invariably are susceptible to gentamicin.

- Once the causative agent and its in vitro antimicrobial susceptibility pattern are known, nonmeningeal infections should be treated with ampicillin, an appropriate aminoglycoside, or an extended-spectrum cephalosporin (such as cefotaxime). Many experts would treat nonmeningeal infections caused by *Enterobacter* species, *Serratia* species, or *Pseudomonas* species and some other less commonly occurring gram-negative bacilli with a beta-lactam antimicrobial agent and an aminoglycoside. For ampicillin-susceptible CSF isolates of *E coli*, meningitis can be treated with ampicillin or cefotaxime; meningitis caused by an ampicillin-resistant isolate is treated with cefotaxime with or without an aminoglycoside. Combination therapy with beta-lactam and aminoglycoside antimicrobial agents is used for empiric therapy and until CSF is sterile. Some experts continue combination therapy for a longer duration. Expert advice from an infectious disease specialist can be helpful for management of meningitis.

- The drug of choice for treatment of infections caused by ESBL-producing organisms is meropenem, which is active against gram-negative aerobic organisms with chromosomally mediated ampC beta-lactamases or ESBL-producing strains, except carbapenemase-producing strains, especially some *Klebsiella pneumoniae* isolates. Of the aminoglycosides, amikacin retains the most activity against ESBL-producing strains. An aminoglycoside or cefepime can be used if the organism is susceptible. Expert advice from an infectious disease specialist can help in management of ESBL-producing gram-negative infections in neonates.

- All infants with gram-negative meningitis should undergo repeat lumbar puncture to ensure sterility of the CSF after 24 to 48 hours of therapy. If CSF remains culture positive, choice and doses of antimicrobial agents should be evaluated and another lumbar puncture should be performed.

- Duration of therapy is based on clinical and bacteriologic response of the patient and the site(s) of infection; the usual duration of therapy for uncomplicated bacteremia is 10 to 14 days, and for meningitis, minimum duration is 21 days.

- All infants with gram-negative meningitis should undergo careful follow-up examinations, including testing for hearing loss, neurologic abnormalities, and developmental delay.

ISOLATION OF THE HOSPITALIZED PATIENT: Standard precautions are recommended. Exceptions include hospital nursery epidemics, infants with *Salmonella* infection, and infants with infection caused by gram-negative bacilli that are resistant to multiple antimicrobial agents, including ESBL-producing strains and carbapenemase-producing *Enterobacteriaceae*; in these situations, contact precautions also are indicated.[1]

CONTROL MEASURES: Infection control personnel should be aware of pathogens causing infections in infants so that clusters of infections are recognized and investigated appropriately. Several cases of infection caused by the same genus and species of bacteria

---

[1] Centers for Disease Control and Prevention. Guidance for control of infections with carbapenem-resistant or carbapenemase-producing *Enterobacteriaceae* in acute care facilities. *MMWR Morb Mortal Wkly Rep.* 2009;58(10):256–260

occurring in infants in physical proximity or caused by an unusual pathogen indicate the need for an epidemiologic investigation (see Infection Control for Hospitalized Children, p 160). Periodic review of in vitro antimicrobial susceptibility patterns of clinically important bacterial isolates from newborn infants, especially infants in the neonatal intensive care unit, can provide useful epidemiologic and therapeutic information. IGIV therapy of newborn infants receiving antimicrobial agents for suspected or proven serious infection has been shown to have no effect on outcomes measured.

Escherichia coli Diarrhea
(Including Hemolytic-Uremic Syndrome)

CLINICAL MANIFESTATIONS: At least 5 pathotypes of diarrhea-producing *Escherichia coli* strains have been identified. Clinical features of disease caused by each pathotype are summarized as follows (also see Table 3.5, p 325):

- Shiga toxin-producing *E coli* (STEC) organisms are associated with diarrhea, hemorrhagic colitis, and hemolytic-uremic syndrome (HUS). The term thrombotic thrombocytopenic purpura (TTP) sometimes is used incorrectly for adults with STEC-associated HUS. STEC O157:H7 is the most consistently virulent STEC serotype, but other serotypes increasingly are being associated with illness. STEC illness typically begins with nonbloody diarrhea caused by virulent STEC serotypes, including O157:H7. Stools usually become bloody after 3 or 4 days. Severe abdominal pain is typical; fever occurs in less than one third of cases. Severe infection can result in hemorrhagic colitis. In people with presumptive diagnoses of intussusception, appendicitis, inflammatory bowel disease, or ischemic colitis, disease caused by *E coli* O157:H7 and other STEC should be considered.

- Diarrhea caused by enteropathogenic *E coli* (EPEC) is watery. Although usually mild, diarrhea can result in dehydration and even death. Illness occurs almost exclusively in children younger than 2 years of age and predominantly in resource-limited countries, either sporadically or in epidemics. Chronic EPEC diarrhea can result in growth retardation.

- Diarrhea caused by enterotoxigenic *E coli* (ETEC) is a 1- to 5-day, self-limited illness of moderate severity, typically with watery stools and abdominal cramps. ETEC is common in infants in resource-limited countries and in travelers to those countries. ETEC infection rarely is diagnosed in the United States. Outbreaks and studies with small numbers of patients have demonstrated that ETEC infection occurs among nontravelers in the United States.

- Diarrhea caused by enteroinvasive *E coli* (EIEC) is similar clinically to diarrhea caused by *Shigella* species. Although dysentery can occur, diarrhea usually is watery without blood or mucus. Patients often are febrile, and stools can contain leukocytes.

- Enteroaggregative *E coli* (EAEC) organisms cause watery diarrhea and are common in people of all ages in industrialized as well as resource-limited countries. EAEC has been associated with prolonged diarrhea (14 days or longer). Asymptomatic infection can be accompanied by subclinical inflammatory enteritis, which can cause growth disturbances.

    Sequelae of STEC Infection. HUS is a serious sequela of STEC enteric infection. *E coli* O157:H7 is the STEC serotype most commonly associated with HUS, defined by the triad of microangiopathic hemolytic anemia, thrombocytopenia, and acute renal dysfunction.

Table 3.5. Classification of *Escherichia coli* Associated With Diarrhea

Pathotype	Epidemiology	Type of Diarrhea	Mechanism of Pathogenesis
Shiga toxin-producing *E coli* (STEC)	Hemorrhagic colitis and hemolytic-uremic syndrome in all ages	Bloody or nonbloody	Shiga toxin production, large bowel attachment, coagulopathy
Enteropathogenic *E coli* (EPEC)	Acute and chronic endemic and epidemic diarrhea in infants	Watery	Small bowel adherence and effacement
Enterotoxigenic *E coli* (ETEC)	Infant diarrhea in resource-limited countries and travelers' diarrhea in all ages	Watery	Small bowel adherence, heat stable/heat-labile enterotoxin production
Enteroinvasive *E coli* (EIEC)	Diarrhea with fever in all ages	Bloody or nonbloody; dysentery	Adherence, mucosal invasion and inflammation of large bowel
Enteroaggregative *E coli* (EAEC)	Acute and chronic diarrhea in all ages	Watery, occasionally bloody	Small and large bowel adherence, enterotoxin and cytotoxin production

HUS occurs in up to 15% of STEC-infected children. The illness is serious and typically develops 7 days (up to 3 weeks) after onset of diarrhea. More than 50% of children require dialysis, and 3% to 5% die. Patients with HUS can develop neurologic complications (eg, seizures, coma, or cerebral vessel thrombosis). Children presenting with an elevated white blood cell count ($>20 \times 10^9$ per mL) or hematocrit less than 23% and with oligoanuria are at higher risk of poor outcome. One or more years after HUS, patients with normal creatinine clearance and without proteinuria or hypertension have a good prognosis.

ETIOLOGY: Five pathotypes of diarrhea-producing *E coli* have been distinguished by pathogenic and clinical characteristics. Each pathotype comprises characteristic serotypes, indicated by somatic (O) and flagellar (H) antigens. However, some serotypes are found in more than one pathotype group.

EPIDEMIOLOGY: Transmission of most diarrhea-associated *E coli* strains is from food or water contaminated with human or animal feces or from infected symptomatic people. STEC is shed in feces of cattle and, to a lesser extent, sheep, deer, and other ruminants. Human infection is acquired via contaminated food or water or via direct contact with an infected person, a fomite, or a carrier animal or its environment. Many food vehicles have caused *E coli* O157 outbreaks, including undercooked ground beef (a major source), raw leafy greens, and unpasteurized milk and juice. Outbreak investigations also have implicated petting zoos, drinking water, and ingestion of recreational water. The infectious dose is low; thus, person-to-person transmission is common in households and has occurred in child care centers. Less is known about the epidemiology of STEC strains other than O157:H7. The non-O157 STEC strains most commonly linked to illness in the United States are O26, O45, O103, O111, O121, and O145. Among children younger than 5 years of age, the incidence of HUS is highest in 1-year-old children and lowest in infants. An outbreak in Germany of HUS and bloody diarrhea caused by a virulent *E coli* strain O104:H4 with virulence profiles combining STEC and EAEC loci infected a large number of children and adults, with a high proportion of patients developing HUS.

With the exception of EAEC, non-STEC pathotypes most commonly are associated with disease in resource-limited countries, where food and water supplies commonly are contaminated and facilities and supplies for hand hygiene are suboptimal. Diarrhea attributable to ETEC occurs in people of all ages but especially is frequent and severe in infants in resource-limited countries. ETEC is a major cause of travelers' diarrhea. EAEC increasingly is recognized as a cause of diarrhea in the United States.

The **incubation period** for most *E coli* strains is 10 hours to 6 days; for *E coli* O157:H7, the incubation period usually is 3 to 4 days (range, 1–8).

DIAGNOSTIC TESTS: Diagnosis of infection caused by diarrhea-associated *E coli* other than STEC is difficult, because tests are not widely available to distinguish these pathotypes from normal *E coli* strains present in stool flora. Several sensitive, specific, and rapid enzyme immunoassays for detection of Shiga toxins in stool or broth culture of stool specimens are available commercially. These tests are necessary to detect non-O157 STEC infections. All stool specimens submitted for routine testing from patients with acute community-acquired diarrhea (regardless of patient age, season, or presence or absence of blood in the stool) should be cultured simultaneously for *E coli* O157:H7 and tested with an assay that detects Shiga toxins produced by O157 STEC. Several immunoassays have been approved by the US Food and Drug Administration for diagnosis of STEC infection.[1] Most *E coli* O157:H7 isolates can be identified presumptively when grown on sorbitol-containing selective media, because they cannot ferment sorbitol within 24 hours. Serotyping with specific antisera then can confirm the isolates as *E coli* O157:H7.

STEC also should be sought in stool specimens from all patients diagnosed with postdiarrheal HUS. However, the absence of STEC does not preclude the diagnosis of probable STEC-associated HUS, because HUS typically is diagnosed a week or more after onset of diarrhea, when the organism may not be detectable by conventional methods. Selective enrichment followed by immunomagnetic separation can increase markedly the sensitivity of STEC detection, so this testing especially is useful for patients who were not tested early in their diarrheal illness. The test is available at some state public health laboratories and at the Centers for Disease Control and Prevention (CDC). Additional methods used in reference and research laboratories include DNA probes and polymerase chain reaction assay. Serologic diagnosis using enzyme immunoassay to detect serum antibodies to *E coli* O157 and O111 lipopolysaccharides is available at the CDC for outbreak investigations.

TREATMENT: Orally administered electrolyte-containing solutions usually are adequate to prevent or treat dehydration and electrolyte abnormalities.[2] Antimotility agents should not be administered to children with inflammatory or bloody diarrhea. Careful monitoring of patients with hemorrhagic colitis (including complete blood cell count with smear, blood

---

[1] Centers for Disease Control and Prevention. Recommendations for diagnosis of Shiga toxin-producing *Escherichia coli* infections by clinical laboratories. *MMWR Recomm Rep.* 2009;58(RR-12):1–14

[2] Centers for Disease Control and Prevention. Managing acute gastroenteritis among children: oral rehydration, maintenance, and nutritional therapy. *MMWR Recomm Rep.* 2003;52(RR-16):1–16

urea nitrogen, and creatinine concentrations) is recommended to detect changes suggestive of HUS. If patients have no laboratory evidence of hemolysis, thrombocytopenia, or nephropathy 3 days after resolution of diarrhea, their risk of developing HUS is low.

Antimicrobial Therapy. A meta-analysis did not find that children with hemorrhagic colitis caused by STEC have a greater risk of developing HUS if treated with an antimicrobial agent. However, a controlled trial has not been performed, and a beneficial effect of antimicrobial treatment has not been proven. Most experts advise not prescribing antimicrobial therapy for children with *E coli* O157:H7 enteritis or a clinical or epidemiologic picture strongly suggestive of STEC infection. For an episode of severe watery diarrhea in a traveler to a resource-limited country, therapy can be helpful. Azithromycin or a fluoroquinolone have been the most reliable agents for therapy, although fluoroquinolones are not approved in people younger than 18 years of age for this indication (see Fluoroquinolones, p 800). Whenever possible, an antimicrobial agent should be chosen on the basis of results of susceptibility testing.

ISOLATION OF THE HOSPITALIZED PATIENT: In addition to standard precautions, contact precautions are indicated for patients with all types of *E coli* diarrhea for the duration of illness. Patients with postdiarrheal HUS should be presumed to have STEC infection.

CONTROL MEASURES:

Escherichia coli *O157:H7* and Other STEC Infection. All ground beef should be cooked thoroughly until no pink meat remains and the juices are clear or to an internal temperature of 160°F. Raw milk should not be ingested, and only pasteurized apple juice and cider products should be consumed. Because *E coli* O157:H7 has a low infectious dose and can be waterborne, people with diarrhea caused by *E coli* O157:H7 and non O157 STEC strains should not use recreational water venues (eg, swimming pools, water slides) until 2 weeks after symptoms resolve.

Outbreaks in Child Care Centers. If an outbreak of HUS or diarrhea attributable to STEC occurs in a child care center, immediate involvement of public health authorities is critical. Infection caused by STEC is reportable, and rapid reporting of cases allows interventions to prevent further disease. Ill children should not be permitted to reenter the child care center until diarrhea has resolved and 2 stool cultures (obtained at least 48 hours after antimicrobial therapy has been discontinued) are negative for STEC. Strict attention to hand hygiene is important but can be insufficient to prevent transmission. The child care center should be closed to new admissions during an outbreak, and care should be exercised to prevent transfer of exposed children to other centers.

Nursery and Other Institutional Outbreaks. Strict attention to hand hygiene is essential for limiting spread. Exposed patients should be observed closely, their stools should be cultured for the causative organism, and they should be separated from unexposed infants (also see Children in Out-of-Home Child Care, p 133).

Travelers' Diarrhea. Travelers' diarrhea usually is acquired by ingestion of contaminated food or water and is a significant problem for people traveling in resource-limited countries. Diarrhea commonly is caused by ETEC. Diarrhea attributable to *E coli* O157 is rare in US travelers; a much higher proportion of patients with non-O157 STEC infection have traveled internationally in the previous week. Travelers should be advised to drink only bottled or canned beverages and boiled or bottled water; travelers should avoid ice, raw produce including salads, and fruit that they have not peeled themselves. Cooked foods should be eaten hot. Antimicrobial agents are not recommended for prevention of travelers' diarrhea in children. Antimicrobial therapy generally is recommended for travelers in resource-limited areas when diarrhea is moderate to severe or is associated with fever or bloody stools. Several antimicrobial agents, such as azithromycin, doxycycline, rifaximin, and ciprofloxacin, can be effective in treatment of travelers' diarrhea. The drug of first choice for children is azithromycin and for adults is ciprofloxacin. Treatment for no more than 3 days is advised. Packets of oral rehydration salts can be added to boiled or bottled water and ingested to help maintain fluid balance.

Recreational Water. People with diarrhea caused by these potentially waterborne pathogens should not use recreational water venues (eg, swimming pools, water slides) for 2 weeks after symptoms resolve.

Fungal Diseases

In addition to the mycoses listed by individual agents (aspergillosis, blastomycosis, candidiasis, coccidioidomycosis, cryptococcosis, paracoccidioidomycosis, and sporotrichosis) in section 3, infants and children with immunosuppression or other underlying conditions can become infected by uncommonly encountered fungi. Children can acquire infection with these fungi through inhalation via the respiratory tract or direct inoculation after traumatic disruption of cutaneous barriers. A list of these fungi and the pertinent underlying host conditions, reservoirs or routes of entry, clinical manifestations, diagnostic laboratory tests, and treatments can be found in Table 3.6 (p 329). Taken as a group, few fungal susceptibility data are available on which to base treatment recommendations for these fungal infections, especially in children. Consultation with a pediatric infectious disease specialist experienced in the diagnosis and treatment of invasive fungal infections should be considered when caring for a child infected with one of these mycoses.

Table 3.6. Additional Fungal Diseases

Disease and Agent	Underlying Host Condition(s)	Reservoir(s) or Route(s) of Entry	Common Clinical Manifestations	Diagnostic Laboratory Test(s)	Treatment
Hyalohyphomycosis					
Fusarium species	Granulocytopenia; hematopoietic stem cell transplantation; severe immunocompromise	Respiratory tract; sinuses; skin	Pulmonary infiltrates; cutaneous lesions; sinusitis; disseminated infection	Culture of blood or tissue specimen	Voriconazole or D-AMB (1–1.5 mg/kg per day)[a]
Malassezia species	Immunosuppression; preterm birth; exposure to parenteral nutrition that includes fat emulsions	Skin	Central line-associated bloodstream infection; interstitial pneumonitis; urinary tract infection; meningitis	Culture of blood, catheter tip, or tissue specimen (requires special laboratory handling)	Removal of catheters and temporary cessation of lipid infusion; D-AMB
Penicilliosis					
Penicillium marneffei	Human immunodeficiency virus infection	Respiratory tract	Pneumonitis; invasive dermatitis; disseminated infection	Culture of blood, bone marrow, or tissue; histopathologic examination of tissue	Itraconazole[b] or D-AMB
Phaeohyphomycosis					
Alternaria species	None or trauma or immunosuppression	Respiratory tract; skin	Sinusitis; cutaneous lesions	Culture and histopathologic examination of tissue	Voriconazole or high-dose D-AMB[a]
Bipolaris species	None, trauma, immunosuppression, or chronic sinusitis	Environment	Sinusitis; disseminated infection	Culture and histopathologic examination of tissue	Voriconazole, itraconazole,[b] or D-AMB[a]; surgical excision
Curvularia species	Immunosuppression; altered skin integrity; asthma or nasal polyps; chronic sinusitis	Environment	Allergic fungal sinusitis; invasive dermatitis; disseminated infection	Culture and histopathologic examination of tissue	Allergic fungal sinusitis: surgery and corticosteroids Invasive disease: voriconazole, itraconazole,[b] or D-AMB[a]

Table 3.6. Additional Fungal Diseases, contiuned

Disease and Agent	Underlying Host Condition(s)	Reservoir(s) or Route(s) of Entry	Common Clinical Manifestations	Diagnostic Laboratory Test(s)	Treatment
Exophiala species, Exserohilum species	None or trauma or immunosuppression	Environment	Sinusitis; cutaneous lesions; disseminated infection	Culture and histopathologic examination of tissue	Voriconazole,[c] itraconazole,[b] D-AMB, or surgical excision
Pseudallescheria boydii (Scedosporium boydii) Scedosporium species	None or trauma or immunosuppression	Environment	Pneumonia; disseminated infection; osteomyelitis or septic arthritis; mycetoma (immunocompetent patients); endocarditis	Culture and histopathologic examination of tissue	Voriconazole[d] or itraconazole; surgical excision for pulmonary infection, as feasible
Trichosporonosis					
Trichosporon species	Immunosuppression; central venous catheter	Normal flora of gastrointestinal tract	Bloodstream infection; endocarditis; pneumonitis; disseminated infection	Blood culture; histopathologic examination of tissue; urine culture	D-AMB[a] or voriconazole[d]
Mucormycosis (Zygomycosis)					
Rhizopus; Mucor; Lichtheimia (formerly Absidia); Rhizomucor species	Immunosuppression; hematologic malignant neoplasm; renal failure; diabetes mellitus; iron overload syndromes	Respiratory tract; skin	Rhinocerebral infection; pulmonary infection; disseminated infection; skin and gastrointestinal tract less commonly	Histopathologic examination of tissue and culture	High dose of D-AMB (1.5 mg/kg per day) or posaconazole[e] and surgical excision, as feasible (voriconazole has no activity)

D-AMB indicates deoxycholate amphotericin B; if the patient is intolerant of or refractory to D-AMB, liposomal amphotericin B can be substituted.

[a] Consider use of a lipid-based formulation of amphotericin B.

[b] Itraconazole has been shown to be effective for cutaneous disease in adults, but safety and efficacy have not been established in children younger than 12 years of age.

[c] Voriconazole demonstrates activity in vitro, but no clinical data are available.

[d] Itraconazole may be the treatment of choice, but data on safety and effectiveness in children are limited.

[e] Posaconazole demonstrates activity in vitro, but few clinical data are available for children.

Fusobacterium Infections
(Including Lemierre Disease)

CLINICAL MANIFESTATIONS: *Fusobacterium necrophorum* and *Fusobacterium nucleatum* can be isolated from oropharyngeal specimens in healthy people, are frequent components of human dental plaque, and may lead to periodontal disease. Invasive disease attributable to *Fusobacterium* species has been reported following otitis media, tonsillitis, gingivitis, and oropharyngeal trauma. Ten percent of cases of invasive *Fusobacterium* infections are associated with Epstein-Barr virus infection.

Invasive infection with *Fusobacterium* species can lead to life-threatening disease. Otogenic infection is the most frequent primary source in children younger than 5 years of age and can be complicated by meningitis and thrombosis of dural venous sinuses. Invasive infection following tonsillitis was described early in the 20th century and was referred to as postanginal sepsis or Lemierre disease. Lemierre disease occurs most often in adolescents and young adults and can include internal jugular vein thrombophlebitis or thrombosis (JVT), evidence of septic embolic lesions in lungs or other sterile sites, and isolation of *Fusobacterium* species from blood or other normally sterile sites. Lemierre-like syndromes also have been reported following infection with *Arcanobacterium haemolyticum*, *Bacteroides* species, anaerobic *Streptococcus* species, other anaerobic bacteria, and methicillin-susceptible and resistant strains of *Staphylococcus aureus*. Fever and sore throat are followed by severe neck pain (anginal pain) that can be accompanied by unilateral neck swelling, trismus, and dysphagia. People with classic Lemierre disease have a sepsis syndrome with multiple organ dysfunction, disseminated intravascular coagulation, empyema, pyogenic arthritis, or osteomyelitis. Persistent headache or other neurologic signs indicate the presence of cerebral venous sinus thrombosis (eg, cavernous sinus thrombosis), meningitis, or brain abscess.

JVT can be completely vaso-occlusive. Some children with JVT associated with Lemierre disease have evidence of thrombophilia at diagnosis, which can include presence of antiphospholipid antibodies, abnormal levels of factor VIII, and factor V Leiden. These findings often resolve over several months and can indicate response to the inflammatory, prothrombotic process associated with infection rather than an underlying hypercoagulable state.

ETIOLOGY: *Fusobacterium* species are anaerobic, non–spore-forming, gram-negative bacilli. Human infection usually results from *F necrophorum* subspecies *funduliforme*, but infections with other species including *F nucleatum*, *Fusobacterium gonidiaformans*, *Fusobacterium naviforme*, *Fusobacterium mortiferum*, and *Fusobacterium varium* have been reported. Infection with *Fusobacterium* species, alone or in combination with other oral anaerobic bacteria, may result in Lemierre disease.

EPIDEMIOLOGY: *Fusobacterium* species commonly are found in soil and in the respiratory tracts of animals, including cattle, dogs, fowl, goats, sheep, and horses, and can be isolated from the oropharynx of healthy people. *Fusobacterium* infections are most common in adolescents and young adults, but infections, including fatal cases of Lemierre disease, have been reported in infants and young children. Children with sickle cell disease may be at greater risk of infection, particularly osteomyelitis.

DIAGNOSTIC TESTS: *Fusobacterium* species can be isolated using conventional liquid anaerobic blood culture media. However, the organism grows best on semisolid media for fastidious anaerobic organisms or blood agar supplemented with vitamin K, hemin, menadione, and a reducing agent. Colonies are cream to yellow colored, smooth, and round with a narrow zone of hemolysis on blood agar. Many strains fluoresce chartreuse green under ultraviolet light. Most *Fusobacterium* organisms are indole positive. The accurate identification of anaerobes to the species level has become important with the increasing incidence of microorganisms that are resistant to multiple drugs. Sequencing of the 16S rRNA gene and phylogenetic analysis can identify anaerobic bacteria to the genus or taxonomic group level and frequently to the species level.

Febrile children and adolescents, especially those with sore throat or neck pain who are sufficiently ill to warrant a blood culture, should have an anaerobic blood culture in addition to aerobic blood culture performed to detect invasive *Fusobacterium* species infection. Computed tomography and magnetic resonance imaging are more sensitive than ultrasonography to document thrombosis and thrombophlebitis of the internal jugular vein early in the course of illness.

TREATMENT: *Fusobacterium* species are susceptible to metronidazole, clindamycin, chloramphenicol, carbapenems (meropenem or imipenem), cefoxitin, and ceftriaxone. Metronidazole is the treatment preferred by many experts, because the drug has excellent activity against all *Fusobacterium* species and good tissue penetration. However, metronidazole lacks activity against microaerophilic streptococci that can coinfect some patients. Clindamycin also is an effective agent. *Fusobacterium* species intrinsically are resistant to gentamicin and fluoroquinolone agents. Tetracyclines have limited activity. Up to 50% of *F nucleatum* and 20% of *F necrophorum* isolates produce beta-lactamases, rendering them resistant to penicillin, ampicillin, and some cephalosporins.

Because *Fusobacterium* infections often are polymicrobial, multiple antimicrobial agents frequently are necessary. Therapy has been advocated with a penicillin-beta-lactamase inhibitor combination (piperacillin-tazobactam or ticarcillin-clavulanate) or a carbapenem (meropenem or imipenem) or combination therapy with metronidazole in addition to other agents active against aerobic oral and respiratory tract pathogens (cefotaxime, ceftriaxone, or cefuroxime). Duration of antimicrobial therapy depends on the anatomic location and severity of infection but usually is several weeks. Surgical intervention involving débridement or incision and drainage of abscesses may be necessary. Anticoagulation therapy has been used in both adults and children with JVT and cavernous sinus thrombosis. In cases with extensive thrombosis, anticoagulation therapy may decrease the risk of clot extension and shorten recovery time.

ISOLATION OF THE HOSPITALIZED PATIENT: Standard precautions are recommended. Person-to-person transmission of *Fusobacterium* species has not been documented.

CONTROL MEASURES: Oral hygiene and dental cleanings may reduce density of oral colonization with *Fusobacterium* species, prevent gingivitis and dental caries, and reduce the risk of invasive disease.

Giardia intestinalis (formerly Giardia lamblia and Giardia duodenalis) Infections
(Giardiasis)

CLINICAL MANIFESTATIONS: Symptomatic infection with *Giardia intestinalis* causes a broad spectrum of clinical manifestations. Children can have occasional days of acute watery diarrhea with abdominal pain, or they may experience a protracted, intermittent, often debilitating disease characterized by passage of foul-smelling stools associated with flatulence, abdominal distention, and anorexia. Anorexia combined with malabsorption can lead to significant weight loss, failure to thrive, and anemia. Humoral immunodeficiencies predispose to chronic symptomatic *G intestinalis* infections. Asymptomatic infection is common; approximately 50% to 75% of infected people in outbreaks occurring in child care settings and in the community were asymptomatic.

ETIOLOGY: *Giardia intestinalis* is a flagellate protozoan that exists in trophozoite and cyst forms; the infective form is the cyst. Infection is limited to the small intestine and biliary tract.

EPIDEMIOLOGY: Giardiasis is the most common intestinal parasitic infection of humans identified in the United States and globally with a worldwide distribution. Approximately 20 000 cases are reported in the United States each year, with highest incidence reported among children 1 to 9 years of age, adults 35 to 44 years of age, and residents of northern states. Peak onset of illness occurs annually during early summer through early fall.[1] Humans are the principal reservoir of infection, but *Giardia* organisms can infect dogs, cats, beavers, rodents, sheep, cattle, nonhuman primates, and other animals. People become infected directly from an infected person or through ingestion of fecally contaminated water or food. Most community-wide epidemics have resulted from a contaminated water supply. From 1971 to 2006, 123 drinking water outbreaks resulting in 28 127 cases of giaridiasis were reported in the United States. In 2007 and 2008, there were 2 *Giardia*-associated drinking water outbreaks involving 81 people.[2] Outbreaks resulting from person-to-person transmission occur in child care centers or institutional care settings where staff and family members in contact with infected children or adults become infected. Outbreaks associated with food or food handlers, although less common, also have been reported. Surveys conducted in the United States have identified overall prevalence rates of *Giardia* organisms in stool specimens that range from 5% to 7%, with variations depending on age, geographic location, and seasonality. Duration of cyst excretion is variable but can range from weeks to months. Giardiasis is communicable for as long as the infected person excretes cysts.

The **incubation period** usually is 1 to 3 weeks.

DIAGNOSTIC TESTS: Commercially available, sensitive, and specific enzyme immunoassay (EIA) and direct fluorescence antibody (DFA) assays are becoming the standard for diagnosis of giardiasis in the United States. EIA has a sensitivity of up to 95% and a specificity of 98% to 100% when compared with microscopy. DFA assay has the

---

[1] Centers for Disease Control and Prevention. Giardiasis surveillance—United States, 2006–2008. *MMWR Surveill Summ.* 2010;59(SS-6):15–25

[2] Centers for Disease Control and Prevention. Surveillance for waterborne disease outbreaks associated with drinking water—United States, 2007–2008. *MMWR Surveill Summ.* 2011;60(SS-12):38–68

advantage that organisms are visualized. Laboratories can reduce reagent and personnel costs by pooling specimens from patients before evaluation either by microscopy or EIA. Traditionally, diagnosis has been based on the microscopic identification of trophozoites or cysts in stool specimens. However, this requires an experienced microscopist, and sensitivity can be suboptimal if the specimen contains low numbers of organisms. Stool needs to be examined as soon as possible or placed immediately in a preservative, such as neutral-buffered 10% formalin or polyvinyl alcohol. A single direct smear examination of stool has a sensitivity of 75% to 95%. Sensitivity is higher for diarrheal stool specimens, because they contain higher concentrations of organisms. Sensitivity of microscopy is increased by examining 3 or more specimens collected every other day. Commercially available stool collection kits in childproof containers are convenient for preserving stool specimens collected at home. When giaridiasis is suspected clinically but the organism is not found on repeated stool examination, examination of duodenal contents obtained by direct aspiration or by using a commercially available string test (Enterotest) may be diagnostic. Rarely, duodenal biopsy is required for diagnosis.

TREATMENT: Some infections are self-limited and treatment is not required. Dehydration and electrolyte abnormalities can occur and should be corrected. Tinidazole, metronidazole, and nitazoxanide are the drugs of choice. A 5- to 10-day course of metronidazole has an efficacy of 80% to 100% in pediatric patients. A 1-time dose of tinidazole, a nitroimidazole for children 3 years of age and older, has a median efficacy of 91% in pediatric patients (range, 80%–100%) and has fewer adverse effects than does metronidazole. A 3-day course of nitazoxanide oral suspension has similar efficacy to metronidazole and has the advantage(s) of treating other intestinal parasites and of being approved for use in children 1 year of age and older. Quinacrine and an oral suspension of furazolidone are alternatives but are used more often for combination therapy for refractory disease. Paromomycin, a poorly absorbed aminoglycoside that is 50% to 70% effective, is recommended for treatment of symptomatic infection in pregnant women in the second and third trimester (see Drugs for Parasitic Infections, p 848).

Symptom recurrence after completing antimicrobial treatment can be attributable to reinfection, post-*Giardia* lactose intolerance (occurs in 20%–40% of patients), immunosuppresion, insufficient treatment, or drug resistance. Detailed exposure history and repeat fecal testing is important in determining the cause of recurrence of symptoms. If reinfection is suspected, a second course of the same drug should be effective. Treatment with a different class of drug is recommended for resistant giaridiasis. Other treatment options include combination of a nitroimidazole plus quinacrine for at least 2 weeks or high-dose courses of the original agent.

Patients who are immunocompromised because of hypogammaglobulinemia or lymphoproliferative disease are at higher risk of giardiasis, and it is more difficult to treat in these patients. Patients with acquired immunodeficiency syndrome (AIDS) often respond to standard therapy; however, in some cases, additional treatment is required. If giardiasis is refractory to standard treatment among human immunodeficiency virus (HIV)-infected patients with AIDS, high doses, longer treatment duration, or combination therapy may be appropriate.

Treatment of asymptomatic carriers generally is not recommended. Possible exceptions to prevent transmission are carriers in households of patients with hypogammaglobulinemia or cystic fibrosis.

ISOLATION OF THE HOSPITALIZED PATIENT: In addition to standard precautions, contact precautions for the duration of illness are recommended for diapered and incontinent children.

CONTROL MEASURES:

- *Child care centers:* In child care centers, improved sanitation and personal hygiene should be emphasized (also see Children in Out-of-Home Child Care, p 133). Hand hygiene by staff and children should be emphasized, especially after toilet use or handling of soiled diapers, which is a key preventive action for control of spread of giardiasis. When an outbreak is suspected, the local health department should be contacted, and an epidemiologic investigation should be undertaken to identify and treat all symptomatic children, child care providers, and family members infected with *G intestinalis*. People with diarrhea should be excluded from the child care center until they become asymptomatic. Treatment or exclusion of asymptomatic carriers is not effective for outbreak control and is not recommended.

- *Drinking water:* Waterborne disease can be prevented by combination of adequate filtration of water from surface water sources (eg, lakes, rivers, streams), chlorination, and maintenance of water distribution systems.

- *Camping/hiking:* Where water might be contaminated, travelers, campers, and hikers should be advised of methods to make water safe for drinking, including boiling, chemical disinfection, and filtration. Boiling is the most reliable method to make water safe for drinking. The time of boiling depends on altitude (1 minute at sea level). Chemical disinfection with iodine is an alternative method of water treatment using either tincture of iodine or tetraglycine hydroperiodide tablets. Chlorine in various forms also can be used for chemical disinfection, but germicidal activity is dependent on several factors, including pH, temperature, and organic content of the water. Commercially available portable water filters provide various degrees of protection. Many commercially available filters are marketed as being able to remove *Giardia* and *Cryptosporidium* species from water. Additional information about water purification, including a traveler's guide for buying water filters, can be found at **www.cdc.gov/ crypto/factsheets/filters.html.**

- *Recreational water:* People with diarrhea caused by *Giardia* species should not use recreational water venues (eg, swimming pools, water slides) for 2 weeks after symptoms resolve. More information on giardiasis can be found at **www.cdc.gov/parasites/ giardia/.** Waterborne disease outbreaks associated with recreational water attributable to many enteric pathogens, including *G intestinalis*, have been reported.[1]

---

[1] Centers for Disease Control and Prevention. Surveillance for waterborne disease outbreaks and other health events recreational water—United States, 2007–2008. *MMWR Surveill Summ.* 2011;60(SS-12):1–32

Gonococcal Infections

CLINICAL MANIFESTATIONS: Gonococcal infections in children and adolescents occur in 3 distinct age groups.

- Infection in the **newborn infant** usually involves the eyes. Other possible manifestations of neonatal gonococcal infection include scalp abscess (which can be associated with fetal scalp monitoring) and disseminated disease with bacteremia, arthritis, or meningitis.
- In children beyond the newborn period, including **prepubertal children,** gonococcal infection may occur in the genital tract and almost always is transmitted sexually. Vaginitis is the most common manifestation in prepubertal females. Gonococcal urethritis is possible but uncommon in the prepubertal male. Anorectal and tonsillopharyngeal infection also can occur in prepubertal children and often is asymptomatic.
- In **sexually active adolescents,** as in adults, gonococcal infection of the genital tract in females often is asymptomatic, and common clinical syndromes are urethritis, endocervicitis, and salpingitis. In males, infection often is symptomatic, and the primary site is the urethra. Infection of the rectum and pharynx can occur alone or with genitourinary tract infection in either sex. Rectal and pharyngeal infections often are asymptomatic. Extension from primary genital mucosal sites can lead to epididymitis in males and to bartholinitis, pelvic inflammatory disease (PID) with resultant tubal scarring, and perihepatitis (Fitz-Hugh-Curtis syndrome) in females. Even asymptomatic infection in females can progress to PID, with tubal scarring that can result in ectopic pregnancy or infertility. Infection involving other mucous membranes can produce conjunctivitis, pharyngitis, or proctitis. Hematogenous spread from mucosal sites can involve skin and joints (arthritis-dermatitis syndrome) and occurs in up to 3% of untreated people with mucosal gonorrhea. Bacteremia can result in a maculopapular rash with necrosis, tenosynovitis, and migratory arthritis. Arthritis may be reactive (sterile) or septic in nature. Meningitis and endocarditis occur rarely.

ETIOLOGY: *Neisseria gonorrhoeae* is a gram-negative, oxidase-positive diplococcus.

EPIDEMIOLOGY: Gonococcal infections occur only in humans. The source of the organism is exudate and secretions from infected mucosal surfaces; *N gonorrhoeae* is communicable as long as a person harbors the organism. Transmission results from intimate contact, such as sexual acts, parturition, and rarely, household exposure in prepubertal children. Sexual abuse should be considered strongly when genital, rectal, or pharyngeal colonization or infection are diagnosed in prepubertal children beyond the newborn period. In 2010, a total of 309 341 cases of gonorrhea were reported in the United States, a rate of 99 cases per 100 000 population. *N gonorrhoeae* still is the second most commonly reported notifiable disease in the United States, with *Chlamydia trachomatis* genital tract infection being the most commonly reported. Reported incidence of infection is highest in females 15 through 24 years of age and in males 20 through 24 years of age. In 2009, gonorrhea rates remained highest among black people. Similar to recent years, the rate among black people was 20.5 times higher than the rate among white people. Gonorrhea rates were 4.2 times higher among American Indian/Alaska Native people and 2.2 times higher among Hispanic people than among white people in 2009. Rates among white people were 1.5 times higher than rates among people of Asian/Pacific Island ancestry. Concurrent infection with *C trachomatis* is common.

　　The **incubation period** usually is 2 to 7 days.

DIAGNOSTIC TESTS: Microscopic examination of Gram-stained smears of exudate from the conjunctivae, vagina of prepubertal girls, male urethra, skin lesions, synovial fluid, and when clinically warranted, cerebrospinal fluid (CSF) may be useful in the initial evaluation. Identification of gram-negative intracellular diplococci in these smears can be helpful, particularly if the organism is not recovered in culture. However, because of low sensitivity, a negative result should not be considered sufficient for ruling out infection.

N gonorrhoeae can be isolated from normally sterile sites, such as blood, CSF, or synovial fluid, using nonselective chocolate agar with incubation in 5% to 10% carbon dioxide. Selective media that inhibit normal flora and nonpathogenic *Neisseria* organisms are used for cultures from nonsterile sites, such as the cervix, vagina, rectum, urethra, and pharynx. Specimens for *N gonorrhoeae* culture from mucosal sites should be inoculated immediately onto appropriate agar, because the organism is extremely sensitive to drying and temperature changes.

Caution should be exercised when interpreting the significance of isolation of *Neisseria* organisms, because *N gonorrhoeae* can be confused with other *Neisseria* species that colonize the genitourinary tract or pharynx. At least 2 confirmatory bacteriologic tests involving different biochemical principles should be performed by the laboratory. Interpretation of culture of *N gonorrhoeae* from the pharynx of young children necessitates particular caution because of the high carriage rate of nonpathogenic *Neisseria* species and the serious implications of such a culture result.

Nucleic acid amplification tests (NAATs) are highly sensitive and specific when used on male urethral swab, female endocervical or vaginal swab, and male or female urine specimens. These tests include polymerase chain reaction (PCR), transcription-mediated amplification (TMA), and strand-displacement assay (SDA). Only the TMA assay is approved by the US Food and Drug Administration (FDA) for testing vaginal swabs from postmenarcheal females, and use of other NAATs from vaginal swab specimens may yield false-positive results because of other *Neisseria* species present in the female genital tract. Use of urine specimens increases feasibility of initial testing and follow-up of populations such as adolescents. These techniques also permit dual testing of urine for *C trachomatis* and *N gonorrhoeae*.

Culture is the most widely used test for identifying *N gonorrhoeae* from nongenital sites, and specimens also should be sent for antimicrobial susceptibility testing to aid in management should infection persist following initial therapy. NAATs are not approved by the FDA for use on rectal or pharyngeal swabs; some commercial and public health laboratories offer NAATs of rectal and pharyngeal swab specimens following in-house validation testing. Some NAATs have the potential to cross-react with nongonococcal *Neisseria* that commonly are found in the throat. A limited number of nonculture tests are approved by the FDA for conjunctival specimens.

***Sexual Abuse.*[1]** In all prepubertal children beyond the newborn period and in adolescents who have gonococcal infection but report no prior sexual activity, sexual abuse must be considered to have occurred until proven otherwise. Cultures should be performed on genital, rectal, and pharyngeal swab specimens for all patients before antimicrobial treatment is given. All gonococcal isolates from such patients should be preserved. Nonculture gonococcal tests, including Gram stain, DNA probes, enzyme immunoassays, or NAATs of oropharyngeal, rectal, or genital tract swab specimens in children cannot be relied

---

[1] Kellogg N; American Academy of Pediatrics, Committee on Child Abuse and Neglect. The evaluation of sexual abuse in children. *Pediatrics.* 2005;116(2):506–512

on as the sole method for diagnosis of gonococcal infection for this purpose, because false-positive results can occur. In prepubertal children for whom culture is not available, some experts support use of NAATs on vaginal swabs if a positive result can be verified by a different NAAT. Detection of gonorrhea in a child requires an evaluation for other sexually transmitted infections, such as *C trachomatis* infection, syphilis, and human immunodeficiency virus (HIV) infection. Completion of the series of vaccines for hepatitis B and human papillomavirus should be documented, then offered if not completed and if appropriate for the age group.

TREATMENT[1]**:** Increases in the prevalence of fluoroquinolone resistance among gonococcal isolates in the United States resulted in new treatment recommendations in 2007. Because of the high prevalence of penicillin-, tetracycline-, and quinolone-resistant *N gonorrhoeae*, an extended-spectrum cephalosporin (eg, ceftriaxone, cefixime) is recommended as initial therapy for children and adults (see Table 3.7, p 339).[2] Antimicrobial resistance is widespread in many parts of the world, so treatment recommendations may vary depending on where infection was acquired.

Ceftriaxone is recommended for gonococcal infections of all sites in children and adults. Cefixime is recommended for uncomplicated gonococcal infections of the vagina, pubertal cervix, urethra, and rectum of a prepubertal child. Cefotaxime also can be used for gonococcal ophthalmia, scalp abscesses, and disseminated gonococcal infection in newborn infants.

All patients with presumed or proven gonorrhea should be evaluated for concurrent syphilis, HIV, and *C trachomatis* infections. Completion of the series of vaccines for hepatitis B and human papillomavirus should be documented and then recommended if not completed and if appropriate for the age group. All patients beyond the neonatal period with gonorrhea should be treated presumptively for *C trachomatis* infection (see *Chlamydia trachomatis*, p 276). A single dose of ceftriaxone, spectinomycin, or azithromycin is not effective treatment for concurrent infection with syphilis (see Syphilis, p 690).

Test-of-cure samples are not required in adolescents or adults with uncomplicated gonorrhea who are asymptomatic after being treated with one of the recommended antimicrobial regimens. However, because reinfection by a new or untreated partner is not uncommon, clinicians may consider advising sexually active adolescents and adults with gonorrhea to be retested 3 months after treatment. Children treated with ceftriaxone do not require follow-up cultures unless they remain in an at-risk environment, but if treated with other regimens, then follow-up culture is indicated. Patients who have symptoms that persist after treatment or whose symptoms recur shortly after treatment should be reevaluated by culture for *N gonorrhoeae*, and any gonococci isolated should be tested for antimicrobial susceptibility. Although treatment failure after cephalosporin therapy is rare in the United States, MICs to cephalosporins are increasing.[3] Treatment failures have been reported more frequently from Asian countries. In addition to submission of clinical specimens for culture and susceptibility testing, a history of recent travel or sexual activity

---

[1] Centers for Disease Control and Prevention. Sexually transmitted diseases treatment guidelines, 2010. *MMWR Recomm Rep*. 2010;59(RR-12):1:110

[2] Centers for Disease Control and Prevention. Update to CDC's sexually transmitted disease treatment guidelines, 2006: fluoroquinolones no longer recommended for treatment of gonococcal infections. *MMWR Morb Mortal Wkly Rep*. 2007;56(14):332–336

[3] Centers for Disease Control and Prevention. Cephalosporin susceptibility among *Neisseria gonorrhoeae* isolates—United States, 2000–2010. *MMWR Morb Mortal Wkly Rep*. 2011;60(26):873–877

Table 3.7. Uncomplicated Gonococcal Infection: Treatment of Children Beyond the Newborn Period and Adolescents[a]

Disease[b]	Prepubertal Children Who Weigh Less Than 100 lb (45 kg)	Disease[b]	Patients Who Weigh 100 lb (45 kg) or More and Who Are 8 Years of Age or Older
Uncomplicated vulvo-vaginitis, cervicitis, urethritis, proctitis, or pharyngitis	Ceftriaxone, 125 mg, IM, in a single dose **OR** Cefixime, 8 mg/kg (maximum 400 mg), orally, in a single dose **PLUS[a]** Erythromycin base or ethylsuccinate, 50 mg/kg per day (maximum 2 g/day), orally, in 4 divided doses for 14 days **OR** Azithromycin, 20 mg/kg (maximum 1 g), orally, in a single dose	Uncomplicated endo-cervicitis, urethritis, proctitis, or pharyngitis[c]	Ceftriaxone, 250 mg, IM, in a single dose **OR** Cefixime, 400 mg, orally, in a single dose **PLUS[a]** Azithromycin, 1 g, orally, in a single dose **OR** Doxycycline, 100 mg, orally, twice a day for 7 days

IM indicates intramuscularly.

[a] In addition to the recommended treatment for gonococcal infection, therapy for *Chlamydia trachomatis* is recommended on the presumption that the patient has concomitant infection.

[b] Spectinomycin has been effective in published clinical trials (except for pharyngeal infection) but is not available in the United States.

[c] Alternative regimens include ceftizoxime (500 mg, IM, in a single dose), cefotaxime (500 mg, IM, in a single dose), cefpodoxime (400 mg, orally, in a single dose), or cefoxitin (2 g, IM, administered with probenecid, 1 g, orally). Only ceftriaxone is recommended for pharyngitis; in people who cannot take ceftriaxone, desensitization should be considered, or azithromycin (2 g, orally) is effective, but concerns about ease of development of resistance should restrict its use to limited circumstances (Centers for Disease Control and Prevention. *Neisseria gonorrhoeae* with reduced susceptibility to azithromycin—San Diego County, California, 2009. *MMWR Morb Mortal Wkly Rep.* 2011;60[18]:579–581).

in Asian countries should be elicited in people with treatment failure. Clinicians and laboratory personnel should report treatment failures or resistant gonococcal isolates to the CDC through their state or local health department.

Specific recommendations for management and antimicrobial therapy are as follows:

Neonatal Disease. Infants with clinical evidence of ophthalmia neonatorum, scalp abscess, or disseminated infections attributable to *N gonorrhoeae* should be hospitalized. Cultures of blood, eye discharge, and other potential sites of infection, such as CSF, should be performed on specimens from infants to confirm the diagnosis and to determine antimicrobial susceptibility. Tests for concomitant infection with *C trachomatis*, congenital syphilis, and HIV infection should be performed. Results of the maternal test for hepatitis B surface antigen should be confirmed. The mother and her partner(s) also need appropriate examination and management for *N gonorrhoeae*.

Nondisseminated Neonatal Infections. Recommended antimicrobial therapy, including that for ophthalmia neonatorum, is ceftriaxone (25–50 mg/kg, intravenously or intramuscularly, not to exceed 125 mg) given once. Infants with gonococcal ophthalmia should receive eye irrigations with saline solution immediately and at frequent intervals until discharge is eliminated. Topical antimicrobial treatment alone is inadequate and unnecessary when recommended systemic antimicrobial treatment is given. Infants with gonococcal ophthalmia should be hospitalized and evaluated for disseminated infection (sepsis, arthritis, meningitis).

Disseminated Neonatal Infections. Recommended therapy for arthritis and septicemia is ceftriaxone or cefotaxime for 7 days. Cefotaxime is recommended for infants with hyperbilirubinemia. If meningitis is documented, treatment should be continued for a total of 10 to 14 days.

Gonococcal Infections in Children Beyond the Neonatal Period and Adolescents. Recommendations for treatment of gonococcal infections, by age and weight, are given in Tables 3.7 (p 339) and 3.8 (p 341).

Special Problems in Treatment of Children (Beyond the Neonatal Period) and Adolescents. Patients with uncomplicated infections of the vagina, endocervix, urethra, or anorectum and a history of severe adverse reactions to cephalosporins (anaphylaxis, Stevens-Johnson syndrome, and toxic epidermal necrolysis) should be treated with spectinomycin (40 mg/kg, maximum 2 g, given intramuscularly as a single dose), if available (spectinomycin currently is not available in the United States). Because data are limited regarding alternative regimens for treating gonorrhea among people who have documented severe cephalosporin allergy, consultation with an expert in infectious diseases is recommended. One treatment option is cephalosporin treatment after desensitization. If desensitization is not an option, azithromycin may be considered. Azithromycin (2 g, orally) is effective against uncomplicated gonococcal infection and *C trachomatis* infection, but because of concerns regarding emerging antimicrobial resistance to macrolides, its use should be restricted to limited circumstances.

Patients with uncomplicated pharyngeal gonococcal infection should be treated with ceftriaxone (Table 3.7, p 339) in a single dose. Spectinomycin is approximately 50% effective for treatment of pharyngeal gonorrhea, so it should be used only in people with a history of severe cephalosporin allergy, and a pharyngeal culture should be obtained 3 to 5 days after treatment to verify eradication; spectinomycin currently is not available in the United States. A single dose of ceftriaxone is not effective treatment for concurrent infection with syphilis (see Syphilis, p 690). Spectinomycin is not active against *Treponema pallidum*.

Table 3.8. Complicated Gonococcal Infection: Treatment of Children Beyond the Newborn Period and Adolescents[a]

Disease[b]	Prepubertal Children Who Weigh Less Than 100 lb (45 kg)	Disease[b]	Patients Who Weigh 100 lb (45 kg) or More and Who Are 8 Years of Age or Older
Disseminated gonococcal infection (eg, arthritis-dermatitis syndrome)	Ceftriaxone, 50 mg/kg/day (maximum 1 g/day), IV or IM, once a day for 7 days **PLUS**[a] Erythromycin base or ethylsuccinate 50 mg/kg/day (maximum 2 g), orally, divided into 4 doses daily for 14 days[c]	Disseminated gonococcal infections[d]	Ceftriaxone, 1 g, IV or IM, given once a day for 7 days[e] **PLUS**[a] Azithromycin 1 g, orally, in a single dose **OR** Doxycycline, 100 mg, orally or IV, twice a day for 7 days
Meningitis or endocarditis	Ceftriaxone, 50 mg/kg/day (maximum 2 g/day), IV or IM, given every 12 h; for meningitis, duration is 10–14 days; for endocarditis, duration is at least 28 days **PLUS**[a] Erythromycin base or ethylsuccinate 50 mg/kg/day, orally, divided into 4 doses daily for 14 days[c]	Meningitis or endocarditis	Ceftriaxone, 1–2 g, IV, every 12 h; for meningitis, duration is 10–14 days; for endocarditis, duration is at least 28 days **PLUS**[a] Azithromycin 1 g, orally, in a single dose **OR** Doxycycline, 100 mg, orally or IV, twice a day for 7 days
Conjunctivitis[f]	Ceftriaxone, 50 mg/kg (maximum 125 mg), IM, in a single dose	Conjunctivitis[f]	Ceftriaxone, 1 g, IM, in a single dose **PLUS**[a] Azithromycin, 1 g, orally, in a single dose **OR** Doxycycline, 100 mg, orally, twice daily for 7 days
		Epididymitis	Ceftriaxone, 250 mg, IM, in a single dose **PLUS**[a] Doxycycline, 100 mg, orally, twice daily for 10 days

Table 3.8. Complicated Gonococcal Infection: Treatment of Children Beyond the Newborn Period and Adolescents,[a] continued

Disease[b]	Prepubertal Children Who Weigh Less Than 100 lb (45 kg)	Disease[b]	Patients Who Weigh 100 lb (45 kg) or More and Who Are 8 Years of Age or Older
Conjunctivitis,[f] continued		Pelvic inflammatory disease	See Table 3.43, p 552

IV indicates intravenously; IM, intramuscularly.

[a] Concomitant therapy for *Chlamydia trachomatis* is recommended in addition to the recommended treatment for gonococcal infection.

[b] Hospitalization should be considered, especially for people treated as outpatients whose infection has failed to respond and people who are unlikely to adhere to treatment regimens. Patients with meningitis or endocarditis should be hospitalized.

[c] Limited evidence suggests that azithromycin, 20 mg/kg (maximum 1 g), orally, in a single dose, is an alternative treatment for chlamydia in children who weigh less than 45 kg.

[d] An alternative for people who are allergic to beta-lactam drugs is spectinomycin, 2 g, IM, every 12 hours. Spectinomycin treatment requires a follow-up culture if pharyngeal infection exists. **Spectinomycin currently is not available in the United States.**

[e] Alternatively, parenteral therapy can be discontinued 24 to 48 hours after improvement occurs, at which time therapy can be switched to an oral regimen (cefixime, 400 mg, orally, twice a day), to complete at least a 7-day course.

[f] Eyes should be lavaged with saline solution to clear accumulated secretions.

Adapted from Centers for Disease Control and Prevention. Sexually transmitted diseases treatment guidelines, 2010. *MMWR Recomm Rep.* 2010;59(RR-12):1–109 (see **www.cdc.gov/std/treatment**).

Children or adolescents with HIV infection should receive the same treatment for gonococcal infection as children without HIV infection.

Acute PID. *N gonorrhoeae* and *C trachomatis* are implicated in many cases of PID; most cases have a polymicrobial etiology. No reliable clinical criteria distinguish gonococcal from nongonococcal-associated PID. Hence, broad-spectrum treatment regimens are recommended (see Pelvic Inflammatory Disease, p 548).

Acute Epididymitis. Sexually transmitted organisms, such as *N gonorrhoeae* or *C trachomatis*, can cause acute epididymitis in sexually active adolescents and young adults but rarely if ever cause acute epididymitis in prepubertal children. The recommended regimen for sexually transmitted epididymitis is ceftriaxone plus doxycycline (see Table 3.8, p 341).

ISOLATION OF THE HOSPITALIZED PATIENT: Standard precautions are recommended, including for newborn infants with ophthalmia.

CONTROL MEASURES:

Neonatal Ophthalmia. For routine prophylaxis of infants immediately after birth, 0.5% erythromycin ophthalmic ointment is instilled into each eye; subsequent irrigation should not be performed (see Prevention of Neonatal Ophthalmia, p 880). Also approved for prophylaxis of neonatal ophthalmia are 1% tetracycline ophthalmic ointment and 1% silver nitrate, but these no longer are available in the United States. Prophylaxis may be delayed for as long as 1 hour after birth to facilitate parent-infant bonding. The efficacy of topical prophylaxis in preventing chlamydial ophthalmia is less clear, likely because colonization of the nasopharynx is not prevented.

Infants Born to Mothers With Gonococcal Infections. When prophylaxis is administered correctly, infants born to mothers with gonococcal infection rarely develop gonococcal ophthalmia. However, because gonococcal ophthalmia or disseminated infection occasionally can occur in this situation, infants born to mothers known to have gonorrhea should receive ceftriaxone as a single dose of 25 to 50 mg/kg, to a maximum of 125 mg (see Prevention of Neonatal Ophthalmia, p 880).

Children and Adolescents With Sexual Exposure to a Patient Known to Have Gonorrhea. Exposed people should undergo examination, culture, and the same treatment as people known to have gonorrhea.

Pregnancy. All pregnant women at risk of gonorrhea or living in an area in which the prevalence of *N gonorrhoeae* is high should have an endocervical culture for gonococci at the time of their first prenatal visit. A repeat test in the third trimester is recommended for women at continued risk of gonococcal infection. Recommended therapeutic regimens for patients found to be infected are as described previously for gonococcal infection, except that doxycycline should not be used in pregnant women with PID because of the potential toxic effects on the fetus. Women who are allergic to cephalosporins should be treated with spectinomycin, if available, although spectinomycin is unreliable against pharyngeal gonococcal infection (spectinomycin currently is not available in the United States). Other options for pregnant women with severe cephalosporin allergy include cephalosporin treatment after desensitization or azithromycin (2 g, orally).

Case Reporting and Management of Sexual Partners. All cases of gonorrhea must be reported to local public health officials (see Appendix VI, Nationally Notifiable Infectious Diseases in the United States, p 902). Ensuring that sexual contacts are treated and counseled to use condoms is essential for community control, prevention of reinfection, and prevention of complications in the contact. Recommendations for services provided to partners of people with gonorrhea are available.[1] Cases in prepubertal children must be investigated to determine the source of infection.

For patients with gonorrhea whose partners' treatment cannot be ensured or is unlikely, delivery of antimicrobial therapy (ie, either a prescription or medication) by heterosexual male or female patients to their partners is an option, particularly in states where patient-delivered partner therapy (PDPT) is allowed (**www.cdc.gov/std/ept/**). Use of this approach always should be accompanied by efforts to educate partners about symptoms and to encourage partners to seek clinical evaluation. This approach has not been studied adequately as a part of routine partner management in men who have sex with men (MSM), a population with a high risk of coexisting undiagnosed sexually transmitted infections and HIV infection.

Granuloma Inguinale
(Donovanosis)

CLINICAL MANIFESTATIONS: Initial lesions of this sexually transmitted infection are single or multiple subcutaneous nodules that progress to form painless, highly vascular, beefy red and friable, granulomatous ulcers without regional adenopathy. Lesions usually involve genitalia, but anal infections occur in 5% to 10% of patients; lesions at distant sites (eg, face, mouth, or liver) are rare. Subcutaneous extension into the inguinal area results in induration that can mimic inguinal adenopathy (ie, "pseudobubo"). Fibrosis manifests as sinus tracts, adhesions, and lymphedema, resulting in extreme genital deformity. Urethral obstruction can occur.

ETIOLOGY: The disease, Donovanosis, is caused by *Klebsiella granulomatis* (formerly known as *Calymmatobacterium granulomatis*), an intracellular gram-negative bacillus.

EPIDEMIOLOGY: Indigenous granuloma inguinale occurs rarely in the United States and most industrialized nations. Cases still are reported in Papua, New Guinea, and parts of India, southern Africa, central Australia, and to a much lesser extent, the Caribbean and parts of South America, most notably Brazil. The highest incidence of disease occurs in tropical and subtropical environments. The incidence of infection seems to correlate with sustained high temperatures and high relative humidity. Infection usually is acquired by sexual intercourse, most commonly with a person with active infection but possibly also from a person with asymptomatic rectal infection. Young children can acquire infection by contact with infected secretions. The period of communicability extends throughout the duration of active lesions or rectal colonization.

The **incubation period** is 8 to 80 days.

DIAGNOSTIC TESTS: The causative organism is difficult to culture, and diagnosis requires microscopic demonstration of dark staining intracytoplasmic Donovan bodies on Wright or Giemsa staining of a crush preparation from subsurface scrapings of a lesion or tissue. The microorganism also can be detected by histologic examination of biopsy specimens. Lesions should be cultured for *Haemophilus ducreyi* to exclude chancroid. Granuloma inguinale often is misdiagnosed as carcinoma, which can be excluded by histologic examination of tissue or by response of the lesion to antimicrobial agents. Diagnosis by polymerase chain reaction assay and serologic testing is available only in research laboratories.

---

[1] Centers for Disease Control and Prevention. Recommendations for partner services programs for HIV infection, syphilis, gonorrhea, and chlamydial infection. *MMWR Recomm Rep.* 2008;57(RR-9):1–63

TREATMENT: Doxycycline is the treatment of choice. Doxycycline should not be given to children younger than 8 years of age or to pregnant women. Trimethoprim-sulfamethoxazole is an alternative regimen, except in pregnant women. Ciprofloxacin, which is not recommended for use in pregnant or lactating women or children younger than 18 years of age, is effective. Gentamicin can be added if no improvement is evident in several days. Erythromycin or azithromycin is an alternative therapy for pregnant women or women who are infected with human immunodeficiency virus. Antimicrobial therapy is continued for at least 3 weeks or until the lesions have resolved. Partial healing usually is noted within 7 days of initiation of therapy. Relapse can occur, especially if the antimicrobial agent is stopped before the primary lesion has healed completely. Complicated or long-standing infection can require surgical intervention.

Patients should be evaluated for other sexually transmitted infections, such as gonorrhea, syphilis, chancroid, chlamydia, hepatitis B virus, and human immunodeficiency virus infections. Immunization status for hepatitis B and human papillomavirus should be reviewed and documented and then recommended if not complete and appropriate for age.

ISOLATION OF THE HOSPITALIZED PATIENT: Standard precautions are recommended.

CONTROL MEASURES: Sexual partners should be examined, counseled to use condoms, and offered antimicrobial therapy (but only if lesions are present).

Haemophilus influenzae Infections

CLINICAL MANIFESTATIONS: *Haemophilus influenzae* type b (Hib) causes pneumonia, bacteremia, meningitis, epiglottitis, septic arthritis, cellulitis, otitis media, purulent pericarditis, and other less common infections, such as endocarditis, endophthalmitis, osteomyelitis, peritonitis, and gangrene. Non-type b encapsulated strains can cause disease similar to type b infections. Nontypable strains more commonly cause infections of the respiratory tract (eg, otitis media, sinusitis, pneumonia, conjunctivitis) and, less often, bacteremia, meningitis, chorioamnionitis, and neonatal septicemia.

ETIOLOGY: *H influenzae* is a pleomorphic gram-negative coccobacillus. Encapsulated strains express 1 of 6 antigenically distinct capsular polysaccharides (a through f); nonencapsulated strains lack capsule genes and are designated nontypable.

EPIDEMIOLOGY: The major reservoir of Hib is young infants and toddlers, who carry the organism in the upper respiratory tract, which is the natural habitat of *H influenzae* in humans. The mode of transmission is person-to-person by inhalation of respiratory tract droplets or by direct contact with respiratory tract secretions. In neonates, infection is acquired intrapartum by aspiration of amniotic fluid or by contact with genital tract secretions containing the organism. Pharyngeal colonization by *H influenzae* is relatively common, especially with nontypable and nontype b capsular type strains.

Before introduction of effective Hib conjugate vaccines, Hib was the most common cause of bacterial meningitis in children in the United States. The peak incidence of invasive Hib infections occurred between 6 and 18 months of age. In contrast, the peak age for Hib epiglottitis was 2 to 4 years of age.

Unimmunized children younger than 4 years of age are at increased risk of invasive Hib disease. Factors that predispose to invasive disease include sickle cell disease, asplenia, human immunodeficiency virus (HIV) infection, certain immunodeficiency syndromes, and malignant neoplasms. Historically, invasive Hib was more common in boys; black, Alaska Native, Apache, and Navajo children; child care attendees; children living in crowded conditions; and children who were not breastfed.

Since introduction of Hib conjugate vaccines in the United States, the incidence of invasive Hib disease has decreased by 99% to fewer than 2 cases per 100 000 children younger than 5 years of age. In the United States, invasive Hib disease occurs primarily in underimmunized children and among infants too young to have completed the primary immunization series. Hib remains an important pathogen in many resource-limited countries where Hib vaccines are not available routinely. The epidemiology of invasive *H influenzae* disease in the United States has shifted in the postvaccination era. Nontypable *H influenzae* now causes the majority of invasive *H influenzae* disease in all age groups. From 1999 through 2008, the annual incidence of invasive nontypable *H influenzae* disease was 1.73/100 000 in children younger than 5 years of age and 4.08/100 000 in adults 65 years of age and older.

Nontypable *H influenzae* causes approximately 30% to 50% of episodes of acute otitis media and sinusitis in children and is a common cause of recurrent otitis media. These infections are twice as frequent in boys and peak in the late fall.

The **incubation period** is unknown.

DIAGNOSTIC TESTS: The diagnosis of invasive disease is established by growth of *H influenzae* from cerebrospinal fluid (CSF), blood, synovial fluid, pleural fluid, or pericardial fluid. Gram stain of an infected body fluid specimen can facilitate presumptive diagnosis. All *H influenzae* isolates associated with invasive infection should be serotyped. Although the potential for suboptimal sensitivity and specificity exists with slide agglutination serotyping (SAST) depending on reagents used, SAST or genotyping by polymerase chain reaction (PCR) are acceptable methods for capsule typing. If PCR capsular typing is not available locally, isolates can be submitted to the state health department or to a reference laboratory for testing.

Otitis media attributable to *H influenzae* is diagnosed by culture of tympanocentesis fluid; cultures of other respiratory tract swab specimens (eg, throat, ear drainage) are not indicative of middle-ear culture results.

TREATMENT:
- Initial therapy for children with meningitis possibly caused by Hib is cefotaxime or ceftriaxone. Meropenem is an alternative empiric agent. Ampicillin can be substituted if the Hib isolate is susceptible to ampicillin. Treatment of other invasive *H influenzae* infections is similar. Therapy is continued at least 10 days by the intravenous route and longer in complicated infections.
- Dexamethasone may be beneficial for treatment of infants and children with Hib meningitis to diminish the risk of hearing loss, if given before or concurrently with the first dose of antimicrobial agent(s).
- Epiglottitis is a medical emergency. An airway must be established promptly with an endotracheal tube or by tracheostomy.
- Infected pleural or pericardial fluid should be drained.
- For empiric treatment of acute otitis media in children younger than 2 years of age or in children 2 years of age or older with severe disease, oral amoxicillin (see details in Pneumococcal Infections, p 571, and Appropriate Use of Antimicrobial Agents, p 802) is rec-

ommended.[1] Duration of therapy is 5 to 10 days. The 5- to 7-day course is considered for children 2 years of age and older. In the United States, approximately 30% to 40% of *H influenzae* isolates produce beta-lactamase, necessitating a beta-lactamase–resistant agent, such as amoxicillin-clavulanate; an oral cephalosporin, such as cefdinir, cefuroxime, or cefpodoxime; or azithromycin for children with beta-lactam antibiotic allergy. In vitro susceptibility testing of isolates from middle-ear fluid specimens help guide therapy in complicated or persistent cases.

ISOLATION OF THE HOSPITALIZED PATIENT: In patients with invasive Hib disease, droplet precautions are recommended for 24 hours after initiation of effective antimicrobial therapy.

CONTROL MEASURES (FOR INVASIVE HIB DISEASE):

Care of Exposed People. Careful observation of exposed, unimmunized, or incompletely immunized children who are household, child care, or nursery school contacts of patients with invasive Hib disease is essential. Exposed children in whom febrile illness develops should receive prompt medical evaluation.

Chemoprophylaxis. The risk of invasive Hib disease is increased among unimmunized household contacts younger than 4 years of age. Rifampin eradicates Hib from the pharynx in approximately 95% of carriers and decreases the risk of secondary invasive illness in exposed household contacts. Nursery and child care center contacts also may be at increased risk of secondary disease. Secondary disease in child care contacts is rare when all contacts are older than 2 years of age.

Indications and guidelines for chemoprophylaxis in different circumstances are summarized in Table 3.9 (p 348).

- **Household.** Chemoprophylaxis is not recommended for contacts of people with invasive disease caused by nontype b *H influenzae* strains, because secondary disease is rare. In households with a person with invasive Hib disease and at least 1 household member who is younger than 48 months of age and unimmunized or incompletely immunized against Hib, rifampin prophylaxis is recommended for all household contacts, regardless of age. In households with a contact who is an immunocompromised child, even if the child is older than 48 months of age and fully immunized, all members of the household should receive rifampin because of the possibility that immunization may not have been effective. Similarly, in households with a contact younger than 12 months of age who has not received the 2- or 3-dose primary series of Hib conjugate vaccine, depending on vaccine product, all household members should receive rifampin prophylaxis. Given that most secondary cases in households occur during the first week after hospitalization of the index case, when indicated, prophylaxis (see Table 3.9, p 348) should be initiated as soon as possible. Because some secondary cases occur later, initiation of prophylaxis 7 days or more after hospitalization of the index patient still may be of some benefit.

- **Child care and preschool.** When 2 or more cases of invasive Hib disease have occurred within 60 days and unimmunized or incompletely immunized children attend the child care facility or preschool, rifampin prophylaxis for all attendees (irrespective of their age and vaccine status) and child care providers should be considered. In addition to these recommendations for chemoprophylaxis, unimmunized or incompletely

[1] American Academy of Pediatrics, Subcommittee on Management of Acute Otitis Media. Diagnosis and management of acute otitis media. *Pediatrics.* 2004;113(5):1451–1465

Table 3.9. Indications and Guidelines for Rifampin Chemoprophylaxis for Contacts of Index Cases of Invasive *Haemophilus influenzae* Type b (Hib) Disease

Chemoprophylaxis Recommended

- For all household contacts[a] in the following circumstances:
  - Household with at least 1 contact younger than 4 years of age who is unimmunized or incompletely immunized[b]
  - Household with a child younger than 12 months of age who has not completed the primary Hib series
  - Household with a contact who is an immunocompromised child, regardless of that child's Hib immunization status
- For preschool and child care center contacts when 2 or more cases of Hib invasive disease have occurred within 60 days (see text)
- For index patient, if younger than 2 years of age or member of a household with a susceptible contact and treated with a regimen other than cefotaxime or ceftriaxone, chemoprophylaxis usually is provided just before discharge from hospital

Chemoprophylaxis Not Recommended

- For occupants of households with no children younger than 4 years of age other than the index patient
- For occupants of households when all household contacts 12 through 48 months of age have completed their Hib immunization series and when household contacts younger than 12 months of age have completed their primary series of Hib immunizations
- For preschool and child care contacts of 1 index case
- For pregnant women

[a] Defined as people residing with the index patient or nonresidents who spent 4 or more hours with the index patient for at least 5 of the 7 days preceding the day of hospital admission of the index case.
[b] Complete immunization is defined as having had at least 1 dose of conjugate vaccine at 15 months of age or older; 2 doses between 12 and 14 months of age; or the 2- or 3-dose primary series when younger than 12 months with a booster dose at 12 months of age or older.

immunized children should receive a dose of vaccine and should be scheduled for completion of the recommended age-specific immunization schedule (see Fig 1.1–1.3, p 27–31). Data are insufficient on the risk of secondary transmission to recommend chemoprophylaxis for attendees and child care providers when a single case of invasive Hib disease occurs; the decision to provide chemoprophylaxis in this situation is at the discretion of the local health department.

- **Index case.** Treatment of Hib disease with cefotaxime or ceftriaxone eradicates Hib colonization, eliminating the need for prophylaxis of the index patient. Patients who are treated with ampicillin, meropenem, or another antibiotic regimen and who are younger than 2 years of age should receive rifampin prophylaxis at the end of therapy for invasive infection.
- **Dosage.** Rifampin should be given orally, once a day for 4 days (20 mg/kg; maximum dose, 600 mg). The dose for infants younger than 1 month of age is not established; some experts recommend lowering the dose to 10 mg/kg. For adults, each dose is 600 mg.

Immunization. Two single-antigen (monovalent) Hib conjugate vaccine products and 2 combination vaccine products that contain Hib conjugate are available in the United States (see Table 3.10). The Hib conjugate vaccines consist of the Hib capsular poly-saccharide (polyribosylribotol phosphate [PRP]) covalently linked to a carrier protein. Protective antibodies are directed against PRP. Conjugate vaccines vary in composition and immunogenicity, and as a result, recommendations for their use differ.

Depending on the vaccine, the recommended primary series consists of 3 doses given at 2, 4, and 6 months of age or 2 doses given at 2 and 4 months of age (see Recommendations for Immunization, p 350, and Table 3.11, p 350). The recommended doses can be given as a Hib-hepatitis B (HepB) combination or as a diphtheria and tetanus tox-oids and acellular pertussis (DTaP)-inactivated poliovirus (IPV)/Hib combination vaccine. The regimens in Table 3.11 (p 350) likely are to be equivalent in protection after completion of the recommended primary series. For American Indian/Alaska Native children, opti-mal immune protection is achieved by administration of PRP-OMP (outer membrane protein complex) Hib vaccine (see American Indian/Alaska Native Children, *Haemophilus influenzae* type b, p 94).

Combination Vaccines. Two combination vaccines that contain Hib are licensed in the United States: HepB-Hib combination and DTaP-IPV/Hib combination (see Table 3.10) vaccines. The HepB-Hib combination vaccine is licensed for use at 2, 4, and 12 through 15 months of age and should not be given to infants younger than 6 weeks of age. The DTaP-IPV/Hib combination vaccine is licensed for children 6 weeks through 4 years of age, given as a 4-dose series at 2, 4, 6, and 15 through 18 months of age.

Vaccine Interchangeability. The monovalent Hib conjugate vaccines available in the United States are considered interchangeable for primary and booster immunization.

Table 3.10. *Haemophilus influenzae* Type b (Hib) Conjugate Vaccines Licensed for Use in Infants and Children in the United States[a]

Vaccine	Trade Name	Components	Manufacturer
PRP-T[b]	Hiberix[b]	PRP conjugated to tetanus toxoid	GlaxoSmithKline Biologicals
PRP-OMP	PedvaxHIB	PRP conjugated to OMP	Merck & Co, Inc
PRP-OMP-HepB[c]	Comvax	PRP-OMP + hepatitis B vaccine	Merck & Co, Inc
DTaP-IPV/PRP-T[d]	Pentacel	DTaP-IPV + PRP-T	Sanofi Pasteur

PRP-T indicates polyribosylribotol phosphate-tetanus toxoid; DTaP, diphtheria and tetanus toxoids and acellular pertussis; OMP, outer membrane protein complex from *Neisseria meningitidis;* HepB, hepatitis B vaccine.

[a] Hib conjugate vaccines may be given in combination products or as reconstituted products, provided the combination or reconstituted vaccine is licensed by the US Food and Drug Administration (FDA) for the child's age and administration of the other vaccine component(s) also is justified.

[b] PRP-T (Hiberix), manufactured by GlaxoSmithKline Biologicals, is licensed only for the final (booster) dose of the Hib vaccine series and should not be used for primary immunization in infants at 2, 4, or 6 months of age (Centers for Disease Control and Prevention. Licensure of a *Haemophilus influenzae* type b [Hib] vaccine [Hiberix] and updated recommendations for use of Hib vaccines. *MMWR Morb Mortal Wkly Rep.* 2009;58[36]:1008–1009).

[c] The combination *H influenzae* type b (PRP-OMP) and HepB (Recombivax, 5 μg) vaccine (Comvax) is licensed for use at 2, 4, and 12 through 15 months of age.

[d] The DTaP-IPV liquid component is used to reconstitute a lyophilized ActHIB vaccine component to form Pentacel.

Table 3.11. Recommended Regimens for Routine *Haemophilus influenzae* Type b (Hib) Conjugate Immunization for Children Immunized at 2 Months Through 4 Years of Age[a]

Vaccine Product Monovalent Vaccines	Primary Series	Booster Dose	Catch-up Doses[b]
PRP-T (GlaxoSmithKline)	Not licensed	12 through 15 mo	16 mo through 4 y
PRP-OMP (Merck)[c,d]	2, 4 mo	12 through 15 mo	16 mo through 4 y
Combination vaccines			
PRP-OMP-HepB[c,d]	2, 4 mo	12 through 15 mo	Not licensed
DTaP-IPV/PRP-T	2, 4, 6 mo	12 through 15 mo	16 mo through 4 y

PRP-T indicates polyribosylribotol phosphate-tetanus toxoid; OMP, outer membrane protein complex from *Neisseria meningitidis.*
[a] See text and Table 3.10 (p 349) for further information about specific vaccines and Table 1.8 (p 35) for information about combination vaccines.
[b] See Catch-up Immunization Schedule (Fig 1.3, p 31) for additional information.
[c] If a PRP-OMP vaccine is not administered as both doses in the primary series, a third dose of Hib conjugate vaccine is needed to complete the primary series
[d] Preferred for American Indian/Alaska Native children.

Dosage and Route of Administration. The dose of each Hib conjugate vaccine is 0.5 mL, given intramuscularly.

Children With Immunologic Impairment. Children at increased risk of Hib disease may have impaired anti-PRP antibody responses to conjugate vaccines. Examples include children with HIV infection; children with immunoglobulin deficiency; recipients of hematopoietic stem cell transplants; and children undergoing chemotherapy for a malignant neoplasm. Some children with immunologic impairment may benefit from more doses of conjugate vaccine than usually indicated (see Recommendations for Immunization, below).

Adverse Reactions. Adverse reactions to Hib conjugate vaccines are uncommon. Pain, redness, and swelling at the injection site occur in approximately 25% of recipients, but these symptoms typically are mild and last fewer than 24 hours.

Recommendations for Immunization.

Indications and Schedule

- All children should be immunized with an Hib conjugate vaccine beginning at approximately 2 months of age or as soon as possible thereafter (see Table 3.11). Other general recommendations are as follows:
  - Immunization can be initiated as early as 6 weeks of age.
  - Vaccine can be given during visits for other childhood immunizations (see Simultaneous Administration of Multiple Vaccines, p 33).

- For routine immunization of children younger than 7 months of age, the following guidelines are recommended:
  - **Primary series.** A 3-dose regimen of PRP-T (tetanus toxoid conjugate)-containing or a 2-dose regimen of PRP-OMP-containing vaccine should be administered (see Table 3.11, p 350). Doses are given at approximately 2-month intervals. When sequential doses of different vaccine products are given or uncertainty exists about which products previously were administered, 3 doses of a conjugate vaccine are considered sufficient to complete the primary series, regardless of the regimen used.
  - **Booster immunization at 12 through 15 months of age.** For children who have completed a primary series, an additional dose of conjugate vaccine is recommended at 12 through 15 months of age and at least 2 months after the last dose. Any monovalent or combination Hib conjugate vaccine is acceptable for this dose.
- Children younger than 5 years of age who did not receive Hib conjugate vaccine during the first 6 months of life should be immunized according to the recommended catch-up immunization schedule (see Fig 1.3, p 31, and Table 3.11, p 350). For accelerated immunization in infants younger than 12 months of age, a minimum of a 4-week interval between doses can be used.
- Special circumstances are as follows:
  - **Lapsed immunizations.** Recommendations for children who have had a lapse in the schedule of immunizations are based on limited data. Current recommendations are summarized in Fig 1.3 (p 31).
  - **Preterm infants.** For preterm infants, immunization should be based on chronologic age and should be initiated at 2 months of age according to recommendations in Table 3.11 (p 350).
  - Children with decreased or absent splenic function who have received a primary series of Hib immunizations and a booster dose at 12 months of age or older need not be immunized further. Children who have received a primary series and a booster dose and are undergoing scheduled splenectomy (eg, for Hodgkin disease, spherocytosis, immune thrombocytopenia, or hypersplenism) may benefit from an additional dose of any licensed conjugate vaccine. This dose should be provided at least 7 to 10 days before the procedure. Patients with HIV infection or immunoglobulin (Ig) G2 subclass deficiency and children receiving chemotherapy for malignant neoplasms also are at increased risk of invasive Hib disease. Whether these children will benefit from additional doses after completion of the primary series of immunizations and the booster dose at 12 months of age or later is unknown.

    For children 12 through 59 months of age with an underlying condition predisposing to Hib disease who are not immunized or have received only 1 dose of conjugate vaccine before 12 months of age, 2 doses of any conjugate vaccine, separated by 2 months, are recommended. For children in this age group who received 2 doses before 12 months of age, 1 additional dose of conjugate vaccine is recommended.
  - Unimmunized children with an underlying disease (sickle cell disease, leukemia, or HIV infection, or functional or anatomic asplenia) possibly predisposing to Hib disease who are older than 59 months of age should receive 1 dose of any licensed Hib conjugate vaccine.

♦ Children with Hib invasive infection younger than 24 months of age can remain at risk of developing a second episode of disease. These children should be immunized according to the age-appropriate schedule for unimmunized children and as if they had received no previous Hib vaccine doses (see Table 3.11, p 350, and Table 1.8, p 35). Immunization should be initiated 1 month after onset of disease or as soon as possible thereafter.

Immunologic evaluation should be performed in children who experience invasive Hib disease despite 2 to 3 doses of vaccine and in children with recurrent invasive disease attributable to type b strains.

Reporting. All cases of *H influenzae* invasive disease, including type b, nontype b, and nontypable, should be reported to the Centers for Disease Control and Prevention through the local or state public health department.

Hantavirus Pulmonary Syndrome

CLINICAL MANIFESTATIONS: Hantaviruses in humans cause 2 distinct syndromes: hantavirus pulmonary syndrome (HPS), a noncardiogenic pulmonary edema observed in the New World; and hemorrhagic fever with renal syndrome (HFRS), which occurs worldwide (see Hemorrhagic Fevers and Related Syndromes, p 358). After an incubation period of 1 to 5 weeks, the prodromal illness of HPS is 3 to 7 days and is characterized by fever; chills; headache; myalgia of the shoulders, lower back, and thighs; nausea; vomiting; diarrhea; dizziness; and sometimes cough. Respiratory tract symptoms or signs usually do not occur for the first 3 to 7 days, at which time pulmonary edema and severe hypoxemia appear abruptly after the onset of cough and dyspnea. The disease then progresses over a number of hours. In severe cases, persistent hypotension caused by myocardial dysfunction is present. In fatal cases, death occurs in 1 to 2 days following hospitalization.

Extensive bilateral interstitial and alveolar pulmonary edema and pleural effusions are the result of a diffuse pulmonary capillary leak and appear to be caused by immune response to hantavirus in endothelial cells of the microvasculature. Intubation and assisted ventilation usually are required for only 2 to 4 days, with resolution heralded by onset of diuresis and rapid clinical improvement.

The severe myocardial depression is different from that of septic shock; cardiac indices and stroke volume index are low, pulmonary wedge pressure is normal, and systemic vascular resistance is increased. Poor prognostic indicators include persistent hypotension, marked hemoconcentration, a cardiac index of less than 2, and abrupt onset of lactic acidosis with a serum lactate concentration of >4 mmol/L (36 mg/dL).

The mortality rate for patients with HPS is 30% to 40%. Asymptomatic and mild forms of disease are rare. Limited information suggests that clinical manifestations and prognosis are similar in adults and children. Serious sequelae are uncommon.

ETIOLOGY: Hantaviruses are RNA viruses of the Bunyaviridae family. Within the Hantavirus genus, Sin Nombre virus (SNV) is the major cause of HPS in the 4-corners region of the United States (Arizona, Colorado, New Mexico, Utah). Bayou virus, Black Creek Canal virus, Monongahela virus, and New York virus are responsible for sporadic cases in Louisiana, Texas, Florida, New York, and other areas of the eastern United States (Utah, Colorado, Arizona, and New Mexico). Hantavirus serotypes associated with an HPS syndrome in South America and Panama include Andes virus, Oran virus,

Laguna Negra virus, and Choclo virus. During the past decade, Chile and Argentina have reported most of the HPS cases in the Americas.

EPIDEMIOLOGY: Rodents, the natural hosts for hantaviruses, acquire a lifelong, asymptomatic, chronic infection with prolonged viruria and virus in saliva, urine, and feces. Humans acquire infection through direct contact with infected rodents, rodent droppings, or nests or inhalation of aerosolized virus particles from rodent urine, droppings, or saliva. Rarely, infection may be acquired from rodent bites or contamination of broken skin with excreta. Person-to-person transmission of hantaviruses has not been demonstrated in patients in the United States but has been reported in Chile and Argentina. At-risk activities include handling or trapping rodents; cleaning or entering closed, rarely used rodent-infested structures; cleaning feed storage or animal shelter areas; hand plowing; and living in a home with an increased density of mice in or around the home. For backpackers or campers, sleeping in a structure also inhabited by rodents has been associated with HPS. Weather conditions resulting in exceptionally heavy rainfall and improved rodent food supplies can result in a large increase in the rodent population. Increased rodent population results in more frequent contact between humans and infected mice and may account for increase human incidence. Most cases occur during spring and summer, and geographic location is determined by the habitat of the rodent carrier.

SNV is transmitted by the deer mouse, *Peromyscus maniculatus*; Black Creek Canal virus is transmitted by the cotton rat, *Sigmodon hispidus;* Bayou virus is transmitted by the rice rat, *Oryzomys palustris;* and New York virus is transmitted by the white-footed mouse, *Peromyscus leucopus.*

The **incubation period** may be 1 to 6 weeks after exposure to infected rodents, their saliva, or excreta.

DIAGNOSTIC TESTS: Characteristic laboratory findings include neutrophilic leukocytosis with immature granulocytes, more than 10% immunoblasts (basophilic cytoplasm, prominent nucleoli, and an increased nuclear-cytoplasmic ratio), thrombocytopenia, and increased hematocrit. In fatal cases, SNV has been identified by immunohistochemical staining of capillary endothelial cells of the lungs and almost every organ in the body. SNV RNA has been detected by reverse transcriptase-polymerase chain reaction assay of peripheral blood mononuclear cells and other clinical specimens from the early phase of the disease, frequently before the hospitalization. Viral RNA is not detected readily in bronchoalveolar lavage fluids.

Hantavirus-specific immunoglobulin (Ig) M and IgG antibodies are present at the onset of clinical disease. IgG could be missing in rapid fatal cases. A rapid diagnostic test can facilitate immediate appropriate supportive therapy and early transfer to a tertiary care facility. Enzyme immunoassay (available through many state health departments and the Centers for Disease Control and Prevention) and Western blot are assays that use recombinant antigens and have a high degree of specificity for detection of IgG and IgM antibody. Viral culture is not useful for diagnosis. Diagnosis can be made retrospectively by immunohistochemistry in tissues obtained from autopsy.

TREATMENT: Patients with suspected HPS should be transferred immediately to a tertiary care facility. Supportive management of pulmonary edema, severe hypoxemia, and hypotension during the first 24 to 48 hours is critical for recovery.

Extracorporeal membrane oxygenation (ECMO) may provide particularly important short-term support for the severe capillary leak syndrome in the lungs.

Ribavirin is active in vitro against hantaviruses including SNV. However, 2 clinical studies (1 open-label study and 1 randomized, placebo-controlled, double-blind study) found that intravenous ribavirin probably is ineffective in treatment of HPS in the cardiopulmonary stage. Steroids are being evaluated in South American trials.

ISOLATION OF THE HOSPITALIZED PATIENT: Standard precautions are recommended. HPS has not been associated with health care-associated or person-to-person transmission in the United States.

CONTROL MEASURES:

Care of Exposed People. Serial clinical examinations should be used to monitor people assessed to be at high risk of infection after a high-risk exposure (see Epidemiology, p 353).

Environmental Control. Hantavirus infections of humans occur primarily in adults and are associated with domestic, occupational, or leisure activities bringing humans into contact with infected rodents, usually in a rural setting. Eradicating the host reservoir is not feasible. The best available approach for disease control and prevention is risk reduction through environmental hygiene practices that discourage rodents from colonizing the home and work environment and that minimize aerosolization and contact with virus in saliva and excreta. Measures to decrease exposure in the home and workplace include eliminating food sources available to rodents in structures used by humans, limiting possible nesting sites, sealing holes and other possible entrances for rodents, and using "snap traps" and rodenticides. Before entering areas with potential rodent infestations, doors and windows should be opened to ventilate the enclosure.

Hantaviruses, because of their lipid envelope, are susceptible to most disinfectants, including diluted bleach solutions, detergents, and most general household disinfectants. Dusty or dirty areas or articles should be moistened with a 10% bleach or other disinfectant solution before being cleaned. Brooms and vacuum cleaners should not be used to clean rodent-infested areas. Use of a 10% bleach solution to disinfect dead rodents and wearing rubber gloves before handling trapped or dead rodents are recommended. Gloves and traps should be disinfected after use. The cleanup of areas potentially infested with hantavirus-infected rodents should be carried out by knowledgeable professionals using appropriate personal protective equipment. Potentially infected material removed should be handled according to local regulations as infectious waste.

Chemoprophylaxis measures or vaccines are not available.

Public Health Reporting. Possible occurrence should be reported immediately to local and state public health authorities.

Helicobacter pylori Infections

CLINICAL MANIFESTATIONS: *Helicobacter pylori* causes chronic active gastritis and results in duodenal, and to a lesser extent, gastric ulcers. Persistent infection with *H pylori* increases the risk of gastric cancer. *H pylori* infection can be asymptomatic or can result in gastroduodenal inflammation that can manifest as epigastric pain, nausea, vomiting, hematemesis, and guaiac-positive stools. Symptoms can resolve within a few days or wax and wane despite persistence of the organism for years or for life. *H pylori* infection is not associated with secondary gastritis (eg, autoimmune or chemical with nonsteroidal anti-inflammatory agents).

ETIOLOGY: *H pylori* is a gram-negative, spiral, curved, or U-shaped microaerophilic bacillus that has 2 to 6 sheathed flagella at one end. The organism is catalase, oxidase, and urease positive.

EPIDEMIOLOGY: *H pylori* organisms have been isolated from humans and other primates. An animal reservoir for human transmission has not been demonstrated. Organisms are transmitted from infected humans by the fecal-oral, gastro-oral, and oral-oral routes. Infection rates are low in children in resource-rich, industrialized countries except in children from lower socioeconomic groups. Most infections are acquired in the first 5 years of life and can reach prevalence rates of up to 80% in resource-limited countries. Approximately 70% of infected people are asymptomatic, 20% of people have macroscopic (ie, visual) and microscopic findings of ulceration, and an estimated 1% have features of neoplasia.

The **incubation period** is unknown.

DIAGNOSTIC TESTS: *H pylori* infection can be diagnosed by culture of gastric biopsy tissue on nonselective media (eg, chocolate agar) or selective media (eg, Skirrow agar) at 37°C (98°F) under microaerobic conditions for 3 to 7 days. Organisms usually can be visualized on histologic sections with Warthin-Starry silver, Steiner, Giemsa, or Genta staining. Presence of *H pylori* can be diagnosed but not excluded on the basis of hematoxylin-eosin stains. Because of production of urease by organisms, urease testing of a gastric specimen can give a rapid and specific microbiologic diagnosis. Each of these tests requires endoscopy and biopsy. Noninvasive, commercially available tests for active infection include breath tests that detect labeled carbon dioxide in expired air after oral administration of isotopically labeled urea (^{13}C or ^{14}C); these tests are expensive and are not useful in young children. The US Food and Drug Administration approved the first *H pylori* breath test for children 3 to 17 years of age in 2012. A stool antigen test (monoclonal antibody test) also is available commercially and can be used for children of any age, especially before and after treatment. Each of these commercially available tests for active infection (ie, breath or stool tests) has a high sensitivity and specificity. Serologic testing for *H pylori* infection by detection of immunoglobulin G (IgG) antibodies specific for *H pylori* does not help clarify the current status of infection and is not recommended for screening children.

TREATMENT: Treatment is recommended for infected patients who have peptic ulcer disease (currently or in the past 1–5 years), gastric mucosa-associated lymphoid tissue-type lymphoma, or early gastric cancer. Screening for and treatment of infection, if found, also is recommended for children with one or more primary relatives with gastric cancer, children who are in a high-risk group for gastric cancer (eg, immigrants from resource-limited countries or countries with high rates of gastric cancer) or children who have unexplained iron-deficiency anemia. Treatment is recommended if infection is found at the time of diagnostic endoscopy for gastrointestinal tract symptoms even if gastritis is the only histologic lesion found. Eradication therapy for *H pylori* consists of at least 7 to 14 days of treatment; eradication rates are higher for regimens of 14 days. A number of treatment regimens have been evaluated and are approved for use in adults; the safety and efficacy of these regimens in pediatric patients has not been established. Effective treatment regimens include 2 antimicrobial agents (eg, clarithromycin plus either amoxicillin or metronidazole) plus a proton-pump inhibitor (lansoprazole, omeprazole, esomeprazole, pantoprazole, rabeprazole). These regimens are effective in eliminating the organism, healing the ulcer, and preventing recurrence. Alternate therapies in people 8 years of age and older include bismuth subsalicylate plus metronidazole plus tetracycline plus either a proton-pump inhibitor or an H_2 blocker (eg, cimetidine, famotidine, nizatidine, and ranitidine) or bismuth subcitrate potassium plus metronidazole plus tetracycline plus omeprazole. Tetracycline products are not recommended in patients 8 years of age and younger (see Tetracyclines, p 801). A breath or stool test may be performed as follow-up to document organism eradication after completion of therapy, although the stool antigen test may remain positive for up to 90 days after treatment. Salvage therapies for treatment failure include increasing the duration of therapy (ie, 2 to 4 weeks) or bismuth-based quadruple therapy for 1 to 2 weeks (eg, bismuth subsalicylate plus 2 antibiotics and a proton pump inhibitor).

ISOLATION OF THE HOSPITALIZED PATIENT: Standard precautions are recommended.

CONTROL MEASURES: Disinfection of gastroscopes prevents transmission of the organism between patients.

Hemorrhagic Fevers Caused by Arenaviruses[1]

CLINICAL MANIFESTATIONS: Arenaviruses are responsible for several hemorrhagic fevers (HFs): Bolivian, Argentine, Brazilian, Venezuelan, Lassa, Chapare, and Lujo. Lymphocytic choriomeningitis virus (LCMV) also is an arenavirus but induces generally less severe disease, although it could be responsible for HFs in immunosuppressed patients; LCMV is discussed in a separate chapter (p 481). Disease associated with arenaviruses ranges in severity from mild, acute, febrile infections to severe illnesses in which vascular leak, shock, and multiorgan dysfunction are prominent features. Fever, headache, myalgia, conjunctival suffusion, bleeding, and abdominal pain are common early symptoms in all infections. Thrombocytopenia, axillary petechiae, and encephalopathy usually are present in Argentine HF, Bolivian HF, and Venezuelan HF, and exudative pharyngitis often occurs in Lassa fever. Mucosal bleeding occurs in severe cases as a consequence of vascular damage, thrombocytopenia, and platelet dysfunction. Proteinuria is common, but renal failure is unusual. Increased serum concentrations of aspartate transaminase can indicate a severe or fatal outcome of Lassa fever. Shock develops 7 to 9 days after onset of illness in more severely ill patients with these infections. Upper and lower respiratory tract symptoms can develop in people with Lassa fever. Encephalopathic signs such as tremor, alterations in consciousness, and seizures can occur in South American HFs and in severe cases of Lassa fever.

ETIOLOGY: Arenaviruses are RNA viruses. The major New World arenavirus hemorrhagic fevers occurring in the Western hemisphere are Argentine HF caused by Junin virus, Bolivian HF caused by Machupo virus, and Venezuelan HF caused by Guanarito virus. A fourth arenavirus, Sabia virus, caused 2 unrelated cases of naturally occurring HF in Brazil and 2 laboratory-acquired cases. Chapare virus has been isolated from a human fatal case in Bolivia. The Old World complex of arenaviruses includes Lassa virus, which causes Lassa fever in West Africa; Lujo virus, described in southern Africa during an outbreak characterized by fatal human-to-human transmission; and LCMV (see Lymphocytic Choriomeningitis, p 481) and usually produce less severe infections.

---

[1] Does not include lymphocytic choriomeningitis virus, which is reviewed on p 481.

Several other arenaviruses are known only from their rodent reservoirs in the Old and New World.

EPIDEMIOLOGY: Arenaviruses are maintained in nature by association with specific rodent hosts, in which they produce chronic viremia and viruria. The principal routes of infection are inhalation and contact of mucous membranes and skin (eg, through cuts, scratches, or abrasions) with urine and salivary secretions from these persistently infected rodents. All arenaviruses are infectious as aerosols, and arenaviruses causing HF should be considered highly hazardous to people working with any of the viruses in the laboratory. Laboratory-acquired infections have been documented with Lassa, Machupo, Junin, and Sabia viruses. The geographic distribution and habitats of the specific rodents that serve as reservoir hosts largely determine the areas with endemic infection and populations at risk. Before a vaccine became available in Argentina, several hundred cases of Argentine HF occurred yearly in agricultural workers and inhabitants of the Argentine pampas. The vaccine is not licensed in the United States. Epidemics of Bolivian HF occurred in small towns between 1962 and 1964; sporadic disease activity in the countryside has continued since then. Venezuelan HF first was identified in 1989 and occurs in rural north-central Venezuela. Lassa fever is endemic in most of West Africa, where rodent hosts live in proximity with humans, causing thousands of infections annually. Lassa fever has been reported in the United States in people who have traveled to West Africa.

The **incubation periods** are from 6 to 17 days.

DIAGNOSTIC TESTS: Viral nucleic acid can be detected in acute disease by reverse transcriptase-polymerase chain reaction assay. These viruses may be isolated from blood of acutely ill patients as well as from various tissues obtained postmortem, but isolation should be attempted only under Biosafety level-4 conditions. Virus antigen is detectable by enzyme immunoassay (EIA) in acute specimens and postmortem tissues. Virus-specific immunoglobulin (Ig) M antibodies are present in the serum during acute stages but may be undetectable in rapidly fatal cases. The IgG antibody response is delayed. Diagnosis can be made retrospectively by immunohistochemistry in tissues obtained from autopsy.

TREATMENT: Intravenous ribavirin substantially decreases the mortality rate in patients with severe Lassa fever, particularly if they are treated during the first week of illness. For Argentine HF, transfusion of immune plasma in defined doses of neutralizing antibodies is the standard specific treatment when administered during the first 8 days from onset of symptoms. Intravenous ribavirin initiated 8 days or more after onset of Argentine HF symptoms does not reduce mortality; whether ribavirin treatment initiated early in the course of the disease has a role in the treatment of Argentine HF remains to be seen. Intravenous ribavirin is not available commercially in the United States and can be obtained only under an investigational new drug (IND) application.

ISOLATION OF THE HOSPITALIZED PATIENT: In addition to standard precautions, contact and droplet precautions, including careful prevention of needlestick injuries and careful handling of clinical specimens for the duration of illness, are recommended for all HFs caused by arenaviruses. A negative-pressure ventilation room is recommended for patients with prominent cough or severe disease, and people entering the room should wear personal protection respirators. Additional viral HF-specific isolation precautions have been recommended in the event that a viral HF virus is used as a weapon of bioterrorism.[1]

---

[1] Centers for Disease Control and Prevention. Update: management of patients with suspected viral hemorrhagic fever—United States. *MMWR Morb Mortal Wkly Rep.* 1995;44(25):475–479

CONTROL MEASURES:

Care of Exposed People. No specific measures are warranted for exposed people unless direct contamination with blood, excretions, or secretions from an infected patient has occurred. If such contamination has occurred, recording body temperature twice daily for 21 days is recommended, with prompt reporting of fever.

Immunoprophylaxis. A live-attenuated Junin vaccine protects against Argentine HF and probably against Bolivian HF. The vaccine is associated with minimal adverse effects in adults; similar findings have been obtained from limited safety studies in children 4 years of age and older. The vaccine is not available in the United States.

Environmental. In town-based outbreaks of Bolivian HF, rodent control has proven successful. Area rodent control is not practical for control of Argentine HF or Venezuelan HF. Intensive rodent control efforts have decreased the rate of peridomestic Lassa virus infection, but rodents eventually reinvade human dwellings, and infection still occurs in rural settings.

Public Health Reporting. Because of the risk of health care-associated transmission, the state health department and the Centers for Disease Control and Prevention should be contacted for specific advice about management and diagnosis of suspected cases.

Hemorrhagic Fevers and Related Syndromes Caused by Viruses of the Family Bunyaviridae[1]

CLINICAL MANIFESTATIONS: These vectorborne infections are severe febrile diseases in which shock and bleeding can be significant and multisystem involvement can occur. In the United States, one of these infections causes an illness marked by acute respiratory and cardiovascular failure (see Hantavirus Pulmonary Syndrome, p 352).

Hemorrhagic fever with renal syndrome (HFRS) is a complex, multiphasic disease characterized by vascular instability and varying degrees of renal insufficiency. Fever, flushing, conjunctival injection, abdominal pain, and lumbar pain are followed by hypotension, oliguria, and subsequently, polyuria. Petechiae are frequent, but more serious bleeding manifestations are rare. Shock and acute renal insufficiency may occur. Nephropathia epidemica (attributable to Puumala virus) occurs in Europe and presents as a milder disease with acute influenza-like illness, abdominal pain, and proteinuria. Acute renal dysfunction also occurs, but hypotensive shock or requirement for dialysis are rare. However, more severe forms of HFRS (ie, attributable to Dobrava virus) also occur in Europe.

Crimean-Congo hemorrhagic fever (CCHF) is a multisystem disease characterized by hepatitis and profuse bleeding. Fever, headache, and myalgia are followed by signs of a diffuse capillary leak syndrome with facial suffusion, conjunctivitis, and proteinuria. Petechiae and purpura often appear on the skin and mucous membranes. A hypotensive crisis often occurs after the appearance of frank hemorrhage from the gastrointestinal tract, nose, mouth, or uterus.

Rift Valley fever (RVF), in most cases, is a self-limited febrile illness. Occasionally, hemorrhagic fever with shock and icterus, encephalitis, or retinitis develops.

---

[1] Does not include hantavirus pulmonary syndrome, which is reviewed on p 352.

ETIOLOGY: Bunyaviridae are segmented, single-stranded RNA viruses with different geographic distributions depending on their vector or reservoir. Hemorrhagic fever syndromes are associated with viruses from 3 genera: hantaviruses, nairoviruses (CCHF virus), and phleboviruses (RVF and sandfly fever viruses). Old World hantaviruses (Hantaan, Seoul, Dobrava, and Puumala viruses) cause HFRS, and New World hantaviruses (Sin Nombre and related viruses) cause hantavirus pulmonary syndrome (see Hantavirus Pulmonary Syndrome, p 352).

EPIDEMIOLOGY: The epidemiology of these diseases mainly is a function of the distribution and behavior of their reservoirs and vectors. All genera except hantaviruses are associated with arthropod vectors, and hantavirus infections are associated with exposure to infected rodents.

Classic HFRS occurs throughout much of Asia and Eastern and Western Europe, with up to 100 000 cases per year. The most severe form of the disease is caused by the prototype Hantaan virus and Dobrava viruses in rural Asia and Europe, respectively; Puumala virus is associated with milder disease (nephropathia epidemica) in Western Europe. Seoul virus is distributed worldwide in association with *Rattus* species and can cause a disease of variable severity. Person-to-person transmission never has been reported with HFRS.

CCHF occurs in much of sub-Saharan Africa, the Middle East, areas in West and Central Asia, and the Balkans. CCHF virus is transmitted by ticks and occasionally by contact with viremic animals at slaughter. Health care-associated transmission of CCHF is a frequent and serious hazard.

RVF occurs throughout sub-Saharan Africa and has caused large epidemics in Egypt in 1977 and 1993–1995, Mauritania in 1987, Saudi Arabia and Yemen in 2000, Kenya in 1997 and 2006–2007, Madagascar in 1990 and 2008, and South Africa in 2010. The virus is arthropodborne and is transmitted from domestic livestock to humans by mosquitoes. The virus also can be transmitted by aerosol and by direct contact with infected aborted tissues or freshly slaughtered infected animal carcasses. Person-to-person transmission has not been reported, but laboratory-acquired cases are well documented.

The **incubation periods** for CCHF and RVF range from 2 to 10 days; for HFRS, incubation periods usually are longer, ranging from 7 to 42 days.

DIAGNOSTIC TESTS: CCHF and RVF viruses can be cultivated readily (restricted to Biosafety level-4 laboratories) from blood and tissue specimens of infected patients. Detection of viral antigen by enzyme immunoassay (EIA) is a useful alternative. Serum immunoglobulin (Ig) M and IgG virus-specific antibodies typically develop early in convalescence in CCHF and RVF but could be absent in rapidly fatal cases of CCHF. In HFRS, IgM and IgG antibodies usually are detectable at the time of onset of illness or within 48 hours, when it is too late for virus isolation and antigen detection. IgM antibodies or rising IgG titers in paired serum specimens, as demonstrated by EIA, are diagnostic; neutralizing antibody tests provide greater virus-strain specificity but rarely are tested. Polymerase chain reaction assay performed with appropriate safety precautions is a useful complement to serodiagnostic assays on samples obtained during the acute phase of CCHF, RVF, or HFRS. Diagnosis can be made retrospectively by immunohistochemistry assay of tissues obtained from necropsy.

TREATMENT: Ribavirin administered intravenously to patients with HFRS within the first 4 days of illness seems effective in decreasing renal dysfunction, vascular instability, and mortality. However, intravenous ribavirin is not available commercially in the United States and can be obtained only under an investigational new drug (IND) application. Supportive therapy for HFRS should include: (1) avoidance of transporting patients; (2) treatment of shock; (3) monitoring of fluid balance; (4) dialysis for complications of renal failure; (5) control of hypertension during the oliguric phase; and (6) early recognition of possible myocardial failure with appropriate therapy.

Oral and intravenous ribavirin given to patients with CCHF has been associated with milder disease, although no controlled studies have been performed. Ribavirin also may be efficacious as postexposure prophylaxis of CCHF. Studies in animals and humans investigating whether ribavirin has potential benefit in treatment of hemorrhagic RVF have been inconclusive, showing an increase of encephalitis.

ISOLATION OF THE HOSPITALIZED PATIENT: In addition to standard precautions, contact and droplet precautions, including careful prevention of needlestick injuries and management of clinical specimens, are indicated for patients with CCHF for the duration for their illness. Airborne isolation also may be required in certain circumstances when patients undergo procedures that stimulate coughing and promote generation of aerosols. Standard precautions should be followed with RVF and HFRS.

CONTROL MEASURES:

Care of Exposed People. People having direct contact with blood or other secretions from patients with CCHF should be observed closely for 14 days with daily monitoring for fever. Immediate therapy with intravenous ribavirin should be considered at the first sign of disease.

Environmental Immunoprophylaxis. Monitoring of laboratory rat colonies and urban rodent control may be effective for ratborne HFRS.

Crimean-Congo Hemorrhagic Fever. Arachnicides for tick control generally have limited benefit but should be used in stockyard settings. Personal protective measures (eg, physical tick removal and protective clothing with permethrin sprays) may be effective for people at-risk (farmers, veterinarians, abattoir workers).

Rift Valley Fever. Regular immunization of domestic animals should have an effect on limiting or preventing RVF outbreaks and protecting humans but is not performed routinely. Personal protective clothing (with permethrin sprays) may be effective for people at risk (farmers, veterinarians, abattoir workers). Mosquito control measures are difficult to implement.

Public Health Reporting. Because of the risk of health care-associated transmission of CCHF and diagnostic confusion with other viral hemorrhagic fevers, the state health department and the Centers for Disease Control and Prevention should be contacted about any suspected diagnosis of viral hemorrhagic fever and the management plan for the patient.

Hepatitis A

CLINICAL MANIFESTATIONS: Hepatitis A characteristically is an acute, self-limited illness associated with fever, malaise, jaundice, anorexia, and nausea. Symptomatic hepatitis A virus (HAV) infection occurs in approximately 30% of infected children younger than 6 years of age; few of these children will have jaundice. Among older children and adults, infection usually is symptomatic and typically lasts several weeks, with jaundice occurring in 70% or more. Signs and symptoms typically last less than 2 months, although 10% to 15% of symptomatic people have prolonged or relapsing disease lasting as long as 6 months. Fulminant hepatitis is rare but is more common in people with underlying liver disease. Chronic infection does not occur.

ETIOLOGY: HAV is an RNA virus classified as a member of the picornavirus family.

EPIDEMIOLOGY: The most common mode of transmission is person to person, resulting from fecal contamination and oral ingestion (ie, the fecal-oral route). In resource-limited countries where infection is endemic, most people are infected during the first decade of life. In the United States, hepatitis A was one of the most frequently reported vaccine-preventable diseases in the prevaccine era, but incidence of disease attributable to HAV has declined significantly since hepatitis A vaccine was licensed in 1995. These declining rates have been accompanied by a shift in age-specific rates. Historically, the highest rates occurred among children 5 to 14 years of age, and the lowest rates occurred among adults older than 40 years of age. Beginning in the late 1990s, national age-specific rates declined more rapidly among children than among adults; as a result, in recent years, rates have been similar among all age groups. In addition, the previously observed unequal geographic distribution of hepatitis A incidence in the United States, with the highest rates of disease occurring in a limited number of states and communities, has disappeared after introduction of targeted immunization in 1999. Continued surveillance is needed to verify that the decline in incidence is sustained.

Among cases of hepatitis A reported to the Centers for Disease Control and Prevention (CDC), recognized risk factors include close personal contact with a person infected with HAV, international travel, household or personal contact with a child who attends a child care center, household or personal contact with a newly arriving international adoptee, a recognized foodborne outbreak, men who have sex with men, and use of illegal drugs. Transmission by blood transfusion or from mother to newborn infant (ie, vertical transmission) is limited to case reports. In approximately two-thirds of reported cases, the source cannot be determined. Fecal-oral spread from people with asymptomatic infections, particularly young children, likely accounts for many of these cases with an unknown source.

Before availability of vaccine, most HAV infection and illness occurred in the context of community-wide epidemics, in which infection primarily was transmitted in households and extended-family settings. However, community-wide epidemics have not been observed in recent years. Common-source foodborne outbreaks occur; waterborne outbreaks are rare. Health care-associated transmission is unusual, but outbreaks have occurred in neonatal intensive care units from neonates infected through transfused blood who subsequently transmitted HAV to other neonates and staff.

In child care centers, recognized symptomatic (icteric) illness occurs primarily among adult contacts of children. Most infected children younger than 6 years of age are asymptomatic or have nonspecific manifestations. Hence, spread of HAV infection within and outside a child care center often occurs before recognition of the index case(s). Outbreaks have occurred most commonly in large child care centers and specifically in facilities that enroll children in diapers.

Patients infected with HAV are most infectious during the 1 to 2 weeks before onset of jaundice or elevation of liver enzymes, when concentration of virus in the stool is highest. The risk of transmission subsequently diminishes and is minimal by 1 week after onset of jaundice. However, HAV can be detected in stool for longer periods, especially in neonates and young children.

The **incubation period** is 15 to 50 days, with an average of 28 days.

DIAGNOSTIC TESTS: Serologic tests for HAV-specific total (ie, immunoglobulin [Ig] G and IgM) antibody (anti-HAV) are available commercially. The presence of serum IgM anti-HAV indicates current or recent infection, although false-positive results may occur. IgM anti-HAV is detectable in up to 20% of vaccinees when measured 2 weeks after hepatitis A immunization. In most infected people, serum IgM anti-HAV becomes detectable 5 to 10 days before onset of symptoms and declines to undetectable concentrations within 6 months after infection. However, people who test positive for IgM anti-HAV more than 1 year after infection have been reported. IgG anti-HAV is detectable shortly after appearance of IgM. A positive total anti-HAV (ie, IgM and IgG) test result and a negative IgM anti-HAV test result indicate past infection and immunity.

TREATMENT: Supportive.

ISOLATION OF THE HOSPITALIZED PATIENT: In general, hospitalization is not required for patients with uncomplicated acute hepatitis A. When hospitalization is necessary, contact precautions are recommended in addition to standard precautions for diapered and incontinent patients for at least 1 week after onset of symptoms.

CONTROL MEASURES[1]:

General Measures. The major methods of prevention of HAV infections are improved sanitation (eg, in food preparation and of water sources) and personal hygiene (eg, hand hygiene after diaper changes in child care settings), immunization with hepatitis A vaccine, and administration of Immune Globulin (IG).

Schools, Child Care, and Work. Children and adults with acute HAV infection who work as food handlers or attend or work in child care settings should be excluded for 1 week after onset of the illness.

Immune Globulin. IG for intramuscular administration, when given within 2 weeks after exposure to HAV, is greater than 85% effective in preventing symptomatic infection. When administered for preexposure prophylaxis, 1 dose of 0.02 mL/kg confers protection against hepatitis A for up to 3 months, and a dose of 0.06 mL/kg protects for 3 to 5 months. Recommended preexposure and postexposure IG doses and duration of protection are given in Tables 3.12 (p 363) and 3.13 (p 363). HAV vaccine is preferred for preexposure protection in all populations unless contraindicated and for postexposure prophylaxis for most people 1 through 40 years of age (see Postexposure Prophylaxis, p 367).

Hepatitis A Vaccine. Two inactivated HAV vaccines, Havrix and Vaqta, are available in the United States. The vaccines are prepared from cell culture-adapted HAV, which is propagated in human fibroblasts, purified from cell lysates, formalin inactivated, and

---

[1] Centers for Disease Control and Prevention. Prevention of hepatitis A through active or passive immunization: recommendations of the Advisory Committee on Immunization Practices (ACIP). *MMWR Recomm Rep.* 2006;55(RR-7):1–23

Table 3.12. Recommendations for Preexposure Immunoprophylaxis of Hepatitis A Virus (HAV) for Travelers[a]

Age	Recommended Prophylaxis	Notes
Younger than 12 mo	IG	0.02 mL/kg[b] protects for up to 3 mo. For trips of 3 mo or longer, 0.06 mL/kg[b] should be given at departure and every 5 mo if exposure to HAV continues.
12 mo through 40 y	HAV vaccine	
41 y or older	HAV vaccine with or without IG	If departure is in less than 2 wk, older adults, immuno-compromised people, and people with chronic liver disease or other chronic medical conditions can receive IG with the initial dose of hepatitis A vaccine to ensure optimal protection.

IG indicates Immune Globulin.
[a] All people 12 months of age or older at high risk of HAV disease should be immunized routinely (see People at Increased Risk, p 366).
[b] IG should be administered deep into a large muscle mass. Ordinarily, no more than 5 mL should be administered in one site in an adult or large child; lesser amounts (maximum 3 mL in one site) should be given to small children and infants.

Table 3.13. Recommendations for Postexposure Immunoprophylaxis of Hepatitis A Virus (HAV)

Time Since Exposure	Age of Patient	Recommended Prophylaxis
2 wk or less	Younger than 12 mo	IG, 0.02 mL/kg[a]
	12 mo through 40 y	HAV vaccine[b]
	41 y or older	IG, 0.02 mL/kg,[a] but HAV vaccine[b] can be used if IG is unavailable[a]
	People of any age who are immuno-compromised or have chronic liver disease	IG, 0.02 mL/kg[a]
More than 2 wk	Younger than 12 mo	No prophylaxis
	12 mo or older	No prophylaxis, but HAV vaccine may be indicated for ongoing exposure[b]

IG indicates Immune Globulin.
[a] IG should be administered deep into a large muscle mass. Ordinarily, no more than 5 mL should be administered in one site in an adult or large child; lesser amounts (maximum 3 mL in one site) should be given to small children and infants.
[b] Dosage and schedule of hepatitis A vaccine as recommended according to age in Table 3.14.

adsorbed to an aluminum hydroxide adjuvant. Both HAV vaccines are formulated without a preservative.

Administration, Dosages, and Schedules (see Table 3.14, p 364). HAV vaccines are licensed for people 12 months of age and older and have pediatric and adult formulations that are administered in a 2-dose schedule. The adult formulations are recommended for people 19 years of age and older. Recommended doses and schedules for these different products and formulations are given in Table 3.14, p 364. A combination HAV/hepatitis B vaccine (Twinrix) is licensed in the United States for people 18 years

Table 3.14. Recommended Doses and Schedules for Inactivated Hepatitis A Virus (HAV) Vaccines[a]

Age	Vaccine	Hepatitis A Antigen Dose	Volume per Dose, mL	No. of Doses	Schedule
12 mo through 18 y	Havrix	720 ELU	0.5	2	Initial and 6–12 mo later
12 mo through 18 y	Vaqta	25 U[b]	0.5	2	Initial and 6–18 mo later
19 y or older	Havrix	1440 ELU	1.0	2	Initial and 6–12 mo later
19 y or older	Vaqta	50 U[b]	1.0	2	Initial and 6–18 mo later
18 y or older	Twinrix[c]	720 ELU	1.0	3 or 4	Initial and 1 and 6 mo later **OR** Initial, 7 and 21–30 days, followed by a dose at 12 mo

ELU indicates enzyme-linked immunosorbent assay units.
[a] Havrix and Twinrix are manufactured by GlaxoSmithKline Biologicals; Vaqta is manufactured and distributed by Merck & Co Inc.
[b] Antigen units (each unit is equivalent to approximately 1 μg of viral protein).
[c] A combination of hepatitis B (Engerix-B, 20 μg) and hepatitis A (Havrix, 720 ELU) vaccine (Twinrix) is licensed for use in people 18 years of age and older in 3-dose and 4-dose schedules.

of age and older and can be administered in a 3-dose schedule or an accelerated 4-dose schedule (see Table 3.14). All HAV-containing vaccines are administered intramuscularly.

Immunogenicity. Available HAV vaccines are highly immunogenic when given in their respective recommended schedules and doses. At least 95% of healthy children, adolescents, and adults have protective antibody concentrations when measured 1 month after receipt of the first dose of either single-antigen vaccine. One month after a second dose, more than 99% of healthy children, adolescents, and adults have protective antibody concentrations.

Available data on the immunogenicity of HAV vaccine in young children indicate high rates of seroconversion, but antibody concentrations are lower in infants with passively acquired maternal anti-HAV in comparison with vaccine recipients lacking anti-HAV. By 12 months of age, passively acquired maternal anti-HAV antibody no longer is detectable in most infants. HAV vaccine is highly immunogenic for children who begin immunization at 12 months of age or older regardless of maternal anti-HAV status.

Efficacy. In double-blind, controlled, randomized trials, the protective efficacy in preventing clinical HAV infection was 94% to 100%.

Efficacy of Postexposure Immunization. A randomized clinical trial conducted among people 2 through 40 years of age comparing postexposure efficacy of IG and HAV vaccine found that the efficacy of a single dose of HAV vaccine was similar to that of IG in preventing symptomatic infection when administered within 14 days after exposure.

Duration of Protection. The need for additional booster doses beyond the 2-dose primary immunization series has not been determined, because long-term efficacy of HAV vaccines has not been established. Detectable antibody persists after a 2-dose series for at least 10 years in adults and 5 to 6 years in children. Kinetic models of antibody decline indicate that protective levels of anti-HAV could be present for 25 years or longer in adults and 14 to 20 years in children.

Vaccine in Immunocompromised Patients. The immune response in immunocompromised people, including people with human immunodeficiency virus infection, may be suboptimal.

Vaccine Interchangeability. The 2 single-antigen HAV vaccines licensed by the US Food and Drug Administration (FDA), when given as recommended, seem to be similarly effective. Studies among adults have found no difference in the immunogenicity of a vaccine series that mixed the 2 currently available vaccines, compared with using the same vaccine throughout the licensed schedule. Therefore, although completion of the immunization regimen with the same product is preferable, immunization with either product is acceptable.

Administration With Other Vaccines. Data indicate that HAV vaccine may be administered simultaneously with other vaccines. Vaccines should be given in a separate syringe and at a separate injection site (see Simultaneous Administration of Multiple Vaccines, p 33).

Adverse Events. Adverse reactions are mild and include local pain and, less commonly, induration at the injection site. No serious adverse events attributed definitively to HAV vaccine have been reported.

Precautions and Contraindications. The vaccine should not be administered to people with hypersensitivity to any of the vaccine components. Safety data in pregnant women are not available, but the risk is considered to be low or nonexistent, because the vaccine contains inactivated, purified, virus particles. Because HAV vaccine is inactivated, no special precautions need to be taken when vaccinating immunocompromised people.

Preimmunization Serologic Testing. Preimmunization testing for anti-HAV generally is not recommended for children because of their expected low prevalence of infection. Testing may be cost-effective for people who have a high likelihood of immunity from previous infection, including people whose childhood was spent in a country with high endemicity, people with a history of jaundice potentially caused by HAV, and people older than 50 years of age.

Postimmunization Serologic Testing. Postimmunization testing for anti-HAV is not indicated because of the high seroconversion rates in adults and children. In addition, some commercially available anti-HAV tests may not detect low but protective concentrations of antibody among immunized people.

RECOMMENDATIONS FOR IMMUNOPROPHYLAXIS:

Preexposure Prophylaxis Against HAV Infection (see Tables 3.12, p 363, and 3.14, p 364). HAV immunization is recommended routinely for children 12 through 23 months of age, for people who are at increased risk of infection, for people who are at increased risk of severe manifestations of hepatitis A if infected, and for any person who wants to obtain immunity.

Children Who Routinely Should Be Immunized or Considered for Immunization. All children in the United States should receive HAV vaccine at 12 through 23 months of age, as recommended in the routine childhood immunization schedule (Fig 1.1, p 27–28). Table 3.14 (p 364) shows FDA-licensed HAV-containing vaccines, doses, and schedules. Children who are not immunized by 2 years of age can be immunized at subsequent visits.

People at Increased Risk of HAV Infection or Its Consequences Who Routinely Should Be Immunized.

- **People traveling internationally.**[1] All susceptible people traveling to or working in countries that have high or intermediate hepatitis A endemicity should be immunized or receive IG before departure (see Table 3.12, p 363). Travelers to Western Europe, Scandinavia, Australia, Canada, Japan, and New Zealand (ie, countries in which endemicity is low) are at no greater risk of HAV infection than are people living in or traveling to the United States. HAV vaccine at the age-appropriate dose is preferred to IG. The first dose of HAV vaccine should be administered as soon as travel is considered.
  - One dose of single-antigen vaccine administered at any time before departure can provide adequate protection for most healthy people. However, no data are available for other populations or other hepatitis A vaccine formulations (eg, the combination HAV-hepatitis B vaccine).
  - Older adults, immunocompromised people, and people with chronic liver disease or other chronic medical conditions who are traveling to an area with endemic infection in 2 weeks or less should receive the initial dose of vaccine and simultaneously can receive IG (0.02 mL/kg) at a separate anatomic site. The vaccine series then should be completed according to the licensed schedule.
  - Travelers who elect not to receive vaccine, are younger than 12 months of age, or are allergic to a vaccine component should receive a single dose of IG (0.02 mL/kg), which provides effective protection for up to 3 months.
- **Close contacts of newly arriving international adoptees.**[2,3] Data from a study conducted at 3 adoption clinics in the United States indicate that 1% to 6% of newly arrived international adoptees have acute HAV infection. The risk of HAV infection among close personal contacts of international adoptees is estimated at 106 (range, 90–819) per 100 000 household contacts of international adoptees within the first 60 days of their arrival in the United States. Therefore, HAV vaccine should be

---

[1] Centers for Disease Control and Prevention. Update: prevention of hepatitis A after exposure to hepatitis A virus and in international travelers. Updated recommendations of the Advisory Committee on Immunization Practices (ACIP). *MMWR Morb Mortal Wkly Rep.* 2007;56(41):1080–1084

[2] Centers for Disease Control and Prevention. Updated recommendations from the Advisory Committee on Immunization Practices (ACIP) for use of hepatitis A vaccine in close contacts of newly arriving international adoptees. *MMWR Morb Mortal Wkly Rep.* 2009;58(36):1006–1007

[3] American Academy of Pediatrics, Committee on Infectious Diseases. Recommendations for administering hepatitis A vaccine to contacts of international adoptees. *Pediatrics.* 2011;128(4):803–804

administered to all previously unvaccinated people who anticipate close personal contact (eg, household contact or regular babysitting) with an international adoptee from a country with high or intermediate endemicity during the first 60 days following arrival of the adoptee in the United States. The first dose of the 2-dose HAV vaccine series should be administered as soon as adoption is planned, ideally 2 or more weeks before the arrival of the adoptee.

- **Men who have sex with men.** Outbreaks of hepatitis A among men who have sex with men have been reported often, including in urban areas in the United States, Canada, and Australia. Therefore, men (adolescents and adults) who have sex with men should be immunized. Preimmunization serologic testing may be cost-effective for older people in this group.
- **Users of injection and noninjection drugs.** Periodic outbreaks among injection and noninjection drug users have been reported in many parts of the United States and in Europe. Adolescents and adults who use illegal drugs should be immunized. Preimmunization serologic testing may be cost-effective for older people in this group.
- **Patients with clotting-factor disorders.** Reported outbreaks of hepatitis A in patients with hemophilia receiving solvent-detergent–treated factor VIII and factor IX concentrates were identified during the 1990s, primarily in Europe, although 1 case was reported in the United States. Therefore, susceptible patients with chronic clotting disorders who receive clotting-factor concentrates should be immunized. Preimmunization testing for anti-HAV may be cost-effective for older people in this group.
- **People at risk of occupational exposure (eg, handlers of nonhuman primates and people working with HAV in a research laboratory setting).** Outbreaks of hepatitis A have been reported among people working with nonhuman primates. These infected primates were born in the wild and were not primates that had been born and raised in captivity. People working with HAV-infected primates or with HAV in a research laboratory setting should be immunized.
- **People with chronic liver disease.** Because people with chronic liver disease are at increased risk of fulminant hepatitis A, susceptible patients with chronic liver disease should be immunized. Susceptible people who are awaiting or have received liver transplants should be immunized.

Postexposure Prophylaxis (see Table 3.13, p 363).[1] People who have been exposed to HAV and previously have not received HAV vaccine should receive a single dose of single-antigen HAV vaccine or IG as soon as possible (see Table 3.13, p 363, for prophylaxis guidance and dosages). The efficacy of IG or vaccine for postexposure prophylaxis when administered more than 2 weeks after exposure has not been established. Information about the relative efficacy of vaccine compared with IG postexposure is limited, and no data are available for people older than 40 years of age or people with underlying medical conditions.

- For healthy people 12 months through 40 years of age, HAV vaccine at the age-appropriate dose is preferred to IG because of vaccine advantages, including long-term protection and ease of administration.

---

[1] Centers for Disease Control and Prevention. Update: prevention of hepatitis A after exposure to hepatitis A virus and in international travelers. Updated recommendations of the Advisory Committee on Immunization Practices (ACIP). *MMWR Morb Mortal Wkly Rep.* 2007;56(41):1080–1084

- For people older than 40 years of age, IG is preferred because of the absence of data regarding vaccine performance in this age group and the increased risk of severe manifestations of hepatitis A with increasing age. However, HAV vaccine can be used if IG is unavailable. The magnitude of risk of HAV transmission should be considered in decisions to use IG or HAV vaccine.
- IG should be used for children younger than 12 months of age, immunocompromised people, people with chronic liver disease, and people for whom HAV vaccine is contraindicated.
- People who are given IG and for whom HAV vaccine also is recommended for other reasons should receive a dose of vaccine simultaneously with IG. For people who receive vaccine, the second dose should be given according to the licensed schedule to complete the series.
- **Household and sexual contacts.** All previously unimmunized people with close personal contact with a person with serologically confirmed HAV infection, such as household and sexual contacts, should receive vaccine or IG within 2 weeks after the most recent exposure (Table 3.13, p 363). Serologic testing of contacts is not recommended, because testing adds unnecessary cost and may delay administration of postexposure prophylaxis.
- **Newborn infants of HAV-infected mothers.** Perinatal transmission of HAV is rare. Some experts advise giving IG (0.02 mL/kg) to an infant if the mother's symptoms began between 2 weeks before and 1 week after delivery. Efficacy in this circumstance has not been established. Severe disease in healthy infants is rare.
- **Child care center staff, employees, and children and their household contacts.** Outbreaks of HAV infection at child care centers have been recognized since the 1970s, but their frequency has decreased as HAV immunization rates in children have increased and as hepatitis A incidence among children has declined. Because infections in children usually are mild or asymptomatic, outbreaks often are identified only when adult contacts (eg, parents) become ill. Serologic testing to confirm HAV infection in suspected cases is indicated.

  HAV vaccine or IG (Table 3.13, p 363) should be administered to all previously unimmunized staff members and attendees of child care centers or homes if (1) one or more cases of hepatitis A are recognized in children or staff members; or (2) cases are recognized in 2 or more households of center attendees. In centers that provide care only to children who do not wear diapers, vaccine or IG need be given only to classroom contacts of an index-case patient. When an outbreak occurs (ie, hepatitis A cases in 2 or more families), vaccine or IG also should be considered for members of households that have children (center attendees) in diapers.

  Children and adults with hepatitis A should be excluded from the center until 1 week after onset of illness, until the postexposure prophylaxis program has been completed in the center, or until directed by the health department. Although precise data concerning the onset of protection after postexposure prophylaxis are not available, allowing prophylaxis recipients to return to the child care center setting immediately after receipt of the vaccine or IG dose seems reasonable.
- **Schools.** Schoolroom exposure generally does not pose an appreciable risk of infection, and postexposure prophylaxis is not indicated when a single case occurs and the source of infection is outside the school. However, HAV vaccine or IG could be used

for unimmunized people who have close contact with the index patient if transmission within the school setting is documented.

- **Hospitals.** Usually, health care-associated HAV in hospital personnel has occurred through spread from patients with acute HAV infection in whom the diagnosis was not recognized. Careful hygienic practices should be emphasized when a patient with jaundice or known or suspected hepatitis A is admitted to the hospital. When outbreaks occur, HAV vaccine or IG is recommended for people in close contact with infected patients (Table 3.13, p 363). There is no recommendation for routine preexposure use of HAV vaccine for hospital personnel.

- **Exposure to an infected food handler.** If a food handler is diagnosed with hepatitis A, HAV vaccine or IG should be provided to other food handlers at the same establishment (Table 3.13, p 363). Food handlers with acute HAV infection should be excluded for 1 week after onset of illness. Because common-source transmission to patrons is unlikely, postexposure prophylaxis with HAV vaccine or IG typically is not indicated but may be considered if the food handler directly handled food during the time when the food handler likely was infectious and had diarrhea or poor hygiene practices and if prophylaxis can be provided within 2 weeks of exposure. Routine HAV immunization of food handlers is not recommended.

- **Common-source exposure.** Postexposure prophylaxis usually is not recommended, because these outbreaks commonly are recognized too late for prophylaxis to be effective in preventing HAV infection in exposed people. HAV vaccine or IG can be considered if it can be administered to exposed people within 2 weeks of an exposure to the HAV-contaminated water or food.

Hepatitis B

CLINICAL MANIFESTATIONS: People acutely infected with hepatitis B virus (HBV) may be asymptomatic or symptomatic. The likelihood of developing symptoms of acute hepatitis is age dependent: less than 1% of infants younger than 1 year of age, 5% to 15% of children 1 through 5 years of age, and 30% to 50% of people older than 5 years of age are symptomatic, although few data are available for adults older than 30 years of age. When symptomatically infected, the spectrum of signs and symptoms is varied and includes subacute illness with nonspecific symptoms (eg, anorexia, nausea, or malaise), clinical hepatitis with jaundice, or fulminant hepatitis. Extrahepatic manifestations, such as arthralgia, arthritis, macular rashes, thrombocytopenia, polyarteritis nodosa, glomerulonephritis, or papular acrodermatitis (Gianotti-Crosti syndrome), can occur early in the course of illness and may precede jaundice. Acute HBV infection cannot be distinguished from other forms of acute viral hepatitis on the basis of clinical signs and symptoms or nonspecific laboratory findings.

Chronic HBV infection is defined as presence of any one of the following: hepatitis B surface antigen (HBsAg), nucleic acid, hepatitis B virus (HBV) DNA, or hepatitis B e antigen (HBeAg) in serum for at least 6 months or by presence of any one of the following: HBsAg, nucleic acid, HBV DNA, or HBeAg in serum from a person who tests negative for antibody of the immunoglobulin (Ig) M subclass to hepatitis B core antigen (IgM anti-HBc).

Age at the time of acute infection is the primary determinant of risk of progressing to chronic infection. More than 90% of infants infected perinatally or in the first year of life will develop chronic HBV infection. Between 25% and 50% of children infected between 1 and 5 years of age become chronically infected, whereas 5% to 10% of acutely infected older children and adults develop chronic HBV infection. Patients who develop acute HBV infection while immunosuppressed or with an underlying chronic illness (eg, end-stage renal disease) have an increased risk of developing chronic infection. In the absence of treatment, up to 25% of infants and children who acquire chronic HBV infection will die prematurely from HBV-related hepatocellular carcinoma or cirrhosis. Risk factors for developing hepatocellular carcinoma include duration of infection, degree of histologic injury, replicative state of the virus (HBV DNA levels), presence of cirrhosis, and concomitant infection with hepatitis C virus (HCV) or human immunodeficiency virus (HIV).

The clinical course of untreated chronic HBV infection varies according to the population studied, reflecting differences in age at acquisition, rate of loss of hepatitis B e antigen (HBeAg), and possibly HBV genotype. Perinatally infected children usually have normal alanine aminotransferase (ALT) concentrations and minimal or mild liver histologic abnormalities, with detectable HBeAg and high HBV DNA concentrations ($\geq$20 000 IU/mL) for years to decades after initial infection ("immune tolerant phase"). Chronic HBV infection acquired during later childhood or adolescence usually is accompanied by more active liver disease and increased serum transaminase concentrations. Patients with detectable HBeAg *(HBeAg-positive chronic hepatitis B)* usually have high concentrations of HBV DNA and HBsAg in serum and are more likely to transmit infection. Because HBV-associated liver injury is thought to be immune-mediated, in people coinfected with HIV and HBV, the return of immune competence with antiretroviral treatment of HIV infection may lead to a reactivation of HBV-related liver inflammation and damage. Over time (years to decades), HBeAg becomes undetectable in many chronically infected people. This transition often is accompanied by development of antibody to HBeAg (anti-HBe) and decreases in serum HBV DNA and serum transaminase concentrations and may be preceded by a temporary exacerbation of liver disease. These patients have *inactive chronic infection* but still may have exacerbations of hepatitis. Serologic reversion (reappearance of HBeAg) is more common if loss of HBeAg is not accompanied by development of anti-HBe; reversion with loss of anti-HBe also can occur.

Some patients who lose HBeAg may continue to have ongoing histologic evidence of liver damage and moderate to high concentrations of HBV DNA *(HBeAg-negative chronic hepatitis B)*. Patients with histologic evidence of chronic HBV infection, regardless of HBeAg status, remain at higher risk of death attributable to liver failure compared with HBV-infected people with no histologic evidence of liver inflammation and fibrosis. Other factors that may influence natural history of chronic infection include gender, race, alcohol use, and coinfection with HCV, hepatitis D virus (HDV), or HIV.

Resolved hepatitis B is defined as clearance of HBsAg, normalization of serum transaminase concentrations, and development of antibody to HBsAg (anti-HBs). Chronically infected adults clear HBsAg and develop anti-HBs at the rate of 1% to 2% annually; during childhood, the annual clearance rate is less than 1%. Reactivation of resolved chronic infection is possible if these patients become immunosuppressed.

ETIOLOGY: Hepatitis B virus is a DNA-containing, 42-nm-diameter hepadnavirus. Important components of the viral particle include an outer lipoprotein envelope containing HBsAg and an inner nucleocapsid consisting of hepatitis B core antigen. Viral polymerase activity can be detected in preparations of plasma containing HBV.

EPIDEMIOLOGY: HBV is transmitted through infected blood or body fluids. Although HBsAg has been detected in multiple body fluids including human milk and saliva, only blood, serum, semen, vaginal secretions, and cerebrospinal, synovial, pleural, pericardial, peritoneal and amniotic fluids are considered the most potentially infectious. People with chronic HBV infection are the primary reservoirs for infection. Common modes of transmission include percutaneous and permucosal exposure to infectious body fluids, sharing or using nonsterilized needles, syringes or glucose monitoring equipment or devices, sexual contact with an infected person, perinatal exposure to an infected mother, and household exposure to a person with chronic HBV infection. Transmission by transfusion of contaminated blood or blood products is rare in the United States because of routine screening of blood donors and viral inactivation of certain blood products before administration (see Blood Safety, p 114).

Perinatal transmission of HBV is highly efficient and usually occurs from blood exposures during labor and delivery. In utero transmission of HBV accounts for less than 2% of perinatal infections in most studies. Without postexposure prophylaxis, the risk of an infant acquiring HBV from an infected mother as a result of perinatal exposure is 70% to 90% for infants born to mothers who are HBsAg and HBeAg positive; the risk is 5% to 20% for infants born to HBsAg-positive but HBeAg-negative mothers.

Person-to-person spread of HBV can occur in settings involving interpersonal contact over extended periods, such as in a household with a person with chronic HBV infection (eg, an adoptee). In regions of the world with a high prevalence of chronic HBV infection, transmission between children in household settings may account for a substantial amount of transmission. The precise mechanisms of transmission from child to child are unknown; however, frequent interpersonal contact of nonintact skin or mucous membranes with blood-containing secretions, open skin lesions, or blood-containing saliva are potential means of transmission. Transmission from sharing inanimate objects, such as razors or toothbrushes, also may occur. HBV can survive in the environment for up to 7 days but is inactivated by commonly used disinfectants, including household bleach diluted 1:10 with water. HBV is not transmitted by the fecal-oral route.

Transmission among children born in the United States is unusual because of high coverage with hepatitis B vaccine starting at birth. The risk of HBV transmission is higher in children who have not completed a vaccine series, children undergoing hemodialysis, institutionalized children with developmental disabilities, and children emigrating from countries with endemic HBV (eg, Southeast Asia, China, Africa). Person-to-person transmission has been reported in child care settings, but risk of transmission in child care facilities in the United States has become negligible as a result of high infant hepatitis B immunization rates.

Acute HBV infection is reported most commonly among adults 30 through 49 years of age in the United States. Since 1990, the incidence of acute HBV infection has declined in all age categories, with a 98% decline in children younger than 19 years of age and a 93% decline in young adults 20 through 29 years of age, with most of the decline among people 20 through 24 years of age. Among acute hepatitis B patients interviewed in 2009, groups at highest risk included users of injection drugs, people with multiple heterosexual partners, men who have sex with men, and people who reported surgery during the 6 weeks to 6 months before onset of symptoms. Others at increased risk include people with occupational exposure to blood or body fluids, staff of institutions and nonresidential child care programs for children with developmental disabilities, patients undergoing hemodialysis, and sexual or household contacts of people with an acute or chronic infection. Approximately 60% of infected people do not have a readily identifiable risk characteristic. HBV infection in adolescents and adults is associated with other sexually transmitted infections, including syphilis and HIV. Investigations have indicated an increased risk of HBV infection among adults with diabetes mellitus. Outbreaks in nonhospital health care settings, including assisted-living facilities and nursing homes, highlighted the increased risk among people with diabetes mellitus undergoing assisted blood glucose monitoring.[1]

The prevalence of HBV infection and patterns of transmission vary markedly throughout the world (see Table 3.15, p 373). Approximately 45% of people worldwide live in regions of high HBV endemicity, where the prevalence of chronic HBV infection is greater than 8%. Historically in these regions, most new infections occurred as a result of perinatal or early childhood infections. In regions of intermediate HBV endemicity, where the prevalence of HBV infection is 2% to 7%, multiple modes of transmission (ie, perinatal, household, sexual, injection drug use, and health care-associated) contribute to the burden of infection. In countries of low endemicity, where chronic HBV infection prevalence is less than 2% (including the United States) and where routine immunization has been adopted, the peak age of new infections increasingly is among unimmunized age groups. Many people born in countries with high endemicity live in the United States. Infant immunization programs in some of these countries have, in recent years, reduced greatly the seroprevalence of HBsAg, but many other countries with endemic HBV have yet to implement widespread routine childhood hepatitis B immunization programs. The **incubation period** for acute infection is 45 to 160 days, with an average of 90 days.

DIAGNOSTIC TESTS: Serologic antigen tests are available commercially to detect HBsAg and HBeAg. Serologic assays also are available for detection of anti-HBs, anti-HBc, IgM anti-HBc, and anti-HBe (see Table 3.16, p 373, and Fig 3.2, p 374). In addition, nucleic acid amplification testing, gene-amplification techniques (eg, polymerase chain reaction assay, branched DNA methods), and hybridization assays are available to detect and quantify HBV DNA. HBsAg is detectable during acute infection. If infection is self-limited, HBsAg disappears in most patients within a few weeks to several months after infection, followed by appearance of anti-HBs. The time between disappearance of HBsAg and appearance of anti-HBs is termed the *window period* of infection. During the window period, the only marker of acute infection is IgM anti-HBc, which is highly specific for establishing the diagnosis of acute infection. However, IgM anti-HBc usually is not present in infants infected perinatally. People with chronic HBV infection have circulating HBsAg and anti-HBc; on rare occasions, anti-HBs also is present. Both anti-HBs and anti-HBc are detected in people with resolved infection, whereas anti-HBs alone is present in people immunized with hepatitis B vaccine. Transient HBsAg antigenemia can occur following

---

[1]Centers for Disease Control and Prevention. Use of hepatitis B vaccination for adults with diabetes mellitus: recommendations of the Advisory Committee on Immunization Practices (ACIP). *MMWR Morb Mortal Wkly Rep.* 2011;60(50):1709–1711

Table 3.15. Estimated International HBsAg Prevalence[a]

Region	Estimated HBsAg Prevalence
North America	0.1%
Mexico and Central America	0.3%
South America	0.7%
Western Europe	0.7%
Australia and New Zealand	0.9%
Caribbean (except Haiti)	1.0%
Eastern Europe and North Asia	2.8%
South Asia	2.8%
Middle East	3.2%
Haiti	5.6%
East Asia	7.4%
Southeast Asia	9.1%
Africa	9.3%
Pacific Islands	12.0%

HBsAg indicates hepatitis B surface antigen.

[a] Centers for Disease Control and Prevention. A comprehensive immunization strategy to eliminate transmission of hepatitis B virus infection in the United States. Recommendations of the Advisory Committee on Immunization Practices (ACIP). Part II: immunization of adults. *MMWR Recomm Rep.* 2006;55(RR-16):1–33.

Table 3.16. Diagnostic Tests for Hepatitis B Virus (HBV) Antigens and Antibodies

Factors To Be Tested	HBV Antigen or Antibody	Use
HBsAg	Hepatitis B surface antigen	Detection of acutely or chronically infected people; antigen used in hepatitis B vaccine
Anti-HBs	Antibody to HBsAg	Identification of people who have resolved infections with HBV; determination of immunity after immunization
HBeAg	Hepatitis B e antigen	Identification of infected people at increased risk of transmitting HBV
Anti-HBe	Antibody to HBeAg	Identification of infected people with lower risk of transmitting HBV
Anti-HBc (total)	Antibody to HBcAg[a]	Identification of people with acute, resolved, or chronic HBV infection (not present after immunization); passively transferred maternal anti-HBc is detectable for as long as 24 months among infants born to HBsAg-positive women
IgM anti-HBc	IgM antibody to HBcAg	Identification of people with acute or recent HBV infections (including HBsAg-negative people during the "window" phase of infection)

HBcAg indicates hepatitis B core antigen; IgM, immunoglobulin M.

[a] No test is available commercially to measure HBcAg.

FIGURE 3.2. VIROLOGIC AND SEROLOGIC RESPONSE FOLLOWING ACUTE HEPATITIS B VIRUS INFECTION.

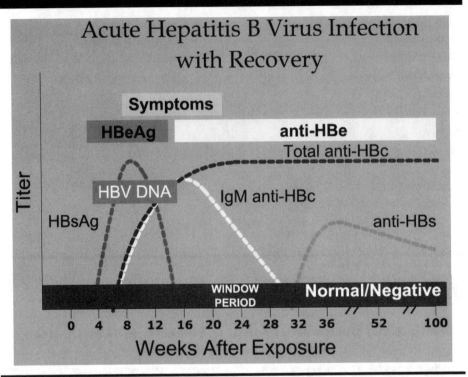

From Centers for Disease Control and Prevention. Viral Hepatitis Resource Center. Online Serology Training: Hepatitis B. Available at: **http://www.cdc.gov/hepatitis/Resources/Professionals/Training/Serology/training.htm#one.**

hepatitis B vaccine, with HBsAg being detected as early as 24 hours after and up to 2 to 3 weeks following administration of the vaccine. The presence of HBeAg in serum correlates with higher concentrations of HBV and greater infectivity. Tests for HBeAg and HBV DNA are useful in selection of candidates to receive antiviral therapy and to monitor response to therapy.

TREATMENT: No specific therapy for *acute* HBV infection is available, and acute HBV infection usually does not warrant referral to a hepatitis specialist. Hepatitis B Immune Globulin (HBIG) and corticosteroids are not effective treatment.

Children and adolescents who have chronic HBV infection are at risk of developing serious liver disease, including primary hepatocellular carcinoma (HCC), with advancing age and should receive hepatitis A vaccine. Although the peak incidence of primary HCC attributable to HBV infection is in the fifth decade of life, HCC occurs in children as young as 6 years of age who become infected perinatally or in early childhood. Several algorithms have been published describing the initial evaluation, monitoring, and criteria for treatment. Children with chronic HBV infection should be screened periodically for hepatic complications using serum liver transaminase tests, alpha-fetoprotein concentration, and abdominal ultrasonography. Definitive recommendations on the frequency and indications for specific tests are not yet available because of lack of data on their reliability in predicting sequelae. Patients with persistently elevated serum ALT concentrations (exceeding twice the upper limit of normal) and patients with an increased serum alpha-fetoprotein concentration or abnormal findings on abdominal ultrasonography should be referred to a specialist in management of chronic HBV infection for further management and treatment.

The goal of treatment in chronic HBV infection is to prevent progression to cirrhosis, hepatic failure, and hepatocellular carcinoma. Current indications for treatment of chronic HBV infection include evidence of ongoing HBV viral replication, as indicated by the presence for longer than 6 months of serum HBV DNA greater than 20 000 IU/mL without HBeAg positivity, greater than 2000 IU/mL with HBeAg positivity, and elevated serum alanine aminotransferase (ALT) concentrations for longer than 6 months or evidence of chronic hepatitis on liver biopsy. Children without necroinflammatory liver disease and children with immunotolerant chronic HBV infection (ie, normal ALT concentrations despite presence of HBV DNA) usually do not warrant antiviral therapy. Treatment response is measured by biochemical, virologic, and histologic response. An important consideration in the choice of treatment is to avoid selection of antiviral-resistant mutations.

The US Food and Drug Administration (FDA) has approved 3 nucleoside analogues (eg, entecavir, lamivudine, and telbivudine), 2 nucleotide analogues (tenofovir and adefovir), and 2 interferon-alfa drugs (interferon alfa-2b and pegylated interferon alfa-2a) for treatment of chronic HBV infection in adults. Tenofovir, entecavir, and pegylated interferon alfa-2a are preferred in adults as first-line therapy in lieu of the lower likelihood of developing antiviral resistance mutations over long-term therapy. Of these, FDA licensure in the pediatric population is as follows: interferon, ≥1 year of age; lamivudine, ≥3 years of age; adefovir, ≥12 years of age; telbivudine, ≥16 years of age; and entecavir, ≥16 years of age. Developments in antiviral therapies of HBV may be found on the American Association for the Study of Liver Diseases Web site (www.aasld.org).

The optimal agent and duration of therapy for chronic HBV infection in children remain unclear. There are few large randomized controlled trials of antiviral therapies for chronic hepatitis B in childhood. Studies indicate that approximately 17% to 58% of children with increased transaminase concentrations who are treated with interferon alfa-2b for 6 months lose HBeAg, compared with approximately 8% to 17% of untreated controls. Response to interferon-alfa is better for children from Western countries (20%–58%) as compared with Asian countries (17%).Children from Asian countries with HBV infection are more likely: (1) to have acquired infection perinatally; (2) to have a prolonged immune tolerant phase of infection; and (3) to be infected with HBV genotype C. All 3 of these factors are associated with lower response rates to interferon-alfa, which is less effective for chronic infections acquired during early childhood, especially if transaminase concentrations are normal. Children with chronic HBV infection who were treated with lamivudine had higher rates of virologic response (loss of detectable HBV DNA and loss of HBeAg) after 1 year of treatment than did children who received placebo (23% vs 13%). Resistance to lamivudine can develop while on treatment and may occur early. The optimal duration of lamivudine therapy is not known, but a minimum of 1 year is required. For those who have not yet seroreverted but do not have resistant virus, therapy beyond 1 year may be beneficial (ie, continued seroreversions).Combination therapy with lamivudine and interferon-alfa has been studied with mixed results as compared with monotherapy with interferon-alfa. Children coinfected with HIV and HBV should receive the lamivudine dose approved for treatment of HIV. Consultation with health care professionals with expertise in treating chronic hepatitis B in children is recommended.

ISOLATION OF THE HOSPITALIZED PATIENT: Standard precautions are indicated for patients with acute or chronic HBV infection. For infants born to HBsAg-positive mothers, no special care in addition to standard precautions, other than removal of maternal blood by a gloved attendant, is necessary.

CONTROL MEASURES:

Strategy for Prevention of HBV Infection. The primary goal of hepatitis B-prevention programs is to eliminate transmission of HBV, thereby decreasing rates of chronic HBV infection and HBV-related chronic liver disease. A secondary goal is prevention of acute HBV infection. In the United States over the past 2 decades, a comprehensive immunization strategy to eliminate HBV transmission has been implemented progressively and now includes the following 4 components[1],[2]: (1) universal immunization of infants beginning at birth; (2) prevention of perinatal HBV infection through routine screening of all pregnant women and appropriate immunoprophylaxis of infants born to HBsAg-positive women and infants born to women with unknown HBsAg status; (3) routine immunization of children and adolescents who previously have not been immunized; and (4) immunization of previously unimmunized adults at increased risk of infection.

Hepatitis B Immunoprophylaxis. Two types of products are available for immunoprophylaxis. Hepatitis B Immune Globulin (HBIG) provides short-term protection (3–6 months) and is indicated only in specific postexposure circumstances (see Care of Exposed People, p 386). HBV vaccine is used for preexposure and postexposure protection and provides long-term protection. Preexposure immunization with HBV vaccine is the most effective means to prevent HBV transmission. Accordingly, HBV immunization is recommended for all infants, children, and adolescents through 18 years of age. Infants should be immunized as part of the routine childhood immunization schedule. All children 11 through 12 years of age should have their immunization records reviewed and should complete the vaccine series if they have not received the vaccine or did not complete the immunization series.

Postexposure immunoprophylaxis with either hepatitis B vaccine and HBIG or hepatitis B vaccine alone effectively prevents most infections after exposure to HBV. Effectiveness of postexposure immunoprophylaxis is related directly to the time elapsed between exposure and administration. Immunoprophylaxis of perinatal infection is most effective if given within 12 hours of birth; data are limited on effectiveness when administered between 25 hours and 7 days of life. Serologic testing of all pregnant women for HBsAg during each pregnancy is essential for identifying women whose infants will require postexposure immunoprophylaxis beginning at birth (see Care of Exposed People, p 386).

---

[1]Centers for Disease Control and Prevention. A comprehensive immunization strategy to eliminate transmission of hepatitis B virus infection in the United States: recommendations of the Advisory Committee on Immunization Practices (ACIP).Part 1: immunization of infants, children, and adolescents. *MMWR Recomm Rep.* 2005;54(RR-16):1–31

[2]Centers for Disease Control and Prevention. A comprehensive immunization strategy to eliminate transmission of hepatitis B virus infection in the United States: recommendations of the Advisory Committee on Immunization Practices (ACIP).Part II: immunization of adults. *MMWR Recomm Rep.* 2006;55(RR-16):1–33

Hepatitis B Immune Globulin.[1] HBIG is prepared from hyperimmunized donors whose plasma is known to contain a high concentration of anti-HBs. Plasma donors have negative serologic and nucleic acid test results for HIV and HCV. Additionally, the processes used to manufacture HBIG products are demonstrated to inactivate HBV, HIV, and HCV. Standard Immune Globulin is not effective for postexposure prophylaxis against HBV infection, because concentrations of anti-HBs are too low.

Hepatitis B Vaccine. Highly effective and safe hepatitis B vaccines produced by recombinant DNA technology are licensed in the United States in single-antigen formulations and as components of combination vaccines. Plasma-derived hepatitis B vaccines no longer are available in the United States but may be used successfully in a few countries. Recombinant vaccines contain 5 to 40 µg of HBsAg protein/mL and result in production of anti-HBs in the recipient, which provides protection. Single-dose (including pediatric) formulations contain no thimerosal as a preservative. Although the concentration of recombinant HBsAg protein differs among vaccine products, rates of seroprotection are equivalent when given to immunocompetent infants, children, adolescents, or young adults in the doses recommended (see Table 3.17, p 378).

HBV vaccine can be given concurrently with other vaccines (see Simultaneous Administration of Multiple Vaccines, p 33).

Vaccine Interchangeability. In general, the various brands of age-appropriate hepatitis B vaccines are interchangeable within an immunization series. The immune response using 1 or 2 doses of a vaccine produced by one manufacturer followed by 1 or more subsequent doses from a different manufacturer is comparable to a full course of immunization with a single product. However, until additional data supporting interchangeability of acellular pertussis-containing hepatitis B combination vaccines are available, vaccines from the same manufacturer should be used, whenever feasible, for at least the first 3 doses in the pertussis series (see Pertussis, p 553). In addition, a 2-dose schedule of the adult formulation of Recombivax HB is licensed for adolescents 11 through 15 years of age (see Table 3.17, p 378).

Routes of Administration. Vaccine is administered intramuscularly in the anterolateral thigh for infants or deltoid area for children and adults (see Vaccine Administration, p 20). Administration in the buttocks or intradermally has been associated with decreased immunogenicity and is not recommended at any age.

Efficacy and Duration of Protection. Hepatitis B vaccines licensed in the United States have a 90% to 95% efficacy for preventing HBV infection and clinical HBV disease among susceptible children and adults. Long-term studies of immunocompetent adults and children indicate that immune memory remains intact for up to 2 decades and protects against symptomatic acute and chronic HBV infection, even though anti-HBs concentrations may become low or undetectable over time. Breakthrough infections (detected by presence of anti-HBc or HBV DNA) have occurred in a limited number of immunized people, but these infections typically are transient and asymptomatic. Chronic HBV infection in immunized people has been documented in dialysis patients whose anti-HBs concentrations fell below 10 mIU/mL and rarely in infants born to HBsAg-positive mothers.

---

[1] Dosages recommended for postexposure prophylaxis are for products licensed in the United States. Because concentration of anti-HBs in other products may vary, different dosages may be recommended in other countries.

Table 3.17. Recommended Dosages of Hepatitis B Vaccines

Patients	Vaccine[a]		Combination Vaccine
	RecombivaxHB[b] Dose, µg (mL)	Engerix-B[c] Dose, µg (mL)	Twinrix[d]
Infants of HBsAg-negative mothers and children and adolescents younger than 20 y of age	5 (0.5)	10 (0.5)	Not applicable
Infants of HBsAg-positive mothers (HBIG [0.5 mL] also is recommended)	5 (0.5)	10 (0.5)	Not applicable
Adults 20 y of age or older	10 (1.0)	20 (1.0)	20 (1.0)
Adults undergoing dialysis and other immunosuppressed adults	40 (1.0)[e]	40 (2.0)[f]	Not applicable

HBsAg indicates hepatitis B surface antigen; HBIG, Hepatitis B Immune Globulin.

[a] Both vaccines are administered in a 3-dose schedule at 0, 1, and 6 months; 4 doses may be administered if a birth dose is given and a combination vaccine is used (at 2, 4, and 6 months) to complete the series. Only single-antigen hepatitis B vaccine can be used for the birth dose. Single-antigen or combination vaccine containing hepatitis B vaccine may be used to complete the series.

[b] Available from Merck & Co Inc.
- A 2-dose schedule, administered at 0 months and then 4 to 6 months later, is licensed for adolescents 11 through 15 years of age using the adult formulation of Recombivax HB (10 µg).
- A combination of hepatitis B (Recombivax, 5 µg) and *Haemophilus influenzae* type b (PRP-OMP) vaccine is recommended for use at 2, 4, and 12 through 15 months of age (Comvax). This vaccine should not be administered at birth, before 6 weeks of age, or after 71 months of age. For additional information, see *Haemophilus influenzae* Infections (p 345).

[c] Available from GlaxoSmithKline Biologicals. The US Food and Drug Administration also has licensed this vaccine for use in an optional 4-dose schedule at 0, 1, 2, and 12 months for all age groups. A 0-, 12-, and 24-month schedule is licensed for children 5 through 16 years of age, and a 0-, 1-, and 6-month schedule is licensed for adolescents 11 through 16 years of age.
- A combination of diphtheria and tetanus toxoids and acellular pertussis (DTaP), inactivated poliovirus (IPV), and hepatitis B (Engerix-B 10 µg) is recommended for use at 2, 4, and 6 months of age (Pediarix). This vaccine should not be administered at birth, before 6 weeks of age, or at 7 years of age or older. For additional information, see Pertussis (p 553).

[d] A combination of hepatitis B (Engerix-B, 20 µg) and hepatitis A (Havrix, 720 enzyme-linked immunosorbent assay units [ELU]) vaccine (Twinrix) is licensed for use in people 18 years of age and older in a 3-dose schedule administered at 0 mo, 1 mo, and 6 or more months later. Alternately, a 4-dose schedule at days 0, 7, and 21 to 30 followed by a booster dose at 12 months may be used.

[e] Special formulation for adult dialysis patients given at 0, 1, and 6 months.

[f] Two 1.0-mL doses given in 1 or 2 injections in a 4-dose schedule at 0, 1, 2, and 6 months of age.

Booster Doses. For children and adults with normal immune status, routine booster doses of hepatitis B vaccine are not recommended. For hemodialysis patients and other immunocompromised people at continued risk of infection, the need for booster doses should be assessed by annual anti-HBs testing, and a booster dose should be given when the anti-HBs concentration is less than 10 mIU/mL.

Adverse Reactions. Adverse effects most commonly reported in adults and children are pain at the injection site, reported by 3% to 29% of recipients, and a temperature greater than 37.7°C (99.8°F), reported by 1% to 6% of recipients. Anaphylaxis is uncommon, occurring in approximately 1 in 600 000 recipients, according to vaccine adverse events passive reporting surveillance systems. Large, controlled epidemiologic studies and review by the Institute of Medicine[1] (see Institute of Medicine Reviews of Adverse Events After Immunization, p 43) show no association between hepatitis B vaccine and sudden infant death syndrome, diabetes mellitus, or demyelinating disease, including multiple sclerosis.

Immunization During Pregnancy or Lactation. No adverse effect on the developing fetus has been observed when pregnant women have been immunized. Because HBV infection may result in severe disease in the mother and chronic infection in the newborn infant, pregnancy is not a contraindication to immunization. Lactation is not a contraindication to immunization.

Serologic Testing. Susceptibility testing before immunization is not indicated routinely for children or adolescents. Testing for past or current infection may be considered for people in risk groups with high rates of HBV infection, including people born in countries with intermediate and high HBV endemicity (even if immunized), users of injection drugs, men who have sex with men, and household and sexual contacts of HBsAg-positive people, provided testing does not delay or impede immunization efforts. A substantial proportion of people with chronic HBV infection are unaware of their infection.

Routine postimmunization testing for anti-HBs is not necessary but is recommended 1 to 2 months after the third vaccine dose for the following specific groups: (1) hemodialysis patients; (2) people with HIV infection; (3) people at occupational risk of exposure from percutaneous injuries or mucosal or nonintact skin exposures (certain health care and public safety workers); (4) immunocompromised patients at risk of exposure to HBV; (5) regular sexual contacts of HBsAg-positive people, and (6) infants born to HBsAg-positive mothers. These infants should have postimmunization testing for HBsAg and anti-HBs performed at 9 to 18 months of age, generally at the next well-child visit after completion of the vaccine series (see Prevention of Perinatal HBV Infection, p 386). Postimmunization testing also should be considered in people 65 years of age or older.

Management of Nonresponders. Vaccine recipients who do not develop a serum anti-HBs response (10 mIU/mL or greater) after a primary vaccine series should be tested for HBsAg and, if HBsAg-negative, reimmunized with an additional 3-dose series. Fewer than 5% of immunocompetent people receiving 6 doses of hepatitis B vaccine administered by the appropriate schedule in the deltoid muscle fail to develop detectable antibody. People who remain anti-HBs negative 1 to 2 months after a reimmunization series are unlikely to respond to additional doses of vaccine and should be considered nonimmune if they are exposed to HBV in the future (Table 3.18, p 380).

Altered Doses and Schedules. Larger vaccine doses are required to induce protective anti-HBs concentrations in adult hemodialysis patients and for immunocompromised adults, including HIV-seropositive people (see Table 3.17, p 378). Humoral immune response to HBV vaccine also may be reduced in children and adolescents who are receiving hemodialysis or are immunocompromised. However, few data exist concerning the response to higher doses of vaccine in children and adolescents, and no specific recommendations can be made. For people with progressive chronic renal failure, hepatitis B vaccine is recommended early in the disease course to provide protection and potentially decrease the need for larger doses once dialysis is initiated.

---

[1]Institute of Medicine. *Adverse Effects of Vaccines: Evidence and Causality.* Washington, DC: National Academies Press; 2011

Table 3.18. Recommendations for Hepatitis B Virus (HBV) Prophylaxis After Percutaneous or Mucosal Exposure to Blood or Body Fluids[a]

	Treatment When Source Is		
Exposed Person	**HBsAg Positive**	**HBsAg Negative**	**Unknown or Not Tested**
Unimmunized	Administer HBIG[b] (1 dose) and initiate HBV series	Initiate HBV series	Initiate HBV vaccine series
Previously immunized			
Known responder	No treatment	No treatment	No treatment
Known nonresponder	HBIG (1 dose) and initiate reimmunization[c] or HBIG (2 doses)	No treatment	If known high-risk source, treat as if source were HBsAg positive
Response unknown	Test exposed person for anti-HBs[d] If adequate, no treatment If inadequate, HBIG × 1 and vaccine booster	No treatment	Test exposed person for anti-HBs[d] • If adequate, no treatment • If inadequate, vaccine booster dose[e]

HBsAg indicates hepatitis B surface antigen; HBIG, Hepatitis B Immune Globulin; anti-HBs, antibody to HBsAg.
[a] Centers for Disease Control and Prevention. Immunization of health-care personnel: recommendations of the Advisory Committee on Immunization Practices (ACIP). *MMWR Recomm Rep.* 2011;60(RR-7):1–45
[b] Dose of HBIG, 0.06 mL/kg, intramuscularly.
[c] The option of giving 1 dose of HBIG (0.06 mL/kg) and reinitiating the vaccine series is preferred for nonresponders who have not completed a second 3-dose vaccine series. For people who previously completed a second vaccine series but failed to respond, 2 doses of HBIG (0.06 mL/kg) are preferred, 1 dose as soon as possible after exposure and the second 1 month later.
[d] Adequate anti-HBs is ≥10 mIU/mL.
[e] The person should be evaluated for antibody response after the vaccine booster dose. For people who receive HBIG, anti-HBs testing should be performed when passively acquired antibody from HBIG no longer is detectable (eg, 4–6 months); for people who did not receive HBIG, anti-HBs testing should be performed 1 to 2 months after the vaccine booster dose. If anti-HBs is inadequate (less than 10 mIU/mL) after the vaccine booster dose, 2 additional doses should be administered to complete a 3-dose reimmunization series, followed by postimmunization testing for anti-HBs and HBsAg.

Preexposure Universal Immunization of Infants, Children, and Adolescents. Hepatitis B immunization is recommended for all infants, children, and adolescents through 18 years of age. Delivery hospitals should develop policies and procedures that ensure administration of a birth dose as part of the routine care of all medically stable infants weighing 2000 g or more at birth, unless there is a physician's order to defer immunization and a report of the negative serologic status of the mother is in the infant's medical record. The hepatitis B vaccine series (3 or 4 doses; see discussion about birth dose in next paragraph) for infants born to HBsAg-negative mothers should be completed by 6 to 18 months of age. All children and adolescents who have not been immunized against HBV should begin the series during any visit.

High seroconversion rates and protective concentrations of anti-HBs (10 mIU/mL or greater) are achieved when hepatitis B vaccine is administered in any of the various recommended schedules, including schedules begun soon after birth in term infants. Only single-antigen hepatitis B vaccine can be used for doses given between birth and 6 weeks of age. Single-antigen or combination vaccine may be used to complete the series; 4 doses of vaccine may be administered if a birth dose is given and a combination vaccine containing a hepatitis B component is used to complete the series.[1] For guidelines for minimum scheduling time between vaccine doses for infants, see Table 1.7 (p 26). The schedule should be chosen to facilitate a high rate of adherence to the primary vaccine series. For immunization of older children and adolescents, doses may be given in a schedule of 0, 1, and 6 months; of 0, 1, and 4 months; or of 0, 2, and 4 months (although shorter intervals between first and last doses result in lower immunogenicity). For older children and adolescents, spacing at 0, 12, and 24 months results in equivalent immunogenicity and can be used when an extended administration schedule is acceptable on the basis of low risk of exposure. A 2-dose schedule for one vaccine formulation is licensed for people 11 through 15 years of age; the schedule is 0 and then 4 to 6 months later (see Table 3.17, p 378).

The recommended schedule for routine hepatitis B immunization of infants born to HBsAg-negative mothers is provided in Fig 1.1 (p 27–28). Age-specific vaccine dosages are provided in Table 3.17 (p 378). Combination products containing HBV vaccine may be given in the United States, provided they are licensed by the FDA for the child's current age and administration of the other vaccine component(s) also is indicated. Children and adolescents who previously have not received hepatitis B vaccine should be immunized routinely at any age with the age-appropriate doses and schedule. Selection of a vaccine schedule should consider the need to achieve completion of the vaccine series. In all settings, immunization should be initiated even though completion of the vaccine series might not be ensured.

Preexposure Immunization of Adults.[2]

- HBV immunization is recommended as a 3-dose series for all unimmunized adults at risk of HBV infection (see Table 3.19, p 382) and for all adults seeking protection from HBV infection. Acknowledgment of a specific risk factor is not a requirement for immunization.

- In settings where a high proportion of adults are likely to have risk factors for HBV infection, all unimmunized adults should be assumed to be at risk and should receive hepatitis B immunization. These settings include: (1) sexually transmitted infection treatment facilities; (2) HIV testing and treatment facilities; (3) facilities providing drug abuse treatment and prevention services; (4) health care settings targeting services to injection drug users; (5) correctional facilities; (6) health care settings serving men who have sex with men; (7) chronic hemodialysis facilities and end-stage renal disease programs; and (8) institutions and nonresidential care facilities for people with developmental disabilities.

---

[1]Centers for Disease Control and Prevention. General recommendations on immunization. Recommendations of the Advisory Committee on Immunization Practices (ACIP). *MMWR Recomm Rep.* 2011;60(RR-2):1–64

[2]Centers for Disease Control and Prevention. A comprehensive immunization strategy to eliminate transmission of hepatitis B virus infection in the United States: recommendations of the Advisory Committee on Immunization Practices (ACIP).Part II: immunization of adults. *MMWR Recomm Rep.* 2006;55(RR-16):1–33

Table 3.19. Adults Recommended to Receive Hepatitis B Virus (HBV) Immunization[a]

People at Risk of Infection by Sexual Exposure
- Sex partners of hepatitis B surface antigen (HBsAg)-positive people
- Sexually active people who are not in a long-term, mutually monogamous relationship (eg, people with more than 1 sex partner during the previous 6 months)
- People seeking evaluation or treatment for a sexually transmitted infection
- Men who have sex with men

People at Risk of Infection by Percutaneous or Mucosal Exposure to Blood
- Current or recent injection-drug users
- Household contacts of HBsAg-positive people
- Residents and staff of facilities for people with developmental disabilities
- Health-care and public safety workers with reasonably anticipated risk of exposure to blood or blood-contaminated body fluids
- People with end-stage renal disease, including predialysis, hemodialysis, peritoneal dialysis, and home dialysis patients
- People with diabetes mellitus 19 through 59 years of age; people with diabetes mellitus 60 years of age and older may be immunized at the discretion of their physician

Others
- International travelers to regions with high or intermediate levels (HBsAg prevalence of 2% or greater) of endemic HBV infection (see Table 3.15, p 373)
- People with chronic liver disease
- People with human immunodeficiency (HIV) infection
- All other people seeking protection from HBV infection

[a] Centers for Disease Control and Prevention. A comprehensive immunization strategy to eliminate transmission of hepatitis B virus infection in the United States: recommendations of the Advisory Committee on Immunization Practices (ACIP). Part II: immunization of adults. *MMWR Recomm Rep.* 2006;55(RR-16):1–33

- Hepatitis B immunization should be administered to unimmunized adults with diabetes mellitus who are 19 through 59 years of age.[1] Hepatitis B immunization may be administered at the discretion of the treating clinician to unimmunized adults with diabetes mellitus who are 60 years of age or older.
- Standing orders should be implemented to identify and immunize eligible adults in primary care and specialty medical settings. If ascertainment of risk for HBV infection is a barrier to immunization in these settings, health care professionals may use alternative immunization strategies, such as offering hepatitis B vaccine to all unimmunized adults in age groups with highest risk of infection (eg, younger than 49 years of age).

Lapsed Immunizations. For infants, children, adolescents, and adults with lapsed immunizations (ie, the interval between doses is longer than that in one of the recommended schedules), the vaccine series can be completed, regardless of the interval from the last dose of vaccine (see Lapsed Immunizations, p 35).

[1] Centers for Disease Control and Prevention. Use of hepatitis B vaccination for adults with diabetes mellitus: recommendations of the Advisory Committee on Immunization Practices (ACIP). *MMWR Morb Mortal Wkly Rep.* 2011;60(50):1709–1711

SPECIAL CONSIDERATIONS:

Infants Weighing <2000 g at Birth. Studies demonstrate that decreased seroconversion rates might occur among certain preterm infants with low birth weight (ie, less than 2000 g) after administration of hepatitis B vaccine at birth. However, by the chronologic age of 1 month, all medically stable preterm infants (see Preterm and Low Birth Weight Infants, p 69), regardless of initial birth weight or gestational age, are as likely to respond to hepatitis B immunization as are term and larger infants.

All infants weighing <2000 g who are born to an HBsAg-positive mother should receive immunoprophylaxis with hepatitis B vaccine and HBIG within 12 hours after birth; the birth dose of hepatitis B vaccine should not be counted toward completion of the HBV vaccine series, and 3 additional doses of hepatitis B vaccine should be administered beginning when the infant is 1 month of age (see Table 3.20, p 384). Only monovalent HBV vaccines should be used from birth to 6 weeks of age.

If maternal HBsAg status is unknown at birth, the infant weighing <2000 g should receive hepatitis B vaccine within 12 hours of birth. The mother's HBsAg status should be determined as quickly as possible. If the infant's birth weight is less than 2000 g and the maternal HBsAg status cannot be determined within 12 hours of life, HBIG should be given, because the less reliable immune response in preterm infants weighing less than 2000 g precludes the option of the 7-day waiting period acceptable for term and larger preterm infants. Only monovalent HBV vaccine should be used from birth through 6 weeks of life.

All infants of HBsAg-negative mothers with a birth weight of less than 2000 g can receive the first dose of hepatitis B vaccine series starting at 1 month of chronologic age or at hospital discharge if before 1 month of chronologic age. Infants born to HBsAg-negative mothers do not need to have postimmunization serologic testing for anti-HBs. Table 3.20 (p 384) provides a summary of the recommendations for immunization of infants on the basis of maternal hepatitis B status and infant birth weight. For information on use of combination vaccines containing hepatitis B vaccine as a component to complete the series, see Table 3.21 (p 386).

Considerations for High-Risk Groups:

Health Care Professionals and Others With Occupational Exposure to Blood. The risk of HBV exposure to a health care professional depends on the tasks the person performs. Health care professionals who have contact with blood or other potentially infectious body fluids should be immunized. Because the risks of occupational HBV infection often are highest during the training of health care professionals, immunization should be initiated as early as possible before or during training and before contact with blood, followed by postimmunization testing for anti-HBs for health care professionals with continuing high risk of exposure. Health care professionals with anti-HBs less than 10 mIU/mL should be reimmunized.

Patients Undergoing Hemodialysis. Immunization is recommended for susceptible patients undergoing hemodialysis. Immunization early in the course of renal disease is encouraged, because response is better than in advanced disease. Specific dosage recommendations have not been made for children undergoing hemodialysis. Some experts recommend increased doses of hepatitis B vaccine for children receiving hemodialysis to increase immunogenicity.

Table 3.20. Hepatitis B Virus (HBV) Immunoprophylaxis Scheme by Infant Birth Weight[a]

Maternal Status	Infant Birth Weight 2000 g or More	Infant Birth Weight Less Than 2000 g
HBsAg positive	Hepatitis B vaccine + HBIG (within 12 h of birth)	Hepatitis B vaccine + HBIG (within 12 h of birth)
	Continue vaccine series beginning at 1–2 mo of age according to recommended schedule for infants born to HBsAg-positive mothers (see Table 3.21)	Continue vaccine series beginning at 1–2 mo of age according to recommended schedule for infants born to HBsAg-positive mothers (see Table 3.21)
		Immunize with 4 vaccine doses; do not count birth dose as part of the 3-dose vaccine series
	Check anti-HBs and HBsAg after completion of vaccine series[b]	Check anti-HBs and HBsAg after completion of vaccine series[b]
	HBsAg-negative infants with anti-HBs levels 10 mIU/mL or greater are protected and need no further medical management	HBsAg-negative infants with anti-HBs levels 10 mIU/mL or greater are protected and need no further medical management
	HBsAg-negative infants with anti-HBs levels less than 10 mIU/mL should be reimmunized with a second 3-dose series and retested	HBsAg-negative infants with anti-HBs levels less than 10 mIU/mL should be reimmunized with a second 3-dose series and retested
	Infants who are HBsAg positive should receive appropriate follow-up, including medical evaluation for chronic liver disease	Infants who are HBsAg positive should receive appropriate follow-up, including medical evaluation for chronic liver disease
HBsAg status unknown	Test mother for HBsAg immediately after admission for delivery	Test mother for HBsAg immediately after admission for delivery
	Hepatitis B vaccine (within 12h of birth)	Hepatitis B vaccine (within 12h of birth)
	Administer HBIG (within 7 days) if mother tests HBsAg positive; if mother's HBsAg status remains unknown, some experts would administer HBIG (within 7 days)	Administer HBIG if mother tests HBsAg positive or if mother's HBsAg result is not available within 12 h of birth
	Continue vaccine series beginning at 1–2 mo of age according to recommended schedule based on mother's HBsAg result (see Table 3.21)	Continue vaccine series beginning at 1–2 mo of age according to recommended schedule based on mother's HBsAg result (see Table 3.21)
		Immunize with 4 vaccine doses; do not count birth dose as part of the 3-dose vaccine series

Table 3.20. Hepatitis B Virus (HBV) Immunoprophylaxis Scheme by Infant Birth Weight,[a] continued

Maternal Status	Infant Birth Weight 2000 g or More	Infant Birth Weight Less Than 2000 g
HBsAg negative	HBV vaccine at birth[c]	Delay first dose of hepatitis B vaccine until 1 mo of age or hospital discharge, whichever is first
	Continue the 3-dose vaccine series beginning at 1–2 mo of age (see Table 3.21)	Continue the 3-dose vaccine series beginning at 2 mo of age (see Table 3.21)
	Follow-up anti-HBs and HBsAg testing not needed	Follow-up anti-HBs and HBsAg testing not needed

HBsAg indicates hepatitis B surface antigen; HBIG, hepatitis B Immune Globulin; anti-HBs, antibody to HBsAg.
[a] Extremes of gestational age and birth weight no longer are a consideration for timing of hepatitis B vaccine doses.
[b] Test at 9 to 18 months of age, generally at the next well-child visit after completion of the primary series. Use testing method that allows determination of a protective concentration of anti-HBs (10 mIU/mL or greater).
[c] The first dose may be delayed until after hospital discharge for an infant who weighs 2000 g or greater and whose mother is HBsAg negative, but only if a physician's order to withhold the birth dose and a copy of the mother's original HBsAg-negative laboratory report are documented in the infant's medical record.

People Born in Countries Where the Prevalence of Chronic HBV Infection Is 2% or Greater. Foreign-born people (including immigrants, refugees, asylum seekers, and internationally adopted children) from countries where the prevalence of chronic HBV infection is 2% or greater (see Table 3.15, p 373) should be screened for HBsAg regardless of immunization status. Previously unimmunized family members and other household contacts should be immunized if a household member is found to be HBsAg positive. In addition, HBsAg positivity is a nationally notifiable disease (see Appendix VI, p 902). People who are HBsAg positive should be reported to the local or state health department and referred for medical management to reduce their risk of chronic liver disease.

Inmates in Juvenile Detention and Other Correctional Facilities. Unimmunized or underimmunized people in juvenile and adult correctional facilities should be immunized. If the length of stay is not sufficient to complete the immunization series, the series should be initiated and follow-up mechanisms with a health care facility should be established to ensure completion of the series (see Hepatitis and Youth in Correctional Settings, p 186).

International Travelers. People traveling to areas where the prevalence of chronic HBV infection is 2% or greater (see Table 3.15, p 373) should be immunized. Immunization should begin at least 4 to 6 months before travel so that a 3-dose regimen can be completed (see Preexposure Universal Immunization, p 380). If immunization is initiated fewer than 4 months before departure, the alternative 4-dose schedule of 0, 1, 2, and 12 months, licensed for one vaccine (see Table 3.17, p 378), should provide protection if the first 3 doses can be administered before travel. Individual clinicians may choose to use an accelerated schedule (eg, doses at days 0, 7, and 21) for travelers who will depart before an approved immunization schedule can be completed. The FDA has not licensed schedules that involve immunization at more than one time point during a single month for hepatitis B vaccine licensed in the United States. People who receive immunization on

Table 3.21. Hepatitis B Vaccine Schedules for Infants by Maternal Hepatitis B Surface Antigen (HBsAg) Status[a,b]

Maternal HBsAg Status	Single-Antigen Vaccine		Single-Antigen + Combination	
	Dose	Age	Dose	Age
Positive	1[c]	Birth (12 h or less)	1[c]	Birth (12 h or less) (Combination vaccine should not be used for birth dose)
	HBIG[d]	Birth (12 h or less)	HBIG[d]	Birth (12 h or less)
	2	1 through 2 mo	2	2 mo
	3[e]	6 mo	3	4 mo
			4[e]	6 mo (Pediarix) or 12 through 15 mo (Comvax)
Unknown[f]	1[c]	Birth (12 h or less)	1[c]	Birth (12 h or less) (Combination vaccine should not be used for birth dose)
	2	1 through 2 mo	2	2 mo
	3[e]	6 mo	3	4 mo
			4[e]	6 mo (Pediarix) or 12 through 15 mo (Comvax)
Negative	1[c,g]	Birth (before discharge)	1[c,g]	Birth (before discharge) (Combination vaccine should not be used for birth dose)
	2	1 through 2 mo	2	2 mo
	3[e]	6 through 18 mo	3	4 mo
			4[e]	6 mo (Pediarix) or 12 through 15 mo (Comvax)

HBIG indicates Hepatitis B Immune Globulin.

[a] Centers for Disease Control and Prevention. A comprehensive immunization strategy to eliminate transmission of hepatitis B virus infection in the United States: recommendations of the Advisory Committee on Immunization Practices (ACIP). Part 1: immunization of infants, children, and adolescents. *MMWR Recomm Rep.* 2005;54(RR-16):1–31.

[b] See Table 3.20 for vaccine schedules for preterm infants weighing less than 2000 g.

[c] Recombivax HB or Engerix-B should be used for the birth dose. Comvax and Pediarix should not be administered at birth or before 6 weeks of age.

[d] HBIG (0.5 mL) administered intramuscularly in a separate site from vaccine.

[e] The final dose in the vaccine series should not be administered before 24 weeks (164 days) of age.

[f] Mothers should have blood drawn and tested for HBsAg as soon as possible after admission for delivery; if the mother is found to be HBsAg positive, the infant should receive HBIG as soon as possible but no later than 7 days of age.

[g] On a case-by-case basis and only in rare circumstances, the first dose may be delayed until after hospital discharge for an infant who weighs 2000 g or more and whose mother is HBsAg negative, but only if a physician's order to withhold the birth dose and a copy of the mother's original HBsAg-negative laboratory report are documented in the infant's medical record.

an accelerated schedule that is not FDA licensed also should receive a dose at 12 months after initiation of the series to promote long-term immunity.

Care of Exposed People (Postexposure Immunoprophylaxis) (Also See Table 3.22, p 387).

Prevention of Perinatal HBV Infection. Transmission of perinatal HBV infection can be prevented in approximately 95% of infants born to HBsAg-positive mothers by early active and passive immunoprophylaxis of the infant (ie, immunization and HBIG administration within 12 hours of birth). Immunization subsequently should be com-

Table 3.22. Guide to Postexposure Immunoprophylaxis of Unimmunized People to Prevent Hepatitis B Virus (HBV) Infection

Type of Exposure	Immunoprophylaxis[a]
Household contact of HBsAg-positive person	Administer hepatitis B vaccine series
Discrete exposure to an HBsAg-positive source[b]:	
• Percutaneous (eg, bite, needlestick, nonintact skin) or mucosal exposure to HBsAg-positive blood or body fluids	Administer hepatitis B vaccine + HBIG; complete vaccine series
• Sexual contact or needle sharing with an HBsAg-positive person	Administer hepatitis B vaccine + HBIG; complete vaccine series
• Victim of sexual assault/abuse by a perpetrator who is HBsAg positive	Administer hepatitis B vaccine + HBIG; complete vaccine series
Discrete exposure to a source with unknown HBsAg status:	
• Percutaneous (eg, bite, needlestick) or mucosal exposure to blood or body fluids with unknown HBsAg status	Administer hepatitis B vaccine series
• Victim of sexual assault/abuse by a perpetrator with unknown HBsAg status	Administer hepatitis B vaccine series

HBsAg indicates hepatitis B surface antigen; HBIG, Hepatitis B Immune Globulin.
[a] Immunoprophylaxis should be administered as soon as possible, preferably within 24 hours after exposure. Studies are limited on the maximum interval after exposure during which postexposure prophylaxis is effective, but the interval is unlikely to exceed 7 days for percutaneous exposures and 14 days for sexual exposures.
[b] If person previously was immunized with hepatitis B vaccine series, administer hepatitis B vaccine booster dose (See Table 3.18).

pleted during the first 6 months of life. HBV immunization alone, initiated at or shortly after birth, also is highly effective for preventing perinatal HBV infections.

Serologic Screening of Pregnant Women. Prenatal HBsAg testing of all pregnant women, regardless of hepatitis B vaccination history, is recommended to identify newborn infants who require immediate postexposure prophylaxis. All pregnant women should be tested during an early prenatal visit with every pregnancy. Testing should be repeated at the time of admission to the hospital for delivery for HBsAg-negative women who are at high risk of HBV infection or who have had clinical HBV infection. Women who are HBsAg-positive should be reported to local health departments for appropriate case management to ensure follow-up of their infants and immunization of sexual and household contacts. In populations where HBsAg testing of pregnant women is not feasible (eg, in remote areas without access to a laboratory), all infants should receive HBV vaccine within 12 hours of birth, the second dose by 2 months of age, and the third dose at 6 months of age. Pregnant women and their contacts who are HBsAg-positive should be referred for medical management to reduce their risk of chronic liver disease.

Management of Infants Born to HBsAg-Positive Women. Infants born to HBsAg-positive mothers, including infants weighing <2000 g, should receive the initial dose of hepatitis B vaccine within 12 hours of birth (see Table 3.17, p 378, for appropriate dosages), and HBIG (0.5 mL) should be given concurrently but at a different anatomic site. The effectiveness of HBIG diminishes the longer after exposure that it is initiated. The interval of effectiveness is unlikely to exceed 7 days. Subsequent doses of vaccine should be given as recommended in Table 3.20 (p 384) and Table 3.21 (p 386). For infants who weigh less than 2000 g at birth, the initial vaccine dose should not be counted in the required 3-dose schedule (a total of 4 doses of hepatitis B vaccine should be administered), and the subsequent 3 doses should be given in accordance with the schedule for immunization of infants weighing <2000 g (see Preterm and Low Birth Weight Infants, p 69).

Infants born to HBsAg-positive women should be tested for anti-HBs and HBsAg at 9 to 18 months of age (generally at the next well-child visit after completion of the immunization series). Testing should not be performed before 9 months of age to avoid detection of anti-HBs from HBIG administered during infancy and to maximize the likelihood of detecting late HBV infections. Testing for HBsAg will identify infants who become infected chronically despite immunization (because of intrauterine infection or vaccine failure) and will aid in their long-term medical management. Testing for IgM anti-HBc is unreliable for infants. Infants with anti-HBs concentrations less than 10 mIU/mL and who are HBsAg negative should receive 3 additional doses of vaccine (see Table 3.20, p 384) followed by testing for anti-HBs 1 to 2 months after the third dose. Alternatively, 1 to 3 additional doses of vaccine can be administered, followed by testing for anti-HBs 1 to 2 months after each dose, to determine whether subsequent doses are needed.

Term Infants (Weighing ≥2000 g at Birth) Born to Mothers Not Tested During Pregnancy for HBsAg. Pregnant women whose HBsAg status is unknown at delivery should undergo blood testing as soon as possible to determine their HBsAg status. While awaiting results, the infant should receive the first hepatitis B vaccine dose within 12 hours of birth as recommended for infants born to HBsAg-positive mothers (see Table 3.17, p 378). Because hepatitis B vaccine, when given at birth, is highly effective for preventing perinatal infection in term infants, the possible added value and the cost of HBIG do not warrant its immediate use in term infants when the mother's HBsAg status is not known. If the woman is found to be HBsAg positive, term infants should receive HBIG (0.5 mL) as soon as possible, but within 7 days of birth, and should complete the hepatitis B immunization series as recommended (see Tables 3.17, p 378, and 3.19, p 382). If HBIG is unavailable, the infant still should receive the 2 subsequent doses of hepatitis B vaccine at 1 to 2, and 6 months of age. If the mother is found to be HBsAg negative, hepatitis B immunization in the dose and schedule recommended for term infants born to HBsAg-negative mothers should be completed (see Table 3.17, p 378). If the mother's HBsAg status remains unknown, some experts would administer HBIG within 7 days of birth and complete the hepatitis B immunization series as recommended for infants born to mothers who are HBsAg positive (Table 3.20, p 384).

Infants Weighing <2000 g Born to Mothers Not Tested During Pregnancy for HBsAg. Maternal HBsAg status should be determined as soon as possible. Infants weighing <2000 g born to mothers whose HBsAg status is unknown should receive hepatitis B vaccine within the first 12 hours of life. Because of the potentially decreased immunogenicity of the hepatitis B vaccine in infants weighing less than 2000 g at birth, these infants should receive HBIG (0.5 mL) if the mother's HBsAg status cannot be determined within the initial 12 hours of birth. In these infants, the initial vaccine dose should not be counted toward the 3 doses of hepatitis B vaccine required to complete the immunization series. The subsequent 3 doses (for a total of 4 doses) are given in accordance with recommendations for immunization of infants with a birth weight less than 2000 g according to the HBsAg status of the mother (see Table 3.20, p 384). Follow-up HBsAg and anti-HBs testing on completion of the immunization series is recommended for all infants weighing <2000 g of HBsAg-positive mothers (see Management of Infants Born to HBsAg-Positive Women, p 387).

Breastfeeding. Breastfeeding of the infant by an HBsAg-positive mother poses no additional risk of acquisition of HBV infection by the infant with appropriate administration of hepatitis B vaccine and HBIG (see Human Milk, p 126).

Household Contacts and Sexual Partners of HBsAg-Positive People.
Household and sexual contacts of HBsAg-positive people (acute or chronic HBV infection) identified through prenatal screening, blood donor screening, or diagnostic or other serologic testing should be immunized.

Children younger than 12 months of age who have close contact with primary caregivers with acute or chronic HBV infection require immunoprophylaxis. If, at the time of exposure, the infant has been immunized fully or has received at least 2 doses of vaccine, the infant should be presumed protected, and HBIG is not required. If only 1 dose of vaccine has been administered, the second dose should be administered if the interval is appropriate, or HBIG should be administered if immunization is not yet due. If immunization has not been initiated, the infant should receive HBIG (0.5 mL), and hepatitis B vaccine should be given in accordance with the routinely recommended 3-dose schedule (see Preexposure Universal Immunization, p 380).

Prophylaxis with HBIG for other unimmunized household contacts of HBsAg-positive people is not indicated unless they have a discrete, identifiable exposure to the index patient (see next paragraph).

Postexposure Prophylaxis for People With Discrete Identifiable Exposures to Blood or Body Fluids.
Management of people with a discrete, identifiable percutaneous (eg, needlestick, laceration, bite or nonintact skin) or mucosal (eg, ocular or mucous membrane) exposure to blood or body fluids includes consideration of whether the HBsAg status of the person who was the source of exposure is known and the hepatitis B immunization and response status of the exposed person (also see Table 3.18, p 380). Immunization is recommended for any person who was exposed but not previously immunized. If possible, a blood specimen from the person who was the source of the exposure should be tested for HBsAg, and appropriate prophylaxis should be administered according to the hepatitis B immunization status and anti-HBs response status (if known) of the exposed person (see Table 3.18, p 380, and Injuries From Discarded Needles in the Community, p 200). Detailed guidelines for management of health care professionals and other people exposed to blood that is or might be HBsAg-positive is provided in the recommendations of the Advisory Committee on Immunization Practices of the Centers for Disease Control and Prevention (CDC).[1]

HBsAg-Positive Source. If the source is HBsAg positive, unimmunized people should receive both HBIG and hepatitis B vaccine as soon as possible after exposure, preferably within 24 hours (see Table 3.18, p 380). The vaccine series should be completed using an age-appropriate dose and schedule. People who are in the process of being immunized but who have not completed the vaccine series should receive the appropriate dose of HBIG and should complete the vaccine series. Children and adolescents who have written documentation of a complete hepatitis B vaccine series and who

---

[1]Centers for Disease Control and Prevention. Immunization of health-care personnel: recommendations of the Advisory Committee on Immunization Practices (ACIP). *MMWR Recomm Rep.* 2011;60(RR-7):1–45

did not receive postimmunization testing should receive a single vaccine booster dose with postimmunization testing 1 to 2 months later (Table 3.18, p 380).

Source With Unknown HBsAg Status. If the HBsAg status of the source is unknown, unimmunized people should begin the hepatitis B vaccine series with the first dose initiated as soon as possible after exposure, preferably within 24 hours (see Table 3.18, p 380). The vaccine series should be completed using an age-appropriate dose and schedule. Children and adolescents with written documentation of a complete hepatitis B vaccine series require no further treatment (Table 3.18, p 380).

Victims of Sexual Assault or Abuse. For unimmunized victims of sexual assault or abuse, active postexposure prophylaxis (ie, vaccine alone) should be initiated, with the first dose of vaccine given as part of the initial clinical evaluation. If the offender is known to be HBsAg positive, HBIG also should be administered. The vaccine series should be completed using an age-appropriate dose and schedule. (For discussion of management of previously immunized people, see Postexposure Prophylaxis for People With Discrete Identifiable Exposures to Blood or Body Fluids That Contain Blood, p 367.)

Child Care. All children, including children who attend child care, should receive hepatitis B vaccine as part of their routine immunization schedule. Immunization not only will decrease the potential for transmission after bites but also will allay anxiety about transmission from attendees who may be HBsAg positive.

Children who are HBsAg positive and who have no behavioral or medical risk factors, such as unusually aggressive behavior (eg, frequent biting), generalized dermatitis, or a bleeding problem, should be admitted to child care without restrictions. Under these circumstances, the risk of HBV transmission in child care settings is negligible, and routine screening for HBsAg is not warranted. Admission of HBsAg-positive children with behavioral or medical risk factors should be assessed on an individual basis by the child's physician, the program director, and public health authorities (for further discussion, see Children in Out-of-Home Child Care, p 133).

Effectiveness of Hepatitis B Prevention Programs. Routine hepatitis B immunization programs have resulted in significant decreases in the prevalence of chronic HBV infection among children in populations with a high incidence of HBV infection. There is an association between higher coverage with hepatitis B vaccine and larger decreases in HBsAg prevalence. The incidence of acute HBV infection among US children younger than 19 years of age decreased by 98% between 1990 and 2010.

Although the long-term sequelae of chronic HBV infection usually are not recognized until adolescence and adulthood, cirrhosis and HCC occur in children. In Taiwan, the average annual incidence of HCC among children 6 to 14 years of age decreased significantly within 10 years of routine infant hepatitis B immunization. Worldwide, routine infant immunization programs and introduction of immunization schedules starting within the first 24 hours of life are expected to decrease significantly the incidence of death from cirrhosis and HCC attributable to HBV infection over the next 30 to 50 years.

The Centers for Disease Control and Prevention Division of Viral Hepatitis maintains a Web site (**www.cdc.gov/hepatitis**) with information on hepatitis for health care professionals and the public.

Hepatitis C

CLINICAL MANIFESTATIONS: Signs and symptoms of hepatitis C virus (HCV) infection are indistinguishable from those of hepatitis A or hepatitis B virus infections. Acute disease tends to be mild and insidious in onset, and most infections are asymptomatic. Jaundice occurs in fewer than 20% of patients, and abnormalities in liver transaminase concentrations generally are less pronounced than abnormalities in patients with hepatitis B virus infection. Persistent infection with HCV occurs in up to 80% of infected children, even in the absence of biochemical evidence of liver disease. Most children with chronic infection are asymptomatic. Although chronic hepatitis develops in approximately 70% to 80% of infected adults, limited data indicate that chronic hepatitis and cirrhosis occur less commonly in children, in part because of the usually indolent nature of infection in pediatric patients. Infection with HCV is the leading indication for liver transplantation among adults in the United States.

ETIOLOGY: HCV is a small, single-stranded RNA virus and is a member of the Flavivirus family. Multiple HCV genotypes and subtypes exist.

EPIDEMIOLOGY: The incidence of acute symptomatic HCV infection in the United States was 0.2 per 100 000 in 2005; after asymptomatic infection and underreporting were considered, approximately 20 000 new cases were estimated to have occurred. For all age groups, the incidence of HCV infection decreased in the United States during the 1990s and has remained low and stable since then. Nevertheless, a substantial burden of disease still exists in the United States because of the propensity of HCV to establish chronic infection and the high incidence of acute HCV infection through the 1980s. The prevalence of HCV infection in the general population of the United States is estimated at 1.3%, equating to an estimated 3.2 million people in the United States who have chronic HCV infection. Seroprevalences vary among populations according to their associated risk factors. Worldwide, the prevalence of chronic HCV infection is highest in Africa.

HCV primarily is spread by parenteral exposure to blood of HCV-infected people. The most common risk factors for acquiring infection are injection drug use, having multiple sexual partners, or having received blood products before 1992. The current risk of HCV infection after blood transfusion in the United States is estimated to be 1 per 2 million units transfused because of exclusion of high-risk donors and of HCV-positive units after antibody testing as well as screening of pools of blood units by some form of nucleic acid amplification test (NAAT; see Blood Safety, p 114). All intravenous and intramuscular Immune Globulin products available commercially in the United States undergo an inactivation procedure for HCV or are documented to be HCV RNA negative before release.

Almost all HCV transmission is by parenteral or percutaneous routes. Approximately 60% of chronic HCV cases reported to public health authorities are in acknowledged injection drug users who have shared needles or injection paraphernalia and, to a lesser extent, in people who received transfusions before 1992, when routine screening of donor blood for HCV began; almost all of these infected people are outside the pediatric age range. Data from recent multicenter, population-based cohort studies indicate that approximately one third of young injection drug users 18 to 30 years of age are infected with HCV. People with sporadic percutaneous exposures, such as health care professionals (approximately 1% of cases), may be infected. Approximately half of the 18 000 people with hemophilia (almost all male) who received transfusions before adoption of heat treatment of clotting factors in 1987 are HCV seropositive. Also, more recently appreciated has been the number of infections acquired in the health care setting, especially nonhospital clinics, in which infection control and needle and intravenous hygienic procedures have not been strict. Prevalence is moderately high among people with frequent but smaller direct percutaneous exposures, such as patients receiving hemodialysis (10%–20%).

Although some have suggested the possibility of HCV being transmitted sexually, the increasing number of lifetime sex partners is associated directly with an increasing likelihood of being an intravenous drug user (an often-unacknowledged risk), and several prospective studies have not been able to demonstrate transmission of HCV sexually between regular heterosexual partners. However, the exception appears to be HCV transmission sexually between or to human immunodeficiency virus (HIV)-infected (presumably immunosuppressed) people. There have been an increasing number of reports of sexual transmission of HCV between HIV-infected men who have sex with men or of HIV-infected heterosexual women.

Transmission among family contacts is uncommon but can occur from direct or inapparent percutaneous or mucosal exposure to blood.

Seroprevalence among pregnant women in the United States has been estimated at 1% to 2%. The risk of perinatal transmission averages 5% to 6%, and transmission occurs only from women who are HCV RNA positive at the time of delivery. Maternal coinfection with HIV has been associated with increased risk of perinatal transmission of HCV, which depends in part on the serologic concentration of HCV RNA in the mother. Serum antibody to HCV (anti-HCV) and HCV RNA have been detected in colostrum, but the risk of HCV transmission is similar in breastfed and bottle-fed infants.

All people with HCV-RNA in their blood are considered to be infectious.

The **incubation period** for HCV disease averages 6 to 7 weeks, with a range of 2 weeks to 6 months. The time from exposure to development of viremia generally is 1 to 2 weeks.

DIAGNOSTIC TESTS: The 2 major types of tests available for laboratory diagnosis of HCV infections are immunoglobulin (Ig) G antibody enzyme immunoassays for HCV and NAATs to detect HCV RNA. Assays for IgM to detect early or acute infection are not available. Third-generation enzyme immunoassays are at least 97% sensitive and more than 99% specific. In June 2010, the US Food and Drug Administration (FDA) approved for use in people 15 years of age and older the OraQuick rapid blood test, which uses a test strip that produces a blue line within 20 minutes if anti-HCV antibodies are present. False-negative results early in the course of acute infection can result from any of the HCV serologic tests because of the prolonged interval between exposure and onset of illness and seroconversion. Within 15 weeks after exposure and within 5 to 6 weeks after onset of hepatitis, 80% of patients will have positive test results for serum anti-HCV antibody. Among infants born to anti-HCV–positive mothers, passively acquired maternal antibody may persist for up to 18 months.

FDA-licensed diagnostic NAATs for qualitative detection of HCV RNA are available. HCV RNA can be detected in serum or plasma within 1 to 2 weeks after exposure to the virus and weeks before onset of liver enzyme abnormalities or appearance of anti-HCV.

Assays for detection of HCV RNA are used commonly in clinical practice to identify anti-HCV–positive patients who have HCV infection, for identifying infection in infants early in life (ie, perinatal transmission) when maternal antibody interferes with ability to detect antibody produced by the infant, and for monitoring patients receiving antiviral therapy. However, false-positive and false-negative results can occur from improper handling, storage, and contamination of test specimens. Viral RNA may be detected intermittently, and thus, a single negative assay result is not conclusive. Quantitative assays for measuring the concentration of HCV RNA are available but are less sensitive than qualitative assays. The clinical value of these quantitative assays appears to be primarily as a prognostic indicator for patients undergoing or about to undergo antiviral therapy.

TREATMENT: Patients diagnosed with HCV infection should be referred to a pediatric hepatitis specialist for clinical monitoring and consideration of antiviral treatment. Therapy is aimed at inhibiting HCV replication, eradicating infection, and improving the natural history of disease. Therapies are expensive and can have significant adverse reactions. Interferon-alfa or peginterferon-alfa alone and peginterferon-alfa in combination with ribavirin are approved by the FDA for treatment of chronic HCV infection in adults. Response to treatment varies depending on the genotype with which the person is infected. Combination therapy with pegylated interferon-alfa and ribavirin is the preferred treatment and results in sustained virologic response, defined as undetectable HCV RNA concentrations 6 or more months after treatment cessation. A sustained viral response occurs in 40% to 45% of treated adult patients infected with genotype 1 and approximately 80% in patients with genotypes 2 or 3. The FDA has approved use of both nonpegylated interferon-alfa–2b in combination with ribavirin and pegylated interferon-alfa-2b combined with ribavirin for treatment of HCV infection in children 3 to 17 years of age. As in adults, pegylated interferon in combination with ribavirin is the preferred treatment with sustained virologic response documented in 55% of pediatric patients infected with HCV genotypes 1 and 4 following 48 weeks of therapy and in 96% of patients infected with HCV genotypes 2 and 3 following 24 weeks of therapy. The few studies of combination therapy in children suggest that children have fewer adverse events compared with adults; however, all treatment regimens are associated with adverse events. Major adverse effects of combination therapy in pediatric patients include influenza-like symptoms, hematologic abnormalities, neuropsychiatric symptoms, thyroid abnormalities, ocular abnormalities including ischemic retinopathy and uveitis, and growth disturbances. Of 107 patients 3 to 17 years of age in a clinical trial of pegylated interferon-alfa-2b plus ribavirin, severely inhibited growth velocity (<3rd percentile) was observed in 70% of the subjects during treatment. Of subjects experiencing severely inhibited growth, 20% had continued inhibited growth velocity (<3rd percentile) after 6 months of follow-up after treatment. Education of patients, their family members, and caregivers about adverse effects and their prospective management is an integral aspect of treatment.

A number of new direct-acting antiviral drugs (DAAs) are in development for treatment of chronic HCV infection. Preliminary results of studies conducted in adults with telaprevir or boceprevir in combination with pegylated interferon-alfa and ribavirin suggest that rates of sustained virologic responses with these new DAAs dramatically are higher, especially in adults with genotype 1 than with current standard of care. In addition, adults with HCV genotype 1 and evidence of rapid virologic response within the first 4 to 8 weeks of treatment may be successfully treated with shorter durations of DAAs plus standard of care therapy. Trials of these oral agents in pediatric patients, in combination with standard therapy, now are starting. All patients with chronic HCV infection should be immunized against hepatitis A and hepatitis B because of the very high rate of severe hepatitis in patients with chronic liver disease from HCV who become coinfected with hepatitis A or B virus.

Management of Chronic HCV Infection. With advancing age, people who have chronic HCV infection are at risk of developing chronic hepatitis and its complications, including cirrhosis and primary hepatocellular carcinoma (HCC). Factors associated with more severe disease in most studies include older age at acquisition, HIV infection, excessive alcohol consumption, and male gender. Among children, liver disease progression appears to be accelerated when comorbid conditions, including childhood cancer, iron overload, thalassemia, or HIV coinfection, are present. Pediatricians need to be alert to concomitant infections and alcohol abuse and careful in prescription of drugs, such as acetaminophen and some antiretroviral agents (such as stavudine), in patients with HCV infection. Children with chronic infection should be followed closely, including sequential monitoring of serum hepatic transaminases, because of potential long-term risk of chronic liver disease. Definitive recommendations on frequency of screening have not been established. The need for screening tests for HCC in HCV-positive children has not been determined. Developments in antiviral therapies for HCV may be found on the American Association for the Study of Liver Diseases Web site **(www.aasld.org).**

ISOLATION OF THE HOSPITALIZED PATIENT: Standard precautions are recommended.

CONTROL MEASURES:

Care of Exposed People.

Immunoprophylaxis. On the basis of lack of clinical efficacy in humans and data from studies using animals, use of Immune Globulin for postexposure prophylaxis against HCV infection is not recommended.

Breastfeeding. Mothers infected with HCV should be advised that transmission of HCV by breastfeeding has not been documented. According to guidelines of the Centers for Disease Control and Prevention (CDC) and the American Academy of Pediatrics, maternal HCV infection is not a contraindication to breastfeeding. Mothers who are HCV positive and choose to breastfeed should consider abstaining if their nipples are cracked or bleeding.

Child Care. Exclusion of children with HCV infection from out-of-home child care is not indicated.

Serologic Testing for HCV Infection.

People Who Have Risk Factors for HCV Infection. Routine serologic testing is recommended for current or former injection drug users, recipients of one or more units of blood or blood products before July 1992, recipients of a solid organ transplant before July 1992, patients receiving long-term hemodialysis, people who received clotting-factor concentrates produced before 1987, people with persistently abnormal alanine transaminase (ALT) concentrations, and people in settings with documented high HCV infection prevalence and where risk-factor ascertainment is poor (eg, inmates of correctional facilities).

Pregnant Women. Routine serologic testing of pregnant women for HCV infection is not recommended.

Children Born to Women With HCV Infection. Children born to women previously identified to be HCV infected should be tested for HCV infection, because approximately 5% of these children will acquire the infection. The duration of presence of passive maternal antibody in infants can be as long as 18 months. Therefore, testing for anti-HCV should not be performed until after 18 months of age. If earlier diagnosis is desired, an NAAT to detect HCV RNA may be performed at or after the infant's first well-child visit at 1 to 2 months of age.

Adoptees. Routine serologic testing of adoptees, either domestic or international, is not recommended. See Medical Evaluation of Internationally Adopted Children for Infectious Diseases (p 191) for specific situations when serologic testing is warranted.

Counseling of Patients With HCV Infection. All people with HCV infection should be considered infectious, should be informed of the possibility of transmission to others, and should refrain from donating blood, organs, tissues, or semen and from sharing toothbrushes and razors.

Infected people should be counseled to avoid hepatotoxic agents, including medications, and should be informed of the risks of excessive alcohol ingestion. All patients with chronic HCV infection should be immunized against hepatitis A and hepatitis B.

Changes in sexual practices of infected people with a steady partner are not recommended; however, they should be informed of the possible risks and use of precautions to prevent transmission. People with multiple sexual partners should be advised to decrease the number of partners and to use condoms to prevent transmission. No data exist to support counseling a woman against pregnancy.

The CDC Division of Viral Hepatitis maintains a Web site (**www.cdc.gov/ hepatitis/HCV**) with information on hepatitis for health care professionals and the public, including specific information for people who have received blood transfusions before 1992. Information also can be obtained from the National Institutes of Health Web site (**www2.niddk.nih.gov/Research/ScientificAreas/ DigestiveDiseases/Liver/VHID.htm**).

Practice guidelines for diagnosis, management, and treatment of hepatitis C are available from the American Association for the Study of Liver Disease and the Infectious Diseases Society of America (**www.aasld.org/practiceguidelines/Documents/ Bookmarked%20Practice%20Guidelines/Diagnosis_of_HEP_C_Update. Aug%20_09pdf.pdf**).

Hepatitis D

CLINICAL MANIFESTATIONS: Hepatitis D virus (HDV) causes infection only in people with acute or chronic hepatitis B virus (HBV) infection; HDV requires HBV as a helper virus and cannot produce infection in the absence of HBV. The importance of HDV infection lies in its ability to convert an asymptomatic or mild chronic HBV infection into fulminant or more severe or rapidly progressive disease. Acute coinfection with HBV and HDV usually causes an acute illness indistinguishable from acute HBV infection alone, except that the likelihood of fulminant hepatitis can be as high as 5%.

ETIOLOGY: HDV measures 36 to 43 nm in diameter and consists of an RNA genome and a delta protein antigen, both of which are coated with hepatitis B surface antigen (HBsAg).

EPIDEMIOLOGY: HDV infection is present worldwide, and an estimated 18 million people are infected with the virus. Over the past 20 years, HDV prevalence has decreased significantly in Europe. At least 8 genotypes of HDV have been described, each with a typical geographic pattern, with genotype I being the predominant type in Europe and North America. HDV can cause an infection at the same time as the initial HBV infection (coinfection), or it can infect a person already chronically infected with HBV (superinfection). Acquisition of HDV is by parenteral, percutaneous, or mucous membrane inoculation. HDV can be acquired from blood or blood products, through injection drug use, or by sexual contact, but only if HBV also is present. Transmission from mother to newborn infant is uncommon. Intrafamilial spread can occur among people with chronic HBV infection. High-prevalence areas include southern Italy and parts of Eastern Europe, South America, Africa, and the Middle East. In the United States, HDV infection is found most commonly in people who abuse injection drugs, people with hemophilia, and people who have emigrated from areas with endemic infection.

The **incubation period** for HDV superinfection is approximately 2 to 8 weeks. When HBV and HDV viruses infect simultaneously, the incubation period is similar to that of HBV (45–160 days; average, 90 days).

DIAGNOSTIC TESTS: People with chronic HBV infection are at risk of HDV coinfection. Accordingly, their care should be supervised by an expert in hepatitis treatment, and consideration should be given to testing for anti-HDV immunoglobulin (Ig) G antibodies using a commercially available test if there is an elevation of transaminases. Anti-HDV may not be present until several weeks after onset of illness, and acute and convalescent sera may be required to confirm the diagnosis. Absence of IgM hepatitis B core antibody (anti-HBc), which is indicative of early HBV infection, suggests that the person has both chronic HBV infection and superinfection with HDV. Presence of anti-HDV IgG antibodies does not prove active infection, and thus, HDV RNA testing should be performed for diagnostic and therapeutic considerations. Patients with circulating HDV RNA should be staged for severity of liver disease, have surveillance for development of hepatocellular carcinoma, and be considered for treatment. Presence of anti-HDV IgM is of lesser utility, because it is present in both acute and chronic HDV infections.

TREATMENT: HDV has proven difficult to treat. However, data suggest pegylated interferon-alpha may result in up to 40% of patients having a sustained response to treatment. Clinical trials suggest at least a year of therapy is associated with the best sustained responses, and longer courses may be warranted if the patient is able to tolerate the adverse events of therapy. Further study of pegylated interferon monotherapy or as combination therapy with a direct acting antiviral agent needs to be performed before treatment of HDV can be advised routinely.

ISOLATION OF THE HOSPITALIZED PATIENT: Standard precautions are recommended.

CONTROL MEASURES: The same control and preventive measures used for HBV infection are indicated. Because HDV cannot be transmitted in the absence of HBV infection, HBV immunization protects against HDV infection. People with chronic HBV infection should take extreme care to avoid exposure to HDV.

Hepatitis E

CLINICAL MANIFESTATIONS: Hepatitis E virus (HEV) infection causes an acute illness with symptoms including jaundice, malaise, anorexia, fever, abdominal pain, and arthralgia. Disease is more common among adults than among children and is more severe in pregnant women, in whom mortality rates can reach 10% to 25% during the third trimester. Chronic HEV infection is rare and has been reported only in recipients of solid organ transplants and people with severe immunodeficiency.

ETIOLOGY: HEV is a spherical, nonenveloped, positive-strand RNA virus. HEV is classified in the genus Hepevirus of the family Hepeviridae. There are 4 major recognized genotypes with a single known serotype.

EPIDEMIOLOGY: Ingestion of fecally contaminated water is the most common route of HEV transmission, and large waterborne outbreaks have been reported in developing countries. Unlike the other agents of viral hepatitis, certain HEV genotypes (genotypes 3 and 4) also have zoonotic hosts, such as swine, and can be transmitted by eating uncooked pork. Person-to-person transmission appears to be much less efficient than with hepatitis A virus but occurs in sporadic and outbreaks settings. Sporadic HEV infection has been reported throughout the world and is common in Africa and the Indian subcontinent, where some studies have shown HEV to be the most common etiology of acute viral hepatitis. Mother-to-infant transmission of HEV occurs frequently and accounts for a significant proportion of fetal loss and infant mortality in countries with endemic infection. In the United States, serologic studies have demonstrated that approximately 20% of the population has immunoglobulin (Ig) G against HEV, with higher prevalence in areas with swine herds. However, symptomatic HEV infection in the United States is uncommon and generally occurs in people who acquire HEV genotype 1 infection after traveling to countries with endemic HEV.

DIAGNOSTIC TESTS: Testing for IgM and IgG anti-HEV is available through some research and commercial reference laboratories. Because anti-HEV assays are not approved by the US Food and Drug Administration and their performance characteristics are not well defined, results should be interpreted with caution, particularly in cases lacking a discrete onset of illness associated with jaundice or with no recent history of travel to a country with endemic infection. Definitive diagnosis may be made by demonstrating viral RNA in serum or stool by means of reverse transcriptase-polymerase chain reaction assay, which is available only in research settings (eg, with prior approval through the Centers for Disease Control and Prevention). Because virus circulates in the body for a relatively short period, the inability to detect HEV in serum or stool does not eliminate the possibility that the person was infected with HEV.

TREATMENT: Supportive.

ISOLATION OF THE HOSPITALIZED PATIENT: In addition to standard precautions, contact precautions are recommended for diapered and incontinent patients for the duration of illness.

CONTROL MEASURES: Provision of safe water is the most effective prevention measure. A recombinant HEV vaccine was evaluated in a phase III clinical trial and was demonstrated to be effective in preventing disease but is not available outside the research setting.

Herpes Simplex

CLINICAL MANIFESTATIONS:

Neonatal. In newborn infants, herpes simplex virus (HSV) infection can manifest as the following: (1) disseminated disease involving multiple organs, most prominently liver and lungs, but in 60% to 75% of cases also involving the central nervous system; (2) localized central nervous system (CNS) disease, with or without skin involvement (CNS disease); or (3) disease localized to the skin, eyes, and/or mouth (SEM disease). Approximately 25% of cases of neonatal HSV manifest as disseminated disease, 30% of cases manifest as CNS disease, and 45% of cases manifest as SEM disease. More than 80% of neonates with SEM disease have skin vesicles; those without have infection limited to the eyes and/ or oral mucosa. Approximately two thirds of neonates with disseminated or CNS disease have skin lesions, but these lesions may not be present at the time of their initial presentation. In the absence of skin lesions, the diagnosis of neonatal HSV infection is difficult. Disseminated infection should be considered in neonates with sepsis syndrome, negative bacteriologic culture results, and severe liver dysfunction. HSV also should be considered as a causative agent in neonates with fever, a vesicular rash, or abnormal cerebrospinal fluid (CSF) findings, especially in the presence of seizures or during a time of year when enteroviruses are not circulating in the community. Although asymptomatic HSV infection is common in older children, it rarely, if ever, occurs in neonates.

Neonatal herpetic infections often are severe, with attendant high mortality and morbidity rates, even when antiviral therapy is administered. Recurrent skin lesions are common in surviving infants and may be associated with CNS sequelae, especially if recurrences are frequent during the first 6 months of life.

Initial signs of HSV infection can occur anytime between birth and approximately 6 weeks of age, although most infected infants develop clinical disease within the first month of life. Infants with disseminated disease and SEM disease have an earlier age of onset, typically presenting between the first and second weeks of life; infants with CNS disease usually present with illness between the second and third weeks of life.

Children Beyond the Neonatal Period and Adolescents. Most primary HSV infections during the period of childhood beyond the neonatal period are asymptomatic. Gingivostomatitis, which is the most common clinical manifestation of HSV during childhood, is caused by HSV type 1 (HSV-1) and is characterized by fever, irritability, tender submandibular adenopathy, and an ulcerative enanthem involving the gingiva and mucous membranes of the mouth, often with perioral vesicular lesions.

Genital herpes, which is the most common manifestation of primary HSV infection in adolescents and adults, is characterized by vesicular or ulcerative lesions of the male or female genital organs, perineum, or both. Genital herpes usually is caused by HSV type 2 (HSV-2), but HSV-1 increasingly is becoming a common cause of genital herpes (20%

to >50% of all cases of genital herpes) in some populations. Most cases of primary genital herpes infection are not recognized as such by the infected person or diagnosed by a health care professional.

Eczema herpeticum with vesicular lesions concentrated in the areas of eczematous involvement can develop in patients with atopic dermatitis who are infected with HSV.

In immunocompromised patients, severe local lesions and, less commonly, disseminated HSV infection with generalized vesicular skin lesions and visceral involvement can occur.

After primary infection, HSV persists for life in a latent form. The site of latency for virus causing herpes labialis is the trigeminal ganglion, and the usual site of latency for genital herpes is the sacral dorsal root ganglia, although any of the sensory ganglia can be involved, depending on the site of primary infection. Reactivation of latent virus most commonly is asymptomatic. When symptomatic, recurrent herpes labialis HSV-1 manifests as single or grouped vesicles in the perioral region, usually on the vermilion border of the lips (typically called "cold sores" or "fever blisters"). Symptomatic recurrent genital herpes manifests as vesicular lesions on the penis, scrotum, vulva, cervix, buttocks, perianal areas, thighs, or back. Recurrences may be heralded by a prodrome of burning or itching at the site of an incipient recurrence, identification of which can be useful in instituting antiviral therapy early.

Conjunctivitis and keratitis can result from primary or recurrent HSV infection. Herpetic whitlow consists of single or multiple vesicular lesions on the distal parts of fingers. HSV infection can be a precipitating factor in erythema multiforme.

HSV encephalitis (HSE) occurs in children beyond the neonatal period or in adolescents and adults and can result from primary or recurrent HSV-1 infection. Symptoms and signs usually include fever, alterations in the state of consciousness, personality changes, seizures, and focal neurologic findings. Encephalitis commonly has an acute onset with a fulminant course, leading to coma and death in untreated patients. HSE usually involves the temporal lobe; thus, temporal lobe abnormalities on imaging studies or electroencephalography in the context of a consistent clinical picture should increase the suspicion of HSE. CSF pleocytosis with a predominance of lymphocytes and some erythrocytes is usual. HSV infection also can cause meningitis with nonspecific clinical manifestations that usually are mild and self-limited. Such episodes of meningitis usually are associated with genital HSV-2 infection. A number of unusual CNS manifestations of HSV have been described, including Bell palsy, atypical pain syndromes, trigeminal neuralgia, ascending myelitis, postinfectious encephalomyelitis, and recurrent (Mollaret) meningitis.

ETIOLOGY: HSVs are enveloped, double-stranded, DNA viruses. Two distinct HSV types exist: HSV-1 and HSV-2. Infections with HSV-1 usually involve the face and skin above the waist; however, an increasing number of genital herpes cases are attributable to HSV-1. Infections with HSV-2 usually involve the genitalia and skin below the waist in sexually active adolescents and adults. However, either type of virus can be found in either area. HSV-2 is the most common cause of herpes disease in neonates (75% of cases). As with all human herpesviruses, HSV-1 and HSV-2 establish latency following primary infection, with periodic reactivation to cause recurrent symptomatic disease or asymptomatic viral shedding.

EPIDEMIOLOGY: HSV infections are ubiquitous and can be transmitted from people who are symptomatic or asymptomatic with primary or recurrent infections.

Neonatal. The incidence of neonatal HSV infection is estimated to range from 1 in 3000 to 1 in 20 000 live births. HSV is transmitted to a neonate most often during birth through an infected maternal genital tract but can be caused by an ascending infection through ruptured or apparently intact amniotic membranes. Intrauterine infections causing congenital malformations have been implicated in rare cases. Other less common sources of neonatal infection include postnatal transmission from a parent or other caregiver, most often from a nongenital infection (eg, mouth or hands) or from another infected infant or caregiver in the nursery, probably via the hands of health care professionals attending the infants.

The risk of HSV transmission to a neonate born to a mother who acquires primary genital infection near the time of delivery is estimated to be 25% to 60%. In contrast, the risk to a neonate born to a mother shedding HSV as a result of reactivation of infection acquired during the first half of pregnancy or earlier is less than 2%. Distinguishing between primary and recurrent HSV infections in women by history or physical examination alone may be impossible, because primary and recurrent genital infections may be asymptomatic or associated with nonspecific findings (eg, vaginal discharge, genital pain, or shallow ulcers). More than three quarters of infants who contract HSV infection have been born to women with no history or clinical findings suggestive of genital HSV infection during or preceding pregnancy.

Children Beyond the Neonatal Period and Adolescents. More than 25% of US children have serologic evidence of HSV-1 infection by 7 years of age. Patients with primary gingivostomatitis or genital herpes usually shed virus for at least 1 week and occasionally for several weeks. Patients with symptomatic recurrences shed virus for a shorter period, typically 3 to 4 days. Intermittent asymptomatic reactivation of oral and genital herpes is common and likely occurs throughout the remainder of a person's life. The greatest concentration of virus is shed during symptomatic primary infections and the lowest concentration of virus is shed during asymptomatic recurrent infections.

Infections with HSV-1 usually result from direct contact with virus shed from visible or microscopic orolabial lesions or in infected oral secretions. Infections with HSV-2 usually result from direct contact with virus shed from visible or microscopic genital lesions or in genital secretions during sexual activity. Genital infections caused by HSV-1 in children can result from autoinoculation of virus from the mouth, but sexual abuse always should be considered in prepubertal children with genital HSV-2 infections. Therefore, genital HSV isolates from children should be typed to differentiate between HSV-1 and HSV-2.

The incidence of HSV-2 infection correlates with the number of sexual partners and with acquisition of other sexually transmitted infections. After primary genital infection, which often is asymptomatic, some people experience frequent clinical recurrences, and others have no clinically apparent recurrences. Genital HSV-2 infection is more likely to recur than is genital HSV-1 infection.

Inoculation of abraded skin occurs from direct contact with HSV shed from oral, genital, or other skin sites. This contact can result in herpes gladiatorum among wrestlers, herpes rugbiaforum among rugby players, or herpetic whitlow of the fingers in any exposed person.

The **incubation period** for HSV infection occurring beyond the neonatal period ranges from 2 days to 2 weeks.

DIAGNOSTIC TESTS: HSV grows readily in cell culture. Special transport media are available that allow transport to local or regional laboratories for culture. Cytopathogenic effects typical of HSV infection usually are observed 1 to 3 days after inoculation. Methods of culture confirmation include fluorescent antibody staining, enzyme immuno-assays (EIAs), and monolayer culture with typing. Cultures that remain negative by day 5 likely will continue to remain negative. Polymerase chain reaction (PCR) assay often can detect HSV DNA in CSF from neonates with CNS infection (neonatal HSV CNS disease) and from older children and adults with HSE and is the diagnostic method of choice for CNS HSV involvement. Histologic examination and viral culture of a brain tissue biopsy specimen is the most definitive method of confirming the diagnosis of HSE. Viral cultures of CSF from a patient with HSE usually are negative.

For diagnosis of neonatal HSV infection, the following specimens should be obtained: (1) swab specimens from the mouth, nasopharynx, conjunctivae, and anus ("surface cultures") for HSV culture (all surface swab specimens can be obtained with a single swab [ending with the anal swab] and placed in 1 viral transport media tube); (2) specimens of skin vesicles and CSF for HSV culture and PCR; (3) whole blood sample for HSV PCR; and (4) whole blood sample for measuring alanine aminotransferase (ALT). Positive cultures obtained from any of the surface sites more than 12 to 24 hours after birth indicate viral replication and, therefore, are suggestive of infant infection rather than merely contamination after intrapartum exposure. As with any PCR assay, false-negative and false-positive results can occur. Whole blood PCR may be of benefit in diagnosis of neonatal HSV disease, but its use should not supplant the standard work-up of such patients (which includes surface cultures and CSF PCR); no data exist to support use of serial blood PCR assay to monitor response to therapy. Rapid diagnostic techniques also are available, such as direct fluorescent antibody (DFA) staining of vesicle scrapings or EIA detection of HSV antigens. These techniques are as specific but slightly less sensitive than culture. Typing HSV strains differentiates between HSV-1 and HSV-2 isolates. Radiographs and clinical manifestations can suggest HSV pneumonitis, and elevated transaminase values can suggest HSV hepatitis; both occur commonly in neonatal HSV disseminated disease. Histologic examination of lesions for presence of multinucleated giant cells and eosino-philic intranuclear inclusions typical of HSV (eg, with Tzanck test) has low sensitivity and should not be performed.

HSV cell culture and PCR are the preferred tests for detecting HSV in genital ulcers or other mucocutaneous lesions consistent with genital herpes. The sensitivity of viral culture is low, especially for recurrent lesions, and declines rapidly as lesions begin to heal. PCR assays for HSV DNA are more sensitive and are increasingly used in many settings. Failure to detect HSV in genital lesions by culture or PCR does not indicate an absence of HSV infection, because viral shedding is intermittent.

Both type-specific and type-common antibodies to HSV develop during the first several weeks after infection and persist indefinitely. Although type-specific HSV-2 antibody usually indicates previous anogenital infection, the presence of HSV-1 antibody does not distinguish anogenital from orolabial infection reliably, because a substantial proportion of initial genital infections are caused by HSV-1 in some populations. Type-specific serologic tests can be useful in confirming a clinical diagnosis of genital herpes. Additionally, these serologic tests can be used to evaluate recurrent or atypical genital tract symptoms with negative HSV cultures and to manage sexual partners of people with genital herpes. There is growing evidence that type-specific antibody avidity testing may prove useful for evaluating risk of neonatal infection. The presence of low-avidity HSV-2 immuno-globulin (Ig) G in serum of near-term pregnant women has been correlated with an elevated risk of neonatal infection. Serologic testing is not useful in neonates.

Several glycoprotein G (gG)-based type-specific assays have been approved by the US Food and Drug Administration (FDA), including at least one that can be used as a point-of-care test. The sensitivities and specificities of these tests for detection of HSV-2 IgG antibody vary from 90% to 100%; false-negative results may occur, especially early after infection, and false-positive results can occur, especially in patients with low likelihood of HSV infection. Therefore, repeat testing or a confirmatory test (eg, an immunoblot assay if the initial test was an EIA) may be indicated in some settings.

TREATMENT: For recommended antiviral dosages and duration of therapy with systemically administered acyclovir, valacyclovir, and famciclovir and with topical penciclovir for different HSV infections, see Antiviral Drugs (p 841). Valacyclovir is an L-valyl ester of acyclovir that is metabolized to acyclovir after oral administration, resulting in higher serum concentrations than are achieved with oral acyclovir and similar serum concentrations as are achieved with intravenous administration of acyclovir. Famciclovir is converted rapidly to penciclovir after oral administration. Table 3.23 (p 403) shows drugs for HSV by type of infection. Valacyclovir has been approved by the FDA for use in children with chickenpox. Instructions for preparing a compounded liquid formulation of valacyclovir are provided in the drug's package insert.

Neonatal. Parenteral acyclovir is the treatment of choice for neonatal HSV infections. Parenteral acyclovir should be administered to all neonates with HSV infection, regardless of manifestations and clinical findings. The best outcome in terms of morbidity and mortality is observed among infants with SEM disease. Although most neonates treated for HSV CNS disease survive, most survivors suffer substantial neurologic sequelae. Approximately 20% of neonates with disseminated disease die despite antiviral therapy. The dosage of acyclovir is 60 mg/kg per day in 3 divided doses, given intravenously for 14 days in SEM disease and for a minimum of 21 days in CNS disease or disseminated disease. Approximately 50% of infants surviving neonatal HSV experience cutaneous recurrences. Use of oral acyclovir suppressive therapy for the 6 months following treatment of acute neonatal HSV disease has been shown to improve neurodevelopmental outcomes in infants with HSV CNS disease and to prevent skin recurrences in infants with any disease classification of neonatal HSV. The dose is 300 mg/m^2/dose, administered 3 times daily for 6 months; absolute neutrophil counts should be assessed at 2 and 4 weeks after initiating suppressive therapy and then monthly during the treatment period.

Infants with ocular involvement attributable to HSV infection should receive a topical ophthalmic drug (1% trifluridine, 0.1% iododeoxyuridine, or 3% vidarabine) as well as parenteral antiviral therapy.

Genital Infection.

Primary. Many patients with first-episode herpes initially have mild clinical manifestations but may go on to develop severe or prolonged symptoms. Therefore, most patients with initial genital herpes should receive antiviral therapy. In adults, acyclovir and valacyclovir decrease the duration of symptoms and viral shedding in primary genital herpes. Oral acyclovir therapy (400 mg, orally, 3 times/day for 10 days; or 200 mg, orally, 5 times/day for 10 days), initiated within 6 days of onset of disease, shortens the duration

Table 3.23. Recommended Therapy for Herpes Simplex Virus Infections[a]

Infection	Drug[b]
Neonatal	Parenteral acyclovir
Keratoconjunctivitis	Trifluridine[c] **OR** Iododeoxyuridine **OR** Vidarabine
Genital	Acyclovir **OR** Famciclovir **OR** Valacyclovir
Mucocutaneous (immunocompromised or primary gingivostomatitis)	Acyclovir **OR** Famciclovir **OR** Valacyclovir
Acyclovir-resistant (severe infections, immunocompromised)	Parenteral foscarnet
Encephalitis	Parenteral acyclovir

[a] See text and Table 4.8 (p 841) for details.
[b] Famciclovir and valacyclovir are approved by the US Food and Drug Administration for treatment of adults.
[c] Treatment of herpes simplex virus ocular infection should involve an ophthalmologist.

of illness and viral shedding by 3 to 5 days. Valacyclovir and famciclovir do not seem to be more effective than acyclovir but offer the advantage of less frequent dosing (famciclovir, 250 mg, orally, 3 times/day for 10 days; valacyclovir, 1 g, orally, 2 times/day for 10 days). Intravenous acyclovir is indicated for patients with a severe or complicated primary infection that requires hospitalization. Topical acyclovir (5%) ointment for primary genital herpes infection is not recommended. Systemic or topical treatment of primary herpetic lesions does not affect the subsequent frequency or severity of recurrences.

Recurrent. Antiviral therapy for recurrent genital herpes can be administered either episodically to ameliorate or shorten the duration of lesions or continuously as suppressive therapy to decrease the frequency of recurrences. Many patients benefit from antiviral therapy; therefore, options for treatment should be discussed with all patients. Oral acyclovir therapy initiated within 1 day of lesion onset or during the prodrome that precedes some outbreaks shortens the mean clinical course by approximately 1 day. If episodic therapy is used, a prescription for the medication should be provided with instructions to initiate treatment immediately when symptoms begin. Valacyclovir and famciclovir also are licensed and efficacious for treatment of adults with recurrent genital herpes.

In adults with frequent genital HSV recurrences, daily oral acyclovir suppressive therapy is effective for decreasing the frequency of symptomatic recurrences and improving quality of life. After approximately 1 year of continuous daily therapy, acyclovir should be discontinued and the recurrence rate should be assessed. If recurrences are observed, additional suppressive therapy should be considered. Acyclovir appears to be safe for adults receiving the drug for more than 15 years, but longer-term effects are unknown. Data also support suppressive therapy in adults with valacyclovir or famciclovir.

Data on long-term use of valacyclovir or famciclovir as suppressive therapy in children are not available. The safety of systemic valacyclovir and famciclovir therapy in pregnant women has not been established. Available data do not indicate an increased risk of major birth defects in comparison with the general population in women treated with acyclovir during the first trimester. Acyclovir may be administered orally to pregnant women with first-episode genital herpes or severe recurrent herpes and should be given intravenously to pregnant women with severe HSV infection. Counseling and education of infected adolescents/adults and their sexual partners, especially on the potential for recurrent episodes and how to reduce transmission to partners, is a critical part of management. Pregnant women or women of childbearing age with genital herpes should be encouraged to inform their health care professionals and those who will care for the newborn infant.

Mucocutaneous.

Immunocompromised Hosts. Intravenous acyclovir is effective for treatment and prevention of mucocutaneous HSV infections. Topical acyclovir also may accelerate healing of lesions in immunocompromised patients. Acyclovir-resistant strains of HSV have been isolated from immunocompromised people receiving prolonged treatment with acyclovir. Under these circumstances, progressive disease may be observed despite acyclovir therapy. Foscarnet is the drug of choice for disease caused by acyclovir-resistant HSV isolates.

Immunocompetent Hosts. Limited data are available on effects of acyclovir on the course of primary or recurrent nongenital mucocutaneous HSV infections in immunocompetent hosts. Therapeutic benefit has been noted in a limited number of children with primary gingivostomatitis treated with oral acyclovir. Slight therapeutic benefit of oral acyclovir therapy has been demonstrated among adults with recurrent herpes labialis. When used as treatment for HSV orolabial disease, a dose of 80 mg/kg per day in 4 divided doses should be used, with a maximum of 3200 mg/day. Topical acyclovir is ineffective. A topical formulation of penciclovir (Denavir) and another drug, docosanol (Abreva), have only limited activity for therapy of herpes labialis and are not recommended.

In a controlled study of a small number of adults with recurrent herpes labialis (6 or more episodes per year), prophylactic acyclovir at a dosage of 400 mg, twice a day, was effective for decreasing the frequency of recurrent episodes. Although no studies of prophylactic therapy have been performed in children, those with frequent recurrences may benefit from continuous oral acyclovir therapy, with reevaluation being performed after 6 months to 1 year of continuous therapy; a dose of 30 mg/kg per day, in 3 divided doses, with a maximum 1000 mg/day is reasonable to begin as suppressive therapy in children. Valacyclovir has been approved for suppression of genital herpes in immunocompetent adults.

Other HSV Infections.

Central Nervous System. Patients with HSE should be treated for 21 days with intravenous acyclovir. Patients who are comatose or semicomatose at initiation of therapy have a poorer outcome. For people with Bell palsy, the combination of acyclovir and prednisone may be considered.

Ocular. Treatment of eye lesions should be undertaken in consultation with an ophthalmologist. Several topical drugs, such as 1% trifluridine, 0.1% iododeoxyuridine, and 3% vidarabine, have proven efficacy for superficial keratitis. Topical corticosteroids, by themselves, are contraindicated in suspected HSV conjunctivitis; however, ophthalmologists may choose to use corticosteroids in conjunction with antiviral drugs to treat locally invasive infections. For children with recurrent ocular lesions, oral suppressive therapy with acyclovir (800 mg/day in 2 divided doses in patients ≥12 years) may be of benefit.

ISOLATION OF THE HOSPITALIZED PATIENT: In addition to standard precautions, the following recommendations should be followed.

Neonates With HSV Infection. Neonates with HSV infection should be hospitalized and managed with contact precautions if mucocutaneous lesions are present.

Neonates Exposed to HSV During Delivery. Infants born to women with active HSV lesions should be managed with contact precautions during the incubation period. Some experts believe that contact precautions are unnecessary if exposed infants were born by cesarean delivery, provided membranes were ruptured for less than 4 hours. The risk of HSV infection in infants born to mothers with a history of recurrent genital herpes who have no genital lesions at delivery is low, and special precautions are not necessary.

One method of infection control for neonates with documented perinatal exposure to HSV is continuous rooming-in with the mother in a private room.

Women in Labor and Postpartum Women With HSV Infection. Women with active HSV lesions should be managed with contact precautions during labor, delivery, and the postpartum period. These women should be instructed about the importance of careful hand hygiene before and after caring for their infants. The mother may wear a clean covering gown to help avoid contact of the infant with lesions or infectious secretions. A mother with herpes labialis or stomatitis should wear a disposable surgical mask when touching her newborn infant until the lesions have crusted and dried. She should not kiss or nuzzle her newborn until lesions have cleared. Herpetic lesions on other skin sites should be covered.

Breastfeeding is acceptable if no lesions are present on the breasts and if active lesions elsewhere on the mother are covered (see Human Milk, p 126).

Children With Mucocutaneous HSV Infection. Contact precautions are recommended for patients with severe mucocutaneous HSV infection. Patients with localized recurrent lesions should be managed with standard precautions.

Patients With HSV Infection of the CNS. Standard precautions are recommended for patients with infection limited to the CNS.

CONTROL MEASURES:

Prevention of Neonatal Infection. Surveillance genital cultures for HSV obtained weekly during pregnancy are not recommended. Women with a history of recurrent genital HSV infection are recognized to be at low risk of transmitting HSV to their infants (see Epidemiology, p 400).

Management of infants exposed to HSV during delivery differs according to the status of the mother's infection, mode of delivery, and expert opinion (see Care of Newborn Infants Whose Mothers Have Active Genital Lesions). Current recommendations for management of pregnant women for prevention of HSV infection include the following:

- **During pregnancy.** During prenatal evaluations, all pregnant women should be asked about past or current signs and symptoms consistent with genital herpes infection in themselves and their sexual partners.

- Although antiviral therapy for women with a history of genital HSV infection is recommended by some obstetricians during the final weeks of pregnancy to suppress maternal recurrence of viral shedding, the safety of antiviral therapy for the fetus and its efficacy in preventing viral shedding or neonatal infection have not been established. Cases of neonatal HSV disease have occurred among women who received antiviral prophylaxis during the latter weeks of pregnancy.

- **Women in labor.** During labor, all women should be asked about recent and current signs and symptoms consistent with genital herpes infection, and they should be examined carefully for evidence of genital infection. Suspicious lesions should be sampled for culture and PCR to assist in subsequent management of the newborn. Cesarean delivery for women who have clinically apparent HSV infection decreases the risk of neonatal HSV infection. In the absence of genital lesions, a maternal history of genital HSV is not an indication for cesarean delivery. Fetal scalp monitors should be avoided, when possible, in infants of women suspected of having active genital herpes infection during labor.

    Care of Newborn Infants Whose Mothers Have Active Genital Lesions at Delivery. Because the risk to infants exposed to HSV during delivery varies in different circumstances (from less than 2% for recurrent genital HSV to 25%–60% for first-episode genital HSV), management of the asymptomatic, exposed neonate is complex. For neonates born vaginally or by cesarean delivery to mothers who have active genital HSV lesions, HSV "surface cultures" should be obtained at 12 to 24 hours of life; sites from which swab specimens are obtained for HSV culture should include the mouth, nasopharynx, conjunctivae, and anus (see Diagnostic Tests, p 401).

For infants born vaginally to mothers with a first-episode genital infection, some experts recommend empiric parenteral acyclovir treatment. HSV cultures should be obtained before starting antiviral therapy. Because neonates do not develop HSV disease following perinatal acquisition for 2 to 3 weeks on average, empiric parenteral acyclovir treatment can be delayed in an asymptomatic infant to approximately 24 hours of life, which allows for surface cultures to reflect more accurately viral replication rather than merely contamination after intrapartum exposure. Most experts would not administer acyclovir as empiric therapy to neonates born to women with active recurrent genital HSV lesions. The infant's parents or caregivers, however, should be educated about the signs and symptoms of neonatal HSV infection during the first 6 weeks of life.

If cultures of samples obtained from the neonate 12 to 24 hours following delivery subsequently grow HSV, HSV infection is confirmed and the infant then should be evaluated for HSV disease. Evaluation should include lumbar puncture for CSF indices and HSV PCR, whole blood for PCR, and determination of serum hepatic transaminases. An infant with no evidence of HSV disease should be treated empirically with intravenous acyclovir for 10 days to prevent HSV infection from progressing to HSV disease. An infant with evidence of SEM disease, CNS disease, or disseminated disease should be managed as described in Treatment, Neonatal (p 402).

If, within the first 6 weeks of life, a neonate born to a woman with active HSV lesions develops clinical findings suggestive of HSV infection, such as skin or scalp rashes (especially vesicular lesions) or unexplained manifestations (such as those of sepsis), cultures and rapid diagnostic tests (eg, CSF PCR) should be performed, and acyclovir therapy should be initiated immediately. The sensitivity of viral cultures for detecting neonatal infection in infants whose mothers were treated with antiviral medication near the end of pregnancy is not known.

Differentiating primary genital infection from recurrent HSV infection in the mother would be helpful for assessing the risk of HSV infection for the exposed infant, but the distinction may be difficult. First-episode clinical infections are not always primary infections. Often, primary infections are asymptomatic, in which case the first symptomatic episode will represent a reactivated recurrent infection. In selected instances, serologic testing can be useful. For example, if a woman with herpetic lesions has no detectable HSV antibodies, she is experiencing a primary infection. Assessment of seropositive women necessitates differentiation of HSV-1 from HSV-2 antibodies using commercially available type-specific serologic assays such as the HerpeSelect Test.

Care of Newborn Infants Whose Mothers Have a History of Genital Herpes But No Active Genital Lesions at Delivery. An infant whose mother has known, recurrent genital infection but no genital lesions at delivery should be observed for signs of infection (eg, vesicular lesions of the skin, respiratory distress, seizures, or signs of sepsis) but should not have specimens for surface cultures for HSV obtained at 12 to 24 hours of life and should not receive empiric parenteral acyclovir. Education of parents and caregivers about the signs and symptoms of neonatal HSV infection during the first 6 weeks of life is prudent.

Infected Health Care Professionals. Transmission of HSV in hospital nurseries from infected health care professionals to newborn infants rarely has been documented. The risk of transmission to infants by health care professionals who have herpes labialis or who are asymptomatic oral shedders of virus is low. Compromising patient care by excluding health care professionals with cold sores who are essential for the operation of the hospital nursery must be weighed against the potential risk of newborn infants becoming infected. Health care professionals with cold sores who have contact with infants should cover and not touch their lesions and should comply with hand hygiene policies. Transmission of HSV infection from health care professionals with genital lesions is not likely as long as they comply with hand hygiene policies. Health care professionals with an active herpetic whitlow should not have responsibility for direct care of neonates or immunocompromised patients and should wear gloves and use hand hygiene during direct care of other patients.

Infected Household, Family, and Other Close Contacts of Newborn Infants. Intrafamilial transmission of HSV to newborn infants has been described but is rare. Household members with herpetic skin lesions (eg, herpes labialis or herpetic whitlow) should be counseled about the risk and should avoid contact of their lesions with newborn infants by taking the same measures as recommended for infected health care professionals as well as avoiding kissing and nuzzling the infant while they have active lip lesions or touching the infant while they have herpetic whitlow. Cases of possible HSV transmission to the genitalia of male neonates have been reported following ritual circumcision involving mouth suction of the site by the performer of the circumcision.

Care of People With Extensive Dermatitis. Patients with dermatitis are at risk of developing eczema herpeticum. If these patients are hospitalized, special care should be taken to avoid exposure to HSV. These patients should not be kissed by people with cold sores or touched by people with herpetic whitlow.

Care of Children With Mucocutaneous Infections Who Attend Child Care or School. Oral HSV infections are common among children who attend child care or school. Most of these infections are asymptomatic, with shedding of virus in saliva occurring in the absence of clinical disease. Only children with HSV gingivostomatitis (ie, primary infection) who do not have control of oral secretions should be excluded from child care. Exclusion of children with cold sores (ie, recurrent infection) from child care or school is not indicated.

Children with uncovered lesions on exposed surfaces pose a small potential risk to contacts. If children are certified by a physician to have recurrent HSV infection, covering the active lesions with clothing, a bandage, or an appropriate dressing when they attend child care or school is sufficient. Additional control measures include avoiding the sharing of respiratory secretions through contact with objects and washing and sanitizing mouthed toys, bottle nipples, and utensils that have come in contact with saliva.

HSV Infections Among Wrestlers and Rugby Players. HSV-1 has been transmitted during athletic competition involving close physical contact and frequent skin abrasions, such as wrestling (herpes gladiatorum) and rugby (herpes rugbiaforum or scrum pox). Competitors often do not recognize or may deny possible infection. Transmission of these infections can be limited or prevented by the following: (1) examination of wrestlers and rugby players for vesicular or ulcerative lesions on exposed areas of their bodies and around their mouths or eyes before practice or competition by a person familiar with the appearance of mucocutaneous infections (including HSV, herpes zoster, and impetigo); (2) exclusion of athletes with these conditions from competition or practice until healing (fully crusted lesions) occurs or a physician's written statement declaring their condition noninfectious is obtained; and (3) cleaning wrestling mats with a freshly prepared solution of household bleach (one quarter cup of bleach in 1 gallon of water) applied for a minimum contact time of 15 seconds at least daily and, preferably, between matches. Consideration of suppressive antiviral therapy should be limited to athletes with a history of recurrent herpes gladiatorum or herpes labialis to reduce the risk of reactivation during wrestling season. Despite these precautions, HSV spread during wrestling and other sports involving close personal contact still can occur through contact with asymptomatic infected people.

Histoplasmosis

CLINICAL MANIFESTATIONS: *Histoplasma capsulatum* causes symptoms in fewer than 5% of infected people. Clinical manifestations are classified according to site (pulmonary or disseminated), duration (acute, subacute, or chronic), and pattern (primary or reactivation) of infection. Most symptomatic patients have acute pulmonary histoplasmosis, a self-limited illness characterized by fever, chills, nonproductive cough, and malaise. Typical radiographic findings include diffuse interstitial or reticulonodular pulmonary infiltrates and hilar or mediastinal adenopathy. Most patients spontaneously recover 2 to 3 weeks after onset of symptoms. Exposure to a large inoculum of conidia can cause more severe pulmonary infection associated with high fevers, hypoxemia, diffuse reticulonodular infiltrates, and acute respiratory distress syndrome (ARDS). Chronic cavitary pulmonary histoplasmosis occurs most often in older adults and can mimic pulmonary tuberculosis. Mediastinal involvement, usually a complication of pulmonary histoplasmosis, includes mediastinal lymphadenitis, which can cause airway encroachment in young children. Inflammatory syndromes (pericarditis and rheumatologic syndromes) also can develop; erythema nodosum can occur in adolescents and adults. Primary cutaneous infections after trauma are rare.

Disseminated histoplasmosis can be either self-limited or progressive. Progressive disseminated histoplasmosis (PDH) can occur in otherwise healthy infants and children younger than 2 years of age. PDH can be a rapidly progressive illness following acute infection or a more chronic, slowly progressive disease. PDH in adults occurs most often in people with underlying immune deficiency (human immunodeficiency virus/acquired immunodeficiency syndrome, solid organ transplant, hematologic malignancy biologic response modifiers including tumor necrosis factor antagonists) or in people older than 65 years of age. Early manifestations of PDH in young children include prolonged fever, failure to thrive, and hepatosplenomegaly; if untreated, malnutrition, diffuse adenopathy, pneumonia, mucosal ulceration, pancytopenia, disseminated intravascular coagulopathy, and gastrointestinal tract bleeding can ensue. Central nervous system involvement is common. Chronic PDH generally occurs in adults with immune suppression and is characterized by prolonger fever, night sweats, weight loss, and fatigue; signs include hepatosplenomegaly, mucosal ulcerations, adrenal insufficiency, and pancytopenia.

ETIOLOGY: *Histoplasma capsulatum* var *capsulatum* is a dimorphic endemic fungus that grows in the environment as a microconidia-bearing mold but converts to yeast phase at body temperature. *H capsulatum* var *duboisii* is the cause of African histoplasmosis and is found only in central and western Africa.

EPIDEMIOLOGY: *Histoplasma capsulatum* is encountered in most parts of the world (including Africa, the Americas, Asia, and Europe) and is endemic in the eastern and central United States, particularly the Mississippi, Ohio, and Missouri River valleys. Infection is acquired through inhalation of conidia from soil, often contaminated with bat guano or bird droppings. The inoculum size, strain virulence, and immune status of the host affect severity of illness. Infections occur sporadically, in outbreaks when weather conditions (dry and windy) predispose to spread of spores or as point-source epidemics after exposure to activities that disturb contaminated soil. Recreational and occupational pursuits, such as playing in hollow trees, caving, mining, construction, excavation, demolition, farming, and cleaning of contaminated buildings, have been associated with histoplasmosis. Person-to-person transmission does not occur. Prior infection confers partial immunity; reinfection can occur but requires a larger inoculum.

The **incubation period** is variable but usually is 1 to 3 weeks.

DIAGNOSTIC TESTS: Culture is the definitive method of diagnosis. *H capsulatum* organisms from bone marrow, blood, sputum, and tissue specimens grow on standard mycologic media in 1 to 6 weeks. The lysis-centrifugation method is preferred for blood cultures. A DNA probe for *H capsulatum* permits rapid identification of cultured isolates.

Demonstration of typical intracellular yeast forms by examination with Gomori methenamine silver or other stains of tissue, blood, bone marrow, or bronchoalveolar lavage specimens strongly supports the diagnosis of histoplasmosis when clinical, epidemiologic, and other laboratory studies are compatible.

Detection of *H capsulatum* antigen in serum, urine, a bronchoalveolar lavage specimen, or cerebrospinal fluid using a quantitative enzyme immunoassay is possible using a rapid, commercially available diagnostic test. Antigen detection in blood and urine specimens is most sensitive for severe, acute pulmonary infections and for progressive disseminated infections. Results often transiently are positive early in the course of acute, self-limited pulmonary infections. A negative test result does not exclude infection. If the result initially is positive, the antigen test also is useful for monitoring treatment response and, after treatment, identifying relapse. Cross-reactions occur in patients with blastomycosis, coccidioidomycosis, paracoccidioidomycosis, and penicilliosis; clinical and epidemiologic circumstances aid in differentiating these infections.

Serologic testing also is available and is most useful in patients with subacute or chronic pulmonary disease. A fourfold increase in either yeast-phase or mycelial-phase titers or a single titer of ≥1:32 in either test is presumptive evidence of active or recent infection. Cross-reacting antibodies can result from *Blastomyces dermatitidis* and *Coccidioides* species infections. The immunodiffusion test is more specific than the complement fixation test, but the complement fixation test is more sensitive.

TREATMENT: Amphotericin B is recommended for severe or disseminated infections (see Drugs for Invasive and Other Serious Fungal Infections, p 835), and itraconazole is recommended for mild to moderate infections that warrant antifungal therapy.[1] Itraconazole is preferred over other azoles by most experts; when used in adults, itraconazole is more effective, has fewer adverse effects, and is less likely to induce resistance than fluconazole. Although safety and efficacy of itraconazole for use in children have not been established, anecdotal experience has found it to be well tolerated and effective. Serum concentrations of itraconazole should be determined to ensure that effective, nontoxic levels are attained.

Immunocompetent children with uncomplicated acute pulmonary histoplasmosis rarely require antifungal therapy, because infection usually is self-limited. If the patient is symptomatic for more than 4 weeks, itraconazole should be given for 6 to 12 weeks, although the effectiveness of this treatment is not well documented. For severe acute pulmonary infections, treatment with amphotericin B is recommended for 1 to 2 weeks. After clinical improvement occurs, itraconazole is recommended for an additional 12 weeks. Methylprednisolone during the first 1 to 2 weeks of therapy can be used if respiratory complications develop.

[1] Wheat LJ, Freifeld AG, Kleiman MB, et al. Clinical practice guidelines for the management of patients with histoplasmosis: 2007 update by the Infectious Diseases Society of America. *Clin Infect Dis.* 2007;45(7):807–825

All patients with chronic pulmonary histoplasmosis should be treated. Mild to moderate cases should be treated with itraconazole for 1 to 2 years. Severe cases initially should be treated with amphotericin B followed by itraconazole for the same duration.

Mediastinal and inflammatory manifestations of infection generally do not need to be treated with antifungal agents. However, mediastinal adenitis that causes obstruction of a bronchus, the esophagus, or another mediastinal structure may improve with a brief course of corticosteroids. In these instances, itraconazole should be used concurrently and continued for 6 to 12 weeks. Dense fibrosis of mediastinal structures without an associated granulomatous inflammatory component does not respond to antifungal therapy, and surgical intervention may be necessary. Pericarditis and rheumatologic syndromes may respond to treatment with nonsteroidal anti-inflammatory agents (indomethacin).

For treatment of progressive disseminated histoplasmosis in a nonimmunocompromised infant or child, amphotericin B is the drug of choice and is given for 4 to 6 weeks. An alternative regimen uses induction with amphotericin B therapy for 2 to 4 weeks and, when there has been substantial clinical improvement and a decline in the serum concentration of histoplasmosis antigen, oral itraconazole is administered for 12 weeks. Longer periods of therapy can be required for patients with severe disease, primary immunodeficiency syndromes, acquired immunodeficiency that cannot be reversed, or patients who experience relapse despite appropriate therapy. After completion of treatment for PDH, urine antigen concentrations should be monitored for 12 months. Stable, low concentrations of urine antigen that are not accompanied by signs of active infection may not necessarily require prolongation or resumption of treatment.

ISOLATION OF THE HOSPITALIZED PATIENT: Standard precautions are recommended.

CONTROL MEASURES: In outbreaks, investigation for a common source of infection is indicated. Exposure to soil and dust from areas with significant accumulations of bird and bat droppings should be avoided, especially by immunocompromised people. If exposure is unavoidable, it should be minimized through use of appropriate respiratory protection (eg, N95 respirator), gloves, and disposable clothing. Old structures likely to have been contaminated with bird or bat droppings should be moistened thoroughly before demolition. Guidelines for preventing histoplasmosis have been designed for health and safety professionals, environmental consultants, and people supervising workers involved in activities in which contaminated materials are disturbed. Additional information about the guidelines is available from the National Institute for Occupational Safety and Health (NIOSH; publication No. 2005-109, available from Publications Dissemination, 4676 Columbia Parkway, Cincinnati, OH 45226-1998; telephone 800-356-4674) and the NIOSH Web site (**www.cdc.gov/niosh/docs/2005-109/pdfs/2005-109.pdf**).

Hookworm Infections
(*Ancylostoma duodenale* and *Necator americanus*)

CLINICAL MANIFESTATIONS: Patients with hookworm infection often are asymptomatic; however, chronic hookworm infection is a common cause of moderate and severe hypochromic, microcytic anemia in people living in tropical developing countries, and heavy infection can cause hypoproteinemia with edema. Chronic hookworm infection in children may lead to physical growth delay, deficits in cognition, and developmental delay. After contact with contaminated soil, initial skin penetration of larvae, often involving the feet, can cause a stinging or burning sensation followed by pruritus and a papulovesicular rash that may persist for 1 to 2 weeks. Pneumonitis associated with migrating larvae is uncommon and usually mild, except in heavy infections. Colicky abdominal pain, nausea, and/or diarrhea and marked eosinophilia can develop 4 to 6 weeks after exposure. Blood loss secondary to hookworm infection develops 10 to 12 weeks after initial infection and symptoms related to serious iron-deficiency anemia can develop in long-standing moderate or heavy hookworm infections. After oral ingestion of infectious *Ancylostoma duodenale* larvae, disease can manifest with pharyngeal itching, hoarseness, nausea, and vomiting shortly after ingestion.

ETIOLOGY: *Necator americanus* is the major cause of hookworm infection worldwide, although *A duodenale* also is an important hookworm in some regions. Mixed infections are common. Both are roundworms (nematodes) with similar life cycles.

EPIDEMIOLOGY: Humans are the only reservoir. Hookworms are prominent in rural, tropical, and subtropical areas where soil contamination with human feces is common. Although the prevalence of both hookworm species is equal in many areas, *A duodenale* is the predominant species in the Mediterranean region, northern Asia, and selected foci of South America. *N americanus* is predominant in the Western hemisphere, sub-Saharan Africa, Southeast Asia, and a number of Pacific islands. Larvae and eggs survive in loose, sandy, moist, shady, well-aerated, warm soil (optimal temperature 23°C–33°C [73°F–91°F]). Hookworm eggs from stool hatch in soil in 1 to 2 days as rhabditiform larvae. These larvae develop into infective filariform larvae in soil within 5 to 7 days and can persist for weeks to months. Percutaneous infection occurs after exposure to infectious larvae. *A duodenale* transmission can occur by oral ingestion and possibly through human milk. Untreated infected patients can harbor worms for 5 years or longer.

The time from exposure to development of noncutaneous symptoms is 4 to 12 weeks.

DIAGNOSTIC TESTS: Microscopic demonstration of hookworm eggs in feces is diagnostic. Adult worms or larvae rarely are seen. Approximately 5 to 8 weeks are required after infection for eggs to appear in feces. A direct stool smear with saline solution or potassium iodide saturated with iodine is adequate for diagnosis of heavy hookworm infection; light infections require concentration techniques. Quantification techniques (eg, Kato-Katz, Beaver direct smear, or Stoll egg-counting techniques) to determine the clinical significance of infection and the response to treatment may be available from state or reference laboratories.

TREATMENT: Albendazole, mebendazole, and pyrantel pamoate all are effective treatments (see Drugs for Parasitic Infections, p 848). Mebendazole is not effective for hookworm when used in a single dose of 500 mg. Although data suggest that these drugs are safe in children younger than 2 years of age, the risks and benefits of therapy should be considered before administration. In 1-year-old children, the World Health Organization recommends reducing the albendazole dose to half of that given to older children and adults. Albendazole is not approved by the US Food and Drug Administration for hookworm infection. Reexamination of stool specimens 2 weeks after therapy to determine whether worms have been eliminated is helpful for assessing response to therapy. Retreatment is indicated for persistent infection. Nutritional supplementation, including iron, is important when severe anemia is present. Severely affected children also may require blood transfusion.

ISOLATION OF THE HOSPITALIZED PATIENT: Only standard precautions are recommended, because there is no direct person-to-person transmission.

CONTROL MEASURES: Sanitary disposal of feces to prevent contamination of soil is necessary in areas with endemic infection. Treatment of all known infected people and screening of high-risk groups (ie, children and agricultural workers) in areas with endemic infection can help decrease environmental contamination. Wearing shoes may not be fully protective, because cutaneous exposure to hookworm larvae over the entire body surface of children could result in infection. Despite relatively rapid reinfection, periodic deworming treatments targeting preschool-aged and school-aged children have been advocated to prevent morbidity associated with heavy intestinal helminth infections.

Human Bocavirus

CLINICAL MANIFESTATIONS: Human bocavirus (HBoV) first was identified in 2005 from a cohort of children with acute respiratory tract symptoms. Cough, rhinorrhea, wheezing, and fever have been attributed to HBoV. HBoV has been identified in 5% to 33% of all children with acute respiratory tract infections in various settings (eg, inpatient facilities, outpatient facilities, child care centers) using many different criteria to identify children for testing. The role of HBoV as a pathogen in human infection is confounded by simultaneous detection of other viral pathogens in patients from whom HBoV is identified, with coinfection rates as high as 80%. Current data have not proven that HBoV is a respiratory tract pathogen rather than simply a colonizing organism. HBoV has been detected in stool samples from children with acute gastroenteritis; however, further studies are needed to better understand the role of HBoV in gastroenteritis. Infection with HBoV appears to be ubiquitous, because nearly all children develop serologic evidence of previous HBoV infection by 5 years of age.

ETIOLOGY: HBoV is a nonenveloped, single-stranded DNA virus classified in the family *Parvoviridae*, genus *Bocavirus*, on the basis of its genetic similarity to the closely related **bo**vine parvovirus 1 and **ca**nine minute virus, from which the name "**boca**virus" was derived. Three distinct genotypes have been described, although there are no data regarding antigenic variation or distinct serotypes.

EPIDEMIOLOGY: Detection of HBoV has been described only in humans. Transmission is presumed to be from respiratory tract secretions, although fecal-oral transmission may be possible on the basis of the finding of HBoV in stool specimens from children, including symptomatic children with diarrhea.

The frequent codetection of other viral pathogens of the respiratory tract in association with HBoV has led to speculation about the role played by HBoV; it may be a true copathogen, it may be shed for long periods after primary infection, or it may reactivate during subsequent viral infections. Extended and intermittent shedding of HBoV has been reported for up to 75 days after initial detection.

HBoV circulates worldwide and throughout the year. In temperate climates, seasonal clustering in the spring associated with increased transmission of other respiratory tract viruses has been reported.

DIAGNOSTIC TESTS: Commercial molecular diagnostic assays for HBoV are available. HBoV polymerase chain reaction and detection of HBoV-specific antibody also are used by research laboratories to detect the presence of virus and infection, respectively.

TREATMENT: No specific therapy is available.

ISOLATION OF THE HOSPITALIZED PATIENT: The presence of virus in respiratory tract secretions and stool suggests that, in addition to standard precautions, contact precautions should be effective in limiting the spread of infection for the duration of the symptomatic illness in infants and young children. However, prolonged shedding of virus in respiratory tract secretions and in stool may occur after resolution of symptoms, particularly in immune-compromised hosts.

CONTROL MEASURES: Although possible health care-associated transmission of HBoV has been described, investigations of transmissibility of HBoV in the community or health care settings have not been published. Appropriate hand hygiene, particularly when handling respiratory tract secretions or diapers of ill children, is recommended. The presence of HBoV in serum also raises the possibility of transmission by transfusion, although this mode of transmission has not been documented.

Human Herpesvirus 6 (Including Roseola) and 7

CLINICAL MANIFESTATIONS: Clinical manifestations of primary infection with human herpesvirus 6 (HHV-6) include roseola (exanthem subitum) in approximately 20% of infected children, undifferentiated febrile illness without rash or localizing signs, and other acute febrile illnesses. HHV-6 infection often is accompanied by cervical and characteristic postoccipital lymphadenopathy, gastrointestinal tract or respiratory tract signs, and inflamed tympanic membranes. Fever usually is high (temperature >39.5°C [103.0°F]) and persists for 3 to 7 days. Approximately 20% of all emergency department visits for febrile children 6 through 12 months of age are attributable to HHV-6. Roseola is distinguished by the erythematous maculopapular rash, which appears once fever resolves and can last hours to days. Febrile seizures are the most common complication and reason for hospitalization among children with primary HHV-6 infection. Approximately 10% to 15% of children with primary HHV-6 illnesses develop febrile seizures, predominantly between the ages of 6 and 18 months. Other neurologic manifestations that may accompany primary infection include a bulging fontanelle and encephalopathy or encephalitis. Hepatitis has been reported as a rare manifestation of initial illness. Congenital HHV-6 infection, which occurs in approximately 1% of newborn infants, generally is asymptomatic at birth. Whether clinical manifestations subsequently develop is unknown.

The frequency and scope of the clinical manifestations occurring with human herpesvirus 7 (HHV-7) infection are unclear. Most primary infections with HHV-7 presumably are asymptomatic or mild and not distinctive. Some initial infections can present as typical roseola and may account for second or recurrent cases of roseola. Febrile illnesses associated with seizures also have been documented to occur during primary HHV-7 infection. Some investigators suggest that the association of HHV-7 with these clinical manifestations results from the ability of HHV-7 to reactivate HHV-6 from latency.

Following primary infection, both HHV-6 and HHV-7 remain in a persistent or latent state and may reactivate. The clinical circumstances and manifestations of reactivation in healthy people are unclear. Illness associated with HHV-6 reactivation has been described primarily among immunocompromised recipients of solid organ and hematopoietic stem cell transplants. Among the clinical findings associated with HHV-6 reactivation in these patients are fever, rash, hepatitis, bone marrow suppression, graft rejection, pneumonia, and encephalitis. A few cases of CNS symptoms have been reported in association with

HHV-7 reactivation in immunocompromised hosts, but clinical findings generally have been reported less frequently with HHV-7 than with HHV-6 reactivation.

ETIOLOGY: HHV-6 and HHV-7 are lymphotropic agents that are closely related members of the Herpesviridae family, which, like all human herpesviruses, establish lifelong infection after initial exposure. HHV-6 strains have 2 distinct subgroups, variants A and B. Essentially all postnatally acquired primary infections in children are caused by variant B strains, except infections in some parts of Africa. Among congenital HHV-6 infections, however, as many as one third may be caused by variant A.

EPIDEMIOLOGY: HHV-6 and HHV-7 cause ubiquitous infections in children worldwide. Humans are the only known natural host. Nearly all children acquire HHV-6 infection within the first 3 years of life, probably resulting from asymptomatic shedding of infectious virus in secretions of a healthy family member or other close contact. During the acute phase of primary infection, HHV-6 and HHV-7 can be isolated from peripheral blood mononuclear cells and from saliva of some children. Viral DNA subsequently may be detected throughout life by polymerase chain reaction (PCR) assay in multiple body sites. Although both HHV-6 and HHV-7 may be detected in blood mononuclear cells, salivary glands, lung and skin, only HHV-6 frequently is found in brain and HHV-7 only in mammary glands. Virus-specific maternal antibody, which is present uniformly in the sera of infants at birth, provides transient partial protection. As the concentration of maternal antibody decreases during the first year of life, the rate of infection increases rapidly, peaking between 6 and 24 months of age. Essentially all children are seropositive for HHV-6B before 4 years of age. Infections occur throughout the year without a seasonal pattern. Secondary cases rarely are identified. Occasional outbreaks of roseola have been reported.

Congenital infection with HHV-6 occurs in approximately 1% of newborn infants as determined by the presence of HHV-6 DNA in cord blood. Most congenital infections appear to result from the germline passage of maternal or paternal chromosomally integrated HHV-6, a unique mechanism of transmission of human viral congenital infection. Transplacental HHV-6 infection also may occur from reinfection or reactivation of maternal HHV-6 infection or from reactivated maternal chromosomally integrated HHV-6. HHV-6 has not been identified in human milk.

HHV-7 infection usually occurs later in childhood compared with HHV-6. By adulthood, the seroprevalence of HHV-7 is approximately 85%. Infectious HHV-7 is present in more than 75% of saliva specimens obtained from healthy adults. Contact with infected respiratory tract secretions of healthy contacts is the probable mode of transmission of HHV-7 to young children. HHV-7 has been detected in human milk, peripheral blood mononuclear cells, cervical secretions, and other body sites. Congenital HHV-7 infection has not been demonstrated by the examination of large numbers of cord blood samples for HHV-7 DNA.

The mean **incubation period** for HHV-6 may be 9 to 10 days. For HHV-7, the incubation period is not known.

DIAGNOSTIC TESTS: Multiple assays for detection of HHV-6 and HHV-7 have been developed, but few are available commercially, and many do not differentiate between new, past, and reactivated infection. Moreover, because laboratory diagnosis of HHV-6 or HHV-7 usually does not influence clinical management (infections among the severely immunocompromised may be an exception), these tests have limited utility in clinical practice. Diagnostic assays include serologic tests, isolation of the virus from tissue culture, and detection of viral DNA by qualitative and quantitative PCR and of RNA by reverse-transcriptase PCR in blood, secretions, and tissues. Most of these assays are available only in research laboratories. Some serologic and DNA detection assays are available commercially.

Serologic tests used include immunofluorescent antibody, neutralization, immunoblot, and enzyme immunoassays (EIAs). A fourfold increase in serum antibody concentration alone does not necessarily indicate new infection. An increase in titer also may occur with reactivation and in association with other infections, especially other beta-herpesvirus infections. However, seroconversion from negative to positive in paired sera is good evidence of recent primary infection. Detection of specific immunoglobulin (Ig) M antibody also is not reliable for diagnosing new infection, because IgM antibodies to HHV-6 and HHV-7 are not always detectable in children with primary infection and also may be present in some asymptomatic previously infected people. These antibody assays do not differentiate HHV-6A from HHV-6B infections. In addition, the diagnosis of primary HHV-7 infection in children with previous HHV-6 infection is confounded by concurrent rise in HHV-6 antibody titer from antigenic cross-reactivity or from reactivation of HHV-6 by a new HHV-7 infection. Detection of low-avidity HHV-6 or HHV-7 antibody with subsequent maturation to high-avidity antibody has been used in such situations to identify recent primary infection. Isolation of HHV-6 or HHV-7 in conjunction with seroconversion or, in the infant with maternal antibodies, a fourfold titer rise confirms primary infection.

Reference laboratories offer diagnostic testing for HHV-6 and HHV-7 infections by detection of viral DNA in blood and cerebrospinal fluid (CSF) specimens. However, detection of HHV-6 DNA or HHV-7 DNA in peripheral blood mononuclear cells, other body fluids, and tissues generally does not differentiate between new infection and persistence of virus from past infection. DNA detection by PCR in plasma and sera has been used to diagnose acute primary infection, but these assays are not reliably sensitive in young children or specific in children with chromosomally integrated HHV-6 infection. Chromosomal integration of HHV-6 is indicated by consistently positive PCR tests for HHV-6 DNA in blood with high viral loads ($\geq$1 copy of HHV-6 DNA per leukocyte) and is confirmed by detection of HHV-6 DNA in hair follicles.

TREATMENT: Supportive. Anecdotal reports suggest that use of ganciclovir or foscarnet may be beneficial for immunocompromised patients with serious HHV-6 disease, but resistance may occur.

ISOLATION OF THE HOSPITALIZED PATIENT: Standard precautions are recommended.

CONTROL MEASURES: None.

Human Herpesvirus 8

CLINICAL MANIFESTATIONS: Human herpesvirus (HHV-8) is the etiologic agent associated with Kaposi sarcoma (KS), primary effusion lymphoma, and multicentric Castleman disease (MCD). In regions with endemic disease, a primary infection syndrome in immunocompetent children has been described, which consists of fever and a maculopapular rash, often accompanied by upper respiratory tract signs. Primary infection among immunocompromised people and men who have sex with men tends to have more severe manifestations that include fever, rash, lymphadenopathy, splenomegaly, diarrhea, arthralgia, and KS. In parts of Africa, among children with and without human immunodeficiency virus (HIV) infection, KS is a frequent, aggressive malignancy. In the United States, KS rarely is observed among children. Most commonly, KS occurs among severely immunocompromised HIV patients in the United States. Among organ transplant recipients and other immunosuppressed patients, KS is an important cause of cancer-related deaths. Primary effusion lymphoma is rare among children. MCD has been described in adolescents, but the proportion of cases attributable to infection with HHV-8 is unknown.

ETIOLOGY: HHV-8 is a member of the family Herpesviridae, the gammaherpesvirus subfamily, and the Rhadinovirus genus and is related closely to herpesvirus saimiri of monkeys and Epstein-Barr virus.

EPIDEMIOLOGY: In regions with high endemicity, the epidemiology of HHV-8 closely reflects that observed for KS. In areas of Africa, the Amazon basin, Mediterranean, and Middle East with endemic disease, seroprevalence ranges from approximately 30% to 60%. Low rates of seroprevalence, generally less than 5%, have been reported in the United States, Northern and Central Europe, and most areas of Asia. Higher rates, however, occur in specific geographic regions, among adolescents and adults with or at high risk of acquiring HIV infection, injection drug users, and internationally adopted children coming from some Eastern European countries.

Acquisition of HHV-8 in areas with endemic infection frequently occurs before puberty, likely by oral inoculation of saliva of close contacts, especially secretions of mothers and siblings. Virus is shed frequently in saliva of infected people and becomes latent for life in peripheral blood mononuclear cells, primarily CD19+ B lymphocytes, and lymphoid tissue. Sexual transmission appears to be the major route of infection among men who have sex with men. Studies from areas with endemic infection have suggested transmission may occur by blood transfusion, but in the United States, such evidence is lacking. Transplantation of infected donor organs has been documented to result in HHV-8 infection. HHV-8 DNA has been detected in blood drawn at birth from infants born to HHV-8 seropositive mothers, suggesting vertical transmission is possible.

The **incubation period** of HHV-8 is unknown.

DIAGNOSTIC TESTS: Nucleic acid amplification testing and serologic assays for HHV-8 are available, and new assays with greater clinical usefulness are being developed. Polymerase chain reaction (PCR) tests may be used on peripheral blood and tissue biopsy specimens of patients with HHV-8–associated disease, such as KS. PCR detection of HHV-8 in peripheral blood specimens has been used in some patients to support the diagnosis of KS and to identify exacerbations of HHV-8-associated diseases, primarily MCD. However, HHV-8 DNA detection in the peripheral blood does not differentiate between latent and active replicating infection.

Currently available serologic assays measuring antibodies to HHV-8 include immunofluorescence assay (IFA), enzyme immunoassays (EIAs), and Western blot assays using recombinant HHV-8 proteins. IFA most frequently is used. These serologic assays can detect both latent and lytic infection but are of limited use in the diagnosis and management of acute clinical disease.

TREATMENT: No antiviral treatment is approved for HHV-8 disease. Several antiviral agents have in vitro activity against HHV-8, but adequate clinical evaluations of these agents have not been conducted. HHV-8 associated malignancies can be treated with radiation and cancer chemotherapies.

ISOLATION OF THE HOSPITALIZED PATIENT: Standard precautions are recommended.

CONTROL MEASURES: None.

Human Immunodeficiency Virus Infection[1]

CLINICAL MANIFESTATIONS: Human immunodeficiency virus (HIV) infection results in a wide array of clinical manifestations and varied natural history. HIV type 1 (HIV-1) is much more common in the United States than is HIV type 2 (HIV-2). Unless otherwise specified, this chapter addresses HIV-1 infection.

Acquired immunodeficiency syndrome (AIDS) is the name given to an advanced stage of HIV infection. The Centers for Disease Control and Prevention (CDC) uses a case definition that comprises AIDS-defining conditions for surveillance (Table 3.24). The CDC classifies all infected children younger than 13 years of age according to clinical stage of disease (Table 3.25, p 420) and immunologic status (Table 3.26, p 422).[2,3] This pediatric classification system emphasizes the importance of the CD4+ T-lymphocyte count and percentage as critical immunologic parameters and as markers of prognosis. Data regarding plasma HIV-1 RNA concentration (viral load) are not included in this classification.

With timely diagnostic testing and appropriate treatment, clinical manifestations of HIV-1 infection and occurrence of AIDS-defining illnesses now are rare among children in the United States and other industrialized countries. Early manifestations of pediatric HIV infection include unexplained fevers, generalized lymphadenopathy, hepatomegaly, splenomegaly, failure to thrive, persistent or recurrent oral and diaper candidiasis, recurrent diarrhea, parotitis, hepatitis, central nervous system (CNS) disease (eg, hyperreflexia, hypertonia, floppiness, developmental delay), lymphoid interstitial pneumonia, recurrent invasive bacterial infections, and other opportunistic infections (OIs) (eg, viral and fungal).[4]

In the era of highly active antiretroviral therapy (HAART), there has been a substantial decrease in frequency of all OIs. The frequency of different OIs in the pre-HAART era varied by age, pathogen, previous infection history, and immunologic status. In the

---

[1] For a complete listing of current policy statements from the American Academy of Pediatrics regarding human immunodeficiency virus and acquired immunodeficiency syndrome, see **http://aappolicy. aappublications.org/.**

[2] Centers for Disease Control and Prevention. 1993 revised classification system for HIV infection and expanded surveillance case definition for AIDS among adolescents and adults. *MMWR Recomm Rep.* 1992;41(RR-17):1–19

[3] Centers for Disease Control and Prevention. 1994 revised classification system for human immunodeficiency virus infection in children less than 13 years of age. Official authorized addenda: human immunodeficiency virus infection codes and official guidelines for coding and reporting ICD-9-CM. *MMWR Recomm Rep.* 1994;43(RR-12):1–19

[4] Centers for Disease Control and Prevention. Guidelines for prevention and treatment of opportunistic infections among HIV-exposed and HIV-infected children. Recommendations from CDC, the National Institutes of Health, the HIV Medicine Association of the Infectious Diseases Society of America, the Pediatric Infectious Diseases Society, and the American Academy of Pediatrics. *MMWR Recomm Rep.* 2009;58(RR-11):1–166. Available at: **http://aidsinfo.nih.gov/Guidelines**

Table 3.24. 1993 Revised Case Definition of AIDS-Defining Conditions for Adults and Adolescents 13 Years of Age and Older[a]

- Candidiasis of bronchi, trachea, or lungs
- Candidiasis, esophageal
- Cervical cancer, invasive
- Coccidioidomycosis, disseminated or extrapulmonary
- Cryptococcosis, extrapulmonary
- Cryptosporidiosis, chronic intestinal (greater than 1 mo duration)
- Cystoisosporiasis (isosporiasis), chronic intestinal (greater than 1 mo duration)
- Cytomegalovirus disease (other than liver, spleen, or nodes)
- Cytomegalovirus retinitis (with loss of vision)
- Encephalopathy, HIV related
- Herpes simplex: chronic ulcer(s) (greater than 1 mo duration) or bronchitis, pneumonitis, or esophagitis
- Histoplasmosis, disseminated or extrapulmonary
- Kaposi sarcoma
- Lymphoma, Burkitt (or equivalent term)
- Lymphoma, immunoblastic (or equivalent term)
- Lymphoma, primary or brain
- *Mycobacterium avium* complex or *Mycobacterium kansasii* infection, disseminated or extrapulmonary
- *Mycobacterium tuberculosis* infection, any site, pulmonary or extrapulmonary
- *Mycobacterium,* other species or unidentified species infection, disseminated or extrapulmonary
- *Pneumocystis jirovecii* pneumonia
- Pneumonia, recurrent
- Progressive multifocal leukoencephalopathy
- *Salmonella* septicemia, recurrent
- Toxoplasmosis of brain
- Wasting syndrome attributable to HIV
- CD4+ T-lymphocyte count less than $200/\mu L$ $(0.20 \times 10^9/L)$ or CD4+ T-lymphocyte percentage less than 15%

AIDS indicates acquired immunodeficiency syndrome; HIV, human immunodeficiency virus.
[a]Modified from Centers for Disease Control and Prevention. 1993 revised classification system for HIV infection and expanded surveillance case definition for AIDS among adolescents and adults. *MMWR Recomm Rep.* 1992;41(RR–17):1–19.

pre-HAART era, the most common OIs observed among children in the United States were infections caused by invasive encapsulated bacteria, *Pneumocystis jirovecii* (previously known as *Pneumocystis carinii),* varicella-zoster virus, cytomegalovirus (CMV), *Herpes simplex* virus, *Mycobacterium avium* complex (MAC), and *Candida* species. Less commonly observed opportunistic pathogens included Epstein-Barr virus (EBV), *Mycobacterium tuberculosis, Cryptosporidium* species, *Cystoisospora* (formerly *Isospora)* species, other enteric pathogens, *Aspergillus* species, and *Toxoplasma gondii.*

Immune reconstitution inflammatory syndrome (IRIS) is a paradoxical clinical deterioration often seen in severely immunosuppressed people that occurs shortly after the initiation of HAART. Local symptoms develop secondary to an inflammatory response as cell-mediated immunity is restored. Underlying infection with mycobacteria (including *Mycobacterium tuberculosis),* herpesviruses, and fungi (including *Cryptococcal* species) predisposes to IRIS.

Table 3.25. Clinical Categories for Children Younger Than 13 Years of Age With Human Immunodeficiency Virus (HIV) Infection[a]

Category N: Not Symptomatic

Children who have no signs or symptoms considered to be the result of HIV infection or have only 1 of the conditions listed in Category A.

Category A: Mildly Symptomatic

- Children with 2 or more of the conditions listed but none of the conditions listed in categories B and C.
- Lymphadenopathy (≥0.5 cm at more than 2 sites; bilateral at 1 site)
- Hepatomegaly
- Splenomegaly
- Dermatitis
- Parotitis
- Recurrent or persistent upper respiratory tract infection, sinusitis, or otitis media

Category B: Moderately Symptomatic

- Children who have symptomatic conditions other than those listed for category A or C that are attributed to HIV infection.
- Anemia (hemoglobin <8 g/dL [<80 g/L]), neutropenia (white blood cell count <1000/μL [<1.0 × 10⁹/L]), and/or thrombocytopenia (platelet count <100 × 10³ μL [<100 × 10⁹/L]) persisting for ≥30 days
- Bacterial meningitis, pneumonia, or sepsis (single episode)
- Candidiasis, oropharyngeal (thrush), persisting (>2 mo) in children older than 6 mo of age
- Cardiomyopathy
- Cytomegalovirus infection, with onset before 1 mo of age
- Diarrhea, recurrent or chronic
- Hepatitis
- Herpes simplex virus (HSV) stomatitis, recurrent (>2 episodes within 1 year)
- HSV bronchitis, pneumonitis, or esophagitis with onset before 1 mo of age
- Herpes zoster (shingles) involving at least 2 distinct episodes or more than 1 dermatome
- Leiomyosarcoma
- Lymphoid interstitial pneumonia or pulmonary lymphoid hyperplasia complex
- Nephropathy
- Nocardiosis
- Persistent fever (lasting >1 mo)
- Toxoplasmosis, onset before 1 mo of age
- Varicella, disseminated (complicated chickenpox)

Category C: Severely Symptomatic

- Serious bacterial infections, multiple or recurrent (ie, any combination of at least 2 culture-confirmed infections within a 2-y period), of the following types: septicemia, pneumonia, meningitis, bone or joint infection, or abscess of an internal organ or body cavity (excluding otitis media, superficial skin or mucosal abscesses, and indwelling catheter-related infections)
- Candidiasis, esophageal or pulmonary (bronchi, trachea, lungs)
- Coccidioidomycosis, disseminated (at site other than or in addition to lungs or cervical or hilar lymph nodes) Cryptococcosis, extrapulmonary
- Cryptosporidiosis or cystoisosporiasis with diarrhea persisting >1 mo
- Cytomegalovirus disease with onset of symptoms after 1 mo of age (at a site other than liver, spleen, or lymph nodes)
- Encephalopathy (at least 1 of the following progressive findings present for at least 2 mo in the absence of a concurrent illness other than HIV infection that could explain the findings): (1) failure to attain or loss of developmental milestones or loss of intellectual ability, verified by standard developmental scale or neuropsychologic tests; (2) impaired brain growth or acquired microcephaly demonstrated by head circumference measurements or brain atrophy demonstrated by computed tomography or magnetic resonance imaging (serial imaging required for children younger than 2 y of age); (3) acquired symmetric motor deficit manifested by 2 or more of the following: paresis, pathologic reflexes, ataxia, or gait disturbance
- HSV infection causing a mucocutaneous ulcer that persists for greater than 1 mo or bronchitis, pneumonitis, or esophagitis for any duration affecting a child older than 1 mo of age
- Histoplasmosis, disseminated (at a site other than or in addition to lungs or cervical or hilar lymph nodes)
- Kaposi sarcoma
- Lymphoma, primary, in brain
- Lymphoma, small, noncleaved cell (Burkitt), or immunoblastic; or large-cell lymphoma of B-lymphocyte or unknown immunologic phenotype
- *Mycobacterium tuberculosis*, disseminated or extrapulmonary
- *Mycobacterium*, other species or unidentified species infection, disseminated (at a site other than or in addition to lungs, skin, or cervical or hilar lymph nodes)
- *Pneumocystis jirovecii* pneumonia
- Progressive multifocal leukoencephalopathy
- *Salmonella* (nontyphoid) septicemia, recurrent
- Toxoplasmosis of the brain with onset at after 1 mo of age
- Wasting syndrome in the absence of a concurrent illness other than HIV infection that could explain the following findings: (1) persistent weight loss >10% of baseline; (2) downward crossing of at least 2 of the following percentile lines on the weight-for-age chart (eg, 95th, 75th, 50th, 25th, 5th) in a child 1 y of age or older; OR (3) <5th percentile on weight-for-height chart on 2 consecutive measurements, ≥30 days apart; PLUS (1) chronic diarrhea (ie, at least 2 loose stools per day for >30 days); OR (2) documented fever (for >30 days, intermittent or constant)

ᵃModified from Centers for Disease Control and Prevention. 1994 revised classification system for human immunodeficiency virus infection in children less than 13 years of age. Official authorized addenda: human immunodeficiency virus infection codes and official guidelines for coding and reporting ICD-9-CM. *MMWR Recomm Rep.* 1994;43(RR-12):1–19

Table 3.26. Pediatric Human Immunodeficiency Virus (HIV) Classification for Children Younger Than 13 Years of Age[a]

Immunologic Definitions	Immunologic Categories						Clinical Classifications[c]			
	Age-Specific CD4+ T-Lymphocyte Count and Percentage of Total Lymphocytes[b]									
	Younger Than 12 mo		1 Through 5 y		6 Through 12 y		N: No Signs or Symptoms	A: Mild Signs and Symptoms	B: Moderate Signs and Symptoms[d]	C: Severe Signs and Symptoms[d]
	µL	%	µL	%	µL	%				
1: No evidence of suppression	≥1500	≥25	≥1000	≥25	≥500	≥25	N1	A1	B1	C1
2: Evidence of moderate suppression	750–1499	15–24	500–999	15–24	200–499	15–24	N2	A2	B2	C2
3: Severe suppression	<750	<15	<500	<15	<200	<15	N3	A3	B3	C3

[a] Modified from Centers for Disease Control and Prevention. 1994 revised classification system for human immunodeficiency virus infection in children less than 13 years of age. Official authorized addenda: human immunodeficiency virus infection codes and official guidelines for coding and reporting ICD-9-CM. *MMWR Recomm Rep.* 1994;43(RR-12);1–19

[b] To convert values in µL to Système International units (× 10^9/L), multiply by 0.001.

[c] Children whose HIV infection status is not confirmed are classified by using this grid with a letter E (for perinatally exposed) placed before the appropriate classification code (eg, EN2).

[d] Lymphoid interstitial pneumonitis in category B or any condition in category C is reportable to state and local health departments as acquired immunodeficiency syndrome (AIDS-defining conditions) (see Table 3.25, p 420, for further definition of clinical categories).

Malignant neoplasms in children with HIV-1 infection are relatively uncommon, but leiomyosarcomas and non-Hodgkin B-cell lymphomas of the Burkitt type (including some that occur in the CNS), occur more commonly in children with HIV infection than in immunocompetent children. Kaposi sarcoma is rare in children in the United States but has been documented in HIV-infected children who have emigrated from sub-Saharan African countries. The incidence of malignant neoplasms in HIV-infected children has decreased during the HAART era.

Prognosis for survival is poor for untreated children who acquired HIV infection through mother-to-child transmission and who have high viral loads (ie, >100 000 copies/mL) and severe suppression of CD4+ T-lymphocyte counts (see Table 3.26, p 422). In these children, AIDS-defining conditions developing during the first 6 months of life, including *P jirovecii* pneumonia (PCP), progressive neurologic disease, and severe wasting, are predictors of a poor outcome. When HAART regimens are begun early, prognosis and survival rates improve dramatically. Although deaths attributable to OIs have declined, non–AIDS-defining infections and multiorgan failure remain major causes of death. In the United States, mortality in HIV-infected children has declined from 7.2/100 person years in 1993 to 0.8/100 person years in 2006. The HIV mortality rate is approximately 30 times higher than for the general US pediatric population.

ETIOLOGY: As noted above, 2 types of HIV cause disease in humans: HIV-1 and HIV-2. These viruses are cytopathic lentiviruses belonging to the family *Retroviridae*, and they are related closely to the simian immunodeficiency viruses (SIVs), agents in African green monkeys and sooty mangabeys. Three distinct genetic groups of HIV-1 exist worldwide: M (major), O (outlier), and N (new). Group M viruses are the most prevalent worldwide and comprise 8 genetic subtypes, or clades, known as A through H. The HIV-1 genome is 10 kb in length and has both conserved and highly variable domains. Three principal genes (*gag, pol,* and *env*) encode the major structural and enzymatic proteins, and 6 accessory genes regulate gene expression and aid in assembly and release of infectious virions. The envelope glycoprotein interacts with the CD4 receptor and with 1 of 2 major coreceptors (CCR5 or CXCR4) on the host cell membrane. HIV-1 is an RNA virus that requires the activity of a viral enzyme, reverse transcriptase, to convert the viral RNA to DNA. A double-stranded DNA copy of the viral genome then can incorporate into the host cell genome, where it persists as a provirus.

HIV-2, the second AIDS-causing virus, predominantly is found in West Africa, with the highest rates of infection in Guinea-Bissau. The prevalence of HIV-2 in the United States is extremely low. HIV-2 is thought to have a milder disease course with a longer time to development of AIDS than HIV-1. Nonnucleoside reverse transcriptase inhibitors (NNRTIs) are not effective against HIV-2, whereas nucleoside reverse transcriptase inhibitors (NRTIs) and protease inhibitors have varying efficacy against HIV-2. CDC guidelines state that HIV-2 serologic testing should be performed in patients who: (1) are from countries of high prevalence, mainly in Western Africa; (2) share needles or have sex partners known to be infected with HIV-2 or are from areas with endemic infection; (3) received transfusions or nonsterile medical care in areas with endemic infection; or (4) are children of women with risk factors for HIV-2 infection. The identification of HIV-2 represents a diagnostic dilemma in the United States. Currently licensed HIV enzyme immunoassays (EIAs) detect HIV-1 and HIV-2 antibodies, but the confirmatory Western blot used by many laboratories will report an indeterminate result or will misclassify the HIV-2 virus as HIV-1 (eg, detection of only p24 and gp160 bands). Therefore, it is vital to notify the laboratory when ordering viral serologic tests for a patient with risk factors for HIV-2. Assays approved by the US Food and Drug Administration (FDA) for determination of viral load are specific for HIV-1; none are approved by the FDA for determination of HIV-2 viral load.

Although B-lymphocyte counts remain normal or somewhat increased, humoral immune dysfunction may precede or accompany cellular dysfunction. Increased serum immunoglobulin (Ig) concentrations of all isotypes, particularly IgG and IgA, are manifestations of the humoral immune dysfunction, but they are not directed necessarily at specific pathogens of childhood. Specific humoral responses to antigens to which the patient previously has not been exposed usually are abnormal; later in disease, recall antibody responses, including responses to vaccine-associated antigens, are slow and diminish in magnitude. A small proportion (less than 10%) of patients will develop panhypogammaglobulinemia. Such patients have a particularly poor prognosis.

EPIDEMIOLOGY: Humans are the only known reservoir for HIV-1 and HIV-2. Latent virus persists in peripheral blood mononuclear cells and in cells of the brain, bone marrow, and genital tract even when plasma viral load is undetectable. Only blood, semen, cervicovaginal secretions, and human milk have been implicated epidemiologically in transmission of infection.

Established modes of HIV transmission include: (1) sexual contact (vaginal, anal, or orogenital); (2) percutaneous blood exposure (from contaminated needles or other sharp instruments); (3) mucous membrane exposure to contaminated blood or other body fluids; (4) mother-to-child transmission during pregnancy, around the time of labor and delivery, and postnatally through breastfeeding; and (5) transfusion with contaminated blood products. Cases of probable HIV transmission from HIV-infected caregiver to their infants through feeding blood-tinged premasticated food have been reported in the United States. As a result of highly effective screening methods, blood, blood components, and clotting factor virtually have been eliminated as a cause of HIV transmission in the United States since 1985. In the United States, transmission of HIV has not been documented with normal household contact. Transmission has been documented after contact of nonintact skin with blood-containing body fluids. Moreover, transmission of HIV has not been documented in schools or child care settings in the United States.

Pediatric AIDS cases account for fewer than 1% of all reported cases of AIDS in the United States. Since the mid 1990s, the number of reported pediatric AIDS cases decreased significantly, primarily because of interruption of mother-to-child transmission of HIV. The decrease in rate of mother-to-child transmission of HIV in the United States was attributable to development and implementation of antenatal HIV testing programs and of interventions to prevent transmission: antiretroviral (ARV) prophylaxis during the antepartum, intrapartum, and postnatal periods; cesarean delivery before labor and before rupture of membranes; and complete avoidance of breastfeeding. Combination ARV regimens during pregnancy have been associated with lower rates of mother-to-child transmission than has zidovudine alone. Currently in the United States, most HIV-infected pregnant women receive 3-drug combination ARV regimens either for treatment of their own HIV infection or, if criteria for treatment are not yet met, for prevention of mother-to-child transmission of HIV (in which case the drugs are stopped after delivery). The CDC estimates that each year, 215 to 370 infants with HIV infection are born in the United States.

The risk of infection for an infant born to an HIV-seropositive mother who did not receive interventions to prevent transmission is estimated to range from 12% to 40% and is thought to average between 21% and 25% in the United States. Most mother-to-child transmission occurs intrapartum, with smaller proportions of transmission occurring in utero and postnatally through breastfeeding. Various risk factors for mother-to-child transmission of HIV have been identified and can be categorized as follows: (1) the amount of virus to which the child is exposed (especially the maternal viral load; a higher maternal viral load is associated with a lower maternal CD4+ T-lymphocyte count and with more advanced maternal clinical disease); (2) the duration of such exposure (eg, duration of ruptured membranes or of breastfeeding, vaginal versus cesarean delivery before labor and before rupture of membranes); and (3) factors that facilitate the transfer of virus from mother to child (eg, maternal breast pathologic lesions, infant oral candidiasis). In addition to these factors, characteristics of the virus and the child's susceptibility to infection are important. Of note, although maternal viral load is a critical determinant affecting the likelihood of mother-to-child transmission of HIV, transmissions have been observed across the entire range of maternal viral loads. The risk of mother-to-child transmission increases with each hour increase in the duration of rupture of membranes, and the duration of ruptured membranes should be considered when evaluating the need for special obstetric interventions. Cesarean delivery performed before onset of labor and before rupture of membranes has been shown to reduce mother-to-child intrapartum transmission. Current US guidelines recommend cesarean delivery before onset of labor and before rupture of membranes for HIV-infected women with a viral load greater than 1000 copies/mL (irrespective of use of ARVs during pregnancy) and for women with unknown viral load near the time of delivery (**http://aidsinfo.nih.gov/ Guidelines/**).

Postnatal transmission to neonates and young infants occurs mainly through breastfeeding. Worldwide, an estimated one third to one half of cases of mother-to-child transmission of HIV occurs as a result of breastfeeding. HIV genomes have been detected in cell-associated and cell-free fractions of human milk. In the United States, HIV-infected mothers are advised not to breastfeed, because safe alternatives to human milk are available readily. Because human milk cell-associated HIV can be detected even in women receiving antiretroviral therapy (ART), replacement (formula) feeding continues to be recommended for US mothers receiving ART. In resource-limited locations, women whose HIV infection status is unknown are encouraged to breastfeed their infants exclusively for the first 6 months of life, because the morbidity associated with formula feeding is unacceptably high. In addition, these women should be offered HIV testing. For HIV-infected mothers, 2010 WHO guidelines recommend that exclusive breastfeeding be provided for the first 6 months of life. The introduction of complimentary foods should occur after 6 months of life, and breastfeeding should continue through 12 months of life. Breastfeeding should be replaced only when a nutritionally adequate and safe diet can be maintained without human milk. In areas where ARVs are available, infants should receive daily nevirapine prophylaxis until 1 week after human milk consumption stops, or mothers should receive ARV prophylaxis (consisting of an ART regimen) for the first 6 months of their infants' lives. For infants known to be HIV-infected, mothers are encouraged to breastfeed exclusively for the first 6 months of life, and after the introduction of complimentary foods, they should continue to breastfeed up to 2 years of age, as per recommendations for the general population.

Although the rate of acquisition of HIV infection among infants has decreased significantly in the United States, the rate of acquisition of HIV during adolescence and young adulthood continues to increase. HIV infection in adolescents occurs disproportionately among youth of minority race or ethnicity. Transmission of HIV among adolescents is attributable primarily to sexual exposure and secondarily to illicit intravenous drug use. Young men who have sex with men particularly are at high risk of acquiring HIV infection. Infection among young women primarily is acquired heterosexually. In 2006, 38% of new HIV infections in males 13 through 29 years of age were in men who have sex with men. From 2005 to 2008, respectively, the absolute number of newly diagnosed HIV infections in the United States decreased from 35 526 to 34 038, but the proportion of all new HIV infections contributed by this age group increased from 14% to 18%. In 2007, in 37 states and 5 dependent areas with confidential named-based HIV infection reporting, 4% of people living with HIV infection were people 13 through 24 years of age.

The ratio of male to female adolescents and young adults with a diagnosis of HIV infection increases with age at diagnosis. In 2007, 31% of people 13 through 19 years of age diagnosed with HIV infection were female, compared with 23% of young adults 20 through 24 years of age and 26% of adults 25 years of age and older. Most HIV-infected adolescents and young adults are asymptomatic and, without testing, remain unaware of their underlying serostatus.

INCUBATION PERIOD: The usual age of onset of symptoms is approximately 12 through 18 months of age for untreated infants in the United States who acquired HIV infection through mother-to-child transmission. However, some HIV-infected infants become ill in the first few months of life, whereas others remain relatively asymptomatic for more than 5 years and, rarely, until early adolescence. Without therapy, a bimodal distribution of symptomatic infection has been described: 15% to 20% of untreated HIV-infected children die before 4 years of age, with a median age at death of 11 months (rapid progressors), and 80% to 85% of untreated HIV-infected children have delayed onset of milder symptoms and survive beyond 5 years of age (slow progressors).

DIAGNOSTIC TESTS[1]: Laboratory diagnosis of HIV-1 infection during infancy is based on detection of the virus or viral nucleic acid (Table 3.27, p 427). Because infants born to HIV-infected mothers acquire maternal antibodies passively, antibody assays are not informative for diagnosis of infection in children younger than 18 months unless assay results are negative. However, in children 18 months of age and older, HIV antibody assays can be used for diagnosis.

In the United States, the preferred test for diagnosis of HIV infection in infants is the HIV DNA polymerase chain reaction (PCR) assay. The DNA PCR assay can detect 1 to 10 DNA copies of proviral DNA in peripheral blood mononuclear cells. Approximately 30% to 40% of HIV-infected infants will have a positive HIV DNA PCR assay result in samples obtained before 48 hours of age. A positive result by 48 hours of age suggests in utero transmission. Approximately 93% of infected infants have detectable HIV DNA by 2 weeks of age, and approximately 95% of HIV-infected infants have a positive HIV

---

[1] Read JS; American Academy of Pediatrics, Committee on Pediatric AIDS. Diagnosis of HIV-1 infection in children younger than 18 months in the United States, *Pediatrics.* 2007;120(6):e1547–e1562. Available at: **http://pediatrics.aappublications.org/cgi/content/full/120/6/e1547**

Table 3.27. Laboratory Diagnosis of HIV Infection[a]

Test	Comment
HIV DNA PCR	Preferred test to diagnose HIV-1 subtype B infection in infants and children younger than 18 months of age; highly sensitive and specific by 2 weeks of age and available; performed on peripheral blood mononuclear cells. False-negative results can occur in non-B subtype HIV-1 infections.
HIV p24 Ag	Less sensitive, false-positive results during first month of life, variable results; not recommended.
ICD p24 Ag	Negative test result does not rule out infection; not recommended.
HIV culture	Expensive, not easily available, requires up to 4 weeks to do test; not recommended.
HIV RNA PCR	Preferred test to identify non-B subtype HIV-1 infections. Similar sensitivity and specificity to HIV DNA PCR in infants and children younger than 18 months of age, but DNA PCR is generally preferred due to greater clinical experience with that assay.

HIV indicates human immunodeficiency virus; PCR, polymerase chain reaction; Ag, antigen; and ICD, immune complex dissociated.

[a] Read JS; American Academy of Pediatrics, Committee on Pediatric AIDS. Diagnosis of HIV-1 infection in children younger than 18 months in the United States, *Pediatrics*. 2007;120(6):e1547–e1562. Available at: **http://pediatrics.aappublications.org/cgi/content/full/120/6/e1547**

DNA PCR assay result by 1 month of age. A single HIV DNA PCR assay has a sensitivity of 95% and a specificity of 97% for samples collected from infected children 1 to 36 months of age.

HIV isolation by culture is less sensitive, less available, and more expensive than the DNA PCR assay. Definitive results may take up to 28 days. This test no longer is recommended for routine diagnosis.

Detection of the p24 antigen (including immune complex dissociated) is less sensitive than the HIV DNA PCR assay or culture. False-positive test results occur in samples obtained from infants younger than 1 month of age. This test generally should not be used, although newer assays have been reported to have sensitivities similar to HIV DNA PCR assays.

Plasma HIV RNA assays also have been used to diagnose HIV infection. However, a false-negative test result may occur in neonates receiving ARV prophylaxis. Although use of ART can reduce plasma viral loads to undetectable levels, results of DNA PCR assay, which detects cell-associated integrated HIV DNA, remain positive even among people with undetectable viral loads.

In the absence of therapy, plasma viral loads among infants who acquired HIV infection through mother-to-child transmission increase rapidly to very high levels (from several hundred thousand to more than 1 million copies/mL) after birth, decreasing only slowly to a "set point" by approximately 2 years of age. This contrasts to infection in adults, in whom a viral load "set point" occurs approximately 6 months after acquisition of infection. An HIV RNA assay with only low-level viral copy number in an HIV-exposed infant may yield a false-positive result, reinforcing the importance of repeating any positive assay result to confirm the diagnosis of HIV infection in infancy. Like HIV DNA PCR assays, the sensitivity of HIV RNA assays for diagnosing infections in the first week of life is low (25%–40%), because transmission usually occurs around the time of delivery. The RNA assays approved by the FDA provide quantitative results used to quantify virus as a predictor of disease progression rather than for routine diagnosis of HIV infection in infants. RNA assays are useful in monitoring changes in viral load during the course of antiretroviral therapy. Diagnostic testing with HIV DNA or RNA assays is recommended at 14 to 21 days of age, and if results are negative, repeated at 1 to 2 months of age and again at 4 to 6 months of age. An infant is considered infected if 2 separate samples test positive by DNA or RNA PCR.[1]

Viral diagnostic testing in the first few days of life (eg, less than 48 hours of age) is recommended by some experts to allow for early identification of infants with presumed in utero infection. If testing is performed at birth, umbilical cord blood should not be used because of possible contamination with maternal blood. Obtaining the sample as early as 14 days of age may facilitate decisions about initiating ARV therapy. If found to be infected, infants would be transitioned from neonatal ARV prophylaxis to ARV treatment. In nonbreastfed children younger than 18 months of age with negative HIV virologic test results, *presumptive* exclusion of HIV infection is based on:

- Two negative HIV DNA or RNA virologic test results, from separate specimens, both of which were obtained at 2 weeks of age or older and one of which was obtained at 4 weeks of age or older; **OR**
- One negative HIV DNA or RNA virologic test result from a specimen obtained at 8 weeks of age or older; **OR**
- One negative HIV antibody test result obtained at 6 months of age or older; **AND**
- No other laboratory or clinical evidence of HIV infection (ie, no subsequent positive results from virologic tests if tests were performed and no AIDS-defining condition for which there is no other underlying condition of immunosuppression).

In nonbreastfed children younger than 18 months of age with negative HIV virologic test results, *definitive* exclusion of HIV is based on:

- At least 2 negative HIV DNA or RNA virologic test results, from separate specimens, both of which were obtained at 1 month of age or older and one of which was obtained at 4 months of age or older;
- At least 2 negative HIV antibody test results from separate specimens obtained at 6 months of age or older; and
- No other laboratory or clinical evidence of HIV infection (ie, no subsequent positive results from virologic tests if tests were performed and no AIDS-defining condition for which there is no other underlying condition of immunosuppression).

In children with 2 negative HIV DNA PCR test results, many clinicians will confirm the absence of antibody (ie, loss of passively acquired natural antibody) to HIV on testing at 12 through 18 months of age ("seroreversion"). A nonbreastfed infant with 2 antibody-negative blood samples drawn at least 1 month apart and which were both obtained after 6 months of age is considered HIV uninfected.

Enzyme immunoassays (EIAs) are used widely as the initial test for serum HIV antibody. These tests are highly sensitive and specific. Repeated EIA testing of initially reactive specimens is common practice and is followed by Western blot analysis to confirm the presence of antibody specific to HIV. A positive HIV antibody test result (EIA

---

[1] Centers for Disease Control and Prevention. Revised surveillance case definitions for HIV infection among adults, adolescents, and children aged <18 months and for HIV infection and AIDS among children aged 18 months to <13 years—United States, 2008. *MMWR Recomm Rep.* 2008;57(RR-10):1–12

followed by Western blot analysis) in a child 18 months of age or older almost always indicates infection, although passively acquired maternal antibody rarely can persist beyond 18 months of age. An HIV antibody test can be performed on samples of blood or oral fluid. Rapid tests for HIV antibodies have been licensed for use in the United States; these tests are used widely throughout the world, particularly to screen mothers of undocumented serostatus in maternity settings. As with standard EIA tests, confirmatory testing is required for a positive rapid test. Results from rapid testing are available within 20 minutes; however, confirmatory Western blot analysis results may take 1 to 2 weeks in some settings.

Infants who acquire HIV infection through mother-to-child transmission commonly have high viral set-points with progressive cellular immune dysfunction and immunosuppression resulting from a decrease in the total number of circulating CD4+ T lymphocytes. Sometimes, T-lymphocyte counts do not decrease until late in the course of infection. Changes in cell populations frequently result in a decrease in the normal CD4+ to CD8+ T-lymphocyte ratio of 1.0 or greater. This nonspecific finding, although characteristic of HIV-1 infection, also occurs with other acute viral infections, including infections caused by cytomegalovirus (CMV) and Epstein-Barr virus (EBV). The risk of OIs correlates with the CD4+ T-lymphocyte percentage and count. The normal values for peripheral CD4+ T-lymphocyte counts are age related, and the lower limits of normal are provided in Table 3.26 (p 422).

Adolescents and HIV Testing. The American Academy of Pediatrics (AAP) recommends that routine screening be offered to all adolescents at least once by 16 through 18 years of age in health care settings when the prevalence of HIV in the patient population is more than 0.1%. In areas of lower community prevalence, routine HIV testing is encouraged for all sexually active adolescents and adolescents with other risk factors for HIV infection.[1]

Consent for Diagnostic Testing. The CDC recommends that diagnostic HIV testing and opt-out HIV screening be part of routine clinical care in all health care settings for patients 13 through 64 years of age, thus preserving the patient's option to decline HIV testing and allowing a provider-patient relationship conducive to optimal clinical and preventive care. Patients or people responsible for the patient's care should be notified orally that testing is planned, advised of the indication for testing and the implications of positive and negative test results, and offered an opportunity to ask questions and to decline testing. With such notification, the patient's general consent for medical care is considered sufficient for diagnostic HIV testing. Although parental involvement in an adolescent's health care usually is desirable, it typically is not required when the adolescent consents to HIV testing. However, laws concerning consent and confidentiality for HIV care differ among states. Public health statutes and legal precedents allow for evaluation and treatment of minors for sexually transmitted infections without parental knowledge or consent, but not every state has explicitly defined HIV infection as a condition for which testing or treatment may proceed without parental consent. Health care professionals should endeavor to respect an adolescent's request for privacy. HIV screening should be discussed with all adolescents and encouraged for adolescents who are sexually active. Repeat HIV antibody testing should be performed for adolescents who remain at risk of HIV infection. Providing information regarding HIV infection, diagnostic testing, transmission, and

---

[1] American Academy of Pediatrics, Committee on Pediatric AIDS. Adolescents and HIV infection: the pediatrician's role in promoting routine testing. *Pediatrics.* 2011;128(5):1023–1029

implications of infection is an essential component of the anticipatory guidance provided to all adolescents as part of primary care.

Access to clinical care, preventive counseling, and support services is essential for people with positive HIV test results.

TREATMENT: Because HIV treatment options and recommendations change with time and vary with occurrence of ARV drug resistance and adverse event profile, consultation with an expert in pediatric HIV infection is recommended in the care of HIV-infected infants, children, and adolescents. Current treatment recommendations for HIV-infected children are available online (**http://aidsinfo.nih.gov**). Whenever possible, enrollment of HIV-infected children in clinical trials should be encouraged. Information about trials for adolescents and children can be obtained by contacting the AIDS Clinical Trials Information Service.[1]

ARV therapy is indicated for most HIV-infected children. The principal objectives of therapy are to suppress viral replication maximally, to restore and preserve immune function, to reduce HIV-associated morbidity and mortality, to minimize drug toxicity, to maintain normal growth and development, and to improve quality of life. Initiation of ARV therapy depends on age of the child and on a combination of virologic, immunologic, and clinical criteria.[2] Data from both observational studies and clinical trials indicate that very early initiation of therapy reduces morbidity and mortality compared with starting treatment when clinically symptomatic or immune suppressed. Effective administration of early therapy will maintain the viral load at low or undetectable concentrations and will reduce viral mutation and evolution.

Initiation of ARV therapy is recommended as follows[2]: (1) HIV-infected infants should receive ARV therapy irrespective of clinical symptoms, immune status, or viral load; (2) children from 1 to <5 years of age should receive ARV therapy: if they have AIDS or significant HIV-related symptoms (CDC clinical categories C and B [except for the following category B condition: single episode of serious bacterial infection]), regardless of CD4+ T-lymphocyte counts or plasma viral load values; if they have a CD4+ T-lymphocyte percentage <25%, regardless of symptoms or viral load; or if they are asymptomatic or mildly symptomatic (CDC clinical category A or N or the following category B condition: single episode of serious bacterial infection) *and* they have a CD4+ T-lymphocyte percentage ≥25% *and* a viral load of ≥100 000 copies/mL; and (3) children ≥5 years of age should receive ARV therapy: if they have AIDS or significant HIV-related symptoms (CDC clinical categories C and B [except for the following category B condition: single episode of serious bacterial infection]); if they have a CD4+ T-lymphocyte count ≤500 cells/mm³; or if they are asymptomatic or mildly symptomatic (CDC clinical category A or N or the following category B condition: single episode of serious bacterial infection) and they have a CD4+ T-lymphocyte count >500 cells/mm³ and a viral load ≥100 000 copies/mL. Starting ARV therapy should be considered[2] for HIV-infected children from 1 to <5 years of age who are asymptomatic or have mild symptoms (clinical category N or A, or the following clinical category B condition: single episode of serious bacterial infection) *and* have a CD4+ T-lymphocyte percentage ≥25%

---

[1] See Appendix I, Directory of Resources, p 883: AIDS Clinical Trials Information Service (available at **http://aidsinfo.nih.gov**).

[2] Panel on Antiretroviral Therapy and Medical Management of HIV-Infected Children. *Guidelines for the Use of Antiretroviral Agents in Pediatric HIV Infection.* August 11, 2011:1–268. Available at **http://aidsinfo.nih.gov/ContentFiles/PediatricGuidelines.pdf**

and a viral load <100 000 copies/mL. Initiation of ARV therapy also should be considered for HIV-infected children ≥5 years of age who are asymptomatic or have mild symptoms (clinical category N or A, or the following clinical category B condition: single episode of serious bacterial infection) and have a CD4+ T-lymphocyte count >500 cells/mm^3 and a viral load <100 000 copies/mL. The child and the child's primary caregiver must be able to adhere to the prescribed regimen.

Initiation of treatment of adolescents[1] generally follows guidelines for adults, for whom initiation of treatment strongly is recommended: if an AIDS-defining illness is present or if the CD4+ T-lymphocyte count is <350 cells/mm^3; if the CD4+ T-lymphocyte count is 350 to 500 cells/mm^3; or regardless of CD4+ T-lymphocyte count in patients with HIV-associated nephropathy or with hepatitis B virus infection when treatment of hepatitis B virus is recommended. ARV treatment should be considered for patients with CD4+ T-lymphocyte counts >500 cells/mm^3. Dosages of ARVs should be prescribed according to Tanner staging of puberty and not only on the basis of age; adolescents in early puberty (Tanner stages I and II) should be prescribed doses based on pediatric schedules, and adolescents in late puberty (Tanner stage V) should be prescribed doses based on adult schedules. In general, combination ARV therapy with at least 3 drugs is recommended for all HIV-infected individuals requiring ARV therapy. Drug regimens most often include 2 NRTIs plus either a protease inhibitor or an NNRTI (**http://aidsinfo.nih.gov**). ARV resistance testing (viral genotyping) is recommended before starting treatment, because infected infants may acquire resistant virus from their mothers. Suppression of virus to undetectable levels is the desired goal. A change in ARV therapy should be considered if there is evidence of disease progression (virologic, immunologic, or clinical), toxicity of or intolerance to drugs, development of resistance, or availability of data suggesting the possibility of a superior regimen.

Immune Globulin Intravenous (IGIV) therapy has been used in combination with ARV therapy for HIV-infected children with hypogammaglobulinemia (IgG <400 mg/dL [4.0 g/L]) and could be considered for HIV-infected children who have recurrent, serious bacterial infections, such as bacteremia, meningitis, or pneumonia. Trimethoprim-sulfamethoxazole prophylaxis may provide comparable protection. Typically, neither form of prophylaxis is necessary for patients receiving effective ARV therapy.

Early prophylaxis, diagnosis, and aggressive treatment of OIs may prolong survival.[2,3] This particularly is true for PCP, which accounts for approximately one third of pediatric AIDS diagnoses overall and may occur early in the first year of life. Because mortality rates are high, chemoprophylaxis should be given to all HIV-exposed infants with indeterminate HIV infection status starting at 4 to 6 weeks of age. If PCP prophylaxis is started

---

[1] Panel on Antiretroviral Guidelines for Adults and Adolescents. Guidelines for the use of antiretroviral agents in HIV-1-infected adults and adolescents. Department of Health and Human Services. October 14, 2011; 1–167. Available at **http://www.aidsinfo.nih.gov/ContentFiles/AdultandAdolescentGL.pdf**

[2] Centers for Disease Control and Prevention. Guidelines for prevention and treatment of opportunistic infections among HIV-exposed and HIV-infected children. Recommendations from CDC, the National Institutes of Health, the HIV Medicine Association of the Infectious Diseases Society of America, the Pediatric Infectious Diseases Society, and the American Academy of Pediatrics. *MMWR Recomm Rep* 2009; 58(RR-11): 1–166. Available at: **http://aidsinfo.nih.gov/contentfiles/Pediatric_OI.pdf**

[3] Centers for Disease Control and Prevention. Guidelines for prevention and treatment of opportunistic infections in HIV-infected adults and adolescents. Recommendations from CDC, the National Institutes of Health, and the HIV Medicine Association of the Infectious Diseases Society of America. *MMWR Early Release.* 2009;58(March 24, 2009):1–207. Available at: **http://www.cdc.gov/mmwr/pdf/rr/rr58e324.pdf**

at 4 to 6 weeks of age in an HIV-exposed infant with indeterminate HIV infection status, prophylaxis can be stopped if the child subsequently meets criteria for presumptive or definitive lack of HIV infection. Prophylaxis is not recommended for infants who meet criteria for presumptive or definitive HIV-uninfected status. Thus, for infants with negative HIV diagnostic test results at 2 and 4 weeks of age (and no positive tests or clinical symptoms and who are, therefore, presumptively not infected with HIV), PCP prophylaxis would not need to be initiated. All infants with HIV infection should receive PCP prophylaxis through 1 year of age regardless of immune status. The need for PCP prophylaxis for HIV-infected children 1 year of age and older is determined by the degree of immunosuppression, as determined by CD4+ T-lymphocyte counts (see *Pneumocystis jirovecii* Infections, p 582).

Guidelines for prevention and treatment of OIs in children, adolescents, and adults provide indications for administration of drugs for infection with MAC, CMV, *T gondii*, and other organisms.[1,2] Successful suppression of HIV replication in the blood to undetectable levels by ART has resulted in relatively normal CD4+ and CD8+ T-lymphocyte counts, leading to a dramatic decrease in the occurrence of most OIs. Limited data on the safety of discontinuing prophylaxis in HIV-infected children receiving ART are available. Prophylaxis should not be discontinued in HIV-infected infants. For older children, many experts consider discontinuing PCP prophylaxis for those who have received at least 6 months of ART on the basis of CD4+ T-lymphocyte count[1]: (1) for children 1 through 5 years of age: CD4+ T-lymphocyte percentage of at least 15% or CD4+ T-lymphocyte absolute count of at least 500 cells/µL for more than 3 consecutive months; and (2) for children 6 years of age or older: CD4+ T-lymphocyte percentage of at least 15% or the CD4+ T-lymphocyte absolute count of at least 200 cells/µL for more than 3 consecutive months. Subsequently, the CD4+ T-lymphocyte absolute count or percentage should be reevaluated at least every 3 months. Prophylaxis should be reinstituted if the original criteria for prophylaxis are reached again.

Immunization Recommendations (also see Immunization in Special Clinical Circumstances, p 69, and Table 1.16, p 75).

All recommended childhood immunizations should be given to HIV-exposed infants. If HIV infection is confirmed, then guidelines for the HIV-infected child should be followed. Children with HIV infection should be immunized as soon as is age appropriate with inactivated vaccines. Trivalent inactivated influenza vaccine (TIV) should be given annually according to the most current recommendations. Additionally, live-virus vaccines (measles-mumps-rubella [MMR] and varicella) can be given to asymptomatic HIV-infected children and adolescents with appropriate CD4+ T-lymphocyte percentages (ie, greater than 15% in children 1 through 5 years of age). Measles-mumps-rubella-varicella (MMRV) vaccine should not be administered to HIV-infected infants because

---

[1] Centers for Disease Control and Prevention. Guidelines for prevention and treatment of opportunistic infections among HIV-exposed and HIV-infected children. Recommendations from CDC, the National Institutes of Health, the HIV Medicine Association of the Infectious Diseases Society of America, the Pediatric Infectious Diseases Society, and the American Academy of Pediatrics. *MMWR Recomm Rep.* 2009;58(RR-11):1–166. Available at: **http://aidsinfo.nih.gov/contentfiles/Pediatric_OI.pdf**

[2] Centers for Disease Control and Prevention. Guidelines for prevention and treatment of opportunistic infections in HIV-infected adults and adolescents. Recommendations from CDC, The National Institutes of Health, and the HIV Medicine Association of the Infectious Diseases Society of America. *MMWR Early Release.* 2009;58(March 24, 2009):1–207. Available at **http://www.cdc.gov/mmwr/pdf/rr/rr58e324.pdf**

of lack of safety data in this population. Rotavirus vaccine may be given to HIV-exposed and HIV-infected infants irrespective of CD4+ T-lymphocyte count. HIV-infected children should all receive a dose of 23-valent polysaccharide pneumococcal vaccine after 24 months of age, with a minimal interval of 8 weeks since the last conjugate pneumococcal vaccine. The suggested schedule for administration of these vaccines is provided in the recommended childhood and adolescent immunization schedule (Fig 1.1–1.3, p 27–31). The immunologic response to these vaccines in HIV-infected infants and children may be less robust and less persistent than in immunocompetent infants and children.

Children Who Are HIV Uninfected Residing in the Household of an HIV-Infected Person. Members of households in which an adult or child has HIV infection can receive MMR vaccine, because these vaccine viruses are not transmitted person to person. To decrease the risk of transmission of influenza to patients with symptomatic HIV infection, all household members 6 months of age or older should receive yearly influenza immunization (see Influenza, p 439). Immunization with varicella vaccine of siblings and susceptible adult caregivers of patients with HIV infection is encouraged to prevent acquisition of wild-type varicella-zoster virus infection, which can cause severe disease in immunocompromised hosts. Transmission of varicella vaccine virus from an immunocompetent host to a household contact is uncommon.

Postexposure Passive Immunization of HIV-Infected Children.

- **Measles** (see Measles, p 489). HIV-infected children with severe immune suppression who are exposed to measles should receive intramuscular Immune Globulin (IG) prophylaxis (0.5 mL/kg, maximum 15 mL), regardless of immunization status, and exposed, asymptomatic HIV-infected patients also should receive intramuscular IG but at a lower dose (0.25 mL/kg). Children who have received IGIV within 2 weeks of exposure do not require additional passive immunization.

- **Tetanus.** HIV-infected children with severe immune suppression who sustain wounds classified as tetanus prone (see Tetanus, p 707, and Table 3.73, p 709) should receive Tetanus Immune Globulin regardless of immunization status.

- **Varicella.** HIV-infected children without a history of previous chickenpox or children who have not received 2 doses of varicella vaccine should receive Varicella-Zoster Immune Globulin, if available, within 10 days of close contact with a person who has chickenpox or shingles (see Varicella-Zoster Infections, p 774). Similar postexposure prophylaxis regimens have been recommended for children with moderate to severe immune compromise who previously have been immunized with varicella vaccine. An alternative to Varicella-Zoster Immune Globulin for passive immunization is IGIV, 400 mg/kg, administered once within 10 days after exposure. Children who have received IGIV within 2 weeks of exposure do not require additional passive immunization.

ISOLATION OF THE HOSPITALIZED PATIENT: Standard precautions should be followed by all health care professionals. The risk to health care professionals of acquiring HIV infection from a patient is minimal, even after accidental exposure from a needlestick injury (see Epidemiology, p 424). Nevertheless, every effort should be made to avoid exposures to blood and other body fluids that could contain HIV. Guidelines for use of occupational postexposure prophylaxis have been published by the CDC and should be started as soon as possible after the exposure but within 72 hours for maximal effectiveness (**http://aidsinfo.nih.gov/contentfiles/HealthCareOccupExpoGL.pdf**).

CONTROL MEASURES:

Interruption of Mother-to-Child Transmission of HIV. Development and implementation of efficacious interventions to prevent mother-to-child transmission of HIV has resulted in a marked decrease in occurrence of cases of mother-to-child transmission of HIV infection in the United States. Recommendations of the US Public Health Service, AAP, and American College of Obstetricians and Gynecologists include the following.[1,2,3]

The AAP and CDC recommend documented, routine HIV testing for all pregnant women in the United States. For women in labor with undocumented HIV infection status during the current pregnancy, immediate maternal HIV testing with opt-out consent, using a rapid HIV antibody test, is recommended. In some states, routinely offering HIV testing during pregnancy is mandated by law. Routine education about HIV infection and testing should be part of a comprehensive program of health care for all women during their childbearing years.

Three efficacious interventions to prevent mother-to-child transmission of HIV are utilized in the United States: ARV prophylaxis, complete avoidance of breastfeeding, and, as indicated, cesarean delivery before labor and before rupture of membranes.[3] The goal is to diagnose HIV infection early in pregnancy to allow antenatal implementation of interventions to prevent transmission (ARV prophylaxis and cesarean delivery before labor and before rupture of membranes). In resource-limited countries where complete avoidance of breastfeeding (replacement feeding) often is not safe, exclusive breastfeeding is associated with a lower risk of postnatal transmission than is mixed breastfeeding and formula feeding. Both maternal and infant ARV prophylaxis during the breastfeeding period are effective in reducing mother-to-child transmission of HIV.

HIV-infected pregnant women should use combination ARV regimens, whether for treatment of the mother's HIV infection or for prevention of mother-to-child transmission of HIV. Detailed recommendations for use of ARVs in HIV-infected pregnant women can be found at **http://aidsinfo.nih.gov.** Women initiating such a regimen during pregnancy should be tested, ideally, for the presence of ARV resistance. However, initiation of ARV prophylaxis should not unduly be delayed, especially if these decisions are being made late in pregnancy. It also is recommended that zidovudine be included in maternal regimens, though a woman already receiving treatment need not have her regimen changed if her viral load is suppressed. The recommendation to include zidovudine is a result of the first clinical trial of ARV prophylaxis for prevention of mother-to-child transmission of HIV. That trial assessed oral administration of zidovudine to pregnant, HIV-infected women beginning at 14 to 34 weeks' gestation and continuing throughout pregnancy, intravenous administration of zidovudine during labor until delivery (ie, intrapartum), and oral administration of zidovudine to the infant for the first 6 weeks of life. This intervention decreased mother-to-child transmission of HIV by two thirds (see Table 3.28, p 435). As noted previously, observational studies suggest that use of

---

[1] For complete listing of current policy statements from the American Academy of Pediatrics regarding human immunodeficiency virus and acquired immunodeficiency syndrome, see **http://aappolicy. aappublications.org/**

[2] American Academy of Pediatrics, American College of Obstetricians and Gynecologists. Human immunodeficiency virus screening. Joint statement of the American Academy of Pediatrics and the American College of Obstetricians and Gynecologists. *Pediatrics.* 1999;104(1 Pt 1):128 (Reaffirmed October 2008)

[3] American Academy of Pediatrics, Committee on Pediatric AIDS. HIV testing and prophylaxis to prevent mother-to-child transmission in the United States. *Pediatrics.* 2008;122(5):1127–1134 (Reaffirmed June 2011)

combination ARV regimens during pregnancy is associated with a lower risk of mother-to-child transmission of HIV than is zidovudine alone. Even though most HIV-infected pregnant women in the United States now receive combination ARV regimens either for treatment of their own HIV infection or for prevention of mother-to-child transmission of HIV, it still is recommended that intravenous zidovudine be given during labor along with other drugs in the antepartum regimen and that the infant subsequently receive 6 weeks of oral zidovudine. Note that efavirenz is classified as a class D teratogen by the FDA and should not be included in maternal regimens begun during the first trimester. If a woman becomes pregnant while virally suppressed on an efavirenz-containing regimen, an attempt should be made to change her regimen. When maternal ARVs are indicated for her treatment, they are continued by the mother postpartum, in contrast to when ARVs are used solely for prophylaxis, in which case they are discontinued postpartum.

Health care professionals who treat HIV-infected pregnant women and their infants should report instances of prenatal exposure to ARVs (either alone or in combination) to the Antiretroviral Pregnancy Registry (1-800-258-4263 or **www.apregistry. com**). Long-term follow-up is recommended for all infants exposed to ARVs in utero or postnatally.

Table 3.28. Zidovudine Regimen for Decreasing the Rate of Mother-to-Child Transmission of HIV[a]

Period of Time	Route	Dosage
During pregnancy, initiate anytime after wk 14 of gestation and continue throughout pregnancy[b]	Oral	200 mg, 3 times per day or 300 mg, 2 times per day
During labor and delivery[c]	Intravenous	2 mg/kg during the first hour, then 1 mg/kg per hour until delivery
For the newborn infant ≥37 weeks' gestation, as soon as possible after birth[d]	Oral	2 mg/kg, 4 times per day, for the first 6 wk of life
For the newborn infant 30 through 36 weeks' gestation, as soon as possible after birth[d]	Oral	2 mg/kg, 2 times per day for the first 2 weeks of life, and then 3 times per day for the next 4 weeks
For the newborn infant <30 weeks' gestation, as soon as possible after birth[d]	Oral	2 mg/kg, 2 times per day for the first 4 weeks of life, and then 3 times per day for the next 2 weeks

[a]Modified from Panel on Treatment of HIV-Infected Pregnant Women and Prevention of Perinatal Transmission: Recommendations for Use of Antiretroviral Drugs in Pregnant HIV-1-Infected Women for Maternal Health and Interventions to Reduce Perinatal HIV Transmission in the United States. September 14, 2011:1–207. Available at: **http://aidsinfo.nih. gov/contentfiles/PerinatalGL.pdf.** Information about other antiretroviral drugs for decreasing the rate of perinatal transmission of HIV can be found online (**http://aidsinfo.nih.gov).**

[b]Most women in industrialized nations are treated with potent combinations of 3 antiretroviral agents (antiretroviral therapy [ART]) started after the first trimester (unless treatment is required for maternal health reasons, in which case the benefit of starting during the first trimester outweighs potential risk to the infant) and continuing to delivery. Oral zidovudine may be used as part of that therapy.

[c]Recommended even for women treated with other antiretroviral agents during pregnancy. Intravenous zidovudine is administered for 3 hours before cesarean delivery.

[d]The effectiveness of antiretroviral agents for prevention of mother-to-child transmission of HIV decreases with delay in initiation after birth. Initiation of postexposure prophylaxis after the first 48 hours of life is not likely to be effective in preventing transmission.

Intrapartum management of HIV-infected women and the immediate postnatal care of their newborn infants are multifaceted. The woman's regular HIV medical subspecialist and the delivering physician should be contacted to discuss the impending delivery and to review the patient's current and postpartum ARV regimen. For women in labor with undocumented HIV infection status, a rapid HIV test should be performed as soon as possible. The HIV-infected woman in labor should receive intravenous zidovudine immediately (regardless of whether she has been taking ARVs before and/or during pregnancy; see Table 3.28, p 435). Her routine oral ARVs should be continued on schedule (with the exception of stavudine [d4T, Zerit], which should not be coadministered with zidovudine). Any procedures that compromise the integrity of fetal skin during labor and delivery (eg, fetal electrodes) or that increase the occurrence of maternal bleeding (eg, instrumented vaginal delivery, episiotomy, vaginal tears) should be avoided when possible. As noted previously, prolonged rupture of membranes is associated with an increased risk of mother-to-child transmission of HIV, whereas cesarean delivery before labor and before rupture of membranes reduces the risk of mother-to-child transmission and is recommended for women with plasma viral loads greater than 1000 copies/mL and women with unknown plasma viral loads around the time of delivery (**http://aidsinfo.nih.gov/Guidelines/**). The newborn infant should be bathed and cleaned of maternal secretions (especially bloody secretions) as soon as possible after birth. Newborn infants should begin ARV prophylaxis as soon as possible after birth, preferably within 12 hours. In the United States, neonatal prophylaxis generally consists of zidovudine for 6 weeks. Among infants whose mothers did not receive any ARVs before onset of labor, neonatal postexposure prophylaxis with a 2- or 3-drug ARV regimen results in a lower rate of mother-to-child transmission of HIV than zidovudine alone. A 2-drug regimen of zidovudine for 6 weeks with 3 doses of nevirapine during the first week of life (at birth and at 48 hours and 96 hours of life) is as effective but less toxic than a 3-drug regimen of zidovudine, lamivudine, and nelfinavir. Therefore, current recommendations for infants of HIV-infected women who did not receive any ARVs before onset of labor are for administration of this 2-drug neonatal prophylaxis regimen. Detailed guidance is available regarding infant ARV prophylaxis regimens.[1] Both mother and infant should have prescriptions for the HIV drugs when they leave the hospital, and the infant should have an appointment for a postnatal visit at 2 to 4 weeks of age to monitor medication adherence and to screen the infant for anemia from zidovudine.

For a newborn infant whose mother's HIV infection status is unknown, the newborn infant's physician should perform rapid HIV antibody testing on the mother or the infant, with appropriate consent as required by state and local law. Test results should be reported to the physician as soon as possible to allow effective ARV prophylaxis to be administered to the infant, ideally within 12 hours. In some states, rapid testing of the neonate is required by law if the mother has refused to be tested.

---

[1] Panel on Treatment of HIV-Infected Pregnant Women and Prevention of Perinatal Transmission. *Recommendations for Use of Antiretroviral Drugs in Pregnant HIV-1-Infected Women for Maternal Health and Interventions to Reduce Perinatal HIV Transmission in the United States.* September 14, 2011:1–207. Available at: **http://aidsinfo. nih.gov/contentfiles/PerinatalGL.pdf**

The newborn infant's physician should be informed of the mother's HIV infection status so that appropriate care and follow-up of the infant can be accomplished. An HIV-infected mother and her infant should be referred to a facility that provides HIV-related services for both adults and children.

Breastfeeding (also see Human Milk, p 126). Transmission of HIV by breastfeeding has been demonstrated, especially from mothers who acquire HIV infection late in pregnancy or during the postpartum period. The rate of late postnatal HIV transmission (after 4 weeks of age) in sub-Saharan African countries is approximately 9 transmissions per 100 child-years of breastfeeding (0.7% transmission/month of breastfeeding) and is relatively constant. Late postnatal transmission is associated with reduced maternal CD4+ T-lymphocyte count, high plasma and human milk viral load, mastitis/breast abscess, and infant oral lesions (eg, oral thrush). Clinical trials in resource-limited settings have demonstrated efficacy of ARV prophylaxis to HIV-infected women while breastfeeding and of ARV prophylaxis to breastfeeding children of HIV-infected women. However, because such prophylaxis cannot be assumed to be completely protective against mother-to-child transmission of HIV, in countries where safe alternative sources of infant feeding readily are available, affordable, and culturally accepted, such as the United States, HIV-infected women should be counseled not to breastfeed their infants or donate to human milk banks. Similarly, women in industrialized countries who are receiving ARV therapy for their own health, even if they have undetectable HIV viral loads, also should be counseled not to breastfeed because of the continued possibility of HIV transmission.

In general, women who are known to be HIV-uninfected should be encouraged to breastfeed. However, women who are HIV-uninfected but who are known to have HIV-infected sex partners or to be active injection drug users should be counseled about the potential risk of acquiring HIV infection themselves and of then transmitting HIV through human milk.

Premastication. Probable transmission of HIV by caregivers who premasticated food for infants has been described in 3 cases in the United States. In 2 of the cases, the caregivers had bleeding gums or sores in their mouths during the time they premasticated the food. Phylogenetic testing was conducted and documented matches of the viral strains in 2 of the caregiver-infant dyads. It is hypothesized that the transmission was via blood-borne virus in the saliva rather than via salivary virus. The CDC recommends that in the United States, where safe alternative methods of feeding are available, HIV-infected caregivers should be asked about whether they practice premastication and counseled not to premasticate food for infants.

HIV in the Athletic Setting. Athletes and staff of athletic programs can be exposed to blood during certain athletic activities. Recommendations have been developed by the AAP for prevention of transmission of HIV and other bloodborne pathogens in the athletic setting (see School Health, Infections Spread by Blood and Body Fluids, p 157).

Sexual Abuse. In cases of proven or suspected sexual abuse, the child should be tested serologically as soon as possible and then periodically for 6 months (eg, at 4–6 weeks, 12 weeks, and 6 months after last known sexual contact) (see Sexually Transmitted Infections, p 176). Serologic evaluation of the perpetrator for HIV infection should be attempted soon after the incident but usually cannot be performed until indictment has occurred. Counseling of the child and family needs to be provided (see Sexually Transmitted Infections, p 176).

Prevention of HIV Transmission Through Adult Behaviors (Sexual Activity). Abstinence from sexual activity is the only certain way to prevent sexual transmission of HIV. Safer sex practices, including use of condoms for all sexual encounters (vaginal, anal, and oral sex), can reduce HIV transmission significantly by reducing exposure to body fluids containing HIV. Recently, ARV therapy has been shown to reduce HIV transmission through sexual activity in select situations. Suppressing HIV viral load to undetectable levels in the blood with ARV combination regimens has resulted in decreases in transmission in discordant couples by as much as 90%. In men who have sex with men, continuous preexposure prophylaxis with ARV therapy (tenofovir and emtricitabine) was associated with reduction in HIV acquisition by 44% in the uninfected partner in a discordant couple. The efficacy of preexposure prophylaxis improved with improved medication compliance. Preexposure prophylaxis has not yet been proven effective in heterosexual couples. Because data on efficacy and long-term safety of preexposure ARV prophylaxis in men who have sex with men is limited, preexposure prophylaxis should be performed using guidelines provided by the CDC (**www.cdc.gov/hiv/prep/pdf/PREPfactsheet.pdf**). ARV-based vaginal microbicides (1% tenofovir gel) have reduced HIV acquisition in uninfected women by 39%. Data from Africa provide evidence that male circumcision can reduce HIV acquisition by uninfected heterosexual males by more than 50%.

Postexposure Prophylaxis for Possible Sexual or Other Nonoccupational Exposure to HIV.[1] Decisions to provide ARVs to people after possible nonoccupational (ie, community) exposure to HIV must balance the potential benefits and risks. Decisions regarding the need for ARV prophylaxis in such instances are predicated on the probability that the source is infected or contaminated with HIV, the likelihood of transmission by the particular exposure, and the interval between exposure and initiation of therapy balanced against expected adverse effects associated with the regimen of drugs.

The risk of transmission of HIV from a puncture wound attributable to a needle found in the community is lower than 0.3%. The actual risks of HIV infection in an infant or child after a needlestick injury or sexual abuse are unknown. To date, there are no confirmed transmissions of HIV from accidental nonoccupational needlestick injuries (needles found in the community). The estimated risk of HIV transmission per episode of receptive penile-anal sexual exposure is 50 per 10 000 exposures, whereas the estimated risk per episode of receptive vaginal exposure is 10 per 10 000 exposures.

All ARVs are associated with adverse effects. In HIV-infected adults receiving combination ARV regimens for treatment of HIV, an estimated 24% to 36% discontinue the drugs because of adverse effects. Adverse effects also are reported by a significant proportion of adults without HIV infection receiving ARV agents as postexposure prophylaxis. Use of daily nevirapine for postexposure prophylaxis is not recommended because of the high incidence of severe (and rarely fatal) adverse effects in adults with normal CD4+ T-lymphocyte counts. Such adverse effects have not been reported with single-dose intrapartum/infant nevirapine used for prevention of mother-to-child transmission of HIV.

---

[1] US Department of Health and Human Services. Antiretroviral postexposure prophylaxis after sexual, injection-drug use, or other nonoccupational exposure to HIV in the United States: recommendations from the US Department of Health and Human Services. *MMWR Recomm Rep.* 2005;54(RR-2):1–20

ARVs generally should not be used if the risk of transmission is low (eg, trivial needle-stick injury with a drug needle from an unknown nonoccupational source) or if care is sought more than 72 hours after the reported exposure.[1] The benefits of postexposure prophylaxis are greatest when risk of infection is high, intervention is prompt, and adherence is likely. Consultation with an experienced pediatric HIV health care professional is essential.

Transition of Adolescents to Adult HIV Health Care Settings. In industrialized countries, it increasingly has become likely that HIV-infected children will survive (and thrive) well into adolescence and young adulthood. Therefore, pediatric and adult HIV programs may benefit from establishment of transition programs to introduce adolescents to the adult health care setting. Successful transition requires careful proactive planning by caregivers in both pediatric and adult venues and a multifaceted, deliberate exercise that pays heed to the medical, psychosocial, life-skills, educational, and family-centered needs of the patient.

The transition period is a convenient time to review the ARV regimen with the adolescent, to recalculate dosages if necessary, and to stress repeatedly the need for adherence. It also is an ideal time to reemphasize topics of contraception, prevention of sexually transmitted infections, and safer sex practices.

Influenza

CLINICAL MANIFESTATIONS: Influenza typically begins with sudden onset of fever, often accompanied by chills or rigors, headache, malaise, diffuse myalgia, and nonproductive cough. Subsequently, respiratory tract signs, including sore throat, nasal congestion, rhinitis, and cough, become more prominent. Conjunctival injection, abdominal pain, nausea, vomiting, and diarrhea less commonly are associated with influenza illness. In some children, influenza can appear as an upper respiratory tract infection or as a febrile illness with few respiratory tract symptoms. Influenza is an important cause of otitis media. Acute myositis characterized by calf tenderness and refusal to walk has been described. In infants, influenza can produce a sepsis-like picture and occasionally can cause croup, bronchiolitis, or pneumonia. Although the large majority of children with influenza recover fully after 3 to 7 days, previously healthy children can have severe symptoms and complications. In the 2010–2011 influenza season, approximately 50% of all children hospitalized with influenza had no known underlying conditions. Neurologic complications associated with influenza range from febrile seizures to severe encephalopathy and encephalitis with status epilepticus, with resulting neurologic sequelae or death. Reye syndrome has been associated with influenza infection. Children with influenza or suspected influenza should not be given aspirin. Death from influenza-associated myocarditis has been reported. Invasive secondary infections or coinfections with group A streptococcus, *Staphylococcus aureus* (including methicillin-resistant *S aureus* [MRSA]), *Streptococcus pneumoniae*, or other bacterial pathogens can result in severe disease and death.

ETIOLOGY: Influenza viruses are orthomyxoviruses of 3 genera or types (A, B, and C). Epidemic disease is caused by influenza virus types A and B, and both influenza A and B virus antigens are included in influenza vaccines. Type C influenza viruses cause sporadic

---

[1] Havens PL; American Academy of Pediatrics, Committee on Pediatric AIDS. Postexposure prophylaxis in children and adolescents for nonoccupational exposure to human immunodeficiency virus. *Pediatrics.* 2003;111(6):1475–1489 (Reaffirmed October 2008)

mild influenza-like illness in children and are not included in influenza vaccines. The virus type or subtype may have an effect on the number of hospitalizations and deaths that season. For example, seasons with influenza A (H3N2) as the predominant circulating strain have had 2.7 times higher average mortality rates than other seasons. The 2009 influenza A (H1N1) pandemic combined both exceptional pediatric virulence and lack of immunity, which resulted in nearly 4 times as many pediatric deaths than previously recorded.

Influenza A viruses are subclassified into subtypes by 2 surface antigens, hemagglutinin (HA) and neuraminidase (NA). Examples of these include H1N1, H1N2, and H3N2 viruses. Specific antibodies to these various antigens, especially to hemagglutinin, are important determinants of immunity. Minor variation within the same influenza B type or influenza A subtypes is called *antigenic drift*. Antigenic drift occurs continuously and results in new strains of influenza A and B viruses, leading to seasonal epidemics. On the basis of ongoing global surveillance data, for only the fourth time in the preceding 25 years, there was no change to any of the influenza vaccine strains for the 2011–2012 season from the previous season. *Antigenic shifts* are major changes in influenza A viruses that result in new subtypes that contain a new HA alone or with a new NA. Antigenic shift occurs only with influenza A viruses and can lead to pandemics if the new strain can infect humans and be transmitted efficiently from person to person in a sustained manner in the setting of little or no preexisting immunity.

From April 2009 to August 2010, the World Health Organization declared such a pandemic caused by influenza A (H1N1) virus. There now have been 4 influenza pandemics caused by antigenic shift in the 20th and 21st centuries. The 2009 pandemic was associated with 2 waves of substantial activity, occurring in the spring and fall of 2009 and extending well into winter 2010. During this time, >99% of virus isolates characterized were the 2009 pandemic influenza A (H1N1) virus. As with previous antigenic shifts, the 2009 pandemic influenza A (H1N1) viral strain has replaced the previously circulating seasonal influenza A (H1N1) strain. During the 2010–2011 influenza season, influenza A (H3N2) was the predominant circulating strain, but weekly virus subtype activity varied regionally. The 2009 pandemic influenza A (H1N1) virus accounted for 34% of activity, cocirculating with the seasonal influenza A subtype H3N2 and/or influenza B virus.

Humans, including children, occasionally are infected with influenza A viruses of swine or avian origin. Human infections with swine viruses have manifested as typical influenza-like illness, and confirmation of infection caused by an influenza virus of swine origin has been discovered retrospectively during routine typing of human influenza isolates. Rare but severe infections with influenza A subtype H5N1 viruses have been identified since 1997 in Asia, Africa, Europe, and the Middle East, areas where these viruses are present in domestic or wild birds. Other influenza subtypes of avian origin, including H7, also are identified occasionally in humans. Infection with a novel influenza A virus now is a nationally reportable disease and should be reported to the Centers for Disease Control and Prevention (CDC) through state health departments.

EPIDEMIOLOGY: Influenza is spread from person to person, primarily by respiratory tract droplets created by coughing or sneezing. Contact with respiratory tract droplet-contaminated surfaces is another possible mode of transmission. During community outbreaks of influenza, the highest incidence occurs among school-aged children. Secondary spread to adults and other children within a family is common. Incidence and disease severity depend, in part, on immunity developed as a result of previous experience (by natural disease) or recent influenza immunization with the circulating strain or a related strain.

Antigenic drift in the circulating strain(s) is associated with seasonal epidemics. In temperate climates, seasonal epidemics usually occur during winter months. Peak influenza activity in the United States can occur anytime from November to May but most commonly occurs in January and February. Community outbreaks can last 4 to 8 weeks or longer. Circulation of 2 or 3 influenza virus strains in a community may be associated with a prolonged influenza season of 3 months or more and bimodal peaks in activity. Influenza is highly contagious, especially among semienclosed institutionalized populations and other ongoing, closed-group gatherings, such as school classrooms. Patients may become infectious during the 24 hours before onset of symptoms. Viral shedding in nasal secretions usually peaks during the first 3 days of illness and ceases within 7 days but can be prolonged in young children and immunodeficient patients. Viral shedding is correlated directly with degree of fever.

Incidence in healthy children generally is 10% to 40% each year, but illness rates as low as 3% also have been reported. Tens of thousands of children visit clinics and emergency departments because of influenza illness each season. Influenza and its complications have been reported to result in a 10% to 30% increase in the number of courses of antimicrobial agents prescribed to children during the influenza season. Although bacterial coinfections with a variety of pathogens, including MRSA, have been reported, medical care encounters for children with influenza are an important cause of inappropriate antimicrobial use.

Hospitalization rates among children younger than 2 years of age are similar to hospitalization rates among people 65 years of age and older. Rates vary among studies (190–480 per 100 000 population) because of differences in methodology and severity of influenza seasons. However, children younger than 24 months of age consistently are at a substantially higher risk of hospitalization than older children. Antecedent influenza infection sometimes is associated with development of pneumococcal or staphylococcal pneumonia in children. Methicillin-resistant staphylococcal community-acquired pneumonia, with a rapid clinical progression and a high fatality rate, has been reported in previously healthy children and adults with concomitant influenza infection. Rates of hospitalization and morbidity attributable to complications, such as bronchitis and pneumonia, are even greater in children with high-risk conditions, including hemoglobinopathies, bronchopulmonary dysplasia, asthma, cystic fibrosis, malignancy, diabetes mellitus, chronic renal disease, and congenital heart disease. Influenza virus infection in neonates also has been associated with considerable morbidity, including a sepsis-like syndrome, apnea, and lower respiratory tract disease.

Fatal outcomes, including sudden death, have been reported in both chronically ill and previously healthy children. Since influenza-related pediatric deaths became nationally notifiable in 2004, the number of deaths among children reported annually ranged from 46 to 83, until the 2009–2010 season, when the number increased to 279. During the entire influenza A (H1N1) pandemic period lasting from April 2009 to August 2010, a total of 344 laboratory-confirmed, influenza-associated pediatric deaths were reported. The 2010–2011 influenza season had at least 114 laboratory-confirmed, influenza-associated pediatric deaths. Most pediatric deaths are attributable to influenza A and occur in children younger than 5 years of age, and approximately 50% of children who died did not have a high-risk condition as defined by the Advisory Committee on Immunization Practices. All influenza-associated pediatric deaths are nationally notifiable and should be reported to the CDC through state health departments.

The **incubation period** usually is 1 to 4 days, with a mean of 2 days.

Influenza Pandemics. A pandemic is defined by emergence and global spread of a new influenza A virus subtype to which the population has little or no immunity and that spreads rapidly from person to person. Pandemics, therefore, can lead to substantially increased morbidity and mortality rates, compared with seasonal influenza. During the 20th century, there were 3 influenza pandemics, in 1918 (H1N1), 1957 (H2N2), and 1968 (H3N2). The pandemic in 1918 killed at least 20 million people in the United States and perhaps as many as 50 million people worldwide. The 2009 influenza A (H1N1) pandemic was the first in the 21st century, lasting from April 2009 to August 2010. It was associated with between 8870 and 18 300 deaths. Pediatric health care professionals should be familiar with national, state, and institutional pandemic plans, including recommendations for vaccine and antiviral drug use, health care surge capacity, and personal protective strategies that can be communicated to patients and families. Public health authorities have developed plans for pandemic preparedness and response to a pandemic in the United States. Up-to-date information on pandemic influenza can be found at **www.pandemicflu.gov.**

DIAGNOSTIC TESTS: Specimens for viral culture or immunofluorescent or rapid diagnostic tests should be obtained, if possible, during the first 72 hours of illness, because the quantity of virus shed decreases rapidly as illness progresses beyond that point. Specimens of nasopharyngeal secretions obtained by swab, aspirate, or wash should be placed in appropriate transport media for culture. After inoculation into eggs or cell culture, influenza virus usually can be isolated within 2 to 6 days. Rapid diagnostic tests for identification of influenza A and B antigens in respiratory tract specimens are available commercially, although their reported sensitivity (44%–97%) and specificity (76%–100%) compared with viral culture are variable and differ by test and specimen type. Additionally, many rapid diagnostic antigen tests cannot distinguish between influenza subtypes, a feature that can be critical during seasons with strains that differ in antiviral susceptibility and/or relative virulence. Direct fluorescent antibody (DFA) and indirect immunofluorescent antibody (IFA) staining for detection of influenza A and B antigens in nasopharyngeal or nasal specimens are available at most hospital-based laboratories and can yield results in 3 to 4 hours. Results of immunofluorescent and rapid diagnostic tests should be interpreted in the context of clinical findings and local community influenza activity. Careful clinical judgment must be exercised, because the prevalence of circulating influenza viruses influences the positive and negative predictive values of these influenza screening tests. False-positive results are more likely to occur during periods of low influenza activity; false-negative results are more likely to occur during periods of peak influenza activity. Serologic diagnosis can be established retrospectively by a fourfold or greater increase in antibody titer in serum specimens obtained during the acute and convalescent stages of illness, as determined by hemagglutination inhibition testing, complement fixation testing, neutralization testing, or enzyme immunoassay (EIA); however, serologic testing rarely is useful in patient management, because 2 serum samples collected 10 to 14 days apart are required. Reverse transcriptase-polymerase chain reaction (RT-PCR) testing of respiratory tract specimens may be available at some institutions. Both RT-PCR and viral culture tests offer potential for high sensitivity as well as specificity and are recommended as the tests of choice.

TREATMENT: Influenza A viruses, including 2 subtypes (H1N1 and H3N2), and influenza B viruses circulate worldwide, but the prevalence of each can vary among communities and within a single community over the course of an influenza season. In the United States, 2 classes of antiviral medications currently are available for treatment or prophylaxis of influenza infections: neuraminidase inhibitors (oseltamivir and zanamivir) and adamantanes (amantadine and rimantadine). Guidelines for use of these 4 antiviral agents are summarized in Table 3.29. Although antiviral medications are not licensed by the US Food and Drug Administration for infants younger than 12 months of age and the 2009 H1N1 pandemic Emergency Use Authorization has expired, recommendations for use of oseltamivir in this young age group still can be followed.

Since 2005, all H3N2 strains in the United States have been resistant to adamantanes. Influenza B viruses intrinsically are resistant to adamantanes. Since January 2006, neuraminidase inhibitors (oseltamivir, zanamivir) have been the only recommended influenza antiviral drugs because of this widespread resistance to the adamantanes and the activity of neuraminidase inhibitors against influenza A and B viruses. In 2007–2008, a significant increase in oseltamivir resistance was reported among influenza A (H1N1) viruses, and in the 2008–2009 influenza season, virtually all H1N1 influenza strains were resistant to oseltamivir. However, the 2009 pandemic influenza A (H1N1) virus, which subsequently replaced the previous influenza A (H1N1) seasonal strain, largely is susceptible to neuraminidase inhibitors (oseltamivir and zanamivir) and resistant to adamantanes (amantadine and rimantadine). Resistance to oseltamivir was documented for 1.3% of all tested 2010–2011 influenza viral samples. These resistance patterns among circulating influenza A virus strains simplify antiviral treatment, as 2009 influenza A (H1N1), influenza A (H3N2), and influenza B all were susceptible to neuraminidase inhibitors and resistant to adamantanes. Enhanced surveillance for influenza antiviral resistance is

Table 3.29. Antiviral Drugs for Influenza[a]

Drug (Trade Name)	Virus	Administration	Treatment Indications[b]	Prophylaxis Indications[b]	Adverse Effects
Oseltamivir (Tamiflu)	A and B	Oral	1 y of age or older	1 y of age or older	Nausea, vomiting
Zanamivir (Relenza)	A and B	Inhalation	7 y of age or older	5 y of age or older	Bronchospasm
Amantadine[c] (Symmetrel)	A	Oral	1 y of age or older	1 y of age or older	Central nervous system, anxiety, gastrointestinal
Rimantadine[c] (Flumadine)	A	Oral	13 y of age or older	1 y of age or older	Central nervous system, anxiety, gastrointestinal

[a]For current recommendations about treatment and chemoprophylaxis of influenza, see **www.cdc.gov/flu/professionals/antivirals/index.htm** or **www.aapredbook.org/flu.**

[b]US Food and Drug Administration (FDA)-approved ages.

[c]High levels of resistance to amantadine and rimantadine persist, and these drugs should not be used unless resistance patterns change significantly. Antiviral susceptibilities of viral strains are reported weekly at **www.cdc.gov/flu/weekly/fluactivitysurv.htm.**

ongoing at the CDC in collaboration with local and state health departments. Each year, options for treatment or chemoprophylaxis of influenza in the United States will depend on influenza strain resistance patterns. Recommendations for influenza chemoprophylaxis and treatment can be found at **www.cdc.gov/flu/professionals/antivirals/index. htm** or **www.aapredbook.org/flu.**

Therapy for influenza virus infection should be offered to any child with presumed influenza or severe, complicated or progressive illness, regardless of influenza-immunization status and for influenza infection of any severity in children with a condition that places them at increased risk. Treatment should be considered for any otherwise healthy child with influenza infection for whom a decrease in duration of clinical symptoms is felt to be warranted by his or her health care professional, particularly if treatment can be initiated within 48 hours of illness onset. Children with severe influenza should be evaluated carefully for possible coinfection with bacterial pathogens (eg, *S aureus*) that might require antimicrobial therapy. Clinicians who want to have influenza isolates tested for susceptibility should contact their state health department.

If antiviral therapy is prescribed, treatment should be started as soon after illness onset as possible and should not be delayed while waiting for a definitive influenza test result, because benefit is greatest when treatment is initiated within 48 hours of onset of symptoms.[1] Treatment should be discontinued approximately 24 to 48 hours after symptoms resolve. The duration of treatment studied was 5 days for both the neuraminidase inhibitors (oseltamivir and zanamivir) and the adamantanes (amantadine and rimantadine). Recommended dosages for drugs approved for treatment and prophylaxis of influenza are provided in Table 4.8 (p 841). Patients with any degree of renal insufficiency should be monitored for adverse events. Only zanamivir, which is administered by inhalation, does not require adjustment for people with severe renal insufficiency.

The most common adverse effects of oseltamivir are nausea and vomiting. Postmarketing reports, mostly from Japan, have noted self-injury and delirium with use of oseltamivir among pediatric patients, but other data suggest that these occurrences were related to influenza disease itself rather than antiviral therapy. Nevertheless, cautioning parents and patients regarding abnormal behavior is advised. Zanamivir use has been associated with bronchospasm in some people and is not recommended for use in patients with underlying airway disease. Both amantadine and rimantadine, but especially amantadine, may cause agitation, which resolves with discontinuation of the drug. An increased incidence of seizures has been reported in children with epilepsy who receive amantadine and, to a lesser extent, rimantadine. Because of a lower incidence of adverse events, rimantadine generally is preferred over amantadine for both prophylaxis and treatment.

Control of fever with acetaminophen or other appropriate antipyretic agents may be important in young children, because fever and other symptoms of influenza could exacerbate underlying chronic conditions. Children and adolescents with influenza should not receive aspirin or any salicylate-containing products because of the potential risk of developing Reye syndrome.

---

[1] Centers for Disease Control and Prevention. Antiviral agents for the treatment and chemoprophylaxis of influenza: recommendations of the Advisory Committee on Immunization Practices (ACIP). *MMWR Recomm Rep.* 2011;60(RR-01):1–24

ISOLATION OF THE HOSPITALIZED PATIENT: In addition to standard precautions, droplet precautions are recommended for children hospitalized with influenza or an influenza-like illness for the duration of illness. Respiratory tract secretions should be considered infectious, and strict hand hygiene procedures should be used.

CONTROL MEASURES:

Influenza Vaccine. Trivalent inactivated influenza vaccine (TIV) and live-attenuated influenza vaccine (LAIV) are multivalent vaccines containing 3 virus strains (one each: A [H3N2], A [H1N1], and B). Quadrivalent influenza vaccine(s) are expected to be available for the 2013–2014 influenza season. Typically, 1 or more strains are changed each year in anticipation of the predominant influenza strains expected to circulate in the United States in the upcoming influenza season. During the past 25 years, there have been only 4 times that the vaccine strains in the influenza vaccine have not changed from the previous year.

TIV distributed in the United States is either subvirion vaccine, prepared by disrupting the lipid-containing membrane of the virus, or purified surface-antigen vaccine. TIV is licensed for use in people 6 months of age or older and is administered via intramuscular (IM) or intradermal (ID) injection. Some influenza vaccines are licensed for use in different age groups of children.

The CDC and FDA reviewed vaccine safety data on febrile seizures in the United States following receipt of 2010–2011 inactivated influenza and pneumococcal conjugate (PCV13) vaccines. The analysis found that febrile seizures following receipt of inactivated influenza and PCV13 vaccines given to this age group did occur but were rare. Febrile seizures were most common in children 12 through 23 months of age when the 2 vaccines were given during the same visit. In this group, approximately 1 additional febrile seizure occurred among every 2225 children immunized. Getting recommended childhood vaccines during a single visit has important benefits of protecting children against many infectious diseases; minimizing the number of visits that parents, caregivers, and children must make; and preventing febrile seizures by protecting children against influenza and pneumococcal infections, both of which can cause fever. After thoroughly evaluating the available information, the AAP and CDC determined that no changes in the childhood immunization schedule are necessary at this time. Studies are ongoing to continue to evaluate this occurrence. Additional information can be found at **www.cdc. gov/vaccinesafety/concerns/FebrileSeizures.html.**

The ID formulation of TIV, introduced in the 2011–2012 season, is licensed for use in people 18 through 64 years of age. This method of delivery involves a microinjection with a needle 90% shorter than needles used for intramuscular administration. The most common adverse events are redness, induration, swelling, pain, and itching at the site of administration and occur at a slightly higher rate than with the IM formulation of TIV. Headache, myalgia, and malaise may occur at the same rate as that with the IM formulation of TIV. There is no preference for IM or ID immunization in people 18 years of age or older. A high-dose influenza vaccine is available for adults 65 years of age and older **(www.cdc.gov/flu/protect/vaccine/qa_fluzone.htm).**

LAIV is a live-attenuated influenza virus vaccine administered by intranasal spray. The 3 vaccine strains are attenuated, cold adapted, temperature sensitive viruses that replicate in the cooler temperature of the upper respiratory tract and stimulate both an IgA and IgG antibody response. LAIV is licensed for people 2 through 49 years of age and is administered via intranasal spray. A quadrivalent LAIV formulation was licensed by the

FDA in 2012 and should be available for the 2013–2014 influenza season as a replacement for trivalent LAIV.

Immunogenicity in Children. Regardless of seasonal epidemiology, children 6 months through 8 years of age who previously have **not** been immunized against influenza require 2 doses of TIV or LAIV administered at least 1 month apart to produce a satisfactory antibody response (see Table 3.30 and Table 3.31, p 447). Significant protection against disease is achieved 1 to 2 weeks after the second dose. In typical seasons in which vaccine strains change, the follow recommendations are routine:

- If a child younger than 9 years of age receives only 1 dose of either TIV or LAIV or if it is unclear whether they received 2 doses in their first season of being immunized, then 2 doses should be given the following influenza season.
- In subsequent seasons, children younger than 9 years of age should receive a single annual dose, regardless of the number of doses previously given.
- Children 9 years of age or older require only 1 dose, regardless of their influenza immunization history.

In seasons in which vaccine strains do not change from the previous year, children 6 months through 8 years of age who received 1 vaccine dose the previous season need to receive only 1 dose in the current season. Recommendations for 2 doses of vaccine will resume for seasons when 1 or more of the vaccine strains change.

Vaccine Efficacy and Effectiveness. The efficacy (ie, prevention of illness among vaccine recipients in controlled trials) and effectiveness (ie, prevention of illness in populations receiving vaccine) of influenza vaccines depend primarily on the age and immunocompetence of vaccine recipients, the degree of similarity between the viruses in the vaccine and those in circulation, and the outcome being measured. Protection against virologically confirmed influenza illness after immunization with TIV in healthy children older than 2 years of age approximately is approximately 70%, with a range of 50% to 95% depending on the closeness of vaccine strain match to the circulating wild strain. Efficacy of LAIV was 86% to 96% against virologically confirmed influenza A (H3N2) virus infection in a large clinical pediatric trial during 1 year. Efficacy of TIV in children 6 through 23 months of age is lower than in older children, although data are limited. Several randomized controlled trials have shown that, among young children, LAIV has a 32% to 55% greater relative efficacy in preventing laboratory-confirmed influenza compared with TIV; however, additional experience over multiple influenza seasons is needed to determine optimal utilization of these 2 vaccines in children. The effectiveness of influenza immunization on acute respiratory tract illness is less evident in pediatric than in adult populations because of the frequency of upper respiratory tract infections and influenza-like illness caused by other viral agents in young children. Antibody titers for seasonal influenza vaccines wane up to 50% of their original levels 6 to 12 months after immunization. An annual dose is critical to maintain protection in all populations.

Coadministration With Other Vaccines. TIV can be administered simultaneously with other live and inactivated vaccines. Although information on how concurrent administration of LAIV with other vaccines affects the safety or efficacy of either LAIV or the simultaneously administered vaccine has not been well studied, inactivated or live vaccines can be administered simultaneously with LAIV. After administration of a live vaccine, at least 4 weeks should pass before another live vaccine is administered.

Table 3.30. Schedule for Trivalent Inactivated Influenza Vaccine (TIV) Dosage by Age[a]

Age	Dose, mL[b]	No. of Doses	Route[c]
6 through 35 mo	0.25	1–2[d]	Intramuscular
3 through 8 y	0.5	1–2[d]	Intramuscular
9 y or older	0.5	1	Intramuscular

[a] Manufacturers include Sanofi Pasteur (Fluzone, split-virus vaccine licensed for people 6 months of age or older), Novartis Vaccine (Fluvirin, purified surface antigen, licensed for people 4 years of age or older), CSL Biotherapies (Afluria, split-virus vaccine licensed for people 18 years of age or older), and GlaxoSmithKline Biologicals (Fluarix and FluLaval, split-virus vaccines licensed for people 18 years of age or older). Age indication for Afluria during the 2011–2012 season, per package insert, is 5 years or older; however, the Advisory Committee on Immunization Practices and American Academy of Pediatrics recommend Afluria not be used in children 6 months through 8 years of age because of increased reports of febrile reactions noted in this age group. If no other age-appropriate, licensed inactivated seasonal influenza vaccine is available for a child 5 through 8 years of age who has a medical condition that increases the child's risk of influenza complications, Afluria can be used; however, providers should discuss with parents or caregivers the benefits and risks of influenza immunization with Afluria before administering this vaccine.

[b] Dosages are those recommended in recent years. Physicians should refer to the product circular each year to ensure that the appropriate dosage is given.

[c] For adults and older children, the recommended site of immunization is the deltoid muscle. For infants and young children, the preferred site is the anterolateral aspect of the thigh.

[d] Two doses administered at least 4 weeks apart are recommended for children younger than 9 years of age who are receiving inactivated trivalent influenza vaccine for the first time. If possible, the second dose should be administered before December.

Table 3.31 Schedule for Live-Attenuated Influenza Vaccine (LAIV)[a]

Age	Dose, mL[b]	No. of Doses	Route
2 through 8 y	0.2	1–2[c]	Intranasal
9 y through 49 y	0.2	1	Intranasal

[a] Manufacturer: MedImmune Vaccines, Inc (FluMist).

[b] Dosage is the one recommended in recent years. Physicians should refer to the product circular each year to ensure that the appropriate dosage is given.

[c] Two doses administered at least 4 weeks apart are recommended for children younger than 9 years of age who are receiving LAIV for the first time. If possible, the second dose should be administered before December.

Recommendations for Influenza Immunization.[1,2] All people 6 months of age and older should receive influenza vaccine annually. Influenza immunization should begin in September or as soon as the vaccine becomes available and continue into March or for as long as vaccine is available. It is recommended that people be immunized even into early spring. People with the following conditions are at increased risk of severe complications from influenza, and it especially is important they receive annual immunization:

- Asthma or other chronic pulmonary diseases, such as cystic fibrosis
- Hemodynamically significant cardiac disease
- Immunosuppressive disorders or therapy (see Special Considerations, p 448)

---

[1] Centers for Disease Control and Prevention. Prevention and control of influenza with vaccines: recommendations of the Advisory Committee on Immunization Practices (ACIP), 2011. *MMWR Morb Mortal Wkly Rep.* 2011;60(33):1128–1132 (for updates, see **www.cdc.gov/flu**)

[2] American Academy of Pediatrics, Committee on Infectious Diseases. Recommendations for prevention and control of influenza in children, 2011–2012. *Pediatrics.* 2011;128(4):813–825 (for updates, see **www.aap.org**)

- Human immunodeficiency virus (HIV) infection (see Human Immunodeficiency Virus Infection, p 418)
- Sickle cell anemia and other hemoglobinopathies
- Diseases requiring long-term salicylate therapy, such as rheumatoid arthritis or Kawasaki disease, which may increase the risk of developing Reye syndrome after influenza illness
- Chronic renal dysfunction
- Chronic metabolic disease, including diabetes mellitus
- Any condition (eg, cognitive dysfunction, spinal cord injuries, seizure disorders, or other neuromuscular disorders) that can compromise respiratory function or handling of respiratory tract secretions or that can increase the risk of aspiration

LAIV Indications. LAIV is indicated for healthy, nonpregnant people 2 through 49 years of age. TIV is preferred for close contacts of severely immunosuppressed people (ie, people requiring care in a protective environment).

People should not receive LAIV if they received other live vaccines within the last 4 weeks, have a moderate to severe febrile illness, are receiving salicylates, have a known or suspected immune deficiency, have a history of Guillain-Barré syndrome (GBS), or have reactive airway disease or other conditions that traditionally would place them in a high-risk category for severe influenza (asthma and other chronic pulmonary disorders or cardiac disorders, pregnancy, chronic metabolic disease including diabetes mellitus, renal dysfunction, hemoglobinopathies, or immunosuppressive therapy).

Special Considerations, LAIV. Clinicians and immunization programs should screen for possible reactive airway disease when considering use of LAIV for children 2 through 4 years of age and avoid use in children with asthma or a recent wheezing episode. Health care professionals should consult the patient's medical record, when available, to identify children 2 through 4 years of age with asthma or recurrent wheezing that might indicate asthma. Some children 2 through 4 years of age have a history of wheezing with respiratory tract illnesses but have not been diagnosed with asthma. Therefore, to identify children who might be at higher risk of asthma and possibly at increased risk of wheezing after receiving LAIV, people administering LAIV also should ask parents/guardians of children 2 through 4 years of age: "In the past 12 months, has a health care professional ever told you that your child had wheezing or asthma?" LAIV is not recommended for children whose parent or guardian answers yes to this question or for children who have had a wheezing episode or asthma diagnosis noted in his or her medical record within the past 12 months. Precaution also should be taken when considering LAIV administration to people with minor acute illness, such as a mild upper respiratory tract infection, with or without fever. Although the vaccine most likely can be given in this case, LAIV should not be administered if nasal congestion will impede delivery of the vaccine to the nasopharyngeal mucosa until the congestion-inducing illness is resolved.

Special Considerations, TIV. Consideration should be given to the potential risks and benefits of administering influenza vaccine to any child with known or suspected immunodeficiency. In children receiving immunosuppressive chemotherapy, influenza immunization may result in a less robust response than in immunocompetent children. The optimal time to immunize children with malignant neoplasms who must undergo chemotherapy is more than 3 weeks after chemotherapy has been discontinued, when the peripheral granulocyte and lymphocyte counts are greater than $1000/\mu L$ ($1.0 \times 10^9/L$).

Children who no longer are receiving chemotherapy generally have high rates of seroconversion. TIV is the influenza vaccine of choice for any child living with a family member or household contact who is immunocompromised severely (ie, in a protected environment). The preference of TIV over LAIV for such people is because of the theoretical risk of infection in an immunocompromised contact of a LAIV-immunized child. As a precautionary measure, people recently immunized with LAIV should restrict contact with severely immunocompromised (ie, in a protected environment) patients for 7 days after LAIV immunization, even though there have been no reports of LAIV transmission between these 2 groups.

Children with hemodynamically unstable cardiac disease constitute a large group potentially at high risk of complications of influenza. The immune response to and safety of TIV in these children are comparable to immune response and safety in healthy children.

Corticosteroids administered for brief periods or every other day seem to have a minimal effect on antibody response to influenza vaccine. Prolonged administration of high doses of corticosteroids (ie, a dose of prednisone of either 2 mg/kg or greater or a total of 20 mg/day or greater or an equivalent) may impair antibody response. Influenza immunization can be deferred temporarily during the time of receipt of high-dose corticosteroids, provided deferral does not compromise the likelihood of immunization before the start of influenza season (see Vaccine Administration, p 20).

Pregnancy. Women, including adolescents, who will be pregnant during influenza season should receive TIV during autumn, because pregnancy increases the risk of complications and hospitalization from influenza. Because the currently available intramuscularly administered TIV is not a live-virus vaccine and rarely is associated with major systemic reactions, most experts consider the vaccine safe during any stage of pregnancy. LAIV is contraindicated during pregnancy. Studies have shown that infants born to women who received influenza vaccine have better influenza-related health outcomes. However, data suggest that no more than half of pregnant women receive seasonal influenza vaccine, even though both pregnant women and their infants are at higher risk of complications. In addition, there is limited evidence that influenza immunization in pregnancy may decrease the risk of preterm birth.

Close Contacts of High-Risk Patients. Immunization of people who are in close contact with children with high-risk conditions or with any child younger than 60 months (5 years) of age is an important means of protection for these children. In addition, immunization of pregnant women may benefit their unborn infants, because transplacentally acquired antibody and human milk may protect infants from infection with influenza virus. Special outreach efforts for annual influenza immunization are recommended for the following people:

- Household contacts, including siblings and care providers, of high-risk children of any age and all healthy children 0 through 59 months of age
- Children who are members of households with high-risk adults (ie, adults with underlying medical conditions that predispose them to severe influenza infection or adults 50 years of age or older), any children younger than 60 months (5 years) of age, and children with HIV infection
- Providers of home care to children 0 through 59 months of age and to other high-risk groups of children and adolescents

- Close contacts of infants younger than 6 months of age (see Recommendations for Influenza Immunization, p 447), because this high-risk group cannot be protected directly by immunization or antiviral prophylaxis

Health Care Personnel. The AAP released a policy statement in fall 2010 recommending a mandatory annual immunization program for all health care personnel.[1] Because voluntary immunization programs have failed to raise coverage rates among health care personnel above an average of 40%, a mandate is necessary to achieve herd immunity, reach Healthy People 2020 objectives, and sufficiently protect people who come in contact with health care personnel. Influenza causes significant morbidity and mortality for both patients and health care personnel. A mandate is expected to cut costs and increase efficiency in health care settings. There is growing support for a mandate among medical organizations, and hospitals that already have implemented mandatory influenza immunization for health care personnel have had enormous success.

Breastfeeding. Breastfeeding is not a contraindication for immunization with either TIV or LAIV.

Timing of Vaccine Administration. Influenza vaccine should be administered as soon as available each year, preferably before the start of influenza season, at the time specified in the annual recommendations of the CDC Advisory Committee on Immunization Practices (**www.cdc.gov/flu/**). The recommended time ranges from the beginning of September to the end of April and longer when vaccine is available and not expired. Influenza vaccine administration throughout the entire season now is recommended, because the influenza season extends into March and April. Immunization throughout the season may protect some people against late outbreaks of influenza. In addition, there may be more than 1 peak of activity during an influenza season, so later immunization still may help protect from a later peak caused by a different strain of influenza virus that same season. The recommended vaccine dose and schedule for different age groups are given in Tables 3.30 (p 447) and 3.31 (p 447).

Annual influenza immunization is recommended, because immunity can decrease during the year after immunization and because in most years, at least one of the vaccine antigens is changed to match ongoing antigenic changes in circulating strains. Strategies to maximize immunization levels include using reminder/recall systems and programs for standing orders. The AAP and CDC recommend vaccine administration at any visit to the medical home during influenza season when it is not contraindicated, at specially arranged "vaccine-only" sessions, and through cooperation with community clinics, schools, and child care centers to provide influenza vaccine. If alternate venues are used, a system of patient record transfer is beneficial to ensuring maintenance of accurate immunization records.

Reactions, Adverse Effects, and Contraindications

Although both TIV and LAIV are produced in eggs, data have shown that TIV administered in a single, age-appropriate dose is well tolerated by nearly all recipients who have egg allergy. More conservative approaches, such as skin testing or a 2-step graded challenge, no longer are recommended. Data are not available to support use of LAIV in people with egg allergy.

---

[1] Bernstein HH; Starke JR; and the American Academy of Pediatrics, Committee on Infectious Diseases. Policy statement: recommendation for mandatory influenza immunization of all health care personnel. *Pediatrics.* 2010;126(4):809–815

Fig 3.3 outlines an approach for administration of TIV to people with presumed egg allergy. As a precaution, clinicians should determine whether the presumed egg allergy is based on a mild or severe reaction (eg, anaphylaxis). Mild reactions are defined as hives alone; severe reactions involve cardiovascular changes, respiratory tract and/or gastrointestinal tract symptoms, or reactions that required use of epinephrine. Clinicians should consult with an allergist for children with a history of severe reaction. Most vaccine administration to people with egg allergy can happen without the need for referral. Data indicate that approximately 1% of children have immunoglobulin E (IgE)-mediated sensitivity to egg, and of those, a very small minority have a severe allergy.

Standard immunization practice should include the ability to respond to acute hypersensitivity reactions.[1] Therefore, influenza vaccine should be given to people with mild egg allergy with the following preconditions:

- Appropriate resuscitative equipment must be readily available.
- The vaccine recipient should be observed in the office for 30 minutes after immunization (the standard observation time for receiving immunotherapy).
- For children who need a second dose, the same product brand is preferred, if possible, but it does not need to be from the same lot as the first dose.

Although a very slight increase in the number of cases of GBS was reported during the "swine flu" vaccine program of 1976, obtaining strong epidemiologic evidence for a possible limited increase in risk of a rare condition with multiple causes is difficult. GBS has an annual background incidence of 10 to 20 cases per 1 million adults, and during the 1976 swine influenza vaccine program, 1 case of GBS was reported per 100 000 people immunized. The risk of influenza vaccine-associated GBS was higher among people 25 years of age or older than among people younger than 25 years of age. If there is an association between seasonal influenza vaccine and GBS, the risk is rare, at no more than 1 to 2 cases per million doses. Whether influenza immunization specifically might increase the risk of recurrence of GBS is unknown. The decision not to immunize should be thoughtfully balanced against the potential morbidity and mortality associated with influenza for that individual.

Immunization of children who have asthma or cystic fibrosis with available TIV is not associated with a detectable increase in adverse events or exacerbations. Because past reports are conflicting, the issue of safety of TIV immunization for children and adults with HIV infection is uncertain. However, experts generally believe that the benefits of immunization with TIV for children with HIV infection far outweigh risks.

Inactivated Influenza Vaccine. TIV contains only killed, noninfectious viruses and, therefore, cannot produce active influenza infection. The most common symptoms associated with TIV administration are soreness at the injection site and fever. Usually occurring 6 to 24 hours after immunization, fever affects approximately 10% to 35% of children younger than 2 years of age. Mild systemic symptoms, such as nausea, lethargy, headache, muscle aches, and chills, also can occur with TIV injection. In children 13 years of age or older, local reactions occur in approximately 10% of recipients.

Live-Attenuated Influenza Vaccine. No statistically significant differences were observed in clinical studies between placebo and LAIV recipients in rates of fever, rhinitis, or nasal congestion. A retrospective analysis of a large pediatric trial in Northern California revealed a statistically significant increase in asthma events among children 12

---

[1] American Academy of Pediatrics, Committee on Pediatric Emergency Medicine. Preparation for emergencies in the offices of pediatricians and pediatric primary care providers. *Pediatrics.* 2007;120(1):200–212

FIGURE 3.3. PRECAUTIONS FOR ADMINISTERING INFLUENZA VACCINE TO PRESUMED EGG ALLERGIC PEOPLE.[a]

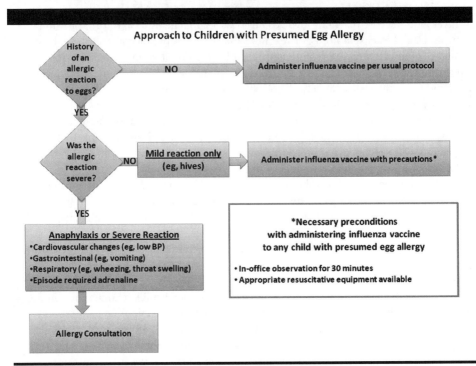

[a]Only applies to TIV.

through 59 months of age after dose 1 of LAIV (relative risk, 3.53; 90% confidence interval, 1.1–15.7). There was no clustering of wheezing events. In a randomized controlled trial conducted among children 6 through 59 months of age, rates of medically significant wheezing were higher among children 6 through 23 months of age who received LAIV (6%) compared with those who received TIV (4%), and rates of hospitalizations attributable to any cause also were significantly higher among LAIV recipients. However, similarly low rates of medically significant wheezing and hospitalizations were observed in children 24 through 59 months of age regardless of the influenza vaccine given.

LAIV should not be administered to people with asthma or children younger than 5 years of age with recurrent wheezing. The risk, if any, of wheezing caused by LAIV among children 2 through 4 years of age with a history of asthma or wheezing is unknown.

LAIV shedding can occur after immunization, although the amount of detectable virus is less than occurs during natural influenza infection. The proposed explanation for the low incidence of transmission is that the vaccine virus is shed for a shorter duration and in a much smaller quantity than are wild-type strains. Further evaluation of transmission of LAIV is being conducted.

Chemoprophylaxis: An Adjunct Method of Protecting Children Against Influenza.
Chemoprophylaxis should not be considered a substitute for immunization in most cases. Influenza vaccine always should be offered if not contraindicated, even when influenza

virus is circulating in the community. However, influenza antiviral drugs are important adjuncts to influenza immunization for control and prevention of influenza disease. Because of high rates of resistance of 2009 pandemic influenza A (H1N1), influenza A (H3N2), and influenza B strains to amantadine or rimantadine, oseltamivir, or zanamivir are recommended. However, recommendations for use of these drugs for chemoprophylaxis may vary by location and season, depending on susceptibility patterns. Providers should inform recipients of antiviral chemoprophylaxis that the risk of influenza is lowered but still remains while taking medication, and susceptibility to influenza returns when medication is discontinued. For current recommendations about chemoprophylaxis against influenza, see **www.cdc.gov/flu/professionals/antivirals/index.htm** or **www.aapredbook.org/flu/.**

Indications for Chemoprophylaxis. Chemoprophylaxis may be considered for the following situations:

- Protection of unimmunized high-risk children or children who were immunized less than 2 weeks before influenza circulation, because adequate immune response develops 2 weeks after immunization
- Protection of children at increased risk of severe infection or complications, such as high-risk children for whom the vaccine is contraindicated
- Protection of unimmunized close contacts of high-risk children
- Protection of immunocompromised children who may not respond to vaccine
- Control of influenza outbreaks in a closed setting, such as an institution with unimmunized high-risk children
- Protection of immunized high-risk children if the vaccine strain poorly matches circulating influenza strains

Chemoprophylaxis does not interfere with the immune response to TIV; however, people immunized with LAIV should not receive antiviral prophylaxis for 14 days after receipt of LAIV, because the vaccine strains are susceptible to antiviral drugs.

Information about influenza surveillance is available through the CDC Voice Information System (influenza update, 888-232-3228) or through **www.cdc.gov/flu/.**

Isosporiasis (now designated as Cystoisosporiasis)

CLINICAL MANIFESTATIONS: Watery diarrhea is the most common symptom and can be profuse and protracted, even in immunocompetent people. Manifestations are similar to those caused by other enteric protozoa (eg, *Cryptosporidium* and *Cyclospora* species) and can include abdominal pain, cramping, anorexia, nausea, vomiting, weight loss, and low-grade fever. Eosinophilia also can occur. The proportion of infected people who are asymptomatic is unknown. Severity of infection ranges from self-limiting in immunocompetent hosts to debilitating and life threatening in immunocompromised patients, particularly people infected with human immunodeficiency virus (HIV). Infections of the biliary system also have been reported.

ETIOLOGY: *Cystoisospora belli* (formerly *Isospora belli*) is a coccidian protozoan; oocysts (rather than cysts) are passed in stools.

EPIDEMIOLOGY: Infection occurs predominately in tropical and subtropical regions of the world and can cause traveler's diarrhea. Infection results from ingestion of sporulated oocysts (eg, in contaminated food and water). Humans are the only known host for *C belli* and shed noninfective oocysts in feces. These oocysts must mature (sporulate) outside the host in the environment to become infective. Under favorable conditions, sporulation can be completed in 1 to 2 days and perhaps more quickly. Oocysts probably are resistant to most disinfectants and can remain viable for prolonged periods in a cool, moist environment.

The **incubation period** is uncertain but ranges from 7 to 12 days in reported cases.

DIAGNOSTIC TESTS: Identification of oocysts in feces or in duodenal aspirates or finding developmental stages of the parasite in biopsy specimens (eg, of the small intestine) is diagnostic. Oocysts in stool are elongate and ellipsoidal (length, 25 to 30 μm). Oocysts can be shed in low numbers, even by people with profuse diarrhea. This constraint underscores the utility of repeated stool examinations, sensitive recovery methods (eg, concentration methods), and detection methods that highlight the organism (eg, oocysts stain bright red with modified acid-fast techniques and autofluoresce when viewed by ultraviolet fluorescent microscopy). Polymerase chain reaction is an emerging and promising tool for diagnosis.

TREATMENT: Trimethoprim-sulfamethoxazole, typically for 7 to 10 days, is the drug of choice (see Drugs for Parasitic Infections, p 848). Immunocompromised patients may need higher doses and longer duration of therapy. Pyrimethamine (plus leucovorin, to prevent myelosuppression) is an alternative treatment for people who cannot tolerate trimethoprim-sulfamethoxazole. Ciprofloxacin is less effective than trimethoprim-sulfamethoxazole. Nitazoxanide also has been reported to be effective, but data are limited. Maintenance therapy to prevent recurrent disease may be indicated for people infected with HIV.

ISOLATION OF THE HOSPITALIZED PATIENT: In addition to standard precautions, contact precautions are recommended for diapered and incontinent people.

CONTROL MEASURES: Preventive measures include avoiding fecal exposure (eg, food, water, skin, and fomites contaminated with stool), practicing hand and personal hygiene, and thorough washing of fruits and vegetables before eating.

Kawasaki Disease

CLINICAL MANIFESTATIONS: Kawasaki disease is a febrile, exanthematous, multisystem vasculitis recognized on all continents. If untreated, approximately 20% of children may develop coronary artery abnormalities, including aneurysms. Approximately 80% of cases of Kawasaki disease occur in children younger than 5 years of age. The illness is characterized by fever and the following clinical features: (1) bilateral bulbar conjunctival injection with limbic sparing and without exudate; (2) erythematous mouth and pharynx, strawberry tongue, and red, cracked lips; (3) a polymorphous, generalized, erythematous rash that can be morbilliform, maculopapular, or scarlatiniform or may resemble erythema multiforme; (4) changes in the peripheral extremities consisting of induration of the hands and feet with erythematous palms and soles, often with later periungual desquamation; and (5) acute, nonsuppurative, usually unilateral, cervical lymphadenopathy with at least one node 1.5 cm in diameter. For diagnosis of classic Kawasaki disease, patients should have fever for at least 5 days (or fever until the date of treatment if given before the fifth day of illness) and at least 4 of the above 5 features without alternative explanation for the findings. The epidemiologic case definition also allows diagnosis of incomplete Kawasaki disease when a person has fewer than 4 principal clinical criteria in the presence of fever and coronary artery abnormalities. Irritability, abdominal pain, diarrhea, and vomiting commonly are associated features. Other findings include urethritis with sterile pyuria (70% of cases), mild anterior uveitis (25%–50%), mild hepatic dysfunction (50%), arthritis or arthralgia (10%–20%), meningismus with cerebrospinal fluid pleocytosis (25%), pericardial effusion of at least 1 mm (less than 5%), gallbladder hydrops (less than 10%), and myocarditis manifested by congestive heart failure (less than 5%). A persistent resting tachycardia and the presence of an S3 gallop often are appreciated. Fine desquamation in the groin area can occur in the acute phase of disease.[1] Inflammation or ulceration may be observed at the inoculation scar of previous bacille Calmette-Guérin immunization. Rarely, Kawasaki disease can present with what appears to be "septic shock" with need for intensive care; these children often have significant thrombocytopenia at admission. Group A streptococcal or *Staphylococcus aureus* toxic shock syndrome should be excluded in such cases.

Incomplete Kawasaki disease can be diagnosed in febrile patients when fever plus fewer than 4 of the characteristic features are present. Patients with fewer than 4 of the characteristic features and who have additional findings not listed above (eg, purulent conjunctivitis) should not be considered to have incomplete Kawasaki disease. The proportion of children with Kawasaki disease with incomplete manifestations is higher among patients younger than 12 months of age. Infants with Kawasaki disease also have a higher risk of developing coronary artery aneurysms than do older children, making diagnosis and timely treatment especially important in this age group. Laboratory findings in incomplete cases are similar to findings in classic cases. Therefore, although laboratory findings in Kawasaki disease are nonspecific, they may prove useful in increasing or decreasing the likelihood of incomplete Kawasaki disease. If coronary artery ectasia or dilatation is evident, diagnosis can be made with certainty. A normal early echocardiographic study is typical and does not exclude the diagnosis but may be useful in evaluation of patients with suspected incomplete Kawasaki disease. Incomplete Kawasaki disease should be considered in any child with unexplained fever for 5 days or longer in association with 2 or more of the principal features of this illness and supportive laboratory data (eg, erythrocyte sedimentation rate [ESR] ≥40 mm/hour or C-reactive protein [CRP] concentration ≥3.0 mg/dL). Fig 3.4 is the American Heart Association algorithm for diagnosis and treatment of suspected incomplete Kawasaki disease.

The average duration of fever in untreated Kawasaki disease is 10 days; however, fever can last 2 weeks or longer. After fever resolves, patients can remain anorectic and/or irritable for 2 to 3 weeks. During this phase, desquamation of the groin, fingers, and toes and fine desquamation of other areas may occur. Recurrent disease occurring months to years later develops in approximately 2% of patients.

Coronary artery abnormalities can be demonstrated with 2-dimensional echocardiography in 20% to 25% of patients who are not treated within 10 days of onset of fever. Increased risk of developing coronary artery aneurysms is associated with male sex; age younger than 12 months or older than 8 years; fever for more than 10 days; high baseline neutrophil (>30 000 cells/mm³) and band count; low hemoglobin concentration (<10 g/dL);

---

[1] For further information on the diagnosis of this disease, see Newburger JW, Takahashi M, Gerber MA, et al. Diagnosis, treatment and long-term management of Kawasaki disease: a statement for health professionals from the Committee on Rheumatic Fever, Endocarditis and Kawasaki Disease, Council on Cardiovascular Disease in the Young, American Heart Association. *Circulation.* 2004;110(17):2747–2771 (also in *Pediatrics.* 2004;114[6]:1708–1733).

FIGURE 3.4. EVALUATION OF SUSPECTED INCOMPLETE KAWASAKI DISEASE (KD).[a]

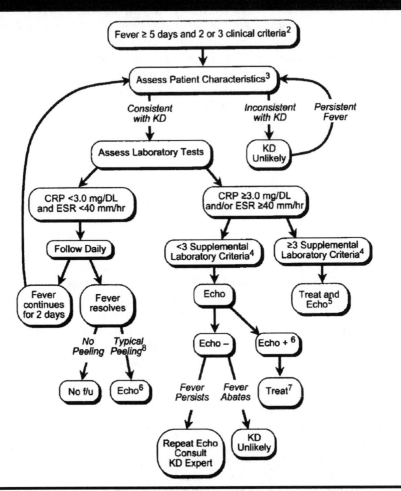

Evaluation of suspected incomplete Kawasaki disease. (1) In the absence of gold standard for diagnosis, this algorithm cannot be evidence based but rather represents the informed opinion of the expert committee. Consultation with an expert should be sought anytime assistance is needed. (2) Infants ≤6 months old on day ≥7 of fever without other explanation should undergo laboratory testing and, if evidence of systemic inflammation is found, an echocardiogram, even if the infants have no clinical criteria. (3) Patient characteristics suggesting Kawasaki disease are provided in text. Characteristics suggesting disease other than Kawasaki disease include exudative conjunctivitis, exudative pharyngitis, discrete intraoral lesions, bullous or vesicular rash, or generalized adenopathy. Consider alternative diagnoses. (4) Supplemental laboratory criteria include albumin ≤3.0 g/dL, anemia for age, elevation of alanine aminotransferase, platelets after 7 d ≥450 000/mm^3, white blood cell count ≥15 000/mm^3, and urine ≥10 white blood cells/high-power field. (5) Can treat before performing echocardiogram. (6) Echocardiogram is considered positive for purposes of this algorithm if any of 3 conditions are met: z score of LAD or RCA ≥2.5, coronary arteries meet Japanese Ministry of Health criteria for aneurysms, or ≥3 other suggestive features exist, including perivascular brightness, lack of tapering, decreased LV function, mitral regurgitation, pericardial effusion, or z scores in LAD or RCA of 2–2.5. (7) If the echocardiogram is positive, treatment should be given to children within 10 d of fever onset and those beyond day 10 with clinical and laboratory signs (CRP, ESR) of ongoing inflammation. (8) Typical peeling begins under nail bed of fingers and then toes.

[a]Reprinted from Newburger JW, Takahashi M, Gerber MA, et al. Diagnosis, treatment and long-term management of Kawasaki disease: a statement for health professionals from the Committee on Rheumatic Fever, Endocarditis and Kawasaki Disease, Council on Cardiovascular Disease in the Young, American Heart Association. *Pediatrics.* 2004;114(6):1705S–1733S.

hypoalbuminemia, hyponatremia, or thrombocytopenia at presentation; fever persisting or occurring after Immune Globulin Intravenous (IGIV) administration; and persistence of elevated ESR or CRP for more than 30 days or recurrent elevations. Hispanic ethnicity also has been associated with an increased risk of coronary artery aneurysms, which may be related to delayed diagnosis and treatment. Aneurysms of the coronary arteries have been demonstrated by echocardiography as early as 5 to 7 days after onset of illness but more typically occur between 1 and 4 weeks after onset of illness; their initial appearance later than 6 weeks is uncommon. Giant coronary artery aneurysms (diameter ≥8 mm) likely are associated with long-term complications. Aneurysms occurring in other medium-sized arteries (eg, iliac, femoral, renal, and axillary vessels) are uncommon and generally do not occur in the absence of significant coronary abnormalities. In addition to coronary artery disease, carditis can involve the pericardium, myocardium, or endocardium, and mitral or aortic regurgitation or both can develop. Carditis generally resolves when fever resolves.

In children with mild coronary artery dilation or ectasia, coronary artery dimensions often return to baseline within 6 to 8 weeks after onset of disease. Approximately 50% of coronary aneurysms (fewer giant aneurysms) regress to normal luminal size within 1 to 2 years, although this process can be accompanied by development of coronary stenosis. In addition, regression of aneurysm(s) may result in a poorly compliant, fibrotic vessel wall.

The current case-fatality rate in the United States and Japan is less than 0.2%. The principal cause of death is myocardial infarction resulting from coronary artery occlusion attributable to thrombosis or progressive stenosis. Rarely, a large coronary artery aneurysm may rupture. The relative risk of mortality is highest within 6 weeks of onset of symptoms, but myocardial infarction and sudden death can occur months to years after the acute episode. There is hypothetical concern that vasculitis of Kawasaki disease may predispose to premature coronary artery disease; longitudinal studies to test this hypothesis, however, have not been performed.

ETIOLOGY: The cause is unknown. Epidemiologic and clinical features suggest an infectious cause or trigger.

EPIDEMIOLOGY: Peak age of occurrence in the United States is between 18 and 24 months. Fifty percent of patients are younger than 2 years of age, and 80% are younger than 5 years of age; children older than 8 years of age less commonly develop the disease. In children younger than 6 months of age, the diagnosis often is delayed, because the symptom complex of Kawasaki disease is incomplete. The prevalence of coronary artery abnormalities is higher when diagnosis and treatment are delayed beyond the 10th day of illness. The male-to-female ratio is approximately 1.5:1. In the United States, 4000 to 5500 cases are estimated to occur each year; the incidence is highest in people of Asian ancestry. Kawasaki disease first was described in Japan, where a pattern of endemic occurrence with superimposed epidemic outbreaks was recognized. A similar pattern of disease occurrence with occasional sharply defined community-wide epidemics has been recognized in North America and Hawaii. Clusters generally occur during winter and spring. No evidence indicates person-to-person or common-source spread, although the incidence is slightly higher in siblings of children with the disease.

The **incubation period** is unknown.

DIAGNOSTIC TESTS: No specific diagnostic test is available. The diagnosis is established by fulfillment of the clinical criteria (see Clinical Manifestations, p 454) and clinical or laboratory exclusion of other possible illnesses, such as staphylococcal or streptococcal toxin-mediated disease; drug reactions (eg, Stevens-Johnson syndrome); measles, adenovirus, parvovirus B19, or enterovirus infections; rickettsial exanthems; leptospirosis; systemic onset juvenile idiopathic arthritis; and reactive arthritis. A greatly increased ESR and serum CRP concentration during the first 2 weeks of illness and an increased platelet count (>450 000/mm^3) on days 10 to 21 of illness almost are universal laboratory features. ESR and platelet count usually are normal within 6 to 8 weeks; CRP concentration returns to normal much sooner.

TREATMENT: Management during the acute phase is directed at decreasing inflammation of the myocardium and coronary artery wall and providing supportive care. Therapy should be initiated when the diagnosis is established or strongly suspected, optimally within the first 10 days of illness. Once the acute phase has passed, therapy is directed at prevention of coronary artery thrombosis. Specific recommendations for therapy include the following measures.

Immune Globulin Intravenous. Therapy with high-dose IGIV and aspirin initiated within 10 days of the onset of fever substantially decreases progression to coronary artery dilatation and aneurysms, compared with treatment with aspirin alone, and results in more rapid resolution of fever and other clinical and laboratory indicators of acute inflammation. Therapy with IGIV should be initiated as soon as possible; its efficacy when initiated later than the 10th day of illness or after detection of aneurysms has been evaluated in only one controlled trial. However, therapy with IGIV and aspirin should be provided for patients diagnosed after day 10 who have manifestations of continuing inflammation (eg, fever or elevated ESR or CRP concentration) or of evolving coronary artery disease. Despite prompt treatment with IGIV and aspirin, 2% to 4% of patients develop coronary artery abnormalities.

Dose. A dose of 2 g/kg as a single dose, given over 10 to 12 hours, has been proven to reduce the risk of coronary artery aneurysm from 17% to 4%. Few complications occur from this regimen, but infusion reactions (fever, chills, hypotension) do occur, and drug-induced aseptic meningitis is seen as a rare complication. ESR becomes elevated as a result of the IGIV infusion.

Retreatment. Many patients have fever in the 24 hours after completing the IGIV infusion. Persistent or recrudescent fever that is present 36 hours after the end of the IGIV infusion is used to define IGIV-resistant cases. Up to 15% of Kawasaki patients can be IGIV resistant. In these situations, the diagnosis of Kawasaki disease should be reevaluated. If Kawasaki disease still is considered to be most likely, retreatment with IGIV (2 g/kg) and continued high-dose aspirin therapy generally is given. For the limited number of patients who are refractory to at least 2 doses of IGIV, infliximab (5 mg/kg as 1 infusion) or intravenous methylprednisolone (usually 30 mg/kg/day for 1 to 3 days) may be administered in attempt to reduce inflammation and improve coronary artery outcomes. Lack of data on use of these modalities precludes definitive recommendations. A chest radiograph should be obtained before administration of infliximab to ensure that the patient does not have active tuberculosis (see Biologic Response Modifiers, p 82). A tuberculin skin test should be placed, but treatment with infliximab should not be delayed awaiting results. The benefit and potential risks of systemic corticosteroids in treatment of Kawasaki disease are controversial.

Aspirin. Aspirin is used for anti-inflammatory and antithrombotic actions, although aspirin alone does not decrease risk of coronary artery abnormalities. The optimal dose or duration of aspirin treatment is unknown. Aspirin is administered in doses of 80 to 100 mg/kg per day in 4 divided doses once the diagnosis is made. Children with acute Kawasaki disease have decreased aspirin absorption and increased clearance and rarely achieve therapeutic serum concentrations. In most children, it is not necessary to monitor aspirin concentrations. The duration of high-dose aspirin therapy varies across institutions. Many centers change from high-dose to low-dose aspirin after the child has been afebrile for 48 to 72 hours. Other clinicians continue high-dose aspirin therapy until day 14 of illness and 48 to 72 hours after fever cessation. Aspirin is discontinued if no coronary artery abnormalities have been detected by 6 to 8 weeks after onset of illness. Low-dose aspirin therapy should be continued indefinitely for people in whom coronary artery abnormalities are present. Because of the theoretical risk of Reye syndrome in patients with influenza or varicella receiving salicylates, parents of children receiving aspirin should be instructed to contact their child's physician promptly if the child develops symptoms of or is exposed to either disease. In general, ibuprofen should be avoided in children with coronary aneurysms taking aspirin for its antiplatelet effects, because ibuprofen antagonizes the platelet inhibition that is induced by aspirin. The child and household contacts should be given influenza vaccine at the time of diagnosis of Kawasaki disease according to seasonal recommendations.

Cardiac Care.[1] An echocardiogram should be obtained at the time of diagnosis and repeated at 2 weeks and 6 to 8 weeks after diagnosis. Children at higher risk—for example, children with persistent or recrudescent fever after initial IGIV or baseline coronary abnormalities—may require more frequent echocardiograms to guide the need for additional therapies. Children also should be assessed during this time for arrhythmias, congestive heart failure, and valvular regurgitation. The care of patients with significant cardiac abnormalities should involve a pediatric cardiologist experienced in management of patients with Kawasaki disease and in assessing echocardiographic studies of coronary arteries in children. Long-term management of Kawasaki disease should be based on the extent of coronary artery involvement. In patients with persistent moderately large coronary artery abnormalities that are not large enough to require anticoagulation, prolonged low-dose aspirin and clopidogrel (1 mg/kg/day) are recommended in combination. Development of giant coronary artery aneurysms (diameter 8 mm or larger) usually requires addition of anticoagulant therapy, such as warfarin or low-molecular weight heparin, to prevent thrombosis. Anticoagulation also sometimes is used in young infants with coronary artery aneurysms measuring less than 8 mm in diameter but for whom the size is equivalent to giant aneurysms when body surface area is considered. For example, a 3-month-old infant with coronary arteries 6 or 7 mm in diameter often would be a candidate for anticoagulation.

Subsequent Immunization. Measles and varicella-containing vaccines should be deferred for 11 months after receipt of high-dose IGIV for treatment of Kawasaki disease, and varicella-containing vaccines should be avoided during aspirin therapy. If the child's risk of exposure to measles or varicella is high, the child should be immunized and then

---

[1] Newburger JW, Takahashi M, Gerber MA, et al. Diagnosis, treatment and long-term management of Kawasaki disease: a statement for health professionals from the Committee on Rheumatic Fever, Endocarditis and Kawasaki Disease, Council on Cardiovascular Disease in the Young, American Heart Association. *Circulation.* 2004;110(17):2747–2771 (also in *Pediatrics.* 2004;114[6]:1708–1733)

reimmunized at least 11 months after administration of IGIV (see Table 1.9, p 38). The schedule for administration of inactivated childhood vaccines should not be interrupted.

ISOLATION OF THE HOSPITALIZED PATIENT: Standard precautions are indicated.

CONTROL MEASURES: None.

Kingella kingae Infections

CLINICAL MANIFESTATIONS: The most common infections associated with *Kingella kingae* are suppurative arthritis, osteomyelitis, and bacteremia. Almost all skeletal infections occur in children younger than 5 years of age. *K kingae* may be a major cause of skeletal infections in children younger than 3 years of age. Pyogenic arthritis caused by *K kingae* generally is monoarticular, most commonly involving the knee, followed in frequency by the hip or ankle. Clinical manifestations of pyogenic arthritis are similar to manifestations associated with infection attributable to other bacterial pathogens in immunocompetent children, although a subacute course may be more common. Osteomyelitis caused by *K kingae* has clinical manifestations similar to *Staphylococcus aureus* osteomyelitis, but epiphyseal infection and a subacute course may be more common. The distal femur is the most common site of osteomyelitis. Bacteremia can occur in previously healthy children and in children with preexisting chronic medical problems; some cases have occurred in adolescents. In addition to fever, children with *K kingae* bacteremia frequently have concurrent findings of respiratory or gastrointestinal tract disease. *K kingae* also has been associated with diskitis, endocarditis in children with underlying heart disease (HACEK group of organisms), meningitis, occult bacteremia, and pneumonia.

ETIOLOGY: *Kingella* organisms are fastidious, gram-negative coccobacilli previously classified as *Moraxella*. Of the 4 species in the genus *Kingella, K kingae* is the species most commonly associated with infection.

EPIDEMIOLOGY: The human oropharynx is the usual habitat of *K kingae*. The organism more frequently colonizes young children than adults and can be transmitted among children in child care centers, generally without causing disease. Infection may be associated with preceding or concomitant stomatitis or upper respiratory tract illness.

The **incubation period** is variable.

DIAGNOSTIC TESTS: *K kingae* can be isolated from blood, synovial fluid, bone exudate, cerebrospinal fluid, respiratory tract secretions, and other sites of infection. Organisms grow better in aerobic conditions with enhanced carbon dioxide. In patients with pyogenic arthritis and osteomyelitis, blood cultures often are negative for *K kingae*. *K kingae* is difficult to isolate on routinely used solid media. Synovial fluid and bone aspirates from patients with suspected *K kingae* infection should be inoculated into Bactec, BacT/Alert, or similar blood culture systems and held for at least 7 days to maximize recovery. Conventional and real-time polymerase chain reaction methods have improved detection of *K kingae* in research studies. *K kingae* should be suspected in young children with culture-negative skeletal infections.

TREATMENT: *K kingae* infrequently produces beta-lactamase. Penicillin is the drug of choice for treatment of invasive infections attributable to beta-lactamase–negative strains of *K kingae*. Strains generally are susceptible to ampicillin-sulbactam, aminoglycosides, ciprofloxacin, erythromycin, chloramphenicol, and oxacillin and are resistant to trimethoprim, clindamycin, and vancomycin. Although *K kingae* are resistant to trimethoprim, most strains are susceptible to trimethoprim-sulfamethoxazole. Gentamicin in combination with penicillin can be useful for the initial treatment of endocarditis. Extended-spectrum cephalosporins cefotaxime or ceftriaxone also may be used to treat endocarditis.

ISOLATION OF THE HOSPITALIZED PATIENT: Standard precautions are recommended.

CONTROL MEASURES: None.

Legionella pneumophila Infections

CLINICAL MANIFESTATIONS: Legionellosis is associated with 2 clinically and epidemiologically distinct illnesses: Legionnaires disease and Pontiac fever. **Legionnaires disease** varies in severity from mild to severe pneumonia characterized by fever, cough, and progressive respiratory distress. Legionnaires disease can be associated with chills, myalgia, gastrointestinal tract, central nervous system, and renal manifestations. Respiratory failure and death can occur. **Pontiac fever** is a milder febrile illness without pneumonia that occurs in epidemics and is characterized by an abrupt onset and a self-limited, influenza-like illness.

ETIOLOGY: *Legionella* species are fastidious aerobic bacilli that stain gram negative after recovery on buffered charcoal yeast extract (BCYE) media. At least 20 different species have been implicated in human disease, but the most common species causing infections in the United States is *Legionella pneumophila*, with most isolates belonging to serogroup 1.

EPIDEMIOLOGY: Legionnaires disease is acquired through inhalation of aerosolized water contaminated with *Legionella pneumophila*. Person-to-person transmission has not been demonstrated. More than 80% of cases are sporadic; the sources of infection can be related to exposure to *L pneumophila*-contaminated water in the home, workplace, or hospitals or other medical facilities or to aerosol-producing devices in public places. Outbreaks have been ascribed to common-source exposure to contaminated cooling towers, evaporative condensers, potable water systems, whirlpool spas, humidifiers, and respiratory therapy equipment. Outbreaks have occurred in hospitals, hotels, and other large buildings as well as on cruise ships. Health care-associated infections can occur and often are related to contamination of the hot water supply. Legionnaires disease occurs most commonly in people who are elderly, are immunocompromised, or have underlying lung disease. Infection in children is rare and usually is asymptomatic or mild and unrecognized. Severe disease has occurred in children with malignant neoplasms, severe combined immunodeficiency, chronic granulomatous disease, organ transplantation, end-stage renal disease, underlying pulmonary disease, and immunosuppression; in children receiving systemic corticosteroids; and as a health care-associated infection in newborn infants.

The **incubation period** for Legionnaires disease (pneumonia) is 2 to 10 days; for Pontiac fever, the incubation period is 1 to 2 days.

DIAGNOSTIC TESTS: Recovery of *Legionella* from respiratory tract secretions, lung tissue, pleural fluid, or other normally sterile fluid specimens by using BCYE media provides definitive evidence of infection, but the sensitivity of culture is laboratory dependent. Detection of *Legionella* antigen in urine by commercially available immunoassays is highly specific. Such tests are sensitive for *L pneumophila* serogroup 1, but these tests rarely detect antigen in patients infected with other *L pneumophila* serogroups or other *Legionella* species. The bacterium can be demonstrated in specimens by direct immunofluorescent assay, but this test is less sensitive, and the specificity is technician dependent and lower than culture or urine immunoassay. Genus-specific polymerase chain reaction-based assays have been developed that detect *Legionella* DNA in respiratory secretions as well as in blood and urine of some patients with pneumonia. For serologic diagnosis, a fourfold increase in titer of antibodies to *L pneumophila* serogroup 1, measured by indirect immunofluorescent antibody (IFA) assay, confirms a recent infection. Convalescent serum samples should be obtained 3 to 4 weeks after onset of symptoms; however, a titer increase can be delayed for 8 to 12 weeks. The positive predictive value of a single titer of 1:256 or greater is low and does not provide definitive evidence of infection. Antibodies to several gram-negative organisms, including *Pseudomonas* species, *Bacteroides fragilis*, and *Campylobacter jejuni*, can cause false-positive IFA test results. Newer serologic assays, such as enzyme immunoassay or tests using *Legionella* antigens other than serogroup 1, are available commercially but have not been standardized adequately.

TREATMENT: Intravenous azithromycin has replaced intravenous erythromycin as the drug of choice. Once the condition of a patient is improving, oral therapy can be substituted. Levofloxacin (or another fluoroquinolone) is the drug of choice for immunocompromised patients, because fluoroquinolone antimicrobial agents are bactericidal and are more effective than macrolides in vitro and in animal models of infection, and limited available observational study data in adults suggest that clinical improvement (resolution of fever and duration of hospitalization) is more rapid with a fluoroquinolone than with a macrolide/azalide. Fluoroquinolones are not approved for this indication in children younger than 18 years of age (see Fluoroquinolones, p 800). Doxycycline and trimethoprim-sulfamethoxazole are alternative drugs. Doxycycline should not be used for pregnant women or for children younger than 8 years of age unless there are no other therapeutic options (see Tetracyclines, p 801). Duration of therapy is 5 to 10 days for azithromycin and 14 to 21 days for other drugs. Longer courses of therapy are recommended for patients who are immunocompromised or who have severe disease.

ISOLATION OF THE HOSPITALIZED PATIENT: Standard precautions are recommended.

CONTROL MEASURES: Monochloramine (rather than free chlorine) treatment of municipal water supplies has been associated with a decrease in health care-associated Legionnaires disease. Hospitals should maintain hot water at the highest temperature allowable by state regulations or codes, preferably 60°C (140°F) or greater, and maintain cold water temperature at less than 20°C (68°F) to minimize waterborne *Legionella* contamination. Occurrence of even a single laboratory-confirmed health care-associated case of legionellosis warrants consideration of an epidemiologic and environmental investigation. Hospitals with transplantation programs (solid organ or hematopoietic stem cell) should maintain a high index of suspicion of legionellosis, use sterile water for the filling and terminal rinsing of nebulization devices, and consider performing periodic culturing for *Legionella* species in the potable water supply of the transplant unit. Some hospitals may choose to perform periodic, routine culturing of water samples from the hospital's potable water system to detect *Legionella* species.

The usual methods for decontaminating potable water supplies to prevent health care-associated cases are hyperchlorination often followed by maintenance of a 1- to 2-mg/L (1- to 2-ppm) free residual chlorine concentration in the heated water or superheating (to 66°C [150°F] or greater) followed by maintenance of a hot water temperature at the faucet of greater than 50°C (122°F). Long-term decontamination of the potable water supply usually requires installation of a permanent disinfection system.

Leishmaniasis

CLINICAL MANIFESTATIONS: The 3 major clinical syndromes are as follows:

- *Cutaneous leishmaniasis.* After inoculation by the bite of an infected female phlebotomine sand fly (approximately 2–3 mm long), parasites proliferate locally in mononuclear phagocytes, leading to an erythematous papule, which typically slowly enlarges to become a nodule and then a shallow painless ulcerative lesion with raised borders. Ulcerative lesions may become dry and crusted or may develop a moist granulating base with an overlying exudate. Lesions can, however, persist as nodules or papules and may be single or multiple. Lesions commonly are located on exposed areas of the body (eg, face and extremities) and may be accompanied by satellite lesions, which appear as sporotrichoid-like nodules, and regional adenopathy. Clinical manifestations of Old World and New World (American) cutaneous leishmaniasis are similar. Spontaneous resolution of lesions may take weeks to years and usually results in a flat atrophic (cigarette paper) scar. Cutaneous leishmaniasis attributable to the *Viannia* subspecies—*Leishmania (Viannia) braziliensis, Leishmania (Viannia) panamensis,* and *Leishmania (Viannia) guyanensis*—seldom heals without treatment.

- *Mucosal leishmaniasis (espundia).* Hematogenous mucocutaneous leishmaniasis (**espundia**) primarily is associated with the *Viannia* subspecies. Mucosal involvement can occur by extension of facial lesions attributable to other species. Mucosal infection is primarily found in the New World. It may become evident clinically from months to years after the cutaneous lesions heal; sometimes mucosal and cutaneous lesions are noted simultaneously. Parasites may disseminate to the naso-oropharyngeal mucosa. Granulomatous inflammation may cause hypertrophy of the nose and lips. In some patients, granulomatous ulceration and necrosis follows, leading to facial disfigurement, secondary infection, and mucosal perforation, which may occur months to years after the initial cutaneous lesion heals.

- *Visceral leishmaniasis (kala-azar).* After cutaneous inoculation of parasites by the sand fly vector, organisms spread throughout the mononuclear macrophage system to the spleen, liver, and bone marrow. The resulting clinical illness typically manifests as fever, anorexia, weight loss, splenomegaly, hepatomegaly, anemia, leukopenia, thrombocytopenia sometimes associated with hemorrhage, hypoalbuminemia, and hypergammaglobulinemia. Peripheral lymphadenopathy is commonly seen in Sudan and East Africa. Kala-azar ("black sickness") refers to hyperpigmentation of skin seen in late-stage disease in patients in the Indian subcontinent. Secondary gram-negative enteric infections and tuberculosis may occur as a result of suppression of the cell-mediated immune response. Untreated fully manifested visceral infection is nearly always fatal. At the other end of the spectrum are patients who are minimally symptomatic but harbor viable parasites lifelong. Reactivation of latent visceral infection can occur in patients who become immunocompromised, including people with concurrent human immunodeficiency virus (HIV) infection and recipients of stem cell or solid organ transplants.

ETIOLOGY: In the human host, *Leishmania* species are obligate intracellular parasites of mononuclear phagocytes. Cutaneous leishmaniasis typically is caused by Old World species *Leishmania tropica, Leishmania major,* and *Leishmania aethiopica* and by New World species *Leishmania mexicana, Leishmania amazonensis, Leishmania braziliensis, Leishmania panamensis, Leishmania guyanensis,* and *Leishmania peruviana.* Mucosal leishmaniasis typically is caused by *Leishmania (V) braziliensis*, *L (V) panamensis*, and *L (V) guyanensis*. Visceral leishmaniasis is caused by *Leishmania donovani* and *Leishmania infantum* (*Leishmania chagasi* is synonymous). *L. donovani* and *L infantum* can cause cutaneous leishmaniasis. However, people with typical cutaneous leishmaniasis caused by these organisms rarely develop visceral leishmaniasis.

EPIDEMIOLOGY: Leishmaniasis typically is a zoonosis with a variety of mammalian reservoir hosts, including canines and rodents. However, the only proven reservoir of *L donovani* in the Indian subcontinent consists of infected humans, and transmission has a large anthroponotic component in East Africa as well. Transmission primarily is vector-borne through the bite of infected female phlebotomine sand flies. Congenital and parenteral transmission also have been reported. Leishmaniasis is endemic in 88 countries, from northern Argentina to southern Texas (not including Uruguay or Chile), in southern Europe, China and Central Asia, the Indian subcontinent, the Middle East, and Africa (particularly East and North Africa, with sporadic cases elsewhere) but not in Australia or Oceania. Overall, visceral leishmaniasis is found in focal areas of approximately 65 countries. Most (>90%) of the world's cases of visceral leishmaniasis occur in the Indian subcontinent (India, Bangladesh, and Nepal), Sudan, and Brazil. The estimated annual number of new cases of cutaneous leishmaniasis is approximately 1.5 million; more than 90% of these occur in Afghanistan, Algeria, Iran, Iraq, Saudi Arabia, and Syria (Old World) and in Brazil and Peru (New World). Approximately 90% of cases of mucosal leishmaniasis occur in 3 countries: Bolivia, Brazil, and Peru. Geographic distribution of cases evaluated in the developed world reflects travel and immigration patterns. The number of cases has increased as a result of increased travel to areas with endemic infection; for example, with ecotourism activities in Central and South America and military activities in Iraq and Afghanistan, the number of imported cases within North America has increased.

The **incubation periods** for the different forms of leishmaniasis range from several days to several years but usually are in the range of several weeks to 6 months. In cutaneous leishmaniasis, primary skin lesions typically appear several weeks after parasite inoculation. In visceral infection, the incubation period typically ranges from 2 to 6 months.

DIAGNOSTIC TESTS: Definitive diagnosis is made by demonstration of the presence of the parasite. A common way of identifying the parasite is by microscopic identification of intracellular leishmanial organisms (amastigotes) on Wright- or Giemsa-stained smears or histologic sections of infected tissues. In cutaneous disease, tissue can be obtained by a 3-mm punch biopsy, by lesion scrapings, or by needle aspiration of the raised non-necrotic edge of the lesion. In visceral leishmaniasis, the organisms can be identified in the spleen and, less commonly, in bone marrow and the liver. The sensitivity is highest for splenic aspiration (approximately 95%), but so is the risk of hemorrhage or bowel perforation. In East Africa in patients with lymphadenopathy, the organisms also can be identified in lymph nodes. Blood cultures, especially of buffy-coat preparations, have been positive in some patients, and organisms occasionally may be observed in blood smears or cultured from buffy-coat preparations in HIV-infected patients. Isolation of parasites (promastigotes) by culture of appropriate tissue specimens in specialized media may take days to several weeks but should be attempted when possible. Knowledge of the infecting species may affect prognosis and influence treatment decisions. Culture media and further information can be provided by the Centers for Disease Control and Prevention (CDC) (**www.cdc.gov/travel**). Investigational polymerase chain reaction assays are available at some reference laboratories.

The diagnosis of some forms of leishmaniasis can be aided by performance of serologic testing, which is available at the CDC. Serologic test results usually are positive in cases of visceral and mucosal leishmaniasis if the patient is immunocompetent but often are negative in cutaneous leishmaniasis. False-positive results may occur in patients with other infectious diseases, especially American trypanosomiasis.

TREATMENT: The decision whether to treat leishmaniasis should be made on an individual basis, with the assistance of infectious disease experts or consultation from the CDC Division of Parasitic Diseases and Malaria: telephone: 770-488-7775; e-mail: parasites@cdc.gov; CDC Emergency Operator (after business hours and on weekends): 770-488-7100. Treatment always is indicated for patients with mucosal or visceral leishmaniasis. Liposomal amphotericin B is the only treatment approved by the US Food and Drug Administration for visceral leishmaniasis and is the most efficacious and least toxic of the antileishmanial drugs available in the United States. Sodium stibogluconate, available through the CDC under an investigational new drug protocol, generally has high efficacy but carries the risk of cardiac and other toxicity. Because of the high prevalence of primary antimonial resistance in India and Nepal, sodium stibogluconate should not be used for patients with visceral leishmaniasis infected in South Asia; liposomal amphotericin B or conventional amphotericin B desoxycholate should be used instead. Paromomycin intramuscular injection is approved for the treatment of visceral leishmaniasis in several countries. Treatment of cutaneous leishmaniasis should be considered, especially if skin lesions are or could become disfiguring or disabling (eg, facial lesions or lesions near joints), are persistent, or are known to be or might be caused by leishmanial species that can disseminate to the naso-oropharyngeal mucosa (see Drugs for Parasitic Infections, p 848). Local wound care and treatment of bacterial superinfection also must be considered in cutaneous leishmaniasis. Miltefosine, the first oral agent for treatment of leishmaniasis, is not licensed or available in the United States but may be used under an individual compassionate use investigational new drug (IND) protocol from the FDA. Miltefosine has demonstrated degrees of efficacy in visceral leishmaniasis and in New and Old World cutaneous lesions but is contraindicated in pregnancy. Meglumine antimoniate by injection is supported by the World Health Organization for treatment of leishmaniasis but is not available in the United States. Paromomycin and azole antifungal drugs also may have some degree of efficacy. Clinical trials of various combination therapies are ongoing. Considerations in HIV-coinfection include monitoring for the immune reconstitution syndrome and secondary prophylaxis.

ISOLATION OF THE HOSPITALIZED PATIENT: Standard precautions are recommended.

CONTROL MEASURES: The best way for travelers to prevent leishmaniasis is by protecting themselves from sand-fly bites. Vaccines and drugs for preventing infection are not available. To decrease risk of being bitten, travelers should:

- Stay in well-screened or air-conditioned areas when feasible. Avoid outdoor activities, especially from dusk to dawn, when sand flies are most active.
- When outside, wear long-sleeved shirts, long pants, and socks.
- Apply insect repellent on uncovered skin and under the ends of sleeves and pant legs. Follow instructions on the label of the repellent. The most effective repellents are those that contain the chemical diethyltoluamide (DEET) (see Prevention of Mosquitoborne Infections, p 209).

- Spray clothing with permethrin-containing insecticides several days before travel and allow them to dry. The insecticide should be reapplied after every 5 washings. Permethrin should never be applied to skin.
- Spray living and sleeping areas with an insecticide.
- If not sleeping in an area that is well screened or air conditioned, a bed net tucked under the mattress is recommended. If possible, a bed net that has been soaked in or sprayed with permethrin should be used. The permethrin will be effective for several months if the bed net is not washed. Sand flies are smaller than mosquitoes and, therefore, can get through smaller holes. Fine-mesh netting (at least 18 holes to the inch) is needed for an effective barrier against sand flies. This particularly is important if the bed net has not been treated with permethrin. However, sleeping under such a closely woven bed net in hot weather can be uncomfortable.
- Bed nets, repellents containing DEET, and permethrin should be purchased before traveling.

Leprosy

CLINICAL MANIFESTATIONS: Leprosy (Hansen disease) is a curable infection involving skin, peripheral nerves, mucosa of the upper respiratory tract, and testes. The clinical forms of leprosy reflect the cellular immune response to *Mycobacterium leprae* and the organism's unique tropism for peripheral nerves. In the United States, the Ridley-Jopling scale is used and has 5 classifications that correlate with histologic findings: (1) polar tuberculoid; (2) borderline tuberculoid; (3) borderline; (4) borderline lepromatous; and (5) polar lepromatous.

The cell-mediated immunity of most patients and their clinical presentation occur between the 2 extremes of tuberculoid and lepromatous forms. Leprosy lesions usually do not itch or hurt; they lack sensation to heat, touch, and pain. The classic presentation of the "leonine facies" and loss of lateral eyebrows (madarosis) occurs in patients with end-stage lepromatous leprosy. A simplified scheme introduced by the World Health Organization, for situations in which there is no doctor, classifies leprosy involving 1 patch of skin as (1) paucibacillary single lesion; (2) paucibacillary (2-5 lesions; usually tuberculous leprosy); and (3) multibacillary (>5 lesions, usually lepromatous leprosy).

Serious consequences of leprosy occur from immune reactions and nerve involvement with resulting anesthesia, which can lead to repeated unrecognized trauma, ulcerations, fractures, and bone resorption. Injuries can have a significant effect on quality of life, because leprosy is a leading cause of permanent physical disability among communicable diseases worldwide. Eye involvement can occur, and patients should be examined by an ophthalmologist. A diagnosis of leprosy should be considered in any patient with hypoesthetic or anesthetic skin rash.

Leprosy Reactions: Acute clinical exacerbations reflect abrupt changes in immunologic balance, especially common during initial years of treatment but can occur in the absence of therapy. Two major types are seen: type 1 (reversal reaction) is predominantly observed in borderline tuberculoid and borderline lepromatous leprosy and is the result of a sudden increase in effective cell-mediated immunity. Acute tenderness and swelling at the site of cutaneous and neural lesions with development of new lesions are major manifestations. Ulcerations can occur. Fever and systemic toxicity are uncommon. Type 2 (erythema nodosum leprosum) occurs in borderline and lepromatous forms as a systemic inflammatory response. Tender, red dermal papules or nodules resembling erythema nodosum along with high fever, migrating polyarthralgia, painful swelling of lymph nodes and spleen, iridocyclitis, and rarely, nephritis can occur.

ETIOLOGY: Leprosy is caused by *M leprae*, an obligate intracellular, acid-fast bacillus that can have variable results on Gram stain. It is weakly acid-fast on standard Ziehl-Nielsen staining and is best identified using the Fite stain. *M leprae* is the only bacterium known to infect nerves.

EPIDEMIOLOGY: Leprosy primarily is a disease of poverty. Approximately 5% of people genetically are susceptible to infection with *M leprae*; several genes now have been identified that are associated with susceptibility to *M leprae*. Accordingly, spouses of leprosy patients are not likely to develop leprosy, but biological parents, children, and siblings who are household contacts of untreated patients with leprosy are at increased risk. The major source of infectious material probably is nasal secretions from patients with untreated infection. Little shedding of *M leprae* from involved intact skin occurs. People with human immunodeficiency virus (HIV) infection do not appear to be at increased risk of becoming infected with *M leprae*. Concomitant HIV infection and leprosy can result in worsening of symptoms of leprosy during HIV treatment as a result of immune reconstitution inflammatory syndrome. There are approximately 6500 leprosy cases in the United States; approximately 3300 require active medical management. As of early 2009, the World Health Organization new case detection rate for the United States was less than 0.1 per 100 000 population. Most cases of leprosy reported were in native-born US citizens from Texas and Louisiana and among immigrants in California, Florida, New York, and Massachusetts. More than 65% of the world's leprosy patients reside in South and Southeast Asia—the majority of these patients reside in India. High endemicity remains in some areas of Angola, Brazil, Central African Republic, Democratic Republic of Congo, India, Madagascar, Mozambique, Nepal, Republic of the Marshall Islands, the Federated States of Micronesia, and the United Republic of Tanzania.

The infectivity of lepromatous patients ceases within 24 hours of the first administration of multidrug therapy, the standard antimicrobial treatment for leprosy.

The **incubation period** ranges from 1 to many years but usually is 3 to 5 years. The incubation period of the tuberculoid form appears to be shorter than that for the lepromatous form. Symptoms can take up to 20 years to develop and are most likely to appear in individuals 20 to 30 years of age.

DIAGNOSTIC TESTS: Histopathologic examination of skin biopsy by an experienced pathologist is the best method of establishing the diagnosis and is the basis for classification of leprosy. These specimens can be sent to National Hansen's Disease (Leprosy) Programs (NHDP) (800-642-2477; **www.hrsa.gov/hansens**) in formalin or embedded in paraffin. Acid-fast bacilli can be found in slit-smears or biopsy specimens of skin lesions but rarely from patients with tuberculoid and indeterminate forms of disease. Organisms have not been cultured successfully in vitro. Molecular tests for mutations causing drug resistance are available through the NHDP.

A polymerase chain reaction (PCR) test for *M leprae* is available on a limited basis after consultation with the NHDP. For early diagnosis, clinical suspicion is vital. Studies from India in early cases indicate that in situ hybridization and in situ PCR techniques are promising and have shown comparable results with in vitro PCR; both allow concomitant histopathologic examination.

TREATMENT: Therapy for patients with leprosy should be undertaken in consultation with an expert in leprosy. The NHDP (800-642-2477) provides medications for leprosy at no charge as well as consultation on clinical and pathologic issues and information about local Hansen disease clinics and clinicians who have experience with the disease.

Leprosy is curable. The primary goal of therapy is prevention of permanent nerve damage, which can be accomplished by early diagnosis and treatment. Combination antimicrobial multidrug therapy (MDT) can be obtained free of charge in the United States from the NHDP and from the World Health Organization in other countries. It is important to treat *M leprae* infections with more than 1 antimicrobial agent to minimize development of antimicrobial-resistant organisms. Adults are treated with dapsone, rifampin, and clofazimine. Resistance to all 3 drugs has been documented but is rare in the United States.

Treatment Regimens Recommended by the NHDP.

Multibacillary leprosy (6 patches or more):
1. Dapsone, 100 mg/day, orally, for 24 months. Pediatric dose: 1 mg/kg, orally, every 24 hours. Maximum dose: 100 mg/day for 24 months; **and**
2. Rifampin, 600 mg/day, orally, for 24 months. Pediatric dose: 10 mg/kg per day for 24 months; **and**
3. Clofazimine, 50 mg/day, orally, for 24 months. Clarithromycin can be used in place of clofazimine for children. Pediatric dose: 7.5 mg/kg per day, orally, for 24 months. Clofazimine is not available commercially; in the United States, it is available only as an investigational drug for treatment of leprosy, and is obtained through the NHDP.

Paucibacillary leprosy (1–5 patches):
1. Dapsone, 100 mg/day, orally, for 12 months. Pediatric dose: 1 to 2 mg/kg, orally, every 24 hours. Maximum dose: 100 mg/day for 12 months; **and**
2. Rifampin, 600 mg/day, orally, for 12 months. Pediatric dose: 10 to 20 mg/kg per day, orally, for 12 months.

Before beginning antimicrobial therapy, patients should be tested for glucose-6-phosphate dehydrogenase deficiency, have baseline complete blood cell counts and liver function test results documented, and be evaluated for any evidence of tuberculosis infection, especially if the patient is infected with HIV. This consideration is important to avoid monotherapy of active tuberculosis with rifampin while treating active leprosy.

Adverse reactions of MDT commonly include darkening of skin caused by daily clofazimine therapy. This will resolve within several months of completing therapy.

Leprosy reactions should be treated aggressively to prevent peripheral nerve damage. Treatment with prednisone, 1 mg/kg per day, orally, can be initiated. The severe type 2 reaction, known as erythema nodosum leprosum (ENL), occurs in patients with multibacillary leprosy. Treatment with thalidomide (100 mg/day for 4 days) is available for ENL under the Celgene S.T.E.P.S. Program (888-771-0141) and is used under strict supervision because of its teratogenicity. Thalidomide is not approved for use in children younger than 12 years of age. Most patients can be treated as outpatients. Rehabilitative measures, including surgery and physical therapy, may be necessary for some patients.

All patients with leprosy should be educated about signs and symptoms of neuritis and cautioned to report signs and symptoms of neuritis immediately so that corticosteroid therapy can be instituted. Patients should receive counseling because of the social and psychological effects of this disease.

Relapse of disease after completing MDT is rare (0.01%–0.14%); the presentation of new skin patches usually is attributable to a late type 1 reaction. Self-examination is critical for any patient with loss of sensitivity in the foot. When it does occur, relapse usually is attributable to reactivation of drug-susceptible organisms. People with relapses of disease require another course of MDT.

ISOLATION OF THE HOSPITALIZED PATIENT: Standard precautions are indicated; isolation is not required.

CONTROL MEASURES: Hand hygiene is recommended for all people in contact with a patient with lepromatous leprosy. Disinfection of nasal secretions, handkerchiefs, and other fomites should be considered until treatment is established. Household contacts, particularly contacts of patients with multibacillary disease, should be examined initially and then annually for 5 years. Postnatal transmission can occur during breastfeeding. Chemoprophylaxis is not recommended. Local public health department regulations for leprosy vary and should be consulted.

A single bacille Calmette-Guérin (BCG) immunization is reported to be from 28% to 60% protective against leprosy. The first commercially available leprosy vaccine was approved in India in January 1998. This vaccine was approved as an immunotherapeutic adjuvant to be used with multidrug therapy; it is not available in the United States. Neither BCG nor the heat-killed leprosy vaccine is recommended for use in household contacts of people with leprosy in the United States.

Newly diagnosed or suspected cases of leprosy in the United States should be reported to local and state public health departments, the Centers for Disease Control and Prevention, and the NHDP.

Leptospirosis

CLINICAL MANIFESTATIONS: Leptospirosis is an acute febrile disease with varied manifestations characterized by vasculitis. The severity of disease ranges from asymptomatic or subclinical to self-limited systemic illness (approximately 90% of patients) to life-threatening illness with jaundice, renal failure, and hemorrhagic pneumonitis. Clinical presentation typically is biphasic, with an acute septicemia phase usually lasting 1 week, followed by a second immune-mediated phase. Regardless of its severity, the acute phase is characterized by nonspecific symptoms, including fever, chills, headache, nausea, vomiting, and a transient rash. The most distinct clinical findings are conjunctival suffusion without purulent discharge (30%–99% of cases) and myalgias of the calf and lumbar regions (40% to 100% of cases). In some patients, the 2 phases are separated by a short-lived abatement of fever (3–4 days). Findings commonly associated with the immune-mediated phase include fever, aseptic meningitis, conjunctival suffusion, uveitis, muscle tenderness, adenopathy, and purpuric rash. Approximately 10% of patients have severe illness, including jaundice and renal dysfunction (Weil syndrome), hemorrhagic pneumonitis, cardiac arrhythmias, or circulatory collapse associated with a case-fatality rate of 5% to 15%. The overall duration of symptoms for both phases of disease varies from less than 1 week to several months. Asymptomatic or subclinical infection with seroconversion is frequent, especially in settings of endemic infection.

ETIOLOGY: Leptospirosis is caused by pathogenic spirochetes of the genus *Leptospira*. Leptospires previously were classified into 2 species, which then were subdivided into more than 200 antigenically defined serovars, grouped into serogroups on the basis of serologic relatedness. Currently, the molecular classification divides the genus into 20 named pathogenic and nonpathogenic genomospecies as determined by DNA-DNA hybridization.

EPIDEMIOLOGY: The reservoirs for *Leptospira* species include a wide range of wild and domestic animals that may shed organisms asymptomatically for years. *Leptospira* organisms excreted in animal urine, amniotic fluid, or placental tissue may remain viable in moist soil or water for weeks to months in warm climates. Humans usually become infected via entry of leptospires through contact of mucosal surfaces or abraded skin with contaminated soil, water, or animal tissues. Infection may be acquired through direct contact with infected animals or their tissues or through contact with infective urine or fluids from carrier animals or urine-contaminated soil or water. People who are predisposed by occupation include abattoir and sewer workers, miners, veterinarians, farmers, and military personnel. Recreational exposures and clusters of disease have been associated with wading, swimming (especially being submerged in or swallowing water), or boating in contaminated water, particularly during flooding or following heavy rainfall. Person-to-person transmission is rare.

The **incubation period** usually is 5 to 14 days, range 2 to 30 days.

DIAGNOSTIC TESTS: *Leptospira* organisms can be isolated from blood or cerebrospinal fluid specimens during the early septicemic phase (first 7–10 days) of illness and subsequently from urine specimens. However, isolation of the organism may be difficult, requiring special media and techniques and incubation for up to 16 weeks. In addition, the sensitivity of culture for diagnosis is low. For these reasons, serum specimens always should be obtained to facilitate diagnosis. Antibodies can develop as early as 5 to 7 days after onset of illness, and can be measured by commercially available immunoassays; however, increases in antibody titer may not be detected until more than10 days after onset, especially if antimicrobial therapy is initiated. Antibody increases can be transient, delayed, or absent in some patients. Microscopic agglutination, the confirmatory serologic test, is performed only in reference laboratories and requires seroconversion demonstrated between acute and convalescent specimens obtained at least 10 days apart. Immunohistochemical techniques can detect leptospiral antigens in infected tissues. Polymerase chain reaction assays for detection of *Leptospira* organisms have been developed but are available only in research laboratories.

TREATMENT: Intravenous penicillin is the drug of choice for patients with severe infection requiring hospitalization and is effective as late as 7 days into the course of illness. Penicillin G decreases the duration of systemic symptoms and persistence of associated laboratory abnormalities and may prevent development of leptospiruria. As with other spirochetal infections, a Jarisch-Herxheimer reaction (an acute febrile reaction accompanied by headache, myalgia, and an aggravated clinical picture lasting less than 24 hours) can develop after initiation of penicillin therapy. Parenteral cefotaxime, doxycycline, and ceftriaxone have been demonstrated in randomized clinical trials to be equal in efficacy to penicillin G for treatment of severe leptospirosis. Severe cases also require appropriate supportive care, including fluid and electrolyte replacement, and often dialysis. For patients with mild disease, oral doxycycline has been shown to shorten the course of illness and decrease occurrence of leptospiruria. Doxycycline should not be used in pregnant women or children younger than 8 years of age unless no other treatment options are available (see Tetracyclines, p 801). Azithromycin has been demonstrated in a clinical trial to be as effective as doxycycline and can be used as an alternative to doxycycline in patients for whom doxycycline is contraindicated.

ISOLATION OF THE HOSPITALIZED PATIENT: In addition to standard precautions, contact precautions are recommended for contact with urine.

CONTROL MEASURES:
- Immunization of animals can prevent clinical disease attributable to infecting serovars contained within the vaccine. However, immunization may not prevent animals from shedding leptospires in their urine and, thus, contaminating environments with which humans may come in contact.
- In areas with known endemic infection, reservoir-control programs may be useful.
- Swimmers should attempt to avoid immersion or swallowing water in potentially contaminated fresh water.
- Protective clothing, boots, and gloves should be worn to decrease risk to people with occupational exposure.
- Doxycycline, 200 mg, administered orally once a week to adults, may provide effective prophylaxis against clinical disease and could be considered for high-risk groups with short-term exposure, but infection may not be prevented. However, indications for prophylactic doxycycline use for children have not been established.

Listeria monocytogenes Infections
(Listeriosis)

CLINICAL MANIFESTATIONS: Listeriosis is a relatively uncommon but severe invasive infection caused by *Listeria monocytogenes*. Listeriosis transmission predominantly is food-borne and occurs most frequently among pregnant women and their fetuses or newborn infants, people of advanced age, and immunocompromised patients. In pregnant women, infections can be asymptomatic or associated with an influenza-like illness with fever, malaise, headache, gastrointestinal tract symptoms, and back pain. Approximately 65% of pregnant women with *Listeria* infection experience a prodromal illness before the diagnosis of listeriosis in their newborn infant. Amnionitis during labor, brown staining of amniotic fluid, or asymptomatic perinatal infection can occur. Neonatal illnesses have early-onset and late-onset syndromes similar to those of group B streptococcal infections. Preterm birth, pneumonia, and septicemia are common in early-onset disease. An erythematous rash with small, pale papules characterized histologically by granulomas, termed "granulomatosis infantisepticum," can occur in severe newborn infection. Late-onset infections occur after the first week of life and usually result in meningitis. Clinical features characteristic of invasive listeriosis outside the neonatal period or pregnancy are septicemia and meningitis with or without parenchymal brain involvement in: (1) immunocompromised patients, including people with organ transplantation, acquired immunodeficiency syndrome, hematologic malignancies, or immunosuppression attributable to corticosteroids; (2) people older than 50 years of age; or (3) patients for whom reports from the laboratory indicate "diphtheroids" on Gram stain or culture from normally sterile sources. *L monocytogenes* also can cause rhombencephalitis (brain stem encephalitis), brain abscess, and endocarditis. Outbreaks of febrile gastroenteritis caused by food contaminated with *L monocytogenes* have been reported.

ETIOLOGY: *L monocytogenes* is a facultative anaerobic, nonspore-forming, motile, gram-positive bacillus that multiplies intracellularly. The organism produces a narrow zone of hemolysis on blood agar medium. *L monocytogenes* serotypes 1/2a, 4b, and 1/2b cause most human cases of invasive listeriosis.

EPIDEMIOLOGY: *L monocytogenes* causes an estimated 2500 cases of invasive disease and 500 deaths annually in the United States. The saprophytic organism is distributed widely in the environment and is an important cause of zoonoses, especially in ruminants. Foodborne transmission causes outbreaks and sporadic infections. Incriminated foods include unpasteurized milk, dairy products, and soft cheeses, including Mexican-style cheese; prepared ready-to-eat deli foods, such as hot dogs, cold cut meats and deli salads, hummus, and pâté; undercooked poultry; precooked seafood and smoked or cured fish; melons and fruit salads; and unwashed raw vegetables. In 2011, a large outbreak of listeriosis occurred in the United States associated with contaminated cantaloupe.[1] The incidence of listeriosis has decreased substantially since 1989, when US regulatory agencies began enforcing rigorous screening guidelines for *L monocytogenes* in ready-to-eat foods. Fetal infection results from transplacental transmission following maternal bacteremia, although some infections can occur through ascending spread from vaginal colonization. Pregnancy-associated infections can result in spontaneous abortion, fetal death, preterm delivery, and neonatal illness or death. Late-onset neonatal infection can result from acquisition of the organism during passage through the birth canal or from environmental sources, followed by hematogenous invasion of the organism from intestine. Health care-associated nursery outbreaks also have been reported. The prevalence of stool carriage of *L monocytogenes* among healthy, asymptomatic adults is estimated to be 1% to 5%.

The **incubation period** is variable, ranging from 1 day to more than 3 weeks.

DIAGNOSTIC TESTS: The organism can be recovered on trypticase soy agar containing 5% sheep, horse, or rabbit blood from cultures of blood, cerebrospinal fluid (CSF), meconium, gastric washings, placental or fetal tissue specimens, amniotic fluid, and other infected tissue specimens, including joint, pleural, or pericardial fluid. Gram stain of gastric aspirate material, placental tissue, biopsy specimens of the rash of early-onset infection, or CSF from an infected patient may demonstrate the organism. *L monocytogenes* can be mistaken for a contaminant because of its morphologic similarity to diphtheroids and streptococci.

TREATMENT:
- Initial therapy with intravenous ampicillin and an aminoglycoside, usually gentamicin, is recommended for severe infections, including meningitis and encephalitis, endocarditis, and infections in neonates and immunocompromised patients. This combination is more effective than ampicillin alone in vitro and in animal models of *L monocytogenes* infection. In immunocompetent patients with mild infections, ampicillin alone can be given. For penicillin-allergic patients, some experts recommend skin testing and desensitization. For patients who fail to respond to therapy or those with a history of anaphylaxis, wheezing, or angioedema, trimethoprim-sulfamethoxazole can be considered. Treatment failures with vancomycin have been reported. Cephalosporins are not active against *L monocytogenes.*

---

[1] Centers for Disease Control and Prevention. Multistate outbreak of listeriosis associated with Jensen farms cantaloupe—United States, August–September 2011. *MMWR Morb Mortal Wkly Rep.* 2011;60(39):1357–1358

- For invasive infections without associated meningitis, treatment for 10 to 14 days usually is sufficient. For *L monocytogenes* meningitis, most experts recommend 14 to 21 days of treatment. Longer courses are needed for patients who are severely ill or who have endocarditis or rhombencephalitis. Diagnostic imaging of the brain near the end of anticipated therapy allows determination of parenchymal involvement of the brain and the need for prolonged therapy in neonates with complicated courses, immocomprised patients, and patients with rhombencepalitis.

ISOLATION OF THE HOSPITALIZED PATIENT: Standard precautions are recommended.

CONTROL MEASURES:

- Antimicrobial therapy for infection diagnosed during pregnancy may prevent fetal or perinatal infection and its consequences.
- General guidelines for preventing listeriosis are similar to those for preventing other foodborne illnesses: (1) thoroughly cook or reheat foods from animal sources until steaming hot (165°F); (2) wash raw vegetables; (3) prevent contamination from fluids of uncooked meats, hot dogs, and packaging onto other foods or food-preparation surfaces by keeping them separate from vegetables, uncooked foods, and ready-to-eat foods; (4) avoid unpasteurized dairy products; and (5) wash hands, knives, utensils, and cutting boards after exposure to uncooked foods. In addition, people at higher risk of listeriosis (pregnant women, older adults, and immunocompromised people) should follow the dietary recommendations in Table 3.32.
- Listerosis is a nationally notifiable disease in the United States. Cases should be reported promptly to the state or local health department to facilitate early recognition and control of common-source outbreaks.

Table 3.32. Dietary Recommendations for People at Higher Risk of Listeriosis[a]

1. Foods to avoid include:
   - Raw or unpasteurized milk, including goat milk.
   - Soft cheeses (eg, feta, goat, Brie, Camembert, Gorgonzola, blue-veined, and Mexican-style queso fresco cheese).
   - Dairy products that contain unpasteurized milk.
   - Foods from delicatessen counters (eg, prepared salads, meats, cheeses) that have not been heated/reheated adequately.
   - Refrigerated pâtés, other meat spreads, and refrigerated, smoked seafood that have not been heated/reheated adequately.
2. Ways to reduce risk include:
   - Cook leftover or ready-to-eat foods (eg, hot dogs) until steaming hot before eating (165°F).
   - Wash raw vegetables.
   - Wash hands, knives, utensils, and cutting boards after exposure to uncooked or ready-to-eat foods.
   - Prevent contamination from fluids of uncooked meats, hot dogs, and packaging onto other foods or food preparation surfaces by keeping them separate from vegetables, uncooked foods, and ready-to-eat foods.
   - Use a refrigerator thermometer to set the refrigerator temperature to 40°F or lower and the freezer temperature to 0°F or lower.

[a] Pregnant women, older adults, and people who are immunocompromised by illness or therapy are at higher risk of invasive listeriosis.

Table 3.32. Dietary Recommendations for People at Higher Risk of Listeriosis,[a] continued

- Clean up all spills in the refrigerator immediately, especially juices from hot dog packages, raw meat, or poultry.
- Clean the inside walls and shelves of your refrigerator with hot water and liquid soap, then rinse. Divide leftovers into shallow containers; cover with airtight lids or enclose in plastic wraps or aluminum foil; use leftovers within 3 to 4 days.
- Use precooked or ready-to-eat food as soon as possible; hot dogs should be eaten within 1 week once the package is opened and within 2 weeks if the package is unopened; deli meat should be eaten within 3 to 5 days once the package is opened and 2 weeks if the package is unopened.

[a]Pregnant women, older adults, and people who are immunocompromised by illness or therapy are at higher risk of invasive listeriosis.

Lyme Disease[1,2]
(Lyme Borreliosis, *Borrelia burgdorferi* Infection)

CLINICAL MANIFESTATIONS: Clinical manifestations of Lyme disease are divided into 3 stages: early localized, early disseminated, and late disease. Early localized disease is characterized by a distinctive rash, erythema migrans, at the site of a recent tick bite. Erythema migrans is the most common manifestation of Lyme disease in children. Only a small proportion of children are diagnosed at the stage of early disseminated or late Lyme disease; most of these children do not have a history of erythema migrans. Erythema migrans begins as a red macule or papule that usually expands over days to weeks to form a large, annular, erythematous lesion that typically increases in size to 5 cm or more in diameter, sometimes with partial central clearing. The lesion usually but not always is painless and not pruritic. Localized erythema migrans can vary greatly in size and shape and may have vesicular or necrotic areas in its center and can be confused with cellulitis. Fever, malaise, headache, mild neck stiffness, myalgia, and arthralgia often accompany the rash of early localized disease.

Approximately 20% of children with Lyme disease come to medical attention with early disseminated disease, most commonly multiple erythema migrans. This rash usually occurs several weeks after an infective tick bite and consists of secondary annular, erythematous lesions similar to but usually smaller than the primary lesion. These lesions reflect spirochetemia with cutaneous dissemination. Other manifestations of early disseminated illness (that may occur with or without rash) are palsies of the cranial nerves (especially cranial nerve VII), ophthalmic conditions (optic neuritis, episcleritis, keratitis, uveitis, conjunctivitis), and lymphocytic meningitis. Systemic symptoms, such as fever, arthralgia, myalgia, headache, and fatigue, also are common during the early disseminated stage. Lymphocytic meningitis can occur and frequently has a more subacute onset

[1] Wormser GP, Dattwyler RJ, Shapiro ED, et al. The clinical assessment, treatment, and prevention of Lyme disease, human granulocytic anaplasmosis, and babesiosis: clinical practice guidelines by the Infectious Diseases Society of America. *Clin Infect Dis.* 2006;43(9):1089–1134

[2] Lantos PM, Charini WA, Medoff G, et al. Final report of the Lyme Disease Review Panel of the Infectious Diseases Society of America. *Clin Infect Dis.* 2010;51(1):1–5

than viral meningitis. Carditis, which usually manifests as various degrees of heart block, occurs rarely in children. Occasionally, people with early Lyme disease have concurrent human granulocytic anaplasmosis or babesiosis, transmitted by the same tick, which may contribute to symptomatology.

Late disease is characterized most commonly by arthritis that usually is pauciarticular and affects large joints, particularly knees. Arthritis can occur without a history of earlier stages of illness (including erythema migrans). Peripheral neuropathy and central nervous system manifestations also can occur rarely during late disease. Children who are treated with antimicrobial agents in the early stage of disease almost never develop late disease.

Because congenital infection occurs with other spirochetal infections, there has been concern that an infected pregnant woman could transmit *Borrelia burgdorferi* to her fetus. No causal relationship between maternal Lyme disease and abnormalities of pregnancy or congenital disease caused by *B burgdorferi* has been documented. No evidence exists that Lyme disease can be transmitted via human milk.

ETIOLOGY: In the United States, Lyme disease is caused by the spirochete *B burgdorferi* sensu stricto. In Eurasia, *B burgdorferi*, *Borrelia afzelii*, and *Borrelia garinii* cause borreliosis.

EPIDEMIOLOGY: Lyme disease occurs primarily in 3 distinct geographic regions of the United States. Most cases occur in southern New England and in the eastern mid-Atlantic states. The disease also occurs, but with lower frequency, in the upper Midwest, especially Wisconsin and Minnesota, and less commonly on the West Coast, especially northern California. The occurrence of cases in the United States correlates with the distribution and frequency of infected tick vectors—*Ixodes scapularis* in the east and Midwest and *Ixodes pacificus* in the west. In Southern states, *Ixodes* ticks feed on reptiles rather than small mammals (as in the northeast). Reptile blood is bacteriostatic for *B burgdorferi*, which explains why the disease is not endemic in the south. Reported cases from states without known enzootic risks may have been acquired in states with endemic infection or may be misdiagnoses resulting from false-positive serologic test results. In addition, a rash similar to erythema migrans known as "southern tick-associated rash illness" or STARI has been reported in south central states without endemic *B burgdorferi* infection; however, the etiology of this condition remains unknown. Most cases of early Lyme disease occur between April and October; more than 50% of cases occur during June and July. People of all ages may be affected, but incidence in the United States is highest among children 5 through 9 years of age and adults 55 through 59 years of age.

The **incubation period** from tick bite to appearance of single or multiple erythema migrans lesions ranges from 1 to 32 days with a median of 11 days. Late manifestations can occur months after the tick bite.

Endemic Lyme disease transmitted by ixodid ticks occurs in Canada, Europe, states of the former Soviet Union, China, and Japan. The primary tick vector in Europe is *Ixodes ricinus*, and the primary tick vector in Asia is *Ixodes persulcatus*. Clinical manifestations of infection vary somewhat from manifestations seen in the United States, probably because of different genomospecies of *Borrelia*.

DIAGNOSTIC TESTS: During the early stages of Lyme disease, the diagnosis is best made clinically by recognizing the characteristic rash, a singular lesion of erythema migrans, because antibodies against *B burgdorferi* are not detectable in most people within the first few weeks after infection. During the first 4 weeks of infection, serodiagnostic tests are insensitive and are not recommended generally. Although cultures of a biopsy specimen of the perimeter of the skin lesion often yield the organism, cultures of *Borrelia* species (which require special media) are not available commercially and are not recommended. Diagnosis in patients with early disseminated disease who have multiple lesions of erythema migrans also is made clinically. Diagnosis of early disseminated disease without rash or late Lyme disease should be made on the basis of clinical findings and serologic test results. Some patients who are treated with antimicrobial agents for early Lyme disease never develop antibodies against *B burgdorferi;* they are cured and are not at risk of late disease. Development of antibodies in patients treated for early Lyme disease do not indicate lack of cure/persistent infection. Most patients with early disseminated disease and virtually all patients with late disease have antibodies against *B burgdorferi.* Once such antibodies develop, they persist for many years and perhaps for life. Consequently, tests for antibodies should not be repeated or used to assess the success of treatment. The results of serologic tests for Lyme disease should be interpreted with careful consideration of the clinical setting and quality of the testing laboratory.

A 2-step approach is recommended for serologic diagnosis of *B burgdorferi.* First, a quantitative screening test for serum antibodies should be performed using a sensitive enzyme immunoassay (EIA) or immunofluorescent antibody assay (IFA). Serum specimens that yield positive or equivocal results then should be tested by a standardized Western immunoblot for presence of antibodies to *B burgdorferi;* serum specimens that yield negative results by EIA or IFA should not be tested further by immunoblot testing. Immunoblot testing should not be performed if the EIA result is negative or instead of or before an EIA; the specificity of immunoblot testing diminishes if this test is performed alone. When testing to confirm early disseminated disease without rash, immunoglobulin (Ig) G and IgM immunoblot assays should be performed. To confirm late disease, only an IgG immunoblot assay should be performed, because false-positive results may occur with the IgM immunoblot. In people with symptoms lasting longer than 1 month, a positive IgM test result alone (ie, with a negative IgG result) is likely to represent a false-positive result and should not be the basis on which to diagnose Lyme disease. A positive result of an IgG immunoblot test requires detection of antibody ("bands") to 5 or more of the following: 18, 23/24, 28, 30, 39, 41, 45, 60, 66, and 93 kDa polypeptides. A positive test result of IgM immunoblot requires detection of antibody to at least 2 of the 23/24, 39, and 41 kDa polypeptides. Two-step testing is needed, because EIA and IFA may yield false-positive results because of the presence of antibodies directed against spirochetes in normal oral flora that cross-react with antigens of *B burgdorferi* or because of cross-reactive antibodies in patients with other spirochetal infections (eg, syphilis, leptospirosis, relapsing fever), certain viral infections (eg, varicella, Epstein-Barr virus), or certain autoimmune diseases (eg, systemic lupus erythematosus).

A licensed, commercially available serologic test (C6) that detects antibody to a peptide of the immunodominant conserved region of the variable surface antigen (VlsE) of *B burgdorferi* appears to have equivalent specificity and sensitivity compared with the 2-step protocol. This assay also detects antibodies to *B garinii* and *B afzelii,* genomospecies that cause Lyme disease in Eurasia. Polymerase chain reaction (PCR) testing (using a laboratory with excellent quality procedures) has been used to detect *B burgdorferi* DNA in joint fluid. Tests of joint fluid for antibody to *B burgdorferi* and urinary antigen detection have no role in diagnosis.

Suspected central nervous system Lyme disease can be confirmed by demonstration of intrathecal production of antibodies against *B burgdorferi*. However, interpretation of results of antibody tests of cerebrospinal fluid is complex, and physicians should seek the advice of a specialist experienced in management of patients with Lyme disease to assist in interpreting results.

The widespread practice of ordering serologic tests for patients with nonspecific symptoms, such as fatigue or arthralgia, who have a low probability of having Lyme disease or because of parental pressure, is discouraged. Almost all positive serologic test results in these patients are false-positive results. In areas with endemic infection, subclinical infection and seroconversion also can occur, and the patient's symptoms merely are coincidental. Patients with acute Lyme disease almost always have objective signs of infection (eg, erythema migrans, facial nerve palsy, arthritis). Nonspecific symptoms commonly accompany these specific signs but almost never are the only evidence of Lyme disease.

TREATMENT: Consensus practice guidelines for assessment, treatment, and prevention of Lyme disease have been published by the Infectious Diseases Society of America.[1,2] Care of children should follow recommendations in Table 3.33, p 478. Antimicrobial therapy for nonspecific symptoms or for asymptomatic seropositivity is discouraged. Additionally, antimicrobial agents administered by other routes of administration or for durations not specified in Table 3.33 are not recommended. Lastly, use of alternative diagnostic approaches or therapies without adequate validation studies and publication in peer-reviewed scientific literature also are discouraged.

Early Localized Disease. Doxycycline is the drug of choice for children 8 years of age and older and, unlike amoxicillin, also treats patients with anaplasmosis (see Tetracyclines, p 801). For children younger than 8 years of age, amoxicillin is recommended. For patients who are allergic to penicillin, the alternative drug is cefuroxime. Erythromycin and azithromycin are less effective. Most experts treat people with early Lyme disease for 14 to 21 days.

Treatment of erythema migrans almost always prevents development of later stages of Lyme disease. Erythema migrans usually resolves within several days of initiating treatment, but other signs and symptoms may persist for several weeks, even in successfully treated patients.

Early Disseminated and Late Disease. Orally administered antimicrobial agents are recommended for treating multiple erythema migrans and uncomplicated Lyme arthritis. Oral agents also are appropriate for treatment of facial nerve palsy without clinical manifestations of meningitis; lumbar puncture is not indicated. If symptoms or signs of other central nervous system involvement, such as meningitis or raised intracranial pressure, are present, lumbar puncture is performed. If cerebrospinal fluid pleocytosis is found, parenterally administered antimicrobial therapy is indicated. Up to one third of patients with arthritis have persistence of synovitis and joint swelling at conclusion of antimicrobial therapy, which almost always resolves without repeating the course of antimicrobial therapy. Some experts would treat a patient who has recurrent or persistent arthritis after treatment with one course of oral antimicrobial therapy with another course of oral

[1] Wormser GP, Dattwyler RJ, Shapiro ED, et al. The clinical assessment, treatment, and prevention of Lyme disease, human granulocytic anaplasmosis, and babesiosis: clinical practice guidelines by the Infectious Diseases Society of America. *Clin Infect Dis*. 2006;43(9):1089–1134

[2] Lantos PM, Charini WA, Medoff G, et al. Final report of the Lyme Disease Review Panel of the Infectious Diseases Society of America. *Clin Infect Dis*. 2010;51(1):1–5

Table 3.33. Recommended Treatment of Lyme Disease in Children

Disease Category	Drug(s) and Dose[a]
Early localized disease[a]	
8 y of age or older	Doxycycline, 4 mg/kg per day, orally, divided into 2 doses (maximum 200 mg/day) for 14–21 days[b]
Younger than 8 y of age or unable to tolerate doxycycline	Amoxicillin, 50 mg/kg per day, orally, divided into 3 doses (maximum 1.5 g/day) for 14–21 days **OR** Cefuroxime, 30 mg/kg per day in 2 divided doses (maximum 1000 mg/day) or 1.0 g/day for 14–21 days
Early disseminated and late disease	
Multiple erythema migrans	Same oral regimen as for early localized disease, but for 21 days
Isolated facial palsy	Same oral regimen as for early localized disease, but for 14–21 days[c,d]
Arthritis	Same oral regimen as for early localized disease, but for 28 days
Persistent or recurrent arthritis[e]	Ceftriaxone sodium, 50–75 mg/kg, IV, once a day (maximum 2 g/day) for 14–28 days Alternatives: Penicillin, 200 000–400 000 U/kg per day, IV, given in divided doses every 4 h (maximum 18–24 million U/day) for 14–28 days **OR** Cefotaxime 150–200 mg/kg per day, IV, divided into 3 or 4 doses (maximum 6 g/day) for 14–28 days **OR** Same oral regimen as for early disease (retreatment) but for 28 days
Atrioventricular heart block or carditis	Oral regimen as for early disease if asymptomatic[f] but for 14–21 days Ceftriaxone or penicillin IV for symptomatic: see persistent or recurrent arthritis for dosing, but for 14–21 days
Meningitis	Ceftriaxone[g] or cefotaxime with alternative of penicillin[g]: see dosing for persistent or recurrent arthritis, for 14 days (range, 10–28 days) **OR** Doxycycline, 4–8 mg/kg per day, orally, divided into 2 doses (maximum 100–200 mg) but for 14 days (range, 10–28 days)[b]
Encephalitis or other late neurologic disease[h]	Ceftriaxone[g] or alternatives of penicillin[g] or cefotaxime[g]: see persistent or recurrent arthritis for dosing, duration also for 14–28 days

IV indicates intravenously.

[a] For patients who are allergic to penicillin, cefuroxime and erythromycin are alternative drugs.

[b] Tetracyclines are contraindicated in pregnancy and in children younger than 8 years of age.

[c] Corticosteroids should not be given.

[d] Treatment has no effect on the resolution of facial nerve palsy; its purpose is to prevent late disease.

[e] Arthritis is not considered persistent or recurrent unless objective evidence of synovitis exists at least 2 months after treatment is initiated. Some experts administer a second course of an oral agent before using an IV-administered antimicrobial agent.

[f] Symptoms for heart block or carditis include syncope, dyspnea, or chest pain.

[g] Ceftriaxone and penicillin should be administered IV for treatment of meningitis or encephalitis.

[h] Other late neurologic manifestations include peripheral neuropathy or encephalopathy.

antimicrobial therapy. Central nervous system infection can be treated with parenterally administered antimicrobial therapy, although there is evidence that orally administered doxycycline may be a suitable alternative. The optimal duration of therapy for manifestations of early disseminated or late disease is not well established, but there is no evidence that children with any manifestation of Lyme disease benefit from prolonged courses of orally or parenterally administered antimicrobial agents. Accordingly, the maximum duration of a single course of therapy is 4 weeks (see Table 3.33).

The Jarisch-Herxheimer reaction (an acute febrile reaction accompanied by headache, myalgia, and an aggravated clinical picture lasting less than 24 hours) can occur when therapy is initiated. Nonsteroidal anti-inflammatory agents may be beneficial, and the antimicrobial agent should be continued.

Pregnancy. Tetracyclines are contraindicated. Otherwise, therapy is the same as recommended for nonpregnant people.

ISOLATION OF THE HOSPITALIZED PATIENT: Standard precautions are recommended.

CONTROL MEASURES:

Ticks. See Prevention of Tickborne Infections (p 207).

Chemoprophylaxis. Many people who seek medical attention for a tick bite have been bitten by a species of tick that does not transmit Lyme disease, or the recovered material is not a tick. The overall risk of infection with B burgdorferi after a recognized deer tick bite is 1% to 3% and, even in areas with high endemicity, is sufficiently low that prophylactic antimicrobial treatment is not indicated routinely. People bitten by an ixodid tick in areas with low incidence of Lyme disease should not receive chemoprophylaxis. The risk is extremely low after brief attachment (eg, a flat, nonengorged deer tick is found) and is higher after engorgement, especially if a nymphal deer tick has been attached for ≥36 hours. Analysis of the tick for spirochete infection has a poor predictive value and is not recommended. On the basis of a study of doxycycline for prevention of Lyme disease after a deer tick bite, some experts recommend a single 200-mg dose (4.4 mg/kg for people weighing less than 45 kg) of doxycycline for people 8 years of age and older who have been bitten in an area with hyperendemic infection (ie, local rate of infection of these ticks with B burgdorferi is 20% or greater) who have found an engorged deer tick, especially if the suspected duration of attachment is ≥36 hours and prophylaxis can be started within 72 hours after the tick was removed. Data are insufficient to recommend amoxicillin prophylaxis.

Blood Donation. Patients with active disease should not donate blood, because spirochetemia occurs in early Lyme disease. Patients who have been treated for Lyme disease can be considered for blood donation.

Vaccines. A Lyme disease vaccine was licensed by the US Food and Drug Administration on December 21, 1998, for people 15 to 70 years of age but was withdrawn in early 2002, reportedly because of poor sales.

Lymphatic Filariasis
(Bancroftian, Malayan, and Timorian)

CLINICAL MANIFESTATIONS: Lymphatic filariasis is caused by infection with adult worms, *Wuchereria bancrofti, Brugia malayi,* or *Brugia timori.* Adult worms cause lymphatic dilatation and dysfunction, which results in abnormal lymph flow and eventually may predispose an infected person to lymphedema in the legs, scrotal area, and arms. Recurrent secondary bacterial infections hasten progression of lymphedema to its advanced stage, known as elephantiasis. Although the initial infection occurs commonly in young children living in areas with endemic infection, chronic manifestations of infection, such as hydrocele and lymphedema, occur infrequently in people younger than 20 years of age. Most filarial infections remain asymptomatic but even then commonly cause subclinical lymphatic dilatation and dysfunction. Lymphadenopathy, most frequently of the inguinal, crural, and axillary lymph nodes, is the most common clinical sign of lymphatic filariasis in children and is associated with living adult worms. Death of the adult worm triggers an acute inflammatory response, which progresses distally (retrograde) along the affected lymphatic vessel, usually in the limbs. If present, systemic symptoms, such as headache or fever, generally are mild. In postpubertal males, adult *W bancrofti* organisms are found most commonly in the intrascrotal lymphatic vessels; thus, inflammation resulting from adult worm death may present as funiculitis (inflammation of the spermatic cord), epididymitis, or orchitis. A tender granulomatous nodule may be palpable at the site of the dead adult worms. Chyluria can occur as a manifestation of bancroftian filariasis. Tropical pulmonary eosinophilia (TPE), characterized by cough, fever, marked eosinophilia, and high serum immunoglobulin E concentrations, is an uncommon manifestation of lymphatic filariasis.

ETIOLOGY: Filariasis is caused by 3 filarial nematodes: *W bancrofti, B malayi,* and *B timori.*

EPIDEMIOLOGY: The parasite is transmitted by the bite of infected species of various genera of mosquitoes, including *Culex, Aedes, Anopheles,* and *Mansonia. W bancrofti,* the most prevalent cause of lymphatic filariasis, is found in Haiti, the Dominican Republic, Guyana, northeast Brazil, sub-Saharan and North Africa, and Asia, extending from India through the Indonesian archipelago to the western Pacific islands. Humans are the only definitive host for the parasite. *B malayi* is found mostly in Southeast Asia and parts of India. *B timori* is restricted to certain islands at the eastern end of the Indonesian archipelago. Live adult worms release microfilariae into the bloodstream, and because adult worms live, on average, for 5 to 8 years and reinfection is common, microfilariae infective for mosquitoes may remain in the patient's blood for decades; individual microfilaria have a lifespan up to 1.5 years. The adult worm is not transmissible from person to person or by blood transfusion, but microfilariae may be transmitted by transfusion.

The **incubation period** is not well established; the period from acquisition to the appearance of microfilariae in blood can be 3 to 12 months, depending on the species of parasite.

DIAGNOSTIC TESTS: Microfilariae generally can be detected microscopically on blood smears obtained at night (10 PM–4 AM), although variations in the periodicity of microfilaremia have been described depending on the parasite and the geographic location of the host. Adult worms or microfilariae can be identified in tissue specimens obtained at biopsy. Serologic enzyme immunoassays are available, but interpretation of results is affected by cross-reactions of filarial antibodies with antibodies against other helminths. Assays for circulating parasite antigen of *W bancrofti* are available commercially but are not licensed by the US Food and Drug Administration. Ultrasonography can be used to visualize adult worms. Lymphatic filariasis often must be diagnosed clinically, because dependable serologic assays are not available uniformly, and in patients with lymphedema, microfilariae no longer may be present.

TREATMENT: The main goal of treatment of an infected person is to kill the adult worm. Diethylcarbamazine citrate (DEC), which is both microfilaricidal and active against the adult worm, is the drug of choice for lymphatic filariasis (see Drugs for Parasitic Infections, p 848). Once lymphedema is established (the late phase of chronic disease), the disease is not affected by chemotherapy. Ivermectin is effective against the microfilariae of *W bancrofti* but has no effect on the adult parasite. In some studies, combination therapy with single-dose DEC-albendazole or ivermectin-albendazole has been shown to be more effective than any one drug alone in suppressing microfilaremia.

Complex decongestive physiotherapy may be effective for treating lymphedema. Chyluria originating in the bladder responds to fulguration; chyluria originating in the kidney usually cannot be corrected. Prompt identification and treatment of bacterial superinfections, particularly streptococcal and staphylococcal infections, and careful treatment of intertriginous and ungual fungal infections are important aspects of therapy for lymphedema.

ISOLATION OF THE HOSPITALIZED PATIENT: Standard precautions are recommended.

CONTROL MEASURES: Control measures have been instituted on the basis of annual community-wide combinations of DEC and albendazole (worldwide except Africa) or albendazole and ivermectin (in Africa) to decrease or possibly eliminate transmission. No vaccine is available for filariasis.

Lymphocytic Choriomeningitis

CLINICAL MANIFESTATIONS: Child and adult infections are asymptomatic in approximately one third of cases. Symptomatic infection may result in a mild to severe influenza-like illness, which includes fever, malaise, myalgia, retro-orbital headache, photophobia, anorexia, and nausea. Initial symptoms may last up to 1 week. A biphasic febrile course is common; after a few days without symptoms, the second phase may occur in up to half of symptomatic patients, consisting of neurologic manifestations that vary from aseptic meningitis to severe encephalitis. Transmission of lymphocytic choriomeningitis (LCM) virus through organ transplantation can result in fatal disseminated infection with multiple organ failure. In the past, LCM virus has caused up to 10% to 15% of all cases of aseptic meningitis, and it was a common cause of aseptic meningitis during winter months. Arthralgia or arthritis, respiratory tract symptoms, orchitis, and leukopenia develop occasionally. Recovery without sequelae is the usual outcome. LCM virus infection should be suspected in presence of: (1) aseptic meningitis or encephalitis during the fall-winter season; (2) febrile illness, followed by brief remission, followed by onset of neurologic illness; and (3) cerebrospinal fluid (CSF) findings of lymphocytosis and hypoglycorrhachia.

Infection during pregnancy has been associated with spontaneous abortion. Congenital infection may cause severe abnormalities, including hydrocephalus, chorioretinitis, intracranial calcifications, microcephaly, and mental retardation. Congenital

LCM etiology should be envisaged when TORCH syndrome is suspected (TOxoplasma, Rubella, Cytomegalovirus, Herpes simplex). Patients with immune abnormalities may experience severe or fatal illness, as observed in patients receiving organs from LCM virus-infected donors.

ETIOLOGY: LCM virus is an arenavirus.

EPIDEMIOLOGY: LCM is a chronic infection of common house mice, which often are infected asymptomatically and chronically shed virus in urine and other excretions. In addition, pet hamsters, laboratory mice, guinea pigs, and colonized golden hamsters can have chronic infection and can be sources of human infection. Humans are infected by aerosol or by ingestion of dust or food contaminated with the virus from the urine, feces, blood, or nasopharyngeal secretions of infected rodents. The disease is observed more frequently in young adults. Human to human transmission has occurred during pregnancy from infected mothers to their fetus and through solid organ transplantation from an undiagnosed, acutely LCM virus-infected organ donor. Several such clusters of cases have been described following transplantation, and 1 case was traced to a pet hamster purchased by the donor. A number of laboratory-acquired LCM virus infections have occurred, both through contaminated tissue culture stocks and infected lab animals.

The **incubation period** usually is 6 to 13 days and occasionally is as long as 3 weeks.

DIAGNOSTIC TESTS: In patients with central nervous system disease, mononuclear pleocytosis often exceeding 1000 cells/μL is present in CSF. Hypoglycorrhachia may occur. LCM virus usually can be isolated from CSF obtained during the acute phase of illness and, in severe disseminated infections, also from blood, urine, and nasopharyngeal secretion specimens. Reverse transcriptase-polymerase chain reaction assays can be used on CSF. Serum specimens from the acute and convalescent phases of illness can be tested for increases in antibody titers by enzyme immunoassays. Demonstration of virus-specific immunoglobulin M antibodies in serum or CSF specimens is useful. In congenital infections, diagnosis usually is suspected at the sequela phase, and diagnosis usually is made by serologic testing. Diagnosis can be made retrospectively by immunohistochemistry assay of tissues obtained from necropsy.

TREATMENT: Supportive. Limited data suggest a role for ribavirin in immunosuppressed patients infected with LCM virus.

ISOLATION OF THE HOSPITALIZED PATIENT: Standard precautions are recommended.

CONTROL MEASURES: Infection can be controlled by preventing rodent infestation in animal and food storage areas. Because the virus is excreted for long periods of time by rodent hosts, attempts should be made to monitor laboratory and wholesale colonies of mice and hamsters for infection. Pet rodents or wild mice in a patient's home should be considered likely sources of infection. Although the risk for LCM virus infection from pet rodents is low, pregnant women should avoid exposure to wild or pet rodents and their aerosolized excreta. Guidelines for minimizing risk of human LCM virus infection associated with rodents are available[1] (also see Diseases Transmitted by Animals, p 215).

---

[1] Centers for Disease Control and Prevention. Update: interim guidance for minimizing risk for human lymphocytic choriomeningitis virus infection associated with pet rodents. *MMWR Morb Mortal Wkly Rep.* 2005;54(32):799–801

Malaria

CLINICAL MANIFESTATIONS: The classic symptoms of malaria are high fever with chills, rigor, sweats, and headache, which may be paroxysmal. If appropriate treatment is not administered, fever and paroxysms may occur in a cyclic pattern. Depending on the infecting species, fever classically appears every other or every third day. Other manifestations can include nausea, vomiting, diarrhea, cough, tachypnea, arthralgia, myalgia, and abdominal and back pain. Anemia and thrombocytopenia are common, and pallor and jaundice caused by hemolysis may occur. Hepatosplenomegaly may be present. More severe disease occurs in people without previous exposure, young children, and people who are pregnant or immunocompromised.

Infection with *Plasmodium falciparum*, 1 of the 5 *Plasmodium* species that infect humans, potentially is fatal and most commonly manifests as a febrile nonspecific illness without localizing signs. Severe disease (most commonly caused by *P falciparum*) may manifest as one of the following clinical syndromes, all of which are medical emergencies and may be fatal unless treated:

- **Cerebral malaria,** which may have variable neurologic manifestations, including generalized seizures, signs of increased intracranial pressure, confusion, and progression to stupor, coma, and death;
- **Hypoglycemia,** which may occur with metabolic acidosis and hypotension associated with hyperparasitemia or be associated with quinine treatment;
- **Renal failure** caused by acute tubular necrosis (rare in children younger than 8 years of age);
- **Respiratory failure and metabolic acidosis,** without pulmonary edema;
- **Severe anemia** attributable to high parasitemia, sequestration and hemolysis associated with hypersplenism; or
- **Vascular collapse and shock** associated with hypothermia and adrenal insufficiency. People with asplenia who become infected may be at increased risk of more severe illness and death.

Syndromes primarily associated with *Plasmodium vivax* and *Plasmodium ovale* infection are as follows:

- **Anemia** attributable to acute parasitemia;
- **Hypersplenism** with danger of late splenic rupture; and
- **Relapse,** for as long as 3 to 5 years after the primary infection, attributable to latent hepatic stages (hypnozoites).

Syndromes associated with *Plasmodium malariae* infection include:

- **Chronic asymptomatic parasitemia** for as long as several years after the last exposure; and
- **Nephrotic syndrome** from deposition of immune complexes in the kidney.

Plasmodium knowlesi is a primate malaria parasite that also can infect humans. *P knowlesi* malaria has been misdiagnosed commonly as the more benign *P malariae* malaria. Disease can be characterized by very rapid replication of the organism and hyperparasitemia resulting in severe disease. Severe disease in patients with *P knowlesi* infection should be treated aggressively, because hepatorenal failure and subsequent death have been reported.

Congenital malaria secondary to perinatal transmission rarely may occur. Most congenital cases have been caused by *P vivax* and *P falciparum; P malariae* and *P ovale* account for fewer than 20% of such cases. Manifestations can resemble those of neonatal sepsis, including fever and nonspecific symptoms of poor appetite, irritability, and lethargy.

ETIOLOGY: The genus *Plasmodium* includes species of intraerythrocytic parasites that infect a wide range of mammals, birds, and reptiles. The 5 species that frequently infect humans are *P falciparum, P vivax, P ovale, P malariae,* and *P knowlesi.* Coinfection with multiple species increasingly is recognized as polymerase chain reaction technology is applied to the diagnosis of malaria.

EPIDEMIOLOGY: Malaria is endemic throughout the tropical areas of the world and is acquired from the bite of the female nocturnal-feeding *Anopheles* genus of mosquito. Half of the world's population lives in areas where transmission occurs. Worldwide, 243 million cases and 863 000 reported deaths occur each year. Most deaths occur in young children. Infection by the malaria parasite poses substantial risks to pregnant women and their fetuses and may result in spontaneous abortion and stillbirth. Malaria also contributes significantly to low birth weight in countries with endemic infection. The risk of malaria is highest, but variable, for travelers to sub-Saharan Africa, Papua New Guinea, the Solomon Islands, and Vanuatu; the risk is intermediate on the Indian subcontinent and is low in most of Southeast Asia and Latin America. The potential for malaria transmission is ongoing in areas where malaria previously was eliminated if infected people return and the mosquito vector is still present. These conditions have resulted in recent cases in travelers to areas such as Jamaica, the Dominican Republic, and the Bahamas. Health care professionals should check an up-to-date source (**wwwn.cdc.gov/travel**) to determine malaria endemicity when providing pretravel malaria advice or evaluating a febrile returned traveler. Transmission is possible in more temperate climates, including areas of the United States where anopheline mosquitoes are present. Nearly all of the approximately 1400 annual reported cases in the United States result from infection acquired abroad.[1] Rarely, mosquitoes in airplanes flying from areas with endemic malaria have been the source of cases in people working or residing near international airports. Local transmission also occurs rarely in the United States. Uncommon modes of malaria transmission are congenital, through transfusions, or through the use of contaminated needles or syringes.

P vivax and *P falciparum* are the most common species worldwide. *P vivax* malaria is prevalent on the Indian subcontinent and in Central America. *P falciparum* malaria is prevalent in Africa, Papua New Guinea, and on the island of Hispaniola (Haiti and the Dominican Republic). *P vivax* and *P falciparum* species are the most common malaria species in southern and Southeast Asia, Oceania, and South America. *P malariae,* although much less common, has a wide distribution. *P ovale* malaria occurs most often in West Africa but has been reported in other areas.

Relapses may occur in *P vivax* and *P ovale* malaria because of a persistent hepatic (hypnozoite) stage of infection. Recrudescence of *P falciparum* and *P malariae* infection occurs when a persistent low-concentration parasitemia causes recurrence of symptoms of the disease or when drug resistance prevents elimination of the parasite. In areas of

---

[1] Centers for Disease Control and Prevention. Malaria surveillance—United States, 2010. *MMWR Surveill Summ.* 2012;61(SS-02):1–17

Africa and Asia with hyperendemic infection, reinfection in people with partial immunity results in a high prevalence of asymptomatic parasitemia.

The spread of chloroquine-resistant *P falciparum* strains throughout the world is of increasing concern. In addition, resistance to other antimalarial drugs also is occurring in many areas where the drugs are used widely. *P falciparum* resistance to sulfadoxine-pyrimethamine is common throughout Africa, mefloquine resistance has been documented in Burma (Myanmar), Laos, Thailand, Cambodia, China, and Vietnam, and emerging resistance to artemisinins has been observed at the Cambodia-Thailand border. Chloroquine-resistant *P vivax* has been reported in Indonesia, Papua New Guinea, the Solomon Islands, Myanmar, India, and Guyana. Malaria symptoms can develop as soon as 7 days after exposure in an area with endemic malaria to as late as several months after departure. More than 80% of cases diagnosed in the United States occur in people who have onset of symptoms after their return to the United States.

DIAGNOSTIC TESTS: Definitive diagnosis relies on identification of the parasite microscopically on stained blood films. Both thick and thin blood films should be examined. The thick film allows for concentration of the blood to find parasites that may be present in small numbers, whereas the thin film is most useful for species identification and determination of the degree of parasitemia (the percentage of erythrocytes harboring parasites). If initial blood smears test negative for *Plasmodium* species but malaria remains a possibility, the smear should be repeated every 12 to 24 hours during a 72-hour period.

Confirmation and identification of the species of malaria parasites on the blood smear is important in guiding therapy. Serologic testing generally is not helpful, except in epidemiologic surveys. Polymerase chain reaction (PCR) assay is available in reference laboratories and some state health departments. DNA probes and malarial ribosomal RNA testing may provide rapid and accurate diagnosis in the future but currently are used in experimental studies only. A new US Food and Drug Administration (FDA)-approved test for antigen detection (a rapid diagnostic test) is available in the United States. It is the only antigen-detection kit available and is approved for use by hospitals and commercial laboratories. However, an evaluation by the World Health Organization (WHO) found that this product had poor sensitivity for detecting low density *P vivax* infections. Rapid diagnostic testing is recommended to be conducted in parallel with routine microscopy to provide further information needed for patient treatment, such as the percentage of erythrocytes harboring parasites. Both positive and negative rapid diagnostic test results should be confirmed by microscopic examination, because low-level parasitemia may not be detected, false-positive results occur, and mixed infections may not be detected accurately. Also, information about the sensitivity of rapid diagnostic tests for the 2 less common species of malaria, *P ovale* and *P malariae*, is limited. More information about rapid diagnostic testing for malaria is available at **www.cdc.gov/malaria/ diagnosis_treatment/index.html**.

TREATMENT: The choice of malaria chemotherapy is based on the infecting species, possible drug resistance, and severity of disease (see Drugs for Parasitic Infections, p 848). Severe malaria is defined as any one or more of the following: parasitemia greater than 5% of red blood cells, signs of central nervous system or other end-organ involvement, shock, acidosis, and/or hypoglycemia. Patients with severe malaria require intensive care and parenteral treatment until the parasite density decreases to less than 1% and they are able to tolerate oral therapy. Exchange transfusion may be warranted when parasitemia exceeds 10% or if there is evidence of complications (eg, cerebral malaria or renal failure) at lower parasite densities. For patients with severe malaria in the United States who do not tolerate or cannot easily access quinidine, intravenous artesunate has become available through a Centers for Disease Control and Prevention (CDC) investigational new drug protocol. Clinicians may contact the physician on call through the CDC malaria hotline (770-488-7788, Monday–Friday, 9:00 AM–5:00 PM Eastern Time; or 777-488-7100 at all other times) for additional information and release of the drug.[1] For patients with *P falciparum* malaria, sequential blood smears to determine percentage of erythrocytes harboring parasites can be useful in monitoring treatment. Assistance with management of malaria is available 24 hours a day through the CDC Malaria Hotline (770-488-7788).

ISOLATION OF THE HOSPITALIZED PATIENT: Standard precautions are recommended.

CONTROL MEASURES: Although there currently is no licensed vaccine against malaria, control of *Anopheles* mosquito populations, protection against mosquito bites, treatment of infected people, and chemoprophylaxis of travelers to areas with endemic infection are effective. Measures to prevent contact with mosquitoes, especially from dusk to dawn (because of the nocturnal biting habits of most female *Anopheles* mosquitoes), through use of bed nets impregnated with insecticide, mosquito repellents containing diethyltoluamide (DEET) (see Prevention of Mosquitoborne Infections, p 209), and protective clothing also are beneficial and should be optimized. The most current information on country-specific malaria transmission, drug resistance, and resulting recommendations for travelers can be obtained by contacting the CDC (**www.cdc.gov/malaria/** or the Malaria Hotline at 770-488-7788).

Chemoprophylaxis for Travelers to Areas With Endemic Malaria.[2] More than 80% of malaria-infected patients reported in the United States did not follow a CDC-recommended prophylaxis regimen. The appropriate chemoprophylactic regimen is determined by the traveler's risk of acquiring malaria in the area(s) to be visited and by the risk of exposure to chloroquine- or mefloquine-resistant *P falciparum* or chloroquine-resistant *P vivax*. Indications for prophylaxis for children are identical to those for adults. Pediatric dosages should be calculated on the basis of the child's current weight; children's dosages never should exceed adult dosages. Drugs used for malaria chemoprophylaxis generally are well tolerated. However, adverse reactions can occur. Minor adverse reactions do not require stopping the drug. Travelers with serious adverse reactions should be advised to contact their physician.

Chemoprophylaxis should begin before arrival in the area with endemic malaria (starting at least 2 weeks before arrival for mefloquine and 1 week before arrival for chloroquine and 1–2 days before arrival for doxycycline and atovaquone-proguanil), allowing time to develop blood concentrations of the drug. If there is desire to ensure tolerance of the antimalarial drug to be used for prophylaxis, then the drug should be started earlier so that there is time to assess any adverse events before departure and time to change

---

[1] Centers for Disease Control and Prevention. Notice to readers: new medication for severe malaria available under an investigational new drug protocol. *MMWR Morb Mortal Wkly Rep.* 2007;56(30):769–770

[2] For further information on prevention of malaria in travelers, see the biennial publication of the US Public Health Service, *Health Information for International Travel,* 2012. Atlanta, GA: US Department of Health and Human Services, Public Health Service, Centers for Disease Control and Prevention, National Center for Infectious Diseases, Division of Global Migration and Quarantine; 2012. Available at: **wwwn.cdc.gov/travel/contentYellowBook.aspx**.

to another effective drug if needed. For example, if there is concern about individual tolerance with mefloquine, then prophylaxis can be started 3 weeks before travel. Most adverse events will occur during the first 3 doses, and if the individual does not tolerate mefloquine, then there still is time to prescribe alternative therapy before travel.

Travelers to areas where chloroquine-resistant malaria species have not been reported should take chloroquine, mefloquine, doxycycline, or atovaquone-proguanil in consultation with their physician. Travelers to areas where chloroquine-resistant *P falciparum* exists should take atovaquone-proguanil, doxycycline, or mefloquine. Adverse reactions that can occur include gastrointestinal tract disturbance, headache, dizziness, blurred vision, insomnia, and pruritus, but these generally are mild and do not require discontinuation of the drug. Drugs for the prevention of malaria currently available in the United States include chloroquine, mefloquine, doxycycline, atovaquone-proguanil, and primaquine.

- A fixed-dose combination of atovaquone-proguanil is approved for prevention and treatment of chloroquine-resistant *P falciparum* malaria. Atovaquone-proguanil is taken daily, starting 1 day before exposure and continuing for the duration of exposure and for 1 week after departure from the area with endemic malaria. A pediatric formulation is available in the United States but is not approved for prophylaxis in children weighing less than 11 kg. However, the CDC suggests that atovaquone-proguanil can be used in children weighing 5 kg or more, when travel to areas where chloroquine-resistant *P falciparum* exists cannot be avoided. Atovaquone-proguanil is contraindicated for pregnant women. The rare adverse effects reported by people using atovaquone-proguanil for chemoprophylaxis are abdominal pain, nausea, vomiting, mouth ulcers, and headache.

- Doxycycline is taken daily, starting 1 to 2 days before exposure, for the duration of exposure and for 4 weeks after departure from the area with endemic malaria. Travelers taking doxycycline should be advised of the need for strict adherence to daily dosing; the advisability of always taking the drug on a full stomach; and the possible adverse effects, including diarrhea, photosensitivity, and increased risk of monilial vaginitis. Use of doxycycline should be avoided for pregnant women and for children younger than 8 years of age because of the risk of dental staining (see Antimicrobial Agents and Related Therapy, Tetracyclines, p 801).

- Mefloquine is taken once weekly, starting at least 2 weeks before travel, continuing weekly during travel, and for 4 weeks after travel has concluded (see Drugs for Parasitic Infections, p 848). Mefloquine is not approved by the FDA for children who weigh less than 5 kg or are younger than 6 months of age. However, the CDC suggests that mefloquine be considered for use in children, regardless of weight or age restrictions, when travel to areas where chloroquine-resistant *P falciparum* exists and cannot be avoided. However, parents should be advised not to travel to countries with endemic malaria with children weighing less than 5 kg or younger than 6 weeks of age because of the risks associated with infection (septicemia or malaria) in young infants. The most common central nervous system abnormalities associated with mefloquine are dizziness, headache, insomnia, and disturbing dreams. Mefloquine has been associated with rare serious adverse events (including psychoses or seizures) at prophylactic doses and no longer is used by the US Army. These reactions are more common with the higher doses used for treatment. Other adverse events that occur with prophylactic doses include gastrointestinal tract disturbances, headache, depression, and anxiety disorders. Mefloquine is contraindicated for use in travelers with a known hypersensitivity to mefloquine; people with active depression or a history of depression; people with general anxiety disorders, psychosis, schizophrenia, or other major psychiatric disturbances; people with a history of seizures (not including febrile seizures); and people with a history of cardiac conduction abnormalities. Although a warning about concurrent use with beta-blockers is given in the product labeling, a review of available data suggests that mefloquine may be used by people concurrently receiving beta-blockers if they have no underlying arrhythmia. Caution should be advised for travelers involved in tasks requiring fine motor coordination and spatial discrimination. Patients in whom mefloquine prophylaxis fails should be monitored closely if they are treated with quinidine or quinine sulfate, because either drug may exacerbate known adverse effects of mefloquine.

The US FDA approved artemether lumefantrine for oral treatment of acute, uncomplicated malaria infections in adults and children weighing at least 5 kg. It has activity against chloroquine-resistant *P falciparum*. Lumefantrine is not approved for treatment of severe malaria nor to prevent malaria. Artemether is the first artemisinin class drug approved in the United States. The artemisinins are derived from the leaves of the *Artemisia annua* plant used to treat malaria.

Primaquine is recommended for prophylaxis in areas with predominantly *P vivax* malaria. Travelers must be tested for glucose-6-phosphate dehydrogenase (G6PD) deficiency and have a documented G6PD in the normal range before primaquine use. Primary primaquine prophylaxis should begin 1 to 2 days before departure to the area with risk of malaria and should be continued once a day while in the area with risk of malaria and daily for 7 days after leaving the area. The drug should not be used during pregnancy or lactation unless the breastfed child has a documented normal G6PD concentration.

Prophylaxis During Pregnancy and Lactation. Malaria in pregnancy carries significant risks of morbidity and mortality for both the mother and fetus. Malaria may increase the risk of adverse outcomes in pregnancy, including abortion, preterm birth, and stillbirth. For these reasons and because no chemoprophylactic regimen completely is effective, women who are pregnant or likely to become pregnant should try to avoid travel to areas where they could contract malaria. Women traveling to areas where drug-resistant *P falciparum* has not been reported may take chloroquine prophylaxis. Harmful effects on the fetus have not been demonstrated when chloroquine is given in the recommended doses for malaria prophylaxis. Pregnancy and lactation, therefore, are not contraindications for malaria prophylaxis with chloroquine.

For pregnant women who travel to areas where chloroquine-resistant *P falciparum* exists, the CDC recommends mefloquine chemoprophylaxis in all trimesters of pregnancy. Consequently, mefloquine is the drug of choice for prophylactic use for women who are pregnant or likely to become pregnant when exposure to chloroquine-resistant *P falciparum* is unavoidable. Lactating mothers of infants weighing more than 5 kg may also use atovaquone-proguanil or mefloquine for prophylaxis when exposure to chloroquine-resistant *P falciparum* is unavoidable.

Reliable Antimalarial Supply While Traveling. Travelers to malaria-endemic settings should seek medical attention immediately if they develop fever. Malaria can be treated effectively early in the course of disease, but delay of appropriate treatment can have serious or even fatal consequences. Travelers who do not take an antimalarial drug for prophylaxis or who are on a less-than-effective regimen or who may be in very remote areas can be given a reliable supply of atovaquone-proguanil or artemether-lumefantrine. If they are diagnosed with malaria while traveling, they will have a medicine that will not interact with their other medications, is of good quality, and is not depleting local resources.

Travelers taking atovaquone-proguanil as their antimalarial drug regimen should not take atovaquone-proguanil for treatment and should use an alternative antimalarial regimen recommended by a travel medicine expert.

Travelers should be advised that any fever or influenza-like illness that develops within 3 months of departure from an area with endemic malaria requires immediate medical evaluation, including blood films to rule out malaria.

Prevention of Relapses. To prevent relapses of *P vivax* or *P ovale* infection after departure from areas where these species are endemic, travelers with prolonged exposure and normal G6PD concentrations should receive presumptive antirelapse therapy (terminal prophylaxis) with primaquine for 14 days. Rarely, travelers exposed to primaquine resistant or tolerant parasites may require high-dose primaquine. Primaquine can cause hemolysis in patients with G6PD deficiency; thus, all patients should be screened for this condition before primaquine therapy is initiated.

Personal Protective Measures. All travelers to areas where malaria is endemic should be advised to use personal protective measures, including the following: (1) using insecticide-impregnated mosquito nets while sleeping; (2) remaining in well-screened areas; (3) wearing protective clothing; and (4) using mosquito repellents containing DEET, picaridin, oil of lemon eucalyptus, or IR3535. To be effective, most repellents require frequent reapplications (see Prevention of Mosquitoborne Infections, p 209, for recommendations regarding prevention of mosquitoborne infections and use of insect repellents).

Measles

CLINICAL MANIFESTATIONS: Measles is an acute viral disease characterized by fever, cough, coryza, conjunctivitis, an erythematous maculopapular rash, and a pathognomonic enanthema (Koplik spots). Complications including otitis media, bronchopneumonia, laryngotracheobronchitis (croup), and diarrhea occur commonly in young children. Acute encephalitis,which often results in permanent brain damage, occurs in approximately 1 of every 1000 cases. In the postelimination era, death, predominantly resulting from respiratory and neurologic complications, has occurred in 1 to 3 of every 1000 cases reported in the United States. Case-fatality rates are increased in children younger than 5 years of age and immunocompromised children, including children with leukemia, human immunodeficiency virus (HIV) infection, and severe malnutrition. Sometimes the characteristic rash does not develop in immunocompromised patients.

Subacute sclerosing panencephalitis (SSPE) is a rare degenerative central nervous system disease characterized by behavioral and intellectual deterioration and seizures that occurs 7 to 10 years after wild-type measles virus infection. Widespread measles immunization has led to the virtual disappearance of SSPE in the United States.

ETIOLOGY: Measles virus is an enveloped RNA virus with 1 serotype, classified as a member of the genus Morbillivirus in the Paramyxoviridae family.

EPIDEMIOLOGY: The only natural hosts of measles virus are humans. Measles is transmitted by direct contact with infectious droplets or, less commonly, by airborne spread. Measles is one of the most highly communicable of all infectious diseases. In temperate areas, the peak incidence of infection usually occurs during late winter and spring. In the prevaccine era, most cases of measles in the United States occurred in preschool- and young school-aged children, and few people remained susceptible by 20 years of age. The childhood and adolescent immunization program in the United States has resulted in a greater than 99% decrease in the reported incidence of measles and interruption of endemic disease transmission since measles vaccine first was licensed in 1963.

From 1989 to 1991, the incidence of measles in the United States increased because of low immunization rates in preschool-aged children, especially in urban areas. Following improved coverage in preschool-aged children and implementation of a routine second dose of MMR vaccine for children, the incidence of measles declined to extremely low levels (<1 case per 1 million population). In 2000, an independent panel of internationally recognized experts reviewed available data and unanimously agreed that measles no longer was endemic (continuous, year-round transmission) in the United States. In the postelimination era, from 2001 through 2010, the incidence of measles in the United States has been low (37–140 cases reported per year), consistent with an absence of endemic transmission. Cases of measles continue to occur, however, as a result of importation of the virus from other countries. Cases are considered international importations if the rash onset occurs within 21 days after entering the United States. During 2011, 222 cases of measles were reported to the Centers for Disease Control and Prevention (CDC) from 30 states—the highest number of reported measles cases since 1996. Seventy-two of the cases were direct importations from 20 to 22 countries, and 17 outbreaks (3 or more cases) occurred. The majority (approximately 85%) of cases were in people who were unimmunized or had unknown immunization status, including 27 cases in infants younger than 12 months of age, some of whom had traveled abroad.

Vaccine failure occurs in as many as 5% of people who have received a single dose of vaccine at 12 months of age or older. Although waning immunity after immunization may be a factor in some cases, most cases of measles in previously immunized children seem to occur in people in whom response to the vaccine was inadequate (ie, primary vaccine failures). This was the main reason a 2-dose vaccine schedule was recommended routinely for children and high-risk adults.

Patients are contagious from 4 days before the rash to 4 days after appearance of the rash. Immunocompromised patients who may have prolonged excretion of the virus in respiratory tract secretions can be contagious for the duration of the illness. Patients with SSPE are not contagious.

The **incubation period** generally is 8 to 12 days from exposure to onset of symptoms. In family studies, the average interval between appearance of rash in the index case and subsequent cases is 14 days, with a range of 7 to 21 days. In SSPE, the mean incubation period of 84 cases reported between 1976 and 1983 was 10.8 years.

DIAGNOSTIC TESTS: Measles virus infection can be diagnosed by a positive serologic test result for measles immunoglobulin (Ig) M antibody, a significant increase in measles IgG antibody concentration in paired acute and convalescent serum specimens by any standard serologic assay, or isolation of measles virus or identification of measles RNA (by reverse transcriptase-polymerase chain reaction assay) from clinical specimens, such as urine, blood or throat or nasopharyngeal secretions. State public health laboratories or the CDC Measles Laboratory will process these viral specimens. The simplest method of establishing the diagnosis of measles is testing for IgM antibody on a single serum specimen obtained during the first encounter with a person suspected of having disease. The sensitivity of measles IgM assays varies by timing of specimen collection and immunization status of the case and may be diminished during the first 72 hours after rash onset. If the result is negative for measles IgM and the patient has a generalized rash lasting more than 72 hours, a second serum specimen should be obtained, and the measles IgM test should be repeated. Measles IgM is detectable for at least 1 month after rash onset in unimmunized people but might be absent or present only transiently in people immunized with 1 or 2 vaccine doses. Therefore, a negative IgM test should not be used to rule out the diagnosis in immunized people. People with febrile rash illness who are seronegative for measles IgM should be tested for rubella using the same specimens. Genotyping of viral isolates allows determination of patterns of importation and transmission, and genome sequencing can be used to differentiate between wild-type and vaccine virus infection in those who have been immunized recently. All cases of suspected measles should be reported immediately to the local or state health department without waiting for results of diagnostic tests. Measles now is on the list of nationally notifiable diseases that should be reported to the CDC within 24 hours.

TREATMENT: No specific antiviral therapy is available. Measles virus is susceptible in vitro to ribavirin, which has been given by the intravenous and aerosol routes to treat severely affected and immunocompromised children with measles. However, no controlled trials have been conducted, and ribavirin is not approved by the US Food and Drug Administration for treatment of measles.

Vitamin A. Vitamin A treatment of children with measles in developing countries has been associated with decreased morbidity and mortality rates. Low serum concentrations of vitamin A also have been found in children in the United States, and children with more severe measles illness have lower vitamin A concentrations. The World Health Organization currently recommends vitamin A for all children with acute measles, regardless of their country of residence. Vitamin A for treatment of measles is administered once daily for 2 days, at the following doses:

- 200 000 IU for children 12 months of age or older;
- 100 000 IU for infants 6 through 11 months of age; and
- 50 000 IU for infants younger than 6 months of age.
- An additional (ie, a third) age-specific dose should be given 2 through 4 weeks later to children with clinical signs and symptoms of vitamin A deficiency.

Parenteral and oral formulations of vitamin A are available in the United States.

ISOLATION OF THE HOSPITALIZED PATIENT: In addition to standard precautions, airborne transmission precautions are indicated for 4 days after the onset of rash in otherwise healthy children and for the duration of illness in immunocompromised patients.

CONTROL MEASURES:

Care of Exposed People.

Use of Vaccine. Available data suggest that measles vaccine, if given within 72 hours of measles exposure, will provide protection in some cases. If the exposure does not result in infection, the vaccine should induce protection against subsequent measles exposures. Immunization is the intervention of choice for control of measles outbreaks in schools and child care centers.

Use of Immune Globulin. Immune Globulin (IG) can be given intramuscularly to prevent or modify measles in a susceptible person within 6 days of exposure. The usual recommended dose is 0.25 mL/kg given intramuscularly; immunocompromised children should receive 0.5 mL/kg intramuscularly (the maximum dose in either instance is 15 mL). IG is indicated for susceptible household or other close contacts of patients with measles, particularly contacts younger than 1 year of age, pregnant women, and immunocompromised people, for whom risk of complications is highest, or other people for whom measles vaccine is contraindicated. IG is not indicated for household or other close contacts who have received 1 dose of vaccine at 12 months of age or older unless they are immunocompromised.

Immune Globulin Intravenous (IGIV) preparations generally contain measles antibodies at approximately the same concentration per gram of protein as IG, although the concentration may vary by lot and manufacturer. For patients who receive IGIV regularly, the usual dose of 400 mg/kg should be adequate for measles prophylaxis after exposures occurring within 3 weeks of receiving IGIV.

For children who receive IG for modification or prevention of measles after exposure, measles vaccine (if not contraindicated) should be administered 5 months (if the dose was 0.25 mL/kg) or 6 months (if the dose was 0.5 mL/kg) after IG administration, provided the child is at least 12 months of age. Intervals between administration of IGIV or other biologic products and measles-containing vaccines vary (see Table 1.9, p 38).

HIV Infection. HIV-infected children who are exposed to measles will require prophylaxis on the basis of immune status and measles vaccine history. HIV-infected children who have serologic evidence of immunity or who received 2 doses of measles vaccine with no or moderate immunosuppression (see Human Immunodeficiency Virus Infection, p 418) should be considered immune and will not require any additional measures to prevent measles. Children with HIV-1 with severe immune suppression who are exposed to measles should receive intramuscular Immune Globulin (IG) prophylaxis (0.5 mL/kg, maximum 15 mL), regardless of immunization status, and exposed, asymptomatic HIV-1-infected patients also should receive intramuscular IG but at a lower dose (0.25 mL/kg) (see Human Immunodeficiency Virus Infection, p 418). Children who have received IGIV within 2 weeks of exposure do not require additional passive immunization.

Health Care Personnel. To decrease health care-associated infection, immunization programs should be established to ensure that all people who work or volunteer in health care facilities who may be in contact with patients with measles have presumptive evidence of immunity to measles (see Health Care Personnel, p 99).

Measles Vaccine. The only measles vaccine licensed in the United States is a live further-attenuated strain prepared in chicken embryo cell culture. Measles vaccines provided through the Expanded Programme on Immunization in developing countries meet the World Health Organization standards and usually are comparable to the vaccine available in the United States. Measles vaccine is available in combination formulations, which include measles-mumps-rubella (MMR) and measles-mumps-rubella-varicella (MMRV) vaccines. Single-antigen measles vaccine no longer is available in the United States. Measles-containing vaccine in a dose of 0.5 mL is administered subcutaneously. Measles-containing vaccines can be given simultaneously with other immunizations in a separate syringe at a separate site (see Simultaneous Administration of Multiple Vaccines, p 33).

Serum measles antibodies develop in approximately 95% of children immunized at 12 months of age and 98% of children immunized at 15 months of age. Protection conferred by a single dose is durable in most people. However, a small proportion (5% or less) of immunized people may lose protection after several years. More than 99% of people who receive 2 doses separated by at least 4 weeks, with the first dose administered on or after their first birthday, develop serologic evidence of measles immunity. Immunization is not deleterious for people who already are immune. Immunized people do not shed or transmit measles vaccine virus.

Improperly stored vaccine may fail to protect against measles. Since 1979, an improved stabilizer has been added to the vaccine that makes it more resistant to heat inactivation. For recommended storage of MMR and MMRV vaccines, see the manufacturers' package labels. MMRV vaccine must be stored frozen between −58°F and +5°F.

Vaccine Recommendations (see Table 3.34, p 494, for summary).

Age of Routine Immunization. The first dose of MMR vaccine should be given at 12 through 15 months of age. Delays in administering the first dose contributed to large outbreaks in the United States from 1989 to 1991. Initial immunization at 12 months of age is recommended for preschool-aged children in high-risk areas, especially large urban areas. The second dose is recommended routinely at school entry (ie, 4 through 6 years of age) but can be given at any earlier age (eg, during an outbreak or before international travel), provided the interval between the first and second doses is at least 28 days. Catch-up second dose immunization should occur for all school children (elementary, middle, high school) who have received only 1 dose, including at the adolescent visit at 11 through 12 years of age and beyond. If a child receives a dose of measles vaccine before 12 months of age, this dose is not considered valid, and 2 doses are required beginning at 12 through 15 months of age and separated by at least 4 weeks.

Use of MMRV Vaccine.[1,2]

- MMRV vaccine is indicated for simultaneous immunization against measles, mumps, rubella, and varicella among children 12 months through 12 years of age; MMRV vaccine is not indicated for people outside this age group. See Varicella-Zoster Infections, p 774, for recommendations for use of MMRV vaccine for the first dose.
- Children with HIV infection also should not receive MMRV vaccine because of lack of safety data in children infected with HIV.
- MMRV vaccine may be administered with other vaccines recommended at 12 through 15 months of age and before or at 4 through 6 years of age (see Fig 1.1, p 27–28).
- At least 28 days should elapse between a dose of measles-containing vaccine, such as MMR vaccine, and a dose of MMRV vaccine. However, the recommended minimal interval between varicella vaccine doses is 90 days.
- Febrile seizures occur in 7 to 9 per 10 000 children receiving the first dose of MMRV vaccine at 12 through 23 months of age and in 3 to 4 per 10 000 children receiving the first dose of MMR and varicella vaccines administered separately at the same visit at 12

---

[1] Centers for Disease Control and Prevention. Use of combination measles, mumps, rubella, and varicella vaccine: recommendations of the Advisory Committee on Immunization Practices (ACIP). *MMWR Recomm Rep.* 2010;59(RR-3):1–12

[2] American Academy of Pediatrics, Committee on Infectious Diseases. Prevention of varicella: update of recommendations for use of quadrivalent and monovalent varicella vaccines in children. *Pediatrics.* 2011;128(3):630–632

Table 3.34. Recommendations for Measles Immunization[a]

Category	Recommendations
Unimmunized, no history of measles (12 through 15 mo of age)	MMR vaccine is recommended at 12 through 15 mo of age; a second dose is recommended at least 28 days after the first dose and usually is given at 4 through 6 y of age
Children 6 through 11 mo of age in epidemic situations[b] or before international travel	Immunize with MMR vaccine, but this dose is not considered valid, and 2 valid doses administered on or after the first birthday are required. The first valid dose should be administered at 12 through 15 mo of age; the second valid dose is recommended at least 28 days later and usually is given at 4 through 6 y of age
Students in kindergarten, elementary, middle, and high school who have received 1 dose of measles vaccine at 12 mo of age or older	Administer the second dose
Students in college and other post-high school institutions who have received 1 dose of measles vaccine at 12 mo of age or older	Administer the second dose
History of immunization before the first birthday	Dose not considered valid; immunize (2 doses)
History of receipt of inactivated measles vaccine or unknown type of vaccine, 1963–1967	Dose not considered valid; immunize (2 doses)
Further attenuated or unknown vaccine given with IG	Dose not considered valid; immunize (2 doses)
Allergy to eggs	Immunize; no reactions likely (see text for details)
Neomycin allergy, nonanaphylactic	Immunize; no reactions likely (see text for details)
Severe hypersensitivity (anaphylaxis) to neomycin or gelatin	Avoid immunization
Tuberculosis	Immunize (see Tuberculosis, p 736); if patient has untreated tuberculosis disease, start antituberculosis therapy before immunizing
Measles exposure	Immunize and/or give IG, depending on circumstances (see text, p 492)
HIV infected	Immunize (2 doses) unless severely immunocompromised (see text, p 498), and give IG if exposed to measles
Personal or family history of seizures	Immunize; advise parents of slightly increased risk of seizures
Immunoglobulin or blood recipient	Immunize at the appropriate interval (see Table 1.9, p 38)

MMR indicates measles-mumps-rubella vaccine; MMRV, measles-mumps-rubella-varicella vaccine; IG, Immune Globulin; HIV, human immunodeficiency virus.

[a] See text for details and recommendations for use of MMRV vaccine.
[b] See Outbreak Control (p 499).

through 23 months of age. Thus, one additional febrile seizure is expected to occur per approximately 2300 to 2600 children 12 through 23 months of age immunized with MMRV vaccine, compared with separate MMR and monovalent varicella vaccines. The period of risk for febrile seizures is from 5 to 12 days following receipt of the vaccine. Febrile seizures do not predispose to epilepsy or neurodevelopmental delays later in life and have no lasting medical consequence. The American Academy of Pediatrics recommends that for the first dose of measles, mumps, rubella, and varicella vaccines at ages 12 through 47 months, either MMR and varicella vaccines or MMRV vaccine be used. Pediatricians should discuss risks and benefits of the vaccine choices with the parents or caregivers. For the first dose of measles, mumps, rubella, and varicella vaccines at ages 48 months and older and for dose 2 at any age (15 months through 12 years), use of MMRV vaccine generally is preferred over separate injections of MMR and varicella vaccines to minimize the number of injections.

Colleges and Other Institutions for Education Beyond High School. Colleges and other institutions should require that all entering students have documentation of evidence of measles immunity: physician-diagnosed measles, serologic evidence of immunity, or receipt of 2 doses of measles-containing vaccines administered at least 28 days apart. Students without documentation of measles immunity should receive MMR vaccine on entry, followed by a second dose 4 weeks later, if not contraindicated.

Immunization During an Outbreak. During an outbreak, MMR vaccine should be offered to all people exposed or in the outbreak setting who lack evidence of immunity. During a community-wide outbreak affecting infants, MMR vaccine may be recommended for infants 6 to 11 months of age (see Outbreak Control, p 499). However, seroconversion rates after MMR immunization significantly are lower in children immunized before the first birthday than are seroconversion rates in children immunized after the first birthday. Doses received prior to the first birthday should not count toward the recommended 2-dose series. Therefore, children immunized before their first birthday should be reimmunized with MMR or MMRV vaccine at 12 through 15 months of age (at least 28 days after the initial measles immunization) and again at school entry (4 through 6 years of age).

International Travel. People traveling internationally should be immune to measles. Infants 6 through 11 months of age should receive 1 dose of MMR vaccine before departure, and then they should receive a measles-containing vaccine at 12 through 15 months of age (at least 28 days after the initial measles immunization) and again at 4 through 6 years of age. Children 12 through 15 months of age should be given their first dose of MMR vaccine before departure and again by 4 through 6 years of age. Children 12 months of age or older who have received 1 dose and are traveling to areas where measles is endemic or epidemic should receive their second dose before departure, provided the interval between doses is 28 days or more.

International Adoptees. The US Department of State requires that internationally adopted children 10 years of age and older receive several vaccines, including MMR, before entry into the United States. Internationally adopted children who are younger than 10 years of age are exempt from Immigration and Nationality Act regulations pertaining to immunization of immigrants before arrival in the United States (see Refugees and Immigrants, p 101); adoptive parents are required to sign a waiver indicating their intention to comply with US immunization recommendations after their child's arrival in the United States.

Health Care Personnel.[1] Adequate presumptive evidence of immunity to measles for people who work in health care facilities is: (1) documented administration of 2 doses of live-virus measles vaccine; (2) laboratory evidence of immunity or laboratory confirmation of disease; or (3) birth before 1957 (see Health Care Personnel, p 99). For recommendations during an outbreak, see Outbreak Control (p 499).

Adverse Events. A temperature of 39.4°C (103°F) or higher develops in approximately 5% to 15% of vaccine recipients, usually between 6 and 12 days after receipt of MMR vaccine; fever generally lasts 1 to 2 days but may last as long as 5 days. Most people with fever otherwise are asymptomatic. Transient rashes have been reported in approximately 5% of vaccine recipients. Febrile seizures 5 to 12 days after immunization occur in 1 in 3000 to 4000 people immunized with MMR vaccine. Transient thrombocytopenia occurs in 1 in 22 000 to 40 000 people after administration of measles-containing vaccines, specifically MMR (see Thrombocytopenia, p 497). There is no evidence that reimmunization increases the risk of adverse events in people already immune to these diseases. Data indicate that only people who are not immune to the viruses in MMR tend to have adverse effects. Thus, events following a second dose of MMR vaccine would be expected to be substantially lower than after a first dose, because most people who received a first dose would be immune.

Rates of most local and systemic adverse events for children immunized with MMRV vaccine are comparable to rates for children immunized with MMR and varicella vaccines administered concomitantly. However, recipients of a first dose of MMRV vaccine have a significantly greater rate of fever 102°F (38.9°C) or higher than do recipients of MMR and varicella administered concomitantly (22% vs 15%, respectively), and measles-like rash is observed in 3% of recipients of MMRV vaccine and 2% of recipients of MMR and varicella vaccines administered concomitantly.

The reported frequency of central nervous system conditions, such as encephalitis and encephalopathy, after measles immunization is less than 1 per million doses administered in the United States. Because the incidence of encephalitis or encephalopathy after measles immunization in the United States is lower than the observed incidence of encephalitis of unknown cause, some or most of the rare reported severe neurologic disorders may be related coincidentally, rather than causally, to measles immunization. Multiple studies, as well as an Institute of Medicine Vaccine Safety Review, refute a causal relationship between autism and MMR vaccine or between inflammatory bowel disease and MMR vaccine. The original 1998 study claiming such a relationship was retracted by the publishing journal in 2010, and the lead author has had his medical license revoked in Great Britain. After reimmunization, reactions are expected to be similar clinically but much less frequent, because most of the vaccine recipients are immune.

Seizures. Risk of febrile seizure following receipt of MMR and MMRV vaccines at 12 through 23 months of age is discussed earlier in the chapter (see Use of MMRV Vaccine, p 493). Children with histories of seizures or children whose first-degree relatives have histories of seizures may be at a slightly increased risk of a seizure but should be immunized with MMR and varicella vaccines, because the benefits greatly outweigh the risks.

---

[1] Centers for Disease Control and Prevention. Immunization of health-care personnel: recommendations of the Advisory Committee on Immunization Practices (ACIP). *MMWR Recomm Rep.* 2011;60(RR-07):1–45

Subacute Sclerosing Panencephalitis. Measles vaccine, by protecting against measles, decreases significantly the possibility of developing SSPE. Vaccine-strain measles virus has never been confirmed in a case of SSPE.

Precautions and Contraindications (also see Table 1.9, p 38).

Febrile Illnesses. Children with minor illnesses, such as upper respiratory tract infections, may be immunized (see Vaccine Safety, p 41). Fever is not a contraindication to immunization. However, if other manifestations suggest a more serious illness, the child should not be immunized until recovered.

Allergic Reactions. Hypersensitivity reactions occur rarely and usually are minor, consisting of wheal and flare reactions or urticaria at the injection site. Reactions have been attributed to trace amounts of neomycin or gelatin or some other component in the vaccine formulation. Anaphylaxis is rare. Measles vaccine is produced in chicken embryo cell culture and does not contain significant amounts of egg white (ovalbumin) cross-reacting proteins. Children with egg allergy are at low risk of anaphylactic reactions to measles-containing vaccines (including MMR and MMRV). Skin testing of children for egg allergy is not predictive of reactions to MMR vaccine and is not required before administering MMR or other measles-containing vaccines. People with allergies to chickens or feathers are not at increased risk of reaction to the vaccine.

People who have had a significant hypersensitivity reaction after the first dose of measles vaccine should: (1) be tested for measles immunity, and if immune, should not be given a second dose; or (2) receive evaluation and possible skin testing before receiving a second dose. People who have had an immediate anaphylactic reaction to previous measles immunization should not be reimmunized but should be tested to determine whether they are immune.

People who have experienced anaphylactic reactions to gelatin or topically or systemically administered neomycin should receive measles vaccine only in settings where such reactions can be managed and after consultation with an allergist or immunologist. Most often, however, neomycin allergy manifests as contact dermatitis, which is not a contraindication to receiving measles vaccine.

Thrombocytopenia. Rarely, MMR vaccine can be associated with thrombocytopenia within 2 months of immunization, with a temporal clustering 2 to 3 weeks after immunization. On the basis of case reports, the risk of vaccine-associated thrombocytopenia may be higher for people who previously experienced thrombocytopenia, especially if it occurred in temporal association with earlier MMR immunization. The decision to immunize these children should be based on assessment of immunity after the first dose and the benefits of protection against measles, mumps, and rubella in comparison with the risks of recurrence of thrombocytopenia after immunization. The risk of thrombocytopenia is higher after the first dose of vaccine than after the second dose. There have been no reported cases of thrombocytopenia associated with receipt of MMR vaccine that have resulted in hemorrhagic complications or death in otherwise healthy people.

Recent Administration of IG. IG preparations interfere with the serologic response to measles vaccine for variable periods, depending on the dose of IG administered. Suggested intervals between IG or blood-product administration and measles immunization are given in Table 1.9 (p 38). If vaccine is given at intervals shorter than those indicated, as may be warranted if the risk of exposure to measles is imminent, the child should be reimmunized at or after the appropriate interval for immunization (and at least 4 weeks after the earlier immunization) unless serologic testing indicates that measles-specific antibodies were produced.

If IG is to be administered in preparation for international travel, administration of vaccine should precede receipt of IG by at least 2 weeks to preclude interference with replication of the vaccine virus.

Tuberculosis. Tuberculin skin testing is not a prerequisite for measles immunization. Antituberculosis therapy should be initiated before administering MMR vaccine to people with untreated tuberculosis infection or disease. Tuberculin skin testing, if otherwise indicated, can be performed on the day of immunization. Otherwise, testing should be postponed for 4 to 6 weeks, because measles immunization temporarily may suppress tuberculin skin test reactivity.

Altered Immunity. Immunocompromised patients with disorders associated with increased severity of viral infections should not be given live-virus measles vaccine (the exception is people with HIV infection, unless they have evidence of severe immunosuppression; see Immunocompromised Children, p 74, and HIV Infection, p 418). The risk of exposure to measles for immunocompromised patients can be decreased by immunizing their close susceptible contacts. Immunized people do not shed or transmit measles vaccine virus. Management of immunodeficient and immunosuppressed patients exposed to measles can be facilitated by previous knowledge of their immune status. If possible, children should receive measles vaccine prior to initiating treatment with biological response modifiers, such as tumor necrosis factor antagonists. Susceptible patients with immunodeficiencies should receive IG after measles exposure (see Care of Exposed People, p 491).

Corticosteroids. For patients who have received high doses of corticosteroids (2 mg/kg or greater than 20 mg/day of prednisone or its equivalent) for 14 days or more and who otherwise are not immunocompromised, the recommended interval before immunization is at least 1 month (see Immunocompromised Children, p 74). In general, inhaled steroids do not cause immunosuppression and are not a contraindication to measles immunization.

HIV Infection. Measles immunization (given as MMR vaccine) is recommended at the usual ages for people with asymptomatic HIV infection and for people with symptomatic infection who are not severely immunocompromised, because measles can be severe and often is fatal in patients with HIV infection (see Human Immunodeficiency Virus Infection, p 418). Severely immunocompromised HIV-infected infants, children, adolescents, and young adults, as defined by low CD4+ T-lymphocyte counts or percentage of total lymphocytes (ie, <750/μL or <15% for infants <12 months of age, <500/μL or <15% for children 1 through 5 years of age, <200/μL or <15% for children 6 through 12 years of age, or <200/μL or <14% for people ≥13 years of age), should not receive measles virus-containing vaccine, because vaccine-related pneumonia has been reported (see Human Immunodeficiency Virus Infection, p 418). All members of the household of an HIV-infected person should receive MMR unless they are HIV infected and severely immunosuppressed, were born before 1957, have had physician-diagnosed measles, have laboratory evidence of measles immunity, have had age-appropriate immunizations, or have a contraindication to measles vaccine. Because measles vaccine virus is not shed after immunization, HIV-infected people are not at risk of measles vaccine virus infection if household members are immunized.

Regardless of immunization status, symptomatic HIV-infected patients who are exposed to measles should receive IG prophylaxis, because immunization may not provide protection (see Care of Exposed People, p 491).

Personal or Family History of Seizures. Children with a personal or family history of seizures should be immunized after parents or guardians are advised that the risk of seizures after measles immunization is increased slightly. Risk of febrile seizure following receipt of MMR and MMRV vaccine at 12 through 23 months of age is discussed earlier in the chapter (see Use of MMRV Vaccine, p 493). Children receiving anticonvulsants should continue such therapy after measles immunization.

Pregnancy. A measles-containing vaccine should not be given to women known to be pregnant. Women who are given MMR vaccine should not become pregnant for at least 28 days. This precaution is based on the theoretical risk of fetal infection, which applies to administration of any live-virus vaccine to women who might be pregnant or who might become pregnant shortly after immunization. No evidence, however, substantiates this theoretical risk. In the immunization of adolescents and young adults against measles, asking women if they are pregnant, excluding women who are, and explaining the theoretical risks to others are recommended precautions.

Outbreak Control. Every suspected measles case should be reported immediately to the local health department, and every effort must be made to obtain laboratory evidence that would confirm that the illness is measles, especially if the illness may be the first case in the community. Subsequent prevention of spread of measles depends on prompt immunization of people at risk of exposure or people already exposed who cannot readily provide documentation of measles immunity, including the date of immunization. People who have not been immunized, including those who have been exempted from measles immunization for medical, religious, or other reasons, should be excluded from school, child care, and health care settings until at least 21 days after the onset of rash in the last case of measles. Extra doses of measles vaccine are not harmful.

Schools and Child Care Facilities. During measles outbreaks in child care facilities, schools, and colleges and other institutions of higher education, all students, their siblings, and personnel born in 1957 or after who cannot provide documentation that they received 2 doses of measles-containing vaccine on or after their first birthday or other evidence of measles immunity should be immunized. People receiving their second dose as well as unimmunized people receiving their first dose as part of the outbreak-control program may be readmitted immediately to the school or child care facility.

Health Care Facilities. If an outbreak occurs in an area served by a hospital or within a hospital, all employees, volunteers, and other personnel who were born in 1957 or after who cannot provide documentation that they have received 2 doses of measles vaccine on or after their first birthday or laboratory evidence of immunity to measles should receive 2 doses of MMR vaccine. Because some health care personnel born before 1957 have acquired measles in health care facilities, immunization with 2 doses of MMR vaccine is recommended for health care personnel without serologic evidence of immunity in this age category during outbreaks. Health care personnel without evidence of immunity who have been exposed should be relieved of direct patient contact from the fifth to the 21st day after exposure, regardless of whether they received vaccine or IG after the exposure. Health care personnel who become ill should be relieved of patient contact for 4 days after rash develops.

Meningococcal Infections

CLINICAL MANIFESTATIONS: Invasive infection usually results in meningococcemia, meningitis, or both. Onset can be insidious and nonspecific but often is abrupt, with fever, chills, malaise, myalgia, limb pain, prostration, and a rash that initially can be macular, maculopapular, petechial, or purpuric. The maculopapular and petechial rash is indistinguishable from the rash caused by some viral infections. Purpura can occur in severe sepsis caused by other bacterial pathogens. In fulminant cases, purpura, limb ischemia, coagulopathy, pulmonary edema, shock (characterized by tachycardia, tachypnea, oliguria, and poor peripheral perfusion, with confusion and hypotension), coma, and death can ensue in hours despite appropriate therapy. Signs and symptoms of meningococcal meningitis are indistinguishable from those associated with acute meningitis caused by other meningeal pathogens (eg, *Streptococcus pneumoniae*). In severe and fatal cases of meningococcal meningitis, raised intracranial pressure is a predominant presenting feature. The overall case-fatality rate for meningococcal disease is 10% and is higher in adolescents. Death is associated with coma, hypotension, leukopenia, thrombocytopenia, and absence of meningitis. Less common manifestations of meningococcal infection include conjunctivitis, pneumonia, febrile occult bacteremia, septic arthritis, and chronic meningococcemia. Invasive infections can be complicated by arthritis, myocarditis, pericarditis, and endophthalmitis. A self-limiting postinfectious inflammatory syndrome occurs in less than 10% of cases 4 or more days after onset of meningococcal infection and most commonly presents as fever and arthritis or vasculitis. Iritis, scleritis, conjunctivitis, pericarditis, and polyserositis are less common manifestations of postinfectious inflammatory syndrome.

Sequelae associated with meningococcal disease occur in 11% to 19% of survivors and include hearing loss, neurologic disability, digit or limb amputations, and skin scarring.

ETIOLOGY: *Neisseria meningitidis* is a gram-negative diplococcus with at least 13 serogroups based on capsule type.

EPIDEMIOLOGY: Strains belonging to groups A, B, C, Y, and W-135 are implicated most commonly in invasive disease worldwide. Serogroup A has been associated frequently with epidemics outside the United States, primarily in sub-Saharan Africa. An increase in cases of serogroup W-135 meningococcal disease has been associated with the Hajj pilgrimage in Saudi Arabia. Since 2002, serogroup W-135 meningococcal disease has been reported in sub-Saharan African countries during epidemic seasons. Prolonged outbreaks of serogroup B meningococcal disease have occurred in New Zealand, France, and Oregon. Serogroup X causes a substantial number of cases of meningococcal disease in parts of Africa but is rare on other continents.

The incidence of meningococcal disease varies over time and by age and location. During the past 60 years, the annual incidence of meningococcal disease in the United States has varied from 0.5 to 1.5 cases per 100 000 population. Incidence cycles have occurred over multiple years. Since the early 2000s, annual incidence rates have decreased and are sustained. The reasons for this decrease, which preceded introduction of meningococcal polysaccharide-protein conjugate vaccine into the immunization schedule, are not known but may be related to immunity of the population to circulating meningococcal strains and to the changes in behavioral risk factors (eg, smoking).

Distribution of meningococcal serogroups in the United States has shifted in the past 2 decades. Serogroups B, C, and Y each account for approximately 30% of reported cases, but serogroup distribution varies by age, location, and time. Approximately three quarters of cases among adolescents and young adults are caused by serogroups C, Y, or W-135 and potentially are preventable with available vaccines. In infants, 50% to 60% of cases are caused by serogroup B and are not preventable with vaccines available in the United States.

Since introduction in the United States of *Haemophilus influenzae* type b and pneumococcal polysaccharide-protein conjugate vaccines for infants, *N meningitidis* has become the leading cause of bacterial meningitis in children and remains an important cause of septicemia. Disease most often occurs in children 2 years of age or younger; the peak incidence occurs in children younger than 1 year of age. Another peak occurs in adolescents and young adults 16 through 21 years of age. Historically, freshman college students who lived in dormitories and military recruits in boot camp had a higher rate of disease compared with people who are the same age and who are not living in such accommodations. Close contacts of patients with meningococcal disease are at increased risk of becoming infected. Patients with persistent complement component deficiencies (eg, C5–C9, properdin, or factor H or factor D deficiencies) or anatomic or functional asplenia are at increased risk of invasive and recurrent meningococcal disease. Patients are considered capable of transmitting the organism for up to 24 hours after initiation of effective antimicrobial treatment. Asymptomatic colonization of the upper respiratory tract provides the source from which the organism is spread. Transmission occurs from person-to-person through droplets from the respiratory tract and requires close contact.

Outbreaks occur in communities and institutions, including child care centers, schools, colleges, and military recruit camps. However, most cases of meningococcal disease are endemic, with fewer than 5% associated with outbreaks. The attack rate for household contacts is 500 to 800 times the rate for the general population. Serologic typing, multilocus sequence typing, multilocus enzyme electrophoresis, and pulsed-field gel electrophoresis of enzyme-restricted DNA fragments can be useful epidemiologic tools during a suspected outbreak to detect concordance among invasive strains.

The **incubation period** is 1 to 10 days, usually less than 4 days.

DIAGNOSTIC TESTS: Cultures of blood and cerebrospinal fluid (CSF) are indicated for patients with suspected invasive meningococcal disease. Cultures of a petechial or purpuric lesion scraping, synovial fluid, and other usually sterile body fluid specimens yield the organism in some patients. A Gram stain of a petechial or purpuric scraping, CSF, and buffy coat smear of blood can be helpful. Because *N meningitidis* can be a component of the nasopharyngeal flora, isolation of *N meningitidis* from this site is not helpful diagnostically. Bacterial antigen detection in CSF supports the diagnosis of a probable case if the clinical illness is consistent with meningococcal disease. A serogroup-specific polymerase chain reaction (PCR) test to detect *N meningitidis* from clinical specimens is used routinely in the United Kingdom and some European countries, where up to 56% of cases are confirmed by PCR testing alone. This test particularly is useful in patients who receive antimicrobial therapy before cultures are obtained. In the United States, PCR-based assays are available in some research and public health laboratories.

Case definitions for invasive meningococcal disease are given in Table 3.35.

Table 3.35. Surveillance Case Definitions for Invasive Meningococcal Disease

Confirmed

A clinically compatible case and isolation of *Neisseria meningitidis* from a usually sterile site, for example:
- Blood
- Cerebrospinal fluid
- Synovial fluid
- Pleural fluid
- Pericardial fluid
- Isolation from skin scraping of petechial or purpuric lesions

Probable

A clinically compatible case with either a positive result of antigen test or immunohistochemistry of formalin-fixed tissue or a positive polymerase chain reaction test of blood or cerebrospinal fluid without a positive sterile site culture

Suspect
- A clinically compatible case and gram-negative diplococci in any sterile fluid, such as cerebrospinal fluid, synovial fluid, or scraping from a petechial or purpuric lesion
- Clinical purpura fulminans without a positive blood culture

---

TREATMENT: The priority in management of meningococcal disease is treatment of shock in meningococcemia and of raised intracranial pressure in severe cases of meningitis. Empiric therapy for suspected meningococcal disease should include an extended-spectrum cephalosporin, such as cefotaxime or ceftriaxone. Once the microbiologic diagnosis is established, definitive treatment with penicillin G (300 000 U/kg/day; maximum, 12 million U/day, divided every 4–6 hours), ampicillin, or an extended-spectrum cephalosporin (cefotaxime or ceftriaxone), is recommended. Some experts recommend susceptibility testing before switching to penicillin. However, susceptibility testing is not standardized, and clinical significance of intermediate susceptibility is unknown. Resistance of *N meningitidis* to penicillin is rare in the United States. Ceftriaxone clears nasopharyngeal carriage effectively after 1 dose and allows outpatient management for completion of therapy when appropriate. For patients with a serious penicillin allergy characterized by anaphylaxis, chloramphenicol is recommended, if available. If chloramphenicol is not available, meropenem can be used, although the rate of cross-reactivity in penicillin-allergic adults is 2% to 3%. For travelers from areas where penicillin resistance has been reported, cefotaxime, ceftriaxone, or chloramphenicol is recommended. Five to 7 days of antimicrobial therapy is adequate. In meningococcemia presenting with shock, early and rapid fluid resuscitation and early use of inotropic and ventilatory support may reduce mortality. In view of the lack of evidence in pediatric populations, adjuvant therapies are not recommended. The postinfectious inflammatory syndromes associated with meningococcal disease often respond to nonsteroidal anti-inflammatory drugs.

ISOLATION OF THE HOSPITALIZED PATIENT: In addition to standard precautions, droplet precautions are recommended until 24 hours after initiation of effective antimicrobial therapy.

CONTROL MEASURES:

Care of Exposed People.

Chemoprophylaxis. Regardless of immunization status, close contacts of all people with invasive meningococcal disease (see Table 3.36), whether endemic or in an outbreak situation, are at high risk and should receive chemoprophylaxis. Currently licensed vaccines are not 100% effective, and some cases will be caused by serogroup B. The decision to give chemoprophylaxis to contacts of people with meningococcal disease is based on risk of contracting invasive disease. Throat and nasopharyngeal cultures are not recommended, because these cultures are of no value in deciding who should receive chemoprophylaxis.

Chemoprophylaxis is warranted for people who have been exposed directly to a patient's oral secretions through close social contact, such as kissing or sharing of toothbrushes or eating utensils, as well as for child care and preschool contacts during the 7 days before onset of disease in the index case. People who frequently slept in the same dwelling as the infected person within this period also should receive chemoprophylaxis. For airline travel lasting more than 8 hours, passengers who are seated directly next to an infected person should receive prophylaxis. Routine prophylaxis is not recommended for health care personnel (Table 3.36) unless they have had intimate exposure to respiratory tract secretions, such as occurs with unprotected mouth-to-mouth resuscitation, intubation, or suctioning before or less than 24 hours after antimicrobial therapy was initiated. Chemoprophylaxis ideally should be initiated within 24 hours after the index patient is identified; prophylaxis given more than 2 weeks after exposure has little value.

Antimicrobial Regimens for Prophylaxis (see Table 3.37, p 504). Rifampin, ceftriaxone, ciprofloxacin, and azithromycin are appropriate drugs for chemoprophylaxis in adults, but neither rifampin nor ciprofloxacin are recommended for pregnant women.

Table 3.36. Disease Risk for Contacts of People With Meningococcal Disease

High risk: chemoprophylaxis recommended (close contacts)
- Household contact, especially children younger than 2 years of age
- Child care or preschool contact at any time during 7 days before onset of illness
- Direct exposure to index patient's secretions through kissing or through sharing toothbrushes or eating utensils, markers of close social contact, at any time during 7 days before onset of illness
- Mouth-to-mouth resuscitation, unprotected contact during endotracheal intubation at any time 7 days before onset of illness
- Frequently slept in same dwelling as index patient during 7 days before onset of illness
- Passengers seated directly next to the index case during airline flights lasting more than 8 hours

Low risk: chemoprophylaxis not recommended
- Casual contact: no history of direct exposure to index patient's oral secretions (eg, school or work)
- Indirect contact: only contact is with a high-risk contact, no direct contact with the index patient
- Health care personnel without direct exposure to patient's oral secretions

In outbreak or cluster
- Chemoprophylaxis for people other than people at high risk should be administered only after consultation with local public health authorities

Table 3.37. Recommended Chemoprophylaxis Regimens for High-Risk Contacts and People With Invasive Meningococcal Disease

Age of Infants, Children, and Adults	Dose	Duration	Efficacy, %	Cautions
Rifampin[a]				
<1 mo	5 mg/kg, orally, every 12 h	2 days		
≥1 mo	10 mg/kg (maximum 600 mg), orally, every 12 h	2 days	90–95	Can interfere with efficacy of oral contraceptives and some seizure and anticoagulant medications; can stain soft contact lenses
Ceftriaxone				
<15 y	125 mg, intramuscularly	Single dose	90–95	To decrease pain at injection site, dilute with 1% lidocaine
≥15 y	250 mg, intramuscularly	Single dose	90–95	To decrease pain at injection site, dilute with 1% lidocaine
Ciprofloxacin[a,b]				
≥1 mo	20 mg/kg (maximum 500 mg), orally	Single dose	90–95	Not recommended routinely for people younger than 18 years of age; use may be justified after assessment of risks and benefits for the individual patient
Azithromycin	10 mg/kg (maximum 500 mg)	Single dose	90	Not recommended routinely; equivalent to rifampin for eradication of *Neisseria meningitidis* from nasopharynx in one study

[a]Not recommended for use in pregnant women.
[b]Use only if fluoroquinolone-resistant strains of *N meningitidis* have not been identified in the community; Centers for Disease Control and Prevention. Emergence of fluoroquinolone-resistant *Neisseria meningitidis*—Minnesota and North Dakota, 2007–2008. *MMWR Morb Mortal Wkly Rep.* 2008;57(7):173–175.

The drug of choice for most children is rifampin (Table 3.37). Rifampin use alters the effectiveness of a number of medications. If antimicrobial agents other than ceftriaxone or cefotaxime (both of which will eradicate nasopharyngeal carriage) are used for treatment of invasive meningococcal disease, the child should receive chemoprophylaxis before hospital discharge to eradicate nasopharyngeal carriage of *N meningitidis*.

Ciprofloxacin, administered to adults in a single oral dose, also is effective in eradicating meningococcal carriage (see Table 3.37). In areas of the United States where ciprofloxacin-resistant strains of *N meningitidis* have been detected, ciprofloxacin should not be used for chemoprophylaxis.[1] Use of azithromycin as a single oral dose has been shown to be effective for eradication of nasopharyngeal carriage and can be used where ciprofloxacin resistance has been detected.

---

[1] Centers for Disease Control and Prevention. Emergence of fluoroquinolone-resistant *Neisseria meningitidis*—Minnesota and North Dakota, 2007–2008. *MMWR Morb Mortal Wkly Rep.* 2008;57(7):173–175

Postexposure Immunoprophylaxis. Because secondary cases can occur several weeks or more after onset of disease in the index case, meningococcal vaccine is an adjunct to chemoprophylaxis when an outbreak is caused by a serogroup prevented by a meningococcal vaccine. For control of meningococcal outbreaks caused by vaccine-preventable serogroups (A, C, Y, and W-135), the preferred vaccine in adults and children 2 years of age and older is a meningococcal conjugate vaccine (see Table 3.38).

Meningococcal Vaccines. Three meningococcal vaccines are licensed in the United States for use in children and adults against serotypes A, C, Y, and W-135.

- Quadrivalent meningococcal polysaccharide vaccine (MPSV4) was licensed in 1981 for use in children 2 years of age and older, is administered **subcutaneously** as a single 0.5-mL dose, and can be given concurrently with other vaccines but at different anatomic sites.
- Two meningococcal conjugate vaccines (MenACWY-D [Menactra, Sanofi Pasteur] and MenACWY-CRM [Menveo, Novartis Vaccines]) are licensed for use in people 2 through 55 years of age. Both meningococcal conjugate vaccines are administered **intramuscularly** as a single 0.5-mL dose and can be given concurrently with other recommended vaccines.
- One meningococcal conjugate vaccine (MenACWY-D) also is licensed for infants as a two dose primary series, 3 months apart, among children 9 through 23 months of age.
- Other meningococcal conjugate vaccines for children younger than 2 years of age may be licensed in the near future.

Table 3.38 Recommended Meningococcal Vaccines for Immunocompetent Children and Adults[a]

Age	Vaccine	Status
9 mo through 10 y	MCV4-D (Menactra, Merck) MCV4-CRM (Menveo, Novartis)[b]	Not routinely recommended; see Table 3.39 (p 507) for people at increased risk
11 through 21 y	MCV4-D or MCV4-CRM	Primary: • 11 through 12 y of age, 1 dose • 13 through 18 y of age, 1 dose if not previously immunized • 19 through 21 y of age, not routinely recommended but may be given as catch-up immunization for those who have not received a dose after their 16th birthday Booster: • 1 dose recommended for adolescents if first dose administered prior to 16th birthday
22 through 55 y	MCV4-D or MCV4-CRM	• Not recommended routinely • Can be used during outbreaks attributable to serogroup in vaccine, travel to countries with hyperendemic or endemic disease or if protection desired
>56 y	MPSV4	

[a] Two vaccines for infants are under investigation: MCV4-CRM and MCV2/Hib (MenHibrix) for use at 2, 4, 6 and 12 through 15 months of age.

[b] Currently licensed by the Food and Drug Administration only for people 2 through 55 years of age.

- No vaccine is available in the United States for prevention of serogroup B meningococcal disease, but clinical trials of several serogroup B vaccines are underway.

Indications for Use of Meningococcal Vaccines (Table 3.38, p 505, and Table 3.39, p 507). Routine childhood immunization with meningococcal conjugate vaccines is not recommended for children 9 months through 10 years of age, because the infection rate is low in this age group; the immune response is less robust than in older children, adolescents, and adults; and duration of immunity is unknown.[1] However, a meningococcal conjugate vaccine is recommended for children and adolescents who are in high-risk groups as a 2-dose series at 9 months through 55 years of age (Table 3.39).[2,3]

Recommendations for use of a meningococcal conjugate vaccine are as follows[3,4,5]:

- Adolescents should be immunized routinely at the 11- through 12-year of age health care visit, when immunization status (see Fig 1.2, p 29–30) and other preventive health services can be addressed (Table 3.38). A booster dose at 16 years of age, is recommended for adolescents immunized at 11 through 12 years of age.
- Adolescents 13 through 18 years of age should be immunized routinely with a meningococcal conjugate vaccine if not previously immunized. Adolescents who receive the first dose at 13 through 15 years of age, should receive a 1-time booster dose at 16 through 18 years of age.
- Adolescents who receive their first dose of meningococcal conjugate vaccine at or after 16 years of age do not need a booster dose unless they have risk factors.
- People at increased risk of invasive meningococcal disease should be immunized with meningococcal conjugate vaccine beginning at 9 months of age. People at increased risk include:
  - Children 9 months of age and older, including adults who have a persistent complement component deficiency (C5–C9, properdin, factor H, or factor D).
  - Children 24 months of age or older including adults who have anatomic or functional asplenia (see Children With Asplenia, p 88). Because of high risk of invasive pneumococcal disease, children with functional or anatomic asplenia should not be immunized with MCV4-D before 2 years of age to avoid interference with the immune response to the PCV series.
  - Children with persistent complement component deficiencies who are vaccinated at 9 through 23 months of age should receive a 2-dose primary series at least 8 weeks apart.

---

[1] Centers for Disease Control and Prevention. Report from the Advisory Committee on Immunization Practices (ACIP): decision not to recommend routine vaccination of all children aged 2–10 years with quadrivalent meningococcal conjugate vaccine (MCV4). *MMWR Morb Mortal Wkly Rep.* 2008;57(17):462–465

[2] Centers for Disease Control and Prevention. Licensure of a meningococcal conjugate vaccine for children aged 2 through 10 years and updated booster dose guidance for adolescents and other persons at increased risk for meningococcal disease—Advisory Committee on Immunization Practices (ACIP), 2011. *MMWR Morb Mortal Wkly Rep.* 2011;60(30):1018–1019

[3] Centers for Disease Control and Prevention. Recommendation of the Advisory Committee on Immunization Practices (ACIP) for use of quadrivalent meningococcal conjugate vaccine (Men-ACWY-D) among children aged 9 through 23 months at increased risk for meningococcal disease. *MMWR Morb Mortal Wkly Rep.* 2011;60(40):1391–1392

[4] Centers for Disease Control and Prevention. Updated recommendations for use of meningococcal conjugate vaccines—Advisory Committee on Immunization Practices (ACIP), 2010. *MMWR Morb Mortal Wkly Rep.* 2011;60(3):72–76

[5] American Academy of Pediatrics, Committee on Infectious Diseases. Meningococcal conjugate vaccines policy update: booster dose recommendations. *Pediatrics.* 2011;128(6):1213–1218

Table 3.39. Recommended Immunization Schedule and Intervals for Children at Risk of Invasive Meningococcal Disease[a]

Age	Subgroup	Primary Immunization	Booster Dose[b]
9 through 23 mo of age, with high-risk conditions[c]	Children who: • have persistent complement deficiencies • travel to or are residents of countries where meningococcal disease is hyperendemic or epidemic • are at risk during a community outbreak attributable to a vaccine serogroup	Two doses of MCV4-D (Menactra), 3 months apart[d]	First dose received at age: • **9 mo to 6 y of age:** Should receive additional dose of MCV4 3 years after primary immunization. Boosters should be repeated every 5 y thereafter • **≥7 y of age:** Should receive additional dose of MCV4 5 years after primary immunization. Boosters should be repeated every 5 y thereafter
2 through 18 y of age, with high-risk conditions and not immunized previously[e,f]	Children who: • have persistent complement deficiencies • have functional or anatomic asplenia • have HIV, if another indication for immunization exists	Two doses of MCV4, 2 mo apart[e]	
	Children who: • travel to or are residents of countries where meningococcal disease is hyperendemic or epidemic • are at risk during a community outbreak attributable to a vaccine serogroup	Single dose of MCV4[e]	

[a] Includes children who have persistent complement deficiencies (eg, C5-C9, properdin, factor H, or factor D), and anatomic or functional asplenia; travelers to or residents of countries in which meningococcal disease is hyperendemic or epidemic; and children who are part of a community outbreak of a vaccine-preventable serogroup.

[b] If child remains at increased risk of meningococcal disease.

[c] Because of high risk of invasive pneumococcal disease (IPD), children with functional or anatomic asplenia should not be immunized with MVC-4 (Menactra) before 2 years of age to avoid interference with the immune response to the pneumococcal conjugate vaccine (PCV) series.

[d] If an infant is receiving the vaccine prior to travel, 2 doses can be administered as early as 2 months apart.

[e] If MCV4-D is used, administer at least 4 weeks after completion of all PCV doses.

[f] Reimmunization with MCV4 every 5 years is recommended for people previously immunized with MCV4 or MPSV4 who remain at increased risk of infection except for children <6 years of age, who should receive a booster dose after 3 years (see Recommended Adult Immunization Schedule, **www.cdc.gov/vaccines/**.

- Children 9 through 23 months of age who travel to or reside in countries in which meningococcal disease is hyperendemic or epidemic should receive a 2 dose primary series at least 8 weeks apart. Children 2 through 10 years of age who travel to or reside in countries in which meningococcal disease is hyperendemic or epidemic should receive 1 dose. Children who remain at increased risk should receive a booster dose 3 years later if the primary dose was given from 9 months through 6 years of age and 5 years after the last dose if the previous dose was given at 7 years of age or older. (CDC Travelers' Health Hotline 877-FYI-TRIP or online at **www.cdc.gov/travel**).
  - Military recruits.
- Because people with human immunodeficiency virus (HIV) infection are likely to be at higher risk of meningococcal disease, although not to the extent that they are at risk of invasive *S pneumoniae* infection, they may be immunized with a meningococcal conjugate vaccine (MCV4). People with HIV infection who are 2 years of age or older should receive a 2-dose primary series at least 8 weeks apart.
- People, including parents of children who wish to decrease their risk of meningococcal disease, may elect to receive MCV4 if they are 9 months of age or older.
- For control of meningococcal outbreaks caused by vaccine-preventable serogroups (A, C, Y, or W-135), MCV4 should be used for people 9 months through 55 years of age. MPSV4 should be used for people older than 55 years of age in outbreak situations.
- Immunization with MCV4 is preferred for children previously immunized with MPSV4 if at least 3 years have elapsed since receiving MPSV4.

Reimmunization. Children previously immunized with either MCV4 or MPSV4 who are at prolonged increased risk for meningococcal disease should be reimmunized with MCV4. In children 2 through 6 years of age, MCV4 should be given as a booster dose 3 years after initial immunization, because concentrations of bactericidal antibodies against serogroups in the vaccine after the first dose are unlikely to provide continued protection for these children at high risk. In children 7 through 10 years of age and in adolescents who have received either MCV4 or MSPV4, a booster dose of a MCV4 is recommended 5 years after the first dose. For children recommended to receive a 2-dose primary series, a booster dose of a MCV4 is recommended 5 years after the primary series regardless of the child's age when the primary series was given.

Adverse Reactions and Precautions. Frequent adverse reactions after MPSV4 and either of the licensed MCV4 immunizations include localized pain, irritability, headache, and fatigue. Fever is reported by 2% to 5% of adolescents who receive either MPSV4 or MCV4. Meningococcal immunization recommendations should not be altered because of pregnancy if a woman is at increased risk of meningococcal disease.

Reporting. All confirmed, presumptive, and probable cases of invasive meningococcal disease must be reported to the appropriate health department (see Table 3.35, p 502). Timely reporting can facilitate early recognition of outbreaks and serogrouping of isolates so that appropriate prevention recommendations can be implemented rapidly.

Counseling and Public Education. When a case of invasive meningococcal disease is detected, the physician should provide accurate and timely information about meningococcal disease and the risk of transmission to families and contacts of the infected person, provide or arrange for prophylaxis, and contact the local public health department. Some experts recommend that patients with invasive meningococcal disease be evaluated for a terminal complement deficiency. If a deficiency is detected, patients should receive a meningococcal conjugate vaccine if 9 months of age or older, and patients and parents should be counseled about the risk of recurrent invasive meningococcal disease. Public health questions, such as whether a mass immunization program is needed, should be referred to the local health department. In appropriate situations, early provision of information in collaboration with the local health department to schools or other groups at increased risk and to the media may help minimize public anxiety and unrealistic or inappropriate demands for intervention.

Human Metapneumovirus

CLINICAL MANIFESTATIONS: Since discovery in 2001, human metapneumovirus (HMPV) has been shown to cause acute respiratory tract illness in patients of all ages. Human metapneumovirus is one of the leading causes of bronchiolitis in infants and also causes pneumonia, asthma exacerbations, croup, and upper respiratory tract infections (URIs) with concomitant acute otitis media in children as well as acute exacerbations of chronic obstructive pulmonary disease (COPD) in adults. Otherwise healthy young children infected with HMPV usually have mild or moderate symptoms, but some young children have severe disease requiring hospitalization. HMPV infection in immunosuppressed hosts also can result in severe disease, and fatalities from HMPV infection have been reported in hematopoietic stem cell or lung transplant recipients. Preterm birth and underlying cardiopulmonary disease likely are risk factors, but the degree of risk associated with these conditions is not defined fully.

Recurrent infection occurs throughout life and, in healthy people, usually is mild or asymptomatic.

ETIOLOGY: HMPV is an enveloped single-stranded negative-sense RNA virus of the family Paramyxoviridae. Four major genotypes of virus have been identified, and these viruses are classified into 2 major antigenic subgroups (designated A and B), which usually cocirculate each year but in varying proportions. Whether the 2 subgroups exhibit pathogenic differences is unknown.

EPIDEMIOLOGY: Humans are the only source of infection. Formal transmission studies have not been reported, but transmission is likely to occur by direct or close contact with contaminated secretions. Health care-associated infections have been reported.

HMPV infections usually occur in annual epidemics during late winter and early spring in temperate climates. Serologic studies suggest that all children are infected at least once by 5 years of age. The population incidence of HMPV hospitalizations is thought to be generally lower than respiratory syncytial virus (RSV), but comparable to influenza and parainfluenza 3 in children younger than 5 years of age. The HMPV season in a community generally coincides with or overlaps the latter half of the RSV season. During this overlapping period, bronchiolitis may be caused by either or both viruses. Sporadic infection may occur throughout the year. In otherwise healthy infants, the duration of viral shedding is 1 to 2 weeks. Prolonged shedding (weeks to months) has been reported in severely immunocompromised hosts.

The **incubation period** is estimated to be 3 to 5 days in most cases.

DIAGNOSTIC TESTS: Rapid diagnostic immunofluorescent assays based on HMPV antigen detection by monoclonal antibodies are available commercially. The reported sensitivity of these assays varies from 65% to 90%. HMPV-specific molecular diagnostic tests using reverse transcriptase-polymerase chain reaction (RT-PCR) amplification of viral genes (both conventional and real time) have been developed, and some (including multiplex PCR assays for multiple respiratory tract viruses) are available commercially and increasingly are being utilized. Serologic testing of acute and convalescent serum specimens is used in research settings to confirm the first episode of infection.

TREATMENT: Treatment is supportive and includes hydration, careful clinical assessment of respiratory status, including measurement of oxygen saturation, use of supplemental oxygen, and if necessary, mechanical ventilation. HMPV is susceptible to ribavirin in vitro, but no controlled clinical data are available to assess therapeutic benefit in people (eg, immunocompromised patients with severe HMPV disease).

Antimicrobial Agents. The rate of bacterial lung infection or bacteremia associated with HMPV infection is not defined, but is suspected to be low. Therefore, antimicrobial agents are not indicated in treatment of infants hospitalized with uncomplicated HMPV bronchiolitis or pneumonia unless evidence exists for the presence of a bacterial infection.

Isolation of the Hospitalized Patient: In addition to standard precautions, contact precautions are recommended for the duration of HMPV-associated illness among infants and young children. Patients with known HMPV infection should be cared for in single rooms or placed in a cohort of HMPV-infected patients.

CONTROL MEASURES: Control of health care-associated HMPV infection depends on adherence to contact precautions. Exposure to HMPV-infected people, including other patients, staff, and family members, may not be recognized, because illness in contacts may be mild.

Preventive measures include limiting exposure to settings where contact with HMPV may occur (eg, child care centers) and emphasis on hand hygiene in all settings, including the home, especially when contacts of high-risk children have respiratory tract infections.

Microsporidia Infections
(Microsporidiosis)

CLINICAL MANIFESTATIONS: Patients with intestinal infection have watery, nonbloody diarrhea, generally without fever. Abdominal cramping also can occur. Data suggest that asymptomatic infection is more common than originally suspected. Symptomatic intestinal infection is most common in immunocompromised people, especially people who are infected with human immunodeficiency virus (HIV) with low CD4+ lymphocyte counts, in whom infection often results in chronic diarrhea. The clinical course can be complicated by malnutrition and progressive weight loss. Chronic infection in immunocompetent people is rare. Other clinical syndromes that can occur in HIV-infected and immunocompromised patients include keratoconjunctivitis, sinusitis, myositis, nephritis, hepatitis, cholangitis, peritonitis, prostatitis, cystitis, disseminated disease, and wasting syndrome.

ETIOLOGY: Microsporidia are obligate intracellular, spore-forming organisms. They have been reclassified from protozoa to fungi. Multiple genera, including *Encephalitozoon, Enterocytozoon, Nosema, Pleistophora, Trachipleistophora, Brachiola,* and *Vittaforma* and *Microsporidium,* have been implicated in human infection, as have unclassified species. *Enterocytozoon bieneusi* and *Encephalitozoon (Septata) intestinalis* are causes of chronic diarrhea in HIV-infected people.

EPIDEMIOLOGY: Most microsporidian infections are transmitted by oral ingestion of spores. Microsporidia spores commonly are found in surface water, and human strains have been identified in municipal water supplies and ground water. Several studies indicate that waterborne transmission occurs. Person-to-person spread by the fecal-oral route also occurs. Spores also have been detected in other body fluids, but their role in transmission is unknown. Data suggest the possibility of zoonotic transmission.

The **incubation period** is unknown.

DIAGNOSTIC TESTS: Infection with gastrointestinal microsporidia can be documented by identification of organisms in biopsy specimens from the small intestine. Microsporidia spores also can be detected in formalin-fixed stool specimens or duodenal aspirates stained with a chromotrope-based stain (a modification of the trichrome stain) and examined by an experienced microscopist. Gram, acid-fast, periodic acid-Schiff, and Giemsa stains also can be used to detect organisms in tissue sections. Organisms often are not noticed, because they are small (1–4 μm), stain poorly, and evoke minimal inflammatory response. Use of stool concentration techniques does not seem to improve the ability to detect *Enterocytozoon bieneusi* spores. Polymerase chain reaction assay also can be used for diagnosis. Identification for classification purposes and diagnostic confirmation of species requires electron microscopy or molecular techniques.

TREATMENT: Restoration of immune function is critical in control of any microsporidian infection. For a limited number of patients, albendazole, fumagillin, metronidazole, atovaquone, and nitazoxanide have been reported to decrease diarrhea but without eradication of the organism. Albendazole is the drug of choice for infections caused by *E intestinalis* but is ineffective against *Enterocytozoon bieneusi* infections, which may respond to fumagillin. However, fumagillin is associated with significant toxicity, and recurrence of diarrhea is common after therapy is discontinued. In HIV-infected patients, antiretroviral therapy, which is associated with improvement in the CD4+ T-lymphocyte cell count, can modify the course of disease favorably. None of these therapies have been studied in children with Microspordia infection.

ISOLATION OF THE HOSPITALIZED PATIENT: In addition to standard precautions, contact precautions are recommended for diapered and incontinent children for the duration of illness.

CONTROL MEASURES: None have been documented. In HIV-infected and other immunocompromised people, decreased exposure may result from attention to hand hygiene, drinking bottled or boiled water, and avoiding unpeeled fruits and vegetables.

Molluscum Contagiosum

CLINICAL MANIFESTATIONS: Molluscum contagiosum is a benign viral infection of the skin with no systemic manifestations. It usually is characterized by 1 to 20 discrete, 2- to 5-mm-diameter, flesh-colored to translucent, dome-shaped papules, some with central umbilication. Lesions commonly occur on the trunk, face, and extremities but rarely are generalized. Molluscum contagiosum is a self-limited infection that usually resolves spontaneously in 6 to 12 months but may take as long as 4 years to disappear completely. An eczematous reaction encircles lesions in approximately 10% of patients. People with eczema, immunocompromising conditions, and human immunodeficiency virus infection tend to have more widespread and prolonged eruptions.

ETIOLOGY: The cause is a poxvirus, which is the sole member of the genus *Molluscipoxvirus.* DNA subtypes can be differentiated, but subtype is not significant in pathogenesis.

EPIDEMIOLOGY: Humans are the only known source of the virus, which is spread by direct contact, including sexual contact, or by fomites. Vertical transmission has been suggested in case reports of neonatal molluscum contagiosum infection. Lesions can be disseminated by autoinoculation. Infectivity generally is low, but occasional outbreaks have been reported, including outbreaks in child care centers. The period of communicability is unknown.

The **incubation period** seems to vary between 2 and 7 weeks but may be as long as 6 months.

DIAGNOSTIC TESTS: The diagnosis usually can be made clinically from the characteristic appearance of the lesions. Wright or Giemsa staining of cells expressed from the central core of a lesion reveals characteristic intracytoplasmic inclusions. Electron microscopic examination of these cells identifies typical poxvirus particles. If questions persist, nucleic acid testing via polymerase chain reaction is available at certain reference centers. Adolescents and young adults with genital molluscum contagiosum should have screening tests for other sexually transmitted infections.

TREATMENT: There is no consensus on management of molluscum contagiosum in children and adolescents. Genital lesions should be treated to prevent spread to sexual contacts. Treatment of nongenital lesions is mainly for cosmetic reasons. Lesions in healthy people typically are self-limited, and treatment may not be necessary. However, therapy may be warranted to: (1) alleviate discomfort, including itching; (2) reduce autoinoculation; (3) limit transmission of the virus to close contacts; (4) reduce cosmetic concerns; and (5) prevent secondary infection. Physical destruction of the lesions is the most rapid and effective means of curing molluscum contagiosum lesions. Modalities available for physical destruction include: curettage, cryotherapy with liquid nitrogen, electrodesiccation, and chemical agents designed to initiate a local inflammatory response (podophyllin, tretinoin, cantharidin, 25% to 50% trichloroacetic acid, liquefied phenol, silver nitrate, tincture of iodine, or potassium hydroxide). Most data available for any of these modalities are anecdotal, and randomized trials usually are limited because of small sample sizes. These options require a trained physician and can result in postprocedural pain, irritation, and scarring. Because physical destruction of the lesions is painful, appropriate local anesthesia is required. Systemic therapy with cimetidine has been tried because of its systemic immunomodulatory effects. However, available data have not supported a benefit. Imiquimod cream is a local immunomodulatory agent that has been reported as a potentially effective topical treatment in several small clinical trials. Cidofovir is a cytosine nucleotide analogue with in vitro activity against molluscum contagiosum; successful intravenous treatment of immunocompromised adults with severe lesions has been reported. However, use of cidofovir should be reserved for severe cases because of potential carcinogenicity and known toxicities (nephrotoxicity, neutropenia) associated with systemic administration of cidofovir. Successful treatment using topical cidofovir, in a combination vehicle, has been reported in both adult and pediatric cases, most of which were immunocompromised. Genital lesions in children usually are not acquired by sexual transmission and do not necessarily denote sexual abuse, as other modes of direct contact with the virus, including autoinoculation, may result in genital disease.

ISOLATION OF THE HOSPITALIZED PATIENT: Standard precautions are recommended.

CONTROL MEASURES: No control measures are known for isolated cases. For outbreaks, which are common in the tropics, restricting direct person-to-person contact and sharing of potentially contaminated fomites, such as towels and bedding, may decrease spread. Molluscum contagiosum should not prevent a child from attending child care, school or from swimming in public pools. When possible, lesions not covered by clothing should be covered by a watertight bandage, especially when participating in contact sports/activities or swimming. The bandage should be changed daily or when soiled.

Moraxella catarrhalis Infections

CLINICAL MANIFESTATIONS: Common infections include acute otitis media, otitis media with effusion, and sinusitis. Bronchopulmonary infection occurs predominantly among patients with chronic lung disease or impaired host defenses. Rare manifestations include bacteremia (sometimes associated with focal infections, such as preseptal cellulitis, osteomyelitis, septic arthritis, abscesses, or rash indistinguishable from that observed in meningococcemia) and conjunctivitis or meningitis in neonates. Unusual manifestations include endocarditis, shunt-associated ventriculitis, and mastoiditis.

ETIOLOGY: *Moraxella catarrhalis* is a gram-negative aerobic diplococcus. Almost 100% of strains produce beta-lactamase that mediates resistance to penicillins.

EPIDEMIOLOGY: *Moraxella catarrhalis* is part of the normal flora of the upper respiratory tract of humans. Two thirds of children are colonized within the first year of life. The mode of transmission is presumed to be direct contact with contaminated respiratory tract secretions or droplet spread. Infection is most common in infants and young children but occurs at all ages. Duration of carriage by infected and colonized children and the period of communicability are unknown.

The **incubation period** is unknown.

DIAGNOSTIC TESTS: The organism can be isolated on blood or chocolate agar culture media after incubation in air or with increased carbon dioxide. Culture of middle ear or sinus aspirates is indicated for patients with unusually severe infection, patients with infection that fails to respond to treatment, and immunocompromised children. Concomitant recovery of *M catarrhalis* with other pathogens (*Streptococcus pneumoniae* or *Haemophilus influenzae*) may indicate mixed infection. Polymerase chain reaction tests for *M catarrhalis* are under development in research laboratories.

TREATMENT: Most strains of *Moraxella* species produce beta-lactamase and are resistant to amoxicillin. When beta-lactamase–producing *M catarrhalis* is isolated from appropriately obtained specimens (middle ear fluid, sinus aspirates, or lower respiratory tract secretions) or when initial therapy with amoxicillin has been unsuccessful, appropriate antimicrobial agents include amoxicillin-clavulanate, cefuroxime, cefdinir, cefpodoxime, azithromycin, trimethoprim-sulfamethoxazole, or in people 18 years of age or older, a fluoroquinolone. If parenteral antimicrobial therapy is needed to treat *M catarrhalis* infection, in vitro data indicate that cefotaxime and ceftriaxone are likely to be effective.

ISOLATION OF THE HOSPITALIZED PATIENT: Standard precautions are recommended.

CONTROL MEASURES: None.

Mumps

CLINICAL MANIFESTATIONS: Mumps is a systemic disease characterized by swelling of one or more of the salivary glands, usually the parotid glands. Approximately one third of infections do not cause clinically apparent salivary gland swelling and may be asymptomatic (subclinical) or may manifest primarily as respiratory tract infection. More than 50% of people with mumps have cerebrospinal fluid pleocytosis, but fewer than 10% have symptoms of viral meningitis. Orchitis is a commonly reported complication after puberty, but sterility rarely occurs. Rare complications include arthritis, thyroiditis, mastitis, glomerulonephritis, myocarditis, endocardial fibroelastosis, thrombocytopenia, cerebellar ataxia, transverse myelitis, encephalitis, pancreatitis, oophoritis, and permanent hearing impairment. In the absence of an immunization program, mumps typically occurs during childhood. Infection occurring among adults is more likely to result in complications. An association between maternal mumps infection during the first trimester of pregnancy and an increase in the rate of spontaneous abortion or intrauterine fetal death has been reported in some studies but not in others. Although mumps virus can cross the placenta, no evidence exists that this results in congenital malformation.

ETIOLOGY: Mumps is an RNA virus in the Paramyxoviridae family. Other infectious causes of parotitis include Epstein-Barr virus, cytomegalovirus, parainfluenza virus types 1 and 3, influenza A virus, enteroviruses, lymphocytic choriomeningitis virus, human immunodeficiency virus (HIV), nontuberculous mycobacterium, and less often, gram-positive and gram-negative bacteria.

EPIDEMIOLOGY: Mumps occurs worldwide, and humans are the only known natural hosts. The virus is spread by contact with infectious respiratory tract secretions and saliva. Mumps virus is the only known cause of epidemic parotitis. Historically, the peak incidence of mumps was between January and May and among children younger than 10 years of age. Mumps vaccine was licensed in the United States in 1967 and recommended for routine childhood immunization in 1977. After implementation of the 1-dose mumps vaccine recommendation, the incidence of mumps in the United States declined from an incidence of 50 to 251 per 100 000 in the prevaccine era to 2 per 100 000 in 1988. After implementation of the 2-dose measles-mumps-rubella (MMR) vaccine recommendation in 1989 for measles control, mumps further declined to extremely low levels, with an incidence of 0.1/100 000 by 1999. From 2000 to 2005, seasonality no longer was evident, and there were fewer than 300 reported cases per year (incidence of 0.1/100 000), representing a greater than 99% reduction in disease incidence since the prevaccine era. In early 2006, a large-scale mumps outbreak occurred in the Midwestern United States, with 6584 reported cases (incidence of 2.2/100 000). Most of the cases occurred among people 18 through 24 years of age, many of whom were college students who had received 2 doses of mumps vaccine. Another outbreak in 2009–2010 affected more than 3500 people, primarily members of traditional observant communities in New York and New Jersey.[1] Because 2 doses of mumps-containing vaccine are not 100% effective, in settings of high immunization coverage such as the United States, most mumps cases likely will occur in people who have received 2 doses. The period of maximum communicability is considered to be several days before and after parotitis

---

[1] Centers for Disease Control and Prevention. Update: mumps outbreak—New York and New Jersey, June 2009–January 2010. *MMWR Morb Mortal Wkly Rep.* 2010;59(5):125–129

onset. The recommended isolation period for mumps is 5 days after onset of parotid swelling. Virus has been isolated from saliva from 7 days before through 8 days after onset of swelling.

The **incubation period** usually is 16 to 18 days, but cases may occur from 12 to 25 days after exposure.

DIAGNOSTIC TESTS: Despite the outbreaks in 2006 and 2009–2010, mumps is an uncommon infection in the United States, and parotitis has other etiologies, including other infectious agents. People with parotitis without other apparent cause should undergo diagnostic testing to confirm mumps virus as the cause or to diagnose other etiologies (eg, influenza A virus, parainfluenza viruses 1 and 3, and bacterial causes). Mumps can be confirmed by isolation of mumps virus or detection of mumps virus nucleic acid by reverse transcriptase-polymerase chain reaction (RT-PCR) in specimens from buccal swabs (Stenson duct exudates), throat washings, saliva, or spinal fluid; by detection of mumps-specific immunoglobulin (Ig) M antibody; or by a significant increase between acute and convalescent titers in serum mumps IgG antibody titer determined by standard quantitative or semi-quantitative serologic assay (most commonly, semi-quantitative enzyme immunoassay). With the availability of RT-PCR assays, culture rarely is performed anymore.

Confirming the diagnosis of mumps in highly immunized populations is challenging, because the IgM response may be absent or short lived; acute IgG titers already might be high, so no significant increase can be detected between acute and convalescent specimens; and mumps virus might be present in clinical specimens only during the first few days after illness onset. Emphasis should be placed on obtaining clinical specimens within 1 to 3 days after onset of symptoms (usually parotitis). In immunized cases, a negative IgM result does not rule out the diagnosis.

TREATMENT: Supportive.

ISOLATION OF THE HOSPITALIZED PATIENT: In addition to standard precautions, droplet precautions are recommended until 5 days after onset of parotid swelling.

CONTROL MEASURES:

School and Child Care. Children should be excluded for 5 days from onset of parotid gland swelling.[1]

Exclusion. When determining means to control outbreaks, exclusion of students without evidence of immunity who refuse immunization from affected schools and schools judged by local public health authorities to be at risk of transmission should be considered. Excluded students can be readmitted immediately after immunization. Students who continue to be exempted from mumps immunization because of medical, religious, or other reasons should be excluded until at least 26 days after onset of parotitis in the last person with mumps in the affected school.

Care of Exposed People. Mumps vaccine has not been demonstrated to be effective in preventing infection after exposure. However, MMR vaccine can be given after exposure, because immunization will provide protection against subsequent exposures. Immunization during the incubation period presents no increased risk.

---

[1] Centers for Disease Control and Prevention. Updated recommendations for isolation of persons with mumps. *MMWR Morb Mortal Wkly Rep.* 2008;57(40):1103–2205

During an outbreak, the first dose of MMR vaccine should be offered to all unimmunized people 12 months of age and older, and a second dose of MMR vaccine should be offered to school and post-high school students and health care personnel born during or after 1957 who have only received 1 dose of MMR vaccine. A second dose may be considered for preschool-aged children and other adults depending on outbreak epidemiology. Health care personnel born before 1957 without a history of MMR immunization should obtain a mumps antibody titer to document their immune status and, if negative, should receive 2 appropriately spaced doses of MMR vaccine. A third dose of MMR vaccine for outbreak control for people who have received 2 doses has not been recommended but is being evaluated.

Immune globulin (IG) preparations are not effective as postexposure prophylaxis for mumps.

Mumps Vaccine. Live-attenuated mumps vaccine has been licensed in the United States since 1967. Vaccine is administered by subcutaneous injection of 0.5 mL of measles-mumps-rubella (MMR) vaccine (licensed for people 12 months of age or older) or measles-mumps-rubella-varicella (MMRV) vaccine (licensed for children 12 months through 12 years of age). Monovalent mumps vaccine no longer is available in the United States. Postlicensure data indicate that the effectiveness of 1 dose of mumps vaccine has been approximately 80% (range, 62%–91%), and on the basis of fewer studies globally, 2-dose vaccine effectiveness has been somewhat higher (range, 79%–95%). Some studies and investigations conducted during the mumps outbreaks in the late 1980s and in 2006 indicate that vaccine-induced immunity might wane, possibly explaining the recent occurrence of mumps in the 15- through 24-year age group.

Vaccine Recommendations.

- The first dose of MMR or MMRV vaccine (see MMRV vaccine recommendations in Varicella-Zoster Infections, p 774) should be given routinely to children at 12 through 15 months of age, with a second dose of MMR or MMRV vaccine administered at 4 through 6 years of age. The second dose of MMR or MMRV vaccine may be administered before 4 years of age, provided at least 28 days have elapsed since the first dose and the interval between varicella vaccine doses is at least 90 days. Administration of MMR or MMRV vaccine is not harmful if given to a person already immune to one or more of the viruses from previous infection or immunization.

- People should be immunized unless they have acceptable evidence of mumps immunity; written documentation of adequate immunization (2 doses of MMR or live mumps vaccine administered ≥28 days apart), physician-diagnosed mumps (except for health care personnel), laboratory evidence of immunity or laboratory confirmation of disease, or birth before 1957. Adequate immunization is 2 doses of mumps-containing vaccine for school-aged children and adults at high risk (ie, health care personnel, students at post-high school educational institutions, and international travelers), and a single dose of mumps-containing vaccine for other adults born in or after 1957. Additionally, health care personnel born before 1957 should consider receiving 1 dose of MMR vaccine unless they have laboratory evidence of immunity or disease.

- Because mumps is endemic throughout most of the world, unless they have other evidence of immunity, people 12 months of age or older should be offered 2 doses of MMR vaccine according to vaccine policy (see above) before beginning travel. Children younger than 12 months of age need not be given mumps vaccine before travel, but they may receive it as MMR vaccine if measles immunization is indicated.

- Any live mumps vaccine dose administered before the first birthday is not considered valid. Unless they have other acceptable evidence of immunity to mumps, these children should receive 2 appropriately spaced doses of MMR or MMRV vaccine.
- A mumps-containing vaccine may be given with other vaccines at different injection sites and with separate syringes (see Simultaneous Administration of Multiple Vaccines, p 33).

Adverse Reactions. Adverse reactions associated with the mumps component of US-licensed MMR or MMRV vaccines are rare. Orchitis, parotitis, and low-grade fever have been reported rarely after immunization. Temporally related reactions, including febrile seizures, nerve deafness, aseptic meningitis, encephalitis, rash, pruritus, and purpura, may follow immunization rarely; however, causality has not been established. Allergic reactions also are rare (see Measles, Precautions and Contraindications [p 497], and Rubella, Precautions and Contraindications [p 634]). Other reactions that occur after immunization with MMR or MMRV vaccine may be attributable to other components of the vaccines (see Measles, p 489, Seizures, p 496, Rubella, p 629, and Varicella-Zoster Infections, p 774).

Reimmunization with MMR vaccine is not associated with an increased incidence of reactions, and postlicensure data on MMRV vaccine are limited.

Precautions and Contraindications. See Measles, p 489, Rubella, p 629, and Varicella-Zoster Infections, p 774, if MMRV is used.

Febrile Illness. Children with minor illnesses with or without fever, such as upper respiratory tract infections, may be immunized (see Vaccine Safety, p 41). Fever is not a contraindication to immunization. However, if other manifestations suggest a more serious illness, the child should not be immunized until recovered.

Allergies. Hypersensitivity reactions occur rarely and usually are minor, consisting of wheal and flare reactions or urticaria at the injection site. Reactions have been attributed to trace amounts of neomycin or gelatin or some other component in the vaccine formulation. Anaphylaxis is rare; MMR and MMRV vaccines are produced in chicken embryo cell culture and do not contain significant amounts of egg white (ovalbumin) cross-reacting proteins. Children with egg allergy are at low risk of anaphylactic reactions to MMR or MMRV vaccine. Skin testing of children for egg allergy is not predictive of reactions to MMR or MMRV vaccine and is not required before administering MMR vaccine. People with allergies to chickens or feathers are not at increased risk of reaction to the vaccine. People who have experienced anaphylactic reactions to gelatin or topically or systemically administered neomycin should receive mumps vaccine only in settings where such reactions could be managed and after consultation with an allergist or immunologist. Most often, however, neomycin allergy manifests as contact dermatitis, which is not a contraindication to receiving mumps vaccine (see Table 1.9, p 38).

Recent Administration of IG. Although the effect of IG administration on the immune response to mumps vaccine is unknown, MMR vaccine should be given at least 2 weeks before administration of IG, blood transfusion, or other blood products because of the theoretical possibility that antibody will neutralize vaccine virus and interfere with successful immunization. The delay in administration of MMR or MMRV is dependent on the dose of IG (such as doses given for treatment of Kawasaki disease) and varies from 3 to 12 months (see Measles, p 489).

Altered Immunity. Patients with immunodeficiency diseases and people receiving immunosuppressive therapy (eg, patients with leukemia, lymphoma, or generalized malignant disease), including high doses of systemically administered corticosteroids, alkylating agents, antimetabolites, or radiation, or people who otherwise are immunocompromised should not receive live-attenuated MMR or MMRV vaccine (see Immunocompromised Children, p 74). Exceptions are patients with HIV infection who are not immunocompromised severely (age-specific CD4+ T-lymphocyte percentages of 15% or greater); these patients should be immunized with MMR but not MMRV vaccine (see Human Immunodeficiency Virus Infection, p 418). The risk of mumps exposure for patients with altered immunity can be decreased by immunizing their close susceptible (ie, household) contacts. Immunized people do not transmit mumps vaccine virus.

After cessation of immunosuppressive therapy, MMR immunization should be deferred for at least 3 months (with the exception of corticosteroid recipients [see the next paragraph]). This interval is based on the assumptions that immunologic responsiveness will have been restored in 3 months and the underlying disease for which immunosuppressive therapy was given is in remission or under control. However, because the interval can vary with the intensity and type of immunosuppressive therapy, radiation therapy, underlying disease, and other factors, a definitive recommendation for an interval after cessation of immunosuppressive therapy when mumps vaccine (as MMR) can be administered safely and effectively often is not possible.

Corticosteroids. For patients who have received high doses of corticosteroids (2 mg/kg/day or greater or greater than 20 mg/day of prednisone or equivalent) for 14 days or more and who otherwise are not immunocompromised, the recommended interval is at least 1 month after corticosteroids are discontinued (see Immunocompromised Children, p 74).

Pregnancy. Conception should be avoided for 28 days after mumps immunization because of the theoretical risk associated with live-virus vaccine. Susceptible postpubertal females should not be immunized if they are known to be pregnant. Mumps immunization during pregnancy has not been associated with congenital malformations (see Measles, p 489, and Rubella, p 629).

Mycoplasma pneumoniae and Other *Mycoplasma* Species Infections

CLINICAL MANIFESTATIONS: *Mycoplasma pneumoniae* is a frequent cause of upper and lower respiratory tract infections in children, including pharyngitis, acute bronchitis, and pneumonia. Acute otitis media is uncommon. Bullous myringitis, once considered pathognomonic for mycoplasma, now is known to occur with other pathogens as well. Coryza, sinusitis, and croup are rare. Symptoms are variable and include cough, malaise, fever, and occasionally, headache. Acute bronchitis and upper respiratory tract illness caused by *M pneumoniae* generally are mild and self-limited. Approximately 10% of infected school-aged children will develop pneumonia with cough and widespread rales on physical examination within days after onset of constitutional symptoms. Cough often initially is nonproductive but later can become productive. Cough can persist for 3 to 4 weeks and can be accompanied by wheezing. Approximately 10% of children with *M pneumoniae* infection will exhibit a rash, which most often is maculopapular. Radiographic abnormalities are variable. Bilateral diffuse infiltrates or focal abnormalities, such as consolidation, effusion, or hilar adenopathy can occur.

Unusual manifestations include nervous system disease (eg, aseptic meningitis, encephalitis, acute disseminated encephalomyelitis, cerebellar ataxia, transverse myelitis, peripheral neuropathy) as well as myocarditis, pericarditis, polymorphous mucocutaneous eruptions (including classic and atypical Stevens-Johnson syndrome), hemolytic anemia, and arthritis. In patients with sickle cell disease, Down syndrome, immunodeficiencies, and chronic cardiorespiratory disease, severe pneumonia with pleural effusion may develop. Acute chest syndrome and pneumonia have been associated with *M pneumoniae* in patients with sickle cell disease. It also has been associated with exacerbations of asthma.

Several other *Mycoplasma* species colonize mucosal surfaces of humans and can produce disease in children. *Mycoplasma hominis* infection has been reported in neonates (especially at scalp electrode monitor site) and children (both immunocompetent and immunocompromised). Intra-abdominal abscesses, septic arthritis, endocarditis, pneumonia, meningoencephalitis, brain abscess, and surgical wound infections all have been reported. The diagnosis should be considered in children with a bacterial culture-negative purulent infection.

ETIOLOGY: Mycoplasmas, including *M pneumoniae*, are pleomorphic bacteria that lack a cell wall. Mycoplasmas cannot be detected using light microscopy.

EPIDEMIOLOGY: Mycoplasmas are ubiquitous in animals and plants, but *M pneumoniae* causes disease only in humans. *M pneumoniae* is transmissible by respiratory droplets during close contact with a symptomatic person. Outbreaks have been described in hospitals, military bases, colleges, and summer camps. Occasionally *M pneumoniae* causes ventilator-associated pneumonia. *M pneumoniae* is a leading cause of pneumonia in school-aged children and young adults and less frequently causes pneumonia in children younger than 5 years of age. Infections occur throughout the world, in any season, and in all geographic settings. In family studies, approximately 30% of household contacts develop pneumonia. Asymptomatic carriage after infection may occur for weeks to months. Immunity after infection is not long lasting.

The **incubation period** usually is 2 to 3 weeks (range, 1–4 weeks).

DIAGNOSTIC TESTS: When Gram stain of colonies is performed, no bacteria are noted. *M pneumoniae* can be grown in special enriched broth followed by passage to SP4 agar media or on commercially-available mixed liquid broth/agar slant media, but most clinical facilities lack the capacity to perform this culture. Isolation takes up to 21 days. Polymerase chain reaction (PCR) tests for *M pneumoniae* increasingly are available and have been used as diagnostic tests at many medical centers and some reference laboratories. Where available, PCR has replaced other tests, because PCR enables more rapid diagnosis in acutely ill patients. Identification of *M pneumoniae* by PCR or in culture from a patient with compatible clinical manifestations suggests causation. PCR kits and testing are available commercially in the United States; sensitivity and specificity are between 80% and 100%. Performance characteristics of individual institutions' non–FDA-approved PCR tests, using different primer sequences and targeting different genes, are not generalizable.

Attributing a nonclassic clinical disorder to *Mycoplasma* on the basis of PCR test or culture results is problematic, because *M pneumoniae* can colonize the respiratory tract for several weeks after acute infection, even after appropriate antimicrobial therapy.

Immunofluorescent tests and enzyme immunoassays that detect *M pneumoniae*-specific immunoglobulin (Ig) M and IgG antibodies in sera are available commercially. IgM antibodies generally are not detectable within the first 7 days after onset of symptoms. Although the presence of IgM antibodies may indicate recent *M pneumoniae* infection, false-positive test results occur, and antibodies persist in serum for several months and may not indicate current infection. Conversely, IgM antibodies may not be elevated in older children and adults who have had recurrent *M pneumoniae* infection. Serologic diagnosis is best made by demonstrating a fourfold or greater increase in antibody titer between acute and convalescent serum specimens. Complement-fixation assay results should be interpreted cautiously, because the assay is both less sensitive and less specific than is immunofluorescent assay or enzyme immunoassay. IgM antibody titer peaks at approximately 3 to 6 weeks and persists for 2 to 3 months after infection. False-positive IgM test results occur frequently, particularly when results are near the threshold for positivity. False-negative results also occur frequently with single specimen testing, with sensitivity ranging from 50% to 60%.

Serum cold hemagglutinin titers traditionally were considered a marker of *M pneumoniae* infection but are positive in only 50% of patients with pneumonia caused by *M pneumoniae*. Serum cold hemagglutinin titers also are nonspecific, particularly at titers <1:64, because titers can be increased during viral infections caused by a variety of agents.

The diagnosis of mycoplasma-associated central nervous system disease (acute or postinfectious) is controversial because of the lack of a reliable cerebrospinal fluid test for *Mycoplasma*. No single test has adequate sensitivity or specificity to establish this diagnosis.

PCR assay of body fluids for *Mycoplasma hominis* is available at reference laboratories and may be helpful diagnostically.

TREATMENT: Observational data indicate that children with pneumonia attributable to *M pneumoniae* have shorter duration of symptoms and fewer relapses when treated with an antimicrobial agent active against *M pneumoniae*. There is no evidence that treatment of upper respiratory tract or nonrespiratory tract disease with antimicrobial agents alters the course of illness. Routine antimycoplasma therapy for asthma is inappropriate unless specific findings of pneumonia are present. Because mycoplasmas lack a cell wall, they inherently are resistant to beta-lactam agents. Macrolides, including erythromycin, azithromycin, and clarithromycin, are the preferred antimicrobial agents for treatment of pneumonia in children younger than 8 years of age. Tetracycline and doxycycline also are effective and may be used for children 8 years of age and older (see Tetracyclines, p 801). Fluoroquinolones are effective but are not recommended as first-line agents for children (see Fluoroquinolones, p 800).

M hominis usually is resistant to erythromycin and azithromycin but generally is susceptible to clindamycin, tetracyclines, and fluoroquinolones.

ISOLATION OF THE HOSPITALIZED PATIENT: In addition to standard precautions, droplet precautions are recommended for the duration of symptomatic illness.

CONTROL MEASURES: Hand hygiene decreases household transmission of respiratory pathogens and should be encouraged.

Tetracycline or azithromycin prophylaxis for close contacts has been shown to limit transmission in family and institutional outbreaks. However, antimicrobial prophylaxis for asymptomatic exposed contacts is not recommended routinely, because most secondary illnesses will be mild and self-limited. Prophylaxis with a macrolide or tetracycline can be considered for people at increased risk of severe illness with *M pneumoniae*, such as children with sickle cell disease who are close contacts of a person who is acutely ill with *M pneumoniae*.

Nocardiosis

CLINICAL MANIFESTATIONS: Immunocompetent children typically develop cutaneous or lymphocutaneous disease with pustular or ulcerative lesions that remain localized after soil contamination of a skin injury. Invasive disease occurs most commonly in immunocompromised patients, particularly people with chronic granulomatous disease, organ transplantation, human immunodeficiency virus infection, or disease requiring long-term systemic corticosteroid therapy. In these children, infection characteristically begins in the lungs, and illness can be acute, subacute, or chronic. Pulmonary disease commonly manifests as rounded nodular infiltrates that can undergo cavitation. Hematogenous spread may occur from the lungs to the brain (single or multiple abscesses), in skin (pustules, pyoderma, abscesses, mycetoma), or occasionally in other organs. Some experts recommend neuroimaging in patients with pulmonary disease attributable to the frequency of concurrent central nervous system (CNS) disease, which initially can be asymptomatic. *Nocardia* organisms can be recovered from patients with cystic fibrosis, but their role as a lung pathogen in these patients is not clear.

ETIOLOGY: *Nocardia* species are aerobic actinomycetes, a large and diverse group of gram-positive bacteria, which include *Actinomyces israelii* (the cause of actinomycosis), *Rhodococcus equi*, and *Tropheryma whipplei* (formerly *Tropheryma whippelii*) (Whipple disease). Pulmonary or disseminated disease most commonly is caused by the *Nocardia asteroides* complex, which includes *Nocardia cyriacigeorgica*, *Nocardia farcinica*, and *Nocardia nova*. Primary cutaneous disease most commonly is caused by *Nocardia brasiliensis*. *Nocardia pseudobrasiliensis* is associated with pulmonary, CNS, or systemic nocardiosis. Other pathogenic species include *Nocardia abscessus*, *Nocardia otitidiscaviarum*, *Nocardia transvalensis*, and *Nocardia veterana*.

EPIDEMIOLOGY: Found worldwide, *Nocardia* species are ubiquitous environmental saprophytes living in soil, organic matter, and water. Lungs are the portals of entry for pulmonary or disseminated disease. Direct skin inoculation occurs, often as the result of contact with contaminated soil after trauma. Person-to-person and animal-to-human transmission do not occur.

The **incubation period** is unknown.

DIAGNOSTIC TESTS: Isolation of *Nocardia* organisms from body fluid, abscess material, or tissue specimens provides a definitive diagnosis. Stained smears of sputum, body fluids, or pus demonstrating beaded, branched, weakly gram-positive, variably acid-fast rods suggest the diagnosis. Brown and Brenn and methenamine silver stains are recommended to demonstrate microorganisms in tissue specimens. *Nocardia* organisms are slow growing but grow readily on blood and chocolate agar in 3 to 5 days. Cultures from normally sterile sites should be maintained for 3 weeks in an appropriate liquid medium. Serologic tests for *Nocardia* species are not useful.

TREATMENT: Trimethoprim-sulfamethoxazole or a sulfonamide alone (eg, sulfisoxazole or sulfamethoxazole) has been the drug of choice for mild infections. Sulfonamides that are less urine soluble, such as sulfadiazine, should be avoided. A high mortality rate with sulfonamide monotherapy in immunocompromised patients and patients with severe disease, disseminated disease, or central nervous system involvement has led to use of combination therapy for the first 4 to 12 weeks based on results of antimicrobial susceptibility testing and clinical improvement. Suggested combinations include amikacin plus ceftriaxone or amikacin plus meropenem or imipenem. Immunocompetent patients with primary lymphocutaneous disease usually respond after 6 to 12 weeks of therapy. Drainage of abscesses is beneficial. Immunocompromised patients and patients with serious disease should be treated for 6 to 12 months and for at least 3 months after apparent cure because of the tendency for relapse. Patients with acquired immunodeficiency syndrome may need even longer therapy, and low-dose maintenance therapy should be continued for life. Patients with meningitis or brain abscess should be monitored with serial neuroimaging studies.

If infection does not respond to trimethoprim-sulfamethoxazole, other agents, such as clarithromycin *(N nova)*, amoxicillin-clavulanate *(N brasiliensis* and *N abscessus)*, imipenem, or meropenem may be beneficial. Linezolid is highly active against all *Nocardia* species in vitro; case series including a small number of patients demonstrated that linezolid may be effective for treatment of some invasive infections. Drug susceptibility testing is recommended by the Clinical and Laboratory Standards Institute for isolates from patients with invasive disease and patients who are unable to tolerate a sulfonamide as well as patients who fail sulfonamide therapy.

ISOLATION OF THE HOSPITALIZED PATIENT: Standard precautions are recommended.

CONTROL MEASURES: None.

Onchocerciasis
(River Blindness, Filariasis)

CLINICAL MANIFESTATIONS: The disease involves skin, subcutaneous tissues, lymphatic vessels, and eyes. Subcutaneous, nontender nodules that can be up to several centimeters in diameter containing adult worms develop 6 to 12 months after initial infection. In patients in Africa, nodules tend to be found on the lower torso, pelvis, and lower extremities, whereas in patients in Central and South America, the nodules more often are located on the upper body (the head and trunk) but may occur on the extremities. After the worms mature, microfilariae are produced that migrate to the dermis and may cause a papular dermatitis. Pruritus often is highly intense, resulting in patient-inflicted excoriations over the affected areas. After a period of years, skin can become lichenified and hypo- or hyperpigmented. Microfilariae may invade ocular structures, leading to inflammation of the cornea, iris, ciliary body, retina, choroid, and optic nerve. Loss of visual acuity and blindness can result if the disease is untreated.

ETIOLOGY: *Onchocerca volvulus* is a filarial nematode.

EPIDEMIOLOGY: *O volvulus* has no significant animal reservoir. Microfilariae in human skin infect *Simulium* species flies (black flies) when they take a blood meal and then in 10 to 14 days develop into infectious larvae that are transmitted with subsequent bites. Black flies breed in fast-flowing streams and rivers (hence, the colloquial name of the disease, "river blindness"). The disease occurs primarily in equatorial Africa, but small foci are found in southern Mexico, Guatemala, northern South America, and Yemen. Prevalence is greatest among people who live near vector breeding sites. The infection is not transmissible by person-to-person contact or blood transfusion.

The **incubation period** from larval inoculation to microfilariae in the skin usually is 6 to 18 months but can be as long as 3 years.

DIAGNOSTIC TESTS: Direct examination of a 1- to 2-mg shaving or biopsy specimen of the epidermis and upper dermis (usually taken from the posterior iliac crest area) can reveal microfilariae. Microfilariae are not found in blood. Adult worms may be demonstrated in excised nodules that have been sectioned and stained. A slit-lamp examination of the anterior chamber of an involved eye may reveal motile microfilariae or "snowflake" corneal lesions. Eosinophilia is common. Specific serologic tests and polymerase chain reaction techniques for detection of microfilariae in skin are available only in research laboratories, including those of the National Institutes of Health.

TREATMENT: Ivermectin, a microfilaricidal agent, is the drug of choice for treatment of onchocerciasis. Treatment decreases dermatitis and the risk of developing severe ocular disease but does not kill the adult worms (which can live for more than a decade) and, thus, is not curative. One single oral dose of ivermectin (150 μg/kg) should be given every 6 to 12 months until asymptomatic. Adverse reactions to treatment are caused by death of microfilariae and can include rash, edema, fever, myalgia, and rarely, asthma exacerbation and hypotension. Such reactions are more common in people with higher skin loads of microfilaria and decrease with repeated treatment in the absence of reexposure. Precautions to ivermectin treatment include pregnancy (class C drug), central nervous system disorders, and high levels of circulating *Loa loa* microfilariaemia (determined by examining a Giemsa stained thick blood smear between 10 AM and 2 PM). Treatment of patients with high levels of circulating *L loa* microfilariaemia with ivermectin sometimes can result in fatal encephalopathy. The American Academy of Pediatrics notes that the drug usually is compatible with breastfeeding. Because low levels of drug are found in human milk after maternal treatment, some experts recommend delaying maternal treatment until the infant is 7 days of age, but risk versus benefit should be considered. Safety and effectiveness in pediatric patients weighing less than 15 kg have not been established. A 6-week course of doxycycline (100–200 mg/day) also is being used to kill adult worms through depletion of the endosymbiotic rickettsia-like bacteria, which appear to be required for survival of *O volvulus*. This approach may provide adjunctive therapy for children 8 years of age or older and nonpregnant adults (see Antimicrobial Agents and Related Therapy, Tetracyclines, p 801). This treatment should be initiated several days after treatment with ivermectin, because there are no studies of the safety of simultaneous treatment. Diethylcarbamazine is contraindicated, because it may cause adverse ocular reactions.

ISOLATION OF THE HOSPITALIZED PATIENT: Standard precautions are recommended.

CONTROL MEASURES: Repellents and protective clothing (long sleeves and pants) can decrease exposure to bites from black flies, which bite by day. Treatment of vector breeding sites with larvicides has been effective for controlling black fly populations, particularly in West Africa. A highly successful initiative being led by the World Health Organization has mass distributed hundreds of millions of ivermectin treatments (donated by the drug manufacturer for this purpose) to communities with severe endemic disease from onchocerciasis.

Human Papillomaviruses

CLINICAL MANIFESTATIONS: Most human papillomavirus (HPV) infections are inapparent clinically. However, HPVs can cause benign epithelial proliferation (warts) of the skin and mucous membranes and are associated with cervical, anogenital, and oropharyngeal dysplasias and cancers. Cutaneous nongenital warts include common skin warts, plantar warts, flat warts, thread-like (filiform) warts, and epidermodysplasia verruciformis. Warts also occur on the mucous membranes, including the anogenital, oral, nasal, and conjunctival areas and the respiratory tract, where respiratory papillomatosis occurs.

Common **skin warts** are dome-shaped with conical projections that give the surface a rough appearance. They usually are painless and multiple, occurring commonly on the hands and around or under the nails. When small dermal vessels become thrombosed, black dots appear in the warts. Plantar warts on the foot may be painful and are characterized by marked hyperkeratosis, sometimes with black dots.

Flat warts ("juvenile warts") commonly are found on the face and extremities of children and adolescents. They usually are small, multiple, and flat topped; seldom exhibit papillomatosis; and rarely cause pain. Filiform warts occur on the face and neck. Cutaneous warts are benign.

Anogenital warts, also called **condylomata acuminata,** are skin-colored warts with a cauliflower-like surface that range in size from a few millimeters to several centimeters. In males, these warts may be found on the penis, scrotum, or anal and perianal area. In females, these lesions may occur on the vulva or perianal areas and less commonly in the vagina or on the cervix. Anogenital warts often are multiple and attract attention because of their appearance. Warts usually are painless, although they may cause itching, burning, local pain, or bleeding.

Persistent anogenital HPV infection may be associated with clinically apparent dysplastic lesions, particularly in the female genital tract (cervix and vagina). Abnormal cells associated with these lesions often are detected during Papanicolaou (Pap) testing of the cervix and are classified morphologically as representing low- or high-grade squamous intraepithelial lesions (L-SIL or H-SIL, respectively). On biopsy, these precursor lesions are classified as low-grade cervical intraepithelial neoplasia (CIN 1) or high-grade cervical intraepithelial neoplasia (CIN 2 or 3). Similar dysplastic lesions can develop at other genital and anal mucosal sites. Over 1 to 2 decades, persistent HPV infection with high-risk HPV types can undergo neoplastic progression and lead to invasive cancers of the cervix, vagina, vulva, penis, anus, or oropharynx.

Juvenile recurrent respiratory papillomatosis is a rare condition characterized by recurring papillomas in the larynx or other areas of the upper respiratory tract. This condition is diagnosed most commonly in children between 2 and 5 years of age and manifests as a voice change, stridor, or abnormal cry. Respiratory papillomas can cause respiratory tract obstruction in young children. Adult onset also has been described.

Epidermodysplasia verruciformis (EV) is a rare, inherited disorder believed to be a consequence of a deficiency of cell-mediated immunity resulting in an abnormal susceptibility to certain HPV types and manifesting as chronic cutaneous HPV infection and frequent development of skin cancer. Lesions may resemble flat warts but often are similar to tinea versicolor, covering the torso and upper extremities. Most appear during the first decade of life, but malignant transformation, which occurs in 30% to 60% of affected people, usually is delayed until adulthood. EV-like HPV disease also can occur in people with impaired cellular immunity because of human immunodeficiency virus (HIV) infection.

ETIOLOGY: HPVs are members of the *Papillomavirus* family and are DNA viruses. More than 100 types have been identified. These viruses are grouped into cutaneous and mucosal types on the basis of their tendency to infect particular types of epithelium. Most often, HPV types found in nongenital warts will be cutaneous types, and those in respiratory papillomatosis, anogenital warts, dysplasias, or cancers will be mucosal types. More than 40 HPV types can infect the genital tract. On the basis of their epidemiologic association with cancers, mucosal HPVs are divided into low-risk and high-risk types. More than 14 high-risk types are recognized, with types 16 and 18 most frequently being associated with cervical cancer and type 16 most frequently being associated with other anogenital cancers and oropharyngeal cancers. Types 6 and 11 frequently are associated with condylomata acuminata, recurrent respiratory papillomatosis, and conjunctival papillomas.

EPIDEMIOLOGY: Papillomaviruses are distributed widely among mammals and are species-specific. Cutaneous warts occur commonly among school-aged children; the prevalence rate is as high as 50%. HPV infections are transmitted from person to person by close contact. Nongenital warts are acquired through contact with HPV and minor trauma to the skin. An increase in the incidence of plantar warts has been associated with swimming in public pools. The intense and often widespread appearance of cutaneous warts in patients with compromised cellular immunity (particularly patients who have undergone transplantation and people with human immunodeficiency virus infection) suggests that alterations in immunity predispose to reactivation of latent intraepithelial infection.

Anogenital HPV infection is the most common sexually transmitted infection in the United States. Most infections are subclinical and clear spontaneously within 2 years. Persistent infection with high-risk types of HPV is associated with development of cervical cancer, with more than 12 000 new cases and 4000 deaths attributed to HPV annually in the United States, and with vulvar, vaginal, penile, and anal cancers and a significant percentage of oropharyngeal cancers. The risk of development of dysplastic cancer precursor lesions is greater in people with HIV infection and people with cellular immune deficiencies.

Rarely, infection is transmitted to a child through the birth canal during delivery or transmitted from nongenital sites. Respiratory papillomatosis is believed to be acquired by aspiration of infectious secretions during passage through an infected birth canal. When anogenital warts are identified in a child who is beyond infancy but is prepubertal, sexual abuse must be considered.

The **incubation period** is unknown but is estimated to range from 3 months to several years. Papillomavirus acquired by a neonate at the time of birth may never cause clinical disease or may become apparent over several years (eg, respiratory papillomatosis). Anogenital and pharyngeal malignant neoplasias are rare long-term sequelae of chronic persistent infection, usually occurring more than 10 years after infection.

DIAGNOSTIC TESTS: Most cutaneous and anogenital warts are diagnosed through clinical inspection. Respiratory papillomatosis is diagnosed using endoscopy and biopsy. Cervical dysplasias may be detected via (1) cytologic examination of exfoliated cells in a Pap test, either by conventional or liquid-based cytologic methods; or (2) histologic examination of cervical tissue biopsy. Cervical biopsy can show HPV-associated lesions, such as warts, dysplasias, and carcinomas. Although characteristic cytologic and histologic changes may suggest the presence of HPV, diagnosing infection requires a molecular test.

Although HPV can be propagated under special laboratory conditions, HPV cannot be isolated from patient samples; therefore, a definitive diagnosis of HPV infection is based on detection of viral nucleic acid (DNA or RNA) or capsid protein. Three tests that detect high-risk types of HPV DNA in exfoliated cells obtained from the cervix are available for clinical use (Digene HC2 High-Risk HPV DNA test [Qiagen Inc, Valencia, CA], Cervista HPV HR test [Hologic, Bedford, MA], and cobas HPV test [Roche Molecular Diagnostics]). The tests detect any of 13 to 14 high-risk HPV types known to be associated with cervical cancer, and the result is reported as negative or positive. Two tests detect type-specific infection, the Cervista HPV 16/18 and the cobas test, which in addition to reporting presence of any of 14 HPV types also reports detection of HPV 16 and/or 18. These tests are recommended by some organizations for use in combination with Pap testing in women 30 years of age or older and for triage of women 20 years of age or older in specific circumstances to help determine whether further assessments, such as colposcopy, are necessary (American Society for Colposcopy and Cervical Pathology guidelines, 2006 algorithm **[www.asccp.org/consensus.shtml]**). However, these tests are not recommended for routine use in adolescents.

TREATMENT[1]: Serologic testing does not inform clinical decisions and is not indicated. Treatment of HPV infection is directed toward eliminating lesions that result from the infection rather than HPV itself. Treatment of anogenital warts may differ from treatment of cutaneous nongenital warts, so treatment options for these warts should be discussed with a health care professional. Spontaneous regression of genital warts occurs within months in some cases. The optimal treatment for genital warts that do not resolve spontaneously has not been identified. Most nongenital warts eventually regress spontaneously but can persist for months or years. Most methods of treatment use chemical or physical destruction of the infected epithelium, including application of salicylic acid products, cryotherapy with liquid nitrogen, or laser or surgical removal of warts. Daily treatment with tretinoin has been useful for widespread flat warts in children. Care must be taken to avoid a deleterious cosmetic result with therapy. Pharmacologic treatments for refractory warts, including cimetidine, have been used with varied success.

Treatments are characterized as patient applied or administered by health care professionals and include ablational/excisional treatments, antiproliferative methods, and immune-modulating therapy. Many of the agents used for treatment have not been tested for safety and efficacy in children, and some agents are contraindicated in pregnancy. Although most forms of therapy are successful for initial removal of warts, treatment may not eradicate HPV infection from the surrounding tissue. Recurrences are common and may be attributable to reactivation rather than reinfection. Patients should be followed-up

---

[1] Centers for Disease Control and Prevention. Sexually transmitted diseases treatment guidelines—2010. *MMWR Recomm Rep.* 2010;59(RR-12):1–110

during and after treatment for genital warts, because many treatments can result in local symptoms or adverse effects.

Cervical cancer screening. HPV infection of the cervix is common in sexually active adolescents and can be associated with epithelial dysplasia, which commonly are low-grade lesions. However, the vast majority of HPV infections eventually clear, and cervical cancer is rare in adolescence. A variety of professional organizations offer guidance on cervical cancer screening, including the American College of Obstetricians and Gynecologists (ACOG **[www.acog.org]**), American Cancer Society (**www.cancer. org)**, and US Preventive Services Task Force (**www.ahrq.gov/clinic/uspstfix.htm**). The ACOG[1,2] and other organizations no longer recommend routine cervical cytologic testing (Pap testing) in otherwise healthy sexually active adolescents. The ACOG and other professional organizations recommend that Pap testing be initiated at 21 years of age for all otherwise healthy women, regardless of their sexual history. This approach recognizes the importance of avoiding unnecessary treatment for cervical dysplasia, which can have substantial economic, emotional, and reproductive adverse effects, including higher risk of preterm birth. Female adolescents with a recent diagnosis of HIV infection should undergo cervical Pap test screening twice in the first year after diagnosis and annually thereafter. Sexually active female adolescents who have had an organ transplant or are receiving long-term corticosteroid therapy also should undergo similar cervical Pap test screening. If cytologic screening has been initiated before 21 years of age, patients with abnormal Pap test results should be cared for by a physician who is knowledgeable in the management of cervical dysplasia. The American Society for Colposcopy and Cervical Pathology's 2006 Consensus Guidelines include algorithms for management of abnormal Pap test results that are specific for adolescence (**www.asccp.org/ consensus/cytological.shtml**).

Respiratory papillomatosis is difficult to treat and is best managed by an otolaryngologist. Local recurrence is common, and repeated surgical procedures for removal often are necessary. Extension or dissemination of respiratory papillomas from the larynx into the trachea, bronchi, or lung parenchyma can result in increased morbidity and mortality; rarely, carcinoma can occur. Intralesional interferon, indole-3-carbinole, photodynamic therapy, and intralesional cidofovir have been used as investigational treatments and may be of benefit for patients with frequent recurrences.

Oral warts can be removed through cryotherapy, electrocautery, or surgical excision.

ISOLATION OF THE HOSPITALIZED PATIENT: Standard precautions are recommended.

CONTROL MEASURES AND CARE OF EXPOSED PEOPLE: Suspected child abuse should be reported to the appropriate local agency if anogenital warts are found in a child who is beyond infancy but is prepubertal.

Sexual abstinence, monogamous relationships, delayed sexual debut, and minimizing the number of sex partners are modes of reducing risk of anogenital HPV infection. Consistent and correct use of latex condoms can decrease risk of anogenital HPV infection when infected areas are covered or protected by the condom. In addition, use of latex condoms has been associated with a decrease in the risk of genital warts and

---

[1] American College of Obstetricians and Gynecologists. ACOG Committee Opinion No. 463: cervical cancer in adolescents: screening, evaluation, and management. *Obstet Gynecol.* 2010;116(2Pt1):469–472

[2] American College of Obstetricians and Gynecologists. ACOG Committee Opinion No. 436: evaluation and management of abnormal cervical cytology and histology in adolescents. *Obstet Gynecol.* 2009;113(6):1422–1425

cervical cancer. The degree and duration of contagiousness in patients with a history of genital infection is unknown. Sex partners of people with genital warts may benefit from examination to assess for the presence of anogenital warts or other sexually transmitted infections.

Although infection with HPV types 6 and 11 leading to respiratory papillomatosis is believed to be acquired during passage through the birth canal, this condition has occurred in infants born by cesarean delivery. Because the preventive value of cesarean delivery is unknown, it should not be performed solely to prevent transmission of HPV to the newborn infant.

HPV Vaccines. Two HPV vaccines are available for use in the United States. A quadrivalent vaccine (HPV4 [types 6, 11, 16, and 18], Gardasil [Merck & Co Inc]) was licensed by the US Food and Drug Administration (FDA) for use in females 9 through 26 years of age in 2006 and in males 9 through 26 years of age in 2009. A bivalent vaccine (HPV2 [types 16 and 18], Cervarix [GlaxoSmithKline]) was licensed for use in females 10 through 25 years of age in 2009.

Although a successful immunization program holds promise for reduction in the incidence of cervical cancer, women who have received an HPV vaccine must continue to have regular Pap test screening. HPV vaccines do not provide protection against all HPV types associated with development of cancer, and vaccines do not alter the progression of HPV infection acquired before immunization.

Immunogenicity. More than 99% of healthy vaccine recipients develop HPV antibodies 1 month after receipt of the third dose. For HPV4 vaccine, antibody responses in young adolescent females as well as males 9 through 15 years of age were higher than antibody responses in females and males 16 through 26 years of age. For HPV2 vaccine, antibody responses in young adolescent females 10 through 14 years of age were higher than antibody responses in females 15 through 25 years of age.

Antibody concentrations decrease over time after the third dose but plateau by 18 to 24 months after receipt of the third dose for either vaccine. In continuing studies of vaccine recipients, antibody concentrations remain well above those associated with naturally acquired HPV infection. However, the clinical significance of antibody levels is not clear, because a serologic correlate of protection has not been established.

Efficacy. HPV4 and HPV2 vaccines are highly effective in preventing HPV16- and 18-related cervical precancerous lesions in females. HPV4 vaccine is highly effective in preventing HPV6- and 11-related genital warts in females and males. HPV4 vaccine also has been shown to be effective in preventing anal precancerous lesions in males. Vaccines offer no protection against progression of infection to disease from HPV acquired before immunization. Therefore, HPV vaccines are most effective for both males and females when given before exposure to HPV through sexual contact.

Studies through 5 years for HPV4 vaccine and 6.4 years for HPV2 vaccine have shown no waning of protection. Long-term follow-up studies are being conducted to determine the duration of efficacy for both vaccines.

Vaccine Recommendations.[1,2,3,4] The American Academy of Pediatrics and the Advisory Committee on Immunization Practices (ACIP) of the Centers for Disease Control and Prevention recommend HPV4 or HPV2 vaccine for routine immunization of females 11 or 12 years of age (although the series can be started at 9 years of age). Vaccine also is recommended for females 13 through 26 years of age not previously immunized. HPV4 is recommended for routine immunization of males at 11 or 12 years of age (although the series can be started at 9 years of age) and also is recommended for males 13 through 21 years of age not previously immunized. Males 22 through 26 years of age may be immunized. Vaccine is recommended for men who have sex with men and males who are immunocompromised (including those with HIV infection) through 26 years of age.[5] The vaccines are not licensed for use in people older than 26 years of age.

- **Dosage and Administration.** The recommended dose and administration schedule for HPV4 and HPV2 vaccines are the same. The vaccines are given in three 0.5-mL doses, administered intramuscularly, preferably in a deltoid muscle. The second dose should be administered 1 to 2 months after the first dose, and the third dose should be administered 6 months after the first dose. The minimum interval between doses 1 and 2 is 4 weeks. The minimum interval between doses 2 and 3 is 12 weeks (and at least 24 weeks after the first dose).
- Dose(s) of vaccine received after a shorter-than-recommended interval should be repeated.
- If the vaccine schedule is interrupted, the vaccine series does not need to be restarted.
- Vaccine recipients should be seated and observed for 15 minutes after immunization because of the risk of syncope in adolescents receiving injections.[6]
- Whenever feasible, in females, the same HPV vaccine should be used for the entire immunization series, because no studies address interchangeability of HPV vaccines. However, if the vaccine provider does not know which HPV vaccine was previously administered, then either vaccine can be used to complete the series to provide protection against HPV types 16 and 18 in females. HPV2 vaccine is not recommended for males.

[1] Centers for Disease Control and Prevention. Quadrivalent human papillomavirus vaccine: recommendations of the Advisory Committee on Immunization Practices (ACIP). *MMWR Recomm Rep.* 2007;56(RR-2):1–24. Available at: **http://www.cdc.gov/mmwr/PDF/rr/rr5602.pdf**

[2] American Academy of Pediatrics, Committee on Infectious Diseases. HPV vaccine recommendations. *Pediatrics.* 2012;129(3):602–605

[3] Centers for Disease Control and Prevention. FDA Licensure of quadrivalent human papillomavirus vaccine (HPV4, Gardasil) for use in males and guidance from the Advisory Committee on Immunization Practices (ACIP). 2010;59(20):630-632. Available at: **http://www.cdc.gov/mmwr/preview/mmwrhtml/mm5920a5.htm?s_cid=mm5920a5_e**

[4] Centers for Disease Control and Prevention. FDA licensure of bivalent human papillomavirus vaccine (HPV2, Cervarix) for use in females and updated HPV vaccination recommendations from the Advisory Committee on Immunization Practices (ACIP). 2010;59(20):626–629. Available at: **http://www.cdc.gov/mmwr/preview/mmwrhtml/mm5920a4.htm?s_cid=mm5920a4_e**

[5] Centers for Disease Control and Prevention. Recommendations on use of quadrivalent human papillomavirus vaccine in males: Advisory Committee on Immunization Practices (ACIP), 2011. *MMWR Morb Mortal Wkly Rep.* 2011;60(50):1705–1708

[6] Centers for Disease Control and Prevention. Syncope after vaccination—United States, January 2005–July 2007. *MMWR Morb Mortal Wkly Rep.* 2008;57(17):457–460

- Both vaccines are available in single-dose vials and prefilled syringes and contain no antimicrobial agents or preservative.
- HPV vaccines should be stored at 2°C to 8°C (36°F–46°F) and not frozen.
- HPV vaccine can be coadministered with any live or inactivated vaccine indicated at the same visit.
- People through 26 years of age with evidence of current HPV infection, such as cervical dysplasia, a positive HPV DNA test result, or anogenital warts or a history of anogenital warts, should receive immunization, because infection with all vaccine HPV types is unlikely and the vaccine could provide protection against HPV infection with types not already acquired.

   Recommendations for special populations. HPV vaccines are not live vaccines and can be administered to people who are immunocompromised as a result of infection (including HIV), disease, or medications. The immune response and vaccine efficacy in immunocompromised people might be less than that in immunocompetent people.

Precautions and Contraindications.

- HPV vaccines can be administered to people with minor acute illnesses.
- Immunization of people with moderate or severe acute illnesses should be deferred until after the patient improves.
- HPV vaccines are contraindicated in people with a history of immediate hypersensitivity to any vaccine component (HPV2 and HPV4) and to yeast (HPV4). HPV2 vaccine in the prefilled syringe formulation should not be administered to latex-sensitive individuals, because the rubber stopper contains latex.
- HPV vaccines are not recommended for use during pregnancy. The health care professional should inquire about pregnancy in sexually active patients, but a pregnancy test is not required before starting the immunization series. If a vaccine recipient becomes pregnant, subsequent doses should be postponed until the postpartum period. If a dose has been administered inadvertently during pregnancy, no action is recommended. Limited data show no definitive evidence of adverse effect of HPV4 or HPV2 vaccine on pregnancy, although further studies are being conducted for HPV2 vaccine to follow rates of spontaneous abortion in pregnancies which occurred inadvertently around the time of vaccination. For a pregnant woman who inadvertently receives either of the HPV vaccines, separate vaccine-in-pregnancy registries have been established (1-800-986-8999 for HPV4 and 1-888-452-9622 for HPV2) to monitor outcomes of exposure during pregnancy.
- HPV4 vaccine may be administered to lactating women. The HPV2 vaccine has not been studied in lactating women.

Paracoccidioidomycosis
(South American Blastomycosis)

CLINICAL MANIFESTATIONS: Disease occurs primarily in adults, in whom the site of initial infection is the lungs. Clinical patterns are categorized as an acute-subacute form that predominates in childhood and a chronic form that is the typical clinical pattern in adults. In both forms, constitutional symptoms, such as fever, malaise, and weight loss, are common. In the acute-subacute form, the initial pulmonary infection usually is asymptomatic, and manifestations are related to dissemination of infection to the reticuloendothelial system, resulting in enlarged lymph nodes and involvement of liver, spleen, and bone marrow. Involvement of bones, joints, skin, and mucous membranes is less common. Occasionally, enlarged lymph nodes coalesce and form abscesses or fistulas. The chronic form of the illness can be localized to the lungs or can disseminate. Oral, upper respiratory tract and gastrointestinal tract granulomatous or ulcerative mucosal lesions are less common manifestations of disease in children than in adults. Infection can be latent for years before causing illness.

ETIOLOGY: *Paracoccidioides brasiliensis* is a thermally dimorphic fungus with yeast and mycelia phases.

EPIDEMIOLOGY: The infection occurs in Latin America, from Mexico to Argentina. The natural reservoir is unknown, although soil is suspected. The mode of transmission is unknown; person-to-person transmission does not occur.

The **incubation period** is highly variable, ranging from 1 month to many years.

DIAGNOSTIC TESTS: Round, multiple-budding cells with a distinguishing pilot's wheel appearance can be seen in 10% potassium hydroxide preparations of sputum, bronchoalveolar lavage specimens, scrapings from ulcers, and material from lesions or in tissue biopsy specimens. The organism can be cultured on most enriched media, including blood agar at 37°C (98°F) and Mycosel or Sabouraud dextrose agar (with antibiotics and cycloheximide) at 24°C (75°F). A number of serologic tests are available; quantitative immunodiffusion is the preferred test. The antibody titer by immunodiffusion usually is ≥1:32 in acute infection.

TREATMENT: Amphotericin B is preferred by many experts for initial treatment of severe paracoccidioidomycosis (see Drugs for Invasive and Other Serious Fungal Infections, p 835). An alternative is intravenous trimethoprim-sulfamethoxazole (8–10 mg/kg/day of the trimethoprim component divided into 3 daily doses). Children treated initially by the intravenous route can transition to orally administered therapy after clinical improvement has been observed, usually after 3 to 6 weeks.

Oral therapy with itraconazole (5 mg/kg once daily; maximum dose 100 mg, once or twice daily) is the treatment of choice for less severe or localized infection and to complete treatment when amphotericin B is used initially. Prolonged therapy for 6 to 12 months is necessary to minimize the relapse rate. Children with severe disease can require a longer course. Itraconazole is associated with fewer adverse effects and a lower relapse rate (3%–5%) than ketoconazole, which now uncommonly is used for treatment. Voriconazole is as well tolerated and effective as itraconazole in adults, but data for its use in children with paracoccidioidomycosis are not available. Trimethoprim-sulfamethoxazole orally (10 mg/kg/day of the trimethoprim component divided into 2 doses daily) is an alternative but treatment must be continued for 2 years or longer to lessen the risk of relapse, which occurs in 10% to 15% of optimally treated patients.

Serial serologic testing by quantitative immunodiffusion is useful for monitoring the response to therapy. The expected response is a progressive decline in titers after 1 to 3 months of treatment with stabilization at a low titer.

ISOLATION OF THE HOSPITALIZED PATIENT: Standard precautions are recommended.

CONTROL MEASURES: None.

Paragonimiasis

CLINICAL MANIFESTATIONS: There are 2 major forms of paragonimiasis: (1) disease attributable to *Paragonimus westermani, Paragonimus heterotremus, Paragonimus africanus,* and *Paragonimus uterobilateralis,* causing primary pulmonary disease with or without extrapulmonary manifestations; and (2) disease attributable to other species of *Paragonimus,* most notably *Paragonimus skrjabini,* for which humans are accidental hosts and manifestations generally are extrapulmonary, resulting in a larva migrans syndrome. The disease has an insidious onset and a chronic course. Pulmonary disease is associated with chronic cough and dyspnea, but most infections probably are inapparent or result in mild symptoms. Heavy infestations cause paroxysms of coughing, which often produce blood-tinged sputum that is brown because of the presence of *Paragonimus* species eggs. Hemoptysis can be severe. Pleural effusion, pneumothorax, bronchiectasis, and pulmonary fibrosis with clubbing can develop. Extrapulmonary manifestations also may involve liver, spleen, abdominal cavity, intestinal wall, intra-abdominal lymph nodes, skin, and central nervous system, with meningoencephalitis, seizures, and space-occupying tumors attributable to invasion of the brain by adult flukes, usually occurring within a year of pulmonary infection. Symptoms tend to subside after approximately 5 years but can persist for as many as 20 years.

Extrapulmonary paragonimiasis is associated with migratory allergic subcutaneous nodules containing juvenile worms. Pleural effusion is common, as is invasion of the brain.

ETIOLOGY: In Asia, classical paragonimiasis is caused by adult flukes and eggs of *P westermani* and *P heterotremus.* In Africa, the adult flukes and eggs of *P africanus and P uterobilateralis* produce the disease. The adult flukes of *P westermani* are up to 12 mm long and 7 mm wide and occur throughout the Far East. A triploid parthenogenetic form of *P westermani,* which is larger, produces more eggs, and elicits greater disease, has been described in Japan, Korea, Taiwan, and parts of eastern China. *P heterotremus* occurs in Southeast Asia and adjacent parts of China. Extrapulmonary paragonimiasis is caused by larval stages of *P skrjabini* and *Paragonimus miyazakii.* The worms rarely mature. *P skrjabini* occurs in China, and *P miyazakii* occurs in Japan. *Paragonimus mexicanus* and *Paragonimus ecuadoriensis* occur in Mexico, Costa Rica, Ecuador, and Peru. *Paragonimus kellicotti,* a lung fluke of mink and opossums in the United States, also can cause a zoonotic infection in humans.

EPIDEMIOLOGY: Transmission occurs when raw or undercooked freshwater crabs or crayfish containing larvae (metacercariae) are ingested. The metacercariae excyst in the small intestine and penetrate the abdominal cavity, where they remain for a few days before migrating to the lungs. *P westermani* and *P heterotremus* mature within the lungs over 6 to 10 weeks, when they then begin egg production. Eggs escape from pulmonary capsules into the bronchi and exit from the human host in sputum or feces. Eggs hatch in freshwater within 3 weeks, giving rise to miracidia. Miracidia penetrate freshwater snails and emerge several weeks later as cercariae, which encyst within the muscles and viscera of freshwater crustaceans before maturing into infective metacercariae. Transmission also occurs when humans ingest raw pork, usually from wild pigs, containing the juvenile stages of *Paragonimus* species (described as occurring in Japan).

Humans are accidental ("dead-end") hosts for *P skrjabini* and *P miyazakii.* These flukes cannot mature in humans and, hence, do not produce eggs.

Paragonimus species also infect a variety of other mammals, such as canids, mustelids, felids, and rodents, which can serve as animal reservoir hosts.

The **incubation period** is variable; egg production begins approximately 8 weeks after ingestion of *P westermani* metacercariae.

DIAGNOSTIC TESTS: Microscopic examination of stool, sputum, pleural effusion, cerebrospinal fluid, and other tissue specimens may reveal eggs. A Western blot serologic antibody test based on *P westermani* antigen, available at the Centers for Disease Control and Prevention (CDC), is sensitive and specific; antibody levels detected by immunoblot decrease slowly after the infection is cured by treatment. Charcot-Leyden crystals and eosinophils in sputum are useful diagnostic elements. Chest radiographs may appear normal or resemble radiographs from patients with tuberculosis. Misdiagnosis is likely unless paragonimiasis is suspected.

TREATMENT: Praziquantel in a 2-day course is the treatment of choice and is associated with high cure rates as demonstrated by disappearance of egg production and radiographic lesions in the lungs. The drug also is effective for some extrapulmonary manifestations. Bithionol, available from the CDC, is an alternative drug (see Drugs for Parasitic Infections, p 848).

ISOLATION OF THE HOSPITALIZED PATIENT: Standard precautions are recommended.

CONTROL MEASURES: Cooking of crabs and crayfish for several minutes until the meat has congealed and turned opaque kills metacercariae. Similarly, meat from wild pigs should be well cooked before eating. Control of animal reservoirs is not possible.

Parainfluenza Viral Infections

CLINICAL MANIFESTATIONS: Parainfluenza viruses are the major cause of laryngotracheobronchitis (croup), but they also commonly cause upper respiratory tract infection, pneumonia, and/or bronchiolitis.[1] Parainfluenza virus types 1 and 2 are the most common pathogens associated with croup, and parainfluenza virus type 3 most commonly is associated with bronchiolitis and pneumonia in infants and young children. Rarely, parotitis, aseptic meningitis, and encephalitis have been associated with type 3 infections. Parainfluenza virus infections can exacerbate symptoms of chronic lung disease and asthma in children and adults. Severe and persistent infections occur in immunodeficient children and are associated most commonly with type 3 virus. Infections with type 4 parainfluenza virus are not as well characterized, but studies using reverse transcriptase-polymerase chain reaction assays suggest that they may be more common than previously appreciated. Parainfluenza infections do not confer complete protective immunity; therefore, reinfections can occur with all serotypes and at any age, but reinfections usually cause a mild illness limited to the upper respiratory tract.

ETIOLOGY: Parainfluenza viruses are enveloped RNA viruses classified in the family *Paramyxoviridae*. Four antigenically distinct types—1, 2, 3, and 4 (with 2 subtypes, 4A and 4B)—have been identified.

---

[1] American Academy of Pediatrics, Subcommittee on Diagnosis and Management of Bronchiolitis. Diagnosis and management of bronchiolitis. *Pediatrics.* 2006;118(4):1774–1793

EPIDEMIOLOGY: Parainfluenza viruses are transmitted from person to person by direct contact and exposure to contaminated nasopharyngeal secretions through respiratory tract droplets and fomites. Parainfluenza virus infections can be sporadic or associated with outbreaks of acute respiratory tract disease. Seasonal patterns of infection are distinct, predictable, and cyclic. Different serotypes have distinct epidemiologic patterns. Type 1 virus tends to produce outbreaks of respiratory tract illness, usually croup, in the autumn of every other year. A major increase in the number of cases of croup in the autumn usually indicates a parainfluenza type 1 outbreak. Type 2 virus also can cause outbreaks of respiratory tract illness in the autumn, often in conjunction with type 1 outbreaks, but type 2 outbreaks tend to be less severe, irregular, and less common. Parainfluenza type 3 virus usually is prominent during spring and summer in temperate climates but often continues into autumn, especially in years when autumn outbreaks of parainfluenza virus types 1 or 2 are absent. Infections with type 4 parainfluenza virus are recognized less commonly and can be associated with mild to severe illnesses.

The age of primary infection varies with serotype. Primary infection with all types usually occurs by 5 years of age. Infection with type 3 virus more often occurs in infants and is a prominent cause of lower respiratory tract illnesses in this age group. By 12 months of age, 50% of infants have acquired type 3 parainfluenza infection. Infections between 1 and 5 years of age are more commonly associated with type 1 and, to a lesser extent, type 2 parainfluenza viruses. Age at acquisition of type 4 parainfluenza infection is not as well defined. Rates of parainfluenza virus hospitalizations for children younger than 5 years of age are estimated to be 1 per 1000, with the highest rates in infants 0 to 5 months of age (3 per 1000).

Immunocompetent children with primary parainfluenza infection may shed virus for up to 1 week before onset of clinical symptoms and for 1 to 3 weeks after symptoms have disappeared, depending on serotype. Severe lower respiratory tract disease with prolonged shedding of the virus can develop in immunodeficient people. In these patients, infection may spread beyond the respiratory tract to liver and lymph nodes.

The **incubation period** ranges from 2 to 6 days.

DIAGNOSTIC TESTS: Rapid antigen identification techniques, including immunofluorescent assays and enzyme immunoassays, can be used to detect the virus in nasopharyngeal secretions, but sensitivities of the tests vary. Virus may be isolated from nasopharyngeal secretions usually within 4 to 7 days of culture inoculation or earlier by using centrifugation of the specimen onto a monolayer of susceptible cells with subsequent staining for viral antigen (shell vial assay). Highly sensitive and specific reverse transcriptase-polymerase chain reaction (RT-PCR) assays are available for detection and differentiation of parainfluenza viruses, and they are becoming the standard diagnostic approach for these viruses. Serologic diagnosis, made retrospectively by a significant increase in antibody titer between serum specimens obtained during acute infection and convalescence, is less useful, because infection may not always be accompanied by a significant homotypic antibody response.

TREATMENT: Specific antiviral therapy is not available. Most infections are self-limited and require no treatment. Monitoring for hypoxia and hypercapnia in more severely affected children with lower respiratory tract disease may be helpful. The following treatment recommendations apply to laryngotracheobronchitis. Racemic epinephrine aerosol commonly is given to severely affected, hospitalized patients with laryngotracheobronchitis to decrease airway obstruction. Parenteral dexamethasone in high doses, oral dexamethasone, and nebulized corticosteroids have been demonstrated to lessen the severity and duration of symptoms and hospitalization in patients with moderate to severe laryngotracheobronchitis. Oral dexamethasone also is effective for outpatients with less severe croup. Management otherwise is supportive. Antimicrobial agents should be reserved for documented secondary bacterial infections.

ISOLATION OF THE HOSPITALIZED PATIENT: In addition to standard precautions, contact precautions are recommended for hospitalized infants and young children for the duration of illness. Strict adherence to infection-control procedures, including prevention of environmental contamination by respiratory tract secretions and careful hand hygiene, should control health care-associated spread. Hospitalized immunocompromised patients with type 3 parainfluenza infection should be isolated to prevent spread to other patients.

CONTROL MEASURES: Efforts should be aimed at decreasing health care-associated infection. Hand hygiene should be emphasized.

Parasitic Diseases

Many parasitic diseases traditionally have been considered exotic and, therefore, frequently are not included in differential diagnoses of patients in the United States, Canada, and Europe. Nevertheless, a number of these organisms are endemic in industrialized countries, and overall, parasites are among the most common causes of morbidity and mortality in various and diverse geographic locations worldwide. Outside the tropics and subtropics, parasitic diseases particularly are common among tourists returning to their own countries, immigrants from areas with highly endemic infection, and immunocompromised people. Some of these infections disproportionately affect impoverished populations, such as black and Hispanic people living in the United States, and aboriginal people living in Alaska and the Canadian Arctic. Physicians and clinical laboratory personnel need to be aware of where these infections may be acquired, their clinical presentations, and methods of diagnosis and should advise people how to prevent infection. Table 3.40 (p 536) gives details on some infrequently encountered parasitic diseases.

Consultation and assistance in diagnosis and management of parasitic diseases are available from the Centers for Disease Control and Prevention (CDC), state health departments, and university departments or divisions of geographic medicine, tropical medicine, pediatric infectious diseases, international health, and public health.

Through authorized investigational new drug mechanisms, the CDC distributes several drugs that are not available commercially in the United States for treatment of parasitic diseases. These drugs are indicated by footnotes in Table 4.12, Manufacturers of Some Antiparasitic Drugs (p 868). To request these drugs, a physician must contact the CDC Parasitic Diseases Public Inquiries office (see Appendix I, Directory of Resources, p 883; 770-488-7775; e-mail: parasites@cdc.gov). Consultation with a medical officer from the CDC is required before a drug is distributed.

Important human parasitic infections are discussed in individual chapters in section 3; the diseases are arranged alphabetically, and the discussions include recommendations for drug treatment. Tables 4.9 (p 849), 4.10 (p 862), 4.11 (p 866), and 4.12 (p 868), reproduced from *The Medical Letter* (see Drugs for Parasitic Infections, p 848), provide dosage recommendations and other relevant information for specific antiparasitic drugs. Although the

Table 3.40. Parasitic Diseases Not Covered Elsewhere[a]

Disease and/or Agent	Where Infection May Be Acquired	Definitive Host	Intermediate Host	Modes of Human Infection	Directly Communicable (Person to Person)	Diagnostic Laboratory Tests in Humans	Causative Form of Parasite	Manifestations in Humans
Angiostrongylus cantonensis (neurotropic disease)	Widespread in the tropics, particularly Pacific Islands, Southeast Asia, and Central and South America	Rats	Snails and slugs	Eating improperly cooked infected mollusks or food contaminated by mollusk secretions containing larvae	No	Eosinophils in CSF; rarely, identification of larvae in CSF or at autopsy; serologic test	Larval worms	Eosinophilia, meningoencephalitis
Angiostrongylus costaricensis (gastrointestinal tract disease)	Central and South America	Rodents	Snails and slugs	Eating improperly cooked infected mollusks or, food contaminated by mollusk secretions containing larvae	No	Gel diffusion; identification of larvae and eggs in tissue	Larval worms	Abdominal pain, eosinophilia
Anisakiasis	Cosmopolitan, mainly Japan	Marine mammal	Certain saltwater fish, squid, and octopus	Eating uncooked infected fish	No	Identification of recovered larvae in granulomas or vomitus	Larval worms	Acute gastrointestinal tract disease

Table 3.40. Parasitic Diseases Not Covered Elsewhere,[a] continued

Disease and/ or Agent	Where Infection May Be Acquired	Definitive Host	Intermediate Host	Modes of Human Infection	Directly Communicable (Person to Person)	Diagnostic Laboratory Tests in Humans	Causative Form of Parasite	Manifestations in Humans
Clonorchis sinensis, Opisthorchis viverrini, Opisthorchis felineus (flukes)	East Asia, Eastern Europe, Russian Federation	Humans, cats, dogs, other mammals	Certain freshwater snails	Eating uncooked infected freshwater fish	No	Eggs in stool or duodenal fluid	Larvae and mature flukes	Abdominal pain; hepatobiliary disease
Dracunculiasis (Dracunculus medinensis) (guinea worm)	Foci in Africa	Humans	Crustacea (copepods)	Drinking infested water	No	Identification of emerging or adult worm in subcutaneous tissues	Adult female worm	Emerging roundworm; inflammatory response; systemic and local blister or ulcer in skin
Fasciolopsiasis (Fasciolopsis buski)	East Asia	Humans, pigs, dogs	Certain freshwater snails, plants	Eating uncooked infected plants	No	Eggs or worm in feces or duodenal fluid	Larvae and mature worms	Diarrhea, constipation, vomiting, anorexia, edema of face and legs, ascites

Table 3.40. Parasitic Diseases Not Covered Elsewhere,[a] continued

Disease and/ or Agent	Where Infection May Be Acquired	Definitive Host	Intermediate Host	Modes of Human Infection	Directly Communicable (Person to Person)	Diagnostic Laboratory Tests in Humans	Causative Form of Parasite	Manifestations in Humans
Intestinal capillariasis (*Capillaria philippinensis*)	Philippines, Thailand	Humans, fish-eating birds	Fish	Ingestion of uncooked infected fish	Uncertain	Eggs and parasite in feces	Larvae and mature worms	Protein-losing enteropathy, diarrhea, malabsorption, ascites, emaciation

CSF indicates cerebrospinal fluid.

[a]For recommended drug treatment, see Drugs for Parasitic Infections (p 848).

recommendations for administration of these drugs given in the disease-specific chapters are similar, they may not be identical in all instances because of differences of opinion among experts. Both sources should be consulted.

Parvovirus B19
(Erythema Infectiosum, Fifth Disease)

CLINICAL MANIFESTATIONS: Infection with parvovirus B19 is recognized most often as erythema infectiosum (EI), or fifth disease, which is characterized by a distinctive rash that may be preceded by mild systemic symptoms, including fever in 15% to 30% of patients. The facial rash can be intensely red with a "slapped cheek" appearance that often is accompanied by circumoral pallor. A symmetric, macular, lace-like, and often pruritic rash also occurs on the trunk, moving peripherally to involve the arms, buttocks, and thighs. The rash can fluctuate in intensity and recur with environmental changes, such as temperature and exposure to sunlight, for weeks to months. A brief, mild, non-specific illness consisting of fever, malaise, myalgia, and headache often precedes the characteristic exanthema by approximately 7 to 10 days. Arthralgia and arthritis occur in fewer than 10% of infected children but commonly occur among adults, especially women. Knees are involved most commonly in children, but a symmetric polyarthropathy of knees, fingers, and other joints is common in adults.

Human parvovirus B19 also can cause an asymptomatic infection. Other manifestations (Table 3.41, p 540), include a mild respiratory tract illness with no rash, a rash atypical for EI that may be rubelliform or petechial, papulopurpuric gloves-and-socks syndrome (PPGSS; painful and pruritic papules, petechiae, and purpura of hands and feet, often with fever and an enanthem), polyarthropathy syndrome (arthralgia and arthritis in adults in the absence of other manifestations of EI), chronic erythroid hypoplasia with severe anemia in immunodeficient patients (eg, HIV-infected patients, patients receiving immune suppressive therapy), and transient aplastic crisis lasting 7 to 10 days in patients with hemolytic anemias (eg, sickle cell disease and autoimmune hemolytic anemia) and other conditions associated with low hemoglobin concentrations, including hemorrhage, severe anemia, and thalassemia. Patients with transient aplastic crisis may have a prodromal illness with fever, malaise, and myalgia, but rash usually is absent. The B19-associated red blood cell aplasia is related to caspase-10 mediated apoptosis of erythrocyte precursors. In addition, parvovirus B19 infection sometimes has been associated with decreases in numbers of platelets, lymphocytes, and neutrophils.

Parvovirus B19 infection occurring during pregnancy can cause fetal hydrops, intrauterine growth retardation, isolated pleural and pericardial effusions, and death, but parvovirus B19 is not a proven cause of congenital anomalies. The risk of fetal death is between 2% and 6% when infection occurs during pregnancy. The greatest risk appears to occur during the first half of pregnancy.

ETIOLOGY: Human parvovirus B19 is a small, nonenveloped, single-stranded DNA virus in the family *Parvoviridae*, genus *Erythrovirus*. Three major genetic variants of the virus have been described. Parvovirus B19 replicates in human erythrocyte precursors, which accounts for some of the clinical manifestations following infection.

EPIDEMIOLOGY: Parvovirus B19 is distributed worldwide and is a common cause of infection in humans, who are the only known hosts. Modes of transmission include contact with respiratory tract secretions, percutaneous exposure to blood or blood products,

Table 3.41. Clinical Manifestations of Human Parvovirus B19 Infection

Conditions	Usual Hosts
Erythema infectiosum (fifth disease)	Immunocompetent children
Polyarthropathy syndrome	Immunocompetent adults (more common in women)
Chronic anemia/pure red cell aplasia	Immunocompromised hosts
Transient aplastic crisis	People with hemolytic anemia (ie, sickle cell anemia)
Hydrops fetalis/congenital anemia	Fetus (first 20 weeks of pregnancy)

and vertical transmission from mother to fetus. Since 2002, plasma derivatives have been screened using nucleic acid amplification tests (NAATs) to decrease the risk of parvovirus B19 transmission. Parvovirus B19 infections are ubiquitous, and cases of EI can occur sporadically or in outbreaks in elementary or junior high schools during late winter and early spring. Secondary spread among susceptible household members is common, with infection occurring in approximately 50% of susceptible contacts in some studies. The transmission rate in schools is less, but infection can be an occupational risk for school and child care personnel, with approximately 20% of susceptible contacts becoming infected. In young children, antibody seroprevalence generally is 5% to 10%. In most communities, approximately 50% of young adults and often more than 90% of elderly people are seropositive. The annual seroconversion rate in women of childbearing age has been reported to be approximately 1.5%. Timing of the presence of parvovirus B19 DNA in serum and respiratory tract secretions indicates that people with EI are most infectious before rash onset and are unlikely to be infectious after onset of the rash and/or joint symptoms. In contrast, patients with aplastic crises are contagious from before the onset of symptoms through at least the week after onset. Symptoms of the PPGSS occur in association with viremia and before development of antibody response, and affected patients should be considered infectious.

The **incubation period** from acquisition of parvovirus B19 to onset of initial symptoms usually is between 4 and 14 days but can be as long as 21 days. Rash and joint symptoms occur 2 to 3 weeks after infection.

DIAGNOSTIC TESTS: Parvovirus B19 cannot be propagated in standard cell culture. In the immunocompetent host, detection of serum parvovirus B19-specific immunoglobulin (Ig) M antibody is the preferred diagnostic test. A positive IgM test result indicates that infection probably occurred within the previous 2 to 4 months. On the basis of enzyme immunoassay results, antibody may be detected in 90% or more of patients at the time of the EI rash and by the third day of illness in patients with transient aplastic crisis. Serum IgG antibody appears by approximately day 7 of EI and persists for life; therefore, presence of parvovirus B19 IgG is not necessarily indicative of acute infection. These assays are available through commercial laboratories and through some state health department and research laboratories. However, their sensitivity and specificity may vary, particularly for IgM antibody. The optimal method for detecting chronic infection in the immunocompromised patient is demonstration of virus by polymerase chain reaction

(PCR) assays, because parvovirus B19 antibody is present variably in persistent infection. Because parvovirus B19 DNA can be detected at low levels by PCR assay in serum for up to 9 months after the acute viremic phase, detection does not necessarily indicate acute infection. Parvovirus DNA has been detected by PCR in tissues (skin, heart, cerebellum), independent of disease.

TREATMENT: For most patients, only supportive care is indicated. Patients with aplastic crises may require transfusion. For treatment of chronic infection in immunodeficient patients, Immune Globulin Intravenous (IGIV) therapy often is effective and should be considered. Some cases of parvovirus B19 infection concurrent with hydrops fetalis have been treated successfully with intrauterine blood transfusions.

ISOLATION OF THE HOSPITALIZED PATIENT: In addition to standard precautions, droplet precautions are recommended for hospitalized children with aplastic crises, children with PPGSS, or immunosuppressed patients with chronic infection and anemia for the duration of hospitalization. For patients with transient aplastic or erythrocyte crisis, these precautions should be maintained for 7 days. Neonates who had hydrops attributable to parvovirus B19 in utero do not require isolation if the hydrops is resolved at the time of birth.

Pregnant health care professionals should be informed of the potential risks to the fetus from parvovirus B19 infections and about preventive measures that may decrease these risks, for example, attention to strict infection control procedures and not caring for immunocompromised patients with chronic parvovirus infection or patients with parvovirus B19-associated aplastic crises, because patients in both groups are likely to be contagious.

CONTROL MEASURES:

- Women who are exposed to children at home or at work (eg, teachers or child care providers) are at increased risk of infection with parvovirus B19. However, because school or child care center outbreaks often indicate wider spread in the community, including inapparent infection, women are at some degree of risk of exposure from other sources at home or in the community. In view of the high prevalence of parvovirus B19 infection, the low incidence of adverse effects on the fetus, and the fact that avoidance of child care or classroom teaching can decrease but not eliminate the risk of exposure, routine exclusion of pregnant women from the workplace where EI is occurring is not recommended. Women of childbearing age who are concerned can undergo serologic testing for IgG antibody to parvovirus B19 to determine their susceptibility to infection.
- Pregnant women who discover that they have been in contact with children who were in the incubation period of EI or with children who were in aplastic crisis should have the relatively low potential risk of infection explained to them, and the option of serologic testing should be offered. Fetal ultrasonography may prove useful in these situations.
- Children with EI may attend child care or school, because they no longer are contagious once the rash appears.
- Transmission of parvovirus B19 is likely to be decreased through use of routine infection-control practices, including hand hygiene and proper disposal of used facial tissues.

Pasteurella Infections

CLINICAL MANIFESTATIONS: The most common manifestation in children is cellulitis at the site of a scratch or bite of a cat, dog, or other animal. Cellulitis typically develops within 24 hours of the injury and includes swelling, erythema, tenderness, and serous or sanguinopurulent discharge at the site. Regional lymphadenopathy, chills, and fever can occur. Local complications, such as septic arthritis, osteomyelitis, and tenosynovitis, are common. Less common manifestations of infection include septicemia, meningitis, endocarditis, respiratory tract infections (eg, pneumonia, pulmonary abscesses, pleural empyema), appendicitis, hepatic abscess, peritonitis, urinary tract infection, and ocular infections (eg, conjunctivitis, corneal ulcer, endophthalmitis). People with liver disease or underlying host defense abnormalities are predisposed to bacteremia attributable to *Pasteurella multocida*.

ETIOLOGY: Species of the genus *Pasteurella* are nonmotile, facultative anaerobic, gram-negative coccobacilli that are primary pathogens in animals. The most common human pathogen is *P multocida*. Most human infections are caused by the following species or sub-species: *P multocida* subspecies *multocida*, *P multocida* subspecies *septica*, *P multocida* subspecies *gallicida*, *Pasteurella canis*, *Pasteurella stomatis*, *Pasteurella dagmatis*, and *Pasteurella haemolytica*.

EPIDEMIOLOGY: *Pasteurella* species are found in the oral flora of 70% to 90% of cats, 25% to 50% of dogs, and many other animals. Transmission can occur from the bite or scratch of a cat or dog or, less commonly, from another animal. Respiratory tract spread from animals to humans also occurs. In a significant proportion of cases, no animal exposure can be identified. Human-to-human spread has been documented vertically from mother to neonate, horizontally from colonized humans, and by contaminated blood products.

The **incubation period** usually is less than 24 hours.

DIAGNOSTIC TESTS: The isolation of *Pasteurella* species from skin lesion drainage or other sites of infection (eg, blood, joint fluid, cerebrospinal fluid, sputum, pleural fluid, or suppurative lymph nodes) is diagnostic. Although *Pasteurella* species resemble several other organisms morphologically and grow on many culture media at 37°C (98°F), laboratory differentiation is not difficult.

TREATMENT: The drug of choice is penicillin. Other effective oral agents include ampicillin, amoxicillin, cefuroxime, cefixime, cefpodoxime, doxycycline, and fluoroquinolones. For patients who are allergic to beta-lactam agents, azithromycin or trimethoprim-sulfamethoxazole are alternative choices, but clinical experience with these agents is limited. Doxycycline is effective but should be avoided in children younger than 8 years of age (see Tetracyclines, p 801). Fluoroquinolones are effective but are not recommended for this use in patients younger than 18 years of age (see Fluoroquinolones, p 800). For suspected polymicrobial infection, oral amoxicillin-clavulanate or, for severe infection, intravenous ampicillin-sulbactam, ticarcillin-clavulanate, or piperacillin-tazobactam can be given. Alternative agents for systemic infection include ceftriaxone or a carbapenem. Isolates usually are resistant to vancomycin, clindamycin, and erythromycin. The duration of therapy usually is 7 to 10 days for local infections and 10 to 14 days for more severe infections. Antimicrobial therapy should be continued for 4 to 6 weeks for bone and joint infections. Wound drainage or débridement may be necessary.

Penicillin resistance is rare, but beta-lactamase–producing strains have been recovered, especially from adults with pulmonary disease.

ISOLATION OF THE HOSPITALIZED PATIENT: Standard precautions are recommended.

CONTROL MEASURES: Limiting contact with wild animals and education about appropriate contact with domestic animals can help to prevent *Pasteurella* infections (see Bite Wounds, p 203). Animal bites and scratches should be irrigated, cleansed, and débrided promptly. Antimicrobial prophylaxis for children with an animal bite wound should be initiated according to the recommendations in Table 2.18, p 204.

Pediculosis Capitis[1]
(Head Lice)

CLINICAL MANIFESTATIONS: Itching is the most common symptom of head lice infestation, but many children are asymptomatic. Adult lice or eggs (nits) are found on the hair and are most readily apparent behind the ears and near the nape of the neck. Excoriations and crusting caused by secondary bacterial infection may occur and often are associated with regional lymphadenopathy. Head lice usually deposit their eggs on a hair shaft 4 mm or less from the scalp. Because hair grows at a rate of approximately 1 cm per month, the duration of infestation can be estimated by the distance of the nit from the scalp.

ETIOLOGY: *Pediculus humanus capitis* is the head louse. Both nymphs and adult lice feed on human blood.

EPIDEMIOLOGY: In the United States, head lice infestation is most common in children attending child care and elementary school. Head lice infestation is not a sign of poor hygiene. All socioeconomic groups are affected. In the United States, infestations are less common in black children than in children of other races. Head lice infestation is not influenced by hair length or frequency of shampooing or brushing. Head lice are not a health hazard, because they are not responsible for spread of any disease. Head lice only are able to crawl; therefore, transmission occurs mainly by direct head-to-head contact with hair of infested people. Transmission by contact with personal belongings, such as combs, hair brushes, and hats, is uncommon. Away from the scalp, head lice survive less than 2 days at room temperature, and their eggs generally become nonviable within a week and cannot hatch at a lower ambient temperature than that near the scalp.

The **incubation period** from the laying of eggs to hatching of the first nymph usually is about 8 to 9 days but can vary from 7 to 12 days, being somewhat shorter in hot climates and longer in cold climates. Lice mature to the adult stage approximately 9 to 12 days later. Adult females then may lay eggs (nits), but these will develop only if the female has mated.

DIAGNOSTIC TESTS: Identification of eggs (nits), nymphs, and lice with the naked eye is possible; diagnosis can be confirmed by using a hand lens or microscope. Nymphal and adult lice shun light and move rapidly and conceal themselves. Wetting hair with water, oil, or a conditioner and using a fine-tooth comb may improve the ability to diagnose infestation and shorten examination time. It is important to differentiate nits from dandruff, benign hair casts (a layer of follicular cells that may slide easily off the hair shaft), plugs of desquamated cells, external hair debris, and fungal infections of the hair.

---

[1] American Academy of Pediatrics, Committee on School Health and Committee on Infectious Diseases. Clinical report: head lice. *Pediatrics.* 2010;126(2):392–403

Because nits remain affixed to the hair firmly, even if dead or hatched, the mere presence of nits is not a sign of an active infestation.

TREATMENT: A number of effective pediculicidal agents are available to treat head lice infestation (see Drugs for Parasitic Infections, p 848). Safety is a major concern with pediculicides, because the infestation itself presents minimal risk to the host. Pediculicides should be used only as directed and with care. Instructions on proper use of any product should be explained carefully. Therapy can be started with over-the-counter 1% permethrin or with a pyrethrin combined with piperonyl butoxide product, both of which have good safety profiles. However, resistance to these compounds has been documented in the United States. For treatment failures not attributable to improper use of an over-the-counter pediculicide, malathion, benzyl alcohol lotion, or spinosad suspension should be used. When lice are resistant to all topical agents, ivermectin may be used, although it is not approved by the Food and Drug Administration (FDA) as a pediculicide. No drug truly is ovicidal, but of the available topical agents, only malathion has ovicidal activity. Drugs that have residual activity may kill nymphs as they emerge from eggs. Pediculicides usually require more than one application. Ideally, retreatment should occur after the eggs that are present at the time of initial treatment have hatched but before any new eggs have been produced.

- ***Permethrin (1%).*** Permethrin is available without a prescription in a 1% lotion that is applied to the scalp and hair for 10 minutes after shampooing with a nonconditioning shampoo and towel drying the hair. Permethrin has a low potential for toxic effects and a high cure rate. Although activity of permethrin can continue for 2 weeks or more after application, some experts advise a second treatment 9 to 10 days after the first treatment, especially if hair is washed within a week after the first treatment. Product labeling recommends a second treatment 7 or more days after the first application if live lice are seen. Permethrin is not approved by the FDA for use on children younger than 2 years of age.

- ***Pyrethrin-based products.*** Pyrethrins are natural extracts from the chrysanthemum and are available (usually formulated with the synergist piperonyl butoxide) without a prescription as shampoos or mousse preparations (both to be applied to dry hair). Pyrethrins have no residual activity, and repeated application 7 to 10 days after the first application is necessary to kill newly hatched lice. Resistance to permethrin renders pyrethrin-based products ineffective. Pyrethrins are contraindicated in people who are allergic to chrysanthemums or ragweed.

- ***Malathion (0.5%).*** This organophosphate pesticide that is both pediculicidal and partially ovicidal is available only by prescription as a lotion and is highly effective as formulated in the United States. The safety and effectiveness of malathion lotion have not been assessed by the FDA in children younger than 6 years of age. Malathion lotion is applied to dry hair, left to dry naturally, and then removed 8 to 12 hours later by washing and rinsing the hair. The product should be reapplied 7 to 9 days later only if live lice still are present at that time. The alcohol base of the lotion is flammable; therefore, the lotion or wet hair during treatment should not be exposed to lighted cigarettes, open flames, or electric heat sources, such as hair dryers or curling irons. The product, if ingested, can cause severe respiratory distress. Malathion is contraindicated in children younger than 2 years of age because of the possibility of increased scalp permeability and absorption.

- **Benzyl alcohol lotion (5%).** Benzyl alcohol is available by prescription in a lotion formulated with mineral oil and is highly effective as a pediculicide. This agent has been evaluated by the FDA for use in children 6 months of age or older. When applied, sufficient amounts should be used on dry hair to saturate the scalp and entire length of the hair, and then washed off after 10 minutes. Retreatment after 9 days is recommended to kill any newly hatched lice. Benzyl alcohol use in neonates has been associated with neonatal gasping syndrome, and its use should, therefore, be avoided in this group.
- **Spinosad suspension (0.9%).** This product, which contains benzyl alcohol and spinosad as the active compound, was approved by the FDA in 2011 for treatment of head lice infestation in children. Enough of the suspension is used to completely cover dry hair completely, starting with the scalp, and is left on for 10 minutes. Safety in children younger than 4 years of age has not been established. Because of the benzyl alcohol, this product should not be used in infants younger than 6 months of age. A second treatment is given at 7 days if live lice are seen.
- **Ivermectin lotion (0.5%).** Ivermectin interferes with the function of invertebrate nerve and muscle cells. It is used widely as an anthelmintic agent. The 0.5% lotion was approved by the FDA in 2012 as a single-application, topical treatment of head lice in people 6 months of age and older. The lotion is applied to dry hair, starting with the scalp, in an amount sufficient to coat the hair and scalp thoroughly. After a 10-minute application, the lotion is rinsed off with water.
- **Oral ivermectin.** Oral ivermectin has not been evaluated by the FDA as a pediculicide. Ivermectin may be effective against head lice if sufficient concentration is present in the blood at the time a louse feeds. It has been given as a single oral dose of 200 μg/kg or 400 μg/kg, with a second dose given after 9 to 10 days. Fewer failures occur at the 400 μg/kg dose. Because it blocks essential neural transmission if it crosses the blood-brain barrier and young children may be at higher risk of this adverse drug reaction, currently, ivermectin should not be used in children weighing less than 15 kg (33 pounds).
- **Lindane shampoo, 1%.** Because of safety concerns and availability of other treatments, lindane shampoo no longer is recommended for treatment of pediculosis capitis.

Other off-label treatments are detailed in the AAP clinical report on head lice published in 2010.[1] With the products available today and limited data on effectiveness of these other treatments, it is unlikely that any would be used.

Data are lacking to determine whether suffocation of lice by application of some occlusive agents, such as petroleum jelly, olive oil, butter, or fat-containing mayonnaise, is as effective as a method of treatment. Because pediculicides kill lice shortly after application, detection of living lice on scalp inspection 24 hours or more after treatment suggests incorrect use of pediculicide, hatching of lice after treatment, reinfestation, or resistance to therapy. In such situations, after excluding incorrect use, immediate retreatment with a different pediculicide followed by a second application 7 to 10 days later is recommended. Itching or mild burning of the scalp caused by inflammation of the skin in response to topical therapeutic agents can persist for many days after lice are killed and is not a reason for retreatment. Topical corticosteroid and oral antihistamine agents may be beneficial for relieving these signs and symptoms. Manual removal of nits after successful treatment

---

[1] American Academy of Pediatrics, Committee on School Health and Committee on Infectious Diseases. Clinical report: head lice. *Pediatrics.* 2010;126(2):392–403

with a pediculicide is helpful, because none of the pediculicides are 100% ovicidal. Fine-toothed nit combs designed for this purpose are available. Removal of nits is tedious and time consuming but may be attempted for aesthetic reasons, to decrease diagnostic confusion, or to improve efficacy.

ISOLATION OF THE HOSPITALIZED PATIENT: In addition to standard precautions, contact precautions are recommended until the patient has been treated with an appropriate pediculicide.

CONTROL MEASURES: Household and other close contacts should be examined and treated if infested. Bedmates of infested people should be treated prophylactically at the same time as the infested household members and contacts. Prophylactic treatment of other noninfested people is not recommended. Children should not be excluded or sent home early from school because of head lice. Parents of children with infestation (ie, at least 1 live, crawling louse) should be notified and informed that their child should be treated. The presence of nits alone does not justify treatment.

"No-nit" policies requiring that children be free of nits before they return to a child care facility or school have not been effective in controlling head lice transmission and are not recommended. Egg cases farther from the scalp are easier to discover, but these tend to be empty (hatched) or nonviable and, thus, are of no consequence.

Supplemental measures generally are not required to eliminate an infestation. Head lice only rarely are transferred via fomites from shared headgear, clothing, combs, or bedding. Special handling of such items is not likely to be useful. If desired, hats, bedding, clothing, and towels worn or used by the infested person in the 2-day period just before treatment is started can be machine-washed and dried using the hot water and hot air cycles, because lice and eggs are killed by exposure for 5 minutes to temperatures greater than 53.5°C (128.3°F). Vacuuming furniture and floors can remove an infested person's hairs that might have viable nits attached. Environmental insecticide sprays increase chemical exposure of household members and have not been helpful in the control of head lice. Treatment of dogs, cats, or other pets is not indicated, because they do not play a role in transmission of human head lice.

Pediculosis Corporis
(Body Lice)

CLINICAL MANIFESTATIONS: Intense itching, particularly at night, is common with body lice infestations. Bites manifest as small erythematous macules, papules, and excoriations primarily on the trunk. In heavily bitten areas, typically around the mid-section, the skin can become thickened and discolored. Secondary bacterial infection of the skin caused by scratching is common.

ETIOLOGY: *Pediculus humanus corporis* (or *humanus*) is the body louse. Nymphs and adult lice feed on human blood.

EPIDEMIOLOGY: Body lice generally are restricted to people living in crowded conditions without access to regular bathing or changes of clothing (refugees, victims of war or natural disasters, homeless people). Under these conditions, body lice can spread rapidly through direct contact or contact with contaminated clothing or bedding. Body lice live in clothes or bedding, lay their eggs on or near the seams of clothing, and move to the skin to feed. Body lice cannot survive away from a blood source for longer than approximately

5 to 7 days at room temperature. In contrast with head lice, body lice are well-recognized vectors of disease (eg, epidemic typhus, trench fever, epidemic relapsing fever, and bacillary angiomatosis).

The **incubation period** from laying eggs to hatching of the first nymph is approximately 1 to 2 weeks, depending on ambient temperature. Lice mature and are capable of reproducing 9 to 19 days after hatching, depending on whether infested clothing is removed for sleeping.

DIAGNOSTIC TESTS: Identification of eggs, nymphs, and lice with the naked eye is possible; diagnosis can be confirmed by using a hand lens or microscope. Adult and nymphal body lice seldom are seen on the body, because they generally are sequestered in clothing.

TREATMENT: Treatment consists of improving hygiene and regular changes of clean clothes and bedding. Infested materials can be decontaminated by washing in hot water (at least 130° F), by machine drying at hot temperatures, by dry cleaning, or by pressing with a hot iron. Temperatures exceeding 53.5°C (128.3°F) for 5 minutes are lethal to lice and eggs. Pediculicides usually are not necessary if materials are laundered at least weekly (see Drugs for Parasitic Infections, p 848). Some people with much body hair may require full-body treatment with a pediculicide, because lice and eggs may adhere to body hair.

ISOLATION OF THE HOSPITALIZED PATIENT: In addition to standard precautions, contact precautions are recommended until the patient has been treated.

CONTROL MEASURES: The most important factor in the control of body lice infestation is the ability to change and wash clothing. Close contacts should be examined and treated appropriately; clothing and bedding should be laundered.

Pediculosis Pubis
(Pubic Lice, Crab Lice)

CLINICAL MANIFESTATIONS: Pruritus of the anogenital area is a common symptom in pubic lice infestations ("crabs" or "pthiriasis"). The parasite most frequently is found in the pubic region, but infestation can involve the eyelashes, eyebrows, beard, axilla, perianal area, and rarely, the scalp. A characteristic sign of heavy pubic lice infestation is the presence of bluish or slate-colored macules (maculae ceruleae) on the chest, abdomen, or thighs.

ETIOLOGY: *Pthirus pubis* is the pubic or crab louse. Nymphs and adult lice feed on human blood.

EPIDEMIOLOGY: Pubic lice infestations are more prevalent in adults and usually are transmitted through sexual contact. Transmission by contaminated items, such as towels, is uncommon. Pubic lice on the eyelashes or eyebrows of children may be evidence of sexual abuse, although other modes of transmission are possible. Infested people should be examined for other sexually transmitted infections (see Sexually Transmitted Infections in Adolescents and Children, p 176). Adult pubic lice can survive away from a host for up to 36 hours, and their eggs can remain viable for up to 10 days under suitable environmental conditions.

The **incubation period** from the laying of eggs to the hatching of the first nymph is approximately 6 to 10 days. Adult lice become capable of reproducing approximately 2 to 3 weeks after hatching.

DIAGNOSTIC TESTS: Identification of eggs (nits), nymphs, and lice with the naked eye is possible; the diagnosis can be confirmed by using a hand lens or microscope.

TREATMENT: All areas of the body with coarse hair should be examined for evidence of pubic lice infestation. Lice and their eggs can be removed manually, or the hairs can be shaved to eliminate infestation immediately. Caution should be used when inspecting, removing or treating lice on or near the eyelashes. Pediculicides used to treat other kinds of louse infestations are effective for treatment of pubic lice (see Pediculosis Capitis, p 543). Retreatment is recommended as for head lice. Topical pediculicides should not be used for treatment of pubic lice infestation of eyelashes; an ophthalmic-grade petrolatum ointment applied to the eyelashes 2 to 4 times daily for 8 to 10 days is effective.

ISOLATION OF THE HOSPITALIZED PATIENT: In addition to standard precautions, contact precautions are recommended until the patient has been treated with an appropriate pediculicide.

CONTROL MEASURES: All sexual contacts should be examined and treated, as needed. Patients should be advised to avoid sexual contact until they and their sex partner have been treated successfully. Bedding, towels, and clothing can be decontaminated by laundering in hot water and machine drying using a hot cycle or by dry cleaning.

Pelvic Inflammatory Disease[1]

CLINICAL MANIFESTATIONS: Pelvic inflammatory disease (PID) comprises a spectrum of inflammatory disorders of the female upper genital tract, including any combination of endometritis, parametritis, salpingitis, oophoritis, tubo-ovarian abscess, and pelvic peritonitis. PID typically manifests as dull, continuous, unilateral or bilateral lower abdominal or pelvic pain that may range from indolent to severe. Additional manifestations may include fever, vomiting, abnormal vaginal discharge, and irregular vaginal bleeding (signaling endometritis). Occasionally, some patients present with sharp right upper abdominal quadrant pain that may be a result of perihepatitis.

Examination findings vary but may include fever, lower abdominal tenderness, vaginal discharge, tenderness on lateral motion of the cervix, unilateral or bilateral adnexal tenderness, and adnexal fullness. Pyuria, white cells on microscopy, leukocytosis, an elevated erythrocyte sedimentation rate, elevated C-reactive protein concentration, and/or an adnexal mass demonstrated by abdominal or transvaginal ultrasonography may be laboratory or imaging findings useful to support the diagnosis.

No single symptom, sign, or laboratory finding is sensitive and specific for the diagnosis of acute PID. Adnexal tenderness in a patient who has been sexually active has been described as the most sensitive finding for PID. Many episodes of PID go unrecognized by patients and/or health care professionals, because patients may be relatively asymptomatic ("silent PID") and do not seek care or because symptoms are mild and nonspecific. Diagnostic criteria recommended currently by the Centers for Disease Control and Prevention (CDC) are presented in Table 3.42 (p 549).

Complications of PID may include perihepatitis (Fitz-Hugh-Curtis syndrome) and tubo-ovarian abscess. Important long-term sequelae are recurrent infection, chronic pelvic pain, a sevenfold increase in incidence of ectopic pregnancy, and infertility resulting

---

[1] Centers for Disease Control and Prevention. Sexually transmitted diseases treatment guidelines, 2010. *MMWR Recomm Rep.* 2010;59(RR-12):1–110

Table 3.42. Criteria for Clinical Diagnosis of Pelvic Inflammatory Disease (PID)[a]

Minimum Criteria

Empiric treatment of PID should be initiated in sexually active young women and other women at risk of STIs if they are experiencing pelvic or lower abdominal pain and if the following **minimum criteria** are present and no other cause(s) for the illness can be identified:

- Uterine tenderness
- Adnexal tenderness
- Cervical motion tenderness

Additional Criteria

More elaborate diagnostic evaluation often is needed, because incorrect diagnosis and management might cause unnecessary morbidity. These additional criteria may be used to enhance the specificity of the minimum criteria listed previously. Additional criteria that support a diagnosis of PID include the following:

- Oral temperature greater than 38.3°C (101°F)
- Mucopurulent cervical or vaginal discharge
- Presence of white blood cells (WBCs) on saline microscopy of vaginal secretions
- Increased erythrocyte sedimentation rate
- Increased C-reactive protein concentration
- Laboratory documentation of cervical infection with *Neisseria gonorrhoeae* or *Chlamydia trachomatis*

Most women with PID have mucopurulent cervical discharge **or** evidence of WBCs on a microscopic evaluation of a saline preparation of vaginal fluid. If the cervical discharge appears normal **and** no WBCs are found on the wet preparation, the diagnosis of PID is unlikely, and alternative causes of pain should be sought.

The **most specific criteria** for diagnosing PID include the following:

- Endometrial biopsy with histopathologic evidence of endometritis
- Transvaginal ultrasonography or magnetic resonance imaging techniques showing thickened, fluid-filled tubes with or without free pelvic fluid or tubo-ovarian complex, or ultrasonographic studies suggesting pelvic infection (eg, tubal hyperemia) or
- Laparoscopic abnormalities consistent with PID
- A diagnostic evaluation that includes some of these more extensive studies may be warranted in selected cases.

STIs indicates sexually transmitted infections.

[a]Adapted from the Centers for Disease Control and Prevention. Sexually transmitted diseases treatment guidelines, 2010. *MMWR Recomm Rep* 2010;59(RR–12):1–110 (see **www.cdc.gov/std/treatment**).

from tubal occlusion. Risk of tubal infertility is estimated to be 12% after a single episode of PID and more than 50% after 3 or more episodes. Factors that may increase the likelihood of infertility are delay in diagnosis, younger age at time of infection, chlamydial disease, delayed initiation of antimicrobial therapy, and PID determined to be severe by laparoscopic examination.

ETIOLOGY: Sexually transmitted organisms, especially *Neisseria gonorrhoeae* and *Chlamydia trachomatis*, are implicated in less than 50% of cases of PID. Other organisms, such as anaerobes, including *Bacteroides* species and *Peptostreptococcus* species; facultative anaerobes, including *Gardnerella vaginalis, Haemophilus influenzae, Streptococcus* species, and enteric gram-negative bacilli; genital tract mycoplasmas, including *Mycoplasma hominis* and *Ureaplasma* *urealyticum;* and cytomegalovirus, also are associated with PID. Polymicrobial infection is common.

EPIDEMIOLOGY: As is true for other sexually transmitted infections (STIs), the incidence of PID is highest among adolescents and young adults. Risk factors for PID include numerous recent sexual partners, multiple lifetime sexual partners, douching, and previous episodes of PID. Latex condoms may reduce the risk of PID. Other barrier contraceptive methods, such as the contraceptive sponge and diaphragm, also have been shown to be effective in preventing transmission of STIs. Use of oral contraceptive pills has been demonstrated to decrease the likelihood of PID in the face of gonococcal cervicitis. Ascending pelvic infection rarely, if ever, has been shown to be a complication of gonococcal vaginitis in prepubertal girls.

An **incubation period** for PID is undefined.

DIAGNOSTIC TESTS: The diagnosis of PID usually is made on the basis of clinical findings (see Table 3.42, p 549) and can be supported by findings of bacterial vaginosis, a preponderance of leukocytes in vaginal discharge, leukocytosis, an increased C-reactive protein concentration or erythrocyte sedimentation rate, or presence of *N gonorrhoeae* or *C trachomatis* or both at the endocervix (see Gonococcal Infections, p 336, and *Chlamydia trachomatis,* p 276). Urine or vaginal or endocervical swab specimens to test for *N gonorrhoeae* and *C trachomatis* should be obtained before treatment is begun, but treatment should not be delayed pending results of tests if clinical suspicion is high for PID. Transvaginal ultrasonography and laparoscopy are useful when appendicitis, ruptured ovarian cyst, or ectopic pregnancy are possible differential diagnoses. Laparoscopy also permits bacteriologic specimens to be obtained directly from tubal exudate or the cul-de-sac. However, laparoscopy cannot detect endometritis and is not indicated for diagnosis in most cases of PID. Endometrial biopsy may demonstrate histopathologic evidence and may be the only sign of PID in some women. Because PID and ectopic pregnancy both can produce abdominal pain and irregular bleeding, a pregnancy test is indicated in the diagnostic evaluation of the adolescent with suspected PID or lower abdominal pain regardless of menstrual history.

TREATMENT: Because the clinical diagnosis of PID, even in the most experienced hands, is imprecise and because consequences of untreated infection are substantial, most experts provide antimicrobial therapy to patients who fulfill minimum criteria rather than limiting therapy to patients who fulfill additional criteria for the diagnosis of PID (Table 3.42, p 549). To minimize risks of progressive infection and subsequent infertility, treatment should be instituted as soon as the clinical diagnosis is made and before results of culture are available. All people who are diagnosed with PID should be tested for *N gonorrhoeae* and *C trachomatis;* however, a number of other organisms also have been associated with PID.

Observation and treatment in the hospital rather than outpatient treatment are suggested in the following circumstances:
- a surgical emergency, such as ectopic pregnancy or appendicitis, cannot be excluded;
- adherence to or tolerance of an outpatient treatment regimen and follow-up within 72 hours cannot be ensured;
- the patient's illness is severe (eg, nausea, vomiting, severe pain, overt peritonitis, or high fever);
- a tubo-ovarian abscess is present;
- the patient is pregnant;

- the patient has failed to respond clinically to outpatient therapy; or
- another serious condition cannot be excluded.

Increasingly, women with PID are treated in the outpatient setting. Physicians should consider that adolescents are at risk of recurrent disease and related longitudinal sequelae and have difficulty adhering to outpatient treatment recommendations. Caution should be used when determining management site, because the value of hospitalization has not been determined in young and middle adolescence. Current data are insufficient to determine whether more aggressive interventions are indicated for women with PID and human immunodeficiency virus (HIV) infection.

An antimicrobial regimen for treatment of PID should be empiric and broad spectrum and should provide coverage directed against the most common causative agents. Antimicrobial regimens consistent with those recommended by the CDC are summarized in Table 3.43 (p 552). Clinical outcome data are limited regarding use of cephalosporins other than cefotetan and cefoxitin (such as ceftriaxone, cefotaxime, or ceftizoxime). Some experts believe that these agents can be used to replace cefoxitin or cefotetan for inpatient treatment of PID; however, cefoxitin and cefotetan are more active against anaerobic bacteria. Regimens used to treat PID should be effective against *N gonorrhoeae* and *C trachomatis*. Because of antimicrobial resistance, a fluoroquinolone no longer is recommended for treatment of *N gonorrhoeae*.[1] Empiric therapy for anaerobic pathogens should be provided for patients with tubo-ovarian abscess, recurrent PID, or recent pelvic surgery. In patients treated orally or parenterally, clinical improvement can be expected within 72 hours after initiation of treatment. Accordingly, outpatients should be reevaluated routinely on the third or fourth day of treatment. Because the risk of IUD-associated PID primarily is within the first 3 weeks of insertion, there is insufficient evidence to recommend IUD be removed in women with a diagnosis of PID, unless diagnosis occurs within that time frame.

ISOLATION OF THE HOSPITALIZED PATIENT: Standard precautions are recommended.

CONTROL MEASURES[2]:
- Male sexual partners of patients with PID should receive diagnostic evaluation for gonococcal and chlamydial urethritis and then should be treated presumptively for both infections if they had sexual contact with the patient during the 60 days preceding onset of symptoms in the patient. A large proportion of these males will be asymptomatic.
- The patient should abstain from sexual intercourse until she and her partner(s) have completed treatment.
- The patient and her partner(s) should be encouraged to use condoms consistently and correctly.
- The patient should be tested for syphilis and HIV infection, and a Papanicolaou test should be performed when appropriate (see CDC guidelines[3]).

---

[1] Centers for Disease Control and Prevention. Update to CDC's sexually transmitted disease treatment-guidelines, 2006: fluoroquinolones no longer recommended for treatment of gonococcal infections. *MMWR Morb Mortal Wkly Rep.* 2007;56(14):332–336

[2] Centers for Disease Control and Prevention. Recommendations for partner services programs for HIV infection, syphilis, gonorrhea, and chlamydial infection. *MMWR Recomm Rep.* 2008;57(RR-9):1–63

[3] Centers for Disease Control and Prevention. Sexually transmitted diseases treatment guidelines, 2010. *MMWR Recomm Rep.* 2010;59(RR–12):1–110

Table 3.43. Recommended Treatment of Pelvic Inflammatory Disease (PID)[a]

Parenteral: Regimen A[b]

Cefotetan, 2 g, IV, every 12 h

OR

Cefoxitin, 2 g, IV, every 6 h

PLUS

Doxycycline, 100 mg, orally or IV, every 12 h to complete 14 days[c]

OR

Parenteral: Regimen B[d]

Clindamycin, 900 mg, IV, every 8 h

PLUS

Gentamicin: loading dose, IV or IM (2 mg/kg), followed by maintenance dose (1.5 mg/kg) every 8 h. Single daily dosing (3–5 mg/kg) can be substituted.

NOTE

Parenteral therapy may be discontinued 24 h after a patient improves clinically; continuing oral therapy should consist of doxycycline (100 mg, orally, twice a day) or clindamycin (450 mg, orally, 4 times a day) to complete a total of 14 days of therapy. Clindamycin should be used if tubo-ovarian abscess is present.

Ambulatory: Regimen[e]

Ceftriaxone, 250 mg, IM, once

OR

Cefoxitin, 2 g, IM, and **probenecid,** 1 g, orally, in a single dose concurrently, once

OR

Other parenteral extended-spectrum **cephalosporin**[f] (eg, **ceftizoxime** or **cefotaxime**),

PLUS

Doxycycline, 100 mg, orally, twice a day for 14 days

WITH or WITHOUT

Metronidazole, 500 mg, orally, twice a day for 14 days

Alternative Ambulatory Regimens

If parenteral cephalosporin therapy is not feasible, use of fluoroquinolones may be considered if community prevalence and individual risk of gonorrhea is low (see **www.cdc.gov/std/treatment**). Tests for gonorrhea must be performed before instituting therapy and management as follows if the test is positive:

- GC NAAT positive: parenteral cephalosporin recommended
- GC culture positive: treatment based on susceptibility results
- GC isolate: quinolone resistant or susceptibility cannot be assessed, parenteral cephalosporin recommended

IV indicates intravenous; IM, intramuscular; NAAT, nucleic acid amplification test; GC, gonococcal.

[a] For further alternative treatment regimens, see Centers for Disease Control and Prevention. Sexually transmitted infections treatment guidelines, 2010. *MMWR Recomm Rep.* 2010;59(RR-11):1–110 (see **www.cdc.gov/std/treatment**).

[b] Hospitalization and parenteral treatment is recommended if patient has severe illness such as tubo-ovarian abscess, is pregnant, or is unable to tolerate or follow ambulatory regimens.

[c] When tubo-ovarian abscess is present, use of clindamycin or metronidazole is added for anaerobic coverage.

[d] Alternative parenteral regimens include ampicillin-sulbactam (3 g, IV, every 6 hours) plus doxycycline (100 mg, IV or PO, every 12 hours).

[e] Patients with inadequate response to outpatient therapy after 72 hours should be reevaluated for possible misdiagnosis and should receive parenteral therapy. Because of widespread fluoroquinolone-resistant gonococci, fluoroquinolones are not recommended for PID in the United States.

[f] Data to indicate whether expanded-spectrum cephalosporins (ceftizoxime, cefotaxime, ceftriaxone) can replace cefoxitin or cefotetan are limited. Many authorities believe they also are effective therapy for PID, but they are less active against anaerobes.

- Unimmunized or incompletely immunized patients should begin or complete the immunization series for human papillomavirus (9 through 26 years of age) and hepatitis B (see Recommended Childhood and Adolescent Immunization Schedule, p 27–31).
- Because of the high risk of reinfection, some experts recommend that patients with PID whose initial test result for *N gonorrhoeae* and *C trachomatis* was positive be retested 3 months after completing treatment to screen for the possibility of reinfection by an untreated or new infection by a new partner.
- The diagnosis of PID provides an opportune time to educate the adolescent about prevention of STIs, including abstinence, consistent use of barrier methods of protection, and the importance of receiving periodic screening for STIs.

Pertussis (Whooping Cough)

CLINICAL MANIFESTATIONS: Pertussis begins with mild upper respiratory tract symptoms similar to the common cold (catarrhal stage) and progresses to cough and then usually to paroxysms of cough (paroxysmal stage), characterized by inspiratory whoop and commonly followed by vomiting. Fever is absent or minimal. Symptoms wane gradually over weeks to months (convalescent stage). Cough illness in immunized children and adults can range from typical to mild and unrecognized. The duration of classic pertussis is 6 to 10 weeks. Approximately half of adolescents with pertussis cough for 10 weeks or longer. Complications among adolescents and adults include syncope, sleep disturbance, incontinence, rib fractures, and pneumonia; amongst adults, complications increase with age. Pertussis is most severe when it occurs during the first 6 months of life, particularly in preterm and unimmunized infants. Disease in infants younger than 6 months of age can be atypical with a short catarrhal stage, gagging, gasping, bradycardia, or apnea as prominent early manifestations; absence of whoop; and prolonged convalescence. Sudden unexpected death can be caused by pertussis. Complications among infants include pneumonia (22%), seizures (2%), encephalopathy (less than 0.5%), hernia, subdural bleeding, conjunctival bleeding, and death. Case-fatality rates are approximately 1% in infants younger than 2 months of age and less than 0.5% in infants 2 through 11 months of age.

ETIOLOGY: Pertussis is caused by a fastidious, gram-negative, pleomorphic bacillus, *Bordetella pertussis*. Other causes of sporadic prolonged cough illness include *Bordetella parapertussis*, *Mycoplasma pneumoniae*, *Chlamydia trachomatis*, *Chlamydophila pneumoniae*, *Bordetella bronchiseptica*, and certain respiratory tract viruses, particularly adenoviruses and respiratory syncytial viruses.

EPIDEMIOLOGY: Humans are the only known hosts of *B pertussis*. Transmission occurs by close contact with cases via aerosolized droplets. Cases occur year round, typically with a late summer-autumn peak. Neither infection nor immunization provides lifelong immunity. Lack of natural booster events and waning immunity since childhood immunization were responsible for the increase in cases of pertussis in people older than 10 years of age noted before use of the adolescent booster immunization. Additionally, waning maternal immunity and reduced transplacental antibody led to an increase in pertussis in very young infants. A total of 27 550 cases of pertussis were reported in the United States in 2010. As many as 80% of immunized household contacts of symptomatic cases acquire infection, mainly because of waning immunity, with symptoms varying from asymptomatic infection to classic pertussis. Older siblings (including adolescents) and adults with mild or unrecognized atypical disease are important sources of pertussis for infants and young children. Infected people are most contagious during the catarrhal stage and the first 2 weeks after cough onset. Factors affecting the length of communicability include age, immunization status or previous infection, and appropriate antimicrobial therapy.

The **incubation period** is 7 to 10 days, with a range of 5 to 21 days.

DIAGNOSTIC TESTS: Culture is considered the "gold standard" for laboratory diagnosis of pertussis. Although culture is 100% specific, *B pertussis* is a fastidious organism. Culture requires collection of an appropriate nasopharyngeal specimen, obtained either by aspiration or with Dacron (polyethylene terephthalate) or calcium alginate swabs. Specimens must be placed into special transport media (such as Regan-Lowe) immediately and not allowed to dry while being transported promptly to the laboratory. Culture can be negative if taken from a previously immunized person, if antimicrobial therapy has been started, if more than 3 weeks has elapsed since cough onset, or if the specimen is not handled appropriately.

Polymerase chain reaction (PCR) assay increasingly is used for detection of *B pertussis* because of its improved sensitivity and more rapid turnaround time. The PCR test requires collection of an adequate nasopharyngeal specimen using a Dacron swab or nasopharyngeal wash or aspirate. Calcium alginate swabs are inhibitory to PCR and should not be used for PCR tests. The PCR test lacks sensitivity in previously immunized people but still may be more sensitive than culture. Unacceptably high rates of false-positive results are reported from some laboratories and a pseudo-outbreak linked to contaminated specimens also has been reported.[1] No Food and Drug Administration (FDA)-licensed PCR test is available, but the Centers for Disease Control and Prevention (CDC) has released a "best practices" document to guide PCR assays (**www.cdc.gov/pertussis/clinical/diagnostic-testing/diagnosis-pcr-bestpractices.html**) as well as video of optimal specimen collection. Multiple DNA target sequences are required to distinguish between *Bordetella* species. Direct fluorescent antibody (DFA) testing no longer is recommended.

Commercial serologic tests for pertussis infection can be helpful for diagnosis, especially later in illness. However, no commercial kit is licensed by the FDA for diagnostic use. Cutoff points for diagnostic values of immunoglobulin (Ig) G antibody to pertussis toxin (PT) have not been established by the FDA, and IgA and IgM assays lack adequate sensitivity and specificity. In the absence of recent immunization, an elevated serum IgG antibody to PT after 2 weeks of onset of cough is suggestive of recent *B pertussis* infection. An increasing titer or a single IgG anti-PT value of approximately 100 IU/mL or greater (using standard reference sera as a comparator) can be used for diagnosis.

An increased white blood cell count attributable to absolute lymphocytosis is suggestive of pertussis in infants and young children but often is absent in adolescents and adults with pertussis and can be only mildly abnormal in young infants at the time of presentation.

TREATMENT: Antimicrobial agents administered during the catarrhal stage may ameliorate the disease. After the cough is established, antimicrobial agents have no discernible effect on the course of illness but are recommended to limit spread of organisms to others. Azithromycin, erythromycin, or clarithromycin are appropriate first-line agents

---

[1] Mandal S, Tatti KM, Woods-Stout D, et al. Pertussis pseudo-outbreak linked to specimens contaminated by Bordetella pertussis DNA from clinic surfaces. *Pediatrics.* 2012;129(2):e424–e430

for treatment and prophylaxis (see Table 3.44, p 556).[1] Resistance of *B pertussis* to macrolide antimicrobial agents has been reported rarely. Penicillins and first- and second-generation cephalosporins are not effective against *B pertussis.*

Antimicrobial agents for infants younger than 6 months of age require special consideration. The FDA has not approved azithromycin or clarithromycin for use in infants younger than 6 months of age. An association between orally administered erythromycin and infantile hypertrophic pyloric stenosis (IHPS) has been reported in infants younger than 1 month of age. Although substantial use of azithromycin in infants younger than 1 month of age without IHPS has been reported, cases of IHPS in such infants following use of azithromycin have been reported. Until additional information is available, azithromycin is the drug of choice for treatment or prophylaxis of pertussis in infants younger than 1 month of age, in whom the risk of developing severe pertussis and life-threatening complications outweighs the potential risk of IHPS with azithromycin. All infants younger than 1 month of age (and preterm infants until a similar postconceptional age) who receive any macrolide should be monitored for development of IHPS during and for 1 month after completing the course (see Table 3.44, p 556). Cases of IHPS should be reported to MedWatch (see MedWatch, p 869).

Trimethoprim-sulfamethoxazole is an alternative for patients older than 2 months of age who cannot tolerate macrolides or who are infected with a macrolide-resistant strain. Studies evaluating trimethoprim-sulfamethoxazole as treatment for pertussis are limited.

Young infants are at increased risk of respiratory failure attributable to apnea or secondary bacterial pneumonia and are at risk of cardiopulmonary failure from pulmonary hypertension. Hospitalized young infants with pertussis should be managed in a setting/facility where these complications can be recognized and managed emergently.

ISOLATION OF THE HOSPITALIZED PATIENT: In addition to standard precautions, droplet precautions are recommended for 5 days after initiation of effective therapy, or if appropriate antimicrobial therapy is not given, until 3 weeks after onset of cough.

CONTROL MEASURES:

Care of Exposed People.

Household and Other Close Contacts. Close contacts who are unimmunized or underimmunized should have pertussis immunization initiated or continued using age-appropriate products according to the recommended schedule as soon as possible; this includes use of tetanus toxoid, reduced-content diphtheria, and acellular pertussis vaccine (Tdap) in children 7 through 10 years of age who did not complete the diphtheria and tetanus toxoids and acellular pertussis vaccine (DTaP) series (see Table 3.45, p 557).

Chemoprophylaxis is recommended for all household contacts of the index case and other close contacts, including children in child care. If the contact lives in a household with a person at high risk of severe pertussis (eg, young infant, pregnant woman, person who has contact with infants) or is at high risk himself or herself, chemoprophylaxis should be given, even if the contact is fully immunized. Early use of chemoprophylaxis in household contacts may limit secondary transmission. If 21 days have elapsed since onset of cough in the index case, chemoprophylaxis has limited value but should be considered for households with high-risk contacts. The agents, doses, and duration of prophylaxis are the same as for treatment of pertussis (see Table 3.44, p 556).

---

[1] Centers for Disease Control and Prevention. Recommended antimicrobial agents for the treatment and postexposure prophylaxis of pertussis: 2005 CDC guidelines. *MMWR Recomm Rep.* 2005;54(RR–14):1–16

Table 3.44. Recommended Antimicrobial Therapy and Postexposure Prophylaxis for Pertussis in Infants, Children, Adolescents, and Adults[a]

| Age | Recommended Drugs | | | Alternative |
	Azithromycin	Erythromycin	Clarithromycin	TMP-SMX
Younger than 1 mo	10 mg/kg/day as a single dose for 5 days[b]	40 mg/kg/day in 4 divided doses for 14 days	Not recommended	Contraindicated at younger than 2 mo of age
1 through 5 mo	See above	See above	15 mg/kg per day in 2 divided doses for 7 days	2 mo of age or older: TMP, 8 mg/kg/day; SMX, 40 mg/kg/day in 2 doses for 14 days
6 mo or older and children	10 mg/kg as a single dose on day 1 (maximum 500 mg), then 5 mg/kg/day as a single dose on days 2 through 5 (maximum 250 mg/day)	40 mg/kg/day in 4 divided doses for 7–14 days (maximum 1–2 g/day)	15 mg/kg/day in 2 divided doses for 7 days (maximum 1 g/day)	See above
Adolescents and adults	500 mg as a single dose on day 1, then 250 mg as a single dose on days 2 through 5	2 g/day in 4 divided doses for 7–14 days	1 g/day in 2 divided doses for 7 days	TMP, 320 mg/day; SMX, 1600 mg/day in 2 divided doses for 14 days

TMP indicates trimethoprim; SMX, sulfamethoxazole.

[a]Centers for Disease Control and Prevention. Recommended antimicrobial agents for the treatment and postexposure prophylaxis of pertussis: 2005 CDC guidelines. *MMWR Recomm Rep.* 2005;54(RR-14):1–16

[b]Preferred macrolide for this age because of risk of idiopathic hypertrophic pyloric stenosis associated with erythromycin.

Table 3.45. Composition and Recommended Use of Vaccines With Tetanus Toxoid, Diphtheria Toxoid, and Acellular Pertussis Components Licensed in the United States[a]

Pharmaceutical	Manufacturer	Pertussis Antigens	Recommended Use
DTaP Vaccine for Children Younger Than 7 Years of Age			
DTaP (Infanrix)	GlaxoSmithKline Biologicals	PT, FHA, pertactin	**All 5 doses,** children 6 wk through 6 y of age
DTaP (Daptacel)	Sanofi Pasteur	PT, FHA, pertactin, fimbriae types 2 and 3	**All 5 doses,** children 6 wk through 6 y of age
DTaP-hepatitis B-IPV (Pediarix)	GlaxoSmithKline Biologicals	PT, FHA, pertactin	**First 3 doses** at 6- to 8-wk intervals beginning at 2 mo of age; then 2 doses of DTaP are needed to complete the 5-dose series before 7 y of age
DTaP-IPV/Hib (Pentacel)	Sanofi Pasteur	PT, FHA, pertactin, fimbriae types 2 and 3	**First 4 doses** at 2, 4, 6, and 15 through 18 mo of age
DTaP-IPV (Kinrix)	GlaxoSmithKline Biologicals	PT, FHA, pertactin	Booster dose for **fifth dose** of DTaP and **fourth dose** of IPV at 4 through 6 y of age
Tdap Vaccines for Adolescents			
Tdap (Boostrix)	GlaxoSmithKline Biologicals	PT, FHA, pertactin	Single dose at 11 through 12 y of age instead of Td (see text for additional recommendations)
Tdap (Adacel)	Sanofi Pasteur	PT, FHA, pertactin, fimbriae types 2 and 3	Single dose at 11 through 12 y of age instead of Td (see text for additional recommendations)

DTaP indicates pediatric formulation of diphtheria and tetanus toxoids and acellular pertussis vaccines; PT, pertussis toxoid; FHA, filamentous hemagglutinin; Hib, *Haemophilus influenzae* type b vaccine; IPV, inactivated poliovirus; Tdap, adolescent/adult formulation of tetanus toxoid, reduced diphtheria toxoid, and acellular pertussis vaccine; Td, tetanus and reduced diphtheria toxoids (for children 7 years of age or older and adults).

[a] DTaP recommended schedule is 2, 4, 6, and 15 through 18 months and 4 through 6 years of age. The fourth dose can be given as early as 12 months, provided 6 months have elapsed since the third dose was given. The fifth dose is not necessary if the fourth dose was given on or after the fourth birthday. Refer to manufacturers' product information for comprehensive product information regarding indications and use of the vaccines listed.

People who have been in contact with an infected person should be monitored closely for respiratory tract symptoms for 21 days after last contact with the infected person. Close contacts with cough should be evaluated and treated for pertussis when appropriate.

Child Care. Pertussis immunization and chemoprophylaxis should be given as recommended for household and other close contacts. Child care providers and exposed children, especially incompletely immunized children, should be observed for respiratory tract symptoms for 21 days after last contact with the index case while infectious. Children and child care providers who are symptomatic or who have confirmed pertussis should be excluded from child care pending physician evaluation and completion of 5 days of the recommended course of antimicrobial therapy if pertussis is suspected. Untreated children and providers should be excluded until 21 days have elapsed from cough onset.

Schools. Students and staff members with pertussis should be excluded from school until they have completed 5 days of the recommended course of antimicrobial therapy. People who do not receive appropriate antimicrobial therapy should be excluded from school for 21 days after onset of symptoms. Public health officials should be consulted for further recommendations to control pertussis transmission in schools. The immunization status of children should be reviewed, and age-appropriate vaccines should be given, if indicated, as for household and other close contacts. Parents and employees should be notified about possible exposures to pertussis. Exclusion of exposed people with cough illness should be considered pending evaluation by a physician.

Health Care Settings.[1] Health care facilities should maximize efforts to immunize all health care professionals (HCPs) with Tdap and to prevent transmission of *B pertussis*. All HCPs should observe respiratory precautions when examining a patient with a cough illness suspected or confirmed to be pertussis.

People exposed to a patient with pertussis who did not take proper infection-control precautions should be evaluated by infection-control personnel for postexposure management and follow-up. The CDC recommends the following:

- Data on the need for postexposure antimicrobial prophylaxis in Tdap-immunized HCPs are inconclusive. Some immunized HCPs still are at risk of *B pertussis* infection. Tdap may not preclude the need for postexposure antimicrobial prophylaxis administration.
- Postexposure antimicrobial prophylaxis is recommended for all HCPs (even if immunized with Tdap) who have unprotected exposure to pertussis and are likely to expose a patient at risk of severe pertussis (eg, hospitalized neonates and pregnant women). Other HCPs should either receive postexposure antimicrobial prophylaxis or be monitored daily for 21 days after pertussis exposure and treated at the onset of signs and symptoms of pertussis.
- Other people (patients, caregivers) defined as close contacts or high-risk contacts of a patient or HCP with pertussis should be given chemoprophylaxis (and immunization when indicated), as recommended for household contacts (see Table 3.44, p 556).
- HCPs with symptoms of pertussis (or HCPs with a cough illness within 21 days of exposure to pertussis) should be excluded from work for at least the first 5 days of the recommended course of antimicrobial therapy. HCPs with symptoms of pertussis who cannot take, or who object to, antimicrobial therapy should be excluded from work for 21 days from onset of cough. Use of a respiratory mask is not sufficient protection during this time.

---

[1] Centers for Disease Control and Prevention. Immunization of health-care personnel. Recommendations of the Advisory Committee on Immunization Practices (ACIP). *MMWR Recomm Rep.* 2011;60(RR-07):1–45

Immunization.

Vaccine Products. Purified acellular-component pertussis vaccines replaced previously used diphtheria, tetanus, and whole-cell pertussis vaccine (DTP) exclusively in 1997 and contain 3 or more immunogens derived from *B pertussis* organisms: inactivated pertussis toxin (toxoid), filamentous hemagglutinin, and fimbrial proteins (agglutinogens) and pertactin (an outer membrane 69-kd protein; see Table 3.45 for products). Acellular pertussis vaccines are adsorbed onto aluminum salts and must be administered intramuscularly. All pertussis vaccines in the United States are combined with diphtheria and tetanus toxoids. DTaP products may be formulated as combination vaccines containing one or more of inactivated poliovirus vaccine, hepatitis B vaccine, and *Haemophilus influenzae* type b vaccine. Recommendations for the series of DTaP for children younger than 7 years of age are shown in Fig 1.1 (p 27–28). Tdap vaccines contain reduced quantities of diphtheria toxoid and some pertussis antigens compared with DTaP. A single dose is recommended universally for people 11 of age and older, including adults, in place of a decennial tetanus and diphtheria vaccine (Td). The preferred schedule is to administer Tdap at the 11- or 12- year-old preventive visit, with catch up of older adolescents. Uses of DTaP and Tdap in special circumstances are shown subsequently.

Dose and Route. Each 0.5-mL dose of DTaP or Tdap is given intramuscularly. Use of a decreased volume of individual doses of pertussis vaccines or multiple doses of decreased-volume (fractional) doses is not recommended.

Interchangeability of Acellular Pertussis Vaccines. Insufficient data exist on the safety, immunogenicity, and efficacy of DTaP vaccines from different manufacturers when administered interchangeably for the primary series in infants to make recommendations. In circumstances in which the type of DTaP product(s) received previously is not known or the previously administered product(s) is not readily available, any DTaP vaccine licensed for use in the primary series may be used. There is no need to match Tdap vaccine manufacturer with DTaP vaccine manufacturer used for earlier doses.

Recommendations for Routine Childhood Immunization With DTaP. Six doses of pertussis-containing vaccine are recommended: 4 doses of DTaP before 2 years of age, 1 booster dose before school entry, and 1 dose of Tdap at 11 or 12 years of age. The first dose of DTaP is given at 2 months of age, followed by 2 additional doses at intervals of approximately 2 months. The fourth dose of DTaP is recommended at 15 through 18 months of age, and the fifth dose of DTaP is given before school entry (kindergarten or elementary school) at 4 through 6 years of age. If the fourth dose of pertussis vaccine is delayed until after the fourth birthday, the fifth dose is not recommended.

Other recommendations are as follows:

- For the fourth dose, DTaP may be administered as early as 12 months of age if the interval between the third and fourth doses is at least 6 months.
- Simultaneous administration of DTaP and all other recommended vaccines is acceptable. Vaccines should not be mixed in the same syringe unless the specific combination is licensed by the FDA (see Simultaneous Administration of Multiple Vaccines, p 33, and *Haemophilus influenzae* Infections, p 345).
- If pertussis is prevalent in the community, immunization can be started as early as 6 weeks of age, and doses 2 and 3 in the primary series can be given at intervals as short as 4 weeks.

- Children younger than 7 years of age who have begun but not completed their primary immunization schedule with DTP (eg, outside the United States) should receive DTaP to complete the pertussis immunization schedule.
- DTaP is not licensed or recommended for people 7 years of age or older.
- Children between 7 and 10 years of age who have not completed their primary immunization schedule or have an unknown vaccine history should receive a single dose of Tdap. If they require additional tetanus and diphtheria toxoid doses, Td should be used.
- Children who have a contraindication to pertussis immunization should receive no further doses of a pertussis-containing vaccine (see Contraindications and Precautions to DTaP Immunization, p 562).

Combined Vaccines. Several pertussis-containing combination vaccines are licensed for use (see Table 3.45, p 557) and may be used when feasible and when any components are indicated and none is contraindicated.

Recommendations for Scheduling Pertussis Immunization for Children Younger Than 7 Years of Age in Special Circumstances.

- For the child whose pertussis immunization schedule is resumed after deferral or interruption of the recommended schedule, the next dose in the sequence should be given, regardless of the interval since the last dose—that is, the schedule is not reinitiated (see Lapsed Immunizations, p 35).
- For children who have received fewer than the recommended number of doses of pertussis vaccine but who have received the recommended number of diphtheria and tetanus toxoid (DT) vaccine doses for their age (ie, children started on DT, then given DTaP), DTaP should be given to complete the recommended pertussis immunization schedule. However, the total number of doses of diphtheria and tetanus toxoids (as DT, DTaP, or DTP) should not exceed 6 before the seventh birthday.
- Although it is well-documented that pertussis confers short-term protection against infection, the duration of protection is unknown. DTaP (or a single dose of Tdap in underimmunized people 7 years of age or older) should be given to complete the immunization series.

Medical Records. Charts of children for whom pertussis immunization has been deferred should be flagged, and the immunization status of these children should be assessed periodically to ensure that they are immunized appropriately.

Adverse Events After DTaP Immunization in Children Younger Than 7 Years of Age.

- **Local and febrile reactions.** Reactions to DTaP most commonly include redness, swelling, induration, and tenderness at the injection site as well as drowsiness; less common reactions include fretfulness, anorexia, vomiting, crying, and slight to moderate fever. These local and systemic manifestations after pertussis immunization occur within several hours of immunization and subside spontaneously within 48 hours without sequelae. Swelling involving the entire thigh or upper arm has been reported in 2% to 3% of vaccinees after administration of the fourth and fifth doses of a variety of acellular pertussis vaccines. Limb swelling can be accompanied by erythema, pain, and fever; it is not an infection. Although thigh swelling may interfere with walking, most children have no limitation of activity; the condition resolves spontaneously and has no sequelae. The pathogenesis is unknown. It may be helpful to inform parents preemptively of the increase in reactogenicity that has been reported after the fourth and fifth doses of DTaP vaccine.

- Entire limb swelling after a fourth dose of DTaP is associated with a modestly increased risk of a similar reaction or an injection-site reaction >5 cm after the fifth dose. Entire limb swelling is not a contraindication to further DTaP, Tdap, or Td immunization.

- A review by the Institute of Medicine (IOM) based on case-series reports found evidence of a rare yet causal relationship between receipt of tetanus toxoid-containing vaccines and brachial neuritis. However, the frequency of this event has not been determined. Brachial neuritis is listed in the Vaccine Injury Table (see Appendix V, p 897).

- Bacterial or sterile abscess at the site of the injection is rare. Bacterial abscess indicates contamination of the product or nonsterile technique and should be reported (see Reporting of Adverse Events, p 44). Sterile abscesses probably are hypersensitivity reactions. Their occurrence does not contraindicate further doses of DTaP or of subsequent doses of Tdap.

- **Allergic reactions.** The rate of anaphylaxis to DTP was estimated to be approximately 2 cases per 100 000 injections; the incidence of allergic reactions after immunization with DTaP is unknown. The Institute of Medicine report titled "Adverse Effects of Vaccines: Evidence and Causality" links tetanus-containing vaccines to anaphylaxis.[1] Severe anaphylactic reactions and resulting deaths, if any, are rare after pertussis immunization. Transient urticarial rashes that occur occasionally after pertussis immunization, unless appearing immediately (ie, within minutes), are unlikely to be anaphylactic (IgE mediated) in origin.

- **Seizures.** The incidence of seizures occurring within 48 hours of administration of DTP was estimated to be 1 case per 1750 doses administered. Seizures have been reported substantially less often after DTaP. Seizures associated with pertussis-containing vaccines usually are febrile seizures. These seizures have not been demonstrated to result in subsequent development of recurrent afebrile seizures (ie, epilepsy) or other neurologic sequelae.

- **Hypotonic-hyporesponsive episodes.** A hypotonic-hyporesponsive episode (HHE) (also termed "collapse" or "shock-like state") was reported to occur at a frequency of 1 per 1750 doses of DTP administered, although reported rates varied widely. HHEs occur significantly less often after immunization with DTaP. A follow-up study of a group of children who experienced an HHE following DTP immunization demonstrated no evidence of subsequent serious neurologic sequelae or intellectual impairment.

- **Temperature 40.5°C (104.8°F) or higher.** After administration of DTP, approximately 0.3% of recipients were reported to develop temperature of 40.5°C (104.8°F) or higher within 48 hours. The rate after administration of DTaP is significantly lower.

- **Prolonged crying.** Persistent, severe, inconsolable screaming or crying for 3 or more hours was observed in up to 1% of infants within 48 hours of immunization with DTP. The frequency of inconsolable crying for 3 or more hours is significantly lower after immunization with DTaP. The significance of persistent crying is unknown. It has been noted after receipt of immunizations other than pertussis vaccine and is not known to be associated with sequelae.

---

[1] Institute of Medicine. *Adverse Effects of Vaccines: Evidence and Causality*. Washington, DC: The National Academies Press; 2011

Evaluation of Adverse Events Temporally Associated With Pertussis Immunization. Appropriate diagnostic studies should be performed to establish the cause of serious adverse events occurring temporally with immunization, rather than assuming that they are caused by the vaccine. The CDC has established independent Clinical Immunization Safety Assessment (CISA) centers to assess people with selected adverse events and offer recommendations for management. Nonetheless, the cause of events temporally related to immunization, even when unrelated to the immunization received, cannot always be established, even after extensive diagnostic and investigative studies. Genetic testing of several cases of encephalopathy temporally associated with DTP revealed genetic defect in neuronal sodium channels (Dravet syndrome); fever associated with DTP likely unmasked the genetic condition and was not the cause of encephalopathy.

The preponderance of evidence does not support a causal relationship between immunization with DTP and sudden infant death syndrome, infantile spasms, or serious acute neurologic illness resulting in permanent neurologic injury. Active surveillance performed by the IMPACT network of Canadian pediatric centers screening more than 12 000 admissions for neurologic disorders between 1993 and 2002 found no case of encephalopathy attributable to DTaP after administration of more than 6.5 million doses.

Contraindications and Precautions to DTaP Immunization.[1]

Contraindications and precautions to immunization with DTaP have been identified. A contraindication is a condition in a recipient that increases the risk for a serious adverse reaction. A vaccine should not be administered when a contraindication is present. The only contraindication applicable to all vaccinees is a history of a severe allergic reaction (ie, anaphylaxis) after a previous dose of the vaccine or to a vaccine component (unless the recipient has been desensitized). Children who experienced encephalopathy within 7 days after administration of a previous dose of diphtheria and tetanus toxoids and pertussis vaccine (DTP, DTaP, or Tdap) not attributable to another identifiable cause should not receive additional doses of a vaccine that contains pertussis. Children in the first year of life with an evolving neurologic disorder generally have DTaP immunization deferred temporarily. Such children should not receive DT, because in the United States, the risk of acquiring diphtheria or tetanus by children younger than 1 year of age is remote. On or before the first birthday, the decision to give DTaP or DT should be made to ensure that the child is at least completely immunized against diphtheria and tetanus; as children become ambulatory, their risk of tetanus-prone wounds increases. For children who begin deferral of DTaP immunization after 1 year of age, DT immunization should be completed according to the recommended schedule (see Diphtheria, p 307, and/or Tetanus, p 707).

A precaution is a condition in a recipient that might increase the risk of a serious adverse reaction or that might compromise the ability of the vaccine to produce immunity. In general, immunizations should be deferred when a precaution is present. However, immunization might be indicated in the presence of a precaution if the benefit of protection from the vaccine outweighs the risk for an adverse reaction. For example, Guillain-Barré syndrome within 6 weeks after a previous dose of tetanus toxoid containing vaccine is a precaution to further doses. A dose of DTaP (or Tdap, if indicated by age), however, should be considered for a person in a community with a pertussis

---

[1] Centers for Disease Control and Prevention. General recommendations on immunization: recommendations of the Advisory Committee on Immunization Practices (ACIP). *MMWR Recomm Rep*. 2011;60 (RR-02):1–60

outbreak even if that person previously developed Guillain-Barré syndrome after a dose. The presence of a moderate or severe acute illness with or without a fever is a precaution to administration of all vaccines. Preterm birth is not a reason to defer immunization (see Preterm and Low Birth Weight Infants, p 69). Preterm birth is associated with increased risk of complications and death from pertussis in infancy. Children with a stable neurologic condition (well-controlled seizures, a history of seizure disorder, cerebral palsy) should receive pertussis immunization on schedule. Children with a family history of a seizure disorder or adverse events after receipt of a pertussis-containing vaccine in a family member should receive pertussis immunization on schedule. Because the majority of contraindications and precautions are temporary, immunizations often can be administered later.

Recommendations for Routine Adolescent Booster Immunization With Tdap[1,2]

- Adolescents 11 years of age and older should receive a single dose of Tdap instead of Td for booster immunization against tetanus, diphtheria, and pertussis. The preferred age for Tdap immunizations is 11 through 12 years of age.
- Adolescents 11 years of age and older who received Td but not Tdap should receive a single dose of Tdap to provide protection against pertussis. Tdap can be administered regardless of time since receipt of last tetanus- or diphtheria-containing vaccine.
- Simultaneous administration of Tdap and all other recommended vaccines is recommended when feasible. Vaccines should not be mixed in the same syringe. Other indicated vaccine(s) that are not available and therefore cannot be given at the time of administration of Tdap can be given at any time thereafter.

Recommendations for Scheduling Tdap in Children 7 through 10 Years of Age Who Did Not Complete Recommended DTaP Doses Before 7 Years of Age.

- Children 7 through 10 years of age who have not completed their immunization schedule with DTaP before 7 years of age (see above) or who have an unknown vaccine history should receive a single dose of Tdap. If further dose(s) of tetanus and diphtheria toxoids are needed in a catch-up schedule, Td is used. The preferred schedule is Tdap followed by Td (if needed) at 2 months and 6 to 12 months, but a single dose of Tdap could be substituted for any dose in the series. Children who receive Tdap at 7 through 10 years of age should not be given the standard Tdap booster at 11 or 12 years of age but should be given Td 10 years after their last Tdap/Td dose.[3]

Recommendations for Adolescent and Adult Immunization With Tdap in Special Situations.[1] Special situations for use of Tdap are provided below. Currently, only 1 lifetime dose of Tdap should be administered to an adolescent or adult.

---

[1] Centers for Disease Control and Prevention. Updated recommendations for the use of tetanus toxoid, reduced diphtheria toxoid and acellular pertussis (Tdap) vaccine from the Advisory Committee on Immunization Practices, 2010. *MMWR Morb Mortal Wkly Rep*. 2011;60(1):13–15

[2] Centers for Disease Control and Prevention. Prevention of pertussis, tetanus, and diphtheria among pregnant and postpartum women and their infants: recommendations of the Advisory Committee on Immunization Practices. *MMWR*. 2011;60(41):1424–1426

[3] Centers for Disease Control and Prevention. Updated recommendations for the use of tetanus toxoid, reduced diphtheria toxoid and acellular pertussis (Tdap) vaccine from the Advisory Committee on Immunization Practices, 2010. *MMWR Morb Mortal Wkly Rep*. 2011;60(1):13–15

- **Use of Tdap in Pregnancy.** Physicians who provide health care to women should implement a Tdap immunization program for pregnant women who previously have not received Tdap. Physicians should administer Tdap during pregnancy, preferably during the third or late-second trimester (after 20 weeks' gestation), or if not administered during pregnancy, Tdap should be administered immediately postpartum. Both Tdap manufacturers have established pregnancy registries for women immunized with Tdap during pregnancy. Health care professionals are encouraged to report Tdap immunization during pregnancy to the following registries: Boostrix, to GlaxoSmithKline Biologicals at 1-888-825-5249; and Adacel, to Sanofi Pasteur at 1-800-822-2463.
- **Protection of Young Infants: the Cocoon Strategy.** The American Academy of Pediatrics, CDC, and American College of Obstetricians and Gynecologists recommend the cocoon strategy to protect mothers and families against pertussis through immunization to decrease their likelihood of acquisition and subsequent transmission of *B pertussis* to young infants who have high risk of severe or fatal pertussis.[1] Immunizing parents or other adult family contacts in the pediatric office setting could increase immunization coverage for this population to protect themselves as well as children to whom they provide care.[2]
  - Underimmunized children younger than 7 years of age should be given DTaP, and underimmunized children 7 years through 10 years of age should be given Tdap (see above).
  - Adolescents and adults who have or anticipate having close contact with an infant younger than 12 months of age (eg, parents, siblings, grandparents, child care providers, and health care professionals) and who previously have not received Tdap should receive a single dose of Tdap to protect against pertussis. Ideally, these adolescents and adults should receive Tdap at least 2 weeks before beginning close contact with the infant. There is no minimum interval suggested or required between Tdap and prior tetanus or diphtheria-toxoid containing vaccine.
  - Cough illness in contacts of neonates should be investigated and managed aggressively, with consideration given for azithromycin prophylaxis for the neonate if pertussis in a contact is likely (see Control Measures).
- **Special Situations**
  - *Pregnant women due for tetanus booster.* If tetanus and diphtheria booster immunization is indicated during pregnancy for a woman who previously has not received Tdap (ie, more than 10 years since previous Td), then Tdap should be administered during pregnancy, preferably during the third or late-second trimester (after 20 weeks' gestation).
  - *Wound management for pregnant women.* As part of standard wound management care to prevent tetanus, a tetanus toxoid-containing vaccine might be recommended for wound management in a pregnant woman if 5 years or more have elapsed since

---

[1] Centers for Disease Control and Prevention. Prevention of pertussis, tetanus, and diphtheria among pregnant and postpartum women and their infants: recommendations of the advisory committee on Immunization Practices. *MMWR*. 2011;60(41):1424–1426

[2] Lessin HR; Edwards KM; American Academy of Pediatrics, Committee on Practice and Ambulatory Medicine, Committee on Infectious Diseases. Immunizing parents and other close family contacts in the pediatric office setting. *Pediatrics*. 2012;129(2):e247–e253

previous Td immunization. If a Td booster is indicated for a pregnant woman who previously has not received Tdap, then Tdap should be administered.

- *Pregnant women with unknown or incomplete tetanus vaccination.* To ensure protection against maternal and neonatal tetanus, pregnant women who never have been immunized against tetanus should receive 3 doses of vaccines containing tetanus and reduced diphtheria toxoids during pregnancy. The recommended schedule is 0, 4 weeks, and 6 to 12 months. Tdap should replace 1 dose of Td, preferably during the third or late-second trimester of pregnancy (after 20 weeks' gestation).

Health Care Professionals.[1]

- The CDC recommends a single booster dose of Tdap as soon as is feasible for HCPs of any age who previously have not received Tdap. There is no minimum interval suggested or required between Tdap and prior receipt of any tetanus or diphtheria toxoid-containing vaccine.
- Tdap is not licensed for multiple administrations. After receipt of Tdap, HCPs should receive routine decennial booster immunization against tetanus and diphtheria according to previously published guidelines.
- Hospitals and ambulatory-care facilities should provide Tdap for HCPs and use approaches that maximize immunization rates (eg, education about the benefits of immunization or mandatory requirement, convenient access, and provision of Tdap at no charge).

Recommendations for Adult Booster Immunization With Tdap.[2] The CDC recommends administration of a single dose of Tdap universally to replace 1 decennial Td booster and to replace Td for wound prophylaxis for adults of any age who did not receive Tdap previously. Adults of any age who previously have not received Tdap, including adults who have or anticipate having close contact with an infant younger than 12 months of age, should be given a single dose of Tdap, with no minimum interval suggested or required between Tdap and prior receipt of a tetanus- or diphtheria-toxoid containing vaccine.

Adverse Events After Administration of Tdap. Local adverse events after administration of Tdap in adolescents and adults are common but usually are mild. Systemic adverse events also are common but usually are mild (eg, any fever, 3%–14%; any headache, 40%–44%; tiredness, 27%–37%). Postmarketing data suggest that these events occur at approximately the same rate and severity as following Td.

Syncope can occur after immunization, is more common among adolescents and young adults, and can result in serious injury if a vaccine recipient falls. Vaccinees should be seated and observed for 15 minutes after immunization. If syncope occurs, patients should be observed until symptoms resolve.

---

[1] Centers for Disease Control and Prevention. Immunization of health-care personnel: recommendations of the Advisory Committee on Immunization Practices (ACIP) and supported by the Healthcare Infection Control Practices Advisory (HICPAC). *MMWR Recomm Rep.* 2011;60(RR-07):1–45

[2] Centers for Disease Control and Prevention. Updated recommendations for the use of tetanus toxoid, reduced diphtheria toxoid and acellular pertussis (Tdap) vaccine from the Advisory Committee on Immunization Practices, 2010. *MMWR Morb Mortal Wkly Rep.* 2011;60(1):13–15

Contraindications, Precautions, and Deferral of Use of Tdap in Adolescents and Adults.
(See Contraindications and Precautions for DTaP). A history of immediate anaphylactic reaction after any component of the vaccine is a contraindication to Tdap (see Tetanus, p 707, for additional recommendations regarding tetanus immunization). History of Guillain-Barré syndrome within 6 weeks of a dose of a tetanus toxoid vaccine is a precaution to Tdap immunization. If decision is made to continue tetanus toxoid immunization, Tdap is preferred if indicated.

A history of severe Arthus hypersensitivity reaction after a previous dose of a tetanus or diphtheria toxoid-containing vaccine administered less than 10 years previously should lead to deferral of Tdap or Td immunization for 10 years after administration of the tetanus or diphtheria toxoid-containing vaccine.

Conditions That Are NOT Contraindications or Precautions to Tdap in Adolescents and Adults

The following conditions are NOT contraindications or precautions for Tdap:
- History of an extensive limb-swelling reaction after pediatric DTP/DTaP or Td immunization that was not an Arthus hypersensitivity reaction.
- Stable neurologic disorder, including well-controlled seizures, a history of seizure disorder, and cerebral palsy.
- Brachial neuritis.
- Latex allergy other than anaphylactic allergies. The tip and rubber plunger of the Boostrix needleless syringe contain latex. This product should not be administered to people with a history of an anaphylactic reaction to latex but may be administered to people with less severe allergies (eg, contact allergy to latex gloves). The Boostrix single-dose vial and Adacel Tdap preparations do not contain latex.
- Breastfeeding.
- Immunosuppression, including people with human immunodeficiency virus infection. The immunogenicity of Tdap in people with immunosuppression has not been studied adequately, but there is no safety risk.

Pinworm Infection
(Enterobius vermicularis)

CLINICAL MANIFESTATIONS: Although some people are asymptomatic, pinworm infection (enterobiasis) may cause pruritus ani and, rarely, pruritus vulvae. Bacterial superinfections can result from scratching and excoriation of the area. Pinworms have been found in the lumen of the appendix, but most evidence indicates that they do not cause acute appendicitis. Many clinical findings, such as grinding of teeth at night, weight loss, and enuresis, have been attributed to pinworm infections, but proof of a causal relationship has not been established. Urethritis, vaginitis, salpingitis, or pelvic peritonitis may occur from aberrant migration of an adult worm from the perineum.

ETIOLOGY: *Enterobius vermicularis* is a nematode or roundworm.

EPIDEMIOLOGY: Enterobiasis occurs worldwide and commonly clusters within families. Prevalence rates are higher in preschool- and school-aged children, in primary caregivers of infected children, and in institutionalized people; up to 50% of these populations may be infected.

Egg transmission occurs by the fecal-oral route either directly or indirectly via contaminated hands or fomites such as shared toys, bedding, clothing, toilet seats, and baths. Female pinworms usually die after depositing up to 10 000 fertilized eggs within 24 hours on the perianal skin. Reinfection occurs either by autoinfection or by infection following ingestion of eggs from another person. A person remains infectious as long as female nematodes are discharging eggs on perianal skin. Eggs remain infective in an indoor environment usually for 2 to 3 weeks. Humans are the only known natural hosts; dogs and cats do not harbor *E vermicularis*.

The **incubation period** from ingestion of an egg until an adult gravid female migrates to the perianal region is 1 to 2 months or longer.

DIAGNOSTIC TESTS: Diagnosis is made when adult worms are visualized in the perianal region, which is best examined 2 to 3 hours after the child is asleep. No egg shedding occurs inside the intestinal lumen; thus, very few ova are present in stool, so examination of stool specimens for ova and parasites is not recommended. Alternatively, diagnosis is made by touching the perianal skin with transparent (not translucent) adhesive tape to collect any eggs that may be present; the tape is then applied to a glass slide and examined under a low-power microscopic lens. Specimens should be obtained on 3 consecutive mornings when the patient first awakens, before washing. Eosinophilia is unusual and should not be attributed to pinworm infection. Serologic testing is not available or useful for diagnosis.

TREATMENT: Because pinworms largely are innocuous, the risk versus benefit of treatments should be weighed. Drugs of choice for treatment (see Drugs for Parasitic Infections, p 848) are pyrantel pamoate and albendazole (not approved for this use by the US Food and Drug Administration), both of which are given in a single dose and repeated in 2 weeks, because none of these drugs completely are effective against the egg or developing larvae stages. Mebendazole no longer is available in the United States. Pyrantel pamoate is available without prescription. For children younger than 2 years of age, in whom experience with these drugs is limited, risks and benefits should be considered before drug administration. Reinfection with pinworms occurs easily; prevention should be discussed when treatment is given. Infected people should bathe in the morning; bathing removes a large proportion of eggs. Frequently changing the infected person's underclothes, bedclothes, and bed sheets may decrease the egg contamination of the local environment and risk of reinfection. Specific personal hygiene measures (eg, exercising hand hygiene before eating or preparing food, keeping fingernails short, avoiding scratching of the perianal region, and avoiding nail biting) may decrease risk of autoinfection and continued transmission. Repeated infections should be treated by the same method as the first infection. All household members should be treated as a group in situations in which multiple or repeated symptomatic infections occur. Vaginitis is self-limited and does not require separate treatment.

ISOLATION OF THE HOSPITALIZED PATIENT: Standard precautions are indicated.

CONTROL MEASURES: Control is difficult in child care centers and schools, because the rate of reinfection is high. In institutions, mass and simultaneous treatment, repeated in 2 weeks, can be effective. Hand hygiene is the most effective method of prevention. Bed linen and underclothing of infected children should be handled carefully, should not be shaken (to avoid spreading ova into the air), and should be laundered promptly.

Pityriasis Versicolor
(Tinea Versicolor)

CLINICAL MANIFESTATIONS: Pityriasis versicolor (formerly tinea versicolor) is a common superficial yeast infection of the skin characterized by multiple scaling, oval, and patchy macular lesions usually distributed over upper portions of the trunk, proximal areas of the arms, and neck. Facial involvement particularly is common in children. Lesions can be hypopigmented or hyperpigmented (fawn colored or brown), and both types of lesions can coexist in the same person. Lesions fail to tan during the summer and during the winter are relatively darker, hence the term *versicolor.* Common conditions confused with this disorder include pityriasis alba, postinflammatory hypopigmentation, vitiligo, melasma, seborrheic dermatitis, pityriasis rosea, pityriasis lichenoides, and dermatologic manifestations of secondary syphilis.

ETIOLOGY: The cause of pityriasis versicolor is *Malassezia* species, a group of lipid-dependent yeasts that exist on healthy skin in yeast phase and cause clinical lesions only when substantial growth of hyphae occurs. Moist heat and lipid-containing sebaceous secretions encourage rapid overgrowth.

EPIDEMIOLOGY: Pityriasis versicolor occurs worldwide but is more prevalent in tropical and subtropical areas. Although primarily a disorder of adolescents and young adults, pityriasis versicolor also may occur in prepubertal children and infants. *Malassezia* species commonly colonize the skin in the first year of life and usually are harmless commensals. *Malassezia* infection can be associated with bloodstream infections, especially in neonates receiving total parenteral nutrition with lipids.

The **incubation period** is unknown.

DIAGNOSIS: Clinical appearance usually is diagnostic. Involved areas are fluorescent-yellow under Wood light examination. Skin scrapings examined microscopically in a potassium hydroxide wet mount preparation or stained with methylene blue or May-Grünwald-Giemsa stain disclose the pathognomonic clusters of yeast cells and hyphae ("spaghetti and meatball" appearance). Growth of this yeast in culture requires a source of long-chain fatty acids, which may be provided by overlaying Sabouraud dextrose agar medium with sterile olive oil.

TREATMENT: Topical treatment with selenium sulfide as 2.5% lotion or 1% shampoo has been the traditional treatment of choice. The lotion, which is approved by the US Food and Drug Administration (FDA) for treatment of tinea versicolor, should be applied in a thin layer covering the body surface from the face to the knees for 10 minutes daily for 7 days. Off-label, monthly applications for 3 months may help prevent recurrences. In adults, topical ketoconazole 2% shampoo used as a single application is effective and approved by the FDA. Other FDA-approved topical treatments for tinea versicolor include ciclopirox (cream, lotion, suspension; apply twice daily for 2 weeks), econazole (cream; apply daily for 2 weeks), oxiconazole (cream, lotion; apply once daily for 2 weeks). Other topical preparations with off-label therapeutic efficacy include sodium hyposulfite or thiosulfate in 15% to 25% concentrations (eg, Tinver lotion) applied twice a day for 2 to 4 weeks. Small focal infections may be treated off-label with topical antifungal agents, such as clotrimazole, ketoconazole (formulations other than the 2% shampoo), miconazole, naftifine, or terbinafine (see Topical Drugs for Superficial Fungal Infections, p 836). Because *Malassezia* species are part of normal flora, relapses are common. Multiple topical treatments may be necessary.

Oral antifungal therapy has advantages over topical therapy, including ease of administration and shorter duration of treatment, but oral therapy is more expensive and associated with a greater risk of adverse reactions. A single dose of ketoconazole (400 mg, orally) or fluconazole (400 mg, orally) or a 5-day course of itraconazole (200 mg, orally, once a day) has been effective in adults. Some experts recommend that children receive 3 days of ketoconazole therapy rather than the single dose given to adults. For pediatric dosage recommendations for ketoconazole, fluconazole, and itraconazole, see Recommended Doses of Parenteral and Oral Antifungal Drugs, p 831. These drugs have not been studied extensively in children for this purpose and are not approved by the US Food and Drug Administration for this indication. Exercise to increase sweating and skin concentrations of medication may enhance the effectiveness of systemic therapy.

Patients should be advised that repigmentation may not occur for several months after successful treatment.

ISOLATION OF THE HOSPITALIZED PATIENT: Standard precautions are recommended.

CONTROL MEASURES: Infected people should be treated.

Plague

CLINICAL MANIFESTATIONS: Naturally acquired plague most commonly manifests in the **bubonic form,** with acute onset of fever and painful swollen regional lymph nodes (buboes). Buboes develop most commonly in the inguinal region but also occur in axillary or cervical areas. Less commonly, plague manifests in the **septicemic form** (hypotension, acute respiratory distress, purpuric skin lesions, intravascular coagulopathy, organ failure) or as **pneumonic plague** (cough, fever, dyspnea, and hemoptysis) and **rarely as** meningeal, pharyngeal, ocular, or gastrointestinal plague. Abrupt onset of fever, chills, headache, and malaise are characteristic in all cases. Occasionally, patients have symptoms of mild lymphadenitis or prominent gastrointestinal tract symptoms, which may obscure the correct diagnosis. When left untreated, plague often will progress to overwhelming sepsis with renal failure, acute respiratory distress syndrome, hemodynamic instability, diffuse intravascular coagulation, necrosis of distal extremities, and death. Plague has been referred to as the Black Death.

ETIOLOGY: Plague is caused by *Yersinia pestis,* a pleomorphic, bipolar-staining, gram-negative coccobacillus.

EPIDEMIOLOGY: Plague is a zoonotic infection primarily maintained in rodents and their fleas. Humans are incidental hosts who develop bubonic or primary septicemic manifestations typically through the bite of infected fleas carried by a rodent or rarely other animals or through direct contact with contaminated tissues. Secondary pneumonic plague arises from hematogenous seeding of the lungs with *Y pestis* in patients with untreated bubonic or septicemic plague. Primary pneumonic plague is acquired by inhalation of respiratory tract droplets from a human or animal with pneumonic plague. Only the pneumonic form has been shown to be transmitted person-to-person, and the last known case of person-to-person transmission in the United States occurred in 1924. Rarely, humans can develop primary pneumonic plague following exposure to domestic cats with respiratory tract plague infections. Plague occurs worldwide with enzootic foci in parts of

Asia, Africa, and the Americas. Most human plague cases are reported from rural, under-developed areas and mainly occur as isolated cases or in focal clusters. Since 2000, more than 95% of the approximately 22 000 cases reported to the World Health Organization have been from countries in sub-Saharan Africa. In the United States, plague is endemic in western states, with most (approximately 85%) of the 37 cases reported from 2006 through 2010 being from New Mexico, Colorado, Arizona, and California. Cases of peripatetic plague have been identified in states without endemic plague, such as Connecticut (2008) and New York (2002).

The **incubation period** is 2 to 8 days for bubonic plague and 1 to 6 days for primary pneumonic plague.

DIAGNOSTIC TESTS: Diagnosis of plague usually is confirmed by culture of *Y pestis* from blood, bubo aspirate, sputum, or another clinical specimen. The organism has a bipolar (safety-pin) appearance when viewed with Wayson or Gram stains. A positive fluorescent antibody test result for the presence of *Y pestis* in direct smears or cultures of blood, bubo aspirate, sputum, or another clinical specimen provides presumptive evidence of *Y pestis* infection. A single positive serologic test result by passive hemagglutination assay or enzyme immunoassay in an unimmunized patient who previously has not had plague also provides presumptive evidence of infection. Seroconversion, defined as a fourfold difference in antibody titer between 2 serum specimens obtained at least 2 weeks apart, also confirms the diagnosis of plague. Polymerase chain reaction assay and immunohistochemical staining for rapid diagnosis of *Y pestis* are available in some reference or public health laboratories. In regions with endemic plague with limited laboratory capacity, a rapid dipstick (immunostrip) test, which uses monoclonal antibodies to detect F1 antigen, may be used to test a bubo aspirate or sputum specimen for case confirmation, per World Health Organization recommendations. Isolates suspected as *Y pestis* should be reported immediately to the state health department and submitted to the Division of Vector-Borne Infectious Diseases of the Centers for Disease Control and Prevention (CDC).

TREATMENT: For children, gentamicin and streptomycin administered intramuscularly or intravenously appear to be equally effective. Tetracycline, doxycycline, chloramphenicol, trimethoprim-sulfamethoxazole, and ciprofloxacin are alternative drugs. Fluoroquinolone or chloramphenicol is appropriate treatment for plague meningitis. Trimethoprim-sulfamethoxazole should not be considered a first-line treatment option when treating bubonic plague and should not be used as monotherapy to treat pneumonic or septicemic plague, because some studies have shown higher treatment failure rates and delayed treatment responses. Fluoroquinolones also have been found to be effective in treating plague in animal and in vitro studies but are not approved by the US Food and Drug Administration for this indication. The usual duration of antimicrobial treatment is 7 to 10 days or until several days after lysis of fever.

Drainage of abscessed buboes may be necessary; drainage material is infectious until effective antimicrobial therapy has been administered.

ISOLATION OF THE HOSPITALIZED PATIENT: For patients with bubonic plague, standard precautions are recommended. For patients with suspected pneumonic plague, respiratory droplet precautions should be initiated immediately and continued for 48 hours after initiation of effective antimicrobial treatment.

CONTROL MEASURES:

Care of Exposed People. All people with exposure to a known or suspected plague source, such as *Y pestis*-infected fleas or infectious tissues, in the previous 6 days should be offered antimicrobial prophylaxis or be cautioned to report fever greater than 38.5°C (101.0°F) or other illness to their physician. People with close exposure (less than 2 m) to a patient with pneumonic plague should receive antimicrobial prophylaxis, but isolation of asymptomatic people is not recommended. Pneumonic transmission typically occurs in the end stage of disease in patients with hemoptysis, thereby placing caregivers and health care professionals at high risk. For people 8 years of age or older, doxycycline or ciprofloxacin is recommended. For children younger than 8 years of age, doxycycline, tetracycline, chloramphenicol, ciprofloxacin, or trimethoprim-sulfamethoxazole are alternative drugs (see Tetracyclines, p 801, and Fluoroquinolones, p 800). The benefits of prophylactic therapy should be weighed against the risks. Prophylaxis is given for 7 days from the time of last exposure and in the usual therapeutic doses.

Other Measures. State public health authorities should be notified immediately of any suspected cases of human plague. The public should be educated about risk factors for plague, measures to prevent disease, and signs and symptoms of infection. People living in areas with endemic plague should be informed about the importance of eliminating sources of rodent food and harborage near residences, the role of dogs and cats in bringing plague-infected rodent fleas into peridomestic environments, the need for flea control and confinement of pets, and the importance of avoiding contact with sick and dead animals. Other preventive measures include surveillance of rodent populations, use of insecticides and insect repellents, and rodent control measures by health authorities when surveillance indicates the occurrence of plague epizootics. Rodent-control measures never should be employed without prior or concurrent use of insecticides.

Vaccine. Previously, an inactivated whole-cell *Y pestis* vaccine was available and recommended for people whose occupation regularly placed them at high risk of exposure to *Y pestis* or plague-infected rodents (eg, some field biologists and laboratory workers). Currently, there is no commercially available vaccine for plague in the United States. Development is in progress of a recombinant fusion protein vaccine (rF1V) that provides protection from aerosolized plague. Information concerning the availability of plague vaccines is available from the CDC Division of Vector-Borne Infectious Diseases.

Pneumococcal Infections[1,2]

CLINICAL MANIFESTATIONS: *Streptococcus pneumoniae* is a common cause of invasive bacterial infections in children, including febrile bacteremia. Pneumococci also are a common cause of acute otitis media, sinusitis, community-acquired pneumonia, pleural empyema, and conjunctivitis. *S pneumoniae* and *Neisseria meningitidis* are the 2 most common causes of bacterial meningitis and subdural hygromas in infants and children in the United States. Pneumococci occasionally cause mastoiditis, periorbital cellulitis, endocarditis,

---

[1] American Academy of Pediatrics, Committee on Infectious Diseases. Policy statement: recommendations for the prevention *Streptococcus pneumoniae* infections in infants and children: use of 13-valent pneumococcal conjugate vaccine (PCV13) and pneumococcal polysaccharide vaccine (PPSV23). *Pediatrics*. 2010;126(1):186–190

[2] Centers for Disease Control and Prevention. Prevention of pneumococcal disease among infants and children—use of 13-valent pneumococcal conjugate vaccine and 23-valent pneumococcal polysaccharide vaccine. *MMWR Recomm Rep*. 2010;59(RR-11):1–18

osteomyelitis, pericarditis, peritonitis, pyogenic arthritis, soft tissue infection, overwhelming septicemia in patients with splenic dysfunction, and neonatal septicemia. Hemolytic-uremic syndrome can accompany complicated invasive disease (eg, pneumonia with pleural empyema).

ETIOLOGY: *S pneumoniae* organisms (pneumococci) are lancet-shaped, gram-positive catalase-negative diplococci. More than 90 pneumococcal serotypes have been identified on the basis of unique polysaccharide capsules. Before implementation of routine immunization in infants with heptavalent pneumococcal conjugate vaccine (PCV7) in 2000, serotypes 4, 6B, 9V, 14, 18C, 19F, and 23F caused most invasive childhood pneumococcal infections in the United States; these 7 types are contained in PCV7. Serotypes 6A, 6B, 9V, 14, 19A, 19F, and 23F were the most common serotypes associated with resistance to penicillin. Serotype 19A was the most common cause of invasive disease in PCV7-immunized children. The 13-valent pneumococcal conjugate vaccine (PCV13) includes types 1, 3, 5, 6A, 7F, and 19A in addition to the seven PCV7 components.

EPIDEMIOLOGY: Pneumococci are ubiquitous, with many people having transient colonization of the upper respiratory tract. In children, nasopharyngeal carriage rates range from 21% in industrialized countries to more than 90% in resource-limited countries. Transmission is from person to person by respiratory droplet contact. The period of communicability is unknown and may be as long as the organism is present in respiratory tract secretions but probably is less than 24 hours after effective antimicrobial therapy is begun. Among young children who acquire a new pneumococcal serotype in the nasopharynx, illness (eg, otitis media) occurs in approximately 15%, usually within a few days of acquisition. Viral upper respiratory tract infections, including influenza, can predispose to pneumococcal infection and transmission. Pneumococcal infections are most prevalent during winter months. Rates of infection are highest in infants, young children, elderly people, and black, Alaska Native, and some American Indian populations. The incidence and severity of infections are increased in people with congenital or acquired humoral immunodeficiency, human immunodeficiency virus (HIV) infection, absent or deficient splenic function (eg, sickle cell disease, congenital or surgical asplenia), or abnormal innate immune responses. Children with cochlear implants have high rates of pneumococcal meningitis, as do children with congenital or acquired cerebrospinal fluid (CSF) leaks.[1] Other categories of children at presumed high risk or at moderate risk of developing invasive pneumococcal disease are outlined in Table 3.46 (p 573). Since introduction of the heptavalent conjugate vaccine, racial disparities have diminished.

From 1998 (before PCV7 was introduced in 2000) to 2007, the incidence of vaccine-type invasive pneumococcal infections decreased by 99%, and the incidence of all invasive pneumococcal disease (IPD) decreased by 76% in children younger than 5 years of age. In adults 65 years of age and older, IPD caused by PCV7 serotypes decreased 92% compared with baseline and all serotype invasive disease by 37%. The reduction in cases in these latter groups indicates the significant indirect benefits of PCV7 immunization by interruption of transmission of pneumococci from children to adults.

---

[1] American Academy of Pediatrics, Committee on Infectious Diseases. Policy statement: cochlear implants in children: surgical site infections and prevention and treatment of acute otitis media and meningitis. *Pediatrics.* 2010;126(2):381–391

Table 3.46. Underlying Medical Conditions That Are Indications for Pneumococcal Immunization Among Children, by Risk Group[a]

Risk group	Condition
Immunocompetent children	Chronic heart disease[b]
	Chronic lung disease[c]
	Diabetes mellitus
	Cerebrospinal fluid leaks
	Cochlear implant
Children with functional or anatomic asplenia	Sickle cell disease and other hemoglobinopathies
	Chronic or acquired asplenia, or splenic dysfunction
Children with immuno-compromising conditions	HIV infection
	Chronic renal failure and nephrotic syndrome
	Diseases associated with treatment with immunosuppressive drugs or radiation therapy, including malignant neoplasms, leukemias, lymphomas, and Hodgkin disease; or solid organ transplantation
	Congenital immunodeficiency[d]

[a] Centers for Disease Control and Prevention. Licensure of a 13-valent pneumococcal conjugate vaccine (PCV13) and recommendations for use among children. Advisory Committee on Immunization Practices (ACIP). *MMWR Morb Mortal Wkly Rep.* 2010;59(9):258–261.
[b] Particularly cyanotic congenital heart disease and cardiac failure.
[c] Including asthma if treated with prolonged high-dose oral corticosteroids.
[d] Includes B- (humoral) or T-lymphocyte deficiency; complement deficiencies, particularly C_1, C_2, C_3, and C_4 deficiency; and phagocytic disorders (excluding chronic granulomatous disease).

The **incubation period** varies by type of infection but can be as short as 1 to 3 days.

DIAGNOSTIC TESTS: Recovery of *S pneumoniae* from a suppurative focus or from blood confirms the diagnosis. The finding of lancet-shaped gram-positive organisms and white blood cells in expectorated sputum or pleural exudate suggests pneumococcal pneumonia in older children and adults. Recovery of pneumococci by culture of an upper respiratory tract swab specimen is not sufficient to assign an etiologic diagnosis of pneumococcal disease involving the middle ear, lower respiratory tract, or sinus. Real-time polymerase chain reaction using *lyt*A is investigational but may be specific and significantly more sensitive than culture of pleural fluid, CSF and blood, particularly in patients who have received recent antimicrobial therapy.

Susceptibility Testing. All *S pneumoniae* isolates from normally sterile body fluids (eg, CSF, blood, middle ear fluid, pleural or joint fluid) should be tested for antimicrobial susceptibility to determine the minimum inhibitory concentration (MIC) of penicillin and cefotaxime or ceftriaxone. CSF isolates also should be tested for susceptibility to vancomycin and meropenem. *Nonsusceptible* includes both *intermediate* and *resistant* isolates. Breakpoints vary depending on whether an isolate is from a nonmeningeal or meningeal source. Accordingly, current definitions by the Clinical and Laboratory Standards Institute (CLSI) for susceptibility and nonsusceptibility are provided in Table 3.47 for nonmeningeal and meningitis isolates.

For patients with meningitis caused by an organism that is nonsusceptible to penicillin, susceptibility testing of rifampin also should be performed. If the patient has a nonmeningeal infection caused by an isolate that is nonsusceptible to penicillin, cefotaxime, and ceftriaxone, susceptibility testing to clindamycin, erythromycin, rifampin, trimethoprim-sulfamethoxazole, linezolid, meropenem, and vancomycin should be considered.

Quantitative MIC testing using reliable methods, such as broth microdilution or antimicrobial gradient strips, should be performed on isolates from children with invasive infections. When quantitative testing methods are not available or for isolates from noninvasive infections, the qualitative screening test using a 1-µg oxacillin disk on an agar plate reliably identifies all penicillin-*susceptible* pneumococci using meningitis breakpoints (ie, disk-zone diameter of 20 mm or greater). Organisms with an oxacillin disk-zone size of less than 20 mm potentially are nonsusceptible for treatment of meningitis and require quantitative susceptibility testing. The oxacillin disk test is used as a screening test for resistance to beta-lactam drugs (ie, penicillins and cephalosporins).

TREATMENT: *S pneumoniae* strains that are nonsusceptible to penicillin G, cefotaxime, ceftriaxone, and other antimicrobial agents using meningitis breakpoints have been identified throughout the United States and worldwide but are uncommon using nonmeningeal breakpoints.

Recommendations for treatment of pneumococcal infections are as follows.

Bacterial Meningitis Possibly or Proven to Be Caused by S pneumoniae. Combination therapy with vancomycin and cefotaxime or ceftriaxone should be administered initially to all children 1 month of age or older with definite or probable bacterial meningitis because of the increased prevalence of *S pneumoniae* resistant to penicillin, cefotaxime, and ceftriaxone.

Table 3.47. Clinical and Laboratory Standards Institute Definitions of In Vitro Susceptibility and Nonsusceptibility of Nonmeningeal and Meningeal Pneumococcal Isolates[a,b]

Drug and Isolate Location	Susceptible, µg/mL	Nonsusceptible, µg/mL	
		Intermediate	Resistant
Penicillin (oral)[c]	≤0.06	0.12–1.0	≥2.0
Penicillin (intravenous)[d]			
Nonmeningeal	≤2.0	4.0	≥8.0
Meningeal	≤0.06	None	≥0.12
Cefotaxime **OR** ceftriaxone			
Nonmeningeal	≤1.0	2.0	≥4.0
Meningeal	≤0.5	1.0	≥2.0

[a] Clinical and Laboratory Standards Institute. *Performance Standards for Antimicrobial Susceptibility Testing: 18th Informational Supplement.* CLSI Publication No. M100-S21. Wayne, PA: Clinical and Laboratory Standards Institute; 2011

[b] Centers for Disease Control and Prevention. Effects of new penicillin susceptibility breakpoints for *Streptococcus pneumoniae*— United States, 2006–2007. *MMWR Morb Mortal Wkly Rep.* 2008;57(50):1353–1355

[c] Without meningitis.

[d] Treated with intravenous penicillin.

For children with serious hypersensitivity reactions to beta-lactam antimicrobial agents (ie, penicillins and cephalosporins), the combination of vancomycin and rifampin should be considered. Vancomycin should not be given alone, because bactericidal concentrations in CSF are difficult to sustain, and clinical experience to support use of vancomycin as monotherapy is minimal. Rifampin also should not be given as monotherapy, because resistance can develop during therapy. Meropenem also can be given as an alternative drug. A repeat lumbar puncture should be considered after 48 hours of therapy in the following circumstances:

- the organism is penicillin nonsusceptible by oxacillin disk or quantitative (MIC) testing, and results from cefotaxime and ceftriaxone quantitative susceptibility testing are not yet available;
- the patient's condition has not improved or has worsened; or
- the child has received dexamethasone, which can interfere with the ability to interpret the clinical response, such as resolution of fever.

Once results of susceptibility testing are available, therapy should be modified according to the guidelines in Table 3.48. Vancomycin should be discontinued and penicillin should be continued if the organism is susceptible to penicillin; if the isolate is penicillin nonsusceptible, cefotaxime or ceftriaxone should be continued. Vancomycin should be continued only if the organism is nonsusceptible to penicillin and to cefotaxime or ceftriaxone.

Addition of rifampin to vancomycin after 24 to 48 hours of therapy should be considered if the organism is susceptible to rifampin and (1) after 24 to 48 hours, despite therapy with vancomycin and cefotaxime or ceftriaxone, the clinical condition has worsened;

Table 3.48. Antimicrobial Therapy for Infants and Children With Meningitis Caused by *Streptococcus pneumoniae* on the Basis of Susceptibility Test Results

Susceptibility Test Results	Antimicrobial Management[a]
• *Susceptible* to penicillin	**Discontinue vancomycin** **AND** Begin penicillin (and discontinue cephalosporin) **OR** Continue cefotaxime or ceftriaxone alone[b]
• *Nonsusceptible* to penicillin (*intermediate* or *resistant*) **AND** *Susceptible* to cefotaxime and ceftriaxone	**Discontinue vancomycin** **AND** Continue cefotaxime or ceftriaxone
• *Nonsusceptible* to penicillin (*intermediate* or *resistant*) **AND** *Nonsusceptible* to cefotaxime and ceftriaxone (*intermediate* or *resistant*) **AND** *Susceptible* to rifampin	Continue vancomycin and high-dose cefotaxime or ceftriaxone **AND** Rifampin may be added in selected circumstances (see text)

[a] See Table 3.49, p 576, for dosages. Some experts recommend the maximum dosages. Initial therapy of nonallergic children older than 1 month of age should be vancomycin and cefotaxime or ceftriaxone. See Bacterial Meningitis Possibly or Proven to Be Caused by *S pneumoniae*, p 574.

[b] Some physicians may choose this alternative for convenience and cost savings but only in treatment of meningitis.

(2) the subsequent culture of CSF indicates failure to eradicate or to decrease substantially the number of organisms; or (3) the organism has an unusually high cefotaxime or ceftriaxone MIC (≥4 µg/mL). Consultation with an infectious disease specialist should be considered in such circumstances.

Dexamethasone. For infants and children 6 weeks of age and older, adjunctive therapy with dexamethasone may be considered after weighing the potential benefits and possible risks. Some experts recommend use of corticosteroids in pneumococcal meningitis, but this issue is controversial and data are not sufficient to make a routine recommendation for children. If used, dexamethasone should be given before or concurrently with the first dose of antimicrobial agents.

Nonmeningeal Invasive Pneumococcal Infections Requiring Hospitalization. For nonmeningeal invasive infections in previously healthy children who are not critically ill, antimicrobial agents currently used to treat infections with *S pneumoniae* and other potential pathogens should be initiated at the usually recommended dosages (see Table 3.49).

For critically ill infants and children with invasive infections potentially attributable to *S pneumoniae,* vancomycin in addition to usual antimicrobial therapy (eg, cefotaxime or ceftriaxone or others) can be considered for strains that possibly are nonsusceptible to penicillin, cefotaxime, or ceftriaxone. Such patients include those with myopericarditis or severe multilobar pneumonia with hypoxia or hypotension. If vancomycin is administered, it should be discontinued as soon as antimicrobial susceptibility test results demonstrate effective alternative agents.

If the organism has in vitro resistance to penicillin, cefotaxime, and ceftriaxone by CLSI standards, therapy should be modified on the basis of clinical response, susceptibility to other antimicrobial agents, and results of follow-up cultures of blood and other infected body fluids. Consultation with an infectious disease specialist should be considered.

Table 3.49. Dosages of Intravenous Antimicrobial Agents for Invasive Pneumococcal Infections in Infants and Children[a]

Antimicrobial Agent	Meningitis		Nonmeningeal Infections	
	Dose/kg per day	Dose Interval	Dose/kg per day	Dose Interval
Penicillin G	250 000–400 000 U[b]	4–6 h	250 000–400 000 U[b]	4–6 h
Cefotaxime	225–300 mg	8 h	75–100 mg	8 h
Ceftriaxone	100 mg	12–24 h	50–75 mg	12–24 h
Vancomycin	60 mg	6 h	40–45 mg	6–8 h
Rifampin[c]	20 mg	12 h	Not indicated	...
Chloramphenicol[d]	75–100 mg	6 h	75–100 mg	6 h
Clindamycin	Not indicated	...	25–40 mg	6–8 h
Meropenem[e]	120 mg	8 h	60 mg	8 h

[a] Doses are for children 1 month of age or older.
[b] Because 1 U = 0.6 µg/mL, this range is equal to 150 to 240 mg/kg per day.
[c] Indications for use are not defined completely.
[d] Drug should be considered only for patients with life-threatening allergic response after administration of beta-lactam antimicrobial agents.
[e] Drug is approved for pediatric patients 3 months of age and older.

For children with severe hypersensitivity to beta-lactam antimicrobial agents (ie, penicillins and cephalosporins), initial management should include vancomycin or clindamycin in addition to antimicrobial agents for other potential pathogens, as indicated. Vancomycin should not be continued if the organism is susceptible to other appropriate non–beta-lactam antimicrobial agents. Consultation with an infectious disease specialist should be considered.

Nonmeningeal Invasive Pneumococcal Infections in the Immunocompromised Host. The preceding recommendations for management of possible pneumococcal infections requiring hospitalization also apply to immunocompromised children. Vancomycin should be discontinued as soon as antimicrobial susceptibility test results indicate that effective alternative antimicrobial agents are available.

Dosages. The recommended dosages of intravenous antimicrobial agents for treatment of invasive pneumococcal infections are given in Table 3.49 (p 576).

Acute Otitis Media.[1] According to clinical practice guidelines of the American Academy of Pediatrics (AAP) and the American Academy of Family Physicians (AAFP) on acute otitis media (AOM), amoxicillin (80–90 mg/kg/day) is recommended, except in select cases in which the option of observation without antimicrobial therapy is warranted. Optimal duration of therapy is uncertain. For younger children and children with severe disease at any age, a 10-day course is recommended; for children 6 years of age and older with mild or moderate disease, duration of 5 to 7 days is appropriate.

Patients who fail to respond to initial management should be reassessed at 48 to 72 hours to confirm the diagnosis of AOM and exclude other causes of illness. If AOM is confirmed in the patient managed initially with observation, amoxicillin should be given. If the patient has failed initial antibacterial therapy, a change in antibacterial agent is indicated. Suitable alternative agents should be active against penicillin-nonsusceptible pneumococci as well as beta-lactamase–producing *Haemophilus influenzae* and *Moraxella catarrhalis*. Such agents include high-dose oral amoxicillin-clavulanate; oral cefdinir, cefpodoxime, or cefuroxime; or intramuscular ceftriaxone in a 3-day course. Amoxicillin-clavulanate should be given at 80 to 90 mg/kg per day of the amoxicillin component in the 14:1 formulation to decrease the incidence of diarrhea. Patients who continue to fail therapy with one of the aforementioned oral agents should be treated with a 3-day course of parenteral ceftriaxone. Clarithromycin and azithromycin are appropriate alternatives for initial therapy in patients with a type I (immediate, anaphylactic) reaction to a beta-lactam agent, although macrolide resistance among *S pneumoniae* is high. For patients with a history of non-type I allergic reaction to penicillin, agents such as cefdinir, cefuroxime, or cefpodoxime can be used orally.

Myringotomy or tympanocentesis should be considered for children failing to respond to second-line therapy and for severe cases to obtain cultures to guide therapy. For multidrug-resistant strains of *S pneumoniae*, use of clindamycin, rifampin, or other agents should be considered in consultation with an expert in infectious diseases.

Sinusitis. Antimicrobial agents effective for treatment of AOM also are likely to be effective for acute sinusitis and are recommended.

ISOLATION OF THE HOSPITALIZED PATIENT: Standard precautions are recommended, including for patients with infections caused by drug-resistant *S pneumoniae*.

---

[1] American Academy of Pediatrics, Clinical Practice Guideline. Subcommittee on Management of Acute Otitis Media. Diagnosis and management of acute otitis media. *Pediatrics.* 2004;113(5):1451–1465

CONTROL MEASURES:

Active Immunization. Two pneumococcal vaccines are available for use in children in the United States: PCV13 and 23-valent pneumococcal polysaccharide vaccine (PPSV23). PCV13 has replaced PCV7 and is licensed for use in infants and children from 6 weeks through 71 months of age. PCV13 is composed of the 7 purified capsular polysaccharide serotypes that were in PCV7 (4, 6B, 9V, 14, 18C, 19F, and 23F) plus another 6 (1, 3, 5, 6A, 7F, and 19A) individually conjugated to a nontoxic variant of diphtheria toxin carrier protein, CRM_{197} (~34 µg). PCV13 is available in single-dose, prefilled syringes that do not contain latex or preservative but do contain 0.02% polysorbate 80, 0.125 mg of aluminum (as aluminum phosphate adjuvant), and 5 mM succinate buffer. PPSV23 is licensed for use in children 2 years of age and older and adults. PPSV23 is composed of 23 capsular polysaccharides in isotonic saline solution containing 0.25% phenol as preservative. Each available vaccine is recommended in a dose of 0.5 mL to be administered intramuscularly. Immunization with PPSV23 does not induce immunologic memory or boosting with subsequent doses, and no effects on nasopharyngeal carriage or indirect protection of unimmunized groups have been documented.

Routine Immunization With Pneumococcal Conjugate Vaccine. PCV13 is recommended for all infants and children 2 through 59 months of age. For infants, the vaccine should be administered at 2, 4, 6, and 12 through 15 months of age; catch-up immunization is recommended for all children 59 months of age or younger, and the schedule is the same as previously published for PCV7, with PCV13 replacing PCV7 for all doses (Table 3.50, p 579). Infants should begin the PCV13 immunization series in conjunction with other recommended vaccines at the time of the first regularly scheduled health maintenance visit after 6 weeks of age. Infants of very low birth weight (1500 g or less) should be immunized when they attain a chronologic age of 6 to 8 weeks, regardless of their gestational age at birth. PCV13 can be administered concurrently with all other age-appropriate childhood immunizations using a separate syringe and a separate injection site.

Supplemental Dose Recommendation. A single supplemental dose of PCV13 is recommended for all healthy children 14 through 59 months of age fully immunized with PCV7; this should be given at least 8 weeks after the last dose of PCV7. For fully immunized children 14 through 71 months of age who have an underlying medical condition (Table 3.46, p 573) that increases their risk of pneumococcal disease or complications, a single supplemental dose of PCV13 is recommended.

Immunization of Children Unimmunized or Incompletely Immunized With PCV13. PCV13 is recommended for all children younger than 72 months of age who are at high risk or presumed high risk of acquiring invasive pneumococcal infection, as defined in Table 3.46 (p 573). For toddlers 2 through 71 months of age who have not received PCV13 or need "catch up" immunization, the schedule is the same as previously published for PCV7, with PCV13 replacing PCV7 for all doses (Table 3.50, p 579).

Immunization of Children 6 Through 18 Years of Age With High-Risk Conditions. A single dose of PCV13 may be administered to children 6 through 18 years of age who are at increased risk of IPD because of sickle cell disease, HIV infection, or other immunocompromising conditions; cochlear implant; or CSF leaks, regardless of whether they previously have received PCV7 or PPSV23. PCV13 is licensed by the Food and Drug Administration for children 6 weeks through 71 months of age. On the basis of limited safety data for a single dose of PCV7 in older children, PCV13 is likely to be safe and effective, although additional studies are needed. If both PCV13 and PPSV23 are used,

Table 3.50. Recommended Schedule for Doses of PCV13, Including Catch-up Immunizations in Previously Unimmunized and Partially Immunized Children

Age at Examination	Immunization History	Recommended Regimen[a,b]
2 through 6 mo	0 doses	3 doses, 2 mo apart; fourth dose at 12 through 15 mo of age
	1 dose	2 doses, 2 mo apart; fourth dose at 12 through 15 mo of age
	2 doses	1 dose, 2 mo after the most recent dose; fourth dose at 12 through 15 mo of age
7 through 11 mo	0 doses	2 doses, 2 mo apart; third dose at 12 mo of age
	1 or 2 doses before age 7 mo	1 dose at age 7 through 11 mo, with another dose at 12 through 15 mo of age (≥2 mo later)
12 through 23 mo	0 doses	2 doses, ≥2 mo apart
	1 dose at <12 mo	2 doses, ≥2 mo apart
	1 dose at ≥12 mo	1 dose, ≥2 mo after the most recent dose
	2 or 3 doses at <12 mo	1 dose, ≥2 mo after the most recent dose
24 through 59 mo[c] Healthy children	Any incomplete schedule	1 dose, ≥2 mo after the most recent dose[c]
24 through 71 mo Children with underlying medical conditions[d]	Any incomplete schedule of <3 doses	2 doses, one ≥2 mo after the most recent dose and another dose ≥2 mo later
	Any incomplete schedule of 3 doses	1 dose, ≥2 mo after the most recent dose

PCV13 indicates 13-valent pneumococcal conjugate vaccine.

[a]For children immunized at younger than 12 months of age, the minimum interval between doses is 4 weeks. Doses administered at 12 months of age or older should be at least 8 weeks apart.

[b]Centers for Disease Control and Prevention. Licensure of a 13-valent pneumococcal conjugate vaccine (PCV13) and recommendations for use among children. Advisory Committee on Immunization Practices (ACIP). *MMWR Morb Mortal Wkly Rep*. 2010;59(RR-11):1–18

[c]A single dose should be administered to all healthy children 24 through 59 months of age with any incomplete schedule.

[d]Children with sickle cell disease, asplenia, chronic heart or lung disease, diabetes mellitus, cerebrospinal fluid leak, cochlear implant, human immunodeficiency virus infection, or another immunocompromising condition (see Table 3.46, p 573). PPV23 also is indicated. See Table 3.51, p 580.

PCV13 should be administered first, and the administration of PPSV23 should follow at an interval of at least 8 weeks.

Immunization of Children 2 Through 18 Years of Age Who Are at Increased Risk of IPD With PPSV23 After PCV7 or PCV13. Children 2 years of age or older with an underlying medical condition increasing the risk of IPD should receive PPSV23 as soon as possible after a diagnosis is made. Doses of PCV13 should be completed before PPSV23 is administered, with a minimum interval of 8 weeks between the last dose of PCV13 and the first dose of PPSV23. If a child previously has received PPSV23, the child should also receive the recommended doses of PCV13. A second dose of PPSV23 is recommended 5 years after the first dose in children with sickle cell disease or functional or anatomic asplenia, HIV

Table 3.51. Recommendations for Pneumococcal Immunization with PCV13 or PPSV23 Vaccine for Children at High Risk or Presumed High Risk of Pneumococcal Disease, as Defined in Table 3.46 (p 573)

Age	Previous Dose(s) of Any Pneumococcal Vaccine	Recommendations
23 mo or younger	None	PCV13, as in Table 3.50 (p 579)
24 through 71 mo	4 doses of PCV13	1 dose of PPSV23 vaccine at 24 mo of age, at least 8 wk after last dose of PCV13
		1 dose of PPSV23, 5 y after the first dose of PPV7[a]
24 through 71 mo	3 previous doses of PCV7 before 24 mo of age	1 dose of PCV13
		1 dose of PPSV23, ≥8 wk after the last dose of PCV7
		1 dose of PPSV23, 5 y after the first dose of PPSV23[a]
24 through 71 mo	<3 doses of PCV7 before 24 mo of age	2 doses of PCV13, at least 8 wk after last dose of PCV13 (if applicable)
		1 dose of PPSV23 vaccine, ≥8 wk after the last dose of PCV13
		1 dose of PPSV23 vaccine, 5 y after the first dose of PPSV23 vaccine[a]
24 through 71 mo	1 dose of PPSV23	2 doses of PCV13, 8 wk apart, beginning at 6–8 wk after last dose of PPSV23
		1 dose of PPSV23 vaccine, 5 y after the last dose of PPV23 and at least 8 wk after PCV13[a]

PCV13 indicates 13-valent pneumococcal conjugate vaccine; PPSV23, 23-valent pneumococcal polysaccharide vaccine.
[a] A second dose of PPSV23 5 years after the first dose is recommended only for children who have sickle cell disease, functional or anatomic asplenia, HIV infection, or other immunocompromising conditions (Table 3.46). No more than 2 doses of PPSV23 are recommended. All other children with underlying medical conditions should receive 1 dose of PPSV23.

infection, or other immunocompromising conditions, but no more than 2 total doses of PPSV23 are recommended.

Control of Transmission of Pneumococcal Infection and Invasive Disease Among Children Attending Out-of-Home Child Care. Before routine use of PCV7, children attending out-of-home child care were twofold to threefold more likely to acquire invasive pneumococcal infection than were healthy children of the same age not enrolled in out-of-home child care. PPSV23 has not been shown to decrease nasopharyngeal carriage of pneumococci. In contrast, PCV7 reduces carriage of pneumococcal serotypes in the vaccine, and PCV13 is expected to have a similar effect. Available data are insufficient to recommend any antimicrobial regimen for preventing or interrupting the carriage or transmission of pneumococcal infection in out-of-home child care settings. Antimicrobial chemoprophylaxis is not recommended for contacts of children with invasive pneumococcal disease, regardless of their immunization status.

General Recommendations for Use of Pneumococcal Vaccines.

- Either PPSV23 or PCV13 can be given concurrently with other vaccines, except MCV4-D should not be administered concomitantly with or within 4 weeks of administration of PCV13 because of potential interference with the immune response to PCV13. Pneumococcal vaccine should be injected with a separate syringe in a separate injection site.
- When elective splenectomy is performed for any reason, immunization with PCV13 should be completed at least 2 weeks before splenectomy. Immunization also should precede initiation of immune-compromising therapy or placement of a cochlear implant by at least 2 weeks. PPSV23 can be given 8 or more weeks after PCV13.
- Generally, pneumococcal vaccines should be deferred during pregnancy, because it is unknown whether pneumococcal vaccines can cause fetal harm when administered to a pregnant woman. However, inactivated or killed vaccines, including licensed polysaccharide vaccines, have been administered safely during pregnancy. The risk of severe pneumococcal disease in a pregnant woman who has an underlying medical condition increasing risk of IPD should prompt immunization with PPSV23 if not previously administered within the previous 5 years.

Case Reporting. Cases of invasive pneumococcal disease in children younger than 5 years of age and drug-resistant infection in all ages should be reported according to state standards. Before introduction of PCV13, approximately 99% of invasive disease cases were caused by non-PCV7 serotypes. Therefore, the overwhelming majority of invasive pneumococcal disease cases occurring among unimmunized children have not represented vaccine failures. Early evidence suggests that IPD caused by PCV13 serotypes is decreasing. To differentiate PCV13 failure in an immunized child from disease caused by a serotype not included in PCV13, the isolate would need to be serotyped (**www.cdc. gov/ncidod/biotech/strep/references.htm**). A protocol for identifying pneumococcal serotypes using polymerase chain reaction is available for state public health laboratories on the CDC Web site (**www.cdc.gov/ncidod/biotech/strep/pcr.htm**). If the isolate is a serotype included in the vaccine, an evaluation of the patient's HIV status and immunologic function should be considered.

Adverse Reactions to Pneumococcal Vaccines. Adverse reactions after administration of polysaccharide or conjugate vaccines generally are mild and limited to local reactions of redness or swelling. Fever may occur within the first 1 to 2 days after injections, particularly after use of conjugate vaccine.

Passive Immunization. Immune Globulin Intravenous administration is recommended for preventing pneumococcal infection in patients with congenital or acquired immunodeficiency diseases, including people with HIV infection who have recurrent pneumococcal infections (see Human Immunodeficiency Virus Infection, p 418).

Chemoprophylaxis. Daily antimicrobial prophylaxis is recommended for children with functional or anatomic asplenia, regardless of their immunization status, for prevention of pneumococcal disease on the basis of results of a large, multicenter study (see Children With Asplenia, p 88). Oral penicillin V (125 mg, twice a day, for children younger than 5 years of age; 250 mg, twice a day, for children 5 years of age and older) is recommended. The study, performed before routine use of PCV7 in the United States, demonstrated that oral penicillin V given to infants and young children with sickle cell disease decreased the incidence of pneumococcal bacteremia by 84% compared with the placebo control group. Although overall incidence of invasive pneumococcal infection is decreased after penicillin prophylaxis, cases of penicillin-resistant invasive pneumococcal infections and nasopharyngeal carriage of penicillin-resistant strains in patients with sickle cell disease have increased in recent years. Parents should be informed that penicillin prophylaxis may not be effective in preventing all cases of invasive pneumococcal infections. In children with suspected or proven penicillin allergy, erythromycin is an alternative agent for prophylaxis.[1]

The age at which prophylaxis is discontinued is an empiric decision. Most children with sickle cell disease who have received all recommended pneumococcal vaccines for age and who had received penicillin prophylaxis for prolonged periods, who are receiving regular medical attention, and who have not had a previous severe pneumococcal infection or a surgical splenectomy safely may discontinue prophylactic penicillin at 5 years of age. However, they must be counseled to seek medical attention for all febrile events. The duration of prophylaxis for children with asplenia attributable to other causes is unknown. Some experts continue prophylaxis throughout childhood.

Pneumocystis jirovecii Infections

CLINICAL MANIFESTATIONS: Infants and children develop a characteristic syndrome of subacute diffuse pneumonitis with dyspnea, tachypnea, oxygen desaturation, nonproductive cough, and fever. However, the intensity of these signs and symptoms can vary, and in some immunocompromised children and adults, onset can be acute and fulminant. Chest radiographs often show bilateral diffuse interstitial or alveolar disease; rarely, lobar, miliary, cavitary, and nodular lesions or even no lesions are seen. Most children with *Pneumocystis* pneumonia are hypoxic with low arterial oxygen pressure. The mortality rate in immunocompromised patients ranges from 5% to 40% in patients treated and approaches 100% without therapy.

ETIOLOGY: Nomenclature for *Pneumocystis* species has evolved. Originally considered a protozoan, *Pneumocystis* now is classified as a fungus on the basis of DNA sequence analysis. Because of this, human *Pneumocystis* now is called *Pneumocystis jirovecii*, reflecting the fact that *Pneumocystis carinii* only infects rats. *P carinii* or *P carinii f* sp *hominis* sometimes still are used to refer to human *Pneumocystis*. *P jirovecii* is an atypical fungus, with several morphologic and biologic similarities to protozoa, including susceptibility to a number of antiprotozoal agents but resistance to most antifungal agents. In addition, the organism exists as 2 distinct morphologic forms: the 5- to 7-μm-diameter cysts, which contain up to 8 intracystic bodies, and the smaller, 1- to 5-μm-diameter trophozoite or trophic form.

EPIDEMIOLOGY: *Pneumocystis* species are ubiquitous in mammals worldwide, particularly rodents, and have a tropism for growth on respiratory tract epithelium. *Pneumocystis* isolates recovered from mice, rats, and ferrets differ genetically from each other and from human *P jirovecii*. Infections are species-specific, and cross-species infections are not known to occur. Asymptomatic human infection occurs early in life, with more than 85% of healthy children acquiring antibody by 20 months of age. In resource-limited countries and in times of famine, *P jirovecii* pneumonia (PCP) can occur in epidemics, primarily affecting malnourished infants and children. Epidemics also have occurred among preterm infants. In industrialized countries, PCP occurs almost entirely in

---

[1] American Academy of Pediatrics, Committee on Genetics. Health supervision for children with sickle cell disease. *Pediatrics* 2002;109(3):526–535 (Reaffirmed January 2011)

immunocompromised people with deficient cell-mediated immunity, particularly people with human immunodeficiency virus (HIV) infection, recipients of immunosuppressive therapy after organ transplantation or treatment for malignant neoplasm, and children with congenital immunodeficiency syndromes. Although decreasing in frequency because of effective prophylaxis and antiretroviral therapy, PCP remains one of the most common serious opportunistic infections in infants and children with perinatally acquired HIV infection. Although onset of disease can occur at any age, including rare instances during the first month of life, PCP most commonly occurs in HIV-infected children in the first year of life, with peak incidence at 3 through 6 months of age. The mode of transmission is unknown. Animal studies have demonstrated animal-to-animal transmission by the airborne route; evidence suggests airborne transmission among humans. Evidence also exists for vertical transmission. Although reactivation of latent infection with immunosuppression has been proposed as an explanation for disease after the first 2 years of life, animal models of PCP do not support the existence of latency. Studies of patients with acquired immunodeficiency syndrome (AIDS) with more than one episode of PCP suggest reinfection rather than relapse. In patients with cancer, the disease can occur during remission or relapse. The period of communicability is unknown.

The **incubation period** is unknown, but reports of human outbreaks of PCP in transplant recipients have demonstrated a median of 53 days from exposure to clinically apparent infection.

DIAGNOSTIC TESTS: A definitive diagnosis of PCP is made by visualization of organisms in lung tissue or respiratory tract secretion specimens. The most sensitive and specific diagnostic procedures involve specimen collection from open lung biopsy and, in older children, transbronchial biopsy. However, bronchoscopy with bronchoalveolar lavage, induction of sputum in older children and adolescents, and intubation with deep endotracheal aspiration are less invasive, can be diagnostic, and are sensitive in patients with HIV infection who have a large number of *Pneumocystis* organisms. Methenamine silver, toluidine blue O, calcofluor white, and fluorescein-conjugated monoclonal antibody are the most useful stains for identifying the thick-walled cysts of *P jirovecii*. Extracystic trophozoite forms are identified with Giemsa stain, modified Wright-Giemsa stain, and fluorescein-conjugated monoclonal antibody stain. The sensitivity of all microscopy-based methods depends on the skill of the laboratory technician. Polymerase chain reaction assays for detecting *P jirovecii* infection have been shown to be sensitive even with noninvasive isolates, such as oral wash or expectorated sputum, but are not yet available commercially.

TREATMENT[1]: The drug of choice is intravenous trimethoprim-sulfamethoxazole (TMP-SMX) (see Drugs for Parasitic Infections, p 848), usually administered intravenously. Oral therapy should be reserved for patients with mild disease who do not have malabsorption or diarrhea or for patients with a favorable clinical response to initial intravenous therapy. Duration of therapy is 21 days. The rate of adverse reactions to TMP-SMX (eg, rash, neutropenia, anemia, thrombocytopenia, renal toxicity, hepatitis, nausea, vomiting, and diarrhea) is higher in HIV-infected children than in non–HIV-infected patients. It is not necessary to discontinue therapy for most mild adverse reactions. At least half of the

---

[1] Centers for Disease Control and Prevention. Guidelines for prevention and treatment of opportunistic infections among HIV-exposed and HIV-infected children. Recommendations from CDC, the National Institutes of Health, the HIV Medicine Association of the Infectious Diseases Society of America, the Pediatric Infectious Disease Society, and the American Academy of Pediatrics. *MMWR Recomm Rep*. 2009;58 (RR-11):1–166. Available at: **http://aidsinfo.nih.gov/contentfiles/Pediatric_OI.pdf**

patients with more severe reactions (excluding anaphylaxis) requiring interruption of therapy subsequently will tolerate TMP-SMX if rechallenged after the reaction resolves.

Intravenously administered pentamidine is an alternative drug for children and adults who cannot tolerate TMP-SMX or who have severe disease and have not responded to TMP-SMX after 5 to 7 days of therapy. The therapeutic efficacy of intravenous pentamidine in adults with PCP is similar to that of TMP-SMX. Pentamidine is associated with a high incidence of adverse reactions, including pancreatitis, diabetes mellitus, renal toxicity, electrolyte abnormalities, hypoglycemia, hyperglycemia, hypotension, cardiac arrhythmias, fever, and neutropenia. If a recipient of didanosine requires pentamidine, didanosine should not be administered until 1 week after pentamidine therapy has been completed because of overlapping toxicities.

Atovaquone is approved for oral treatment of mild to moderate PCP in adults who are intolerant of TMP-SMX. Experience with use of atovaquone in children is limited. Adverse reactions to atovaquone are limited to rash, nausea, and diarrhea. Other potentially useful drugs in adults include clindamycin with primaquine (adverse reactions are rash, nausea, and diarrhea), dapsone with trimethoprim (associated with neutropenia, anemia, thrombocytopenia, methemoglobinemia, rash, and transaminase elevation), and trimetrexate with leucovorin. Experience with the use of these combinations in children is limited.

In patients with AIDS, prophylaxis should be initiated at the end of therapy for acute infection and should be continued until 6 months after CD4+ T-lymphocyte cell count and percentage exceed the values designated as requiring prophylaxis (see Table 3.52, p 585) or lifelong if CD4+ T-lymphocyte cells do not exceed these thresholds in response to antiretroviral therapy.

Corticosteroids appear to be beneficial in treatment of HIV-infected adults with moderate to severe PCP (as defined by an arterial oxygen pressure [PaO_2] of less than 70 mm Hg in room air or an arterial-alveolar gradient of more than 35 mm Hg). For adolescents older than 13 years of age and adults, the recommended dose of oral prednisone is 80 mg/day in 2 divided doses for the first 5 days of therapy; 40 mg, once daily, on days 6 through 10; and 20 mg, once daily, on days 11 through 21. Studies have shown that use of corticosteroids can lead to reduced acute respiratory failure, decreased need for ventilation, and reduced mortality in children with PCP. Although no controlled studies of the use of corticosteroids in young children have been performed, most experts would recommend corticosteroids as part of therapy for children with moderate to severe PCP disease. On the basis of limited available data, a recommended regimen of oral prednisone for children younger than 13 years of age is 1 mg/kg/dose, twice daily for the first 5 days of therapy; 0.5 mg/kg/dose, twice daily on days 6 through 10; and 0.5 mg/kg, once daily on days 11 through 21.

Chemoprophylaxis. Chemoprophylaxis is highly effective in preventing PCP among some high-risk groups. Prophylaxis against a first episode of PCP is indicated for many patients with significant immunosuppression, including people with HIV infection (see Human Immunodeficiency Virus Infection, p 418) and people with primary or acquired cell-mediated immunodeficiency.

In HIV-infected children, risk of PCP is associated with age-specific CD4+ T-lymphocyte cell counts and percentages that define severe immunosuppression (Immune Category 3 [see Table 3.26, p 422]). Because CD4+ T-lymphocyte cell counts and percentages can decline rapidly in HIV-infected infants, prophylaxis for PCP is

Table 3.52. Recommendations for *Pneumocystis jirovecii* Pneumonia (PCP) Prophylaxis for Human Immunodeficiency Virus (HIV)-Exposed Infants and Children, by Age and HIV Infection Status[a]

Age and HIV Infection Status	PCP prophylaxis[b]
Birth through 4 to 6 wk of age, HIV exposed or HIV infected	No prophylaxis
4 to 6 wk through 12 mo of age	
HIV infected or indeterminate	Prophylaxis
HIV infection presumptively or definitively excluded[c]	No prophylaxis
1 through 5 y of age, HIV infected	Prophylaxis if: CD4+ T-lymphocyte count is less than 500 cells/μL or percentage is less than 15%[d]
6 y of age or older, HIV infected	Prophylaxis if: CD4+ T-lymphocyte count is less than 200 cells/μL or percentage is less than 15%[d]

[a]Centers for Disease Control and Prevention. Guidelines for prevention and treatment of opportunistic infections in HIV-exposed and HIV-infected children. Recommendations from CDC, the National Institutes of Health, the HIV Medicine Association of the Infectious Diseases Society of America, the Pediatric Infectious Diseases Society, and the American Academy of Pediatrics. *MMWR Recomm Rep.* 2009;58(RR-11):1–166. Available at: **http://aidsinfo.nih.gov/contentfiles/Pediatric_OI.pdf**

[b]Children who have had PCP should receive lifelong ("secondary") PCP prophylaxis unless/until their CD4+ T-lymphocyte cell counts and percentages achieve and maintain designated age-specific values greater than those indicative of severe immunosuppression (Immune Category 3) for at least 6 months (see Human Immunodeficiency Virus Infection, Table 3.26, p 422).

[c] In nonbreastfeeding HIV-exposed infants with no positive virologic test results or other laboratory or clinical evidence of HIV infection, HIV presumptively can be excluded on the basis of 2 negative virologic test results, 1 performed at 2 weeks of age or older and 1 performed at 4 weeks of age or older, on 1 negative virologic test result performed at 8 weeks of age or older, or on 1 negative HIV antibody test performed at 6 months of age or older. HIV definitively can be excluded on the basis of 2 negative virologic test results, 1 performed at 4 weeks of age or older and 1 performed at 4 months of age or older, or on 2 negative HIV antibody test results from 2 separate specimens obtained at 6 months of age or older (see Human Immunodeficiency Virus Infection, p 418).

[d]Prophylaxis should be considered on a case-by-case basis for children who might otherwise be at risk of PCP, such as children with rapidly declining CD4+ T-lymphocyte cell counts or percentages or children with Clinical Category C status of HIV infection.

recommended for all infants born to HIV-infected women with indeterminate HIV status beginning at 4 to 6 weeks of age and continuing until 12 months of age unless a diagnosis of HIV has been excluded presumptively or definitively, in which case prophylaxis should be discontinued (see Table 3.52). Children who are HIV infected or whose HIV status is indeterminate should continue prophylaxis throughout the first year of life.

For HIV-infected children 12 months of age or older, PCP prophylaxis should be continued or initiated in the following circumstances: (1) any CD4+ T-lymphocyte cell count or percentage that indicates severe immunosuppression for age (Immune Category 3 [see Table 3.26, p 422, and Table 3.52]); (2) a rapidly decreasing CD4+ T-lymphocyte cell count or percentage; or (3) severely symptomatic HIV disease (Clinical Category C; see Human Immunodeficiency Virus Infection, p 418, and Table 3.52]). Indications for PCP prophylaxis are the same for children and adolescents, except for different age-specific definitions of severely suppressed CD4+ T-lymphocyte cell counts and percentages warranting prophylaxis (see Table 3.26, p 422, and Table 3.52). PCP prophylaxis also is recommended for adolescent and adults with a history of oropharyngeal candidiasis.

Primarily on the basis of demonstrated low risk of PCP in adults and adolescents who discontinue primary or secondary (ie, initiated following an episode of PCP) PCP prophylaxis following reconstitution of their CD4+ T-lymphocyte cell counts and percentages to designated threshold values in response to antiretroviral therapy, discontinuation of PCP prophylaxis also should be considered for children who achieve and maintain designated age-specific minimum CD4+ T-lymphocyte cell counts and percentages that exceed values indicative of severe immunosuppression for at least 3 months (see Table 3.52, p 585).

HIV-infected children older than 1 year of age who are not receiving PCP prophylaxis (eg, children not previously identified as infected or children whose PCP prophylaxis was discontinued) should begin or resume prophylaxis if their CD4+ T-lymphocyte cell counts and percentages indicate severe immunosuppression (see Table 3.52, p 585).

Prophylaxis for PCP is recommended for children who have received hematopoietic stem cell transplants (HSCTs)[1] or solid organ transplants; children with hematologic malignancies (eg, leukemia or lymphoma) and some nonhematologic malignancies; children with severe cell-mediated immunodeficiency, including children who received adrenocorticotropic hormone for treatment of infantile spasm; and children who otherwise are immunosuppressed and who have had a previous episode of PCP. In general, for this diverse group of immunocompromised hosts, the risk of PCP increases with duration and intensity of chemotherapy, other immunosuppressive therapies, and neutropenia as well as with coinfection with immunosuppresive viruses (eg, cytomegalovirus) and rates of PCP for similar patients in a given locale. Consequently, the recommended duration of PCP prophylaxis will vary depending on individual circumstances. Guidelines for allogeneic HSCT recipients[1] recommend that PCP prophylaxis be initiated at engraftment (or before engraftment, if engraftment is delayed) and administered for at least 6 months. It should be continued for more than 6 months in all children receiving ongoing or intensified immunosuppressive therapy (eg, prednisone or cyclosporin) or in children with chronic graft-versus-host disease. Guidelines for PCP prophylaxis for solid organ transplant recipients are less definitive, but some authorities suggest durations ranging from 6 months to 1 year for renal transplants and from 1 year to life for heart, lung, and liver transplants.

The recommended drug regimen for PCP prophylaxis for all immunocompromised patients is TMP-SMX administered orally on 3 consecutive days each week (see Table 3.53, p 587). Alternatively, TMP-SMX can be administered daily, 7 days a week. For patients who cannot tolerate TMP-SMX, alternative choices include oral atovaquone or dapsone. Atovaquone is effective and safe but expensive. Dapsone is effective and inexpensive but associated with more serious adverse effects than atovaquone. Aerosolized pentamidine is recommended for children who cannot tolerate TMP-SMX, atovaquone, or dapsone and are old enough to use a Respirgard II nebulizer. Intravenous pentamidine has been used but is more toxic than other regimens and is not recommended for prophylaxis. Other drugs with potential for prophylaxis include pyrimethamine plus dapsone plus leucovorin or pyrimethamine-sulfadoxine. Experience with these drugs in adults and children for this indication is limited. These agents should be considered only in situations in which recommended regimens are not tolerated or cannot be used for other reasons.

---

[1] Centers for Disease Control and Prevention. Guidelines for preventing opportunistic infections among hematopoietic stem cell transplant recipients. Recommendations of CDC, the Infectious Diseases Society of America, and the American Society of Blood and Marrow Transplantation. *MMWR Recomm Rep.* 2000;49(RR-10):1–128. Also see **www.aidsinfo.nih.gov/**

Table 3.53. Drug Regimens for *Pneumocystis jirovecii* Pneumonia Prophylaxis for Children 4 Weeks of Age and Older[a]

Recommended regimen:

Trimethoprim-sulfamethoxazole (trimethoprim, 150 mg/m^2 [or 5 mg/kg] per day, with sulfamethoxazole, 750 mg/m^2 [or 25 mg/kg] per day), orally, in divided doses twice a day, 3 times per week on consecutive days (eg, Monday-Tuesday-Wednesday)

Acceptable alternative trimethoprim-sulfamethoxazole dosage schedules:

- Trimethoprim (150 mg/m^2 per day) with sulfamethoxazole (750 mg/m^2 per day), orally, **as a single daily dose,** 3 times per week on consecutive days (eg, Monday-Tuesday-Wednesday)
- Trimethoprim (150 mg/m^2 per day) with sulfamethoxazole (750 mg/m^2 per day), orally, in divided doses, twice a day, and **administered 7 days per week**
- Trimethoprim (150 mg/m^2 per day) with sulfamethoxazole (750 mg/m^2 per day), orally, in divided doses twice a day, and administered 3 times per week on alternate days (eg, Monday-Wednesday-Friday)

Alternative regimens if trimethoprim-sulfamethoxazole is not tolerated:

- **Dapsone (children 1 mo of age or older)**
  2 mg/kg (maximum 100 mg), orally, once a day or 4 mg/kg (maximum 200 mg), orally, every week
- **Aerosolized pentamidine (children 5 y of age or older)**
  300 mg, inhaled monthly via Respirgard II nebulizer
- **Atovaquone**
  - **children 1 through 3 mo of age and older than 24 mo through 12 y of age:** 30 mg/kg (maximum 1500 mg), orally, once a day
  - **children 4 through 24 mo of age:** 45 mg/kg (maximum 1500 mg), orally, once a day
  - **children older than 12 y:** 1500 mg, orally, once a day

[a]Centers for Disease Control and Prevention. Guidelines for prevention and treatment of opportunistic infections in HIV-exposed and HIV-infected children. Recommendations from CDC, the National Institutes of Health, the HIV Medicine Association of the Infectious Diseases Society of America, the Pediatric Infectious Diseases Society, and the American Academy of Pediatrics. *MMWR Recomm Rep.* 2009;58(RR-11):1–166. Available at: **http://aidsinfo.nih.gov/contentfiles/Pediatric_OI.pdf**

ISOLATION OF THE HOSPITALIZED PATIENT: Standard precautions are recommended. Some experts recommend that patients with PCP not share a room with other immunocompromised patients, especially patients who are not receiving chemoprophylaxis, although data are insufficient to support this recommendation as standard practice.

CONTROL MEASURES: Appropriate therapy for infected patients and prophylaxis in immunocompromised patients are the only available means of control. Detailed guidelines for children, adolescents, and adults infected with HIV have been issued by the Centers for Disease Control and Prevention and the Infectious Diseases Society of America.[1,2]

[1] Centers for Disease Control and Prevention. Guidelines for prevention of opportunistic infections in HIV-infected adults and adolescents: recommendations from the CDC, the National Institutes of Health, and the HIV Medicine Association of the Infectious Diseases Society of America. *MMWR Recomm Rep.* 2009;58(RR-4):1–207

[2] Centers for Disease Control and Prevention. Guidelines for prevention and treatment of opportunistic infections in HIV-exposed and HIV-infected children. Recommendations from CDC, the National Institutes of Health, the HIV Medicine Association of the Infectious Diseases Society of America, the Pediatric Infectious Diseases Society, and the American Academy of Pediatrics. *MMWR Recomm Rep.* 2009;58(RR-11):1–166. Available at: **http://aidsinfo.nih.gov/contentfiles/Pediatric_OI.pdf**

Poliovirus Infections

CLINICAL MANIFESTATIONS: Approximately 72% of poliovirus infections in susceptible children are asymptomatic. Nonspecific illness with low-grade fever and sore throat (minor illness) occurs in 24% of people who become infected. Aseptic meningitis, sometimes with paresthesias, occurs in 1% to 5% of patients a few days after the minor illness has resolved. Rapid onset of asymmetric acute flaccid paralysis with areflexia of the involved limb occurs in fewer than 1% of infections, and residual paralytic disease involving the motor neurons (paralytic poliomyelitis) occurs in approximately two thirds of people with acute motor neuron disease. Cranial nerve involvement (bulbar poliomyelitis, often showing a tripod sign) and paralysis of respiratory tract muscles can occur. Findings in cerebrospinal fluid (CSF) are characteristic of viral meningitis with mild pleocytosis and lymphocytic predominance.

Adults who contracted paralytic poliomyelitis during childhood may develop the noninfectious postpolio syndrome 15 to 40 years later. Postpolio syndrome is characterized by slow and irreversible exacerbation of weakness most likely occurring in those muscle groups involved during the original infection. Muscle and joint pain also are common manifestations. The prevalence and incidence of postpolio syndrome is unclear. Studies estimate the range of postpolio syndrome in poliomyelitis survivors is from 25% to 40%.

ETIOLOGY: Polioviruses are group C RNA enteroviruses and consist of serotypes 1, 2, and 3.

EPIDEMIOLOGY: Poliovirus infections occur only in humans. Spread is by the fecal-oral and respiratory routes. Infection is more common in infants and young children and occurs at an earlier age among children living in poor hygienic conditions. In temperate climates, poliovirus infections are most common during summer and autumn; in the tropics, the seasonal pattern is less pronounced.

The last reported case of poliomyelitis attributable to indigenously acquired, wild-type poliovirus in the United States occurred in 1979 during an outbreak among unimmunized people that resulted in 10 paralytic cases. The only identified imported case of paralytic poliomyelitis since 1986 occurred in 1993 in a child transported to the United States for medical care. Since 1986, all other cases acquired in the United States have been vaccine-associated paralytic poliomyelitis (VAPP) occurring in vaccine recipients or their contacts and attributable to oral poliovirus (OPV) vaccine. From 1980 to 1997, the average annual number of cases of VAPP reported in the United States was 8. Fewer VAPP cases were reported in 1998 and 1999, after a shift in United States immunization policy from use of OPV to a sequential inactivated poliovirus (IPV) vaccine beginning in 1997. Implementation of an all-IPV vaccine schedule in 2000 essentially ended the occurrence of VAPP cases in the United States. In 2005, however, a healthy, unimmunized young adult from the United States acquired VAPP abroad during a study program in Central America, most likely from an infant grandchild of the host family who recently had been immunized with OPV. In 2005, a type 1 vaccine-derived poliovirus was identified in the stool of an asymptomatic, unimmunized, immunodeficient child in Minnesota. Subsequently, poliovirus infections in 7 other unimmunized children (35% of all children tested) within the index patient's community were documented. None of the infected children had paralysis. Phylogenetic analysis suggested that the vaccine-derived poliovirus circulated in the community for approximately 2 months before the infant's infection was detected and that the initiating OPV dose had been given (likely in another country) before the index child's birth. In 2009, a woman with longstanding common-variable immunodeficiency was diagnosed with VAPP and died of polio-associated complications. Molecular characterization of the poliovirus isolated suggested that the infection likely occurred approximately 12 years earlier, coinciding with OPV immunization of her child. Circulation of indigenous wild-type poliovirus strains ceased in the United States several decades ago, and the risk of contact with imported wild-type polioviruses has decreased, in parallel with the success of the global eradication program.

Communicability of poliovirus is greatest shortly before and after onset of clinical illness, when the virus is present in the throat and excreted in high concentration in feces. Virus persists in the throat for approximately 2 weeks after onset of illness and is excreted in feces for 3 to 6 weeks. Patients potentially are contagious as long as fecal excretion persists. In recipients of OPV vaccine, virus persists in the throat for 1 to 2 weeks and is excreted in feces for several weeks, although in rare cases, excretion for more than 2 months can occur. Immunocompromised patients with significant B-lymphocyte immune deficiencies have excreted virus for periods of more than 20 years.

The **incubation period** of nonparalytic poliomyelitis is 3 to 6 days. For the onset of paralysis in paralytic poliomyelitis, the incubation period usually is 7 to 21 days.

DIAGNOSTIC TESTS: Poliovirus can be detected in specimens from the pharynx, feces, urine, and rarely, cerebrospinal fluid by isolation in cell culture or polymerase chain reaction (PCR). Two or more stool and throat swab specimens for enterovirus isolation should be obtained at least 24 hours apart from patients with suspected paralytic polio-myelitis as early in the course of illness as possible, ideally within 14 days of onset of symptoms. Fecal material is most likely to yield virus in cell culture. However, in immuno-compromised patients, poliovirus may be excreted intermittently, and a negative test does not rule out infection.

Because OPV vaccine no longer is available in the United States, the chance of expo-sure to vaccine-type polioviruses has become remote. Therefore, if a poliovirus is isolated in the United States, the isolate should be reported promptly to the state health depart-ment and sent to the Centers for Disease Control and Prevention through the state health department for further testing. The diagnostic test of choice for confirming poliovirus dis-ease is viral culture of stool specimens and throat swab specimens obtained as early in the course of illness as possible. Interpretation of acute and convalescent serologic test results can be difficult.

TREATMENT: Supportive.

ISOLATION OF THE HOSPITALIZED PATIENT: In addition to standard precautions, contact precautions are indicated for infants and young children for the duration of hospitalization.

CONTROL MEASURES:

Immunization of Infants and Children.

Vaccines. The 2 types of poliovirus vaccines are IPV vaccine, administered parenterally (subcutaneously or intramuscularly), and live OPV vaccine, administered orally. IPV is the only poliovirus vaccine available in the United States. IPV vaccine contains the 3 types of poliovirus grown in Vero cells and inactivated with formaldehyde. IPV vaccine also is available in combination with other childhood vaccines (see Table 1.8, p 35). OPV vac-cine contains attenuated poliovirus types 1, 2, and 3 produced in monkey kidney cells or human diploid cells.

Immunogenicity and Efficacy. Both IPV and OPV vaccines in their recommended schedules are highly immunogenic and effective in preventing poliomyelitis. Administration of IPV vaccine results in seroconversion in 95% or more of vaccine recipients to each of the 3 serotypes after 2 doses and results in seroconversion in 99% to 100% of recipients after 3 doses. Immunity probably is lifelong. Following exposure to live polioviruses, most IPV-immunized children will excrete virus from stool but not from the oropharynx. Stool excretion quantities and duration are reduced compared with shedding from unimmunized people. Immunization with 3 or more doses of OPV vaccine induces excellent serum antibody responses and a variable degree of intestinal immunity against poliovirus reinfection. A 3-dose series of OPV vaccine, as formerly used in the United States, results in sustained, probably lifelong immunity.

Administration With Other Vaccines. Either IPV or OPV vaccine may be given concurrently with other routinely recommended childhood vaccines (see Simultaneous Administration of Multiple Vaccines, p 33). For administration of combination vaccines containing IPV (see Table 1.8, p 35) with other vaccines and interchangeability of the combined vaccine with other vaccine products, see Pertussis (p 553), Hepatitis B (p 369), *Haemophilus influenzae* (p 345), and *Streptococcus pneumoniae* infections (p 668).

Adverse Reactions. No serious adverse events have been associated with use of IPV vaccine. Because IPV vaccine may contain trace amounts of streptomycin, neomycin, and polymyxin B, allergic reactions are possible in recipients with hypersensitivity to one or more of these antimicrobial agents.

OPV vaccine can cause VAPP. Before exclusive use of IPV vaccine in the United States, the overall risk of VAPP associated with OPV vaccine was approximately 1 case per 2.4 million doses of OPV vaccine distributed. The rate of VAPP after the first dose, including vaccine recipient and contact cases, was approximately 1 case per 750 000 doses.

Schedule.[1,2] Four doses of IPV vaccine are recommended for routine immunization of all infants and children in the United States.

- The first 2 doses of the 4-dose IPV vaccine series should be given at 2-month intervals beginning at 2 months of age (minimum age, 6 weeks), and a third dose is recommended at 6 through 18 months of age. Doses may be given at 4-week intervals when accelerated protection is indicated.
- Administration of the third dose at 6 months of age has the potential advantage of enhancing the likelihood of completion of the primary series and does not compromise seroconversion.
- A fourth and final dose in the series should be administered at 4 years of age or older and at a minimum interval of 6 months from the third dose.
- The final dose in the IPV vaccine series should be administered at 4 years of age or older regardless of the number of previous doses; a fourth dose is not necessary if the third dose was given at 4 years of age or older and a minimum of 6 months after the second dose.

---

[1] Centers for Disease Control and Prevention. Updated recommendations of the Advisory Committee on Immunization Practices (ACIP) regarding routine poliovirus vaccination. *MMWR Morb Mortal Wkly Rep.* 2009;58(30):829–830

[2] American Academy of Pediatrics, Committee on Infectious Diseases. Poliovirus. *Pediatrics.* 2011;128(4):805–808

- When IPV vaccine is given in combination with other vaccines at 2, 4, 6, and 12 through 15 months of age, it is necessary to administer a fifth and final dose of IPV vaccine at 4 years of age or older. The minimum interval from dose 4 to dose 5 should be at least 6 months.
- If a child misses an IPV vaccine dose at 4 through 6 years of age, the child should receive a booster dose as soon as feasible.

OPV vaccine remains the vaccine of choice for global eradication, although IPV vaccine may be adopted more widely to augment OPV vaccine in areas where poliomyelitis has been difficult to control. OPV vaccine no longer is licensed or available in the United States.

Children Incompletely Immunized. Children who have not received the recommended doses of poliovirus vaccines on schedule should receive sufficient doses of IPV vaccine to complete the immunization series for their age (see Fig 1.3, p 31).

Vaccine Recommendations for Adults. Most adults residing in the United States are presumed to be immune as a result of previous immunization and have a small risk of exposure to wild-type poliovirus in the United States. Immunization is recommended only for certain adults who are at a greater risk of exposure to wild-type polioviruses than the general population, including the following:

- Travelers to areas or countries where poliomyelitis is or may be epidemic or endemic;
- Members of communities or specific population groups with disease caused by wild-type polioviruses;
- Laboratory workers handling specimens that may contain wild-type polioviruses; and
- Health care personnel in close contact with patients who may be excreting wild-type polioviruses.

For unimmunized adults, primary immunization with IPV vaccine is recommended. Two doses of IPV vaccine should be given at intervals of 1 to 2 months (4–8 weeks); a third dose is given 6 to 12 months after the second dose unless the risk of exposure is increased, such as when traveling to areas where wild-type poliovirus is known to be circulating. If time does not allow 3 doses of IPV vaccine to be given according to the recommended schedule before protection is required, the following alternatives are recommended:

- If protection is not needed until 8 weeks or more, 3 doses of IPV vaccine should be administered at least 4 weeks apart.
- If protection is not needed for 4 to 8 weeks, 2 doses of IPV vaccine should be administered at least 4 weeks apart.
- If protection is needed in fewer than 4 weeks, a single dose of IPV vaccine should be administered.

The remaining doses of IPV vaccine to complete the primary immunization schedule should be given subsequently at the recommended intervals if the person remains at an increased risk.

Recommendations in other circumstances are as follows:

- **Incompletely immunized adults.** Adults who previously received less than a full primary course of OPV or IPV vaccine should be given the remaining required doses of IPV vaccine regardless of the interval since the last dose and the type of vaccine that was received previously.

- **Adults who are at an increased risk of exposure to wild-type poliovirus and who previously completed primary immunization with OPV or IPV vaccine.** These adults can receive a single dose of IPV vaccine.

Precautions and Contraindications to Immunization.

Immunocompromised People. Immunocompromised patients, including people with human immunodeficiency virus (HIV) infection; combined immunodeficiency; abnormalities of immunoglobulin synthesis (ie, antibody deficiency syndromes); leukemia, lymphoma, or generalized malignant neoplasm; or people receiving immunosuppressive therapy with pharmacologic agents (see Immunocompromised Children, p 74) or radiation therapy should receive IPV vaccine. A protective immune response to IPV vaccine in an immunocompromised patient cannot be ensured.

Household Contacts of Immunocompromised People or People With Altered Immune States, Immunosuppression Attributable to Therapy for Other Disease, or Known HIV Infection. IPV vaccine is recommended for these people, and OPV vaccine should not be used. If OPV vaccine inadvertently is introduced into a household of an immunocompromised or HIV-infected person, close contact between the patient and the OPV vaccine recipient should be minimized for approximately 4 to 6 weeks after immunization. Household members should be counseled on practices that will minimize exposure of the immunocompromised or HIV-infected person to excreted poliovirus vaccine. These practices include exercising hand hygiene after contact with the child by all and avoiding diaper changing by the immunosuppressed person.

Pregnancy. Immunization during pregnancy generally should be avoided for reasons of theoretical risk, although no convincing evidence indicates that rates of adverse reactions to IPV vaccine are increased in pregnant women or in their developing fetuses. If immediate protection against poliomyelitis is needed, IPV vaccine is recommended.

Hypersensitivity or Anaphylactic Reactions to IPV Vaccine or Antimicrobial Agents Contained in IPV. The IPV vaccine is contraindicated for people who have experienced an anaphylactic reaction after a previous dose of IPV vaccine or to streptomycin, neomycin, or polymyxin B.

Breastfeeding and mild diarrhea are not contraindications to IPV or OPV vaccine administration.

Reporting of Adverse Events After Immunization. All cases of VAPP and other serious adverse events associated temporally with poliomyelitis vaccine should be reported (see Reporting of Adverse Events, p 44).

Case Reporting and Investigation. A suspected case of poliomyelitis or isolation of a poliovirus should be reported promptly to the state health department and should result in an immediate epidemiologic investigation. Poliomyelitis should be considered in the differential diagnosis of all cases of acute flaccid paralysis, including Guillain-Barré syndrome and transverse myelitis. If the course is compatible clinically with poliomyelitis, specimens should be obtained for virologic studies (see Diagnostic Tests, p 589). If evidence implicates wild-type or a genetically drifted vaccine-derived poliovirus infection, an intensive investigation will be conducted, and a public health decision will be made about the need for supplementary immunizations, choice of vaccine, and other action.

Polyomaviruses (BK Virus and JC Virus)

CLINICAL MANIFESTATIONS: BK virus (BKV) and JC virus (JCV) infections in immunocompetent children generally are asymptomatic. However, because of the tropism of BKV for the genitourinary tract epithelium, it may cause asymptomatic hematuria or cystitis in healthy children. In immunocompromised people, BKV is more likely to cause disease, including hemorrhagic cystitis in hematopoietic stem cell transplant recipients, and interstitial nephritis and ureteral stenosis in renal transplant recipients. The primary symptom of BKV-associated hemorrhagic cystitis is painful hematuria. Passage of blood clots in the urine and secondary obstructive nephropathy can occur in patients with BKV-associated hemorrhagic cystitis. BKV-associated nephropathy occurs in 3% to 8% of renal transplant recipients and less frequently in other solid organ transplant recipients. BKV-associated nephropathy should be suspected in any renal transplant patient with allograft dysfunction. More than 50% of patients with BKV-associated nephropathy experience renal allograft loss.

JCV is the cause of progressive multifocal leukoencephalopathy (PML) that occurs in severely immune-compromised patients, including patients with acquired immunodeficiency syndrome (AIDS), patients receiving intensive chemotherapy, and patients receiving various monoclonal antibody therapies for immune suppression. PML, the only known disease caused by JCV, occurs in approximately 5% of untreated adults with AIDS but is rare in children with AIDS. PML is a demyelinating disease of the central nervous system. Symptoms include cognitive disturbance, hemiparesis, ataxia, cranial nerve dysfunction, and aphasia. Lytic infection of oligodendrocytes by JCV is the primary mechanism of pathogenesis for PML. In the absence of restored T-lymphocyte function, PML almost always is fatal. PML is an AIDS-defining illness in human immunodeficiency virus (HIV)-infected people.[1]

Simian virus 40 (SV40) is a polyomavirus of Asian macaque monkeys and was a contaminant of some lots of Sabin and Salk poliovirus vaccines between 1955 and 1963. Recently, 7 additional polyomaviruses have been detected in humans. The KI polyomavirus (KIPyV) and WU polyomavirus (WUPyV) have been identified in respiratory tract secretions, primarily in association with known pathogenic viruses of the respiratory tract. The Merkel cell polyomavirus (MCPyV) has been detected in >80% of Merkel cell carcinomas, which are rare neuroendocrine tumors of the skin. Human polyomaviruses 6 and 7 (HPyV6 and HPyV7) have been detected as asymptomatic inhabitants of human skin. The trichodysplasia spinulosa-associated polyomavirus (TSPyV) has been identified in tissue from patients with trichodysplasia spinulosa, a rare follicular disease of immunocompromised patients that primarily affects the face. Human polyomavirus 9 (HPyV9) has been detected in the serum of some renal transplant recipients. The natural history, prevalence, and pathogenic potential of these recently discovered human polyomaviruses have not yet been established.

---

[1] Centers for Disease Control and Prevention. Guidelines for prevention and treatment of opportunistic infections among HIV-exposed and HIV-infected children. Recommendations from CDC, the National Institutes of Health, the HIV Medicine Association of the Infectious Diseases Society of America, the Pediatric Infectious Diseases Society, and the American Academy of Pediatrics. *MMWR Recomm Rep.* 2009;58(RR-11):1–166. Available at: **http://aidsinfo.nih.gov/contentfiles/Pediatric_OI.pdf**

ETIOLOGY: Nine known human polyomaviruses belong to the family Polyomaviridae. They are nonenveloped viruses with a circular dsDNA genome with icosahedral symmetry ranging 40 to 50 nm in diameter. The genome of the polyomaviruses is approximately 5 kilobase pairs in length and encodes 5 major proteins—3 for capsid proteins VP1, VP2, and VP3 and 2 for large T and small t antigens. One of the biological characteristics of polyomavirus is the maintenance of a chronic viral infection in their host with little or no symptoms. Diseases caused by human polyomavirus infections are most common among immunosuppressed people.

EPIDEMIOLOGY: Humans are the only known natural hosts for BKV and JCV. The mode of transmission of BKV and JCV is uncertain, but respiratory route and oral route by water or food have been postulated for their transmission. BKV and JCV are ubiquitous in the human population, with BKV infection occurring in early childhood and JCV infection occurring primarily in adolescence and adulthood. BKV persists in the kidney, gastrointestinal tract, and leukocytes of healthy subjects, with urinary excretion occurring in 3% to 5% of healthy adults. JCV persists in the kidney and brain of healthy people. The prevalence of urinary excretion of JCV increases with age.

DIAGNOSTIC TESTS: Antibody assays commonly are used to detect the presence of specific antibodies against individual viruses, and nucleic acid-based polymerase chain reaction assays are the most sensitive tools for rapid viral screening for polyomaviruses and quantification of viral load. Detection of BKV T-antigen by immunohistochemical analysis of renal biopsy material is the gold standard for diagnosis of BKV-associated nephropathy. Visualization of BKV particles in a renal biopsy specimen by electron microscopy is a sensitive alternative to immunohistochemical analysis. Prospective monitoring of BK viral load in plasma commonly is used after renal transplantation. Detection of BKV nucleic acid in plasma by polymerase chain reaction (PCR) assay is associated with an increased risk of BKV-associated nephropathy, especially when BKV viral loads exceed 10 000 genomes/mL. However, detection of BKV in urine of renal transplant recipients is common and does not predict BKV disease after renal transplantation.

The diagnosis of BKV-associated hemorrhagic cystitis is made clinically when other causes of urinary tract bleeding are excluded. Among hematopoietic stem cell transplant recipients, detection of BKV in urine is common (more than 50%), but BKV-associated hemorrhagic cystitis is much less common (10%–15%). Prolonged urinary shedding of BKV and detection of BKV in plasma after hematopoietic stem cell transplantation has been associated with increased risk of developing BKV-associated hemorrhagic cystitis. Urine cytologic testing may suggest urinary shedding of BKV on the basis of presence of decoy cells, which resemble renal carcinoma cells. However, decoy cells do not have high sensitivity or specificity for BKV disease.

A confirmed diagnosis of PML requires a compatible clinical syndrome and magnetic resonance imaging or computed tomographic findings showing lesions in the brain coupled with brain biopsy findings. JCV can be demonstrated by in situ hybridization, electron microscopy, or immunohistochemistry. Diagnosis of PML can be facilitated when JCV DNA is detected in cerebrospinal fluid by a nucleic acid amplification test, which may obviate the need for a brain biopsy. Early in the course of PML, false-negative PCR assay results have been reported, so repeat testing is warranted when clinical suspicion of PML is high. Measurement of JCV DNA concentrations in cerebrospinal fluid samples may be a useful marker for managing PML in patients with AIDS who are receiving antiretroviral therapy (ART).

TREATMENT: There have been no controlled clinical trials of antiviral agents active against BKV or JCV. In patients with biopsy-confirmed BKV-associated nephropathy, reduction of immune suppression may prevent allograft loss. Treatment of adult renal transplant recipients with BKV-associated nephropathy with cidofovir is being evaluated in a National Institutes of Health study being conducted by the Collaborative Antiviral Study Group; leflunomide also has been used as a therapeutic agent in this population, albeit with limited clinical evaluation. The role of Immune Globulin Intravenous (IGIV) in the treatment of BKV-associated nephropathy is uncertain. In renal transplant patients with BKV plasma viral loads greater than 10 000 genomes/mL, judicious reduction of immune suppression has been shown to prevent development of BKV-associated nephropathy without increasing the risk of rejection.

Most patients with BKV-hemorrhagic cystitis after hematopoietic stem cell transplantation require only supportive care, because restoration of immune function by stem cell engraftment ultimately will control BKV replication. Cidofovir and leflunomide have been used in hematopoietic stem cell transplant recipients who have prolonged BKV hemorrhagic cystitis attributable to failure of engraftment. In severe cases, surgical intervention may be required to stop bladder hemorrhage.

Restoration of immune function (eg, ART for patients with AIDS) is necessary for survival of patients with PML. Cidofovir sometimes is used but has not been shown to be effective in producing clinical improvement.

ISOLATION OF THE HOSPITALIZED PATIENT: Standard precautions are recommended.

CONTROL MEASURES: None.

Prion Diseases:
Transmissible Spongiform Encephalopathies

CLINICAL MANIFESTATIONS: Transmissible spongiform encephalopathies (TSEs or prion diseases) constitute a group of rare, rapidly progressive, universally fatal neurodegenerative diseases of humans and animals that are characterized by neuronal degeneration, spongiform change, gliosis, and accumulation of abnormal misfolded protease-resistant amyloid protein (protease-resistant prion protein [PrP^{res}], variably called scrapie prion protein [PrP^{sc}] or, as suggested by the World Health Organization [WHO], TSE-associated PrP [PrP^{TSE}]) that is distributed diffusely throughout the brain and sometimes also in discrete plaques.

Human TSEs include several diseases: Creutzfeldt-Jakob disease (CJD), Gerstmann-Sträussler-Scheinker disease, fatal familial and sporadic insomnia, kuru, and variant CJD (vCJD, caused by the agent of bovine spongiform encephalopathy, popularly called "mad cow" disease). Classic CJD can be sporadic (approximately 85% of cases), familial (approximately 15% of cases), or iatrogenic (fewer than 1% of cases). Sporadic CJD most commonly is a disease of older adults (median age of death, 68 years in the United States) but also rarely has been described in adolescents older than 13 years of age and young adults. Iatrogenic CJD has been acquired through intramuscular injection of contaminated cadaveric pituitary hormones (growth hormone and human gonadotropin), dura mater allografts, corneal transplantation, and contaminated instrumentation of the brain at neurosurgery or depth-electrode electroencephalographic recording. In 1996, an outbreak of vCJD linked to exposure to tissues from BSE-infected cattle was reported in the

United Kingdom. Since the end of 2003, 4 presumptive cases of transfusion-transmitted vCJD have been reported: 3 clinical cases as well as 1 probable asymptomatic transfusion-transmitted vCJD infection in which prion protein was detected in spleen and lymph node but not brain. A fifth iatrogenic vCJD infection in the UK, also preclinical, was attributed to treatment with plasma-derived coagulation factor VIII. The best-known TSEs affecting animals include scrapie of sheep, BSE, and a chronic wasting disease of North American deer, elk, and moose (**www.cdc.gov/ncidod/dvrd/cwd/**). Except for vCJD, thought to result from infection with the BSE agent, no other human TSE has been attributed convincingly to infection with an agent of animal origin.

CJD manifests as a rapidly progressive, dementia-causing illness with defects in memory, personality, and other higher cortical functions. At presentation, approximately one third of patients have cerebellar dysfunction, including ataxia and dysarthria. Iatrogenic CJD also may manifest as dementia with cerebellar signs. Myoclonus develops in at least 80% of affected patients at some point in the course of disease. Death usually occurs in weeks to months (median, 4–5 months); approximately 10% to 15% of patients with sporadic CJD survive for more than 1 year.

vCJD is distinguished from classic CJD by younger age of onset, early "psychiatric" manifestations, and other features, such as painful sensory symptoms, delayed onset of overt neurologic signs, absence of diagnostic electroencephalographic changes, and a more prolonged duration of illness. In vCJD, the neuropathologic examination reveals numerous "florid" plaques (surrounded by vacuoles) and exceptionally striking accumulation of PrP^{TSE} in the brain. In addition, PrP^{TSE} often is detectable in lymphoid tissues of patients with vCJD. In vCJD, but not in classic CJD, a high proportion of people exhibit high signal abnormalities on T2-weighted brain magnetic resonance imaging in the pulvinar region of the posterior thalamus (known as the "pulvinar sign").

ETIOLOGY: The infectious particle or prion responsible for human and animal prion diseases is thought by many authorities to be the abnormal form of normal ubiquitous PrP glycoprotein, without a nucleic acid component. Proponents of the prion hypothesis postulate that sporadic CJD arises from a rare spontaneous structural change of the normal "cellular" protease-sensitive host-encoded glycoprotein (PrP^C or PrP^{sen}) found on the surface of neurons and many other cells in both humans and animals. Conformational changes are postulated to be propagated by a "recruitment" reaction (the nature of which is unknown), in which abnormal PrP^{TSE} serves as a template or lattice for the conversion of neighboring PrP^C molecules.

EPIDEMIOLOGY: Classic CJD is rare, occurring at a rate of approximately 1 case per million people annually. The onset of disease peaks in the 60- through 74-year age group. Familial CJD illnesses, which are associated with a variety of mutations of the PrP-encoding gene (PRNP) on chromosome 20, occur at approximately one sixth the frequency of sporadic CJD, with onset of disease approximately 10 years earlier than sporadic CJD. Case-control studies of sporadic CJD have not identified any consistent environmental risk factor. No statistically significant increase in cases of sporadic CJD has been observed in people previously treated with blood, blood components, or plasma derivatives (see Blood Safety: Reducing the Risk of Transfusion-Transmitted Infections, p 114). The incidence of sporadic CJD is not increased in patients with several diseases associated with frequent exposure to blood or blood products, specifically hemophilia A and B, thalassemia, and sickle cell disease, suggesting that the risk of transfusion transmission of classic CJD, if any, is very low and appropriately regarded as theoretical. CJD has not been reported in infants born to infected mothers.

As of November 2011 (**www.cjd.ed.ac.uk/vcjdworld.htm**), the total number of primary cases of vCJD reported was 173 patients in the United Kingdom, 25 in France, 5 in Spain, 4 in Ireland, 3 in the United States, 3 in the Netherlands, 2 in Portugal, 2 in Italy, 2 in Canada, and 1 each in Taiwan, Japan, and Saudi Arabia. Two of the 3 patients in the United States, 2 of the 4 in Ireland, and 1 each of the patients in France and Canada are believed to have acquired vCJD during prolonged residence in the United Kingdom. The Centers for Disease Control and Prevention has concluded that the third vCJD patient in the United States probably was infected during his prolonged residence as a child in Saudi Arabia. Authorities suspect that the Japanese patient was infected during a short visit of 24 days to the United Kingdom, 12 years before the onset of vCJD. Most patients with vCJD were younger than 30 years of age, and several were adolescents. All but 5 of the 174 United Kingdom patients with noniatrogenic vCJD died before 60 years of age, and all but 15 died before 50 (median age at death is 28 years and 87% of cases died before age 40). On the basis of animal inoculation studies, comparative PrP immunoblotting, and epidemiologic investigations, almost all cases of vCJD are believed to have resulted from exposure to tissues from cattle infected with BSE. As noted, 4 patients are believed to have been infected with vCJD through blood transfusion and 1 from injections of human plasma-derived clotting factor.

The **incubation period** for iatrogenic CJD varies by route of exposure and ranges from 1.5 to more than 30 years.

DIAGNOSTIC TESTS: The diagnosis of human prion diseases can be made with certainty only by neuropathologic examination of affected brain tissue, best obtained at autopsy. In most patients with classic CJD, a characteristic 1-cycle to 2-cycles per second triphasic sharp-wave discharge on electroencephalographic tracing has been described. The likelihood of finding this abnormality is enhanced when serial electroencephalographic recordings are obtained. A protein assay that detects the 14-3-3 protein in cerebrospinal fluid (CSF) has been reported to be reasonably sensitive, although not specific, as a marker for CJD. Measurement of the Tau protein level in addition to the detection of 14-3-3 protein in the CSF has been reported to increase the specificity of CSF testing for CJD. No validated blood test is available. A progressive neurologic syndrome in a person bearing a known pathogenic mutation of the PRNP gene (not a normal polymorphism) is presumed to be prion disease. Because no unique nucleic acid has been detected in the infectious particles of TSEs, genome amplification studies, such as PCR, are not possible. Consideration of brain biopsies for patients with possible CJD should be given when some other potentially treatable disease remains in the differential diagnosis. Complete postmortem examination of the brain is encouraged to confirm the clinical diagnosis and to detect emerging forms of CJD, such as vCJD. State-of-the-art diagnostic testing, including assays of 14-3-3 and Tau proteins in CSF, PRNP gene sequencing, Western blot analysis to identify and characterize PrP^{TSE}, and histologic processing of brain tissues with expert neuropathologic consultation are offered free of charge by the National Prion Disease Pathology Surveillance Center (telephone, 216-368-0587; **www.cjdsurveillance.com**).

TREATMENT: No treatment has been shown in humans to slow or stop the progressive neurodegeneration in prion diseases. Experimental treatments are being studied. Supportive therapy is necessary to manage dementia, spasticity, rigidity, and seizures occurring during the course of the illness. Psychological support may help families of affected people. Genetic counseling is indicated in familial disease, taking into account that penetrance has been variable in some kindreds in which people with a PRNP mutation survived to an advanced age without neurodegenerative disease. A family support and patient advocacy group, the CJD Foundation (telephone 330-665-5590; **www.cjdfoundation.org**), offers helpful information and advice.

ISOLATION OF THE HOSPITALIZED PATIENT: Standard precautions are recommended. Available evidence indicates that even prolonged intimate contact with CJD-infected people has not resulted in transmission of disease. Tissues associated with high levels of infectivity (eg, brain, eyes, and spinal cord of affected people) and instruments in contact with those tissues are considered biohazards; incineration, prolonged autoclaving at high temperature and pressure after thorough cleaning, and especially exposure to a solution of 1 N or greater sodium hydroxide or a solution of 5.25% or greater sodium hypochlorite (undiluted household chlorine bleach) for 1 hour has been reported to decrease infectivity of contaminated surgical instruments.[1] Detailed CJD infection-control recommendations, distribution of infectivity in various tissues, and specific decontamination protocols are available at **www.cdc.gov/ncidod/dvrd/cjd/qa_cjd_infection_control.htm.** Person-to-person transmission of classic CJD by blood, milk, saliva, urine, or feces has not been reported. These body fluids should be handled using standard infection control procedures; universal blood precautions should be sufficient to prevent bloodborne transmission.

CONTROL MEASURES: Immunization against prion diseases is not available, and no protective immune response to infection has been demonstrated. Iatrogenic transmission of CJD through cadaveric pituitary hormones has been obviated by use of recombinant products. Recognition that CJD can be spread by transplantation of infected dura and corneas and that vCJD can be spread by blood transfusion has led to more stringent donor-selection criteria and improved collection protocols. Health care professionals should follow their state's prion disease reporting requirements, and any suspected or confirmed diagnosis of CJD (eg, suspected iatrogenic disease or vCJD) should be reported promptly to the appropriate state or local health departments and to the Centers for Disease Control and Prevention (telephone, 404-639-3091; **www.cdc.gov/ncidod/dvrd/prions/**). Current precautionary policies of the US Food and Drug Administration to reduce the risk of transmitting CJD by human blood or blood products are accessible on the Internet at **www.fda.gov/downloads/BiologicsBloodVaccines/GuidanceComplianceRegulatoryInformation/Guidances/UCM213415.pdf.** General information about BSE is available from the FDA at **www.fda.gov/AnimalVeterinary/ResourcesforYou/AnimalHealthLiteracy/ucm136222.htm,** from the USDA at **www.fsis.usda.gov/Fact_Sheets/Bovine_Spongiform_Encephalopathy_Mad_Cow_Disease/index.asp,** and from the World Organisation for Animal Health at **www.oie.int/en/animal-health-in-the-world/bse-portal/.**

---

[1] **www.cdc.gov/ncidod/dvrd/prions**

Q Fever

CLINICAL MANIFESTATIONS: Although approximately 50% of infections are asymptomatic, symptomatic Q fever occurs in 2 forms: acute and chronic; each form can present as fever of undetermined origin. Q fever in children typically is characterized by abrupt onset of fever often accompanied by chills, headache, weakness, cough, and other nonspecific systemic symptoms. Illness typically is self-limited, although a relapsing febrile illness lasting for several months has been documented in children. Gastrointestinal tract symptoms, such as diarrhea, vomiting, abdominal pain, and anorexia, are reported in 50% to 80% of children. Rash, although uncommon, can occur in young children. Q fever pneumonia usually manifests as mild cough, respiratory distress, and chest pain. Chest radiographic patterns are variable. More severe manifestations of acute Q fever are rare but include hepatitis, hemolytic-uremic syndrome, myocarditis, pericarditis, cerebellitis, encephalitis, meningitis, hemophagocytosis, lymphadenitis, acalculous cholecystitis, and rhabdomyolysis. Chronic Q fever is rare in children but can present as blood culture-negative endocarditis, chronic relapsing or multifocal osteomyelitis, or chronic hepatitis. Children who are immunocompromised or have underlying valvular heart disease may be a higher risk for chronic Q fever.

ETIOLOGY: *Coxiella burnetii,* the cause of Q fever, formerly was considered to be a *Rickettsia* organism but is an obligate gram-negative intracellular bacterium that belongs to the order Legionellaceae. The infectious form of *C burnetii* is highly resistant to heat, desiccation, and disinfectant chemicals and can persist for long periods of time in the environment. *C burnetii* is classified in the gamma subgroup of Proteobacteria. *C burnetii* is a potential agent of bioterrorism.

EPIDEMIOLOGY: Q fever is a zoonotic infection that has been reported worldwide, including the United States. In animals, *C burnetii* infection usually is asymptomatic. The most common reservoirs for human infection are domestic farm animals (eg, sheep, goats, and cows). Cats, dogs, rodents, marsupials, other mammalian species, and some wild and domestic bird species also may serve as reservoirs. Tick vectors may be important for maintaining animal and bird reservoirs but are not thought to be important in transmission to humans. Humans typically acquire infection by inhalation of *C burnetii* in fine-particle aerosols generated from birthing fluids of infected animals during animal parturition or through inhalation of dust contaminated by these materials. Infection also can occur by exposure to contaminated materials, such as wool, straw, bedding, or laundry. Windborne particles containing infectious organisms can travel a half-mile or more, contributing to sporadic cases for which no apparent animal contact can be demonstrated. Unpasteurized dairy products can contain the organism. Seasonal trends occur in farming areas with predictable frequency, and the disease often coincides with the lambing season in early spring.

The **incubation period** usually is 14 to 22 days, with a range from 9 to 39 days, depending on the inoculum size. Chronic Q fever can develop months or years after initial infection.

DIAGNOSTIC TESTS: Isolation of *C burnetii* from blood can be performed only in special laboratories because of the potential hazard to laboratory workers. The diagnosis of Q fever is established through serologic testing. Serologic evidence of a fourfold increase in phase II immunoglobulin (Ig) G by indirect immunofluorescent antibody (IFA) assay between paired sera taken 2 to 4 weeks apart establishes the diagnosis of acute infection. A single high serum phase II IgG titer ($\geq$1:128) by IFA may be considered evidence of probable infection. Acute Q fever also is diagnosed by detection of *C burnetii* in infected tissues by using immunohistochemical staining or DNA detection methods. Confirmation of chronic Q fever is based on an increasing phase 1 IgG titer (typically $\geq$1:800) that is often is higher than phase II IgG *and* an identifiable nidus of infection (eg, endocarditis, vascular infection, osteomyelitis, chronic hepatitis). The FDA has approved a nucleic acid amplification test to diagnose early stages of Q fever infections in military personnel serving overseas.

TREATMENT: Acute Q fever generally is a self-limited illness, and many patients recover without antimicrobial therapy. Doxycycline (2 mg/kg every 12 hours; maximum 100 mg/dose) is the drug of choice for severe infections in patients of any age and treatment is recommended for 14 days (see Tetracyclines, p 801). Appropriate therapy, if initiated within 3 days of illness onset, can lessen the severity of illness and hasten recovery. Children younger than 8 years of age with mild illness, pregnant women, and patients allergic to doxycycline can be treated with trimethoprim-sulfamethoxazole. Chronic Q fever is much more difficult to treat, and relapses can occur despite appropriate therapy, necessitating repeated courses of therapy. The recommended therapy for chronic Q fever endocarditis is a combination of doxycycline and hydroxychloroquine for a minimum of 18 months. Surgical replacement of the infected valve may be necessary in some patients.

ISOLATION OF THE HOSPITALIZED PATIENT: Standard precautions are recommended.

CONTROL MEASURES: Strict adherence to proper hygiene when handling parturient animals can help decrease the risk of infection in the farm setting as can ensuring consumption of pasteurized milk and milk products. Improved prescreening of animal herds used by research facilities may decrease the risk of infection. Special safety practices are recommended for nonpropagative laboratory procedures involving *C burnetii* and for all propagative procedures, necropsies of infected animals, and manipulation of infected human and animal tissues. Vaccines for domestic animals and people working in high-risk occupations have been developed but are not licensed in the United States. Q fever is a nationally reportable disease, and all human cases should be reported to the state health department. For additional information about Q fever, see **www.cdc.gov/qfever/index.html** or **www.bt.cdc.gov/agent/qfever/clinicians/index.asp.**

Rabies[1]

CLINICAL MANIFESTATIONS: Infection with rabies virus and other lyssaviruses characteristically produces an acute illness with rapidly progressive central nervous system manifestations, including anxiety, radicular pain, dysesthesia or pruritus, hydrophobia, and dysautonomia. Some patients may have paralysis. Illness almost invariably progresses to death. Three unimmunized people have recovered from clinical rabies in the United States.[2] The differential diagnosis of acute encephalitic illnesses of unknown cause

---

[1] For further information, see Centers for Disease Control and Prevention. Human rabies prevention: United States, 2008. Recommendations of the Advisory Committee on Immunization Practices. *MMWR Recomm Rep.* 2008;57(RR-3):1–28

[2] Centers for Disease Control and Prevention. Recovery of a patient from clinical rabies—California, 2011. *MMWR Morb Mortal Wkly Rep.* 2012;61(4):61–65

with atypical focal neurologic signs or with features of Guillain-Barré syndrome should include rabies.

ETIOLOGY: Rabies virus is an RNA virus classified in the Rhabdoviridae family, Lyssavirus genus.

EPIDEMIOLOGY: Understanding the epidemiology of rabies has been aided by viral variant identification using monoclonal antibodies and nucleotide sequencing. In the United States, human cases have decreased steadily since the 1950s, reflecting widespread immunization of dogs and the availability of effective prophylaxis after exposure to a rabid animal. Between 2000 and 2009, 24 of 31 cases of human rabies reported in the United States were acquired indigenously. Among the 24 indigenously acquired cases, 18 were associated with bat rabies virus variants, and 4 had a history of bat exposure and had rabies virus antibodies in serum or cerebrospinal fluid (CSF) samples but had no rabies virus antigens detected. Despite the large focus of rabies in raccoons in the eastern United States, only 1 human death has been attributed to the raccoon rabies virus variant. Historically, 2 cases of human rabies were attributable to probable aerosol exposure in laboratories, and 2 unusual cases have been attributed to possible airborne exposures in caves inhabited by millions of bats, although alternative infection routes cannot be discounted. Transmission also has occurred by transplantation of organs, corneas, and other tissues from patients dying of undiagnosed rabies. Person-to-person transmission by bite has not been documented in the United States, although the virus has been isolated from saliva of infected patients.

Wildlife rabies perpetuates throughout all of the 50 United States except Hawaii, which remains "rabies free." Wildlife, including bats, raccoons, skunks, foxes, coyotes, and bobcats, are the most important potential sources of infection for humans and domestic animals in the United States. Rabies in small rodents (squirrels, hamsters, guinea pigs, gerbils, chipmunks, rats, and mice) and lagomorphs (rabbits, pikas, and hares) is rare. Rabies may occur in woodchucks or other large rodents in areas where raccoon rabies is common. The virus is present in saliva and is transmitted by bites or, rarely, by contamination of mucosa or skin lesions by saliva or other potentially infectious material (eg, neural tissue). Worldwide, most rabies cases in humans result from dog bites in areas where canine rabies is enzootic. Most rabid dogs, cats, and ferrets may shed virus for a few days before there are obvious signs of illness. No case of human rabies in the United States has been attributed to a dog, cat, or ferret that has remained healthy throughout the standard 10-day period of confinement.

The **incubation period** in humans averages 1 to 3 months but ranges from days to years.

DIAGNOSTIC TESTS: Infection in animals can be diagnosed by demonstration of virus-specific fluorescent antigen in brain tissue. Suspected rabid animals should be euthanized in a manner that preserves brain tissue for appropriate laboratory diagnosis. Virus can be isolated in suckling mice or in tissue culture from saliva, brain, and other specimens and can be detected by identification of viral antigens or nucleotides in affected tissues. Diagnosis in suspected human cases can be made postmortem by either immunofluorescent or immunohistochemical examination of brain tissue. Antemortem diagnosis can be made by fluorescent microscopy of skin biopsy specimens from the nape of the neck, by isolation of the virus from saliva, by detection of antibody in serum in unimmunized people or in CSF, and by detection of viral nucleic acid in saliva, skin, or other affected tissues. No single test sufficiently is sensitive. Laboratory personnel should be consulted before submission of specimens to the Centers for Disease Control and Prevention so that appropriate collection and transport of materials can be arranged.

TREATMENT: Once symptoms have developed, neither rabies vaccine nor Rabies Immune Globulin (RIG) improves the prognosis. There is no specific treatment. Very few patients with human rabies have survived, even with intensive supportive care. Since 2004, 2 adolescent females and an 8-year-old girl, all of whom had not received rabies postexposure prophylaxis, survived rabies after receipt of a combination of sedation and intensive medical intervention.[1] Details of the protocol used can be found at **www.mcw. edu/rabies.**

ISOLATION OF THE HOSPITALIZED PATIENT: Standard precautions are recommended for the duration of illness. If the patient has bitten another person or the patient's saliva has contaminated an open wound or mucous membrane, the involved area should be washed thoroughly and postexposure prophylaxis should be administered (see Care of Exposed People, p 604).

CONTROL MEASURES: In the United States, animal rabies is common. Education of children to avoid contact with stray or wild animals is of primary importance. Inadvertent contact of family members and pets with potentially rabid animals, such as raccoons, foxes, coyotes, and skunks, may be decreased by securing garbage and pet food outdoors to decrease attraction of domestic and wild animals. Similarly, chimneys and other potential entrances for wildlife, including bats, should be identified and covered. Bats should be excluded from human living quarters. International travelers to areas with endemic canine rabies should be warned to avoid exposure to stray dogs, and if traveling to an area with enzootic infection where immediate access to medical care and biologic agents is limited, preexposure prophylaxis is indicated.

Exposure Risk and Decisions to Give Prophylaxis. Exposure to rabies results from a break in the skin caused by the teeth of a rabid animal or by contamination of scratches, abrasions, or mucous membranes with saliva or other potentially infectious material, such as neural tissue, from a rabid animal. The decision to immunize a potentially exposed person should be made in consultation with the local health department, which can provide information on risk of rabies in a particular area for each species of animal and in accordance with the guidelines in Table 3.54, p 603. In the United States, all mammals are believed to be susceptible, but bats, raccoons, skunks, and foxes are more likely to be infected than are other animals. Coyotes, cattle, dogs, cats, ferrets, and other animals occasionally are infected. Bites of rodents (such as squirrels, mice, and rats) or lagomorphs (rabbits, hares, and pikas) rarely require prophylaxis. Additional factors must be considered when deciding whether immunoprophylaxis is indicated. An unprovoked attack may be more suggestive of a rabid animal than a bite that occurs during attempts to feed or handle an animal. Properly immunized dogs, cats, and ferrets have only a minimal chance of developing rabies. However, in rare instances, rabies has developed in properly immunized animals.

Postexposure prophylaxis for rabies is recommended for all people bitten by wild mammalian carnivores or bats or by high-risk domestic animals that may be infected. Postexposure prophylaxis is recommended for people who report an open wound, scratch,

---

[1] Centers for Disease Control and Prevention. Recovery of a patient from clinical rabies—California, 2011. *MMWR Morb Mortal Wkly Rep.* 2012;61(4):61–65

Table 3.54. Rabies Postexposure Prophylaxis Guide

Animal Type	Evaluation and Disposition of Animal	Postexposure Prophylaxis Recommendations
Dogs, cats, and ferrets	Healthy and available for 10 days of observation	Prophylaxis only if animal develops signs of rabies[a]
	Rabid or suspected of being rabid[b]	Immediate immunization and RIG[c]
	Unknown (escaped)	Consult public health officials for advice
Bats, skunks, raccoons, foxes, and most other carnivores; woodchucks	Regarded as rabid unless geographic area is known to be free of rabies or until animal proven negative by laboratory tests[b]	Immediate immunization and RIG[c]
Livestock, rodents, and lagomorphs (rabbits, hares, and pikas)	Consider individually	Consult public health officials; bites of squirrels, hamsters, guinea pigs, gerbils, chipmunks, rats, mice and other rodents, rabbits, hares, and pikas almost never require antirabies prophylaxis

RIG indicates Rabies Immune Globulin.

[a] During the 10-day observation period, at the first sign of rabies in the biting dog, cat, or ferret, prophylaxis of the exposed person with RIG (human) and vaccine should be initiated. The animal should be euthanized immediately and tested.

[b] The animal should be euthanized and tested as soon as possible. Holding for observation is not recommended. Immunization is discontinued if immunofluorescent test result for the animal is negative.

[c] See text.

or mucous membrane that has been contaminated with saliva or other potentially infectious material (eg, brain tissue) from a rabid animal. Because the injury inflicted by a bat bite or scratch may be small and not readily evident or the circumstances of contact may preclude accurate recall (eg, a bat in a room of a sleeping person or previously unattended child), prophylaxis may be indicated for situations in which a bat physically is present in the same room if a bite or mucous membrane exposure cannot reliably be excluded, unless prompt testing of the bat has excluded rabies virus infection. Prophylaxis should be initiated as soon as possible after bites by known or suspected rabid animals.

Postexposure prophylaxis is recommended for people who report a possibly infectious exposure (eg, bite, scratch, or open wound or mucous membrane contaminated with saliva or other infectious material, such as CSF or brain tissue) to a human with rabies. Rabies virus transmission after exposure to a human with rabies has not been documented convincingly in the United States, except after tissue or organ transplantation from donors who died of unsuspected rabies encephalitis. Casual contact with an infected person (eg, by touching a patient) or contact with noninfectious fluids or tissues (eg, blood or feces) alone does not constitute an exposure and is not an indication for prophylaxis (see Care of Hospital Contacts, below).

Handling of Animals Suspected of Having Rabies. A dog, cat, or ferret that is suspected of having rabies and has bitten a human should be captured, confined, and observed by a veterinarian for 10 days. Any illness in the animal should be reported immediately to the local health department. If signs of rabies develop, the animal should be euthanized in a manner to allow its head to be removed and shipped under refrigeration (not frozen, which would delay testing) to a qualified laboratory for examination.

Other biting animals that may have exposed a person to rabies should be reported immediately to the local health department. Management of animals depends on the species, the circumstances of the bite, and the epidemiology of rabies in the area. Previous immunization of an animal may not preclude the necessity for euthanasia and testing. Because clinical manifestations of rabies in a wild animal cannot be interpreted reliably, a wild mammal suspected of having rabies should be euthanized at once, and its brain should be examined for evidence of rabies virus infection. The exposed person need not receive prophylaxis if the result of rapid examination of the brain by the direct fluorescent antibody test is negative for rabies virus infection.

Care of Hospital Contacts. Immunization of hospital contacts of a patient with rabies should be reserved for people who were bitten or whose mucous membranes or open wounds have come in contact with saliva, CSF, or brain tissue of a patient with rabies (see Care of Exposed People). Other hospital contacts of a patient with rabies do not require prophylaxis.

Care of Exposed People.

Local Wound Care. The immediate objective of postexposure prophylaxis is to prevent virus from entering neural tissue. Prompt and thorough local treatment of all lesions is essential, because virus may remain localized to the area of the bite for a variable time. All wounds should be flushed thoroughly and cleaned with soap and water. Quaternary ammonium compounds (such as benzalkonium chloride) no longer are considered superior to soap. The need for tetanus prophylaxis and measures to control bacterial infection also should be considered. The wound, if possible, should not be sutured.

Prophylaxis (see Table 3.54, p 603). After wound care is completed, concurrent use of passive *and* active prophylaxis is optimal, with the exceptions of people who previously have received complete immunization regimens (preexposure or postexposure) with a cell culture vaccine and people who have been immunized with other types of rabies vaccines and previously have had a documented rabies virus-neutralizing antibody titer; these people should receive only vaccine. Prophylaxis should begin as soon as possible after exposure, ideally within 24 hours. However, a delay of several days or more may not compromise effectiveness, and prophylaxis should be initiated if reasonably indicated, regardless of the interval between exposure and initiation of therapy. In the United States, only the human product RIG is available for passive immunization. Licensed tissue culture rabies vaccine should be used for active immunization. Physicians can obtain expert counsel from their local or state health departments.

Active Immunization (Postexposure). The immunization schedule has been shortened.[1] Three rabies vaccines are licensed commercially for prophylaxis in the United States: human diploid cell vaccine (HDCV), rabies vaccine adsorbed (RVA), and purified chicken embryo cell vaccine (PCECV), but only HDCV and PCECV are available for use in the United States (see Table 3.55, p 605). A 1.0-mL dose of vaccine is given intramuscularly in the deltoid area or anterolateral aspect of the thigh on the first day of postexposure prophylaxis (day 0), and repeated doses are given on days 3, 7, and 14 after

[1] Rupprecht CE, Briggs D, Brown CM, et al. Use of a reduced (4-dose) vaccine schedule for postexposure prophylaxis to prevent human rabies: recommendations of the Advisory Committee on Immunization Practices. *MMWR Recomm Rep.* 2010;59(RR-2):1–9

Table 3.55. US Food and Drug Administration-Licensed Rabies Vaccines[a] and Rabies Immune Globulin Products

Category	Product	Manufacturer	Dose and Route of Administration
Human rabies vaccine	Human diploid cell vaccine (HDCV) (Imovax)	Sanofi Pasteur	1 mL, IM
	Purified chicken embryo cell vaccine (PCECV) (RabAvert)	Novartis Vaccines and Diagnostics	1 mL, IM
Rabies Immune Globulin	Imogam Rabies-HT	Sanofi Pasteur	20 IU/kg, infiltrate around wound[b]
	HyperRab S/D	Talecris Biotherapeutics	20 IU/kg, infiltrate around wound[b]

IM indicates intramuscular.
[a] Rabies vaccine adsorbed (RVA) is licensed in the United States but no longer is distributed in the United States.
[b] Any remaining volume should be administered IM.

the first dose, for a total of 4 doses. Ideally, an immunization series should be initiated and completed with 1 vaccine product unless serious allergic reactions occur. Clinical studies evaluating efficacy or frequency of adverse reactions when the series is completed with a second product have not been conducted. The volume of the dose is not decreased for children. The number of doses recommended for people with altered immunocompetence has not changed; for such people, postexposure prophylaxis should be continued to comprise a 5-dose vaccination regimen with 1 dose of RIG. Serologic testing to document seroconversion after administration of a rabies vaccine series is unnecessary but occasionally has been advised for recipients who may be immunocompromised. Testing will not be useful if RIG also was administered, unless sufficient time has elapsed since RIG administration.

Care should be taken to ensure that the vaccine is administered intramuscularly. Intradermal vaccine is not advised for postexposure prophylaxis in the United States, although for reasons of cost and availability, intradermal regimens are used in some countries. Because virus-neutralizing antibody responses in adults who received vaccine in the gluteal area sometimes have been less than in those who were injected in the deltoid muscle, the deltoid site always should be used except in infants and young children, in whom the anterolateral thigh is the appropriate site.

- **Adverse reactions and precautions with HDCV and PCECV.** Reactions are uncommon in children. In adults, local reactions, such as pain, erythema, and swelling or itching at the injection site, are reported in 15% to 25%, and mild systemic reactions, such as headache, nausea, abdominal pain, muscle aches, and dizziness, are reported in 10% to 20% of recipients. Several cases of neurologic illness resembling Guillain-Barré syndrome that resolved without sequelae in 12 weeks and an acute, generalized, transient neurologic syndrome temporally associated with HDCV have been reported but are not thought to be related causally. A case of acute disseminated encephalomyelitis resulting in death has been reported after immunization with HDCV.

  Immune complex-like reactions in people receiving booster doses of HDCV have been observed, possibly because of interaction between propiolactone contained in the vaccine and human albumin. The reaction, characterized by onset 2 to 21 days after inoculation, begins with generalized urticaria and can include arthralgia, arthritis, angioedema, nausea, vomiting, fever, and malaise. The reaction is not life threatening, occurs in as many as 6% of adults receiving booster doses as part of a preexposure immunization regimen, and is rare in people receiving primary immunization with HDCV. Similar allergic reactions with primary or booster doses have been reported with PCECV.

If the patient has a serious allergic reaction to HDCV, PCECV may be given according to the same schedule as HDCV, and vice-versa. All suspected serious, systemic, neuroparalytic, or anaphylactic reactions to the rabies vaccine should be reported immediately to the Vaccine Adverse Events Reporting System (see Reporting of Adverse Events, p 44).

Although safety of rabies vaccine during pregnancy has not been studied specifically in the United States, pregnancy should not be considered a contraindication to use of vaccine after exposure.

- *Nerve tissue vaccines.* Inactivated nerve tissue vaccines are not licensed in the United States but are available in many areas of the world. These preparations induce neuroparalytic reactions in 1 in 2000 to 1 in 8000 recipients. Immunization with nerve tissue vaccine should be discontinued if meningeal or neuroparalytic reactions develop. Corticosteroids should be used only for life-threatening reactions, because they increase the risk of rabies in experimentally inoculated animals.

Passive Immunization. Human RIG should be used concomitantly with the first dose of vaccine for postexposure prophylaxis to bridge the time between possible infection and antibody production induced by the vaccine (see Table 3.55, p 605). If vaccine is not available immediately, RIG should be administered alone, and immunization should be started as soon as possible. If RIG is not available immediately, vaccine should be administered and RIG administered subsequently if obtained within 7 days after initiating immunization. If administration of both vaccine and RIG is delayed, both should be used regardless of the interval between exposure and treatment, within reason.

The recommended dose of RIG is 20 IU/kg. As much of the dose as possible should be used to infiltrate the wound(s), if present. The remainder is given intramuscularly. In cases of multiple severe wounds in which RIG is insufficient for infiltration, dilution in saline solution to an adequate volume (twofold or threefold) has been recommended to ensure that all wound areas receive infiltrate. For children with a small muscle mass, it may be necessary to administer RIG at multiple sites. Human RIG is supplied in 2-mL (300 IU) and 10-mL (1500 IU) vials. Passive antibody can inhibit the response to rabies vaccines; therefore, the recommended dose should not be exceeded. Vaccine never should be administered in the same parts of the body or with the same syringe used to give RIG. Hypersensitivity reactions to RIG are rare.

Purified equine RIG containing rabies antibodies may be available outside the United States and generally is accompanied by a low rate of serum sickness (less than 1%). Equine RIG is administered at a dose of 40 IU/kg, and desensitization may be required.

Administration of RIG is not recommended for the following exposed people: (1) people who received postexposure prophylaxis with HDCV, RVA, or PCECV for a previous exposure; (2) people who received a 3-dose, intramuscular, preexposure regimen of HDCV, RVA, or PCECV; (3) people who received a 3-dose, intradermal, preexposure regimen of HDCV with the product used in the United States; and (4) people who have a documented adequate rabies virus antibody titer after previous immunization with any other rabies vaccine. These people should receive two 1.0-mL booster doses of HDCV or PCECV; 1 dose is given on the day of exposure, and the second dose is given 3 days later.

Preexposure Control Measures, Including Immunization. The relatively low frequency of reactions to HDCV and PCECV has made provision of preexposure immunization practical for people in high-risk groups, including veterinarians, animal handlers, certain laboratory workers, and people moving to areas where canine rabies is common. Others, such as spelunkers (cavers), who may have frequent exposures to bats and other wildlife, also should be considered for preexposure prophylaxis.

HDCV and PCECV are licensed for intramuscular administration. Previously, intradermal (0.1 mL) dosage formulations of HDCV were available for preexposure use. The preexposure immunization schedule is three 1-mL intramuscular injections each, given on days 0, 7, and 21 or 28. This series of immunizations has resulted in development of rabies virus-neutralizing antibodies in all people properly immunized. Therefore, routine serologic testing for antibody immediately after primary immunization is not indicated.

Serum antibodies usually persist for 2 years or longer after the primary series is administered intramuscularly. Preexposure booster immunization with 1.0 mL of HDCV or PCEC intramuscularly will produce an effective anamnestic response. Rabies virus-neutralizing antibody titers should be determined at 6-month intervals for people at continuous risk of infection (rabies research laboratory workers, rabies biologics production workers). Titers should be determined approximately every 2 years for people with risk of frequent exposure (rabies diagnostic laboratory workers, spelunkers/cavers, veterinarians and staff, animal-control and wildlife workers in rabies-enzootic areas, and all people who frequently handle bats). A single booster dose of vaccine should be administered only as appropriate to maintain adequate antibody concentrations. The Centers for Disease Control and Prevention currently specifies complete viral neutralization at a titer 1:5 or greater by the rapid fluorescent-focus inhibition test as acceptable; the World Health Organization specifies 0.5 IU/mL or greater as acceptable.

Public Health. A variety of approved public health measures, including immunization of dogs, cats, and ferrets and management of stray dogs and selected wildlife, are used to control rabies in animals.[1] In regions where oral immunization of wildlife with recombinant rabies vaccine is undertaken, the prevalence of rabies among foxes, coyotes, and raccoons may be decreased. Unimmunized dogs, cats, ferrets, or other pets bitten by a known rabid animal should be euthanized immediately. If the owner is unwilling to allow the animal to be euthanized, the animal should be placed in strict isolation for 6 months and immunized 1 month before release. If the exposed animal has been immunized within 1 to 3 years, depending on the vaccine administered and local regulations, the animal should be reimmunized and observed for 45 days.

Case Reporting. All suspected cases of rabies should be reported promptly to public health authorities.

---

[1] National Association of State Public Health Veterinarians Inc. Compendium of animal rabies prevention and control, 2011. *MMWR Recomm Rep.* 2011;60(RR-6):1–15

Rat-Bite Fever

CLINICAL MANIFESTATIONS: Rat-bite fever is caused by *Streptobacillus moniliformis* or *Spirillum minus*. *S moniliformis* infection (streptobacillary fever or Haverhill fever) is characterized by fever, rash, and arthritis. There is an abrupt onset of fever, chills, muscle pain, vomiting, headache, and occasionally, lymphadenopathy. A maculopapular or petechial rash develops, predominantly on the extremities including the palms and soles, typically within a few days of fever onset. The bite site usually heals promptly and exhibits no or minimal inflammation. Nonsuppurative migratory polyarthritis or arthralgia follows in approximately 50% of patients. Untreated infection usually has a relapsing course for a mean of 3 weeks. Complications include soft tissue and solid-organ abscesses, septic arthritis, pneumonia, endocarditis, myocarditis, and meningitis. The case-fatality rate is 7% to 10% in untreated patients, and fatal cases have been reported in young children. With *S minus* infection ("sodoku"), a period of initial apparent healing at the site of the bite usually is followed by fever and ulceration at the site, regional lymphangitis and lymphadenopathy, and a distinctive rash of red or purple plaques. Arthritis is rare. Infection with *S minus* is rare in the United States.

ETIOLOGY: The causes of rat-bite fever are *S moniliformis,* a microaerophilic, gram-negative, pleomorphic bacillus, and *S minus,* a small, gram-negative, spiral organism with bipolar flagellar tufts.

EPIDEMIOLOGY: Rat-bite fever is a zoonotic illness. The natural habitat of *S moniliformis* and *S minus* is the upper respiratory tract of rodents. *S moniliformis* is transmitted by bites or scratches from or exposure to oral secretions of infected rats (eg, kissing the rodent); other rodents (eg, mice, gerbils, squirrels, weasels) and rodent-eating animals, including cats and dogs, also can transmit the infection. Haverhill fever refers to infection after ingestion of unpasteurized milk, water, or food contaminated with *S moniliformis. S minus* is transmitted by bites of rats and mice. *S moniliformis* infection accounts for most cases of rat-bite fever in the United States; *S minus* infections occur primarily in Asia.

The incubation period for *S moniliformis* usually is 3 to 10 days but can be as long as 3 weeks; for *S minus,* the incubation period is 7 to 21 days.

DIAGNOSTIC TESTS: *S moniliformis* is a fastidious, slow-growing organism isolated from specimens of blood, synovial fluid, aspirates from abscesses, or material from the bite lesion by inoculation into bacteriologic media enriched with blood. Cultures should be held up to 3 weeks if *S moniliformis* is suspected. Sodium polyanetholsulfonate (SPS), present in most blood culture media, is inhibitory to *S moniliformis;* therefore, SPS-free media should be used, and the laboratory should be alerted to hold the culture for a longer period of time. *S moniliformis* has been detected using a nucleic acid amplification-based assay. *S minus* has not been recovered on artificial media but can be visualized by darkfield microscopy in wet mounts of blood, exudate of a lesion, and lymph nodes. Blood specimens also should be viewed with Giemsa or Wright stain. *S minus* can be recovered from blood, lymph nodes, or local lesions by intraperitoneal inoculation of mice or guinea pigs.

TREATMENT: Penicillin G procaine administered intramuscularly or penicillin G administered intravenously for 7 to 10 days is the treatment for rat-bite fever caused by either agent. Initial intravenous penicillin G therapy for 5 to 7 days followed by oral penicillin V for 7 days also has been successful. Limited experience exists for ampicillin, cefuroxime, and cefotaxime. Doxycycline or streptomycin or gentamicin can be substituted when a patient has a serious allergy to penicillin. Doxycycline should not be given to children younger than 8 years of age unless the benefits of therapy are greater than the risks of dental staining (see Tetracyclines, p 801). Patients with endocarditis should receive intravenous high-dose penicillin G for at least 4 weeks. The addition of streptomycin or gentamicin for initial therapy may be useful.

ISOLATION OF THE HOSPITALIZED PATIENT: Standard precautions are recommended.

CONTROL MEASURES: Exposed people should be observed for symptoms. Because the occurrence of *S moniliformis* after a rat bite is approximately 10%, some experts recommend postexposure administration of penicillin. Rat control is important in the control of disease. People with frequent rodent exposure should wear gloves and avoid hand-to-mouth contact during animal handling. Regular hand hygiene should be practiced.

Respiratory Syncytial Virus

CLINICAL MANIFESTATIONS: Respiratory syncytial virus (RSV) causes acute respiratory tract infections in people of all ages and is one of the most common diseases of early childhood. Most infants are infected during the first year of life, with virtually all having been infected at least once by the second birthday. Most RSV-infected infants experience upper respiratory tract symptoms, and 20% to 30% develop lower respiratory tract disease (eg, bronchiolitis and/or pneumonia) with their first infection. Signs and symptoms of bronchiolitis may include tachypnea, wheezing, cough, crackles, use of accessory muscles, and nasal flaring. During the first few weeks of life, particularly among preterm infants, infection with RSV may produce minimal respiratory tract signs. Lethargy, irritability, and poor feeding, sometimes accompanied by apneic episodes, may be presenting manifestations in these infants. Most previously healthy infants who develop RSV bronchiolitis do not require hospitalization, and most who are hospitalized improve with supportive care and are discharged in fewer than 5 days. Approximately 1% to 3% of all children in the first 12 months of life will be hospitalized because of RSV lower tract disease. Factors that increase the risk of severe RSV lower respiratory tract illness include preterm birth; cyanotic or complicated congenital heart disease (CHD), especially conditions causing pulmonary hypertension; chronic lung disease of prematurity (CLD [formerly called bronchopulmonary dysplasia]); and immunodeficiency disease or therapy causing immunosuppression at any age. Approximately 400 deaths in young children are attributable to complications of RSV infection annually.

The association between RSV bronchiolitis early in life and subsequent asthma remains poorly understood. RSV bronchiolitis may be associated with short-term or long-term complications that include recurrent wheezing and abnormalities in pulmonary function. This association may reflect an underlying predisposition to asthma rather than a direct consequence of RSV infection.

Reinfection with RSV throughout life is common. RSV infection in older children and adults usually manifests as upper respiratory tract illness. More serious disease involving the lower respiratory tract may develop in older children and adults, especially in immunocompromised patients, the elderly, and in people with cardiopulmonary disease.

ETIOLOGY: RSV is an enveloped, nonsegmented, negative strand RNA virus of the family *Paramyxoviridae*. The virus uses attachment (G) and fusion (F) surface glycoproteins for virus entry; these surface proteins lack neuraminidase and hemagglutinin activities. There is only 1 serotype, but variations in the surface proteins (especially the attachment protein) result in the classification of viruses in 2 major subgroups, designated A and B. Numerous genotypes have been identified in each subgroup, and strains of both subgroups often circulate concurrently in a community. The clinical and epidemiologic significance of strain variation has not been determined, but evidence suggests that antigenic differences may affect susceptibility to infection and that some strains may be more virulent than others.

EPIDEMIOLOGY: Humans are the only source of infection. Transmission usually is by direct or close contact with contaminated secretions, which may occur from exposure to large-particle droplets at short distances (typically <3 feet) or fomites. RSV can persist on environmental surfaces for several hours and for a half-hour or more on hands. Infection among health care personnel and others may occur by hand to eye or hand to nasal epithelium self-inoculation with contaminated secretions. Enforcement of infection-control policies is important to decrease the risk of health care-associated transmission of RSV. Health care-associated spread of RSV to hematopoietic stem cell or solid organ transplant recipients or patients with cardiopulmonary abnormalities or immunocompromised conditions has been associated with severe and fatal disease in children and adults. Children with human immunodeficiency virus (HIV) infection experience extended virus shedding and sometimes prolonged illness but usually do not exhibit greatly enhanced disease.

RSV usually occurs in annual epidemics during winter and early spring in temperate climates. Spread among household and child care contacts, including adults, is common. The period of viral shedding usually is 3 to 8 days, but shedding may last longer, especially in young infants and in immunosuppressed people, in whom shedding may continue for as long as 3 to 4 weeks.

The **incubation period** ranges from 2 to 8 days; 4 to 6 days is most common.

DIAGNOSTIC TESTS: Rapid diagnostic assays, including immunofluorescent and enzyme immunoassay techniques for detection of viral antigen in nasopharyngeal specimens, are available commercially and generally are reliable in infants and young children. In children, the sensitivity of these assays in comparison with culture varies between 53% and 96%, with most in the 80% to 90% range. The sensitivity may be lower in older children and is quite poor in adults, because adults typically shed low concentrations of RSV. As with all antigen detection assays, the predictive value is high during the peak season, but false-positive test results are more likely to occur when the incidence of disease is low, such as in the summer in temperate areas. Therefore, antigen detection assays should not be the only basis on which the beginning and end of monthly immunoprophylaxis is determined. In most outpatient settings, specific viral testing has little effect on management.

One disadvantage of antigen detection relative to virologic assessment (culture or reverse transcriptase-polymerase chain reaction [RT-PCR] assay) is that coinfections may not be detected. Young children with bronchiolitis are often infected with more than one virus. Up to 20% of children with RSV bronchiolitis may be coinfected with another respiratory tract virus, such as human metapneumovirus or rhinovirus. Whether children with bronchiolitis who are coinfected with more than one virus experience more severe disease is not clear.

Viral isolation from nasopharyngeal secretions in cell culture requires 1 to 5 days (shell vial techniques can produce results within 24 to 48 hours), but results and sensitivity vary among laboratories. Experienced viral laboratory personnel should be consulted for optimal methods of collection and transport of specimens, which may include keeping specimens cold and protected from light, rapid specimen processing, and stabilization in virus transport media. Conventional serologic testing of acute and convalescent serum specimens cannot be relied on to confirm infection in young infants in whom sensitivity may be low. Molecular diagnostic tests using RT-PCR assays are commercially available and have increased RSV detection rates substantially over viral isolation or antigen detection. These tests should be interpreted with caution, because they detect viral RNA that may persist in the airway for many weeks after cessation of shedding of detectable infectious virus.

TREATMENT: Primary treatment is supportive and should include hydration, careful clinical assessment of respiratory status, measurement of oxygen saturation, use of supplemental oxygen as needed, suction of the upper airway, and if necessary, intubation and mechanical ventilation.[1] Continuous measurement of oxygen saturation may detect transient fluctuations in oxygenation; supplemental oxygen is recommended when oxyhemoglobin saturation persistently falls below 90% in a previously healthy infant.[1] Ribavirin has in vitro antiviral activity against RSV, and aerosolized ribavirin therapy has been associated with a small but statistically significant increase in oxygen saturation during the acute infection in several small studies. However, a consistent decrease in need for mechanical ventilation, decrease in length of stay in the pediatric intensive care unit, or reduction in days of hospitalization among ribavirin recipients has not been demonstrated. The aerosol route of administration, concern about potential toxic effects among exposed health care personnel, and conflicting results of efficacy trials have led to infrequent use of this drug. Ribavirin is not recommended for routine use but may be considered for use in selected patients with documented, potentially life-threatening RSV infection.

Beta-adrenergic Agents. Beta-adrenergic agents are not recommended for routine care of first-time wheezing associated with RSV bronchiolitis. Some physicians elect to use bronchodilator therapy because of concern that reactive airway disease may be misdiagnosed as bronchiolitis. Repeat doses of an inhaled bronchodilator may be continued in a minority of infants with well-documented improvement in respiratory function soon after the first dose, but its use is unlikely to alter the clinical course of RSV disease or to permit earlier hospital discharge.

Corticosteroid Therapy. In most randomized clinical trials of hospitalized infants as well as outpatients with RSV bronchiolitis, corticosteroid therapy has been found to have no effect on disease severity, need for hospitalization among outpatients, or length of stay among inpatients. As such, corticosteroid treatment is not recommended for RSV bronchiolitis. Administration of corticosteroids has been associated with prolonged RSV shedding in some studies.

Antimicrobial Therapy. Intravenous antimicrobial therapy is not indicated in infants hospitalized with RSV bronchiolitis or pneumonia unless there is evidence of secondary bacterial infection. Bacterial lung infections and bacteremia are uncommon in this setting. Otitis media caused by RSV or bacterial superinfection occurs in infants with RSV bronchiolitis, but oral antimicrobial agents can be used if therapy for otitis media is necessary.

---

[1] American Academy of Pediatrics, Subcommittee on Diagnosis and Management of Bronchiolitis. Diagnosis and management of bronchiolitis. *Pediatrics.* 2006;118(4):1774–1793

Other Therapies. Limited data suggest nebulized, hypertonic saline may be associated with improvement in clinical scores and decrease length of hospitalization. The roles of other therapies such as helium/oxygen, nasal continuous positive pressure, and surfactant are under investigation, but these are not recommended at this time.

Prevention of RSV Infections. Palivizumab, a humanized mouse monoclonal antibody, is the only licensed product available to reduce the risk of RSV lower respiratory tract disease in infants and children with CLD, with a history of preterm birth (less than 35 weeks' gestation), or with congenital heart disease. Palivizumab is administered intramuscularly at a dose of 15 mg/kg once every 30 days. An attempt should be made to maintain compliance with monthly administration. In some reports, palivizumab administration in a home-based program has been shown to improve compliance and to reduce exposure to microbial pathogens compared with administration in office- or clinic-based settings. Additional doses of palivizumab should not be given to any patient with a history of a severe allergic reaction following a previous dose. Palivizumab is not effective in treatment of RSV disease and is not approved or recommended for this indication.

Respiratory Syncytial Virus Immune Globulin Intravenous (RSV-IGIV), a hyperimmune, polyclonal globulin prepared from donors selected for high serum titers of RSV neutralizing antibody, previously was used for prophylaxis but no longer is available.

Cost Considerations. Immunoprophylaxis with palivizumab is an effective, although costly, intervention that reduces RSV hospitalization rates by 39% to 82% among high-risk infants. Optimal cost benefit from immunoprophylaxis is achieved during peak outbreak months when most RSV hospitalizations occur. If prophylaxis is initiated after widespread RSV circulation has begun, high-risk infants may not receive the full benefit of protection. Conversely, early initiation or continuation of monthly immunoprophylaxis during months when RSV is not circulating widely is not cost-effective and provides little benefit to recipients.

The primary benefit of immunoprophylaxis is a decrease in the rate of RSV-associated hospitalization. No prospective, randomized clinical trial has demonstrated a significant decrease in the rate of mortality attributable to RSV or in the rate of recurrent wheezing following RSV infection among infants who receive prophylaxis. The rate of RSV-associated mortality in the United States is quite low because of the high level of intensive care available. Economic analyses fail to demonstrate overall savings in health care dollars because of the high cost if all at-risk infants receive prophylaxis.

Initiation and Termination of Immunoprophylaxis. In the temperate climates of North America, peak RSV activity typically occurs between November and March, whereas in equatorial countries, RSV seasonality patterns vary and may occur throughout the year. The inevitability of the RSV season is predictable, but the severity of the season, the time of onset, the peak of activity, and the end of the season cannot be predicted precisely. Substantial variation in timing of community outbreaks of RSV disease from year to year exists in the same community and between communities in the same year, even in the same region. These variations occur within the overall pattern of RSV outbreaks, usually beginning in November or December, peaking in January or February, and ending by the end of March or sometime in April. Communities in the southern United States, particularly some communities in the state of Florida, tend to experience the earliest onset of RSV activity. In recent years, the national median duration of the RSV season has been 19 weeks or less. Results from clinical trials indicate that palivizumab trough serum concentrations more than 30 days after the fifth dose will be well above the protective concentration for most infants. Five monthly doses of palivizumab will provide more than 20 weeks of protective serum antibody concentration. In the continental United States, a total of 5 monthly doses for infants and young children with congenital heart disease, CLD, or preterm birth before 32 weeks' gestation (31 weeks, 6 days and younger) will provide an optimal balance of benefit and cost, even with variation in season onset and end.

For infants who qualify for 5 doses, initiation of immunoprophylaxis in November and continuation for a total of 5 monthly doses will provide protection into April and is recommended for most areas of the United States. If prophylaxis is initiated in October, the fifth and final dose should be administered in February.

Data from the Centers for Disease Control and Prevention (CDC) have identified variations in the onset and offset of the RSV season in the state of Florida that should affect the timing of palivizumab administration. Northwest Florida has an onset in mid-November, which is consistent with other areas of the United States. In north central and southwest Florida, the onset of RSV season typically is late September to early October. The RSV season in southeast Florida (Miami-Dade County) typically has its onset in July. Despite varied onsets, the RSV season is of equal duration in the different regions of Florida. Children who qualify for palivizumab prophylaxis for the entire RSV season (infants and children with CLD or congenital heart disease or preterm infants born before 32 weeks' gestation) should receive palivizumab only during the 5 months following the onset of RSV season in their region (maximum of 5 doses), which should provide coverage during the peak of the season, when prophylaxis is most effective (Table 3.56).

Specific groups of American Indian/Alaska Native children in certain geographic regions may experience more severe RSV disease and a longer RSV season. RSV hospitalizations for Navajo and White Mountain Apache infants and young children may be 2 to 3 times those of children of similar ages in the United States population. However, the timing and duration of the RSV season is similar to the remainder of the United States (November through March), so standard recommendations for children with congenital heart disease, CLD, or preterm birth (31 weeks, 6 days gestation and younger) still are appropriate. Alaska Native infants in southwestern Alaska experience not only higher RSV hospitalization rates but also a longer RSV season. Pediatricians in this area of Alaska may wish to use CDC-generated RSV hospitalization data to assist in determining the onset and offset of RSV season for the appropriate timing of palivizumab administration (**http://www.cdc.gov/surveillance/nrevss/rsv**).

Infants and children with congenital heart disease or CLD or preterm infants born at or before 31 weeks, 6 days' gestation who initiate palivizumab prophylaxis after start of the RSV season will not require all 5 doses (see Table 3.57, p 614).

Table 3.56. Palivizumab Prophylaxis for Infants and Young Children With Chronic Lung Disease of Prematurity or Congenital Heart Disease

Geographic Location	Earliest Date for Initiation of 5 Monthly Doses
Southeast Florida	July 1
North central and southwest Florida	September 15
Most other areas of United States	November 1

Table 3.57. Maximum Number of Monthly Doses of Palivizumab for Respiratory Syncytial Virus Prophylaxis

Infants Eligible for a Maximum of 5 Doses	Infants Eligible for a Maximum of 3 Doses
Infants younger than 24 months of age with chronic lung disease and requiring medical therapy	Preterm infants with gestational age of 32 weeks, 0 days to 34 weeks, 6 days with at least 1 risk factor and born 3 months before or during RSV season.
Infants younger than 24 months of age and requiring medical therapy for congenital heart disease	
Preterm infants born at or before 31 weeks, 6 days of gestation	
Certain infants with neuromuscular disease or congenital abnormalities of the airways	

ELIGIBILITY CRITERIA FOR PROPHYLAXIS OF HIGH-RISK INFANTS AND YOUNG CHILDREN.

- **Infants with CLD.** Palivizumab prophylaxis may be considered for infants and children younger than 24 months of age who receive medical therapy (supplemental oxygen, bronchodilator, diuretic or chronic corticosteroid therapy) for CLD within 6 months before the start of the RSV season. These infants and young children should receive a maximum of 5 doses. Patients with the most severe CLD who continue to require medical therapy may benefit from prophylaxis during a second RSV season. Data are limited regarding the effectiveness of palivizumab during the second year of life. Individual patients may benefit from decisions made in consultation with neonatologists, pediatric intensivists, pulmonologists, or infectious disease specialists.
- **Infants born before 32 weeks' gestation (at or before 31 weeks, 6 days of gestation) (see Table 3.58, p 615).** Infants in this category may benefit from RSV prophylaxis, even if they do not have CLD. For these infants, major risk factors to consider include gestational age and chronologic age at the start of the RSV season. Infants born at or before 28 weeks, 6 days' gestation may benefit from prophylaxis during the RSV season, whenever that occurs during the first 12 months of life. Infants born at 29 weeks, 0 days through 31 weeks, 6 days of gestation may benefit most from prophylaxis up to 6 months of age. However, once an infant qualifies for initiation of prophylaxis at the start of the RSV season, administration should continue throughout the season and should not stop when the infant reaches either 6 months or 12 months of age. A maximum of 5 monthly doses is recommended for infants in this category.
- **Infants born at 32 to less than 35 weeks' gestation (defined as 32 weeks, 0 days through 34 weeks, 6 days of gestation).** Numerous factors have been proposed as increasing the risk of acquiring RSV infection among infants in this gestational age group. Other factors have been associated with an increased risk of severe disease and hospitalization. Certain factors (CHD, prematurity, CLD) are well-established risk factors for hospitalization, because they consistently are present across numerous studies. In contrast, other reported risk factors either are found inconsistently,

Table 3.58. Maximum Number of Palivizumab Doses for RSV Prophylaxis of Preterm Infants Without Chronic Lung Disease, on the Basis of Birth Date, Gestational Age, and Presence of Risk Factors (Shown for Geographic Areas Beginning Prophylaxis on November 1)

Month of Birth	Maximum No. of Doses for Season Beginning November 1		
	≤28 Weeks, 6 Days of Gestation and <12 Months of Age at Start of Season	29 Weeks, 0 Days Through 31 Weeks, 6 Days of Gestation and <6 Months of Age at Start of Season	32 Weeks, 0 Days Through 34 Weeks, 6 Days of Gestation and With Risk Factor[a]
November 1– March 31 of previous RSV season	5[b]	0[c]	0[d]
April	5	0[c]	0[d]
May	5	5	0[d]
June	5	5	0[d]
July	5	5	0[d]
August	5	5	1[e]
September	5	5	2[e]
October	5	5	3[e]
November	5	5	3[e]
December	4	4	3[e]
January	3	3	3[e]
February	2	2	2[e]
March	1	1	1[e]

If infant is discharged from the hospital during RSV season, fewer doses may be required.

[a]Risk factors: (1) infant attends child care; or (2) infant has sibling younger than 5 years of age.

[b]Some of these infants may have received 1 or more doses of palivizumab in the previous RSV season if discharged from the hospital during that season; if so, they still qualify for up to 5 doses during their second RSV season.

[c]Zero doses, because infant will be older than 6 months of age at start of RSV season.

[d]Zero doses, because infant will be older than 90 days of age at start of RSV season.

[e]On the basis of the age of patients at the time of discharge from the hospital, fewer doses may be required, because these infants will receive 1 dose every 30 days until they are 90 days of age.

even in studies by the same authors, or increase the risk of hospitalization by a relatively small factor (less than twofold to threefold). A risk-scoring tool developed from a Canadian prospective study of infants born at 33 through 35 weeks' gestation revealed that multiple risk factors needed to be present before a significant increase in hospitalization risk was seen. Available data do not allow for definition of a subgroup of infants who are at risk of prolonged hospitalization and admission to the intensive care unit. Therefore, although current recommendations were designed to be consistent with the US Food and Drug Administration's approval for marketing of palivizumab for the prevention of serious RSV lower respiratory tract disease, they specifically target infants in this group with consistently identified risk factors for RSV hospitalization during the period of greatest risk, which is the first 3 months of life. Palivizumab prophylaxis should be limited to infants in this group at greatest risk of hospitalization attributable to RSV infection, namely infants younger than 3 months of age at the start of the RSV season or who are born during the RSV season and who are likely to have an increased risk of exposure to RSV. Epidemiologic data suggest that RSV infection is more likely to occur and more likely to lead to hospitalization for infants in this gestational age group when at least 1 of the following 2 risk factors is present:

+ The infant attends child care, defined as a home or facility where care is provided for any number of infants or young toddlers; or

+ One or more older siblings younger than 5 years of age or other children younger than 5 years of age lives permanently in the same household. Multiple births younger than 1 year of age do not qualify as fulfilling this risk factor.

Prophylaxis may be considered for infants born at 32 through less than 35 weeks' gestation (defined as 32 weeks, 0 days through 34 weeks, 6 days of gestation) who are born less than 3 months before the onset of or during the RSV season and for whom at least 1 of the 2 risk factors is present. Infants in this gestational age category should receive prophylaxis only until they reach 3 months of age and should receive a maximum of 3 monthly doses; many will receive only 1 or 2 doses before they reach 3 months of age. Once an infant has passed 90 days of age, the risk of hospitalization attributable to RSV lower respiratory tract disease is reduced. Administration of palivizumab is not recommended after 3 months of age for patients in this category (Tables 3.56 and 3.57).

• **Additional preventive measures for all high-risk infants.** Infants, especially those at high risk, never should be exposed to tobacco smoke. Tobacco smoke is a known risk factor for many adverse health-related outcomes. However, in published studies, passive household exposure to tobacco smoke has not been associated with an increased risk of RSV hospitalization on a consistent basis. Exposure to tobacco smoke must be controlled by families with infants, especially with infants who are at increased risk of RSV disease. Such preventive measures will be far less costly than palivizumab prophylaxis. In contrast to the well-documented beneficial effect of breastfeeding against many viral illnesses, existing data are conflicting regarding the specific protective effect of breastfeeding against RSV infection. Breastfeeding should be encouraged for all infants in accordance with recommendations of the American Academy of Pediatrics. High-risk infants should be kept away from crowds and from situations in which exposure to infected people cannot be controlled. Participation in group child care should be restricted during the RSV season for high-risk infants whenever feasible. Parents should be instructed on the importance of careful hand hygiene. In addition, all infants (beginning at 6 months of age) and their contacts (beginning when the child is born) should receive influenza vaccine as well as other recommended age-appropriate immunizations.

• **Infants with congenital abnormalities of the airway or neuromuscular disease.** Immunoprophylaxis may be considered for infants who have either congenital abnormalities of the airway or a neuromuscular condition that compromises handling of respiratory secretions. Infants and young children in this category should receive a maximum of 5 doses of palivizumab during the first year of life.

• **Infants and children with CHD.** Children who are 24 months of age or younger with hemodynamically significant cyanotic or acyanotic CHD may benefit from palivizumab prophylaxis. Decisions regarding prophylaxis with palivizumab in children with

CHD should be made on the basis of the degree of physiologic cardiovascular compromise. Children younger than 24 months of age with CHD who are most likely to benefit from immunoprophylaxis include:

- Infants who are receiving medication to control congestive heart failure;
- Infants with moderate to severe pulmonary hypertension; and
- Infants with cyanotic heart disease.

Because a mean decrease in palivizumab serum concentration of 58% was observed after surgical procedures that use cardiopulmonary bypass, for children who still require prophylaxis, a postoperative dose of palivizumab (15 mg/kg) should be considered as soon as the patient is medically stable.

The following groups of infants are not at increased risk of RSV and generally should not receive immunoprophylaxis:

- Infants and children with hemodynamically insignificant heart disease (eg, secundum atrial septal defect, small ventricular septal defect, pulmonic stenosis, uncomplicated aortic stenosis, mild coarctation of the aorta, and patent ductus arteriosus)
- Infants with lesions adequately corrected by surgery, unless they continue to require medication for congestive heart failure
- Infants with mild cardiomyopathy who are not receiving medical therapy for the condition

Dates for initiation and termination of prophylaxis should be based on the same considerations as for high-risk infants with CLD.

- **Immunocompromised children.** Palivizumab prophylaxis has not been evaluated in randomized trials in immunocompromised children. Although specific recommendations for immunocompromised patients cannot be made, infants and young children with severe immunodeficiencies (eg, severe combined immunodeficiency or advanced acquired immunodeficiency syndrome) may benefit from prophylaxis.
- **Patients with cystic fibrosis.** Limited studies suggest that some patients with cystic fibrosis may be at increased risk of RSV infection. Whether RSV infection exacerbates the chronic lung disease of cystic fibrosis is not known. In addition, insufficient data exist to determine the effectiveness of palivizumab use in this patient population. Therefore, a recommendation for routine prophylaxis in patients with cystic fibrosis cannot be made.
- **Special situations.**
  - If an infant or child who is receiving palivizumab immunoprophylaxis experiences a breakthrough RSV infection, monthly prophylaxis should continue until a maximum of 3 doses have been administered to infants in the 32 weeks, 0 days' through 34 weeks, 6 days' gestation group, or until a maximum of 5 doses have been administered to infants with CHD, CLD, or preterm birth before 32 weeks' gestation. This recommendation is based on the observation that high-risk infants may be hospitalized more than once in the same season with RSV lower respiratory tract disease and the fact that more than 1 RSV strain often cocirculates in a community.
  - Hospitalized infants who qualify for prophylaxis during the RSV season should receive the first dose of palivizumab 48 to 72 hours before discharge or promptly after discharge.
  - Infants who have begun palivizumab prophylaxis earlier in the season and are hospitalized on the date when the next monthly dose is due should receive that dose as scheduled while they remain in the hospital.

- RSV is known to be transmitted in the hospital setting and to cause serious disease in infants at high risk. Among hospitalized infants, the major means to reduce RSV transmission is strict observance of infection-control practices, including prompt initiation of precautions for RSV-infected infants. If an RSV outbreak occurs in a high-risk unit (eg, pediatric or neonatal intensive care unit or hematopoietic stem cell transplantation unit), primary emphasis should be placed on proper infection-control practices, especially hand hygiene. No data exist to support palivizumab use in controlling outbreaks of health care-associated disease, and palivizumab use is not recommended for this purpose.
- Palivizumab does not interfere with response to vaccines.

ISOLATION OF THE HOSPITALIZED PATIENT: In addition to standard precautions, contact precautions are recommended for the duration of RSV-associated illness among infants and young children, including patients treated with ribavirin. The effectiveness of these precautions depends on compliance and necessitates scrupulous adherence to appropriate hand hygiene practices. Patients with RSV infection should be cared for in single rooms or placed in a cohort.

CONTROL MEASURES: The control of health care-associated RSV transmission is complicated by the continuing chance of introduction through infected patients, staff, and visitors. During the peak of the RSV season, many infants and children hospitalized with respiratory tract symptoms will be infected with RSV and should be cared for with contact precautions (see Isolation of the Hospitalized Patient, above). Early identification of RSV-infected patients (see Diagnostic Tests, p 610) is important so that appropriate precautions can be instituted promptly. During community outbreaks of RSV, a variety of measures have been demonstrated to reduce the risk of health care-associated transmission, including: (1) laboratory screening of symptomatic patients for RSV infection; (2) cohorting of infected patients and staff; (3) excluding visitors with current or recent respiratory tract infections; (4) excluding staff with respiratory tract illness or RSV infection from caring for susceptible infants; (5) using gowns and gloves and possibly goggles or masks for protecting the eyes of health care personnel; (6) emphasizing hand hygiene before and after direct contact with patients, after contact with inanimate objects in the direct vicinity of patients, and after glove removal; and (7) limiting young sibling visitation during the RSV season.

A critical aspect of RSV prevention among high-risk infants is education of parents and other caregivers about the importance of decreasing exposure to and transmission of RSV. Preventive measures include limiting, where feasible, exposure to contagious settings (eg, child care centers) and emphasis on hand hygiene in all settings, including the home, especially during periods when contacts of high-risk children have respiratory tract infections.

Rhinovirus Infections

CLINICAL MANIFESTATIONS: Rhinoviruses are the most frequent causes of the common cold or rhinosinusitis. Rhinoviruses also can be associated with pharyngitis and otitis media and can cause lower respiratory tract infections (eg, bronchiolitis, pneumonia) in children. In children with asthma, rhinoviruses are detected in approximately half of all acute exacerbations, and even more in the fall and spring. Sore throat frequently is the first sign of infection, followed by nasal discharge that initially is watery and clear at the onset but often becomes mucopurulent and viscous after a few days and may persist for 10 to 14 days. Malaise, headache, myalgia, and low-grade fever also may occur.

ETIOLOGY: Rhinoviruses are single positive-stranded RNA viruses classified as 3 species (A, B, C) in the family *Picornaviridae*, genus *Enterovirus*. Approximately 100 antigenic serotypes have been identified by neutralization with type-specific antisera, and many additional types have been identified by molecular methods. Infection with one type confers some type-specific immunity, but immunity is of variable degree and brief duration and offers little protection against other serotypes.

EPIDEMIOLOGY: Transmission occurs predominantly by person-to-person contact, with self-inoculation by contaminated secretions on hands and/or aerosol spread. Infections occur throughout the year, but peak activity occurs during autumn and spring. Multiple serotypes circulate simultaneously, and the prevalent serotypes circulating in a given population change from season to season. By adulthood, antibodies to many serotypes have developed. Viral shedding from nasopharyngeal secretions is most abundant during the first 2 to 3 days of infection and usually ceases by 7 to 10 days. However, virus shedding may continue for as long as 3 weeks.

The **incubation period** usually is 2 to 3 days but occasionally is up to 7 days.

DIAGNOSTIC TESTS: Inoculation of nasopharyngeal secretions in appropriate cell cultures using specialized growth conditions for viral isolation has been the primary means to diagnose infection but is insensitive for many strains. Polymerase chain reaction (PCR) detection methods have become the preferred way to identify rhinoviruses infection and the only way to detect species C viruses that that have not been isolated successfully in cell culture. Commercial molecular diagnostic assays for rhinoviruses are available. Serologic diagnosis of rhinovirus infection is impractical because of the large number of antigenic types.

TREATMENT: In 2008, the US Food and Drug Administration (FDA) issued a safety warning that over-the-counter cold medications should be avoided in children younger than 4 years of age. Use of such medications also is discouraged for children younger than 6 years of age because of lack of efficacy and concerns regarding safety. Antimicrobial agents are not indicated for people with a common cold caused by a rhinovirus or other virus, because antimicrobial agents do not prevent secondary bacterial infection and their use may promote the emergence of resistant bacteria and complicate treatment for a bacterial infection (see Antimicrobial Stewardship: Appropriate and Judicious Use of Antimicrobial Agents, p 802).

ISOLATION OF THE HOSPITALIZED PATIENT: In addition to standard precautions, droplet precautions are recommended for hospitalized infants and children for the duration of illness.

CONTROL MEASURES: Frequent hand hygiene, respiratory hygiene, and general hygienic measures in schools, households, and other settings where transmission is common may help decrease the spread of rhinoviruses.

Rickettsial Diseases

Rickettsial diseases comprise infections caused by bacteria of the genera *Rickettsia* (endemic and epidemic typhus and spotted fever group rickettsioses), *Orientia* species (scrub typhus), *Ehrlichia* species (ehrlichiosis), and *Anaplasma* species (anaplasmosis).

CLINICAL MANIFESTATIONS: Rickettsial infections have many features in common, including the following:

- Fever, rash (especially in spotted fever and typhus group rickettsiae), headache, myalgia, and respiratory tract symptoms are prominent features.
- Local primary eschars occur with some rickettsial diseases, particularly spotted fever rickettsioses, rickettsialpox, and scrub typhus.
- Systemic capillary and small vessel endothelial damage (ie, vasculitis) with increased microvascular permeability is the primary pathologic feature of spotted fever and typhus group rickettsial infections.
- Rickettsial diseases rapidly can become life threatening. Risk factors for severe disease include glucose-6-phosphate dehydrogenase deficiency, male sex, and use of sulfonamides.

Immunity against reinfection by the same agent after natural infection usually is of long duration, except in the case of scrub typhus. Among the 4 groups of rickettsial diseases, some cross-immunity usually is conferred by infections within groups but not between groups. Reinfection of humans with *Ehrlichia* species and *Anaplasma* species has not been described.

ETIOLOGY: The rickettsiae causing human disease include: *Rickettsia* species, *Orientia tsutsugamushi*, *Ehrlichia* species, and *Anaplasma* species. Rickettsiae are small, coccobacillary gram-negative bacteria that are obligate intracellular pathogens and cannot be grown in cell-free media. They grow in different cellular compartments: *Orientia* and *Rickettsia* organisms in the cytoplasm and *Ehrlichia* and *Anaplasma* organisms in different nonacidified modified phagosomes.

EPIDEMIOLOGY: Rickettsial diseases have arthropod vectors including ticks, fleas, mites, and lice. Humans are incidental hosts, except for epidemic (louseborne) typhus, for which humans are the principal reservoir and the human body louse is the vector. Rickettsia life cycles typically involve arthropod and mammalian reservoirs, and transmission occurs as a result of environmental or occupational exposure. Geographic and seasonal occurrence of rickettsial disease is related to arthropod vector life cycles, activity, and distribution.

The **incubation periods** vary according to organism (see specific chapters).

DIAGNOSTIC TESTS: Group-specific antibodies are detectable in the serum of many people 7 to 14 days after onset of illness but slower antibody responses occur commonly in some diseases. Various serologic tests for detecting antirickettsial antibodies are available. The indirect immunofluorescent antibody assay is recommended in most circumstances because of its relative sensitivity and specificity; however, it cannot determine the causative agent to the species level. Treatment early in the course of illness can blunt or delay serologic responses. Polymerase chain reaction (PCR) assays can detect rickettsiae in whole blood or tissues collected during the acute stage of illness and before administration of antimicrobial agents; availability of these tests is limited to reference and research laboratories. In laboratories with experienced personnel, immunohistochemical staining and PCR testing of skin biopsy specimens from patients with rash or eschar can help to diagnose rickettsial infections early in the course of disease. The Weil-Felix test is insensitive and nonspecific and no longer is recommended. The Weil-Felix test will not detect infections caused by *Ehrlichia* species and *Anaplasma* species.

TREATMENT: Prompt and specific therapy is important for optimal outcome. The drug of choice for rickettsioses is doxycycline. Although older tetracycline-class antimicrobial agents generally are not given to children younger than 8 years of age because of the risk of dental staining, doxycycline has not been demonstrated clearly to have the same effect on developing dentition (see Tetracyclines, p 801). The duration of treatment is 7 to 14 days. Antimicrobial treatment is most effective when children are treated during the first week of illness. If the disease remains untreated during the second week, therapy is less effective in preventing complications. Because confirmatory laboratory tests primarily are retrospective, treatment decisions should be made on the basis of clinical findings and epidemiologic data and should not be delayed until test results are known.

CONTROL MEASURES: Control measures primarily involve prevention of vector transmission of rickettsial agents to humans (see Prevention of Tickborne Infections, p 207).

Several rickettsial diseases, including Rocky Mountain spotted fever and ehrlichiosis, are nationally notifiable diseases and should be reported to state and local health departments.

For more details, the following chapters on rickettsial diseases should be consulted:
- *Ehrlichia* Infections (Human Ehrlichiosis), p 312 (or **www.cdc.gov/ehrlichiosis/**).
- Rickettsialpox, p 622.
- Rocky Mountain Spotted Fever, p 623 (or **www.cdc.gov/rmsf/**).
- Endemic Typhus (Murine Typhus), p 770.
- Epidemic Typhus (Louseborne or Sylvatic Typhus), p 771.

OTHER RICKETTSIAL SPOTTED FEVER INFECTIONS: A number of other epidemiologically distinct but clinically similar tickborne spotted fever infections caused by rickettsiae have been recognized (also see **www.cdc.gov/otherspottedfever/index.html**). Many of them present with an eschar at the site of the tick bite. The causative agents of some of these infections share the same group antigen as *Rickettsia rickettsii*. These include:
- *Rickettsia africae,* the causative agent of African tick bite fever that is endemic in sub-Saharan Africa and some Caribbean Islands;
- *Rickettsia conorii,* the causative agent of boutonneuse fevers (Mediterranean spotted fever, India tick typhus, Marseilles fever, Israeli tick typhus, and Astrakhan spotted fever) that is endemic in southern Europe, Africa, the Middle East, and the Indian subcontinent;
- *Rickettsia parkeri,* the causative agent of maculatum infection in the Americas;
- *Rickettsia sibirica,* the causative agent of Siberian tick typhus, endemic in central Asia;
- *Rickettsia australis,* the causative agent of North Queensland tick typhus, endemic in eastern Australia;
- *Rickettsia japonica,* the causative agent of Japanese spotted fever, endemic in Japan;
- *Rickettsia honei,* the causative agent of Thai tick typhus and Flinders Island spotted fever;
- *Rickettsia slovaca,* the causative agent of tickborne lymphadenopathy, endemic in European countries;
- *Rickettsia felis,* the causative agent of cat flea rickettsiosis that occurs worldwide;

- *Rickettsia aeschlimannii,* reported from Africa;
- *Rickettsia heilongjiangensis,* reported from the Russian Far East; and
- *Rickettsia helvetica, Rickettsia massiliae,* and *R sibirica* subspecies *mongolotimonae,* reported from European countries.

Each of these infections has some clinical and pathologic features similar to those of Rocky Mountain spotted fever. Diagnosis is confirmed using serologic assays. Demonstration of a fourfold or greater increase in specific antibodies (immunoglobulin G) in acute and convalescent serum samples taken 2 to 3 weeks apart is diagnostic of spotted fever rickettsioses; however, some PCR and amplicon sequencing assays on DNA from acute whole blood or skin biopsy provide accurate identification of the etiologic agent. These diseases are of importance among people traveling to or returning from areas where these agents are endemic and among people living in these areas.

Rickettsialpox

CLINICAL MANIFESTATIONS: Rickettsialpox is a febrile, eschar-associated illness that is characterized by generalized, relatively sparse, erythematous, papulovesicular eruptions on the trunk, face, and extremities (less often on palms and soles) or mucous membranes of the mouth. The rash develops 1 to 4 days after onset of fever and 3 to 10 days after appearance of an eschar at the site of the bite of a house mouse mite. Regional lymph nodes in the area of the primary eschar typically become enlarged. Without specific antimicrobial therapy, systemic disease lasts approximately 7 to 10 days; manifestations include fever, headache, malaise, and myalgia. Less frequent manifestations include anorexia, vomiting, conjunctivitis, nuchal rigidity, and photophobia. The disease is mild compared with Rocky Mountain spotted fever, and no rickettsialpox-associated deaths have been described; however, disease occasionally is severe enough to warrant hospitalization.

ETIOLOGY: Rickettsialpox is caused by *Rickettsia akari,* a gram-negative intracellular bacillus which is classified with the spotted fever group rickettsiae and related antigenically to other members of that group.

EPIDEMIOLOGY: The natural host for *R akari* in the United States is *Mus musculus,* the common house mouse. The disease is transmitted by the house mouse mite, *Liponyssoides sanguineus.* Disease risk is heightened in areas infested with mice and rats. The disease can occur wherever the hosts, pathogens, and humans coexist but most often erupts in large urban settings. In the United States, rickettsialpox has been described predominantly in northeastern metropolitan centers, especially in New York City. It also has been confirmed in many other countries, including Croatia, Ukraine, Turkey, Russia, South Korea, and Mexico. All age groups can be affected. No seasonal pattern of disease occurs. The disease is not communicable but occurs occasionally among families or people cohabiting a house mouse mite-infested dwelling. In Mexico, *R akari* was detected in the brown dog tick, *Rhipicephalus sanguineus.*

The **incubation period** is 6 to 15 days.

DIAGNOSTIC TESTS: *R akari* can be isolated in cell culture from blood and eschar biopsy specimens during the acute stage of disease, but culture is not attempted routinely. Because antibodies to *R akari* have extensive cross-reactivity with antibodies against *Rickettsia rickettsii* (the cause of Rocky Mountain spotted fever), an indirect immunofluorescent antibody assay for *R rickettsii* (the cause of Rocky Mountain spotted fever) can demonstrate a fourfold or greater change in antibody titers between acute and convalescent serum specimens taken 4 to 6 weeks apart. Use of *R akari* antigen is recommended for accurate serologic diagnosis. Direct fluorescent antibody or immunohistochemical testing of formalin-fixed, paraffin-embedded eschars or papulovesicle biopsy specimens can detect rickettsiae in the samples and are useful diagnostic techniques. Use of polymerase chain reaction for detection of rickettsial DNA also has been used.

TREATMENT: Doxycycline is the drug of choice in all age groups and is effective when given for 3 to 5 days (see Tetracyclines, p 801). Doxycycline will shorten the course of disease; symptoms resolve typically within 12 to 48 hours after initiation of therapy. Relapse is rare. Fluoroquinolones and chloramphenicol are alternative drugs, although fluoroquinolones are not approved for this use in children younger than 18 years of age (see Fluoroquinolones, p 800). Untreated rickettsialpox usually will resolve within 2 to 3 weeks.

ISOLATION OF THE HOSPITALIZED PATIENT: Standard precautions are recommended.

CONTROL MEASURES: Application of residual acaricides can be used in heavily mite-infested environments to eliminate the vector. Rodent-control measures are important in limiting or eliminating spread of rickettsialpox; however, they should be conducted only in conjunction with acaricide application to ensure vector control. No specific management of exposed people is necessary.

Rocky Mountain Spotted Fever

CLINICAL MANIFESTATIONS: Rocky Mountain spotted fever (RMSF) is a systemic, small-vessel vasculitis that often involves a characteristic rash. Fever, myalgia, severe headache, nausea, vomiting, and anorexia are typical presenting symptoms. Abdominal pain and diarrhea often are present and can obscure the diagnosis. The rash usually begins within the first 6 days of symptoms as erythematous macules or maculopapules. Rash usually appears first on the wrists and ankles, often spreading within hours proximally to the trunk and involves the palms and soles. Although early development of a rash is a useful diagnostic sign, rash can be atypical or absent in up to 20% of cases. It may be difficult to visualize in patients with dark skin. A petechial rash typically is a late finding and indicates progression to severe disease. Lack of a typical rash is a risk factor for misdiagnosis and poor outcome. Thrombocytopenia of varying severity and hyponatremia develop in many cases. White blood cell count typically is normal, but leukopenia and anemia can occur. If not treated, illness can last as long as 3 weeks and can be severe, with prominent central nervous system, cardiac, pulmonary, gastrointestinal tract, and renal involvement; disseminated intravascular coagulation; and shock leading to death. RMSF can progress rapidly, even in previously healthy people, and the median time to death is 8 days. Delay in appropriate antimicrobial treatment is associated with severe disease and poor outcomes. Case-fatality rates of untreated RMSF range from 20% to 80%. Significant long-term sequelae are common in patients with severe RMSF, including neurologic (paraparesis; hearing loss; peripheral neuropathy; bladder and bowel incontinence; and cerebellar, vestibular, and motor dysfunction) and nonneurologic (disability from limb or digit amputation). Patients treated early in the course of symptoms may have a mild illness, with fever resolving in the first 48 hours of treatment.

ETIOLOGY: *Rickettsia rickettsii,* an obligate, intracellular, gram-negative bacillus and a member of the spotted fever group of rickettsiae, is the causative agent. The primary targets of infection in mammalian hosts are endothelial cells lining the small blood vessels of all major tissues and organs.

EPIDEMIOLOGY: The pathogen is transmitted to humans by the bite of a tick of the Ixodidae family (hard ticks). Ticks and their small mammal hosts serve as reservoirs of the pathogen in nature. Other wild animals and dogs have been found with antibodies to *Rickettsia rickettsii,* but their role as natural reservoirs is not clear. In ticks, the organism is transmitted transstadially from one life stage to the next and transovarially to the eggs and resulting new generation. People with occupational or recreational exposure to the tick vector (eg, pet owners, animal handlers, and people who spend more time outdoors) are at increased risk of acquiring the organism. People of all ages can be infected. The period of highest incidence in the United States is from April to September, although RMSF can occur year round in certain areas with endemic disease. Laboratory-acquired infection occasionally has resulted from accidental inoculation and aerosol contamination. Transmission has occurred on rare occasions by blood transfusion. Mortality is highest in males, people older than 50 years of age, children 5 to 9 years of age, and people with no recognized tick bite or attachment. In approximately half of pediatric RMSF cases, there is no recall of a recent tick bite. Delay in disease recognition and initiation of antirickettsial therapy after the fifth day of symptoms increase the risk of death. Factors contributing to delayed diagnosis include absence of rash, initial presentation before the fourth day of illness, and onset of illness during months of low incidence.

RMSF is widespread in the United States. Most cases are reported in the south Atlantic, southeastern, and south central states, although most states in the contiguous United States record cases each year. The principal recognized vectors of *R rickettsii* are *Dermacentor variabilis* (the American dog tick) in the eastern and central United States and *Dermacentor andersoni* (the Rocky Mountain wood tick) in the western United States. Another common tick throughout the world that feeds on dogs, *Rhipicephalus sanguineus* (the brown dog tick) has been confirmed as a vector of *R rickettsii* in Arizona and Mexico and may play a role in other regions. Transmission parallels the tick season in a given geographic area. RMSF also occurs in Canada, Mexico, Central America, and South America.

The **incubation period** is approximately 1 week (range, 2–14 days).

DIAGNOSTIC TESTS: The gold standard for serologic diagnosis of RMSF is a fourfold or greater change in immunoglobulin (Ig) G-specific antibody titer between acute and convalescent serum specimens determined by indirect immunofluorescence antibody (IFA) assay. The acute sample should be taken early in the course of illness, preferably in the first week of symptoms, and the convalescent sample should be taken 2 to 3 weeks later. Both IgG and IgM antibodies begin to increase around day 7 to 10 after onset of symptoms; therefore, an elevated acute titer may represent past exposure rather than acute infection. Elevated antibody titers can be an incidental finding in a significant proportion of the general population in some regions; thus, a fourfold rise in antibodies is more specific for acute RMSF than a single elevated titer. IgM antibodies may remain elevated for months and are not highly specific for acute RMSF. Currently, commercially available enzyme immunoassays are not quantitative, cannot be used to evaluate changes in IgG titer, and should not be used for monitoring titer changes.

During the first few days of symptoms, *R rickettsii* can be detected by immunohisto-chemical staining or polymerase chain reaction (PCR) of skin punch biopsy specimens taken from rash sites. Sensitivity of skin biopsy testing decreases greatly after the first 24 hours of appropriate treatment. In severe or fatal cases in which a patient is highly rickettsemic, other tissue specimens or blood samples may be used for PCR testing at the Centers for Disease Control and Prevention or other reference laboratories.

TREATMENT: Doxycycline is the treatment of choice for RMSF in patients of any age and should be started as soon as RMSF is suspected (see Tetracyclines, p 801). The doxycy-cline dose for RMSF is 4 mg/kg per day, divided every 12 hours, intravenously or orally (maximum 100 mg/dose). Treatment is most effective if started in the first few days of symptoms, and treatment started after the fifth day of symptoms is less likely to prevent death or other adverse outcomes. Therefore, physicians always should treat empirically and should not postpone treatment while awaiting laboratory confirmation or classic symptoms such as petechiae to appear. Chloramphenicol sometimes is listed as an alterna-tive treatment; however, its use is associated with a higher risk of fatal outcome. In addi-tion, chloramphenicol carries a risk of serious adverse events and is not available as an oral formulation in the United States. Use of chloramphenicol should be considered only in rare cases, such as severe doxycycline allergies or during pregnancy. If the mother's life is in danger, doxycycline may be considered and the theoretical risk to the fetus should be discussed with the patient. These exceptions should be considered on a case-by-case basis, and the risks and benefits should be discussed with the patient. Antimicrobial treatment should be continued until the patient has been afebrile for at least 3 days and has demon-strated clinical improvement; the usual duration of therapy is 7 to 10 days. The dose and duration of doxycycline used to treat RMSF has not been proven to cause cosmetic stain-ing of adult teeth and can be recommended to treat children of any age safely.

ISOLATION OF THE HOSPITALIZED PATIENT: Standard precautions are recommended.

CONTROL MEASURES: Control of ticks in their natural habitat is difficult. Avoidance of tick-infested areas (eg, grassy areas, areas that border wooded regions) is the best preven-tive measure. If a tick-infested area is entered, people should wear protective clothing and apply tick or insect repellents to clothes and exposed body parts for added protection. All pets should be treated for ticks according to veterinary guidelines and untreated animals should be excluded to prevent the yard and home from becoming a suitable habitat for ticks. Adults should be taught to inspect themselves, their children (bodies and clothing), and pets thoroughly for ticks after spending time outdoors during the tick season and to remove ticks promptly and properly (see Prevention of Tickborne Infections, p 207).

There is no role for prophylactic antimicrobial agents in preventing RMSF. No licensed *R rickettsii* vaccine is available in the United States. For additional information, see **www.cdc.gov/rmsf/.**

Rotavirus Infections

CLINICAL MANIFESTATIONS: Infection begins with acute onset of fever and vomiting followed 24 to 48 hours later by watery diarrhea. Symptoms generally persist for 3 to 8 days. In moderate to severe cases, dehydration, electrolyte abnormalities, and acidosis may occur. In certain immunocompromised children, including children with severe congenital immunodeficiencies or children who are hematopoietic stem cell or solid organ transplant recipients, persistent infection and diarrhea can develop.

ETIOLOGY: Rotaviruses are segmented, double-stranded RNA viruses belonging to the family Reoviridae, with at least 7 distinct antigenic groups (A through G). Group A viruses are the major causes of rotavirus diarrhea worldwide. Serotyping is based on the 2 surface proteins, VP7 glycoprotein (G) and VP4 protease-cleaved hemagglutinin (P). Prior to introduction of the rotavirus vaccine, G types 1 through 4 and 9 and P types 1A[8] and 1B[4] were most common in the United States.

EPIDEMIOLOGY: Before rotavirus vaccine was introduced in the United States, rotavirus was the most common cause of health care-associated diarrhea in young children and was an important cause of acute gastroenteritis in children attending child care. Rotavirus is present in high titer in stools of infected patients several days before and several days after onset of clinical disease. Transmission is believed to be by the fecal-oral route. Rotavirus can be found on toys and hard surfaces in child care centers, indicating that fomites may serve as a mechanism of transmission. Respiratory transmission likely plays a minor role in disease transmission. Spread within families and institutions is common. Rarely, common-source outbreaks from contaminated water or food have been reported.

In temperate climates, rotavirus disease is most prevalent during the cooler months. Before licensure of rotavirus vaccines in North America in 2006 and 2008, the annual epidemic usually started during the autumn in Mexico and the southwest United States and moved eastward, reaching the northeast United States and Canada by spring. The seasonal pattern of disease is less pronounced in tropical climates, with rotavirus infection being more common during the cooler, drier months.

The epidemiology of rotavirus disease in the United States has changed dramatically since rotavirus vaccines became available in 2006. The rotavirus season now is shorter and relatively delayed, peaking in late spring, and the overall burden of rotavirus disease has declined dramatically. In the first 2 years after the RV5 vaccine became available, emergency department visits and hospitalizations for rotavirus decreased by 85%, such that in the 2008 season, there were an estimated 40 000–60 000 fewer gastroenteritis hospitalizations among children younger than 5 years of age compared with prevaccine seasons. There also were substantial reductions in office visits for gastroenteritis during this time period.

The **incubation period** ranges from 1 to 3 days.

DIAGNOSTIC TESTS: It is not possible to diagnose rotavirus infection by clinical presentation or nonspecific laboratory tests. Enzyme immunoassays (EIAs), immunochromotography, and latex agglutination assays for group A rotavirus antigen detection in stool are available commercially. EIAs are used most widely because of their high sensitivity and specificity. Rotavirus also can be identified in stool by electron microscopy, by electrophoresis and silver staining, and by reverse transcriptase-polymerase chain reaction (RT-PCR) assay for detection of viral genomic RNA.

TREATMENT: No specific antiviral therapy is available. Oral or parenteral fluids and electrolytes are given to prevent or correct dehydration. Orally administered Human Immune Globulin, administered as an investigational therapy in immunocompromised patients with prolonged infection, has decreased viral shedding and shortened the duration of diarrhea.

ISOLATION OF THE HOSPITALIZED PATIENT: In addition to standard precautions, contact precautions are indicated for diapered or incontinent children for the duration of illness.

CONTROL MEASURES:

Child Care. General measures for interrupting enteric transmission in child care centers are available (see Children in Out-of-Home Child Care, p 133). Surfaces should be washed with soap and water. A 70% ethanol solution or other disinfectants will inactivate rotavirus and may help prevent disease transmission resulting from contact with environmental surfaces. In general, breastfeeding is associated with milder rotavirus disease and should be encouraged.

Vaccines. Two rotavirus vaccines are licensed for use among infants in the United States. In February 2006, a live, oral human-bovine reassortant pentavalent rotavirus (RV5 [RotaTeq, Merck & Co Inc]) vaccine was licensed as a 3-dose series for use among infants in the United States. In April 2008, a live, oral human attenuated monovalent rotavirus (RV1 [Rotarix, GlaxoSmithKline]) vaccine was licensed as a 2-dose series for infants in the United States. The products differ in composition and schedule of administration. The American Academy of Pediatrics and the Centers for Disease Control and Prevention do not express a preference for either vaccine.

In 2010, porcine circovirus or porcine circovirus DNA was detected in both rotavirus vaccines. There is no evidence that this virus is a safety risk or causes illness in humans.

Some studies performed outside the United States have detected a low level of increased risk of intussusception following rotavirus immunization shortly after the first dose. The level of risk observed in these postmarketing studies is substantially lower than the risk of intussusception after immunization with RotaShield, the previous rotavirus vaccine. Although an increased risk of intussusception from rotavirus vaccine has not been documented in the United States, data currently available cannot exclude a risk as low as that detected in other locations. The benefits of rotavirus immunization include prevention of hospitalization for severe rotavirus disease in the United States and of death in other parts of the world. Currently, the benefits of these vaccines, which are known, far outweigh the rare potential risks.

Following are recommendations for use of these rotavirus vaccines[1,2] (see Table 3.59, p 628):

- Infants in the United States routinely should be immunized with 3 doses of RV5 vaccine administered orally at 2, 4, and 6 months of age or 2 doses of RV1 vaccine administered orally at 2 and 4 months of age.

---

[1] American Academy of Pediatrics, Committee on Infectious Diseases. Prevention of rotavirus disease: updated guidelines for use of rotavirus vaccine. *Pediatrics.* 2009;123(5):1412–1420

[2] Centers for Disease Control and Prevention. Prevention of rotavirus gastroenteritis among infants and children. Recommendations of the Advisory Committee on Immunization Practices (ACIP). *MMWR Recomm Rep.* 2009;58(RR-2):1–25

Table 3.59. Recommended Schedule for Administration of Rotavirus Vaccine

Recommendation	RV5 (RotaTeq [Merck])	RV1 (Rotarix [GlaxoSmithKline])
Number of doses in series	3	2
Recommended ages for doses	2, 4, and 6 months of age	2 and 4 months of age
Minimum age for first dose	6 weeks of age	6 weeks of age
Maximum age for first dose	14 weeks, 6 days of age	14 weeks, 6 days of age
Minimum interval between doses	4 weeks	4 weeks
Maximum age for last dose	8 months, 0 days of age	8 months, 0 days of age

- The first dose of rotavirus vaccine should be administered from 6 weeks through 14 weeks, 6 days of age (the maximum age for the first dose is 14 weeks, 6 days). Immunization should not be initiated for infants 15 weeks, 0 days of age or older.
- The minimum interval between doses of rotavirus vaccine is 4 weeks.
- All doses of rotavirus vaccine should be administered by 8 months, 0 days of age.
- The rotavirus vaccine series should be completed with the same product whenever possible. However, immunization should not be deferred if the product used for previous doses is not available or is unknown. In this situation, the health care professional should continue or complete the series with the product available.
- If any dose in the series was RV5 vaccine or the product is unknown for any dose in the series, a total of 3 doses of rotavirus vaccine should be given.
- Rotavirus vaccine can be administered concurrently with other childhood vaccines.
- Infants with transient, mild illness with or without low-grade fever may receive rotavirus vaccine.
- Preterm infants may be immunized if the infant is at least 6 weeks of postnatal age and is clinically stable. Preterm infants should be immunized on the same schedule and with the same precautions as recommended for full-term infants. The first dose of vaccine should be given at the time of discharge or after the infant has been discharged from the nursery.
- Infants living in households with pregnant women or immunocompromised people can be immunized. Transmission of vaccine virus strains from vaccinees to unimmunized contacts has been observed in postmarketing studies but is uncommon. The potential risk of transmission of vaccine virus should be weighed against the risk of acquiring and transmitting natural rotavirus.
- Rotavirus vaccine should not be administered to infants who have a history of a severe allergic reaction (eg, anaphylaxis) after a previous dose of rotavirus vaccine or to a vaccine component. Latex rubber is contained in the RV1 vaccine oral applicator, so infants with a severe (anaphylactic) allergy to latex should not receive RV1. The RV5 vaccine dosing tube is latex free.
- Severe combined immune deficiency (SCID) and history of intussusception are contraindications for use of both rotavirus vaccines. Gastroenteritis, including severe diarrhea and prolonged shedding of vaccine virus, have been reported in infants who were administered live, oral rotavirus vaccines and later identified as having SCID.

- Precautions for administration of rotavirus vaccine include manifestations of altered immunocompetence (other than SCID, which is a contraindication); moderate to severe illness, including gastroenteritis; preexisting chronic intestinal tract disease; and spina bifida or bladder extrophy.
- Rotavirus vaccine may be administered at any time before, concurrent with, or after administration of any blood product, including antibody-containing blood products.
- Breastfeeding infants should be immunized according to the same schedule as non-breastfed infants.
- If an infant regurgitates, spits out, or vomits during or after vaccine administration, the vaccine dose should not be repeated.
- If a recently immunized infant is hospitalized for any reason, no precautions other than standard precautions need to be taken to prevent spread of vaccine virus in the hospital setting.
- Infants who have had rotavirus gastroenteritis before receiving the full series of rotavirus immunization should begin or complete the schedule following the standard age and interval recommendations.

Rubella

CLINICAL MANIFESTATIONS:

Postnatal Rubella. Many cases of postnatal rubella are subclinical. Clinical disease usually is mild and characterized by a generalized erythematous maculopapular rash, lymphadenopathy, and slight fever. The rash starts on the face, becomes generalized in 24 hours, and lasts a median of 3 days. Lymphadenopathy, which may precede rash, often involves posterior auricular or suboccipital lymph nodes, can be generalized, and lasts between 5 and 8 days. Conjunctivitis and palatal enanthem have been noted. Transient polyarthralgia and polyarthritis rarely occur in children but are common in adolescents and adults, especially females. Encephalitis (1 in 6000 cases) and thrombocytopenia (1 in 3000 cases) are complications.

Congenital Rubella Syndrome. Maternal rubella during pregnancy can result in miscarriage, fetal death, or a constellation of congenital anomalies (congenital rubella syndrome [CRS]). The most commonly described anomalies/manifestations associated with CRS are ophthalmologic (cataracts, pigmentary retinopathy, microphthalmos, and congenital glaucoma), cardiac (patent ductus arteriosus, peripheral pulmonary artery stenosis), auditory (sensorineural hearing impairment), or neurologic (behavioral disorders, meningoencephalitis, microcephaly, and mental retardation). Neonatal manifestations of CRS include growth restriction, interstitial pneumonitis, radiolucent bone disease, hepatosplenomegaly, thrombocytopenia, and dermal erythropoiesis (so-called "blueberry muffin" lesions). Mild forms of the disease can be associated with few or no obvious clinical manifestations at birth. Congenital defects occur in up to 85% if maternal infection occurs during the first 12 weeks of gestation, 50% during the first 13 to 16 weeks of gestation, and 25% during the end of the second trimester.

ETIOLOGY: Rubella virus is an enveloped, positive-stranded RNA virus classified as a Rubivirus in the Togaviridae family.

EPIDEMIOLOGY: Humans are the only source of infection. Postnatal rubella is transmitted primarily through direct or droplet contact from nasopharyngeal secretions. The peak incidence of infection is during late winter and early spring. Approximately 25% to 50%

of infections are asymptomatic. Immunity from wild-type or vaccine virus usually is prolonged, but reinfection on rare occasions has been demonstrated and rarely has resulted in CRS. Although volunteer studies have demonstrated rubella virus in nasopharyngeal secretions from 7 days before to 14 days after onset of rash, the period of maximal communicability extends from a few days before to 7 days after onset of rash. A small number of infants with congenital rubella continue to shed virus in nasopharyngeal secretions and urine for 1 year or more and can transmit infection to susceptible contacts. Rubella virus has been recovered in high titer from lens aspirates in children with congenital cataracts for several years.

Before widespread use of rubella vaccine, rubella was an epidemic disease, occurring in 6- to 9-year cycles, with most cases occurring in children. In the vaccine era, most cases in the mid-1970s and 1980s occurred in young unimmunized adults in outbreaks on college campuses and in occupational settings. More recent outbreaks have occurred in people born in other countries or underimmunized people. The incidence of rubella in the United States has decreased by more than 99% from the prevaccine era.

The United States was determined no longer to have endemic rubella in 2004, and since that time, fewer than 16 US cases have been reported annually. A national serologic survey from 1999-2004 indicated that rubella seroprevalence in the US population remained above the postulated threshold for elimination. Among children and adolescents 6 through 19 years of age, seroprevalence was approximately 95%; however, approximately 10% of adults 20 through 49 years of age lacked antibodies to rubella, although 92% of women were seropositive. In addition, epidemiologic studies of rubella and CRS in the United States have identified that seronegativity is higher among people born outside the United States or from areas with poor vaccine coverage. The risk of CRS is highest in infants of women born outside the United States, because these women are more likely to be susceptible to rubella.

In 2003, the Pan American Health Organization (PAHO) adopted a resolution calling for elimination of rubella and CRS in the Americas by the year 2010. All countries in the Americas implemented the recommended PAHO strategy by the end of 2008, and the last confirmed endemic rubella case in the Americas was diagnosed in Argentina in February 2009. In September 2010, PAHO announced that the region of the Americas had achieved the rubella and CRS elimination goals on the basis of surveillance data, but documentation of elimination is ongoing.

The incubation period for postnatally acquired rubella ranges from 14 to 21 days, usually 16 to 18 days.

DIAGNOSTIC TESTS: Detection of rubella-specific immunoglobulin (Ig) M antibody usually indicates recent postnatal infection or congenital infection in a newborn infant, but both false-negative and false-positive results occur. Most postnatal cases are IgM-positive by 5 days after symptom onset, and most congenital cases are IgM-positive at birth to 3 months of age. For diagnosis of postnatally acquired rubella, a fourfold or greater increase in antibody titer or seroconversion between acute and convalescent IgG serum titers also indicates infection. Congenital infection also can be confirmed by stable or increasing serum concentrations of rubella-specific IgG over the first 7 to 11 months of life. The hemagglutination-inhibition rubella antibody test, which previously was the most commonly used method of serologic screening for rubella infection, generally has been supplanted by a number of equally or more sensitive assays for determining rubella immunity, including enzyme immunoassays and latex agglutination tests. Diagnosis of congenital rubella infection in children older than 1 year of age is difficult; serologic testing usually is not diagnostic, and viral isolation, although confirmatory, is possible in only a small proportion of congenitally infected children of this age.

A false-positive IgM test result may be caused by rheumatoid factor, parvovirus IgM, and heterophile antibodies. The presence of high-avidity IgG or lack of increase in IgG titers can be useful in identifying false-positive rubella IgM results. Low-avidity IgG is associated with recent primary rubella infection, whereas high-avidity IgG is associated with past infection or reinfection. The avidity assay is not a routine test and should be performed in reference laboratories.

Rubella virus can be isolated most consistently from throat or nasal specimens (and less consistently, urine) by inoculation of appropriate cell culture. Detection of rubella virus RNA by reverse-transcriptase polymerase chain reaction from a throat/nasal swab or urine sample with subsequent genotyping of strains may be valuable for diagnosis and molecular epidemiology. Most postnatal cases are positive virologically on the day of symptom onset, and most congenital cases are positive virologically at birth. Laboratory personnel should be notified that rubella is suspected, because specialized testing is required to detect the virus. Blood, urine, and cataract specimens also may yield virus, particularly in infants with congenital infection. With the successful elimination of indigenous rubella and CRS in the United States, molecular typing of viral isolates is critical in defining a source in outbreak scenarios and for sporadic cases.

TREATMENT: Supportive.

ISOLATION OF THE HOSPITALIZED PATIENT: In addition to standard precautions, for postnatal rubella, droplet precautions are recommended for 7 days after onset of the rash. Contact isolation is indicated for children with proven or suspected congenital rubella until they are at least 1 year of age, unless 2 cultures of clinical specimens obtained 1 month apart after 3 months of age are negative for rubella virus.

CONTROL MEASURES:

School and Child Care. Children with postnatal rubella should be excluded from school or child care for 7 days after onset of the rash. During an outbreak, children without evidence of immunity should be immunized or excluded. Children with CRS should be considered contagious until they are at least 1 year of age, unless 2 cultures of clinical specimens obtained 1 month apart are negative for rubella virus after 3 months of age; infection-control precautions should be considered in children up to 3 years of age who are hospitalized for congenital cataract extraction. Caregivers of these infants should be made aware of the potential hazard of the infants to susceptible pregnant contacts.

Surveillance for Congenital Infections. Accurate diagnosis and reporting of CRS are extremely important in assessing control of rubella. All birth defects in which rubella infection is suspected etiologically should be investigated thoroughly and reported to the Centers for Disease Control and Prevention through local or state health departments.

Care of Exposed People. When a pregnant woman is exposed to rubella, a blood specimen should be obtained as soon as possible and tested for rubella antibody (IgG and IgM). An aliquot of frozen serum should be stored for possible repeated testing at a later time. The presence of rubella-specific IgG antibody in a properly performed test at the time of exposure indicates that the person most likely is immune. If antibody is not detectable, a second blood specimen should be obtained 2 to 3 weeks later and tested concurrently with the first specimen. If the second test result is negative, another blood specimen should be obtained 6 weeks after the exposure and also tested concurrently with the first specimen; a negative test result in both the second and third specimens indicates that infection has not occurred, and a positive test result in the second or third specimen but not the first (seroconversion) indicates recent infection.

Immune Globulin. Immune Globulin (IG) does not prevent rubella infection after exposure and is not recommended for that purpose. Although administration of IG after exposure to rubella will not prevent infection or viremia, it may modify or suppress symptoms and create an unwarranted sense of security. Therefore, IG is not recommended for routine postexposure prophylaxis of rubella in early pregnancy or any other circumstance. Infants with CRS have been born to women who received IG shortly after exposure. Administration of IG should be considered only if a pregnant woman who has been exposed to rubella will not consider termination of pregnancy under any circumstance. Administration of IG eliminates the value of IgG antibody testing to detect maternal infection. IgM antibody can be used to detect maternal infection after exposure, even after receipt of IG.

Vaccine. Although live-virus rubella vaccine administered after exposure has not been demonstrated to prevent illness, vaccine theoretically could prevent illness if administered within 3 days of exposure. Immunization of exposed nonpregnant people may be indicated, because if the exposure did not result in infection, immunization will protect these people in the future. Immunization of a person who is incubating natural rubella or who already is immune is not associated with an increased risk of adverse effects.

Rubella Vaccine. The live-virus rubella vaccine distributed in the United States is the RA 27/3 strain grown in human diploid cell cultures. Vaccine is administered by subcutaneous injection as a combined vaccine containing measles-mumps-rubella (MMR) or measles-mumps-rubella-varicella (MMRV). Single-antigen rubella vaccine no longer is available in the United States. Vaccine can be given simultaneously with other vaccines (see Simultaneous Administration of Multiple Vaccines, p 33). Serum antibody to rubella is induced in more than 95% of recipients after a single dose at 12 months of age or older. Clinical efficacy and challenge studies have demonstrated that 1 dose confers long-term immunity against clinical and asymptomatic infection in more than 90% of immunized people. However, both symptomatic and asymptomatic reinfection has occurred.

Because of the 2-dose recommendations for measles- and mumps-containing vaccine (as MMR) and varicella vaccine (as MMRV), 2 doses of rubella vaccine now are given routinely. This provides an added safeguard against primary vaccine failures.

Vaccine Recommendations. At least 1 dose of live-attenuated rubella-containing vaccine is recommended for people 12 months of age or older. In the United States, rubella vaccine is recommended to be administered in combination with measles and mumps vaccines (MMR) or MMRV, which also contains varicella, when a child is 12 through 15 months of age, with a second dose of MMR or MMRV at school entry at 4 through 6 years of age or sooner, according to recommendations for routine measles, mumps, rubella, and varicella immunization. People who have not received the dose at school entry should receive their second dose as soon as possible but optimally no later than 11 through 12 years of age (see Measles, p 489).

Special emphasis must continue to be placed on the immunization of at-risk postpubertal males and females, especially college students, military recruits, recent immigrants, health care professionals, teachers, and child care providers. People who were born in 1957 or after and have not received at least 1 dose of vaccine or who have no serologic evidence of immunity to rubella are considered susceptible and should be immunized with MMR vaccine. Clinical diagnosis of infection is unreliable and should not be accepted as evidence of immunity.

Specific recommendations are as follows:

- Postpubertal females without documentation of presumptive evidence of rubella immunity should be immunized unless they are known to be pregnant. Postpubertal females should be advised not to become pregnant for 28 days after receiving a rubella-containing vaccine (see Precautions and Contraindications, p 634, for further discussion). Routine serologic testing of nonpregnant postpubertal women before immunization is unnecessary and is a potential impediment to protection against rubella, because it requires 2 visits.
- During annual health care examinations, premarital and family planning visits, and visits to sexually transmitted infection clinics, postpubertal females should be assessed for rubella susceptibility and, if deemed susceptible, should be immunized with MMR vaccine.
- Routine prenatal screening for rubella immunity should be undertaken. If a woman is found to be susceptible, rubella vaccine should be administered during the immediate postpartum period before discharge.
- Breastfeeding is not a contraindication to postpartum immunization of the mother (for additional information, see Human Milk, p 126).
- All susceptible health care personnel who may be exposed to patients with rubella or who take care of pregnant women, as well as people who work in educational institutions or provide child care, should be immunized to prevent infection for themselves and to prevent transmission of rubella to pregnant patients.[1]

Adverse Reactions.

- Of susceptible children who receive MMR or MMRV vaccines, fever develops in 5% to 15% from 6 to 12 days after immunization. Rash occurs in approximately 5% of immunized people. Mild lymphadenopathy occurs commonly. Febrile seizures occur more frequently among children 12 through 23 months of age after administration of MMRV vaccine compared with MMR and varicella given as separate injections during the same visit (see Measles, p 489).
- Joint pain, usually in small peripheral joints, has been reported in approximately 0.5% of young children. Arthralgia and transient arthritis tend to be more common in susceptible postpubertal females, occurring in approximately 25% and 10%, respectively, of vaccine recipients. Joint involvement usually begins 7 to 21 days after immunization and generally is transient. The incidence of joint manifestations after immunization is lower than that after natural infection at the corresponding age.
- Transient paresthesia and pain in the arms and legs also have been reported, although rarely.
- Central nervous system manifestations have been reported, but no causal relationship with rubella vaccine has been established.
- Other reactions that occur after immunization with MMR or MMRV are associated with the measles, mumps, and varicella components of the vaccine (see Measles, p 489, Mumps, p 514, and Varicella-Zoster Infections, p 774).

---

[1] Centers for Disease Control and Prevention. Immunization of health-care personnel: recommendations of the Advisory Committee on Immunization Practices (ACIP). *MMWR Recomm Rep.* 2011;60(RR-7):1–45

Precautions and Contraindications.

- **Pregnancy.** Rubella vaccine should not be administered to pregnant women. If vaccine is administered inadvertently or if pregnancy occurs within 28 days of immunization, the patient should be counseled on the theoretical risks to the fetus. The maximal theoretical risk for occurrence of congenital rubella is estimated to be 1.3% on the basis of data accumulated by the Centers for Disease Control and Prevention from more than 200 susceptible women who received the current rubella vaccine (the RA27/3 strain) from 1 to 2 weeks before to 4 to 6 weeks after conception. Of the offspring, 2% had subclinical infection but none had congenital defects. In view of these observations, receipt of rubella vaccine during pregnancy is not an indication for termination of pregnancy.

- **Children of pregnant women.** Immunizing susceptible children whose mothers or other household contacts are pregnant does not cause a risk. Most immunized people intermittently shed small amounts of virus from the pharynx 7 to 28 days after immunization, but no evidence of transmission of the vaccine virus from immunized children has been found.

- **Febrile illness.** Children with minor illnesses, such as upper respiratory tract infection, may be immunized (see Vaccine Safety, p 41). Fever is not a contraindication to immunization. However, if other manifestations suggest a more serious illness, the child should not be immunized until recovery has occurred.

- **Recent administration of IG.** IG preparations interfere with immune response to measles vaccine, and they theoretically may interfere with the serologic response to rubella vaccine (see p 37). If rubella vaccine is indicated postpartum for a woman who has received anti-Rho (D) IG or blood products, suggested intervals are the same as used between IG administration and measles immunization (see Table 1.9, p 38).

- **Altered immunity.** Immunocompromised patients with disorders associated with increased severity of viral infections should not receive live-virus rubella vaccine (see Immunocompromised Children, p 74). Exceptions are patients with human immunodeficiency virus infection who are not severely immunocompromised; these patients may be immunized against rubella with MMR vaccine (see Human Immunodeficiency Virus Infection, p 418). If possible, children receiving biologic response modifiers, such as anti-tumor necrosis factor-alpha (see Biologic Response Modifiers, p 82), should be immunized prior to initiating treatment.

- **Household contacts of immunocompromised people.** The risk of rubella exposure for patients with altered immunity can be decreased by immunizing their close susceptible contacts. Although small amounts of virus are shed after immunization, no evidence of transmission of vaccine virus from immunized children has been found. Precautions and contraindications appropriate for the measles, mumps, and varicella components of MMR or MMRV also should be reviewed before administration (see Measles, p 489, Mumps, p 514, and Varicella-Zoster Infections, p 774).

  Corticosteroids. For patients who have received high doses of corticosteroids (2 mg/kg or greater or more than 20 mg/day) for 14 days or more and who otherwise are not immunocompromised, the recommended interval before immunization is at least 1 month (see Immunocompromised Children, p 74) after steroids have been discontinued.

Salmonella Infections

CLINICAL MANIFESTATIONS: Nontyphoidal *Salmonella* organisms cause a spectrum of illness ranging from asymptomatic gastrointestinal tract carriage to gastroenteritis, bacteremia, and focal infections, including meningitis, brain abscess, and osteomyelitis. The most common illness associated with nontyphoidal *Salmonella* infection is gastroenteritis, in which diarrhea, abdominal cramps, and fever are common manifestations. The site of infection usually is the distal small intestine as well as the colon. Sustained or intermittent bacteremia can occur, and focal infections are recognized in as many as 10% of patients with nontyphoidal *Salmonella* bacteremia.

Salmonella enterica serotypes Typhi, Paratyphi A, Paratyphi B, and certain other uncommon serotypes can cause a protracted bacteremic illness referred to, respectively, as typhoid and paratyphoid fever and collectively as enteric fevers. The onset of enteric fever typically is gradual, with manifestations such as fever, constitutional symptoms (eg, headache, malaise, anorexia, and lethargy), abdominal pain and tenderness, hepatomegaly, splenomegaly, dactylitis, rose spots, and change in mental status. In infants and toddlers, invasive infection with enteric fever serotypes can manifest as a mild, nondescript febrile illness accompanied by self-limited bacteremia, or invasive infection can occur in association with more severe clinical symptoms and signs, sustained bacteremia, and meningitis. Constipation can be an early feature.

ETIOLOGY: *Salmonella* organisms are gram-negative bacilli that belong to the family *Enterobacteriaceae*. More than 2500 *Salmonella* serotypes have been described; most serotypes causing human disease are classified within O serogroups A through E. *Salmonella* serotype Typhi is classified in O serogroup D, along with many other common serotypes including serotype Enteritidis. In 2009, the most commonly reported human isolates in the United States were *Salmonella* serotypes Enteritidis, Typhimurium, Newport, Javiana, and Heidelberg; these 5 serotypes generally account for nearly half of all *Salmonella* infections in the United States (**www.cdc.gov/narms**). The current *Salmonella* nomenclature is shown in Table 3.60.

EPIDEMIOLOGY: The principal reservoirs for nontyphoidal *Salmonella* organisms include birds, mammals, reptiles, and amphibians. The major food vehicles of transmission to humans include food of animal origin, such as poultry, beef, eggs, and dairy products. Other food vehicles (eg, fruits, vegetables, peanut butter, frozen pot pies, powdered infant formula, cereal, and bakery products) have been implicated in outbreaks, presumably when the food was contaminated by contact with an infected animal product or a human carrier. Other modes of transmission include ingestion of contaminated water; contact with infected reptiles or amphibians (eg, pet turtles, iguanas, lizards, snakes, frogs, toads, newts, salamanders) and rodents or other mammals.

Unlike nontyphoidal *Salmonella* serotypes, the enteric fever serotypes (*Salmonella* serotypes Typhi, Paratyphi A, Paratyphi B) are restricted to human hosts, in whom they cause clinical and subclinical infections. Chronic human carriers (mostly involving chronic infection of the gall bladder but occasionally involving infection of the urinary tract) constitute the reservoir in areas with endemic infection. Infection with enteric fever serovars implies ingestion of a food or water vehicle contaminated by a chronic carrier or person with acute infection. Although typhoid fever (300–400 cases annually) and paratyphoid fever (~150 cases annually) are uncommon in the United States, these

Table 3.60. Nomenclature for *Salmonella* Organisms

Complete Name[a]	Serotype[b]	Antigenic Formula
S enterica [a] subspecies *enterica* serotype Typhi	Typhi	9,12,[Vi]:d:-
S enterica subspecies *enterica* serotype Typhimurium	Typhimurium	[1],4,[5],12:i:1,2
S enterica subspecies *enterica* serotype Newport	Newport	6,8,[20]:e,h:1,2
S enterica subspecies *enterica* serotype Paratyphi A	Paratyphi A	[1],2,12:a:[1,5]
S enterica subspecies *enterica* serotype Enteritidis	Enteritidis	[1],9,12:g,m:-

[a] Species and subspecies are determined by biochemical reactions. Serotype is determined based on antigenic make-up. In the current taxonomy, only 2 species are recognized, *Salmonella enterica* and *Salmonella bongori*. *S enterica* has 6 subspecies, of which subspecies I (*enterica*) contains the overwhelming majority of all *Salmonella* pathogens that affect humans, other mammals, and birds.

[b] Many *Salmonella* pathogens that previously were considered species (and, therefore, were written italicized with a small case first letter) now are considered serotypes (also called serovars). Serotypes are now written nonitalicized with a capital first letter (eg, Typhi, Typhimurium, Enteritidis). The serotype of *Salmonella* is determined by its O (somatic) and H (flagellar) antigens and whether Vi is expressed.

infections are highly endemic in many resource-limited countries, particularly in Asia. Consequently, typhoid fever and paratyphoid fever infections in residents of the United States usually are acquired during international travel.

Age-specific incidences for nontyphoidal *Salmonella* infection are highest in children younger than 4 years of age. Rates of invasive infections and mortality are higher in infants, elderly people, and people with immunosuppressive conditions, hemoglobinopathies (including sickle cell disease), malignant neoplasms, and human immunodeficiency virus (HIV) infection. Most reported cases are sporadic, but widespread outbreaks, including health care-associated and institutional outbreaks, have been reported. The incidence of nontyphoidal *Salmonella* gastroenteritis has diminished little in recent years, in contrast to other enteric infections of bacterial etiologies.

Every year, nontyphoidal *Salmonella* organisms are one of the most common causes of laboratory-confirmed cases of enteric disease reported by the Foodborne Diseases Active Surveillance Network (FoodNet **[www.foodsafety.gov and www.cdc.gov/foodnet]**).

A potential risk of transmission of infection to others persists for as long as an infected person excretes nontyphoidal *Salmonella* organisms. Twelve weeks after infection with the most common nontyphoidal *Salmonella* serotypes, approximately 45% of children younger than 5 years of age excrete organisms, compared with 5% of older children and adults; antimicrobial therapy can prolong excretion. Approximately 1% of adults continue to excrete *Salmonella* organisms for more than 1 year.

The **incubation period** for nontyphoidal *Salmonella* gastroenteritis usually is 12 to 36 hours (range, 6–72 hours). For enteric fever, the incubation period usually is 7 to 14 days (range, 3–60 days).

DIAGNOSTIC TESTS: Isolation of *Salmonella* organisms from cultures of stool, blood, urine, bile (including duodenal fluid containing bile), and material from foci of infection is diagnostic. Gastroenteritis is diagnosed by stool culture. Diagnostic tests to detect *Salmonella* antigens by enzyme immunoassay, latex agglutination, and monoclonal antibodies have been developed, as have assays that detect antibodies to antigens of enteric fever serotypes. Gene-based polymerase chain reaction diagnostic tests also are available in research laboratories.

If enteric fever is suspected, blood, bone marrow, or bile culture is diagnostic, because organisms often are absent from stool. The sensitivity of blood culture and bone marrow culture in children with enteric fever is approximately 60% and 90%, respectively. The combination of a single blood culture plus culture of bile (collected from a bile-stained duodenal string) is 90% in detecting *Salmonella* serotype Typhi infection in children with clinical enteric fever.

TREATMENT:

- Antimicrobial therapy usually is not indicated for patients with either asymptomatic infection or uncomplicated (noninvasive) gastroenteritis caused by nontyphoidal *Salmonella* serotypes, because therapy does not shorten the duration of diarrheal disease and can prolong duration of fecal excretion. Although of unproven benefit, antimicrobial therapy is recommended for gastroenteritis caused by nontyphoidal *Salmonella* serotypes in people at increased risk of invasive disease, including infants younger than 3 months of age and people with chronic gastrointestinal tract disease, malignant neoplasms, hemoglobinopathies, HIV infection, or other immunosuppressive illnesses or therapies.

- If antimicrobial therapy is initiated in patients with gastroenteritis, amoxicillin or trimethoprim-sulfamethoxazole is recommended for susceptible strains. Resistance to these antimicrobial agents is becoming more common, especially in resource-limited countries. In areas where ampicillin and trimethoprim-sulfamethoxazole resistance is common, a fluoroquinolone or azithromycin usually is effective. However, fluoroquinolones are not approved for this indication in people younger than 18 years of age (see Fluoroquinolones, p 800).

- For patients with localized invasive disease (eg, osteomyelitis, abscess, meningitis) or bacteremia in people infected with HIV, empiric therapy with ceftriaxone is recommended. Once antimicrobial susceptibility test results are available, ampicillin or ceftriaxone for susceptible strains is recommended for at least 4 to 6 weeks.

- For invasive, nonfocal infections such as bacteremia or septicemia caused by nontyphoidal *Salmonella* or for enteric fever caused by *Salmonella* serotypes Paratyphi A, and Paratyphi B, 10 to 14 days of therapy is recommended, although shorter courses (7–10 days) have been effective; after the patient becomes afebrile, completion of therapy with a fluoroquinolone or azithromycin orally can be considered in patients with uncomplicated infections. Drugs of choice, route of administration, and duration of therapy are based on susceptibility of the organism (if known), knowledge of the antimicrobial susceptibility patterns of prevalent strains, site of infection, host, and clinical response. Multidrug-resistant isolates of *Salmonella* serotypes Typhi and Paratyphi A and strains with decreased susceptibility to fluoroquinolones are common in Asia and are found increasingly in travelers to areas with endemic infection. Invasive salmonellosis attributable to strains with decreased fluoroquinolone susceptibility is associated with greater risk for treatment failure. *Salmonella* serotypes Typhi and Paratyphi A and nontyphoidal *Salmonella* isolates with ciprofloxacin resistance or that produce extended-spectrum beta-lactamases occasionally are reported. Empiric treatment of enteric fever with ceftriaxone or fluoroquinolone is recommended, but once antimicrobial susceptibility results are known, therapy should be changed as necessary. Azithromycin is an effective alternative for people with uncomplicated infections. Relapse of nontyphoidal *Salmonella* infection can occur, particularly in immunocompromised patients, who may require longer duration of treatment and retreatment. Aminoglycosides are not recommended for treatment of invasive *Salmonella* infections.

- The propensity to become a chronic *Salmonella* serotype Typhi carrier (excretion longer than 1 year) following acute typhoid infection correlates with prevalence of choleli-thiasis, increases with age, and is greater in females than males. Chronic carriage in children is uncommon. The chronic carrier state may be eradicated by 4 weeks of oral therapy with ciprofloxacin or norfloxacin, antimicrobial agents that are highly concentrated in bile. High-dose parenteral ampicillin also can be used if 4 weeks of oral fluoroquinolone therapy is not well tolerated (see Fluoroquinolones, p 800). Cholecystectomy may be indicated in some adults if antimicrobial therapy alone fails.

- Corticosteroids may be beneficial in patients with severe enteric fever, which is characterized by delirium, obtundation, stupor, coma, or shock. These drugs should be reserved for critically ill patients in whom relief of manifestations of toxemia may be life saving. The usual regimen is high-dose dexamethasone given intravenously at an initial dose of 3 mg/kg, followed by 1 mg/kg, every 6 hours, for a total course of 48 hours.

ISOLATION OF THE HOSPITALIZED PATIENT: In addition to standard precautions, contact precautions should be used for diapered and incontinent children for the duration of illness. In children with typhoid fever, precautions should be continued until culture results for 3 consecutive stool specimens obtained at least 48 hours after cessation of antimicrobial therapy are negative.

CONTROL MEASURES: Important measures include proper food hygiene practices, treated water supplies, proper hand hygiene, adequate sanitation to dispose of human fecal waste, exclusion of infected people from handling food or providing health care, prohibiting sale of pet turtles and restricting sale of other reptiles for pets, limiting exposure of children younger than 5 years of age and immunocompromised children to reptiles and rodents (see Nontraditional Pets, p 215), reporting cases to appropriate health authorities, and investigating outbreaks. Eggs and other foods of animal origin should be cooked thoroughly. People should not eat raw eggs or foods containing raw eggs. Notification of public health authorities and determination of serotype are of primary importance in detection and investigation of outbreaks.

Child Care. Outbreaks of *Salmonella* illness in child care centers are rare. Specific strategies for controlling infection in out-of-home child care include adherence to hygiene practices, including meticulous hand hygiene and limiting exposure to reptiles and rodents (see Children in Out-of-Home Child Care, p 133).

When nontyphoidal *Salmonella* serotypes are identified in a symptomatic child care attendee or staff member with enterocolitis, older children and staff members do not need to be excluded unless they are symptomatic. Stool cultures are not required for asymptomatic contacts or for return to child care following resolution of illness. Antimicrobial therapy is not recommended for people with asymptomatic nontyphoidal *Salmonella* infection or uncomplicated diarrhea or for people who are contacts of an infected person. When *Salmonella* serotype Typhi infection is identified in a child care staff member, local or state health departments may be consulted regarding regulations for length of exclusion and testing, which may vary by jurisdiction.

Typhoid Vaccine. Resistance to infection with *Salmonella* serotype Typhi is enhanced by typhoid immunization, but currently licensed vaccines do not provide complete protection. Two typhoid vaccines are licensed for use in the United States (see Table 3.61).

The demonstrated efficacy of the 2 vaccines licensed by the US Food and Drug Administration ranges from 50% to 80%, but the duration of protection differs notably between the vaccines. Vaccine is selected on the basis of age of the child, need for booster doses, and possible contraindications (see Precautions and Contraindications, p 640) and reactions (see Adverse Events, p 640).

Indications. In the United States, immunization is recommended only for the following people:

- **Travelers to areas where risk of exposure to *Salmonella* serotype Typhi is recognized.** Risk is greatest for travelers to the Indian subcontinent, Latin America, Asia, the Middle East, and Africa who may have prolonged exposure to contaminated food and drink. Such travelers need to be cautioned that typhoid vaccine is not a substitute for careful selection of food and drink (see **www.cdc.gov/travel**).
- **People with intimate exposure to a documented typhoid fever carrier,** as occurs with continued household contact.
- **Laboratory workers with frequent contact with *Salmonella* serotype Typhi and people living outside the United States in areas with endemic typhoid infection.**

Dosages. For primary immunization, the following dosage is recommended for each vaccine:

- **Typhoid vaccine live oral Ty21a (Vivotif).** Children (6 years of age and older) and adults should take 1 enteric-coated capsule every other day for a total of 4 capsules. Each capsule should be taken with cool liquid, no warmer than 37°C (98°F), approximately 1 hour before a meal. The capsules should be kept refrigerated, and all 4 doses must be taken to achieve maximal efficacy. Immunization should be completed at least 1 week before possible exposure.
- **Typhoid Vi polysaccharide vaccine (Typhim Vi).** Primary immunization of people 2 years of age and older with Vi capsular polysaccharide (ViCPS) vaccine consists of one 0.5-mL (25-μg) dose administered intramuscularly. Vaccine should be given at least 2 weeks before possible exposure.

Table 3.61. Commercially Available Typhoid Vaccines in the United States

Typhoid Vaccine	Type	Route	Minimum Age of Receipt, y	No. of Doses[a]	Booster Frequency, y	Adverse Effects Incidence
Ty21a	Live-attenuated	Oral	6	4	5	Less than 5%
ViCPS	Polysaccharide	Intramuscular	2	1	2	Less than 7%

ViCPS indicates Vi capsular polysaccharide vaccine.

[a]Primary immunization. For further information on dosage, schedules, and adverse events, see text.

- **Protection against *Salmonella* serotypes Paratyphi A and Paratyphi B.** Neither Ty21a nor ViCPS vaccine provides reliable protection against *Salmonella* serotype Paratyphi A. Results of 2 field trials suggest that Ty21a may provide partial cross-protection against *Salmonella* serotype Paratyphi B.

Booster Doses. In circumstances of continued or repeated exposure to *Salmonella* serotype Typhi, periodic reimmunization is recommended to maintain immunity.

Continued efficacy for 7 years after immunization with the oral Ty21a vaccine has been demonstrated; however, the manufacturer of oral Ty21a vaccine recommends reimmunization (completing the entire 4-dose series) every 5 years if continued or renewed exposure to *Salmonella* serotype Typhi is expected. Oral Ty21a (which does not express Vi antigen) and ViCPS (which protects by stimulating serum IgG Vi antibody) vaccines mediate protection by distinct mechanisms.

ViCPS vaccine is a T-independent antigen that does not elicit immunologic memory to allow boosting of serum Vi antibody titers following an initial immunization. The manufacturer of ViCPS vaccine recommends reimmunization every 2 years if continued or renewed exposure is expected.

No data have been reported concerning use of one vaccine administered after primary immunization with the other.

Adverse Events. The oral Ty21a vaccine produces mild adverse reactions that may include abdominal discomfort, nausea, vomiting, fever, headache, and rash or urticaria. Reported adverse reactions to ViCPS vaccine also are minimal and include fever, headache, and local reaction of erythema or induration of 1 cm or greater.

Precautions and Contraindications. No data are available regarding efficacy of typhoid vaccines in children younger than 2 years of age. A contraindication to administration of parenteral ViCPS vaccine is a history of severe local or systemic reactions after a previous dose. No safety data have been reported for typhoid vaccines in pregnant women. The oral Ty21a vaccine is a live-attenuated vaccine and should not be administered to immu-nocompromised people, including people known to be infected with HIV; the parenteral ViCPS vaccine may be an alternative. The oral Ty21a vaccine requires replication in the gut for effectiveness; it should not be administered during gastrointestinal tract illness. Studies have demonstrated that simultaneous administration of either mefloquine or chlo-roquine with oral Ty21a results in an adequate immune response to the vaccine strain. However, if mefloquine is administered, immunization with Ty21a should be delayed for 24 hours. Also, the antimalarial agent proguanil should not be administered simultane-ously with oral Ty21a vaccine but, rather, should be administered 10 or more days after the fourth dose of oral Ty21a vaccine. Atovaquone also can interfere with oral Ty21a immunogenicity. Antimicrobial agents should be avoided for 24 or more hours before the first dose of oral Ty21a vaccine and 7 days after the fourth dose of Ty21a vaccine.

Scabies

CLINICAL MANIFESTATIONS: Scabies is characterized by an intensely pruritic, erythematous, papular eruption caused by burrowing of adult female mites in upper layers of the epidermis, creating serpiginous burrows. Itching is most intense at night. In older children and adults, the sites of predilection are interdigital folds, flexor aspects of wrists, extensor surfaces of elbows, anterior axillary folds, waistline, thighs, navel, genitalia, areolae, abdomen, intergluteal cleft, and buttocks. In children younger than 2 years of age, the eruption generally is vesicular and often occurs in areas usually spared in older children and adults, such as the scalp, face, neck, palms, and soles. The eruption is caused by a hypersensitivity reaction to the proteins of the parasite.

Characteristic scabietic burrows appear as gray or white, tortuous, thread-like lines. Excoriations are common, and most burrows are obliterated by scratching before a patient is seen by a physician. Occasionally, 2- to 5-mm red-brown nodules are present, particularly on covered parts of the body, such as the genitalia, groin, and axilla. These scabies nodules are a granulomatous response to dead mite antigens and feces; the nodules can persist for weeks and even months after effective treatment. Cutaneous secondary bacterial infection can occur and usually is caused by *Streptococcus pyogenes* or *Staphylococcus aureus* (including methicillin-resistant *S aureus* [MRSA]). Studies have demonstrated a correlation between poststreptococcal glomerulonephritis and scabies.

Crusted (Norwegian) scabies is an uncommon clinical syndrome characterized by a large number of mites and widespread, crusted, hyperkeratotic lesions. Crusted scabies usually occurs in debilitated, developmentally disabled, or immunologically compromised people but has occurred in otherwise healthy children after long-term use of topical corticosteroid therapy.

ETIOLOGY: The mite, *Sarcoptes scabiei* subspecies *hominis*, is the cause of scabies. The adult female mite burrows in the stratum corneum of the skin and lays eggs. Larvae emerge from the eggs in 2 to 4 days and molt to nymphs and then to adults, which mate and produce new eggs. The entire cycle takes approximately 10 to 17 days. *S scabiei* subspecies *canis*, acquired from dogs (with clinical mange), can cause a self-limited and mild infestation usually involving the area in direct contact with the infested animal that will, in humans, resolve without specific treatment.

EPIDEMIOLOGY: Humans are the source of infestation. Transmission usually occurs through prolonged, close, personal contact. Because of the large number of mites in exfoliating scales, even minimal contact with a patient with crusted scabies may result in transmission. Infestation acquired from dogs and other animals is uncommon, and these mites do not replicate in humans. Scabies of human origin can be transmitted as long as the patient remains infested and untreated, including during the interval before symptoms develop. Scabies is endemic in many countries and occurs worldwide in cycles thought to be 15 to 30 years long. Scabies affects people from all socioeconomic levels without regard to age, sex, or standards of personal hygiene. Scabies in adults often is acquired sexually.

The **incubation period** in people without previous exposure usually is 4 to 6 weeks. People who previously were infested are sensitized and develop symptoms 1 to 4 days after repeated exposure to the mite; however, these reinfestations usually are milder than the original episode.

DIAGNOSTIC TESTS: Diagnosis is confirmed by identification of the mite or mite eggs or scybala (feces) from scrapings of papules or intact burrows, preferably from the terminal portion where the mite generally is found. Mineral oil, microscope immersion oil, or water applied to skin facilitates collection of scrapings. A broad-blade scalpel is used to scrape the burrow. Scrapings and oil can be placed on a slide under a glass coverslip and examined microscopically under low power. Adult female mites average 330 to 450 μm in length.

TREATMENT: Topical permethrin 5% cream or oral ivermectin both are effective agents for treatment of scabies. Most experts recommend starting with topical 5% permethrin cream as the drug of choice, particularly for infants, young children (not approved for children younger than 2 months of age), and pregnant or nursing women. Permethrin cream should be removed by bathing after 8 to 14 hours. Infested children and adults should apply lotion or cream containing this scabicide over their entire body below the head. Because scabies can affect the face, scalp, and neck in infants and young children, treatment of the entire head, neck, and body in this age group is required. Special attention should be given to trimming fingernails and ensuring application of medication to these areas. A Cochrane review found that ivermectin is effective for treating scabies but less effective than topical permethrin. Because ivermectin is not ovicidal, it is given as 2 doses, 1 week apart. Ivermectin is not approved for treatment of scabies by the US Food and Drug Administration. The safety of ivermectin in children weighing less than 15 kg (33 lb) has not been determined (see Drugs for Parasitic Infections, p 848). Ivermectin is not recommended for women who are pregnant or who are lactating and intend to breastfeed.

Alternative drugs are precipitated sulfur compounded into petrolatum or 10% crotamiton cream or lotion.

Because scabietic lesions are the result of a hypersensitivity reaction to the mite, itching may not subside for several weeks despite successful treatment. The use of oral antihistamines and topical corticosteroids can help relieve this itching. Topical or systemic antimicrobial therapy is indicated for secondary bacterial infections of the excoriated lesions.

Because of safety concerns and availability of other treatments, lindane should not be used for treatment of scabies.

ISOLATION OF THE HOSPITALIZED PATIENT: In addition to standard precautions, contact precautions are recommended until the patient has been treated with an appropriate scabicide.

CONTROL MEASURES:
- Prophylactic therapy is recommended for household members, particularly for household members who have had prolonged direct skin-to-skin contact. Manifestations of scabies infestation can appear as late as 2 months after exposure, during which time patients can transmit scabies. All household members should be treated at the same time to prevent reinfestation. Bedding and clothing worn next to the skin during the 3 days before initiation of therapy should be laundered in a washer with hot water and dried using a hot cycle. Mites do not survive more than 3 days without skin contact. Clothing that cannot be laundered should be removed from the patient and stored for several days to a week to avoid reinfestation.

- Children should be allowed to return to child care or school after treatment has been completed.
- Epidemics and localized outbreaks may require stringent and consistent measures to treat contacts. Caregivers who have had prolonged skin-to-skin contact with infested patients may benefit from prophylactic treatment.
- Environmental disinfestation is unnecessary and unwarranted. Thorough vacuuming of environmental surfaces is recommended after use of a room by a patient with crusted scabies.
- People with crusted scabies and their close contacts must be treated promptly and aggressively to avoid outbreaks.

Schistosomiasis

CLINICAL MANIFESTATIONS: Infections are established by skin penetration of infecting larvae (cercariae, shed by fresh water snails), which may be accompanied by a transient, pruritic, papular rash (cercarial dermatitis). After penetration, the organism enters the bloodstream, migrates through the lungs, and eventually migrates to the venous plexus that drains the intestines or (in the case of *Schistosoma haematobium*) the bladder, where the adult worms reside. Four to 8 weeks after exposure, an acute illness (Katayama fever) can develop that manifests as fever, malaise, cough, rash, abdominal pain, hepatospleno-megaly, diarrhea, nausea, lymphadenopathy, and eosinophilia. The severity of symptoms associated with chronic disease is related to the worm burden. People with low to moderate worm burdens may never develop overt clinical disease or may develop milder manifestations, such as anemia. Higher worm burdens can have a range of symptoms caused primarily by inflammation and fibrosis triggered by the immune response to eggs produced by adult worms. Severe forms of intestinal schistosomiasis (*Schistosoma mansoni* and *Schistosoma japonicum* infections) can result in hepatosplenomegaly, abdominal pain, bloody diarrhea, portal hypertension, ascites, and esophageal varices and hematemesis. Urinary schistosomiasis (*S haematobium* infections) can result in the bladder becoming inflamed and fibrotic. Symptoms and signs include dysuria, urgency, terminal microscopic and gross hematuria, secondary urinary tract infections, hydronephrosis, and nonspecific pelvic pain. *S haematobium* also is associated with lesions of the lower genital tract (vulva, vagina, and cervix) in women, hematospermia in men, and certain forms of bladder cancer. Other organ systems can be involved—for example, eggs can embolize to the lungs, causing pulmonary hypertension. Less commonly, eggs can localize to the central nervous system, notably the spinal cord in *S mansoni* or *S haematobium* infections and the brain in *S japonicum* infection, causing neurologic complications.

Cercarial dermatitis (swimmer's itch) is caused by larvae of nonhuman schistosome species that penetrate human skin but are unable to complete their life cycle and do not cause systemic disease. Manifestations include pruritus at the penetration site a few hours after water exposure, followed in 5 to 14 days by an intermittent pruritic, sometimes papular, eruption. In previously sensitized people, more intense papular eruptions may occur for 7 to 10 days after exposure.

ETIOLOGY: The trematodes (flukes) *S mansoni*, *S japonicum*, *Schistosoma mekongi*, and *Schistosoma intercalatum* cause intestinal schistosomiasis, and *S haematobium* causes urinary tract disease. All species have similar life cycles. Swimmer's itch is caused by multiple avian and mammalian species of *Schistosoma*.

EPIDEMIOLOGY: Persistence of schistosomiasis depends on the presence of an appropriate snail as an intermediate host. Eggs excreted in stool (*S mansoni, S japonicum, S mekongi,* and *S intercalatum*) or urine *(S haematobium)* into fresh water hatch into motile miracidia, which infect snails. After development and asexual replication in snails, cercariae emerge and penetrate the skin of humans in contact with water. Children commonly are first infected when they accompany their mothers to lakes, ponds, and other open fresh water sources. School-aged children commonly are the most heavily infected people in the community and are important in maintaining transmission because of behaviors such as uncontrolled defecation and urination and prolonged wading and swimming in infected waters. Communicability lasts as long as infected snails are in the environment or live eggs are excreted in the urine and feces of humans into fresh water sources with appropriate snails. In the case of *S japonicum,* animals play an important zoonotic role (as a source of eggs) in maintaining the life cycle. Infection is not transmissible by person-to-person contact or blood transfusion.

The distribution of schistosomiasis often is focal, limited by the presence of appropriate snail vectors, infected human reservoirs, and fresh water sources. *S mansoni* occurs throughout tropical Africa, in parts of several Caribbean islands, and in areas of Venezuela, Brazil, Suriname, and the Arabian Peninsula. *S japonicum* is found in China, the Philippines, and Indonesia. *S haematobium* occurs in Africa and the Middle East. *S mekongi* is found in Cambodia and Laos. *S intercalatum* is found in West and Central Africa. Adult worms of *S mansoni* can live as long as 30 years in the human host. Thus, schistosomiasis can be diagnosed in patients many years after they have left an area with endemic infection. Immunity is incomplete, and reinfection occurs commonly. Swimmer's itch can occur in all regions of the world after exposure to fresh water, brackish water, or salt water.

The **incubation period** is variable but is approximately 4 to 6 weeks for *S japonicum,* 6 to 8 weeks for *S mansoni,* and 10 to 12 weeks for *S haematobium.*

DIAGNOSTIC TESTS: Eosinophilia is common and may be intense in Katayama syndrome. Infection with *S mansoni* and other species (except *S haematobium*) is determined by microscopic examination of stool specimens to detect characteristic eggs, but results may be negative if performed too early in the course of infection. In light infections, several stool specimens examined by a concentration technique may be needed before eggs are found, or a biopsy of the rectal mucosa may be necessary. *S haematobium* is diagnosed by examining urine for eggs. Egg excretion in urine often peaks between noon and 3 PM. Biopsy of the bladder mucosa may be necessary. Urine reagent dipsticks commonly will be positive for hematuria. Serologic tests, available through the Centers for Disease Control and Prevention and some commercial laboratories, can detect schistosome infection; additional tests can distinguish between infection with *S mansoni, S haematobium,* or *S japonicum.* Specific serologic tests may be particularly helpful for detecting light infections. Results of these antibody-based tests remain positive for many years and are not useful in differentiating ongoing infection from past infection or reinfection.

Swimmer's itch can be difficult to differentiate from other causes of dermatitis. A skin biopsy may demonstrate larvae, but their absence does not exclude the diagnosis.

TREATMENT: The drug of choice for schistosomiasis caused by any species is praziquantel; the alternative drug for *S mansoni* is oxamniquine, although this drug is not available in the United States but is used in some areas of Brazil (see Drugs for Parasitic Infections, p 848). Praziquantel does not kill developing worms; therapy given within 4 to 8 weeks of exposure should be repeated 1 to 2 months later. Swimmer's itch is a self-limited disease that may require symptomatic treatment of the rash. More intense reactions may require a course of oral corticosteroids.

ISOLATION OF THE HOSPITALIZED PATIENT: Standard precautions are recommended.

CONTROL MEASURES: Elimination of the intermediate snail host is difficult to achieve in most areas. Thus, mass or selective treatment of infected populations, sanitary disposal of human waste, and education about the source of infection are key elements of current control measures. Travelers to areas with endemic infection should be advised to avoid contact with freshwater streams and lakes.

Shigella Infections

CLINICAL MANIFESTATIONS: *Shigella* species primarily infect the large intestine, causing clinical manifestations that range from watery or loose stools with minimal or no constitutional symptoms to more severe symptoms, including high fever, abdominal cramps or tenderness, tenesmus, and mucoid stools with or without blood. *Shigella dysenteriae* serotype 1 often causes a more severe illness than other shigellae with a higher risk of complications, including pseudomembranous colitis, toxic megacolon, intestinal perforation, hemolysis, and hemolytic-uremic syndrome (HUS). Generalized seizures have been reported among young children with shigellosis; although the pathophysiology and incidence are poorly understood, such seizures usually are self-limited and associated with high fever or electrolyte abnormalities. Septicemia is rare during the course of illness and is caused either by *Shigella* organisms or by other gut flora that gain access to the bloodstream through intestinal mucosa damaged during shigellosis. Septicemia occurs most often in neonates, malnourished children, and people with *S dysenteriae* serotype 1 infection. Reactive arthritis (Reiter syndrome) is a rare complication of *Shigella* infection that can develop weeks or months after shigellosis, especially in patients expressing HLA-B27.

ETIOLOGY: *Shigella* species are facultative aerobic, gram-negative bacilli in the family Enterobacteriacecae. Four species (with more than 40 serotypes) have been identified. Among *Shigella* isolates reported in industrialized nations including the United States in 2009, approximately 86% were *Shigella sonnei*, 12% were *Shigella flexneri*, 1% were *Shigella boydii*, and less than 1% were *S dysenteriae* (**www.cdc.gov/narms**). In resource-limited countries, especially in Africa and Asia, *S flexneri* predominates, and *S dysenteriae* often causes outbreaks. Shiga toxin is produced by *S dysenteriae* serotype 1, which enhances virulence at the colonic mucosa and can cause small blood vessel and renal damage (HUS).

EPIDEMIOLOGY: Humans are the natural host for *Shigella* organisms, although other primates can be infected. The primary mode of transmission is fecal-oral, although transmission also can occur via contact with a contaminated inanimate object, ingestion of contaminated food or water, or sexual contact. Houseflies also may be vectors through physical transport of infected feces. Ingestion of as few as 10 organisms, depending on the species, is sufficient for infection to occur. Children 5 years of age or younger in child care settings and their caregivers and people living in crowded conditions are at increased risk of infection. Infections attributable to *S flexneri*, *S boydii*, and *S dysenteriae* are more common in older children and adults than are infections attributable to *S sonnei* in the United States; nonetheless, more than 25% of cases caused by each species are reported among children younger than 5 years of age. Travel to resource-limited countries with inadequate sanitation can place travelers at risk of infection. Even without antimicrobial therapy, the carrier state usually ceases within 1 to 4 weeks after onset of illness; long-term carriage is uncommon and does not correlate with underlying intestinal dysfunction.

The **incubation period** varies from 1 to 7 days, typically 1 to 3 days.

DIAGNOSTIC TESTS: Isolation of *Shigella* organisms from feces or rectal swab specimens containing feces is diagnostic; sensitivity is improved by testing stool as soon as it is passed. The presence of fecal leukocytes on a methylene-blue stained stool smear is sensitive for the diagnosis of colitis but is not specific for *Shigella* species. Although bacteremia is rare, blood should be cultured in severely ill, immunocompromised, or malnourished children. Other tests for bacterial detection, including a fluorescent antibody test, enzyme-linked DNA probes and microassays, are available in research laboratories. Qualitative and quantitative polymerase chain reaction assays are being implemented in some clinical laboratories.

TREATMENT:
- Although severe dehydration is rare with shigellosis, correction of fluid and electrolyte losses, preferably by oral rehydration solutions, is the mainstay of treatment.
- Most clinical infections with *S sonnei* are self-limited (48 to 72 hours), and mild episodes do not require antimicrobial therapy. Available evidence suggests that antimicrobial therapy is somewhat effective in shortening duration of diarrhea and hastening eradication of organisms from feces. Treatment is recommended for patients with severe disease, dysentery, or underlying immunosuppressive conditions; in these patients, empiric therapy should be given while awaiting culture and susceptibility results. Antimicrobial susceptibility testing of clinical isolates is indicated, because resistance to antimicrobial agents is common and susceptibility data can guide appropriate therapy. Plasmid-mediated resistance has been identified in all *Shigella* species. In 2009 in the United States sentinel surveillance system, approximately 46% of *Shigella* species were resistant to ampicillin, 40% were resistant to trimethoprim-sulfamethoxazole, and less than 1% were resistant to ciprofloxacin and to ceftriaxone (**www.cdc.gov/narms**). Ciprofloxacin and ceftriaxone resistance is increasing around the world.
- For cases in which treatment is required and susceptibility is unknown or an ampicillin- and trimethoprim-sulfamethoxazole–resistant strain is isolated, parenteral azithromycin for 3 days, ceftriaxone for 5 days, or a fluoroquinolone (such as ciprofloxacin) for 3 days should be administered. Oral cephalosporins are not useful for treatment. Fluoroquinolones are not approved by the US Food and Drug Administration for use in people younger than 18 years of age with shigellosis, although fluoroquinolones have been shown to be beneficial (see Fluoroquinolones, p 800). For susceptible strains, ampicillin or trimethoprim-sulfamethoxazole is effective; amoxicillin is less effective because of its rapid absorption from the gastrointestinal tract. The oral route of therapy is recommended except for seriously ill patients.
- Antimicrobial therapy typically is administered for 5 days; a 2-day course of ceftriaxone can be used if there is a good clinical response and no extraintestinal infection.
- Antidiarrheal compounds that inhibit intestinal peristalsis are contraindicated, because they can prolong the clinical and bacteriologic course of disease and increase the rate of complications.

- Nutritional supplementation, including vitamin A (200 000 IU) and zinc (10 or 20 mg elemental Zn, orally daily for 10–14 days), can be given to hasten clinical resolution in geographic areas where children are at risk of malnutrition.

ISOLATION OF THE HOSPITALIZED PATIENT: In addition to standard precautions, contact precautions are indicated for the duration of illness.

CONTROL MEASURES:

Child Care Centers. General measures for interrupting enteric transmission in child care centers are recommended (see Children in Out-of-Home Child Care, p 133). Meticulous hand hygiene is the single most important measure to decrease transmission. Waterless hand sanitizers may be an effective option in circumstances where access to soap or clean water is limited and as an adjunct to washing hands with soap. Eliminating access to shared water-play areas and contaminated diapers also can decrease infection rates. Child care staff members who change diapers should not be responsible for food preparation.

When *Shigella* infection is identified in a child care attendee or staff member, stool specimens from symptomatic attendees and staff members should be cultured. The local health department should be notified to evaluate and manage potential outbreaks. Ill children and staff should not be permitted to return to the child care facility until 24 or more hours after diarrhea has ceased and, depending on state regulations, until one or more stool cultures are negative for *Shigella* species.

Institutional Outbreaks. The most difficult outbreaks to control are outbreaks that involve children not yet or recently toilet-trained, adults who are unable to care for themselves (mentally disabled people or skilled nursing facility residents), or an inadequate chlorinated water supply. A cohort system, combined with appropriate antimicrobial therapy, and a strong emphasis on hand hygiene, should be considered until stool cultures no longer yield *Shigella* species. In residential institutions, ill people and newly admitted patients should be housed in separate areas.

General Control Measures. Strict attention to hand hygiene is essential to limit spread. Other important control measures include improved sanitation, a safe water supply through chlorination, proper cooking and storage of food, the exclusion of infected people as food handlers, and measures to decrease contamination of food and surfaces by houseflies. People should refrain from recreational water venues (eg, swimming pools, water parks) for 1 week after symptoms resolve. Breastfeeding provides some protection for infants. Case reporting to appropriate health authorities (eg, hospital infection control personnel and public health departments) is essential.

Smallpox (Variola)

The last naturally occurring case of smallpox occurred in Somalia in 1977, followed by 2 cases in 1978 after a photographer was infected during a laboratory exposure and later transmitted smallpox to her mother in the United Kingdom. In 1980, the World Health Assembly declared that smallpox (variola virus) had been eradicated successfully worldwide. The United States discontinued routine childhood immunization against smallpox in 1972 and routine immunization of health care professionals in 1976. Immunization of US military personnel continued until 1990. Following eradication, 2 World Health Organization reference laboratories were authorized to maintain stocks of variola virus. As a result of terrorism events on September 11, 2001, and concern that the virus and the expertise to use it as a weapon of bioterrorism may have been misappropriated, the smallpox immunization policy was revisited. In 2002, the United States resumed immunization of military personnel deployed to certain areas of the world and initiated a civilian preevent smallpox immunization program in 2003 to facilitate preparedness and response to a smallpox bioterrorism event.

CLINICAL MANIFESTATIONS: People infected with variola major strains develop a severe prodromal illness characterized by high fever (102°F–104°F [38.9°C–40.0°C]) and constitutional symptoms, including malaise, severe headache, backache, abdominal pain, and prostration, lasting for 2 to 5 days. Infected children may suffer from vomiting and seizures during this prodromal period. Most patients with smallpox tend to be severely ill and bedridden during the febrile prodrome. The prodromal period is followed by development of lesions on mucosa of the mouth or pharynx, which may not be noticed by the patient. This stage occurs less than 24 hours before onset of rash, which usually is the first recognized manifestation of infectiousness. With onset of oral lesions, the patient becomes infectious and remains so until all skin crust lesions have separated. The rash typically begins on the face and rapidly progresses to involve the forearms, trunk, and legs, with the greatest concentration of lesions on the face and distal extremities. The majority of patients will have lesions on the palms and soles. With rash onset, fever decreases but does not resolve. Lesions begin as macules that progress to papules, followed by firm vesicles and then deep-seated, hard pustules described as "pearls of pus." Each stage lasts 1 to 2 days. By the sixth or seventh day of rash, lesions may begin to umbilicate or become confluent. Lesions increase in size for approximately 8 to 10 days, after which they begin to crust. Once all the crusts have separated, 3 to 4 weeks after the onset of rash, the patient no longer is infectious. Variola minor strains cause a disease that is indistinguishable clinically from variola major, except that it causes less severe systemic symptoms, more rapid rash evolution, reduced scarring, and fewer fatalities.

Varicella (chickenpox) is the condition most likely to be mistaken for smallpox. Generally, children with varicella do not have a febrile prodrome, but adults may have a brief, mild prodrome. Although the 2 diseases are confused easily in the first few days of the rash, smallpox lesions develop into pustules that are firm and deeply embedded in the dermis, whereas varicella lesions develop into superficial vesicles. Because varicella erupts in crops of lesions that evolve quickly, lesions on any one part of the body will be in different stages of evolution (papules, vesicles, and crusts), whereas all smallpox lesions on any one part of the body are in the same stage of development. The rash distribution of the 2 diseases differs; varicella most commonly affects the face and trunk, with relative sparing of the extremities, and lesions on the palms or soles are rare.

Variola major in unimmunized people is associated with case-fatality rates of ≤30% during epidemics of smallpox. The mortality rate is highest in children younger than 1 year of age and adults older than 30 years of age. The potential for modern supportive therapy to improve outcome is not known.

In addition to the typical presentation of smallpox (90% of cases or greater), there are 2 uncommon forms of variola major: hemorrhagic (characterized either by a hemorrhagic diathesis prior to onset of the typical smallpox rash [early hemorrhagic smallpox] or by hemorrhage into skin lesions and disseminated intravascular coagulation [late hemorrhagic smallpox]) and malignant or flat type (in which the skin lesions do not progress to the pustular stage but remain flat and soft). Each variant occurs in approximately 5% of cases and is associated with a 95% to 100% mortality rate.

ETIOLOGY: Variola is a member of the *Poxviridae* family (genus *Orthopoxvirus*). Other members of this genus that can infect humans include monkeypox virus, cowpox virus, and vaccinia virus. In 2003, an outbreak of monkeypox linked to prairie dogs exposed to rodents imported from Ghana occurred in the United States. Cowpox virus was used by Benjamin Jesty in 1774 and by Edward Jenner in 1798 as material for the first smallpox vaccine. Later, cowpox virus was replaced with vaccinia virus.

EPIDEMIOLOGY: Humans are the only natural reservoir for variola virus (smallpox). Smallpox is spread most commonly in droplets from the oropharynx of infected people, although rare transmission from aerosol spread has been reported. Infection from direct contact with lesion material or indirectly via fomites, such as clothing and bedding, also has been reported. Because most patients with smallpox are extremely ill and bedridden, spread generally is limited to household contacts, hospital workers, and other health care professionals. Secondary household attack rates for smallpox were considerably lower than for measles and similar to or lower than rates for varicella.

The **incubation period** is 7 to 17 days (mean, 12 days).

DIAGNOSTIC TESTS: Variola virus can be detected in vesicular or pustular fluid by a number of different methods, including electron microscopy, immunohistochemistry, culture, or polymerase chain reaction (PCR) assay. Only PCR can definitively diagnose infection with variola virus; all other methods simply screen for orthopoxviruses. Screening is available through state health departments, and final variola-specific laboratory confirmation is available only at the Centers for Disease Control and Prevention (CDC). Diagnostic work-up includes exclusion of varicella-zoster virus or other common conditions that cause a vesicular/pustular rash illness.

TREATMENT: There is no known effective antiviral therapy available to treat smallpox. Infected patients should receive supportive care. Cidofovir has been suggested as having a role in smallpox therapy, but data to support cidofovir use in smallpox are not available. Investigational agents, such as CMX001 (the lipophilic derivative of cidofovir), are being evaluated in animal models. Vaccinia Immune Globulin (VIG) is reserved for certain complications of immunization and has no role in treatment of smallpox.

ISOLATION OF THE HOSPITALIZED PATIENT: On admission, a patient suspected of having smallpox should be placed in a private, airborne infection isolation room equipped with negative-pressure ventilation with high-efficiency particulate air filtration. Standard, contact, and airborne precautions should be implemented immediately, and hospital infection control personnel and the state (and/or local) health department should be alerted at once. After evaluation by the state or local health department, if smallpox laboratory diagnostics are considered necessary, the CDC Emergency Operations Center should be consulted at 770-488-7100.

CONTROL MEASURES:

Care of Exposed People. Cases of febrile rash illness for which smallpox is considered in the differential diagnosis should be reported immediately to local or state health departments.

Use of vaccine. Postexposure immunization (within 3–4 days of exposure) provides some protection against disease and significant protection against a fatal outcome. Except for severely immunocompromised people who are not expected to benefit from live vaccinia vaccine, any person with a significant exposure to a patient with proven smallpox during the infectious stage of illness requires immunization as soon after exposure as possible but within 4 days of first exposure ("ring vaccination"). Because infected people are not contagious until the rash (and/or oral lesions) appears, people exposed only during the prodromal period are not at risk.

Preexposure Immunization.

Smallpox vaccine. The only smallpox vaccine licensed in the United States is ACAM2000, a live-virus vaccine.[1] The vaccine does not contain variola virus but a related virus called vaccinia virus, different from the cowpox virus initially used for immunization by Jesty and Jenner. Vaccinia vaccines are highly effective in preventing smallpox, with protection waning after 5 to 10 years following 1 dose; protection after reimmunization has lasted longer. However, substantial protection against death from smallpox persisted in the past for more than 30 years after immunization during infancy during a time of worldwide smallpox virus circulation and routine smallpox immunization practices. Preexposure smallpox immunization is not recommended for children. Smallpox vaccine had been recommended for adults participating in smallpox response team and for people working with orthopoxviruses. Smallpox reimmunization recommendations can be found at **http://emergency.cdc.gov/agent/smallpox/ revaxmemo.asp.** Information about vaccine administration and adverse events[2] can be found in the vaccine package insert and medication guide at **www.fda.gov/ BiologicsBloodVaccines/Vaccines/ApprovedProducts/ucm180810.htm** or at **www.bt.cdc.gov/agent/smallpox/index.asp.**

Sporotrichosis

CLINICAL MANIFESTATIONS: Sporotrichosis manifests either as cutaneous or extracutaneous disease. The lymphocutaneous manifestation is the most common **cutaneous** form. Inoculation occurs at a site of minor trauma, causing a painless papule that enlarges slowly to become a nodular lesion that can develop a violaceous hue or can ulcerate. Secondary lesions follow the same evolution and develop along the lymphatic distribution proximal to the initial lesion. A localized cutaneous form of sporotrichosis, also called fixed cutaneous form, common in children, presents as a solitary crusted papule or papuloulcerative or nodular lesion in which lymphatic spread is not observed. The extremities and face are the most common sites of infection. A disseminated cutaneous form with multiple lesions is rare, usually occurring in immunocompromised children.

Extracutaneous sporotrichosis is uncommon, with cases occurring primarily in immunocompromised patients. Osteoarticular infection results from hematogenous spread or local inoculation. The most commonly affected joints are the knee, elbow, wrist, and ankle. Pulmonary sporotrichosis clinically resembles tuberculosis and occurs after inhalation or aspiration of aerosolized spores. Disseminated disease generally occurs after hematogenous spread from primary skin or lung infection. Disseminated sporotrichosis can involve multiple foci (eg, eyes, pericardium, genitourinary tract, central nervous system) and occurs predominantly in immunocompromised patients. Pulmonary and disseminated forms of sporotrichosis are uncommon in children.

---

[1] Centers for Disease Control and Prevention. Notice to readers: newly licensed smallpox vaccine to replace old smallpox vaccine. *MMWR Morb Mortal Wkly Rep.* 2008;57(8):207–208

[2] Centers for Disease Control and Prevention. Surveillance guidelines for smallpox vaccine (vaccinia) adverse reactions. *MMWR Recomm Rep.* 2006;55(RR-1):1–16

ETIOLOGY: *Sporothrix schenckii* is a thermally dimorphic fungus that grows as a mold or mycelial form at room temperature and as a yeast at 37°C (98°F) and in host tissues. *S schenckii* is a complex of at least six species. The related species *Sporothrix brasiliensis*, *Sporothrix globosa*, and *Sporothrix mexicana* also cause human infection.

EPIDEMIOLOGY: *S schenckii* is a ubiquitous organism that has worldwide distribution but is most common in tropical and subtropical regions of Central and South America and parts of North America. The fungus is isolated from soil and plants, including hay, straw, thorny plants (especially roses), sphagnum moss, and decaying vegetation. Cutaneous disease occurs from inoculation of debris containing the organism. People engaging in gardening or farming are at risk of infection. Inhalation of spores can lead to pulmonary disease. Zoonotic spread from infected cats or scratches from digging animals, such as armadillos, has led to cutaneous disease.

The **incubation period** is 7 to 30 days after cutaneous inoculation but can be as long as 3 months.

DIAGNOSTIC TESTS: Culture of *Sporothrix* species from a tissue, wound drainage, or sputum specimen is diagnostic. Culture of *Sporothrix* species from a blood specimen suggests the disseminated form of infection associated with immunodeficiency. Histopathologic examination of tissue may not be helpful, because the organism seldom is abundant. Special fungal stains to visualize the oval or cigar-shaped organism are required. Serologic testing and polymerase chain reaction assay show promise for accurate and specific diagnosis but are available only in research laboratories.

TREATMENT[1]: Sporotrichosis usually does not resolve without treatment. Itraconazole (6–10 mg/kg, up to a maximum of 400 mg, orally, daily) is the drug of choice for children with lymphocutaneous and localized cutaneous disease. The duration of therapy is 2 to 4 weeks after all lesions have resolved, usually for a total duration of 3 to 6 months. Alternative therapies include saturated solution of potassium iodide (1 drop, 3 times daily, increasing as tolerated to a maximum of 1 drop/kg of body weight or 40 to 50 drops, 3 times daily, whichever is lowest). Oral fluconazole should only be used if the patient cannot tolerate other agents.

Amphotericin B is recommended as the initial therapy for visceral or disseminated sporotrichosis in children. (See Recommended Doses of Parenteral and Oral Antifungal Drugs, p 831). After clinical response to amphotericin B therapy is documented, itraconazole can be substituted and should be continued for at least 12 months. Serum concentrations of itraconazole should be measured after at least 2 weeks of therapy to ensure adequate drug exposure. Itraconazole may be required for lifelong therapy in children with human immunodeficiency virus infection. Pulmonary and disseminated infections respond less well than cutaneous infection, despite prolonged therapy. Surgical débridement or excision may be necessary to resolve cavitary pulmonary disease.

ISOLATION OF THE HOSPITALIZED PATIENT: Standard precautions are indicated.

CONTROL MEASURES: Use of protective gloves and clothing in occupational and avocational activities associated with infection can decrease risk of disease.

---

[1] Kauffman CA, Bustamante B, Chapman SW, Pappas PG; Infectious Diseases Society of America. Clinical practice guidelines for the management of sporotrichosis: 2007 update by the Infectious Diseases Society of America. *Clin Infect Dis.* 2007;45(10):1255–1265

Staphylococcal Food Poisoning

CLINICAL MANIFESTATIONS: Staphylococcal foodborne illness is characterized by abrupt and sometimes violent onset of severe nausea, abdominal cramps, vomiting, and prostration, often accompanied by diarrhea. Low-grade fever or mild hypothermia can occur. Duration of illness typically is 1 to 2 days, but the intensity of symptoms can require hospitalization. The short incubation period, brevity of illness, and usual lack of fever help distinguish staphylococcal from other types of food poisoning except that caused by *Bacillus cereus*. Chemical food poisoning usually has a shorter incubation period, and *Clostridium perfringens* food poisoning usually has a longer incubation period. Patients with foodborne *Salmonella* or *Shigella* infection usually have fever and a longer incubation period (see Appendix X, Clinical Syndromes Associated With Foodborne Diseases, p 921).

ETIOLOGY: Enterotoxins produced by strains of *Staphylococcus aureus* and, rarely, *Staphylococcus epidermidis* elicit the symptoms of staphylococcal food poisoning. Of the 8 immunologically distinct heat-stable enterotoxins (A, B, C1–3, D, E, and F), enterotoxin A is the most commonly identified cause of staphylococcal food poisoning outbreaks in the United States.

EPIDEMIOLOGY: Illness is caused by ingestion of food containing staphylococcal enterotoxins. Foods usually implicated are those that come in contact with hands of food handlers without food subsequently being cooked or foods that are heated or refrigerated inadequately, such as pastries, custards, salad dressings, sandwiches, poultry, sliced meats, and meat products. When these foods remain at room temperature for several hours, toxin-producing staphylococci multiply and produce heat-stable toxin in the food. The organisms can be of human origin from purulent discharges of an infected finger or eye, abscesses, acneiform facial eruptions, nasopharyngeal secretions, or apparently normal skin. Less commonly, enterotoxins can be of bovine origin, such as contaminated milk or milk products, especially cheese.

The **incubation period** ranges from 30 minutes to 8 hours after ingestion, typically 2 to 4 hours.

DIAGNOSTIC TESTS: Recovery of large numbers of staphylococci or of enterotoxin from stool or vomitus supports the diagnosis, as does the presence of enterotoxin genes detected by polymerase chain reaction or by a commercially available enzyme immunoassay. In an outbreak, demonstration of either enterotoxin or a large number of staphylococci (greater than 10^5 colony-forming units/g of specimen) in an epidemiologically implicated food confirms the diagnosis. Identification (by pulsed-field gel electrophoresis or phage typing) of the same type of *S aureus* from stool or vomitus of 2 or more ill people, from stool or vomitus of an ill person and an implicated food, or stool or vomitus of an ill person and a person who handled the food also confirms the diagnosis. Local health authorities should be notified to help determine the source of the outbreak.

TREATMENT: Treatment is supportive. Antimicrobial agents are not indicated.

ISOLATION OF THE HOSPITALIZED PATIENT: Standard precautions are recommended.

CONTROL MEASURES: Prompt consumption or immediate cooling or refrigeration of cooked or baked foods will help to prevent the illness. Cooked foods should be refrigerated at temperatures less than 5°C (41°F). People with boils, abscesses, and other purulent lesions of the hands, face, or nose should be excluded temporarily from food preparation and handling. Strict hand hygiene before food handling should be enforced.

Staphylococcal Infections

CLINICAL MANIFESTATIONS: *Staphylococcus aureus* causes a variety of localized and invasive suppurative infections and 3 toxin-mediated syndromes: toxic shock syndrome, scalded skin syndrome, and food poisoning (see Staphylococcal Food Poisoning, p 652). Localized infections include hordeola, furuncles, carbuncles, impetigo (bullous and non-bullous), paronychia, mastitis, ecthyma, cellulitis, erythroderma, peritonsillar abscess (Quinsy), omphalitis, parotitis, lymphadenitis, and wound infections. *S aureus* also causes infections associated with foreign bodies, including intravascular catheters or grafts, pacemakers, peritoneal catheters, cerebrospinal fluid shunts, and prosthetic joints, which can be associated with bacteremia. Bacteremia can be complicated by septicemia; endocarditis; pericarditis; pneumonia; pleural empyema; soft tissue, muscle, or visceral abscesses; arthritis; osteomyelitis; septic thrombophlebitis of small and large vessels; and other foci of infection. Primary *S aureus* pneumonia also can occur after aspiration of organisms from the upper respiratory tract and typically is associated with mechanical ventilation or viral infections in the community (eg, influenza). Meningitis is rare unless accompanied by an intradermal foreign body (eg, ventriculoperitoneal shunt) or a congenital or acquired defect in the dura. *S aureus* infections can be fulminant and commonly are associated with metastatic foci and abscess formation, often requiring prolonged antimicrobial therapy, drainage, and foreign body removal to achieve cure. Risk factors for severe *S aureus* infections include chronic diseases, such as diabetes mellitus and cirrhosis, immunodeficiency, nutritional disorders, surgery, and transplantation.

Staphylococcal toxic shock syndrome (TSS), a toxin-mediated disease, usually is caused by strains producing TSS toxin-1 or possibly other related staphylococcal enterotoxins. TSS toxin-1 acts as a superantigen that stimulates production of tumor necrosis factor and other mediators that cause capillary leak, leading to hypotension and multiorgan failure. Staphylococcal TSS is characterized by acute onset of fever, generalized erythroderma, rapid-onset hypotension, and signs of multisystem organ involvement, including profuse watery diarrhea, vomiting, conjunctival injection, and severe myalgia (see Table 3.62, p 654). Although approximately 50% of reported cases of staphylococcal TSS occur in menstruating females using tampons, nonmenstrual TSS cases occur after childbirth or abortion, after surgical procedures, and in association with cutaneous lesions. TSS also can occur in males and females without a readily identifiable focus of infection. Prevailing clones (eg, USA300) of community-associated methicillin-resistant *S aureus* (MRSA) rarely produce TSS toxin. People with TSS, especially menses-associated illness, are at risk of a recurrent episode.

Staphylococcal scalded skin syndrome (SSSS) is a toxin-mediated disease caused by circulation of exfoliative toxins A and B. The manifestations of SSSS are age related and include Ritter disease (generalized exfoliation) in the neonate, a tender scarlatiniform eruption and localized bullous impetigo in older children, or a combination of these with thick white/brown flaky desquamation of the entire skin, especially on the face and neck, in older infants and toddlers. The hallmark of SSSS is the toxin-mediated cleavage of the stratum granulosum layer of the epidermis (ie, Nikolsky sign). Healing occurs without scarring. Bacteremia is rare, but dehydration and superinfection can occur with extensive exfoliation.

Table 3.62. *Staphylococcus aureus* Toxic Shock Syndrome: Clinical Case Definition[a]

Clinical Findings
- Fever: temperature 38.9°C (102.0°F) or greater
- Rash: diffuse macular erythroderma
- Desquamation: 1–2 wk after onset, particularly on palms, soles, fingers, and toes
- Hypotension: systolic pressure 90 mm Hg or less for adults; lower than fifth percentile for age for children younger than 16 years of age; orthostatic drop in diastolic pressure of 15 mm Hg or greater from lying to sitting; orthostatic syncope or orthostatic dizziness
- Multisystem organ involvement: 3 or more of the following:
  1. Gastrointestinal: vomiting or diarrhea at onset of illness
  2. Muscular: severe myalgia or creatinine phosphokinase concentration greater than twice the upper limit of normal
  3. Mucous membrane: vaginal, oropharyngeal, or conjunctival hyperemia
  4. Renal: serum urea nitrogen or serum creatinine concentration greater than twice the upper limit of normal or urinary sediment with 5 white blood cells/high-power field or greater in the absence of urinary tract infection
  5. Hepatic: total bilirubin, aspartate transaminase, or alanine transaminase concentration greater than twice the upper limit of normal
  6. Hematologic: platelet count 100 000/mm³ or less
  7. Central nervous system: disorientation or alterations in consciousness without focal neurologic signs when fever and hypotension are absent

Laboratory Criteria
- *Negative* results on the following tests, if obtained:
  - Blood, throat, or cerebrospinal fluid cultures; blood culture may be positive for *S aureus*
  - Serologic tests for Rocky Mountain spotted fever, leptospirosis, or measles

Case Classification
- **Probable:** a case that meets the laboratory criteria and in which 4 of 5 clinical findings are present
- **Confirmed:** a case that meets laboratory criteria and all 5 of the clinical findings, including desquamation, unless the patient dies before desquamation occurs.

[a]Adapted from Wharton M, Chorba TL, Vogt RL, Morse DL, Buehler JW. Case definitions for public health surveillance. *MMWR Recomm Rep.* 1990;39(RR-13):1–43.

Coagulase-Negative Staphylococci. Most coagulase-negative staphylococci (CoNS) isolates from patient specimens represent contamination of culture material (see Diagnostic Tests, p 658). Of the isolates that do not represent contamination, most come from infections that are associated with health care, in patients who have obvious disruptions of host defenses caused by surgery, medical device insertion, immunosuppression, or developmental maturity (eg, very low birth weight infants). CoNS are the most common cause of late-onset bacteremia and septicemia among preterm infants, typically infants weighing less than 1500 g at birth, and of episodes of health care-associated bacteremia in all age groups. CoNS are responsible for bacteremia in children with intravascular catheters, cerebrospinal fluid shunts, peritoneal catheters, vascular grafts or intracardiac patches, prosthetic cardiac valves, pacemaker wires, or prosthetic joints. Mediastinitis after open-heart surgery, endophthalmitis after intraocular trauma, and omphalitis and scalp abscesses in preterm neonates have been described. CoNS also can enter the bloodstream from the respiratory tract of mechanically ventilated preterm infants or from the gastrointestinal tract of infants with necrotizing enterocolitis. Some species of CoNS are associated with urinary tract infection, including *Staphylococcus saprophyticus* in adolescent females and young adult women, often after sexual intercourse, and *Staphylococcus epidermidis* and *Staphylococcus haemolyticus* in hospitalized patients with urinary tract catheters. In general, CoNS infections have an indolent clinical course in children with intact immune function and even in children who are immunocompromised.

ETIOLOGY: Staphylococci are catalase-positive, gram-positive cocci that appear microscopically as grape-like clusters. There are 32 species that are related closely on the basis of DNA base composition, but only 17 species are indigenous to humans. *S aureus* is the only species that produces coagulase. Of the 16 CoNS species, *S epidermidis*, *S haemolyticus*, *S saprophyticus*, *Staphylococcus schleiferi*, and *Staphylococcus lugdunensis* most often are associated with human infections. Staphylococci are ubiquitous and can survive extreme conditions of drying, heat, and low-oxygen and high-salt environments. *S aureus* has many surface proteins, including the microbial surface components recognizing adhesive matrix molecule (MSCRAMM) receptors, which allow the organism to bind to tissues and foreign bodies coated with fibronectin, fibrinogen, and collagen. This permits a low inoculum of organisms to adhere to sutures, catheters, prosthetic valves, and other devices. Many CoNS produce an exopolysaccharide slime biofilm that makes these organisms, as they bind to medical devices (eg, catheters), relatively inaccessible to host defenses and antimicrobial agents.

EPIDEMIOLOGY:

Staphylococcus aureus. *S aureus*, which is second only to CoNS as a cause of health care-associated bacteremia, is equal to *Pseudomonas aeruginosa* as the most common cause of health care-associated pneumonia in adults and is responsible for most health care-associated surgical site infections. *S aureus* colonizes the skin and mucous membranes of 30% to 50% of healthy adults and children. The anterior nares, throat, axilla, perineum, vagina, or rectum are usual sites of colonization. Rates of carriage of more than 50% occur in children with desquamating skin disorders or burns and in people with frequent needle use (eg, diabetes mellitus, hemodialysis, illicit drug use, allergy shots).

S aureus-mediated TSS was recognized in 1978, and many early cases were associated with tampon use. Although changes in tampon composition and use have resulted in a decreased proportion of cases associated with menses, menstrual and nonmenstrual cases of TSS continue to occur and are reported with similar frequency. Risk factors for TSS include absence of antibody to TSS toxin-1 and focal *S aureus* infection with a TSS toxin-1–producing strain. TSS toxin-1 producing strains can be part of normal flora of the anterior nares or vagina, and colonization at these sites is believed to result in protective antibody in more than 90% of adults. Health care-associated TSS can occur and most often follows surgical procedures. In postoperative cases, the organism generally originates from the patient's own flora.

Transmission of S aureus. *S aureus* is transmitted most often by direct contact in community settings and indirectly from patient to patient via transiently colonized hands of health care professionals in health care settings. Health care professionals and family members who are colonized with *S aureus* in the nares or on skin also can serve as a reservoir for transmission. Contaminated environmental surfaces and objects also can play a role in transmission of *S aureus*, although their contribution to spread probably is minor. Although not transmitted by the droplet route routinely, *S aureus* can be dispersed into the air over short distances. Dissemination of *S aureus* from people, including infants, with nasal carriage is related to density of colonization, and increased dissemination occurs during viral upper respiratory tract infections. Additional risk factors for health care-associated acquisition of *S aureus* include illness requiring care in neonatal or pediatric intensive care or burn units; surgical procedures; prolonged hospitalization; local epidemic of *S aureus* infection; and the presence of indwelling catheters or prosthetic devices.

Staphylococcus aureus *Colonization and Disease.* Nasal, skin, vaginal, and rectal carriage are the primary reservoirs for *S aureus*. Although domestic animals can be colonized, data suggest that colonization is acquired from humans. Adults who carry MRSA in the nose preoperatively are more likely to develop surgical site infections after general, cardiac, orthopedic, or solid organ transplant surgery than are patients who are not carriers. Heavy cutaneous colonization at an insertion site is the single most important predictor of intravenous catheter-related infections for short-term percutaneously inserted catheters. For hemodialysis patients with *S aureus* skin colonization, the incidence of central line-associated bloodstream infection is sixfold higher than for patients without skin colonization. After head trauma, adults who are nasal carriers of *S aureus* are more likely to develop *S aureus* pneumonia than are noncolonized patients.

Health Care-Associated MRSA. MRSA has been endemic in most US hospitals since the 1980s, recently accounting for more than 60% of health care-associated *S aureus* infections in intensive care units reported to the Centers for Disease Control and Prevention (CDC). Health care-associated MRSA strains are resistant to all beta-lactamase–resistant (BLR) beta-lactam antimicrobial agents and cephalosporins as well as to antimicrobial agents of several other classes (multidrug resistance). Methicillin-susceptible *S aureus* (MSSA) strains can be heterogeneous for methicillin resistance (see Diagnostic Tests, p 658).

Risk factors for nasal carriage of health care-associated MRSA include hospitalization within the previous year, recent (within the previous 60 days) antimicrobial use, prolonged hospital stay, frequent contact with a health care environment, presence of an intravascular or peritoneal catheter or tracheal tube, increased number of surgical procedures, or frequent contact with a person with one or more of the preceding risk factors. A discharged patient known to have had colonization with MRSA should be assumed to have continued colonization when rehospitalized, because carriage can persist for years.

MRSA, both health care- and community-associated strains, and methicillin-resistant CoNS are responsible for a large portion of infections acquired in health care settings. A review of 25 pediatric hospitals demonstrated a 10-fold increase in MRSA infections since 1999 without change in the frequency of MSSA infections. Health care-associated MRSA strains are difficult to treat, because they usually are multidrug resistant and predictably susceptible only to vancomycin, linezolid, and agents not approved by the US Food and Drug Administration (FDA) for use in children.

Community-Associated MRSA. Unique clones of MRSA are responsible for community-associated infections in healthy children and adults without typical risk factors for health care-associated MRSA infections. The most frequent manifestation of community-associated (CA) MRSA infections is skin and soft tissue infection, but invasive disease also occurs. Antimicrobial susceptibility patterns of these strains differ from those of health care-associated MRSA strains. Although CA MRSA are resistant to all beta-lactam antimicrobial agents, they typically are susceptible to multiple other antimicrobial agents, including trimethoprim-sulfamethoxazole, gentamicin, and doxycycline; clindamycin susceptibility is variable. A review of prescribing patterns among 25 pediatric hospitals has demonstrated clindamycin to be the most commonly prescribed antimicrobial agent for nonlife-threatening MRSA infections. However, attention to local resistance rates of *S aureus* to clindamycin is imperative, because CA MRSA and MSSA with intrinsic resistance to clindamycin exceeding 20% have been reported by some institutions. CA MRSA infections have occurred in settings where there is crowding; frequent skin-to-skin contact; body piercing; sharing of personal items, such as towels and clothing; and poor personal hygiene, such as occurs among athletic teams, in correctional facilities, and in military training facilities. However, most CA MRSA infections occur in people without direct links to those settings. Transmission of community-associated MRSA from an infected classmate has been described in child care centers and among sports teams. Although CA MRSA arose from the community, in many health care settings, these clones are overtaking health care-associated MRSA strains as a cause of health care-associated MRSA infections, making usefulness of the epidemiologic terms "health care-associated" and "community-associated" of less value.

Vancomycin-Intermediately Susceptible S aureus. Strains of MRSA with intermediate susceptibility to vancomycin (minimum inhibitory concentration [MIC], 4–8 µg/mL) have been isolated from people (historically, dialysis patients) who had received multiple courses of vancomycin for a MRSA infection. Strains of MRSA can be heterogeneous for vancomycin resistance (see Diagnostic Tests, p 658). Extensive vancomycin use allows vancomycin-intermediately susceptible *S aureus* (VISA) strains to grow. These strains may emerge during therapy. Recommended control measures from the CDC have included using proper methods to detect VISA, using appropriate infection-control measures, and adopting measures to ensure appropriate vancomycin use. Although rare, outbreaks of VISA and heteroresistant VISA have been reported in France, Spain, and Japan. Communicability persists as long as lesions or the carrier state are present.

Vancomycin-Resistant S aureus. In 2002, 2 isolates of vancomycin-resistant *S aureus* (VRSA [MIC, 16 µg/mL or greater]) were identified in adults from 2 different states. As of November 2011, VRSA had been isolated from 12 adults from 4 states (**www.cdc. gov/HAI/settings/lab/vrsa_lab_search_containment.html**). Each of these adults with VRSA infections had underlying medical conditions, a history of MRSA infections, and prolonged exposure to vancomycin. No spread of VRSA beyond case patients has been documented. A concern is that most automated antimicrobial susceptibility testing methods commonly used in the United States were unable to detect vancomycin resistance in these isolates.

Coagulase-Negative Staphylococci. CoNS are common inhabitants of the skin and mucous membranes. Virtually all infants have colonization at multiple sites by 2 to 4 days of age. The most frequently isolated CoNS organism is *S epidermidis*. Different species colonize specific areas of the body. *S haemolyticus* is found on areas of skin with numerous apocrine glands. The frequency of health care-associated CoNS infections increased steadily until 2000, when these infections seem to have plateaued. Infants and children in intensive care units, including neonatal intensive care units, have the highest incidence of CoNS bloodstream infections. CoNS can be introduced at the time of medical device placement, through mucous membrane or skin breaks, through loss of bowel wall integrity (eg, necrotizing enterocolitis in very low birth weight neonates), or during catheter manipulation. Less often, health care professionals with environmental CoNS colonization on hands transmit the organism. The roles of the environment or fomites in CoNS transmission are not known.

Methicillin-resistant CoNS. Methicillin-resistant CoNS account for most health care-associated CoNS infections. Methicillin-resistant strains are resistant to all beta-lactam drugs, including cephalosporins, and usually several other drug classes. Once these strains become endemic in a hospital, eradication is difficult, even when strict infection-prevention practices are followed.

The **incubation period** is variable for staphylococcal disease. A long delay can occur between acquisition of the organism and onset of disease. For toxin-mediated SSSS, the **incubation period** usually is 1 to 10 days; for postoperative TSS, it can be as short as 12 hours. Menses-related cases can develop at any time during menses.

DIAGNOSTIC TESTS: Gram-stained smears of material from skin lesions or pyogenic foci showing gram-positive cocci in pairs and clusters can provide presumptive evidence of infection. Isolation of organisms from culture of otherwise sterile body fluid is the method for definitive diagnosis. *S aureus* almost never is a contaminant when isolated from a blood culture. CoNS isolated from a single blood culture commonly are dismissed as "contaminants." In a very preterm neonate, an immunocompromised person, or a patient with an indwelling catheter or prosthetic device, repeated isolation of the same strain of CoNS (by antimicrobial susceptibility results or molecular techniques) from blood cultures or another normally sterile body fluid suggests true infection, but genotyping more strongly supports the diagnosis. For central line-association bloodstream infection, quantitative blood cultures from the catheter will have 5 to 10 times more organisms than cultures from a peripheral blood vessel. Criteria that suggest CoNS as pathogens rather than contaminants include the following:

- 2 or more positive blood cultures from different collection sites;
- a single positive culture from blood and another sterile site (eg, cerebrospinal fluid, joint) with identical antimicrobial susceptibility patterns for each isolate;
- growth in a continuously monitored blood culture system within 15 hours of incubation;
- clinical findings of infection;
- an intravascular catheter that has been in place for 3 days or more; and
- similar or identical genotypes among all isolates.

S aureus-mediated TSS is a clinical diagnosis (Table 3.62, p 654). *S aureus* grows in culture of blood specimens from fewer than 5% of patients. Specimens for culture should be obtained from an identified site of infection, because these sites usually will yield the organism. Because approximately one third of isolates of *S aureus* from nonmenstrual cases produce toxins other than TSS toxin-1, and TSS toxin-1-producing organisms can be present as normal flora, TSS-1 production by an isolate is not useful diagnostically.

Quantitative antimicrobial susceptibility testing should be performed for all staphylococci, including CoNS, isolated from normally sterile sites. Health care-associated MRSA heterogeneous or heterotypic strains appear susceptible by disk testing. However, when a parent strain is cultured on methicillin-containing media, resistant subpopulations are apparent. When these resistant subpopulations are cultured on methicillin-free media, they can continue as stable resistant mutants or revert to susceptible strains (heterogeneous resistance). Cells expressing heteroresistance grow more slowly than the oxacillin-susceptible cells and can be missed at growth conditions above 35°C (95°F).

A large proportion of CA *S aureus* strains are methicillin resistant, and more than 90% of health care-associated *S aureus* as well as CoNS strains are methicillin and multidrug resistant. Because of the high rates of CA MRSA infections in the United States, clindamycin has become an often-used drug for treatment of nonlife-threatening presumed *S aureus* infections. Routine antimicrobial susceptibility testing of *S aureus* strains historically did not include a method to detect strains susceptible to clindamycin that rapidly become clindamycin-resistant when exposed to this agent. This clindamycin-inducible resistance can be detected by the D zone test. When a MRSA isolate is determined to be erythromycin resistant and clindamycin susceptible by routine methods, the D zone test is performed. Patients with MRSA isolates that demonstrate clindamycin-inducible resistance should not receive clindamycin routinely. All *S aureus* strains with an MIC to vancomycin of 4 µg/mL or greater should be confirmed and further characterized. Early detection of VISA is critical to trigger aggressive infection-control measures (see Table 3.63, p 660).

Guidelines for laboratory detection of VISA and VRSA are available at **www.cdc. gov/ncidod/dhqp/ar_visavrsa_lab.html.** *S aureus* and CoNS strain genotyping has become a necessary adjunct for determining whether several isolates from one patient or from different patients are the same. Typing, in conjunction with epidemiologic information, can facilitate identification of the source, extent, and mechanism of transmission in an outbreak. Antimicrobial susceptibility testing is the most readily available method for typing by a phenotypic characteristic. A number of molecular typing methods are available for *S aureus*. Choice of method should consider purpose of typing and available resources. The primary method used currently by the CDC is pulsed-field gel electrophoresis.

TREATMENT: The most frequent manifestation of CA MRSA infection is skin and soft tissue infection. Fig 3.5 shows the initial management of skin and soft tissue infections suspected to be caused by CA MRSA.

Serious MSSA infections require intravenous therapy with a BLR beta-lactam antimicrobial agent, such as nafcillin or oxacillin, because most *S aureus* strains produce beta-lactamase enzymes and are resistant to penicillin and ampicillin (see Table 3.64, p 662). First- or second-generation cephalosporins (eg, cefazolin or cefuroxime) or vancomycin are effective but less so than nafcillin or oxacillin, especially for some sites of infection (eg, endocarditis, meningitis). Furthermore, nafcillin or oxacillin, rather than vancomycin (or clindamycin if the *S aureus* strain is susceptible to this agent), is recommended for treatment of serious MSSA infections to minimize emergence of vancomycin- or clindamycin-resistant strains. Treatment of serious MRSA infections in adults does not support addition of gentamicin or rifampin to vancomycin because of an increase in adverse effects and lack of greater efficacy of the combination versus monotherapy. A patient who has a nonserious allergy to penicillin can be treated with a first- or second-generation cephalosporin, and if the patient is not also allergic to cephalosporins, with vancomycin or with clindamycin, if endocarditis or central nervous system infection is not a consideration and the *S aureus* strain is susceptible.

Intravenous vancomycin is recommended for treatment of serious infections caused by staphylococcal strains resistant to BLR beta-lactam antimicrobial agents (eg, MRSA and all CoNS). For empiric therapy of life-threatening *S aureus* infections, initial therapy should include vancomycin and a BLR beta-lactam antimicrobial agent (eg, nafcillin, oxacillin) if the isolate is MSSA. For hospital-acquired CoNS infections, vancomycin

Table 3.63. Recommendations for Detecting and Preventing Spread of *Staphylococcus aureus* With Decreased Susceptibility to Vancomycin[a]

Definitions:
- **Vancomycin-susceptible *S aureus***
  MIC 2 µg/mL or less
- **Vancomycin-intermediately susceptible *S aureus* (VISA)**
  MIC 4 through 8 µg/mL
  Not transferable to susceptible strains
- **Vancomycin-resistant *S aureus* (VRSA)**
  MIC 16 µg/mL or greater
  Potentially transferable to susceptible strains
- **Confirmation of VISA and VRSA**
  Possible VISA and VRSA isolates should be retested using vancomycin screen plates or a validated MIC method.
  VISA and VRSA isolates should be reported to the local health department or CDC.

Infection control[b]:
- Isolate patient in a private room.
- Minimize numbers of people caring for VISA/VRSA patients.
- Implement appropriate infection-control precautions:
  - Use contact precautions (gown and gloves).
  - Wear mask/eye protection or face shield if performing procedures (eg, wound manipulations, suctioning) likely to generate splash or splatter of VISA/VRSA contaminated materials (eg, blood, body fluids, secretions).
  - Perform hand hygiene using appropriate agent (eg, hand washing with soap and water or alcohol-based hand sanitizer).
  - Dedicate nondisposable items for patient use.
  - Monitor and strictly enforce compliance with contact precautions and other measures.
- Educate and inform health care professionals about the need for contact isolation.
- Consult with state health department and CDC before discharging and/or transferring the patient, and notify receiving institution or unit of presence of VISA and of appropriate precautions.

MIC indicates minimum inhibitory concentration; CDC, Centers for Disease Control and Prevention.
[a]Hageman JC, Patel JB, Carey RC, Tenover FC, McDonald LC. *Investigation and Control of Vancomycin-Intermediate and -Resistant Staphylococcus aureus (VISA/VRSA): A Guide for Health Departments and Infection Control Personnel.* Atlanta, GA: Centers for Disease Control and Prevention; 2006. Available at: **www.cdc.gov/hai/pdfs/visa_vrsa/visa_vrsa_guide.pdf.**
[b]For information regarding control of spread of VISA and vancomycin-resistant *S aureus,* e-mail SEARCH@cdc.gov or visit **www.cdc.gov/ncidod/dhqp.**

is the drug of choice. Subsequent therapy should be determined by antimicrobial susceptibility results.

VISA infection is rare in children. For seriously ill patients with a history of recurrent MRSA infections or for patients failing vancomycin therapy for whom VISA strains are a consideration, initial therapy could include linezolid or trimethoprim-sulfamethoxazole, with or without gentamicin. If antimicrobial susceptibility results document multidrug resistance, alternative agents, such as quinupristin-dalfopristin, daptomycin, or tigecycline, could be considered, but quinupristin-dalfopristin is not approved by the FDA for use in

FIGURE 3.5. ALGORITHM FOR INITIAL MANAGEMENT OF SKIN AND SOFT TISSUE INFECTIONS CAUSED BY COMMUNITY-ASSOCIATED *STAPHYLOCOCCUS AUREUS*

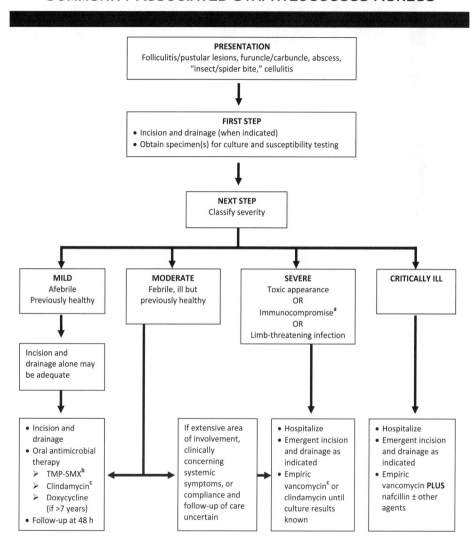

[a]Immunocompromise: any chronic illness except asthma or eczema.
[b]TMP-SMX = trimethoprim-sulfamethoxazole, if group A streptococcus unlikely.
[c]Consider prevalence of clindamycin-susceptible methicillin-susceptible *S aureus* and "D" test-negative community-associated methicillin-resistant *S aureus* strains in the community.

Table 3.64. Parenteral Antimicrobial Agent(s) for Treatment of Bacteremia and Other Serious *Staphylococcus aureus* Infections

Susceptibility	Antimicrobial Agents	Comments
I. Initial empiric therapy (organism of unknown susceptibility)		
Drugs of choice:	Vancomycin (15 mg/kg Q6-H+ nafcillin or oxacillin	For life-threatening infections (ie, septicemia, endocarditis, CNS infection); linezolid could be substituted for vancomycin if the patient has received several recent courses of vancomycin
	Vancomycin (15 mg/kg Q8H)	For nonlife-threatening infection without signs of sepsis (eg, skin infection, cellulitis, osteomyelitis, pyarthrosis) when rates of MRSA colonization and infection in the community are substantial
	Clindamycin	For nonlife-threatening infection without signs of sepsis when rates of MRSA colonization and infection in the community are substantial and prevalence of clindamycin resistance is low
II. Methicillin-susceptible, penicillin-resistant *S aureus* (MSSA)		
Drugs of choice:	Nafcillin or oxacillin[a]	
Alternatives:	Cefazolin	
	Clindamycin	Only for patients with a serious penicillin allergy and clindamycin-susceptible strain
	Vancomycin	Only for patients with a serious penicillin and cephalosporin allergy
	Ampicillin + sulbactam	
III. MRSA (oxacillin MIC, 4 µg/mL or greater)		
A. Health care-associated (multidrug resistant)		
Drugs of choice:	Vancomycin + gentamicin[a]	
Alternatives: suscep-tibility testing results available before alter-native drugs are used	Trimethoprim-sulfamethoxazole Linezolid[b] Quinupristin-dalfopristin[b] Fluoroquinolones	Not recommended for people younger than 18 years of age or as monotherapy (see Fluoroquinolones, p 800)

Table 3.64. Parenteral Antimicrobial Agent(s) for Treatment of Bacteremia and Other Serious *Staphylococcus aureus* Infections, continued

Susceptibility	Antimicrobial Agents	Comments
B. Community-associated (not multidrug resistant)		
Drugs of choice:	Vancomycin + gentamicin	For life-threatening infections
	Clindamycin (if strain susceptible)	For pneumonia, septic arthritis, osteomyelitis, skin or soft tissue infections
	Trimethoprim-sulfamethoxazole	For skin or soft tissue infections
Alternative:	Vancomycin	
IV. Vancomycin-intermediately susceptible *S aureus* (MIC, 4 to 16 µg/mL)[b]		
Drugs of choice:	Optimal therapy is not known	Dependent on in vitro susceptibility test results
	Linezolid[b]	
	Daptomycin[c]	
	Quinupristin-dalfopristin[b]	
	Tigecycline[b]	
Alternatives:	Vancomycin + linezolid ± gentamicin	
	Vancomycin + trimethoprim-sulfamethoxazole[a]	

CNS indicates central nervous system; MRSA, methicillin-resistant *S aureus*; MIC, minimum inhibitory concentration.

[a] One of the adjunctive agents, gentamicin or rifampin, should be added to the therapeutic regimen for life-threatening infections such as endocarditis or CNS infection or infections with a vancomycin-intermediate *S aureus* strain. Consultation with an infectious diseases specialist should be considered to determine which agent to use and duration of use.

[b] Linezolid, quinupristin-dalfopristin, and tigecycline are agents with activity in vitro and efficacy in adults with multidrug-resistant, gram-positive organisms, including *S aureus*. Because experience with these agents in children is limited, consultation with an infectious diseases specialist should be considered before use.

[c] Daptomycin is active in vitro against multidrug-resistant, gram-positive organisms, including *S aureus*, but has not been evaluated in children. Daptomycin is approved by the US Food and Drug Administration only for treatment of complicated skin and skin structure infections and for *S aureus* bloodstream infections. Daptomycin is ineffective for treatment of pneumonia and is not indicated in patients 18 years of age and older.

children younger than 16 years of age, and daptomycin and tigecycline are not approved for use in people younger than 18 years of age.

Duration of therapy for serious MSSA or MRSA infections depends on the site and severity of infection but usually is 4 weeks or more for endocarditis, osteomyelitis, necrotizing pneumonia, or disseminated infection. After initial parenteral therapy and documented clinical improvement, completion of the course with an oral drug can be considered in older children if adherence can be ensured and endocarditis or central nervous system (CNS) infection is not a consideration. For endocarditis and CNS infection, parenteral therapy is recommended for the entire treatment. Drainage of abscesses and removal of foreign bodies is desirable and almost always is required for medical treatment to be effective.

As summarized in Table 3.65, the first priority in management of *S aureus* TSS is aggressive fluid management as well as management of respiratory or cardiac failure, if present. Initial antimicrobial therapy should include a parentally administered beta-lactam antistaphylococcal antimicrobial agent and a protein synthesis-inhibiting drug, such as clindamycin, at maximum dosages. Vancomycin should be substituted for BLR penicillins or cephalosporins in regions where community-associated MRSA infections are common (see Table 3.64, p 662). Once the organism is identified and susceptibility is known, therapy for *S aureus* should be modified, but an active antimicrobial agent should be continued for 10 to 14 days. Administration of antimicrobial agents can be changed to the oral route once the patient is tolerating oral alimentation. The total duration of therapy is based on the usual duration of established foci of infection (eg, pneumonia, osteomyelitis). Aggressive drainage and irrigation of accessible sites of purulent infection should be performed as soon as possible. All foreign bodies, including those recently inserted during surgery, should be removed if possible. Immune Globulin Intravenous (IGIV) can be considered in patients with severe staphylococcal TSS unresponsive to all other therapeutic measures, because IGIV may neutralize circulating toxin. The optimal IGIV regimen is unknown, but 150 to 400 mg/kg per day for 5 days or a single dose of 1 to 2 g/kg has been used. SSSS in infants should be treated with a parenteral BLR beta-lactam antimicrobial agent or, if MRSA is a consideration, vancomycin. In older children, depending on severity, oral agents can be considered. Skin and soft tissue infections, such as impetigo or cellulitis attributable to *S aureus*, can be treated with oral penicillinase-resistant beta-lactam drugs, such as cloxacillin, dicloxacillin, or a first- or second-generation cephalosporin. However, the continued increase in prevalence of CA MRSA throughout the United States may limit the utility of these agents. In this situation, or for the penicillin-allergic patient, trimethoprim-sulfamethoxazole, doxycycline in children 8 years of age and older, or clindamycin can be used if the isolate is susceptible. Trimethoprim-sulfamethoxazole should not be used as a single agent in the initial treatment of cellulitis, because it is not active against group A streptococci.

Duration of therapy for central line-associated bloodstream infections is controversial and depends on consideration of a number of factors, including the organism (*S aureus* vs CoNS), the type and location of the catheter, the site of infection (exit site vs tunnel vs line), the feasibility of using an alternative vessel at a later date, and the presence or absence of a catheter-related thrombus. Infections are more difficult to treat when associated with a thrombus, thrombophlebitis, or intra-atrial thrombus. If a central line can be removed, there is no demonstrable thrombus, and bacteremia resolves promptly, a 3- to

Table 3.65. Management of Staphylococcal Toxic Shock Syndrome

- Fluid management to maintain adequate venous return and cardiac filling pressures to prevent end-organ damage
- Anticipatory management of multisystem organ failure
- Parenteral antimicrobial therapy at maximum doses
  - Kill organism with bactericidal cell wall inhibitor (eg, beta-lactamase–resistant antistaphylococcal antimicrobial agent)
  - Reduce enzyme or toxin production with protein synthesis inhibitor (eg, clindamycin)
- Immune Globulin Intravenous may be considered for infection refractory to several hours of aggressive therapy or in the presence of an undrainable focus or persistent oliguria with pulmonary edema

5-day course of therapy seems appropriate for CoNS infections in the immunocompetent host. A longer course (eg, 7 to 10 days) is suggested if the patient is immunocompromised or the organism is *S aureus;* experts differ on recommended duration, but many suggest 14 days. If the patient needs a new central line, waiting 48 to 72 hours after bacteremia apparently has resolved before insertion is optimal. If a tunneled catheter is needed for ongoing care, in situ treatment of the infection can be attempted. If the patient responds to antimicrobial therapy with immediate resolution of the *S aureus* bacteremia, treatment should be continued for 10 to 14 days parenterally. Antimicrobial lock therapy of tunneled central lines may result in a higher rate of catheter salvage in adults with CoNS infections, but experience with this approach is limited in children. If blood cultures remain positive for staphylococci for more than 3 to 5 days or if the clinical illness fails to improve, the central line should be removed, parenteral therapy should be continued, and the patient should be evaluated for metastatic foci of infection. Vegetations or a thrombus in the heart or great vessels always should be considered when a central line becomes infected. Transesophageal echocardiography, if feasible, is the most sensitive technique for identifying vegetations.

ISOLATION OF THE HOSPITALIZED PATIENT: Standard precautions are recommended for many patients infected or colonized with MSSA, including patients with TSS. However, contact precautions should be used for patients with abscesses or draining wounds that cannot be covered, regardless of staphylococcal strain, and should be maintained until draining ceases or can be contained by a dressing. Patients infected or colonized with MRSA should be managed with contact precautions for the duration of hospitalization and subsequent hospitalizations, because MRSA carriage can persist for years. For MSSA or MRSA pneumonia, droplet precautions are recommended for the first 24 hours of antimicrobial therapy. Droplet precautions should be maintained throughout the illness for MSSA or MRSA tracheitis with a tracheostomy tube in place.

To prevent transmission of VISA and VRSA, the CDC has issued specific infection-control recommendations that should be followed (see Table 3.63, p 660). For CoNS, Standard Precautions are recommended. For known epidemic MRSA strains, Contact Precautions should be used.

CONTROL MEASURES:

Coagulase-Negative Staphylococci. Prevention and control of CoNS infections have focused on prevention of intraoperative contamination by skin flora and sterile insertion of intravascular and intraperitoneal catheters and other prosthetic devices. Prophylactic administration of an antimicrobial agent intraoperatively lowers the incidence of infection after cardiac surgery and implantation of synthetic vascular grafts and prosthetic devices and often has been used at the time of cerebrospinal fluid shunt placement.

Staphylococcus aureus. Measures to prevent and control *S aureus* infections can be considered separately for people and for health care facilities.

Individual Patient. Community-associated *S aureus* infections in immunocompetent hosts usually cannot be prevented, because the organism is ubiquitous and there is no vaccine. However, strategies focusing on hand hygiene and wound care have been effective at limiting transmission of *S aureus* and preventing spread of infections in community settings. Specific strategies include appropriate wound care, minimizing skin trauma and keeping abrasions and cuts covered, optimizing hand hygiene and personal hygiene practices (eg, shower after activities involving skin-to-skin contact), avoiding sharing of personal items (eg, towels, razors, clothing), cleaning shared equipment between uses, and regular cleaning of frequently touched environmental surfaces. For patients who experience recurrent *S aureus* infections or who are predisposed to *S aureus* infections because of disorders of neutrophil function, chronic skin conditions, or obesity, a variety of techniques have been used to prevent infection, including scrupulous attention to skin hygiene and to use of clothing and bed linens that minimize sweating, but none have been shown to be effective in preventing recurrent infections with community-associated MRSA. Another promising technique is the use of bleach in the bath water 2 to 3 times a week ($\frac{1}{4}$ cup per $\frac{1}{4}$ tub or 13 gallons of water) for approximately 3 months; studies are ongoing to determine whether this intervention reduces the incidence of recurrent infections.

Measures to prevent health care-associated *S aureus* infections in individual patients include strict adherence to recommended infection-control precautions and appropriate intraoperative antimicrobial prophylaxis, and in some circumstances, use of antimicrobial regimens to attempt to eradicate nasal carriage in certain patients can be considered.

Child Care or School Settings. Children with *S aureus* colonization or infection should not be excluded routinely from child care or school settings. Children with draining or open abrasions or wounds should have these covered with a clean, dry dressing. Routine hand hygiene should be emphasized for personnel and children in these facilities.

General Measures. Published recommendations of the CDC Healthcare Infection Control Practices Advisory Committee (HICPAC)[1] for prevention of health care-associated pneumonia should be effective for decreasing the incidence of *S aureus* pneumonia. Careful preparation of the skin before surgery, including cleansing of skin before placement of intravascular catheters using barrier methods, will decrease the incidence of *S aureus* wound and catheter infections. Meticulous surgical technique with minimal trauma to tissues, maintenance of good oxygenation, and minimal hematoma and dead space formation will minimize risk of surgical site infection. Appropriate hand hygiene, including before and after use of gloves, by health care professionals and strict adherence to contact precautions are of paramount importance.

---

[1] Centers for Disease Control and Prevention. Guidelines for preventing health-care–associated pneumonia, 2003: recommendations of CDC and the Healthcare Infection Control Practices Advisory Committee. *MMWR Recomm Rep.* 2004;53(RR-3):1–36

Intraoperative Antimicrobial Prophylaxis. The benefits of systemic antimicrobial prophylaxis do not justify the potential risks associated with antimicrobial use in most clean surgical procedures, because the risk of overall infection (most commonly caused by *S aureus*) is only 1% to 2%. Some exceptions apply, such as a person undergoing organ transplantation, neurosurgery, or insertion of a major prosthetic device, such as a prosthetic joint or a heart valve, or a known MRSA carrier undergoing a major surgical procedure. If antimicrobial prophylaxis is used, the agent is administered 30 to 60 minutes before the operation (60–120 minutes for vancomycin), and a total duration of therapy of less than 24 hours is recommended. Staphylococci are the most common pathogens causing surgical site infections, and cefazolin is the most commonly recommended drug.

Eradication of Nasal Carriage. Preprocedure detection and eradication of nasal carriage using mupirocin twice a day for 5 to 7 days before surgery can decrease the incidence of *S aureus* infections in some colonized adult patients after cardiothoracic, general, or neurosurgical procedures. Use of intermittent or continuous intranasal mupirocin for eradication of nasal carriage also has been shown to decrease the incidence of invasive *S aureus* infections in adult patients undergoing long-term hemodialysis or ambulatory peritoneal dialysis. However, eradication of nasal carriage of *S aureus* is difficult, and mupirocin-resistant strains can emerge with repeated or widespread use; therefore, this treatment is not recommended for routine use.

Institutions. Measures to control spread of *S aureus* within health care facilities involve use and careful monitoring of HICPAC guidelines.[1,2] Strategies for controlling spread of MRSA also are found in recommendations for controlling spread of multidrug-resistant organisms (**www.cdc.gov/drugresistance/index.html**). These include general recommendations for all settings and focus on administrative issues; engagement, education, and training of personnel; judicious use of antimicrobial agents; monitoring of prevalence trends over time; use of standard precautions for all patients; and use of contact precautions when appropriate. When endemic rates are not decreasing despite implementation of and adherence to the aforementioned measures, additional interventions, such as use of active surveillance cultures to identify colonized patients and to place them in contact precautions, may be warranted. When a patient or health care professional is found to be a carrier of *S aureus*, attempts to eradicate carriage with topical nasal mupirocin therapy may be useful. Both low-level (MIC, 8–256 µg/mL) and high-level (MIC, greater than 512 µg/mL) resistance to mupirocin have been identified in *S aureus*, with high-level resistance associated with failure of decolonization therapy. Other topical preparations for intranasal application to be considered if mupirocin fails are ointments containing bacitracin and polymyxin B or a povidone-iodine cream. These preparations have not been studied in children. Minimizing prolonged use of vancomycin will decrease emergence of VISA. Recommendations for investigation and control of VISA and VRSA

[1] Hageman JC, Patel JB, Carey RC, Tenover FC, McDonald LC. *Investigation and Control of Vancomycin-Intermediate and -Resistant Staphylococcus aureus (VISA/VRSA): A Guide for Health Departments and Infection Control Personnel.* Atlanta, GA: Centers for Disease Control and Prevention; 2006. Available at: **www.cdc.gov/hai/pdfs/visa_vrsa/visa_vrsa_guide.pdf**

[2] Siegel JD, Rhinehart E, Jackson M, Chianello L, and the Healthcare Infection Control Practices Advisory Committee. 2007 *Guideline for Isolation Precautions: Preventing Transmission of Infectious Agents in Healthcare Settings. Recommendations of the Healthcare Infection Control Practices Advisory Committee.* Atlanta, GA: Centers for Disease Control and Prevention; 2007. Available at: **www.cdc.gov/hicpac/2007IP/2007isolationPrecautions.html**

have been published by the CDC (Table 3.63, p 660). Ongoing review and restriction of vancomycin use is critical in attempts to control the emergence of VISA and VRSA (see Appropriate and Judicious Use of Antimicrobial Agents, p 802). To date, the use of catheters impregnated with various antimicrobial agents or metals to prevent health care-associated infections has not been evaluated adequately in children.

Nurseries. Outbreaks of *S aureus* infections in newborn nurseries require unique measures of control. Hand hygiene should be emphasized to all personnel and visitors. Application of triple dye, iodophor ointment, or 1% chlorhexidine powder to the umbilical stump has been used to delay or prevent *S aureus* colonization. Other measures recommended during outbreaks include reinforcement of hand hygiene, alleviating overcrowding and understaffing, colonization surveillance cultures of newborn infants at admission and periodically thereafter, use of contact precautions for colonized or infected infants, and cohorting of colonized or infected infants and their caregivers. For hand hygiene, soaps containing chlorhexidine or alcohol-based hand rubs are preferred during an outbreak. Colonized health care professionals epidemiologically implicated in transmission should receive decolonization therapy, but eradication of colonization may not occur.

Group A Streptococcal Infections

CLINICAL MANIFESTATIONS: The most common group A streptococcal (GAS) infection is acute pharyngotonsillitis, which may present with a strawberry tongue, which occurs following peeling of a white coating, leaving a red glistening tongue with prominent papillae. Purulent complications of pharyngotonsillitis, including otitis media, sinusitis, peritonsillar and retropharyngeal abscesses, and suppurative cervical adenitis, develop in some patients, usually those who are untreated. Nonsuppurative sequelae include acute rheumatic fever (ARF) and acute glomerulonephritis. The goals of antimicrobial therapy for GAS upper respiratory tract disease are to reduce acute morbidity, nonsuppurative sequelae (acute rheumatic fever and acute glomerulonephritis), and transmission to close contacts.

Scarlet fever occurs most often in association with pharyngitis and, rarely, with pyoderma or an infected wound. Scarlet fever has a characteristic confluent erythematous sandpaper-like rash that is caused by one or more of several erythrogenic exotoxins produced by group A streptococci. Severe scarlet fever occurs rarely. Other than occurrence of rash, the epidemiologic features, symptoms, signs, sequelae, and treatment of scarlet fever are the same as those of streptococcal pharyngitis.

Toddlers (1 through 3 years of age) with GAS respiratory tract infection initially can have serous rhinitis and then develop a protracted illness with moderate fever, irritability, and anorexia (streptococcal fever or streptococcosis). Acute pharyngotonsillitis is uncommon in children younger than 3 years of age.

The second most common site of GAS infection is skin. Streptococcal skin infections (ie, pyoderma or impetigo) can result in acute glomerulonephritis, which occasionally occurs in epidemics. ARF is not a sequela of GAS skin infection.

Other manifestations of GAS infections include erysipelas, perianal cellulitis, vaginitis, bacteremia, pneumonia, endocarditis, pericarditis, septic arthritis, cellulitis, necrotizing fasciitis, purpura fulminans, osteomyelitis, myositis, puerperal sepsis, surgical wound infection, acute otitis media, sinusitis, retropharyngeal abscess, peritonsillar abscess, mastoiditis, and neonatal omphalitis. Invasive GAS infections can be severe, may or may not be associated with an identified focus of local infection, and can be associated with streptococcal toxic shock syndrome (STSS) or necrotizing fasciitis. Severe infection can follow minor or unrecognized trauma. An association between GAS infection and sudden onset of obsessive-compulsive or tic disorders—pediatric autoimmune neuropsychiatric disorders associated with streptococcal infections (PANDAS)—has been proposed but is unproven.

STSS is caused by toxin-producing GAS strains and typically manifests as an acute illness characterized by fever, generalized erythroderma, rapid-onset hypotension, and signs of multiorgan involvement, including rapidly progressive renal failure (see Table 3.66, p 670). Evidence of local soft tissue infection (eg, cellulitis, myositis, or necrotizing fasciitis) associated with severe, rapidly increasing pain is common, but STSS can occur without an identifiable focus of infection. STSS also can be associated with invasive infections, such as bacteremia, pneumonia, pleural empyema, osteomyelitis, pyarthrosis, or endocarditis.

ETIOLOGY: More than 120 distinct serotypes or genotypes of group A beta-hemolytic streptococci *(Streptococcus pyogenes)* have been identified based on M-protein serotype or M-protein gene sequence (*emm* types). Because of a variety of factors, including M nontypability and *emm* sequence variation within given M types, *emm* typing generally is more discriminating than M typing. Epidemiologic studies suggest an association between certain serotypes (eg, types 1, 3, 5, 6, 18, 19, and 24) and rheumatic fever, but a specific rheumatogenic factor has not been identified. Several serotypes (eg, types 49, 55, 57, and 59) are associated with pyoderma and acute glomerulonephritis. Other serotypes (eg, types 1, 6, and 12) are associated with pharyngitis and acute glomerulonephritis. Most cases of STSS are caused by strains producing at least 1 of several different pyrogenic exotoxins, most commonly streptococcal pyrogenic exotoxin A (SPE A). These toxins act as superantigens that stimulate production of tumor necrosis factor and other inflammatory mediators that cause capillary leak and other physiologic changes, leading to hypotension and organ damage.

EPIDEMIOLOGY: Pharyngitis usually results from contact with a person who has GAS pharyngitis. Fomites and household pets, such as dogs, are not vectors of GAS infection. Transmission of GAS infection, including in school outbreaks of pharyngitis, almost always follows contact with respiratory tract secretions. Pharyngitis and impetigo (and their nonsuppurative complications) can be associated with crowding, which often is present in socioeconomically disadvantaged populations. The close contact that occurs in schools, child care centers, contact sports (eg, wrestling), boarding schools, and military installations facilitates transmission. Foodborne outbreaks of pharyngitis occur rarely and are a consequence of human contamination of food in conjunction with improper food preparation or improper refrigeration procedures.

Streptococcal pharyngitis occurs at all ages but is most common among school-aged children and adolescents. GAS pharyngitis and pyoderma are less common in adults than in children.

Geographically, GAS pharyngitis and pyoderma are ubiquitous. Pyoderma is more common in tropical climates and warm seasons, presumably because of antecedent insect bites and other minor skin trauma. Streptococcal pharyngitis is more common during late autumn, winter, and spring in temperate climates, presumably because of close person-to-person contact in schools. Communicability of patients with streptococcal pharyngitis is highest during acute infection and untreated gradually diminishes over a period of weeks.

Table 3.66. Streptococcal Toxic Shock Syndrome: Clinical Case Definition[a]

I. Isolation of group A streptococcus *(Streptococcus pyogenes)*
   A. From a normally sterile site (eg, blood, cerebrospinal fluid, peritoneal fluid, or tissue biopsy specimen)
   B. From a nonsterile site (eg, throat, sputum, vagina, open surgical wound, or superficial skin lesion)
II. Clinical signs of severity
   A. Hypotension: systolic pressure 90 mm Hg or less in adults or lower than the fifth percentile for age in children

AND

   B. Two or more of the following signs:
   • Renal impairment: creatinine concentration 177 μmol/L (2 mg/dL) or greater for adults or at least 2 times the upper limit of normal for age
   • Coagulopathy: platelet count 100 000/mm³ or less or disseminated intravascular coagulation
   • Hepatic involvement: elevated alanine transaminase, aspartate transaminase, or total bilirubin concentrations at least 2 times the upper limit of normal for age
   • Adult respiratory distress syndrome
   • A generalized erythematous macular rash that may desquamate
   • Soft tissue necrosis, including necrotizing fasciitis or myositis, or gangrene

Adapted from The Working Group on Severe Streptococcal Infections. Defining the group A streptococcal toxic shock syndrome: rationale and consensus definition. *JAMA.* 1993;269(3):390–39.

[a] An illness fulfilling criteria IA and IIA and IIB can be defined as a *definite* case. An illness fulfilling criteria IB and IIA and IIB can be defined as a *probable* case if no other cause for the illness is identified.

Patients are not considered to be contagious beginning 24 hours after initiation of appropriate antimicrobial therapy.

Throat culture surveys of healthy asymptomatic children during school outbreaks of pharyngitis have yielded GAS prevalence rates as high as 20%. These surveys identified children who were pharyngeal carriers. Carriage of GAS can persist for months, but risk of transmission to others is low.

The incidence of ARF in the United States decreased sharply during the 20th century. Rates of this nonsuppurative sequela likely still are low, although the true incidence in the United States is unknown, because ARF no longer is a nationally reportable condition. Focal outbreaks of ARF in school-aged children occurred in several areas throughout the 1990s, and small clusters continue to be reported periodically. Although reasons for these focal outbreaks are not completely clear, they most likely relate to increased circulation of rheumatogenic strains, and their occurrence reemphasizes the importance of diagnosing GAS pharyngitis and treating with a recommended antimicrobial regimen.

In streptococcal impetigo, the organism usually is acquired by direct contact from another person with impetigo. GAS colonization of healthy skin usually precedes development of impetigo, but group A streptococci do not penetrate intact skin. Impetiginous lesions occur at the site of breaks in skin (eg, insect bites, burns, traumatic wounds, varicella). After development of impetiginous lesions, the upper respiratory tract often becomes colonized with GAS. Infection of surgical wounds and postpartum (puerperal) sepsis usually result from contact transmission. Anal or vaginal carriers and people with skin infection can transmit GAS to surgical and obstetrical patients, resulting in health care-associated outbreaks. Infections in neonates result from intrapartum or contact transmission; in the latter situation, infection can begin as omphalitis, cellulitis, or necrotizing fasciitis.

The incidence of invasive GAS infections is highest in infants and the elderly. Before use of varicella vaccine, varicella was the most commonly identified predisposing factor in children with GAS infection. Other factors increasing risk for invasive GAS disease among children include exposure to other children and household crowding. The portal of entry is unknown in most invasive GAS infections; and the entry site is presumed to be skin or mucous membranes. Such infections rarely follow symptomatic GAS pharyngitis. Although case reports have suggested a possible temporal association between use of non-steroidal anti-inflammatory drugs and invasive GAS infections in children with varicella, a causal relationship has not been established.

The incidence of GAS-mediated TSS is highest among young children and the elderly, although STSS can occur at any age. Of all cases of invasive streptococcal infections in children, fewer than 5% are associated with documented STSS. Among children, STSS has been reported with focal lesions (eg, varicella, cellulitis, trauma, osteomyelitis), pneumonia, and bacteremia without a defined focus. Mortality rates are substantially lower for children than for adults with GAS-mediated STSS.

The **incubation period** for streptococcal pharyngitis is 2 to 5 days. For impetigo, a 7- to 10-day period between acquisition of group A streptococci on healthy skin and development of lesions has been demonstrated. The incubation period for STSS is not known but has been as short as 14 hours in cases associated with subcutaneous inoculation of organisms (eg, childbirth, penetrating trauma).

DIAGNOSTIC TESTS: Laboratory confirmation of GAS pharyngitis is recommended for children, because accurate clinical differentiation of viral and GAS pharyngitis is difficult, except in children with obvious viral symptoms (eg, rhinorrhea, cough, hoarseness). A specimen should be obtained by vigorous swabbing of both tonsils and the posterior pharynx for culture and/or rapid antigen testing. Culture on sheep blood agar can confirm GAS infection, with latex agglutination differentiating group A streptococci from other beta-hemolytic streptococci. False-negative culture results occur in fewer than 10% of symptomatic patients when an adequate throat swab specimen is obtained and cultured by trained personnel. Recovery of group A streptococci from the pharynx does not distinguish patients with true streptococcal infection (defined by a serologic response to extracellular antigens [eg, streptolysin O]) from streptococcal carriers who have an intercurrent viral pharyngitis. The number of colonies of group A streptococci on an agar culture plate also does not differentiate true infection from carriage. Cultures that are negative for group A streptococci after 18 to 24 hours should be incubated for a second day to optimize recovery of group A streptococci.

Several rapid diagnostic tests for GAS pharyngitis are available. Most are based on nitrous acid extraction of group A carbohydrate antigen from organisms obtained by throat swab. Specificities of these tests generally are high, but the reported sensitivities vary considerably (ie, false-negative results occur). As with throat swab cultures, sensitivity of these tests is highly dependent on the quality of the throat swab specimen, the experience of the person performing the test, and the rigor of the culture method used for comparison. The Food and Drug Administration has approved a variety of rapid tests for use in home settings. Parents should be informed about these tests and told that their use should be discouraged. However, when a child or adolescent suspected of having GAS pharyngitis has a negative rapid streptococcal test result either at home or in the physician's office, a negative result of throat culture can provide more assurance that the patient does not have GAS infection. Because of high specificity of rapid tests, a positive test result does not require throat culture confirmation. Rapid diagnostic tests using techniques such as optical immunoassay and chemiluminescent DNA probes have been developed. These tests may be as sensitive as standard throat cultures on sheep blood agar. The diagnosis of ARF is based on the Jones criteria (Table 3.67, p 673).

Indications for GAS Testing. Factors to be considered in the decision to obtain a throat swab specimen for testing children with pharyngitis are the patient's age; signs and symptoms; season; and family and community epidemiology, including contact with a case of GAS infection or presence in the family of a person with a history of ARF or with poststreptococcal glomerulonephritis. GAS pharyngitis is uncommon in children younger than 3 years of age, but outbreaks of GAS pharyngitis have been reported in young children in child care settings. The risk of ARF is so remote in young children in industrialized countries that diagnostic studies for GAS pharyngitis often are not indicated for children younger than 3 years of age. Children with manifestations highly suggestive of viral infection, such as coryza, conjunctivitis, hoarseness, cough, anterior stomatitis, discrete ulcerative lesions, or diarrhea, are unlikely to have GAS pharyngitis and generally should not be tested. In contrast, children with acute onset of sore throat and clinical signs and symptoms such as pharyngeal exudate, pain on swallowing, fever, and enlarged tender anterior cervical lymph nodes or exposure to a person with GAS pharyngitis are more likely to have GAS infection and should have a rapid antigen test and/or throat culture performed.

Testing Contacts for GAS Infection. Indications for testing contacts for GAS infection vary according to circumstances. Testing asymptomatic household contacts for GAS is not recommended except when contacts are at increased risk of developing sequelae of GAS infection, ARF, or acute glomerulonephritis; if test results are positive, contacts should be treated.

In schools, child care centers, or other environments in which a large number of people are in close contact, the prevalence of GAS pharyngeal carriage in healthy children can be as high as 20% in the absence of an outbreak of streptococcal disease. Therefore, classroom or more widespread culture surveys are not indicated.

Follow-up Throat Cultures. Post-treatment throat swab cultures are indicated only for patients who are at particularly high risk of ARF or have active symptoms compatible with GAS pharyngitis. Repeated courses of antimicrobial therapy are not indicated for asymptomatic patients with GAS-positive cultures; the exceptions are people who have had or whose family members have had ARF or other uncommon epidemiologic circumstances, such as outbreaks of rheumatic fever or acute poststreptococcal glomerulonephritis.

Patients who have repeated episodes of pharyngitis at short intervals and in whom GAS infection is documented by culture or antigen detection test present a special problem. Most often, these people are chronic GAS carriers who are experiencing frequent viral illnesses and for whom repeated testing and use of antimicrobial agents are unnecessary. In assessing such patients, inadequate adherence to oral treatment also should be considered. Although relatively uncommon, macrolide and azalide resistance among GAS strains occurs, resulting in erythromycin, clarithromycin, or azithromycin treatment

Table 3.67. Jones Criteria for Diagnosis of Acute Rheumatic Fever[a]

Major Criteria	Minor Criteria	Supporting Evidence
Carditis	Clinical findings:	Positive throat culture or rapid
Polyarthritis	Fever, arthralgia[b]	test for GAS antigen
Chorea	Laboratory findings:	OR
Erythema marginatum	Elevated acute phase	Elevated or rising streptococcal
Subcutaneous nodules	reactants; prolonged PR	antibody test
	interval	

[a]Diagnosis requires 2 major criteria or 1 major and 2 minor criteria with supporting evidence of antecedent group A streptococcal infection.
[b]Arthralgia is not a minor criterion in a patient with arthritis as a major criterion.

failures. Testing asymptomatic household contacts usually is not helpful. However, if multiple household members have pharyngitis or other GAS infections, simultaneous cultures of all household members and treatment of all people with positive cultures or rapid antigen test results may be of value.

Testing for GAS in Nonpharyngitis Infections. Cultures of impetiginous lesions often yield both streptococci and staphylococci, and determination of the primary pathogen is not possible. Culture is performed when it is necessary to determine susceptibility of the *S aureus*. In suspected invasive GAS infections, cultures of blood and focal sites of possible infection are indicated. In necrotizing fasciitis, imaging studies often delay, rather than facilitate, the diagnosis. Clinical suspicion of necrotizing fasciitis should prompt surgical evaluation with intervention, including débridement of deep tissues with Gram stain and culture of surgical specimens.

STSS is diagnosed on the basis of clinical findings and isolation of group A streptococci (see Table 3.66, p 670). Blood culture results are positive for *S pyogenes* in approximately 50% of patients with STSS. Culture results from a focal site of infections also usually are positive and can remain so for several days after appropriate antimicrobial agents have been initiated. *S pyogenes* uniformly is susceptible to beta-lactam antimicrobial agents, and susceptibility testing is needed only for nonbeta-lactam agents, such as erythromycin or clindamycin, to which *S pyogenes* can be resistant. A significant increase in antibody titers to streptolysin O, deoxyribonuclease B, or other streptococcal extracellular enzymes 4 to 6 weeks after infection can help to confirm the diagnosis if culture results are negative.

TREATMENT:

Pharyngitis.

- Although penicillin V is the drug of choice for treatment of GAS pharyngitis, amoxicillin equally is effective. A clinical GAS isolate resistant to penicillin or cephalosporin never has been documented. Prompt administration of penicillin therapy shortens the clinical course, decreases risk of suppurative sequelae and transmission, and prevents acute rheumatic fever, even when given up to 9 days after illness onset. For all patients with ARF, a complete course of penicillin or another appropriate antimicrobial agent for GAS pharyngitis should be given to eradicate GAS organisms from the throat, even if GAS organisms are not recovered in the initial throat culture.

The dose of orally administered penicillin V is 400 000 U (250 mg), 2 to 3 times per day, for 10 days for children weighing less than 27 kg (60 lb) and 800 000 U (500 mg), 2 to 3 times per day, for heavier children, adolescents, and adults. To prevent ARF, oral treatment with penicillin should be given for the full 10 days, regardless of the promptness of clinical recovery. Although different preparations of oral penicillin vary in absorption, their clinical efficacy is similar. Treatment failures may occur more often with oral penicillin than with intramuscularly administered penicillin G benzathine as a result of inadequate adherence to oral therapy. In addition, short-course treatment (less than 10 days) for GAS pharyngitis, particularly with penicillin V, is associated with inferior bacteriologic eradication rates.

- Orally administered amoxicillin given as a single daily dose (50 mg/kg; maximum, 1000–1200 mg) for 10 days is as effective as orally administered penicillin V or amoxicillin given multiple times per day for 10 days. This approach is an acceptable treatment option if strict adherence to once-daily dosing can be ensured.
- Intramuscular penicillin G benzathine is appropriate therapy. It ensures adequate blood concentrations and avoids the problem of adherence, but administration is painful. For children who weigh less than 27 kg, penicillin G benzathine is given in a single dose of 600 000 U (375 mg); for heavier children and adults, the dose is 1.2 million U (750 mg). Discomfort is less if the preparation of penicillin G benzathine is brought to room temperature before intramuscular injection. Mixtures containing shorter-acting penicillins (eg, penicillin G procaine) in addition to penicillin G benzathine have not been demonstrated to be more effective than penicillin G benzathine alone but are less painful when administered. Although supporting data are limited, the combination of 900 000 U (562.5 mg) of penicillin G benzathine and 300 000 U (187.5 mg) of penicillin G procaine is satisfactory therapy for most children; however, the efficacy of this combination for heavier patients, such as adolescents and adults, has not been demonstrated.
- For some patients who are allergic to penicillin, a 10-day course of a narrow-spectrum (first-generation) oral cephalosporin is indicated. However, as many as 5% to 10% of penicillin-allergic people also are allergic to cephalosporins. Patients with immediate or type I hypersensitivity to penicillin should not be treated with a cephalosporin. Oral clindamycin (20 mg/kg per day in 3 divided doses; maximum, 1.8 g/day) for 10 days is an acceptable alternative to penicillin in people with intermediate or type I hypersensitivity to penicillin.
- An oral macrolide or azalide (eg, erythromycin, clarithromycin, or azithromycin) is acceptable for patients allergic to penicillins. Therapy for 10 days is indicated **except** for azithromycin (12 mg/kg/day [maximum, 500 mg] on day 1, then 6 mg/kg/day [maximum, 250 mg/day]), which is given on days 2 through 5. Erythromycin is associated with substantially higher rates of gastrointestinal tract adverse effects than are these other agents. GAS strains resistant to macrolides or azilides have been highly prevalent in some areas of the world and have resulted in treatment failures. In recent years, macrolide resistance rates in most areas of the United States have been 5% to 8%, but resistance rates need continued monitoring.
- Tetracyclines, sulfonamides (including trimethoprim-sulfamethoxazole), and fluoroquinolones should not be used for treating GAS pharyngitis.

Children who have a recurrence of GAS pharyngitis shortly after completing a full course of a recommended oral antimicrobial agent can be retreated with the same antimicrobial agent, an alternative oral drug, or an intramuscular dose of penicillin G benzathine, especially if inadequate adherence to oral therapy is likely. Alternative drugs include a narrow-spectrum cephalosporin (ie, cephalexin), amoxicillin-clavulanate, clindamycin, a macrolide, or azalide. Expert opinions differ about the most appropriate therapy in this circumstance.

Management of a patient who has repeated and frequent episodes of acute pharyngitis associated with positive laboratory tests for group A streptococci is problematic. To determine whether the patient is a long-term streptococcal pharyngeal carrier who is experiencing repeated episodes of intercurrent viral pharyngitis (which is the situation in most cases), the following should be determined: (1) whether the clinical findings are more suggestive of a GAS or a viral cause; (2) whether epidemiologic factors in the community support a GAS or a viral cause; (3) the nature of the clinical response to the antimicrobial therapy (in true GAS pharyngitis, response to therapy usually is 24 hours or less); (4) whether laboratory test results are positive for GAS infection between episodes of acute pharyngitis; and (5) whether a serologic response to GAS extracellular antigens (eg, antistreptolysin O) has occurred. Serotyping of GAS isolates generally is available only in research laboratories, but if performed, repeated isolation of the same serotype suggests carriage, and isolation of differing serotypes indicates repeated infections.

Pharyngeal Carriers. Antimicrobial therapy is not indicated for most GAS pharyngeal carriers. The few specific situations in which eradication of carriage may be indicated include the following: (1) a local outbreak of ARF or poststreptococcal glomerulonephritis; (2) an outbreak of GAS pharyngitis in a closed or semiclosed community; (3) a family history of ARF; or (4) multiple ("ping-pong") episodes of documented symptomatic GAS pharyngitis occurring within a family for many weeks despite appropriate therapy.

Streptococcal carriage can be difficult to eradicate with conventional antimicrobial therapy. A number of antimicrobial agents, including clindamycin, cephalosporins, amoxicillin-clavulanate, azithromycin, and a combination of rifampin for the last 4 days of treatment with either penicillin V or penicillin G benzathine have been demonstrated to be more effective than penicillin in eliminating chronic streptococcal carriage. Of these drugs, oral clindamycin, given as 20 mg/kg per day in 3 doses (maximum, 1.8 g/day) for 10 days has been reported to be most effective. Documented eradication of the carrier state is helpful in the evaluation of subsequent episodes of acute pharyngitis; however, carriage can recur after reacquisition of GAS infection, as some individuals appear to be "carrier prone."

Nonbullous Impetigo. Local mupirocin or retapamulin ointment may be useful for limiting person-to-person spread of nonbullous impetigo and for eradicating localized disease. With multiple lesions or with nonbullous impetigo in multiple family members, child care groups, or athletic teams, impetigo should be treated with antimicrobial regimens administered systemically. Because episodes of nonbullous impetigo may be caused by *Staphylococcus aureus* or *S pyogenes,* children with nonbullous impetigo usually should be treated with an antimicrobial agent active against both GAS and *S aureus* infections.

Toxic Shock Syndrome. As outlined in Tables 3.68 and 3.69 (p 676), most aspects of management are the same for toxic shock syndrome caused by group A streptococci or by *S aureus.* Paramount are immediate aggressive fluid replacement and management of respiratory and cardiac failure, if present, and aggressive surgical débridement of any deep-seated GAS infection. Because *S pyogenes* and *S aureus* toxic shock syndrome are difficult to distinguish clinically, initial antimicrobial therapy should include an antistaphylococcal agent and a protein synthesis-inhibiting antimicrobial agent, such as clindamycin.

Table 3.68. Management of Streptococcal Toxic Shock Syndrome Without Necrotizing Fasciitis

- Fluid management to maintain adequate venous return and cardiac filling pressures to prevent end-organ damage
- Anticipatory management of multisystem organ failure
- Parenteral antimicrobial therapy at maximum doses with the capacity to:
  - Kill organism with bactericidal cell wall inhibitor (eg, beta-lactamase–resistant antimicrobial agent)
  - Decrease enzyme, toxin, or cytokine production with protein synthesis inhibitor (eg, clindamycin)
- Immune Globulin Intravenous may be considered for infection refractory to several hours of aggressive therapy or in the presence of an undrainable focus or persistent oliguria with pulmonary edema

Table 3.69. Management of Streptococcal Toxic Shock Syndrome With Necrotizing Fasciitis

- Principles outlined in Table 3.68
- Immediate surgical evaluation
  - Exploration or incisional biopsy for diagnosis and culture
  - Resection of all necrotic tissue
- Repeated resection of tissue may be needed if infection persists or progresses

The addition of clindamycin is more effective than penicillin alone for treating well-established GAS infections, because the antimicrobial activity of clindamycin is not affected by inoculum size, has a long postantimicrobial effect, and acts on bacteria by inhibiting protein synthesis. Inhibition of protein synthesis results in suppression of synthesis of the *S pyogenes* antiphagocytic M-protein and bacterial toxins. Clindamycin should not be used alone as initial antimicrobial therapy in life-threatening situations, because in the United States, 1% to 2% of GAS strains are resistant to clindamycin.

Once GAS infection has been identified, antimicrobial therapy can be changed to penicillin and clindamycin. Intravenous therapy should be continued until the patient is afebrile and stable hemodynamically and blood culture results are negative. The total duration of therapy is based on duration established for the primary site of infection.

Aggressive drainage and irrigation of accessible sites of infection should be performed as soon as possible. If necrotizing fasciitis is suspected, immediate surgical exploration or biopsy is crucial to identify deep soft tissue infection that should be débrided immediately.

The use of Immune Globulin Intravenous (IGIV) can be considered as adjunctive therapy of STSS or necrotizing fasciitis if the patient is severely ill, although randomized trials to assess efficacy have not been performed. Various regimens of IGIV, including 150 to 400 mg/kg per day for 5 days or a single dose of 1 to 2 g/kg, have been used, but the optimal regimen is unknown.

Other Infections. Parenteral antimicrobial therapy is required for severe infections, such as endocarditis, pneumonia, septicemia, meningitis, arthritis, osteomyelitis, erysipelas, necrotizing fasciitis, neonatal omphalitis, and streptococcal toxic shock syndrome. Treatment often is prolonged (2–6 weeks).

Prevention of Sequelae. ARF and acute glomerulonephritis are serious nonsuppurative sequelae of GAS infections. During epidemics of GAS infections on military bases in the 1950s, rheumatic fever developed in 3% of untreated patients with acute GAS pharyngitis. The current incidence after endemic infections is not known but is believed to be substantially less than 1%. The risk of ARF virtually can be eliminated by adequate treatment of the antecedent GAS infection; however, rare cases have occurred even after apparently appropriate therapy. The effectiveness of antimicrobial therapy for preventing acute poststreptococcal glomerulonephritis after pyoderma or pharyngitis has not been established. Suppurative sequelae, such as peritonsillar abscesses and cervical adenitis, usually are prevented by treatment of the primary infection.

ISOLATION OF THE HOSPITALIZED PATIENT: In addition to standard precautions, droplet precautions are recommended for children with GAS pharyngitis or pneumonia until 24 hours after initiation of appropriate antimicrobial therapy. For burns with secondary GAS infection and extensive or draining cutaneous infections that cannot be covered or contained adequately by dressings, contact precautions should be used for at least 24 hours after initiation of appropriate therapy.

CONTROL MEASURES: The most important means of controlling GAS disease and its sequelae is prompt identification and treatment of infections.

School and Child Care. Children with streptococcal pharyngitis or skin infections should not return to school or child care until at least 24 hours after beginning appropriate antimicrobial therapy. Close contact with other children during this time should be avoided.

Care of Exposed People. Contacts of documented cases of GAS infection who have recent or current clinical evidence of a GAS infection should undergo appropriate laboratory tests and should be treated if test results are positive. Rates of GAS carriage are higher among sibling contacts of children with GAS pharyngitis than among parent contacts in nonepidemic settings; rates as high as 50% for sibling contacts and 20% for parent contacts have been reported during epidemics. More than half of contacts who acquire GAS infection become ill. Asymptomatic acquisition of group A streptococci may pose some risk of nonsuppurative complications; studies indicate that as many as one third of patients with ARF had no history of recent streptococcal infection and another third had minor respiratory tract symptoms that were not brought to medical attention. However, routine laboratory evaluation of asymptomatic household contacts usually is not indicated except during outbreaks or when contacts are at increased risk of developing sequelae of infection (see Indications for GAS Testing, p 672). In rare circumstances, such as a large family with documented, repeated, intrafamilial transmission resulting in frequent episodes of GAS pharyngitis during a prolonged period, physicians may elect to treat all family members identified by laboratory tests as harboring GAS organisms.

Household contacts of patients with severe invasive GAS disease, including STSS, are at increased risk of developing severe invasive GAS disease compared with the general population. However, the risk is not sufficiently high to warrant routine testing for GAS colonization, and a clearly effective regimen has not been identified to justify routine chemoprophylaxis of all household contacts. However, because of increased risk of sporadic, invasive GAS disease among certain populations and because of increased risk of death in people 65 years of age and older who develop invasive GAS disease, physicians may choose to offer targeted chemoprophylaxis to household contacts who are 65 years of age and older or who are members of other high-risk populations (eg, people with human immunodeficiency virus infection, varicella, or diabetes mellitus). Because of the rarity of subsequent cases and the low risk of invasive GAS infections in children, chemoprophylaxisis is not recommended in schools or child care facilities.

Secondary Prophylaxis for Rheumatic Fever. Patients who have a well-documented history of ARF (including cases manifested solely as Sydenham chorea) and patients who have documented rheumatic heart disease should be given continuous antimicrobial prophylaxis to prevent recurrent attacks (secondary prophylaxis), because asymptomatic and symptomatic GAS infections can result in a recurrence of ARF. Continuous prophylaxis should be initiated as soon as the diagnosis of ARF or rheumatic heart disease is made.

Duration. Secondary prophylaxis should be long-term, perhaps for life, for patients with rheumatic heart disease (even after prosthetic valve replacement), because these patients remain at risk of recurrence of ARF. The risk of recurrence decreases as the interval from the most recent episode increases, and patients without rheumatic heart disease are at a lower risk of recurrence than are patients with residual cardiac involvement. These considerations, as well as the estimate of exposure to GAS infection, influence the duration of secondary prophylaxis in adults but should not alter the practice of secondary prophylaxis for children and adolescents. Secondary prophylaxis for all patients who have had ARF should be continued for at least 5 years or until the person is 21 years of age, whichever is longer (see Table 3.70, p 679). Prophylaxis also should be continued if the risk of contact with people with GAS infection is high, such as for parents with school-aged children and for people in professions that bring them into contact with children, such as teachers.

The drug regimens in Table 3.71 (p 679) are effective for secondary prophylaxis. The intramuscular regimen has been shown to be the most reliable, because the success of oral prophylaxis depends primarily on patient adherence; however, inconvenience and pain of injection may cause some patients to discontinue intramuscular prophylaxis. In non-US populations in which the risk of ARF particularly is high, administration of penicillin G benzathine every 3 weeks is justified and recommended, because drug concentrations in serum can decrease below a protective level before the fourth week after administration of a dose. In the United States, administration every 4 weeks seems adequate, except for people who have had recurrent ARF despite adherence to an every-4-week regimen. Oral sulfadiazine is as effective as oral penicillin for secondary prophylaxis but may not be available readily in the United States. By extrapolating from data demonstrating effectiveness of sulfadiazine, sulfisoxazole has been deemed an appropriate alternative drug.

Allergic reactions to oral penicillin are similar to reactions with intramuscular penicillin but usually are less severe and occur less commonly. These reactions also occur less commonly in children than in adults. Anaphylaxis is rare in patients receiving oral penicillin. Severe allergic reactions in patients receiving continuous penicillin G benzathine prophylaxis also are rare. Rare reports of anaphylaxis and death generally have involved patients older than 12 years of age with severe rheumatic heart disease. Most severe reactions seem to represent vasovagal responses rather than anaphylaxis. Reactions also can include a serum sickness-like reaction characterized by fever and joint pains, which can be mistaken for recurrence of ARF.

Table 3.70. Duration of Prophylaxis for People Who Have Had Acute Rheumatic Fever (ARF): Recommendations of the American Heart Association[a]

Category	Duration
Rheumatic fever without carditis	5 y since last episode of ARF or until 21 y of age, whichever is longer
Rheumatic fever with carditis but without residual heart disease (no valvular disease[b])	10 y since last episode of ARF or until age 21 y, whichever is longer
Rheumatic fever with carditis and residual heart disease (persistent valvular disease[b])	10 y since last episode of ARF or until 40 y of age, whichever is longer; consider lifelong prophylaxis for people with severe valvular disease or likelihood of ongoing exposure to group A streptococcal infection

[a]Modified from Gerber M, Baltimore R, Eaton C, et al. Prevention of rheumatic fever and diagnosis and treatment of acute streptococcal pharyngitis. A scientific statement from the American Heart Association, Rheumatic Fever, Endocarditis, and Kawasaki Disease Committee, Council on Cardiovascular Disease in the Young, and the Quality of Care and Outcomes Research Interdisciplinary Working Group. *Circulation*. 2009;119(11):1541–1551.
[b]Clinical or echocardiographic evidence.

Table 3.71. Chemoprophylaxis for Recurrences of Acute Rheumatic Fever[a]

Drug	Dose	Route
Penicillin G benzathine	1.2 million U, every 4 wk[b]; 600 000 U, every 4 wk for patients weighing less than 27.3 kg (60 lb)	Intramuscular
OR		
Penicillin V	250 mg, twice a day	Oral
OR		
Sulfadiazine or sulfisoxazole	0.5 g, once a day for patients weighing 27 kg (60 lb) or less	Oral
	1.0 g, once a day for patients weighing greater than 27 kg (60 lb)	
For people who are allergic to penicillin and sulfonamide drugs		
Macrolide or azalide	Variable (see text)	Oral

[a]Gerber M, Baltimore R, Eaton C, et al. Prevention of rheumatic fever and diagnosis and treatment of acute streptococcal pharyngitis. A scientific statement from the American Heart Association, Rheumatic Fever, Endocarditis, and Kawasaki Disease Committee, Council on Cardiovascular Disease in the Young, and the Quality of Care and Outcomes Research Interdisciplinary Working Group. *Circulation*. 2009;119(11):1541–1551.
[b]In particularly high-risk situations (usually non-US sites), administration every 3 weeks is recommended.

Reactions to continuous sulfadiazine or sulfisoxazole prophylaxis are rare and usually minor; evaluation of blood cell counts may be advisable after 2 weeks of prophylaxis, because leukopenia has been reported. Prophylaxis with a sulfonamide during late pregnancy is contraindicated because of interference with fetal bilirubin metabolism. Febrile mucocutaneous syndromes (erythema multiforme, Stevens-Johnson syndrome, or toxic epidermal necrolysis) have been associated with penicillin and with sulfonamides. When an adverse event occurs with any of these therapeutic regimens, the drug should be stopped immediately and an alternative drug should be selected. For the rare patient allergic to both penicillins and sulfonamides, erythromycin is recommended. Other macrolides, such as azithromycin or clarithromycin, also should be acceptable; they have less risk of gastrointestinal tract intolerance but increased costs.

Poststreptococcal Reactive Arthritis. After an episode of acute GAS pharyngitis, reactive arthritis may develop in the absence of sufficient clinical manifestations and laboratory findings to fulfill the Jones criteria for diagnosis of ARF. This syndrome has been termed poststreptococcal reactive arthritis (PSRA). The precise relationship of PSRA to ARF is unclear. In contrast with the arthritis of ARF, PSRA does not respond dramatically to nonsteroidal anti-inflammatory agents. Because a very small proportion of patients with PSRA have been reported to develop valvular heart disease later, these patients should be observed carefully for 1 to 2 years for carditis. Some experts recommend secondary prophylaxis for these patients during the observation period. If carditis occurs, the patient should be considered to have had ARF, and secondary prophylaxis should be continued (see Secondary Prophylaxis for Rheumatic Fever, p 678).

Bacterial Endocarditis Prophylaxis.[1] The American Heart Association (AHA) has published updated recommendations regarding use of antimicrobial agents to prevent infective endocarditis (see prevention of Bacterial Endocarditis, p 879). The AHA no longer recommends prophylaxis for patients with rheumatic heart disease. However, use of oral antiseptic solutions and maintenance of optimal oral health remain important components of an overall health care program. For the relatively few patients with rheumatic heart disease in whom infective endocarditis prophylaxis still is recommended (eg, people with prosthetic valves), current AHA recommendations should be followed, recognizing that the agent selected should be one other than a penicillin, because penicillin-resistant alpha-hemolytic streptococci likely are present when penicillin is used for secondary prevention of rheumatic fever.

Group B Streptococcal Infections

CLINICAL MANIFESTATIONS: Group B streptococci are a major cause of perinatal infections, including bacteremia, endometritis, and chorioamnionitis; urinary tract infections in pregnant women; and systemic and focal infections in young infants. Invasive disease in infants is categorized on the basis of chronologic age at onset. Early-onset disease usually occurs within the first 24 hours of life (range, 0–6 days) and is characterized by signs of systemic infection, respiratory distress, apnea, shock, pneumonia, and less often, meningitis (5%–10% of cases). Late-onset disease, which typically occurs at 3 to 4 weeks of age (range, 7–89 days), commonly manifests as occult bacteremia or meningitis; other focal infections, such as osteomyelitis, septic arthritis, necrotizing fasciitis, pneumonia, adenitis, and cellulitis, occur less commonly. Late, late-onset disease occurs beyond 89 days of age, usually in very preterm infants requiring prolonged hospitalization. Group B streptococci also cause systemic infections in nonpregnant adults with underlying medical

---

[1] Wilson W, Taubert KA, Gewitz M, et al. Prevention of infective endocarditis. Recommendations by the American Heart Association. A guideline from the American Heart Association Rheumatic Fever, Endocarditis, and Kawasaki Disease Committee, Council on Cardiovascular Disease in the Young, and the Council on Clinical Cardiology, Council on Cardiovascular Surgery and Anesthesia, and the Quality of Care and Outcomes Research Interdisciplinary Working Group. *Circulation.* 2007;116(15):1736–1754

conditions, such as diabetes mellitus, chronic liver or renal disease, malignancy, or other immunocompromising conditions and in adults 65 years of age and older.

ETIOLOGY: Group B streptococci *(Streptococcus agalactiae)* are gram-positive, aerobic diplococci that typically produce a narrow zone of beta hemolysis on 5% sheep blood agar. These organisms are divided into 10 types on the basis of capsular polysaccharides (Ia, Ib, II, and III through IX). Types Ia, Ib, II, III, and V account for approximately 95% of cases in infants in the United States. Type III is the predominant cause of early-onset meningitis and the majority of late-onset infections in infants. Pilus-like structures are important virulence factors and potential vaccine candidates.

EPIDEMIOLOGY: Group B streptococci are common inhabitants of the human gastrointestinal and genitourinary tracts. Less commonly, they colonize the pharynx. The colonization rate in pregnant women ranges from 15% to 35%. Colonization during pregnancy can be constant or intermittent. Before recommendations for prevention of early-onset group B streptococcal (GBS) disease through maternal intrapartum antimicrobial prophylaxis (see Control Measures, p 683) were made, the incidence was 1 to 4 cases per 1000 live births; early-onset disease accounted for approximately 75% of cases in infants and occurred in approximately 1 to 2 infants per 100 colonized women. Associated with implementation of widespread maternal intrapartum antimicrobial prophylaxis, the incidence of early-onset disease has decreased by approximately 80% to an estimated 0.28 cases per 1000 live births in 2008. The use of intrapartum chemoprophylaxis has had no measurable impact on late-onset GBS disease, which nearly equals that of early-onset disease (an estimated 0.25 cases per 1000 live births in 2008). The case-fatality ratio in term infants ranges from 1% to 3% but is higher in preterm neonates (20% for early-onset disease and 5% for late-onset disease). Approximately 50% of early-onset cases still afflict term neonates.

Transmission from mother to infant occurs shortly before or during delivery. After delivery, person-to-person transmission can occur. Although uncommon, GBS infection can be acquired in the nursery from health care professionals (probably via breaks in hand hygiene) or visitors and more commonly in the community (colonized family members or caregivers). The risk of early-onset disease is increased in preterm infants (less than 37 weeks' gestation), infants born after the amniotic membranes have been ruptured 18 hours or more, and infants born to women with high genital GBS inoculum, intrapartum fever (temperature 38°C [100.4°F] or greater), chorioamnionitis, GBS bacteriuria during the current pregnancy, or a previous infant with invasive GBS disease. A low or an undetectable maternal concentration of type-specific serum antibody to capsular polysaccharide of the infecting strain also is a predisposing factor. Other risk factors are intrauterine fetal monitoring and maternal age younger than 20 years. Black race is an independent risk factor for both early-onset and late-onset disease. Although the incidence of early-onset disease has declined in all racial groups since the 1900s, rates consistently have been higher among black infants (0.52–0.83 cases per 1000 live births from 2002–2007) compared with white infants (0.24–0.33 cases per 1000 live births from 2002–2007), with the highest incidence observed among preterm black infants. The reason for this racial/ethnic disparity is not known. The period of communicability is unknown but can extend throughout the duration of colonization or disease. Infants can remain colonized for several months after birth and after treatment for systemic infection. Recurrent GBS disease affects an estimated 1% to 3% of appropriately treated infants.

The **incubation period** of early-onset disease is fewer than 7 days. In late-onset and late, late-onset disease, the incubation period from GBS acquisition to disease is unknown.

DIAGNOSTIC TESTS: Gram-positive cocci in pairs or short chains by Gram stain of body fluids that typically are sterile (eg, cerebrospinal [CSF], pleural, or joint fluid) provide presumptive evidence of infection. Cultures of blood, CSF, and if present, a suppurative focus are necessary to establish the diagnosis. Rapid tests that identify group B streptococcal antigen in body fluids other than CSF are not recommended for diagnosis because of poor specificity.

TREATMENT:
- Ampicillin plus an aminoglycoside is the initial treatment of choice for a newborn infant with presumptive invasive GBS infection.
- Penicillin G alone can be given when group B streptococcus has been identified as the cause of the infection and when clinical and microbiologic responses have been documented.
- For infants with meningitis attributable to group B streptococcus, the recommended dosage of penicillin G for infants 7 days of age or younger is 250 000 to 450 000 U/kg per day, intravenously, in 3 divided doses; for infants older than 7 days of age, 450 000 to 500 000 U/kg per day, intravenously, in 4 divided doses is recommended. For ampicillin, the recommended dosage for infants with meningitis 7 days of age or younger is 200 to 300 mg/kg per day, intravenously, in 3 divided doses; the recommended dosage for infants older than 7 days of age is 300 mg/kg per day, intravenously, in 4 divided doses.
- For meningitis, some experts believe that a second lumbar puncture approximately 24 to 48 hours after initiation of therapy assists in management and prognosis. If CSF sterility is not achieved, a complicated course (eg, cerebral infarcts) can be expected; also, an increasing protein concentration suggests an intracranial complication (eg, infarction, ventricular obstruction). Additional lumbar punctures and diagnostic imaging studies are indicated if response to therapy is in doubt, neurologic abnormalities persist, or focal neurologic deficits occur. Consultation with a specialist in pediatric infectious diseases often is useful.
- For infants with bacteremia without a defined focus, treatment should be continued for 10 days. For infants with uncomplicated meningitis, 14 days of treatment is satisfactory, but longer periods of treatment may be necessary for infants with prolonged or complicated courses. Septic arthritis or osteomyelitis requires treatment for 3 to 4 weeks; endocarditis or ventriculitis requires treatment for at least 4 weeks.
- Because of the reported increased risk of infection, the sibling of a multiple birth index case with early- or late-onset disease should be observed carefully and evaluated and treated empirically for suspected systemic infection if signs of illness occur.

ISOLATION OF THE HOSPITALIZED PATIENT: Standard precautions are recommended, except during a nursery outbreak of disease attributable to group B streptococci (see Control Measures, Nursery Outbreak, p 684).

CONTROL MEASURES:

Chemoprophylaxis. Recommendations from the Centers for Disease Control and Prevention (CDC)[1] and American Academy of Pediatrics[2] include the following:

- All pregnant women should be screened at 35 to 37 weeks' gestation for vaginal and rectal GBS colonization. The only exceptions to this recommendation for universal culture screening are women with GBS bacteriuria during the current pregnancy or women who have had a previous infant with invasive GBS disease; these women always should receive intrapartum chemoprophylaxis. Intrapartum chemoprophylaxis should be given to all pregnant women identified as carriers of group B streptococci. Colonization during a previous pregnancy is *not* an indication for intrapartum chemoprophylaxis.

- Women with group B streptococci isolated from urine during the current pregnancy should receive intrapartum chemoprophylaxis, because these women usually have a high inoculum of group B streptococci at vaginal sites and are at increased risk of delivering an infant with early-onset GBS disease; culture screening at 35 to 37 weeks' gestation is not necessary.

   If GBS status is not known at onset of labor or rupture of membranes, intrapartum chemoprophylaxis should be administered to *all* women with gestation less than 37 weeks, duration of membrane rupture 18 hours or longer, or intrapartum temperature of 38.0°C (100.4°F) or greater.

- Oral antimicrobial agents should *not* be used to treat women who are found to have GBS colonization during culture screening. If there is GBS bacteriuria, treatment is warranted according to obstetric standards of care. Such treatment is *not* effective in eliminating carriage of group B streptococci or preventing neonatal disease.

- Intrapartum antimicrobial prophylaxis is *not* recommended for cesarean deliveries performed before labor onset in women with intact amniotic membranes. Women expected to undergo cesarean deliveries should undergo routine culture screening, because onset of labor or rupture of membranes can occur before the planned cesarean delivery, and in this circumstance, intrapartum antimicrobial prophylaxis is recommended.

- Penicillin G (5 million U initially, then 2.5 to 3.0 million U, every 4 hours, until delivery) intravenously is the preferred agent for intrapartum chemoprophylaxis because of its efficacy and narrow spectrum of antimicrobial activity. An alternative drug is intravenous ampicillin (2 g initially, then 1 g every 4 hours until delivery).

- Penicillin-allergic women without a history of anaphylaxis, angioedema, respiratory distress, or urticaria following administration of a penicillin or a cephalosporin should receive intravenous cefazolin (2 g initially, then 1 g every 8 hours). Cefazolin is recommended because of its ability to achieve high amniotic fluid concentrations and effectively prevent early-onset GBS disease.

---

[1] Centers for Disease Control and Prevention. Prevention of perinatal group B streptococcal disease. Revised guidelines from CDC, 2010. *MMWR Recomm Rep.* 2010;59(RR–10):1–36

[2] American Academy of Pediatrics, Committee on Infectious Diseases. Recommendations for the prevention of perinatal group B streptococcal (GBS) disease. *Pediatrics.* 2011;128(3):611–616

- Penicillin-allergic women at high risk of anaphylaxis should receive intravenous clinda-mycin (900 mg every 8 hours) *if* their GBS isolate is documented to be susceptible to clindamycin. If clindamycin susceptibility testing has not been performed, intravenous vancomycin (1 g every 12 hours) should be administered. The efficacy of clindamycin or vancomycin is not established.
- Routine use of antimicrobial agents as chemoprophylaxis for neonates born to mothers who have received adequate intrapartum chemoprophylaxis is *not* recom-mended. Antimicrobial therapy is appropriate only for infants with clinically suspected systemic infection.
- An algorithm for management of newborn infants is provided in Fig 3.6. The recom-mendations are intended to help clinicians promptly detect and treat cases of early-onset infections.
- Newborn infants with signs of sepsis should receive a full diagnostic evaluation and initiation of empiric antimicrobial therapy.
- Well-appearing newborn infants whose mothers had suspected chorioamnionitis should undergo a limited evaluation (includes a blood culture and complete blood cell count with differential and platelet counts) and receive empiric antimicrobial therapy pending culture results.
- Well-appearing infants infants whose mothers had no chorioamnionitis and no indica-tion for GBS prophylaxis should receive routine clinical care.
- Well-appearing infants of any gestational age whose mother received adequate intrapartum GBS prophylaxis (≥4 hours of penicillin, ampicillin, or cefazolin before delivery) should be observed for ≥48 hours; diagnostic testing is *not* recommended. All other maternal antimicrobial agents or durations before delivery are considered inadequate for purposes of neonatal management.
- Well-appearing infants ≥37 weeks' gestation born to mothers who had an indication for GBS prophylaxis but received no or inadequate prophylaxis and in whom duration of membrane rupture before delivery was <18 hours should be observed for ≥48 hours, and *no* diagnostic testing is recommended.
- If the infant is well appearing and either <37 weeks' gestation or the duration of mem-brane rupture before delivery was ≥18 hours, then the infant should undergo a limited evaluation and observation for ≥48 hours.

Neonatal Infection Control. Routine cultures to determine whether infants are colonized with group B streptococci are *not* recommended.

Nursery Outbreak. Cohorting of ill and colonized infants and use of contact precau-tions during an outbreak are recommended. Other methods of control (eg, treatment of asymptomatic carriers with penicillin) are ineffective. Routine hand hygiene by health care professionals caring for infants colonized or infected with GBS is the best way to pre-vent spread to other infants.

FIGURE 3.6. MANAGEMENT OF NEONATES FOR PREVENTION OF EARLY-ONSET GROUP B STREPTOCOCCAL (GBS) DISEASE

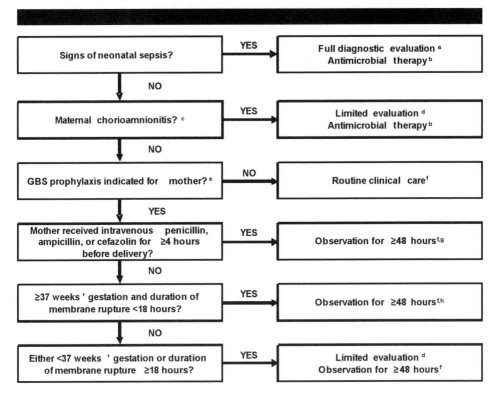

a Full diagnostic evaluation includes complete blood cell (CBC) count with differential, platelets, blood culture, chest radiograph (if respiratory abnormalities are present), and lumbar puncture (if patient stable enough to tolerate procedure and sepsis is suspected).

b Antimicrobial therapy should be directed toward the most common causes of neonatal sepsis, including GBS and other organisms (including gram-negative pathogens), and should take into account local antimicrobial resistance patterns.

c Consultation with obstetric providers is important to determine the level of clinical suspicion for chorioamnionitis. Chorioamnionitis is diagnosed clinically, and some of the signs are nonspecific.

d Limited evaluation includes blood culture (at birth) and CBC count with differential and platelets (at birth and/or at 6–12 hours of life).

e GBS prophylaxis indicated if one or more of the following: (1) mother GBS positive at 35 to 37 weeks' gestation; (2) GBS status unknown with one or more intrapartum risk factors, including <37 weeks' gestation, rupture of membranes ≥18 hours or temperature ≥100.4°F (38.0°C), or intrapartum nucleic acid amplification test results positive for GBS; (3) GBS bacteriuria during current pregnancy; (4) history of a previous infant with GBS disease.

f If signs of sepsis develop, a full diagnostic evaluation should be performed and antimicrobial therapy should be initiated.

g If ≥37 weeks' gestation, observation may occur at home after 24 hours if other discharge criteria have been met, if there is a knowledgeable observer and ready access to medical care.

h Some experts recommend a CBC with differential and platelets at 6 to 12 hours of age.

Non-Group A or B Streptococcal and Enterococcal Infections

CLINICAL MANIFESTATIONS: Streptococci other than Lancefield groups A or B can be associated with invasive disease in infants, children, adolescents, and adults. The principal clinical syndromes of groups C and G streptococci are septicemia, upper and lower respiratory tract infections, skin and soft tissue infections, septic arthritis, meningitis with a parameningeal focus, brain abscess, and endocarditis with various clinical manifestations. Group F is an infrequent cause of invasive infection. Viridans streptococci are the most common cause of bacterial endocarditis in children, especially children with congenital or valvular heart disease, and these organisms have become a common cause of bacteremia in neutropenic patients with cancer. Among the viridans streptococci, organisms from the *Streptococcus anginosus* group often cause localized infections, such as brain or dental abscess or abscesses in other sites, including lymph nodes, liver, and lung. Enterococci are associated with bacteremia in neonates and bacteremia, device-associated infections, intra-abdominal abscesses, and urinary tract infections in older children and adults.

ETIOLOGY: Changes in taxonomy and nomenclature of the *Streptococcus* genus have evolved with advances in molecular technology. Among gram-positive organisms that are catalase negative and display chains by Gram stain, the genera associated most often with human disease are *Streptococcus* and *Enterococcus*. Members of the *Streptococcus* genus that are beta-hemolytic on blood agar plates include *Streptococcus pyogenes* (see Group A Streptococcal Infections, p 668), *Streptococcus agalactiae* (see Group B Streptococcal Infections, p 680) and groups C and G streptococci. *S agalactiae* subspecies *equisimilis* is the group C species most often associated with human infections. Streptococci that are non-beta–hemolytic (alpha-hemolytic or nonhemolytic) on blood agar plates include (1) *Streptococcus pneumoniae*, a member of the *mitis* group (see Pneumococcal Infections, p 571); (2) the *bovis* group; and (3) species of viridans streptococci commonly isolated from humans, which can be divided into 4 groups by use of 16S rRNA gene sequencing (the *anginosus* group, the *mitis* group, the *salivarius* group, and the *mutans* group). The *anginosus* group (*S anginosus*, *Streptococcus constellatus*, and *Streptococcus intermedius*) can have variable hemolysis, and approximately one third possess group A, C, F, or G antigens. Nutritionally variant streptococci, once thought to be viridans streptococci, now are classified in the genera *Abiotrophia* and *Granulicatella*.

The genus *Enterococcus* (previously included with Lancefield group D streptococci) contains at least 18 species, with *Enterococcus faecalis* and *Enterococcus faecium* accounting for most human enterococcal infections. Outbreaks and nosocomial spread in association with *Enterococcus gallinarum* also have occurred occasionally. Nonenterococcal group D streptococci include *Streptococcus bovis* and *Streptococcus equinus*, both members of the *bovis* group.

EPIDEMIOLOGY: The habitats that nongroup A and B streptococci and enterococci occupy in humans include skin (groups C and G), oropharynx (groups C and G and the *mutans* group), gastrointestinal tract (groups C and G, the *bovis* group and *Enterococcus* species), and vagina (groups C, D and G and *Enterococcus* species). Typical human habitats of different species of viridans streptococci are the oropharynx, epithelial surfaces of the oral cavity, teeth, skin, and gastrointestinal and genitourinary tracts. Intrapartum transmission is responsible for most cases of early-onset neonatal infection caused by nongroup A and B streptococci and enterococci. Environmental contamination or transmission via hands of health care professionals can lead to colonization of patients. Groups C and G streptococci have been known to cause foodborne outbreaks of pharyngitis.

The **incubation period** and the period of communicability are unknown.

DIAGNOSTIC TESTS: Diagnosis is established by culture of usually sterile body fluids with appropriate biochemical testing and serologic analysis for definitive identification. Antimicrobial susceptibility testing of isolates from usually sterile sites should be performed to guide treatment of infections caused by viridans streptococci or enterococci. The proportion of vancomycin-resistant enterococci among hospitalized patients can be as high as 30%.

TREATMENT: Penicillin G is the drug of choice for groups C and G streptococci. Other agents with good activity include ampicillin, cefotaxime, vancomycin, and linezolid. The combination of gentamicin with a beta-lactam antimicrobial agent (eg, penicillin or ampicillin) or vancomycin may enhance bactericidal activity needed for treatment of life-threatening infections (eg, endocarditis or meningitis).

Many viridans streptococci remain fully susceptible to penicillin (minimal inhibitory concentration [MIC], ≤ 0.1 μg/mL). Strains with an MIC >0.1 μg/mL and <0.5 μg/mL are considered relatively resistant by criteria in the American Heart Association guidelines for determining treatment of streptococcal endocarditis. Strains with a penicillin MIC ≥ 0.5 μg/mL are considered resistant. The Clinical Laboratory Standards Institute defines susceptible viridans streptococci as having an MIC ≤ 0.12 μg/mL, intermediate isolates as having an MIC of 0.25 μg/mL to 2 μg/mL, and those exhibiting resistance as having an MIC ≥ 4 μg/mL. Nonpenicillin antimicrobial agents with good activity against viridans streptococci include cephalosporins (especially ceftriaxone), vancomycin, linezolid, daptomycin, and tigecycline, although experience with daptomycin and tigecycline is limited, and these are not approved for use in children. *Abiotrophia* and *Granulicatella* organisms can exhibit relative or high-level resistance to penicillin. The combination of high-dose penicillin or vancomycin and an aminoglycoside can enhance bactericidal activity.

Enterococci exhibit uniform resistance to cephalosporins and isolates resistant to vancomycin, especially *E faecium,* are increasing in prevalence. In general, children with a central line-associated bloodstream infection caused by enterococci should have the device removed promptly.

Invasive enterococcal infections, such as endocarditis or meningitis, should be treated with ampicillin if the isolate is susceptible or vancomycin in combination with an aminoglycoside. Gentamicin is the aminoglycoside recommended for achieving synergy. Gentamicin should be discontinued if in vitro susceptibility testing demonstrates high-level resistance, in which case synergy cannot be achieved. The role of combination therapy for treating central line-associated bloodstream infections is uncertain. Linezolid is approved for use in children, including neonates, only for treatment of infections caused by vancomycin-resistant *E faecium*. Isolates of vancomycin-resistant enterococci (VRE) that also are resistant to linezolid have been described. Resistance to linezolid among VRE isolates also can develop during prolonged treatment. Although most vancomycin-resistant isolates of *E faecalis* and *E faecium* are daptomycin susceptible, daptomycin is approved for use only in adults for treatment of infections attributable to vancomycin-resistant *E faecalis.* Limited data suggest that clearance rates of daptomycin are more rapid in young children compared with adolescents and adults. Quinupristin-dalfopristin is approved for use in adults for treatment of infections attributable to vancomycin-resistant

E faecium but is not active against *E faecalis*. Microbiologic and clinical cure has been reported in children infected with vancomycin-resistant *E faecium* who were treated with quinupristin-dalfopristin. Tigecycline is approved for use in adults with infections caused by vancomycin-susceptible *E faecalis*. Tigecycline has good activity in vitro against both vancomycin-resistant *E faecalis* and vancomycin-resistant *E faecium*, but experience in children is limited.

Endocarditis. Guidelines for antimicrobial therapy in adults have been formulated by the American Heart Association and should be consulted for regimens that are appropriate for children and adolescents.[1]

ISOLATION OF THE HOSPITALIZED PATIENT: Standard precautions are recommended. For patients with infection or colonization attributable to VRE, contact as well as standard precautions are indicated. Common practice is to maintain precautions until the patient no longer harbors the organism or is discharged from the health care facility. Criteria of negative culture results from body fluid or tissue specimens from multiple sites (may include stool or rectal swab, perineal area, axilla or umbilicus, wound, and indwelling urinary catheter or colostomy sites, if present) on at least 3 separate occasions obtained after cessation of antimicrobial therapy and more than 1 week apart define resolution of VRE colonization.

CONTROL MEASURES: Patients with a prosthetic valve or prosthetic material used for cardiac valve repair, previous infective endocarditis, or congenital heart disease associated with the highest risk of adverse outcome from endocarditis should receive antimicrobial prophylaxis to prevent endocarditis at the time of dental and other selected surgical procedures (see Prevention of Bacterial Endocarditis, p 879). For these patients, early instruction in proper diet; oral health, including use of dental sealants and adequate fluoride intake; and prevention or cessation of smoking will aid in prevention of dental carries and potentially lower their risk of recurrent endocarditis.[2]

Use of vancomycin and treatment with broad-spectrum antimicrobial agents are risk factors for colonization and infection with VRE. Hospitals should develop institution-specific guidelines for the proper use of vancomycin.[3]

---

[1] Wilson W, Taubert KA, Gewitz M, et al. Prevention of infective endocarditis. Recommendations by the American Heart Association. A guideline from the American Heart Association Rheumatic Fever, Endocarditis, and Kawasaki Disease Committee, Council on Cardiovascular Disease in the Young, and the Council on Clinical Cardiology, Council on Cardiovascular Surgery and Anesthesia, and the Quality of Care and Outcomes Research Interdisciplinary Working Group. *Circulation.* 2007;116(15):1736–1754

[2] Hageman JC, Patel JB, Carey RC, Tenover FC, McDonald LC. *Investigation and Control of Vancomycin-Intermediate and -Resistant Staphylococcus aureus (VISA/VRSA): A Guide for Health Departments and Infection Control Personnel.* Atlanta, GA: Centers for Disease Control and Prevention; 2006. Available at: **www.cdc.gov/hai/pdfs/visa_vrsa/visa_vrsa_guide.pdf**

[3] Centers for Disease Control and Prevention. Surveillance for dental caries, dental sealants, tooth retention, edentulism, and enamel fluorosis—United States, 1988–1994 and 1999–2002. *MMWR Surveill Summ.* 2005;54(SS–3):1–43

Strongyloidiasis
(Strongyloides stercoralis)

CLINICAL MANIFESTATIONS: Most infections with *Strongyloides stercoralis* are asymptomatic. When symptoms occur, they are most often related to larval skin invasion, tissue migration, and/or the presence of adult worms in the intestine. Infective (filariform) larvae are acquired from skin contact with contaminated soil, producing transient pruritic papules at the site of penetration. Larvae migrate to the lungs and can cause a transient pneumonitis or Loeffler-like syndrome. After ascending the tracheobronchial tree, larvae are swallowed and mature into adults within the gastrointestinal tract. Symptoms of intestinal infection include nonspecific abdominal pain, malabsorption, vomiting, and diarrhea. Larval migration from defecated stool can result in migratory pruritic skin lesions in the perianal area, buttocks, and upper thighs, which may present as serpiginous, erythematous tracks called "larva currens." Immunocompromised people, most often those receiving glucocorticoids for underlying malignancy or autoimmune disease, people receiving biologic response modifiers, and people infected with human T-lymphotropic virus 1 (HTLV-1) are at risk of *Strongyloides* hyperinfection syndrome and disseminated disease, in which larvae migrate via the systemic circulation to distant organs including the brain, liver, heart, and skin. This condition, which frequently is fatal, is characterized by fever, abdominal pain, diffuse pulmonary infiltrates, and septicemia or meningitis caused by enteric gram-negative bacilli.

ETIOLOGY: *S stercoralis* is a nematode (roundworm).

EPIDEMIOLOGY: Strongyloidiasis is endemic in the tropics and subtropics, including the southeastern United States, wherever suitable moist soil and improper disposal of human waste coexist. Humans are the principal hosts, but dogs, cats, and other animals can serve as reservoirs. Transmission involves penetration of skin by infective (filariform) larvae from contact with infected soil. Infections rarely can be acquired from intimate skin contact or from inadvertent coprophagy, such as from ingestion of contaminated food or within institutional settings. Adult females release eggs in the small intestine, where they hatch as first-stage (rhabditiform) larvae that are excreted in feces. A small percentage of larvae molt to the infective (filariform) stage during intestinal transit, at which point they can penetrate the bowel mucosa or perianal skin, thus maintaining the life cycle within a single person (autoinfection). Because of this capacity for autoinfection, people can remain infected for decades after leaving a geographic area with endemic infection.

The **incubation period** in humans is unknown.

DIAGNOSTIC TESTS: Strongyloidiasis can be difficult to diagnose in immunocompetent people, because excretion of larvae in feces is highly variable and often of low intensity. At least 3 consecutive stool specimens should be examined microscopically for characteristic larvae (not eggs), but stool concentration techniques may be required to establish the diagnosis. The use of agar plate culture methods may have greater sensitivity than fecal microscopy, and examination of duodenal contents obtained using the string test (Entero-Test), or a direct aspirate through a flexible endoscope also may demonstrate larvae. Eosinophilia (blood eosinophil count greater than $500/\mu L$) is common in chronic infection but may be absent in hyperinfection syndrome. Serodiagnosis is sensitive and should be considered in all people with unexplained eosinophilia.

In disseminated strongyloidiasis, filariform larvae may be isolated from sputum or bronchoalveolar lavage fluid as well as spinal fluid. Gram-negative bacillary meningitis is a common associated finding in disseminated disease and carries a high mortality rate.

TREATMENT: Ivermectin is the treatment of choice for both chronic (asymptomatic) strongyloidiasis and hyperinfection with disseminated disease. Alternative agents include thiabendazole and albendazole, although both drugs are associated with lower cure rates (see Drugs for Parasitic Infections, p 848). Prolonged or repeated treatment may be necessary in people with hyperinfection and disseminated strongyloidiasis, and relapse can occur.

ISOLATION OF THE HOSPITALIZED PATIENT: Standard precautions are recommended.

CONTROL MEASURES: Sanitary disposal of human waste is effective at interrupting transmission of *S stercoralis*. Examination of stool for larvae and serum for antibodies to *S stercoralis* is recommended in patients with unexplained eosinophilia, especially for those who are immunosuppressed or for whom administration of glucocorticoids is planned. If possible, patients should be treated for strongyloidiasis prior to initiation of immunosuppressive therapy.

Syphilis

CLINICAL MANIFESTATIONS:

Congenital Syphilis. Intrauterine infection with *Treponema pallidum* can result in stillbirth, hydrops fetalis, or preterm birth or may be asymptomatic at birth. Infected infants can have hepatosplenomegaly, snuffles (copious nasal secretions), lymphadenopathy, mucocutaneous lesions, pneumonia, osteochondritis and pseudoparalysis, edema, rash, hemolytic anemia, or thrombocytopenia at birth or within the first 4 to 8 weeks of age. Skin lesions or moist nasal secretions of congenital syphilis are highly infectious. However, organisms rarely are found in lesions more than 24 hours after treatment has begun. Untreated infants, regardless of whether they have manifestations in early infancy, may develop late manifestations, which usually appear after 2 years of age and involve the central nervous system (CNS), bones and joints, teeth, eyes, and skin. Some consequences of intrauterine infection may not become apparent until many years after birth, such as interstitial keratitis (5–20 years of age), eighth cranial nerve deafness (10–40 years of age), Hutchinson teeth (peg-shaped, notched central incisors), anterior bowing of the shins, frontal bossing, mulberry molars, saddle nose, rhagades (perioral fissures), and Clutton joints (symmetric, painless swelling of the knees). The first 3 manifestations are referred to as the Hutchinson triad. Late manifestations can be prevented by treatment of early infection.

Acquired Syphilis. Infection with *T pallidum* in childhood or adulthood can be divided into 3 stages. The **primary stage** appears as one or more painless indurated ulcers (chancres) of the skin or mucous membranes at the site of inoculation. Lesions most commonly appear on the genitalia but may appear elsewhere, depending on the sexual contact responsible for transmission (ie, oral). These lesions appear, on average, 3 weeks after exposure (10–90 days) and heal spontaneously in a few weeks. Chancres sometimes are not recognized clinically. The **secondary stage,** beginning 1 to 2 months later, is characterized by rash, mucocutaneous lesions, and lymphadenopathy. The polymorphic maculopapular rash is generalized and typically includes the palms and soles. In moist areas around the vulva or anus, hypertrophic papular lesions (condylomata lata) can occur and can be confused with condyloma acuminata secondary to human papillomavirus (HPV) infection. Generalized lymphadenopathy, fever, malaise, splenomegaly, sore throat, headache, and arthralgia can be present. This stage also resolves spontaneously without treatment in approximately 3 to 12 weeks, leaving the infected person completely asymptomatic. A variable latent period follows but sometimes is interrupted during the first few years by recurrences of symptoms of secondary syphilis. **Latent syphilis** is defined as the period after infection when patients are seroreactive but demonstrate no clinical manifestations of disease. Latent syphilis acquired within the preceding year is referred to as **early latent syphilis;** all other cases of latent syphilis are **late latent syphilis** (greater than 1 year's duration) or **syphilis of unknown duration.** The **tertiary stage** of infection occurs 15 to 30 years after the initial infection and can include gumma formation, cardiovascular involvement, or neurosyphilis. Neurosyphilis is defined as infection of the CNS with *T pallidum.* Manifestations of neurosyphilis can occur at any stage of infection, especially in people infected with human immunodeficiency virus (HIV) and neonates with congenital syphilis.

ETIOLOGY: *T pallidum* is a thin, motile spirochete that is extremely fastidious, surviving only briefly outside the host. The organism has not been cultivated successfully on artificial media.

EPIDEMIOLOGY: Syphilis, which is rare in much of the industrialized world, persists in the United States and in resource-limited countries. The incidence of acquired and congenital syphilis increased dramatically in the United States during the late 1980s and early 1990s but decreased subsequently, and in 2000, the incidence was the lowest since reporting began in 1941. Since 2001, however, the rate of primary and secondary syphilis has increased, primarily among men who have sex with men. Among women, the rate of primary and secondary syphilis has increased since 2005, with a concomitant increase in cases of congenital syphilis. Rates of infection remain disproportionately high in large urban areas and in the southern United States. In adults, syphilis is more common among people with human immunodeficiency virus (HIV) infection. Primary and secondary rates of syphilis are highest in black, non-Hispanic people and in males compared with females.

Congenital syphilis is contracted from an infected mother via transplacental transmission of *T pallidum* at any time during pregnancy or possibly at birth from contact with maternal lesions. Among women with untreated early syphilis, as many as 40% of pregnancies result in spontaneous abortion, stillbirth, or perinatal death. Infection can be transmitted to the fetus at any stage of maternal disease. The rate of transmission is 60% to 100% during primary and secondary syphilis and slowly decreases with later stages of maternal infection (approximately 40% with early latent infection and 8% with late latent infection). The World Health Organization estimates that 1 million pregnancies are affected by syphilis worldwide. Of these, 460 000 will result in stillbirth, hydrops fetalis, abortion, or perinatal death; 270 000 will result in an infant born preterm or with low birth weight; and 270 000 will result in an infant with stigmata of congenital syphilis.

Acquired syphilis almost always is contracted through direct sexual contact with ulcerative lesions of the skin or mucous membranes of infected people. Open, moist lesions of the primary or secondary stages are highly infectious. Relapses of secondary syphilis with infectious mucocutaneous lesions can occur up to 4 years after primary infection. Sexual abuse must be suspected in any young child with acquired syphilis. In most cases, identification of acquired syphilis in children must be reported to state child protective services agencies. Physical examination for signs of sexual abuse and forensic interviews may be conducted under the auspices of a pediatrician with expertise in child abuse or at a local child advocacy center.

The **incubation period** for acquired primary syphilis typically is 3 weeks but ranges from 10 to 90 days.

DIAGNOSTIC TESTS: Definitive diagnosis is made when spirochetes are identified by microscopic darkfield examination or direct fluorescent antibody (DFA) tests of lesion exudate, nasal discharge, or tissue, such as placenta, umbilical cord, or autopsy specimens. Specimens should be scraped from moist mucocutaneous lesions or aspirated from a regional lymph node. Specimens from mouth lesions best are examined by DFA techniques to distinguish *T pallidum* from nonpathogenic treponemes that may be seen on darkfield microscopy. Although such testing can provide definitive diagnosis, in most instances, serologic testing is necessary. Polymerase chain reaction tests and immunoglobulin (Ig) M immunoblotting have been developed but are not yet available commercially.

Presumptive diagnosis is possible using nontreponemal and treponemal serologic tests. Use of only 1 type of test is insufficient for diagnosis, because false-positive nontreponemal test results occur with various medical conditions, and treponemal test results remain positive long after syphilis has been treated adequately and can be falsely positive with other spirochetal diseases.

Standard nontreponemal tests for syphilis include the Venereal Disease Research Laboratory (VDRL) slide test and the rapid plasma reagin (RPR) test. These tests measure antibody directed against lipoidal antigen from *T pallidum,* antibody interaction with host tissues, or both. These tests are inexpensive and performed rapidly and provide semiquantitative results. Quantitative results help define disease activity and monitor response to therapy. Nontreponemal test results (eg, VDRL or RPR) may be falsely negative (ie, nonreactive) with early primary syphilis, latent acquired syphilis of long duration, and late congenital syphilis. Occasionally, a nontreponemal test performed on serum samples containing high concentrations of antibody against *T pallidum* will be weakly reactive or falsely negative, a reaction termed the *prozone* phenomenon. Diluting serum results in a positive test. When nontreponemal tests are used to monitor treatment response, the same specific test (eg, VDRL or RPR) must be used throughout the follow-up period, preferably performed by the same laboratory, to ensure comparability of results.

A reactive nontreponemal test result from a patient with typical lesions indicates a presumptive diagnosis of syphilis and the need for treatment. However, any reactive nontreponemal test result must be confirmed by one of the specific treponemal tests to exclude a false-positive test result. False-positive results can be caused by certain viral infections (eg, Epstein Barr virus infection, hepatitis, varicella, and measles), lymphoma, tuberculosis, malaria, endocarditis, connective tissue disease, pregnancy, abuse of injection drugs, laboratory or technical error, or Wharton jelly contamination when umbilical cord blood specimens are used. Treatment should not be delayed while awaiting the results of the treponemal test results if the patient is symptomatic or at high risk of infection. A sustained fourfold decrease in titer, equivalent to a change of 2 dilutions (eg, from 1:32 to 1:8), of the nontreponemal test result after treatment usually demonstrates adequate therapy, whereas a sustained fourfold increase in titer from 1:8 to 1:32 after treatment suggests reinfection or relapse. The nontreponemal test titer usually decreases fourfold within 6 to 12 months after therapy for primary or secondary syphilis and usually becomes nonreactive within 1 year after successful therapy if the infection (primary or secondary syphilis) was treated early. The patient usually becomes seronegative within

2 years even if the initial titer was high or the infection was congenital. Some people will continue to have low stable nontreponemal antibody titers despite effective therapy. This serofast state is more common in patients treated for latent or tertiary syphilis.

Treponemal tests in use include fluorescent treponemal antibody absorption (FTA-ABS), Microhemagglutination test for antibodies to *T pallidum* (MHA-TP), *T pallidum* enzyme immunoassay (TP-EIA), and *T pallidum* particle agglutination (TP-PA) tests. People who have reactive treponemal test results usually remain reactive for life, even after successful therapy. However, 15% to 25% of patients treated during the primary stage revert to being serologically nonreactive after 2 to 3 years. Treponemal test antibody titers correlate poorly with disease activity and should not be used to assess response to therapy.

Treponemal tests also are not 100% specific for syphilis; positive reactions occur variably in patients with other spirochetal diseases, such as yaws, pinta, leptospirosis, rat-bite fever, relapsing fever, and Lyme disease. Nontreponemal tests can be used to differentiate Lyme disease from syphilis, because the VDRL test is nonreactive in Lyme disease.

The Centers for Disease Control and Prevention (CDC) recommends syphilis serologic screening with a nontreponemal test, such as the RPR or VDRL test, to identify people with possible untreated infection; this screening is followed by confirmation using one of several treponemal tests. Some clinical laboratories and blood banks have begun to screen samples using treponemal enzyme immunoassay (EIA) tests, rather than beginning with a nontreponemal test; the reasons for this change in sequence of the screening relates to cost and manpower issues. However, this "reverse sequence screening" approach is associated with high rates of false-positive results, and in 2011, the CDC reaffirmed its longstanding recommendation that nontreponemal tests be used to screen for syphilis and that treponemal testing be used to confirm syphilis as the cause of nontreponemal reactivity.[1] The traditional algorithm performs well in identifying people with active infection who require further evaluation and treatment while minimizing false-positive results in low prevalence populations.

In summary, nontreponemal antibody tests (VDRL and RPR) are used for screening, and treponemal tests (FTA-ABS, MHA-TP, TP-EIA, and TP-PA) are used to establish a presumptive diagnosis. Quantitative nontreponemal antibody tests are useful in assessing the adequacy of therapy and in detecting reinfection. All patients who have syphilis should be tested for HIV infection.

Cerebrospinal Fluid Tests. For evaluation of possible neurosyphilis, the VDRL test should be performed on cerebrospinal fluid (CSF). The CSF VDRL is highly specific but is insensitive. In addition, evaluation of CSF protein and white blood cell count is used to assess the likelihood of CNS involvement. The CSF leukocyte count usually is elevated in neurosyphilis (greater than 5 white blood cells [WBCs]/mm^3). Although the FTA-ABS test of CSF is less specific than the VDRL test, some experts recommend using the FTA-ABS test, believing it to be more sensitive than the VDRL test. Results from the VDRL test should be interpreted cautiously, because a negative result on a VDRL test of CSF does not exclude a diagnosis of neurosyphilis. Alternatively, a reactive VDRL test in the CSF of neonates can be the result of nontreponemal IgG antibodies that cross the blood-brain barrier. Fewer data exist for the TP-PA test for CSF, and none exist for the RPR test; these tests should not be used for CSF evaluation.

---

[1] Centers for Disease Control. Discordant results from reverse sequence syphilis screening—five laboratories, United States, 2006–2010. *MMWR Morb Mortal Wkly Rep.* 2011;60(5):133–137

Testing During Pregnancy. All women should be screened serologically for syphilis early in pregnancy with a nontreponemal test (eg, RPR or VDRL) and preferably again at delivery.[1] In areas of high prevalence of syphilis and in patients considered at high risk of syphilis, a nontreponemal serum test at the beginning of the third trimester (28 weeks of gestation) and at delivery is indicated. For women treated during pregnancy, follow-up serologic testing is necessary to assess the efficacy of therapy. Low-titer false-positive non-treponemal antibody test results occasionally occur in pregnancy. The result of a positive nontreponemal antibody test should be confirmed with a treponemal antibody test (eg, FTA-ABS, MHA-TP, TP-EIA, or TP-PA). When a pregnant woman has a reactive non-treponemal test result and a persistently negative treponemal test result, a false-positive test result is confirmed. As noted previously, some laboratories are screening pregnant women using an EIA treponemal test, but this reverse sequence screening approach is not recommended. Pregnant women with reactive treponemal EIA screening tests should have confirmatory testing with a nontreponemal test; subsequent evaluation and possible treatment of the infant should follow the infant's RPR or VDRL result, as outlined in Fig 3.7. Any woman who delivers a stillborn infant after 20 weeks' gestation should be tested for syphilis.

Evaluation of Infants for Congenital Infection During the First Month of Age. No newborn infant should be discharged from the hospital without determination of the mother's serologic status for syphilis at least once during pregnancy and also at delivery in communities and populations in which the risk of congenital syphilis is high. Testing of umbilical cord blood or an infant serum sample is inadequate for screening, because these can be nonreactive if the mother's serologic test result is of low titer or if she was infected late in pregnancy. All infants born to seropositive mothers require a careful examination and a nontreponemal syphilis test. The test performed on the infant should be the same as that performed on the mother to enable comparison of titer results. A negative maternal RPR or VDRL test result at delivery does not rule out the possibility of the infant having congenital syphilis, although such a situation is rare. The diagnostic and therapeutic approach to infants being evaluated for congenital syphilis is summarized in Fig 3.7 (p 695) and depends on: (1) identification of maternal syphilis; (2) adequacy of maternal therapy; (3) maternal response to therapy; (4) comparison of maternal and infant serologic titers; and (5) evaluation of results of the infant's nontreponemal serologic test, physical examination, ophthalmologic examination, long-bone and chest radiography, and laboratory tests (liver function tests; complete blood cell [CBC] and platelet counts; and CSF cell count, protein, and quantitative VDRL). Infants born to mothers who are coinfected with syphilis and HIV do not require different evaluation, therapy, or follow-up for syphilis than is recommended for all infants.

Evaluation and Treatment of Older Infants and Children. Children who are identified as having reactive serologic tests for syphilis after the neonatal period (ie, 1 month of age and older) should have maternal serologic test results and records reviewed to assess whether they have congenital or acquired syphilis. The recommended evaluation includes: (1) CSF analysis for VDRL testing, cell count, and protein concentration; (2) CBC, differential, and platelet counts; and (3) other tests as indicated clinically (eg, long-bone

[1] Wolff T, Shelton E, Sessions C, Miller T. Screening for syphilis infection in pregnant women: evidence for the US Preventive Services Task Force reaffirmation recommendation statement. *Ann Intern Med.* 2009;150(10):710–716

FIGURE 3.7. ALGORITHM FOR EVALUATION AND TREATMENT OF INFANTS BORN TO MOTHERS WITH REACTIVE SEROLOGIC TESTS FOR SYPHILIS.

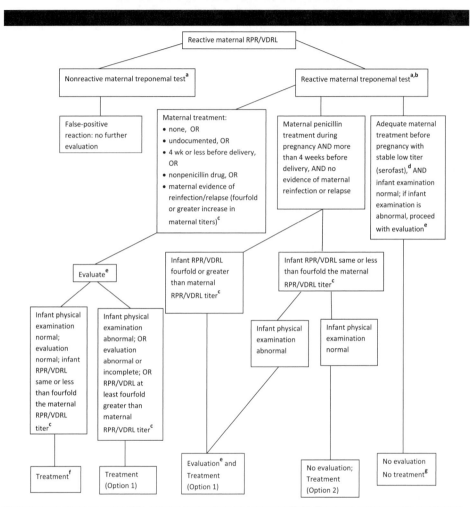

RPR indicates rapid plasma reagin; VDRL, Venereal Disease Research Laboratory; TP-PA, *Treponema pallidum* particle agglutination; FTA-ABS, fluorescent treponemal antibody absorption; TP-EIA, T pallidum enzyme immunoassay; MHA-TP, Microhemagglutination test for antibodies to *T pallidum.*

[a] TP-PA, FTA-ABS, TP-EIA, or MHA-TP.

[b] Test for human immunodeficiency virus (HIV) antibody. Infants of HIV-infected mothers do not require different evaluation or treatment.

[c] A fourfold change in titer is the same as a change of 2 dilutions. For example, a titer of 1:64 is fourfold greater than a titer of 1:16, and a titer of 1:4 is fourfold lower than a titer of 1:16.

[d] Women who maintain a VDRL titer 1:2 or less or an RPR 1:4 or less beyond 1 year after successful treatment are considered serofast.

[e] Complete blood cell (CBC) and platelet count; cerebrospinal fluid (CSF) examination for cell count, protein, and quantitative VDRL; other tests as clinically indicated (eg, chest radiographs, long-bone radiographs, eye examination, liver function tests, neuroimaging, and auditory brainstem response).

[f] Treatment (Option 1 or Option 2, below), with many experts recommending Treatment Option 1. If a single dose of benzathine penicillin G is used, then the infant must be fully evaluated, full evaluation must be normal, and follow-up must be certain. If any part of the infant's evaluation is abnormal or not performed, or if the CSF analysis is rendered uninterpretable, then a 10-day course of penicillin is required.

[g] Some experts would consider a single intramuscular injection of benzathine penicillin (Treatment Option 2), particularly if follow-up is not certain.

Treatment Options:

(1) Aqueous penicillin G, 50 000 U/kg, intravenously, every 12 hours (1 week of age or younger) or every 8 hours (older than 1 week); or procaine penicillin G, 50 000 U/kg, intramuscularly, as a single daily dose for 10 days. If 24 or more hours of therapy is missed, the entire course must be restarted.

(2) Benzathine penicillin G, 50 000 U/kg, intramuscularly, single dose.

or chest radiography, liver function tests, abdominal ultrasonography, ophthalmologic examination, auditory brain stem response testing, and neuroimaging studies).

Cerebrospinal Fluid Testing. Guidance for examination of CSF in the evaluation for possible congenital syphilis is provided under Evaluation of Newborn Infants for Congenital Infection During the First Month of Age (p 694). CSF test results obtained during the neonatal period can be difficult to interpret; normal values differ by gestational age and are higher in preterm infants. Values as high as 18 WBCs/mm³ and/or protein up to 130 mg/dL might occur among normal term neonates; some specialists, however, recommend that lower values (ie, 5 WBCs/mm³ and protein of 40 mg/dL) be considered the upper limits of normal when assessing a term infant for congenital syphilis. Other causes of elevated values should be considered when an infant is being evaluated for congenital syphilis.

CSF should be examined in all patients with neurologic or ophthalmic signs or symptoms, evidence of active tertiary syphilis (eg, aortitis and gumma), treatment failure, or HIV infection with late latent syphilis or syphilis of unknown duration. Abnormalities in CSF in patients with neurosyphilis include increased protein concentration, increased WBC count, and/or a reactive VDRL test result. Some experts also recommend performing the FTA-ABS test on CSF, believing it to be more sensitive but less specific than VDRL testing of CSF for neurosyphilis.

TREATMENT[1]: Parenteral penicillin G remains the preferred drug for treatment of syphilis at any stage. Recommendations for penicillin G use and duration of therapy vary, depending on the stage of disease and clinical manifestations. Parenteral penicillin G is the only documented effective therapy for patients who have neurosyphilis, congenital syphilis, or syphilis during pregnancy and is recommended for HIV-infected patients. Such patients always should be treated with penicillin, even if desensitization for penicillin allergy is necessary.

Penicillin Allergy. Skin testing for penicillin hypersensitivity with the major and minor determinants reliably can identify people at high risk of reacting to penicillin, although only the major determinant (benzylpenicilloyl poly-L-lysine [Pre-Pen]) and penicillin G skin tests have been available commercially. Skin testing without the minor determinant misses 3% to 10% of allergic patients who are at risk of serious or fatal reactions. Thus, a cautious approach to penicillin therapy is advised when a patient cannot be tested with all of the penicillin skin test reagents. If the major determinant is not available for skin testing, all patients with IgE-mediated reactions to penicillin should be desensitized in a hospital setting. In patients with non-IgE–mediated reactions, outpatient oral desensitization or monitored test doses may be considered. An oral or intravenous desensitization protocol for patients with a positive skin test result is available and should be performed in a hospital setting.[2] Oral desensitization is regarded as safer and easier to perform. Desensitization usually can be completed in approximately 4 hours, after which the first dose of penicillin can be given.

[1] Centers for Disease Control and Prevention. Sexually transmitted infection treatment guidelines—United States, 2010. *MMWR Recomm Rep.* 2010;59(RR–12):1–110

[2] Wolff T, Shelton E, Sessions C, Miller T. Screening for syphilis infection in pregnant women: evidence for the US Preventive Services Task Force reaffirmation recommendation statement. *Ann Intern Med.* 2009;150(10):710–716

Congenital Syphilis: Infants in the First Month of Age. The diagnostic and therapeutic approach to neonates delivered to mothers with syphilis is outlined in Fig 3.7 (p 695). Management decisions are based on the 3 possible maternal situations: (1) maternal treatment before pregnancy; (2) adequate maternal treatment and response during pregnancy; or (3) inadequate maternal treatment or inadequate maternal response to treatment (or reinfection) during pregnancy.

For proven or probable congenital syphilis (based on the neonate's physical examination and radiographic and laboratory testing), the preferred treatment is aqueous crystalline penicillin G, administered intravenously. The dosage should be based on chronologic age rather than gestational age and is 50 000 U/kg, intravenously, every 12 hours (1 week of age or younger) or every 8 hours (older than 1 week). Alternatively, procaine penicillin G, 50 000 U/kg, intramuscularly, can be administered as a single daily dose for 10 days; no treatment failures have occurred with this formulation despite its low CSF concentrations. When the neonate is at risk of congenital syphilis because of inadequate maternal treatment or response to treatment (or reinfection) during pregnancy but the neonate's physical examination, radiographic imaging, and laboratory analyses are normal (including infant RPR/VDRL either the same as or less than fourfold the maternal RPR/VDRL), some experts would treat with a single dose of penicillin G benzathine (50 000 U/kg intramuscularly), but most still would prefer 10 days of treatment. If more than 1 day of therapy is missed, the entire course should be restarted. Data supporting use of other antimicrobial agents (eg, ampicillin) for treatment of congenital syphilis are not available. When possible, a full 10-day course of penicillin is preferred, even if ampicillin initially was provided for possible sepsis. Use of agents other than penicillin requires close serologic follow-up to assess adequacy of therapy.

Infants who have a normal physical examination and a serum quantitative nontreponemal serologic titer either the same as or less than fourfold (eg, 1:4 is fourfold lower than 1:16) the maternal titer are at minimal risk of syphilis if (1) they are born to mothers who completed appropriate penicillin treatment for syphilis during pregnancy and more than 4 weeks before delivery; and (2) the mother had no evidence of reinfection or relapse. Although a full evaluation may be unnecessary, these infants should be treated with a single intramuscular injection of penicillin G benzathine, because fetal treatment failure can occur despite adequate maternal treatment during pregnancy. Alternatively, these infants may be examined carefully, preferably monthly, until their nontreponemal serologic test results are negative.

Infants who have a normal physical examination and a serum quantitative nontreponemal serologic titer either the same as or less than fourfold (eg, 1:4 is fourfold lower than 1:16) the maternal titer and (1) whose mother's treatment was adequate before pregnancy; and (2) whose mother's nontreponemal serologic titer remained low and stable before and during pregnancy and at delivery (VDRL less than 1:2; RPR less than 1:4) require no evaluation. Some experts, however, would treat with penicillin G benzathine as a single intramuscular injection if follow-up is uncertain.

Congenital Syphilis: Older Infants and Children. Because establishing the diagnosis of neurosyphilis is difficult, infants older than 1 month of age who possibly have congenital syphilis or who have neurologic involvement should be treated with intravenous aqueous crystalline penicillin for 10 days (see Table 3.72, p 698). This regimen also should be used to treat children older than 2 years of age who have late and previously untreated congenital syphilis. Some experts suggest giving such patients a single dose of penicillin

Table 3.72. Recommended Treatment for Syphilis in People Older Than 1 Month of Age

Status	Children	Adults
Congenital syphilis	Aqueous crystalline penicillin G, 200 000–300 000 U/kg/day, IV, administered as 50 000 U/kg, every 4–6 h for 10 days[a]	
Primary, secondary, and early latent syphilis[b]	Penicillin G benzathine,[c] 50 000 U/kg, IM, up to the adult dose of 2.4 million U in a single dose	Penicillin G benzathine, 2.4 million U, IM, in a single dose **OR** *If allergic to penicillin and not pregnant,* Doxycycline, 100 mg, orally, twice a day for 14 days **OR** Tetracycline, 500 mg, orally, 4 times/day for 14 days
Late latent syphilis[d] or latent syphilis of unknown duration	Penicillin G benzathine, 50 000 U/kg, IM, up to the adult dose of 2.4 million U, administered as 3 single doses at 1-wk intervals (total 150 000 U/kg, up to the adult dose of 7.2 million U)	Penicillin G benzathine, 7.2 million U total, administered as 3 doses of 2.4 million U, IM, each at 1-wk intervals **OR** *If allergic to penicillin and not pregnant,* Doxycycline, 100 mg, orally, twice a day for 4 wk **OR** Tetracycline, 500 mg, orally, 4 times/day for 4 wk
Tertiary	…	Penicillin G benzathine 7.2 million U total, administered as 3 doses of 2.4 million U, IM, at 1-wk intervals *If allergic to penicillin and not pregnant, same as for late latent syphilis*
Neurosyphilis[e]	Aqueous crystalline penicillin G, 200 000–300 000 U/kg/day, IV, every 4–6 h for 10–14 days, in doses not to exceed the adult dose	Aqueous crystalline penicillin G, 18–24 million U per day, administered as 3–4 million U, IV, every 4 h for 10–14 days[f] **OR** Penicillin G procaine,[c] 2.4 million U, IM, once daily **PLUS** probenecid, 500 mg, orally, 4 times/day, both for 10–14 days[f]

IV indicates intravenously; IM, intramuscularly.

[a] If the patient has no clinical manifestations of disease, the cerebrospinal fluid (CSF) examination is normal, and the CSF Venereal Disease Research Laboratory (VDRL) test result is negative, some experts would treat with up to 3 weekly doses of penicillin G benzathine, 50 000 U/kg, IM. Some experts also suggest giving these patients a single dose of penicillin G benzathine, 50 000 U/kg, IM, after the 10-day course of intravenous aqueous penicillin.

[b] Early latent syphilis is defined as being acquired within the preceding year.

[c] Penicillin G benzathine and penicillin G procaine are approved for intramuscular administration only.

[d] Late latent syphilis is defined as syphilis beyond 1 year's duration.

[e] Patients who are allergic to penicillin should be desensitized.

[f] Some experts administer penicillin G benzathine, 2.4 million U, IM, once per week for up to 3 weeks after completion of these neurosyphilis treatment regimens.

G benzathine, 50 000 U/kg, intramuscularly, after the 10-day course of intravenous aqueous crystalline penicillin. If the patient has no clinical manifestations of disease, the CSF examination is normal, and the result of the VDRL test of CSF is negative, some experts would treat with 3 weekly doses of penicillin G benzathine (50 000 U/kg, intramuscularly).

Syphilis in Pregnancy. Regardless of stage of pregnancy, women should be treated with penicillin according to the dosage schedules appropriate for the stage of syphilis as recommended for nonpregnant patients (see Table 3.72, p 698). For penicillin-allergic patients, no proven alternative therapy has been established. A pregnant woman with a history of penicillin allergy should be treated with penicillin after desensitization. Desensitization should be performed in consultation with a specialist and only in facilities in which emergency assistance is available (see Penicillin Allergy, p 696).

Erythromycin, azithromycin, or any other nonpenicillin treatment of syphilis during pregnancy cannot be considered reliable to cure infection in the fetus. Tetracycline is not recommended for pregnant women because of potential adverse effects on the fetus.

Early Acquired Syphilis (Primary, Secondary, Early Latent Syphilis). A single intramuscular dose of penicillin G benzathine is the preferred treatment for children and adults (see Table 3.72, p 698). All children should have a CSF examination before treatment to exclude a diagnosis of neurosyphilis. Evaluation of CSF in adolescents and adults is necessary only if clinical signs or symptoms of neurologic or ophthalmic involvement are present. Neurosyphilis should be considered in the differential diagnosis of neurologic disease in HIV-infected people.

For nonpregnant patients who are allergic to penicillin, doxycycline or tetracycline should be given for 14 days. Children younger than 8 years of age should not be given tetracycline or doxycycline unless the benefits of therapy are greater than the risks of dental staining (see Tetracyclines, p 801). Clinical studies, along with biologic and pharmacologic considerations, suggest ceftriaxone should be effective for early-acquired syphilis. The recommended dose and duration of ceftriaxone therapy are 1 g, once daily, either intramuscularly or intravenously for 10 to 14 days (for adolescents and adults). Because efficacy of ceftriaxone is not well documented, close follow-up is essential. Single-dose therapy with ceftriaxone is not effective. Preliminary data suggest that azithromycin might be effective as a single oral dose of 2 g. However, several cases of azithromycin treatment failures have been reported, and resistance to azithromycin has been documented in several geographic areas. When follow-up cannot be ensured, especially for children younger than 8 years of age, consideration must be given to hospitalization and desensitization followed by administration of penicillin G (see Penicillin Allergy, p 696).

Syphilis of More Than 1 Year's Duration (Late Latent Syphilis, Except Neurosyphilis) or of Unknown Duration. Penicillin G benzathine should be given intramuscularly, weekly for 3 successive weeks (see Table 3.72, p 698). In patients who are allergic to penicillin, doxycycline or tetracycline for 4 weeks should be given only with close serologic and clinical follow-up. Limited clinical studies suggest that ceftriaxone might be effective, but the optimal dose and duration have not been defined. Patients who have syphilis and who demonstrate any of the following criteria should have a prompt CSF examination:
1. Neurologic or ophthalmic signs or symptoms;
2. Evidence of active tertiary syphilis (eg, aortitis, gumma, iritis, uveitis);
3. Treatment failure; or
4. HIV infection with late latent syphilis or syphilis of unknown duration.

If dictated by circumstances and patient or parent preferences, a CSF examination may be performed for patients who do not meet these criteria. Some experts recommend performing a CSF examination on all patients who have latent syphilis and a nontreponemal serologic test result of 1:32 or greater or if the patient is HIV infected and has a serum CD4+ T-lymphocyte count 350 or less. The risk of asymptomatic neurosyphilis in these circumstances is increased approximately threefold. If a CSF examination is performed and the results indicate abnormalities consistent with neurosyphilis, the patient should be treated for neurosyphilis (see Neurosyphilis). Children younger than 8 years of age should not be given tetracycline or doxycycline unless the benefits of therapy are greater than the risks of dental staining (see Tetracyclines, p 801).

Neurosyphilis. The recommended regimen for adults is aqueous crystalline penicillin G, intravenously, for 10 to 14 days (see Table 3.72, p 698). If adherence to therapy can be ensured, patients may be treated with an alternative regimen of daily intramuscular penicillin G procaine plus oral probenecid for 10 to 14 days. Some experts recommend following both of these regimens with penicillin G benzathine, 2.4 million U, intramuscularly, weekly, for 1 to 3 doses. For children, intravenous aqueous crystalline penicillin G for 10 to 14 days is recommended, and some experts recommend additional therapy with intramuscular penicillin G benzathine, 50 000 U/kg per dose (not to exceed 2.4 million U), for up to 3 single weekly doses.

If the patient has a history of allergy to penicillin, consideration should be given to desensitization, and the patient should be managed in consultation with an allergy specialist (see Penicillin Allergy, p 696).

Other Considerations.

- Mothers of infants with congenital syphilis should be tested for other sexually transmitted infections (STIs), including *Neisseria gonorrhoeae, Chlamydia trachomatis*, HIV, and hepatitis B infections. If injection drug use is suspected, the mother also may be at risk of hepatitis C virus infection.
- All recent sexual contacts of people with acquired syphilis should be evaluated for other STIs as well as syphilis (see Control Measures, p 702). Partners who were exposed within 90 days preceding the diagnosis of primary, secondary, or early latent syphilis in the index patient should be treated presumptively for syphilis, even if they are seronegative.
- All patients with syphilis should be tested for other STIs, including HIV, and hepatitis B infection. Patients who have primary syphilis should be retested for HIV after 3 months if the first HIV test result is negative.
- For HIV-infected patients with syphilis, careful follow-up is essential. Patients infected with HIV who have early syphilis may be at increased risk of neurologic complications and higher rates of treatment failure with currently recommended regimens.
- Children with acquired primary, secondary, or latent syphilis should be evaluated for possible sexual assault or abuse.

Follow-up and Management.

Congenital syphilis. All infants who have reactive serologic tests for syphilis or were born to mothers who were seroreactive at delivery should receive careful follow-up evaluations during regularly scheduled well-child care visits at 2, 4, 6, and 12 months of age. Serologic nontreponemal tests should be performed every 2 to 3 months until the nontreponemal test becomes nonreactive or the titer has decreased at least fourfold (eg, 1:16 to 1:4). Nontreponemal antibody titers should decrease by 3 months of age and should be nonreactive by 6 months of age if the infant was infected and adequately treated or was not infected and initially seropositive because of transplacentally acquired maternal antibody. The serologic response after therapy may be slower for infants treated after the neonatal period. Patients with increasing titers or with persistent stable titers 6 to 12 months after initial treatment should be reevaluated, including a CSF examination, and treated with a 10-day course of parenteral penicillin G, even if they were treated previously.

Treponemal tests should not be used to evaluate treatment response, because results for an infected child can remain positive despite effective therapy. Passively transferred maternal treponemal antibodies can persist in an infant until 15 months of age. A reactive treponemal test after 18 months of age is diagnostic of congenital syphilis. If the nontreponemal test is nonreactive at this time, no further evaluation or treatment is necessary. If the nontreponemal test is reactive at 18 months of age, the infant should be evaluated (or reevaluated) fully and treated for congenital syphilis.

Treated infants with congenital neurosyphilis and initially positive results of VDRL tests of CSF or abnormal CSF cell counts and/or protein concentrations should undergo repeated clinical evaluation and CSF examination at 6-month intervals until their CSF examination is normal. A reactive result of VDRL testing of CSF at the 6-month interval is an indication for retreatment. Abnormal CSF indices that cannot be attributed to another ongoing illness also require retreatment. Neuroimaging studies, such as magnetic resonance imaging, should be considered in these children.

Acquired syphilis. Treated pregnant women with syphilis should have quantitative nontreponemal serologic tests repeated at 28 to 32 weeks of gestation, at delivery, and according to the recommendations for the stage of disease. Serologic titers may be repeated monthly in women at high risk of reinfection or in geographic areas where the prevalence of syphilis is high. The clinical and antibody response should be appropriate for stage of disease. Most women will deliver before their serologic response to treatment can be assessed definitively. Therapy should be judged inadequate if the maternal antibody titer has not decreased fourfold by delivery. Inadequate maternal treatment is likely if clinical signs of infection are present at delivery or if maternal antibody titer is fourfold higher than the pretreatment titer. Fetal treatment is considered inadequate if delivery occurs within 28 days of maternal therapy.

Indications for Retreatment.

Primary/secondary syphilis:
- If clinical signs or symptoms persist or recur or if a fourfold increase in titer of a nontreponemal test occurs, evaluate CSF and HIV status and repeat therapy.
- If the nontreponemal titer fails to decrease fourfold within 6 months after therapy, evaluate for HIV; repeat therapy unless follow-up for continued clinical and serologic assessment can be ensured. Some experts recommend CSF evaluation.

Latent syphilis: In the following situations, CSF examination should be performed and retreatment should be provided:

- Titers increase at least fourfold (eg, 1:4 to 1:16);
- An initially high titer (greater than 1:32) fails to decrease at least fourfold (eg, 1:32 to 1:8) within 12 to 24 months; or
- Signs or symptoms attributable to syphilis develop.

In all these instances, retreatment, when indicated, should be performed with 3 weekly injections of penicillin G benzathine, 2.4 million U, intramuscularly, unless CSF examination indicates that neurosyphilis is present, at which time treatment for neurosyphilis should be initiated. Retreated patients should be treated with the schedules recommended for patients with syphilis for more than 1 year. In general, only 1 retreatment course is indicated. The possibility of reinfection or concurrent HIV infection always should be considered when retreating patients with early syphilis, and repeat HIV testing should be performed in such cases.

Patients with neurosyphilis must have periodic serologic testing, clinical evaluation at 6-month intervals, and repeat CSF examinations. If the CSF cell count has not decreased after 6 months or CSF is not entirely normal after 2 years, retreatment should be considered. CSF abnormalities may persist for extended periods of time in HIV-infected people with neurosyphilis. Close follow-up is warranted.

ISOLATION OF THE HOSPITALIZED PATIENT: Standard precautions are recommended for all patients, including infants with suspected or proven congenital syphilis. Because moist open lesions, secretions, and possibly blood are contagious in all patients with syphilis, gloves should be worn when caring for patients with congenital, primary, and secondary syphilis with skin and mucous membrane lesions until 24 hours of treatment has been completed.

CONTROL MEASURES:

- All women should be screened for syphilis early in pregnancy. For communities and populations in which the prevalence of syphilis is high or for patients at high risk, serologic testing also should be performed at 28 to 32 weeks of gestation and at delivery. No newborn infant should leave the hospital without the maternal serologic status having been determined at least once during the pregnancy.
- Education of patients and populations about STIs, treatment of sexual contacts, reporting of each case to local public health authorities for contact investigation and appropriate follow-up, and serologic screening of high-risk populations are indicated.
- All recent sexual contacts of a person with acquired syphilis should be identified, examined, serologically tested, and treated appropriately. Sexual contacts of people with primary, secondary, or early latent syphilis who were exposed within the preceding 90 days may be infected even if seronegative and should be treated for early-acquired syphilis. People exposed more than 90 days previously should be treated presumptively if serologic test results are not available immediately and follow-up is uncertain. For identification of at-risk sexual partners, the periods before treatment are as follows: (1) 3 months plus duration of symptoms for primary syphilis; (2) 6 months plus duration of symptoms for secondary syphilis; and (3) 1 year for early latent syphilis. Recommendations for partner service programs provided to partners of people with syphilis are available.[1]

---

[1] Centers for Disease Control and Prevention. Recommendations for partner service programs for HIV infection, syphilis, gonorrhea, and chlamydial infection. *MMWR Recomm Rep.* 2008;57(RR-9):1–83

- All people, including hospital personnel, who have had close unprotected contact with a patient with early congenital syphilis before identification of the disease or during the first 24 hours of therapy should be examined clinically for the presence of lesions 2 to 3 weeks after contact. Serologic testing should be performed and repeated 3 months after contact or sooner if symptoms occur. If the degree of exposure is considered substantial, immediate treatment should be considered.

Tapeworm Diseases
(Taeniasis and Cysticercosis)

CLINICAL MANIFESTATIONS:

Taeniasis. Infection often is asymptomatic; however, mild gastrointestinal tract symptoms, such as nausea, diarrhea, and pain, can occur. Tapeworm segments can be seen migrating from the anus or in feces.

Cysticercosis. Manifestations depend on the location and number of pork tapeworm larval cysts (cysticerci) and the host response. Cysticerci may be found anywhere in the body. The most common and serious manifestations are caused by cysticerci in the central nervous system. Larval cysts of *Taenia solium* in the brain (neurocysticercosis) can cause seizures, behavioral disturbances, obstructive hydrocephalus, and other neurologic signs and symptoms. In some countries, including parts of the southwest United States, neurocysticercosis is a leading cause of epilepsy. The host reaction to degenerating cysticerci can produce signs and symptoms of meningitis. Cysts in the spinal column can cause gait disturbance, pain, or transverse myelitis. Subcutaneous cysticerci produce palpable nodules, and ocular involvement can cause visual impairment.

ETIOLOGY: Taeniasis is caused by intestinal infection by the adult tapeworm, *Taenia saginata* (beef tapeworm) or *T solium* (pork tapeworm). *Taenia asiatica* causes taeniasis in Asia. Human cysticercosis is caused only by the larvae of *T solium (Cysticercus cellulosae)*.

EPIDEMIOLOGY: These tapeworm diseases have worldwide distribution. Prevalence is high in areas with poor sanitation and human fecal contamination in areas where cattle graze or swine are fed. Most cases of *T solium* infection in the United States are imported from Latin America or Asia. High rates of *T saginata* infection occur in Mexico, parts of South America, East Africa, and central Europe. *T asiatica* is common in China, Taiwan, and Southeast Asia. Taeniasis is acquired by eating undercooked beef *(T saginata)* or pork *(T solium)*. *T asiatica* is acquired by eating viscera of infected pigs that contain encysted larvae. Infection often is asymptomatic.

Cysticercosis in humans is acquired by ingesting eggs of the pork tapeworm *(T solium)*, through fecal-oral contact with a person harboring the adult tapeworm, or by autoinfection. Eggs are found only in human feces, because humans are the obligate definitive host. Eggs liberate oncospheres in the intestine that migrate through the blood and lymphatics to tissues throughout the body, including the central nervous system, the oncospheres develop into cysticerci. Although most cases of cysticercosis in the United States have been imported, cysticercosis can be acquired in the United States from tapeworm carriers who emigrated from an area with endemic infection and still have *T solium* intestinal stage infection.

The **incubation period** for taeniasis (the time from ingestion of the larvae until segments are passed in the feces) is 2 to 3 months. For cysticercosis, the time between infection and onset of symptoms may be several years.

DIAGNOSIS: Diagnosis of taeniasis (adult tapeworm infection) is based on demonstration of the proglottids or ova in feces or the perianal region. However, these techniques are insensitive. Species identification of the parasite is based on the different structures of gravid proglottids and scolex. Diagnosis of neurocysticercosis is made primarily on the basis of computed tomography (CT) scanning or magnetic resonance imaging (MRI) of the brain or spinal cord. Antibody assays that detect specific antibody to larval *T solium* in serum and cerebrospinal fluid (CSF) are the confirmatory tests of choice. In the United States, antibody tests are available through the Centers for Disease Control and Prevention and several commercial laboratories. In general, antibody tests are more sensitive with serum specimens than with CSF specimens. Serum antibody assay results often are negative in children with solitary parenchymal lesions but usually are positive in patients with multiple lesions.

TREATMENT:

Taeniasis. Praziquantel is highly effective for eradicating infection with the adult tapeworm, and niclosamide is an alternative (see Drugs for Parasitic Infections, p 848). Praziquantel is not approved for this indication, but dosing is provided for children older than 4 years of age for some other indications. Niclosamide is not approved for *T solium* but is approved for *T saginata*. However, niclosamide is not available commercially in the United States.

Cysticercosis. Neurocysticercosis treatment should be individualized on the basis of the number and viability of cysticerci as assessed by neuroimaging studies (MRI or CT scan) and where they are located. For patients with only a single nonviable cyst (eg, only calcifications on CT scan), management generally is aimed at symptoms and should include anticonvulsants for patients with seizures and insertion of shunts for patients with hydrocephalus. Two antiparasitic drugs—albendazole and praziquantel—are available. Praziquantel is not approved for this indication, but dosing is provided for children older than 4 years of age for some other indications. Although both drugs are cysticercidal and hasten radiologic resolution of cysts, most symptoms result from the host inflammatory response and may be exacerbated by treatment. In some clinical trials, patients treated with albendazole had better radiologic and clinical responses than patients treated with low doses of praziquantel. Several studies have indicated that patients with single inflamed cysts within brain parenchyma do well without antiparasitic therapy. Most experts recommend therapy with albendazole or praziquantel for patients with nonenhancing or multiple cysticerci. Albendazole is preferred over praziquantel, because it has fewer drug-drug interactions with anticonvulsants. Coadministration of corticosteroids for the first 2 to 3 days of therapy may decrease adverse effects if more extensive viable central nervous system cysticerci are suspected. Arachnoiditis, vasculitis, or diffuse cerebral edema (cysticercal encephalitis) is treated with corticosteroid therapy until cerebral edema is controlled and albendazole or praziquantel therapy is completed.

Seizures may recur for months or years. Anticonvulsant therapy is recommended until there is neuroradiologic evidence of resolution and seizures have not occurred for 1 to 2 years. Calcification of cysts may require prolonged or indefinite use of anticonvulsants. Intraventricular cysts and hydrocephalus usually require surgical therapy. Intraventricular cysticerci often can be removed by endoscopic surgery, which is the treatment of choice. If cysticerci cannot be removed easily, hydrocephalus should be corrected with placement of intraventricular shunts. Adjunctive chemotherapy with antiparasitic agents and corticosteroids may decrease the rate of subsequent shunt failure.

Ocular cysticercosis is treated by surgical excision of the cysticerci. Ocular and spinal cysticerci generally are not treated with anthelmintic drugs, which can exacerbate inflammation. An ophthalmic examination should be performed before treatment to rule out intraocular cysticerci.

ISOLATION OF THE HOSPITALIZED PATIENT: Standard precautions are recommended.

CONTROL MEASURES: Eating raw or undercooked beef or pork should be avoided. People known to harbor the adult tapeworm of *T solium* should be treated immediately. Careful attention to hand hygiene and appropriate disposal of fecal material is important.

Examination of stool specimens obtained from food handlers who recently have emigrated from countries with endemic infection for detection of eggs and proglottids is advisable. To prevent fecal-oral transmission of *T solium* eggs, people traveling to developing countries with high endemic rates of cysticercosis should avoid eating uncooked vegetables and fruits that cannot be peeled.

Other Tapeworm Infections
(Including Hydatid Disease)

Most infections are asymptomatic, but nausea, abdominal pain, and diarrhea have been observed in people who are heavily infected.

ETIOLOGIES, DIAGNOSIS, AND TREATMENT

Hymenolepis nana. This tapeworm, also called dwarf tapeworm because it is the smallest of the adult human tapeworms, can complete its entire cycle within humans. New infection may be acquired by ingestion of eggs passed in feces of infected people or of infected arthropods (fleas). More problematic is autoinfection, which tends to perpetuate infection in the host, because eggs can hatch within the intestine and reinitiate the cycle, leading to development of new worms and a large worm burden. Diagnosis is made by recognition of the characteristic eggs passed in stool. Praziquantel is the treatment of choice, with nitazoxanide as an alternative drug. If infection persists after treatment, retreatment with praziquantel is indicated. Nitazoxanide is an alternative drug. Praziquantel and nitazoxanide are not approved for this indication, but dosing guidelines are available for children 4 years of age and older (praziquantel) and 1 year of age and older (nitazoxanide) for other indications.

Dipylidium caninum. This tapeworm is the most common and widespread adult tapeworm of dogs and cats. *Dipylidium caninum* infects children when they inadvertently swallow a dog or cat flea, which serves as the intermediate host. Diagnosis is made by finding the characteristic eggs or motile proglottids in stool. Proglottids resemble rice kernels. Therapy with praziquantel is effective. Niclosamide is an alternative therapeutic option. Praziquantel and niclosamide are not approved for this indication, but dosing guidelines are available for children 4 years of age and older (praziquantel) and 2 years of age and older (niclosamide) for other indications.

Diphyllobothrium latum *(and related species).* The *Diphyllobothrium latum* tapeworm, also called fish tapeworm, has fish as one of its intermediate hosts. Consumption of infected, raw freshwater fish (including salmon) leads to infection. Three to 5 weeks are needed for the adult tapeworm to mature and begin to lay eggs. The worm sometimes causes mechanical obstruction of the bowel or diarrhea, abdominal pain, or rarely, megaloblastic anemia secondary to vitamin B_{12} deficiency. Diagnosis is made by recognition of the characteristic proglottids or eggs passed in stool. Therapy with praziquantel is effective;

niclosamide is an alternative. Praziquantel is not approved for this indication, but dosing is provided for children 4 years of age and older for other indications.

Echinococcus granulosus *and* Echinococcus multilocularis. The larval forms of these tapeworms are the causes of hydatid disease. The distribution of *Echinococcus granulosus* is related to sheep or cattle herding. Areas of high prevalence include parts of Central and South America, East Africa, Eastern Europe, the Middle East, the Mediterranean region, China, and Central Asia. The parasite also is endemic in Australia and New Zealand. In the United States, small foci of endemic transmission have been reported in Arizona, California, New Mexico, and Utah, and a strain adapted to wolves, moose, and caribou occurs in Alaska and Canada. Dogs, coyotes, wolves, dingoes, and jackals can become infected by swallowing protoscolices of the parasite within hydatid cysts in the organs of sheep or other intermediate hosts. Dogs pass embryonated eggs in their stools, and sheep become infected by swallowing the eggs. If humans swallow *Echinococcus* eggs, they can become inadvertent intermediate hosts, and cysts can develop in various organs, such as the liver, lungs, kidney, and spleen. These cysts usually grow slowly (1 cm in diameter per year) and eventually can contain several liters of fluid. If a cyst ruptures, anaphylaxis and multiple secondary cysts from seeding of protoscolices can result. Clinical diagnosis often is difficult. A history of contact with dogs in an area with endemic infection is helpful. Cystic lesions can be demonstrated by radiography, ultrasonography, or computed tomography of various organs. Serologic tests, available at the Centers for Disease Control and Prevention, are helpful, but false-negative results occur. In uncomplicated cases, treatment of choice is **p**uncture **a**spiration, **i**njection of protoscolicidal agents, and **r**easpiration (PAIR). Contraindications to PAIR include communication of the cyst with the biliary tract (eg, bile staining after initial aspiration), superficial cysts, and heavily septated cysts. Surgical therapy is indicated for complicated cases and requires meticulous care to prevent spillage, including preparations such as soaking of surgical drapes in hypertonic saline. In general, the cyst should be removed intact, because leakage of contents is associated with a higher rate of complications. Patients are at risk of anaphylactic reactions to cyst contents. Treatment with albendazole generally should be initiated days to weeks before surgery or PAIR and continued for several weeks to months afterward.

Echinococcus multilocularis, a species for which the life cycle involves foxes, dogs, and rodents, causes the alveolar form of hydatid disease, which is characterized by invasive growth of the larvae in the liver with occasional metastatic spread. The alveolar form of hydatid disease is limited to the northern hemisphere and usually is diagnosed in people 50 years of age or older. The preferred treatment is surgical removal of the entire larval mass. In nonresectable cases, continuous treatment with albendazole has been associated with clinical improvement.

ISOLATION OF THE HOSPITALIZED PATIENT: Standard precautions are recommended.

CONTROL MEASURES: Preventive measures for *H nana* include educating the public about personal hygiene and sanitary disposal of feces.

Infection with *D caninum* is prevented by keeping dogs and cats free of fleas and worms.

Thorough cooking to an internal temperature of 63°C [145°F], freezing (−35°C [-31°F]) until solid, or irradiation of freshwater fish ensures protection against *D latum*.

Control measures for prevention of *E granulosus* and *E multilocularis* include educating the public about hand hygiene and avoiding exposure to dog feces. Prevention and control of infection in dogs decreases the risk.

Tetanus
(Lockjaw)

CLINICAL MANIFESTATIONS: Tetanus is caused by neurotoxin produced by the anaerobic bacterium *Clostridium tetani* in a contaminated wound and can manifest in 1 of 4 clinical forms: generalized, local, neonatal, and cephalic.

Generalized tetanus (lockjaw) is a neurologic disease manifesting as trismus and severe muscular spasms, including risus sardonicus. Onset is gradual, occurring over 1 to 7 days, and symptoms progress to severe generalized muscle spasms, which often are aggravated by any external stimulus. Severe spasms persist for 1 week or more and subside over several weeks in people who recover.

Local tetanus manifests as local muscle spasms in areas contiguous to a wound. Localized tetanus most often progresses to generalized tetanus.

Neonatal tetanus is a form of generalized tetanus occurring in newborn infants lacking protective passive immunity because their mothers are not immune.

Cephalic tetanus is a dysfunction of cranial nerves associated with infected wounds on the head and neck. Cephalic tetanus can precede generalized tetanus.

ETIOLOGY: *C tetani* is a spore-forming, obligate anaerobic, gram-positive bacillus. This organism is a wound contaminant that causes neither tissue destruction nor an inflammatory response. The vegetative form of *C tetani* produces a potent plasmid-encoded exotoxin (tetanospasmin), which binds to gangliosides at the myoneural junction of skeletal muscle and on neuronal membranes in the spinal cord, blocking inhibitory impulses to motor neurons. The action of tetanus toxin on the brain and sympathetic nervous system is less well documented. *C tetani* also produces tetanolysin, a toxin with hemolytic and cytolytic properties; however, its effect on clinical presentation of tetanus has not been elucidated.

EPIDEMIOLOGY: Tetanus occurs worldwide and is more common in warmer climates and during warmer months, in part because of higher frequency of contaminated wounds associated with those locations and seasons. The organism, a normal inhabitant of soil and animal and human intestines, is ubiquitous in the environment, especially where contamination by excreta is common. Organisms multiply in wounds, recognized or unrecognized, and elaborate toxins in the presence of anaerobic conditions. Contaminated wounds, especially wounds with devitalized tissue and deep-puncture trauma, are at greatest risk. Neonatal tetanus is common in many developing countries where pregnant women are not immunized appropriately against tetanus and nonsterile umbilical cord-care practices are followed. Widespread active immunization against tetanus has modified the epidemiology of disease in the United States, where 40 or fewer cases have been reported annually since 1999. Tetanus is not transmissible from person to person.

The incubation period ranges from 3 to 21 days, with most cases occurring within 8 days. Shorter incubation periods have been associated with more heavily contaminated wounds, more severe disease, and a worse prognosis. In neonatal tetanus, symptoms usually appear from 4 to 14 days after birth, averaging 7 days.

DIAGNOSTIC TESTS: The diagnosis of tetanus is made clinically by excluding other causes of tetanic spasms, such as hypocalcemic tetany, phenothiazine reaction, strychnine poisoning, and conversion disorder. Attempts to culture *C tetani* are associated with poor yield, and a negative culture does not rule out disease. A protective serum antitoxin concentration should not be used to exclude the diagnosis of tetanus.

TREATMENT: Human Tetanus Immune Globulin (TIG), 3000 to 6000 U, given in a single dose, is recommended for treatment; however, the optimal therapeutic dose has not been established. Some experts recommend 500 U, which appears to be as effective as higher doses and causes less discomfort. Available preparations must be given intramuscularly. Infiltration of part of the dose locally around the wound is recommended, although the efficacy of this approach has not been proven. Results of studies on the benefit from intrathecal administration of TIG are conflicting. The TIG preparation in use in the United States is not licensed or formulated for intrathecal or intravenous use.

- In countries where TIG is not available, equine tetanus antitoxin may be available. This product no longer is available in the United States. Equine antitoxin is administered after appropriate testing for sensitivity and desensitization if necessary (see Sensitivity Tests for Reactions to Animal Sera, p 64, and Desensitization to Animal Sera, p 64).
- Immune Globulin Intravenous (IGIV) contains antibodies to tetanus and can be considered for treatment in a dose of 200 to 400 mg/kg if TIG is not available. The US Food and Drug Administration has not licensed IGIV for this use, and antitetanus antibody concentrations are not assessed routinely in IGIV.
- All wounds should be cleaned and débrided properly, especially if extensive necrosis is present. In neonatal tetanus, wide excision of the umbilical stump is not indicated.
- Supportive care and pharmacotherapy to control tetanic spasms are of major importance.
- Oral (or intravenous) metronidazole (30 mg/kg per day, given at 6-hour intervals; maximum, 4 g/day) is effective in decreasing the number of vegetative forms of *C tetani* and is the antimicrobial agent of choice. Parenteral penicillin G (100 000 U/kg per day, given at 4- to 6-hour intervals; maximum 12 million U/day) is an alternative treatment. Therapy for 10 to 14 days is recommended.

ISOLATION OF THE HOSPITALIZED PATIENT: Standard precautions are recommended.

CONTROL MEASURES:

Care of Exposed People (see Table 3.73). After primary immunization with tetanus toxoid, antitoxin persists at protective concentrations in most people for at least 10 years and for a longer time after a booster immunization.

- The use of tetanus toxoid with or without TIG in management of wounds depends on the nature of the wound and the history of immunization with tetanus toxoid, as described in Table 3.73.
- In the unusual circumstance that an infant is born outside the hospital and the umbilical cord likely is contaminated (eg, cut with nonsterile equipment), maternal history of tetanus immunization should be confirmed. If the mother's tetanus immunization status is unknown and she is unlikely to have been immunized, TIG should be administered to the neonate unless tetanus serostatus can be confirmed quickly. Infant diphtheria and tetanus toxoids and acellular pertussis vaccine (DTaP) should be given on the standard schedule.
- For infants younger than 6 months of age who have not received a full 3-dose primary series of tetanus toxoid-containing vaccine, decisions on the need for TIG with wound care should be based on the mother's tetanus toxoid immunization history at the time of delivery, applying the guidelines in Table 3.73.

Table 3.73. Guide to Tetanus Prophylaxis in Routine Wound Management

History of Adsorbed Tetanus Toxoid (Doses)	Clean, Minor Wounds		All Other Wounds[a]	
	DTaP, Tdap, or Td[b]	TIG[c]	DTaP, Tdap, or Td[b]	TIG[c]
Fewer than 3 or unknown	Yes	No	Yes	Yes
3 or more	No if <10 y since last tetanus-containing vaccine dose	No	No[d] if <5 y since last tetanus-containing vaccine dose	No
	Yes if ≥10 y since last tetanus-containing vaccine dose	No	Yes if ≥5 y since last tetanus-containing vaccine dose	No

Tdap indicates booster tetanus toxoid, reduced diphtheria toxoid, and acellular pertussis vaccine; DTaP, diphtheria and tetanus toxoids and acellular pertussis vaccine; Td, adult-type diphtheria and tetanus toxoids vaccine; TIG, Tetanus Immune Globulin (human).
[a] Such as, but not limited to, wounds contaminated with dirt, feces, soil, and saliva; puncture wounds; avulsions; and wounds resulting from missiles, crushing, burns, and frostbite.
[b] DTaP is used for children younger than 7 years of age. Tdap is preferred over Td for underimmunized children 7 years of age and older who have not received Tdap previously.
[c] Immune Globulin Intravenous should be used when TIG is not available.
[d] More frequent boosters are not needed and can accentuate adverse effects.

- Although any open wound is a potential source of tetanus, wounds contaminated with dirt, feces, soil, or saliva are at increased risk. Punctures and wounds containing devitalized tissue, including necrotic or gangrenous wounds, frostbite, crush and avulsion injuries, and burns, particularly are conducive to *C tetani* infection.
- If tetanus immunization is incomplete at the time of wound treatment, a dose of vaccine should be given, and the immunization series should be completed according to the age-appropriate primary immunization schedule. TIG should be administered for tetanus-prone wounds in patients infected with human immunodeficiency virus or other severe immunodeficiency, regardless of the history of tetanus immunizations.
- DTaP is the recommended and preferred vaccine for children 6 weeks through 6 years of age and for catch-up immunization for children 4 months through 6 years of age (see Fig 1.3, p 31). When a booster injection is indicated for wound prophylaxis in a child younger than 7 years of age, DTaP should be used unless pertussis vaccine is contraindicated (see Pertussis, p 553), in which case immunization with diphtheria and tetanus toxoids (DT) vaccine is recommended.
- When tetanus toxoid is required for wound prophylaxis in a child 7 through 10 years of age, use of adult-type diphtheria and tetanus toxoids (Td) vaccine instead of tetanus toxoid alone is advisable so that diphtheria immunity also is maintained. If the child is previously underimmunized for pertussis, tetanus toxoid, reduced diphtheria toxoid, and acellular pertussis vaccine (Tdap) should be administered.
- Adolescents 10 through 18 years of age who require a tetanus toxoid-containing vaccine as part of wound management should receive a single dose of Tdap instead of Td if they have not received Tdap previously (see Pertussis, p 553). People 19 years of age and older who require a tetanus toxoid-containing vaccine as part of wound management should receive Tdap instead of Td if they previously have not received Tdap.

- When TIG is required for wound prophylaxis, it is administered intramuscularly in a dose of 250 U (regardless of age or weight). IGIV or equine tetanus antitoxin is recommended if TIG is unavailable. Equine antitoxin should be administered after appropriate testing of the patient for sensitivity (see Sensitivity Tests for Reactions to Animal Sera, p 64). Equine antitoxin is not available in the United States. If tetanus toxoid and TIG, IGIV, or equine tetanus antitoxin are administered concurrently, separate syringes and sites should be used. Administration of TIG, IGIV, or equine tetanus antitoxin does not preclude initiation of active immunization with adsorbed tetanus toxoid. Efforts should be made to initiate immunization and arrange for its completion. Administration of tetanus toxoid simultaneously or at an interval after receipt of Immune Globulin does not impair development of protective antibody substantially.
- Regardless of immunization status, wounds should be cleaned and débrided properly if dirt or necrotic tissue is present. Wounds should receive prompt surgical treatment to remove all devitalized tissue and foreign material as an essential part of tetanus prophylaxis. It is not necessary or appropriate to débride puncture wounds extensively.

Immunization. Active immunization with tetanus toxoid is recommended for all people. For all appropriate indications, tetanus immunization is administered with diphtheria toxoid-containing vaccines or with diphtheria toxoid- and acellular pertussis-containing vaccines. Vaccine is administered intramuscularly and may be given concurrently with other vaccines (see Simultaneous Administration of Multiple Vaccines, p 33). *Haemophilus influenzae* type b conjugate vaccines containing tetanus toxoid (PRP-T) are not substitutes for tetanus toxoid immunization. Recommendations for use of tetanus toxoid-containing vaccines (summarized in Fig 1.1–1.3 [p 27–31]) are as follows:

- Immunization for children from 6 weeks of age to the seventh birthday (see Fig 1.1, p 27–28, and Fig 1.3, p 31) should consist of 5 doses of tetanus and diphtheria toxoid-containing vaccine. The initial 3 doses are given as DTaP, administered at 2-month intervals beginning at approximately 2 months of age. A fourth dose is recommended 6 to 12 months after the third dose, usually at 15 through 18 months of age (see Pertussis, p 553). The final dose of DTaP is recommended before school entry (kindergarten or elementary school) at 4 through 6 years of age, unless the fourth dose was given after the fourth birthday. DTaP can be given concurrently with other vaccines (see Simultaneous Administration of Multiple Vaccines, p 33).
- For children younger than 7 years of age who have received fewer than the recommended number of doses of pertussis vaccine but who have received the recommended number of DT doses for their age (ie, children in whom immunization was started with DT and who then were given DTaP [or diphtheria and tetanus toxoid and whole-cell pertussis vaccine, DTP, outside the United States]), dose(s) of DTaP should be given to complete the recommended pertussis immunization schedule (see Pertussis, p 553). However, the total number of doses of diphtheria and tetanus toxoids (as DT, DTaP, or DTP) should not exceed 6 before the seventh birthday.
- Immunization against tetanus and diphtheria for children younger than 7 years of age in whom pertussis immunization is contraindicated (see Pertussis, p 553) should be accomplished with DT instead of DTaP, as follows:
  - For children younger than 1 year of age, 3 doses of DT are administered at 2-month intervals; a fourth dose should be administered 6 to 12 months after the third dose, and the fifth dose should be administered before school entry at 4 through 6 years of age.

- For children 1 through 6 years of age who have not received previous doses of DT, DTaP, or DTP, 2 doses of DT approximately 2 months apart should be administered, followed by a third dose 6 to 12 months later to complete the initial series. DT can be given concurrently with other vaccines. An additional dose is recommended before school entry at 4 through 6 years of age unless the preceding dose was given after the fourth birthday.
- For children 1 through 6 years of age who have received 1 or 2 doses of DTaP, DTP, or DT during the first year of life and for whom further pertussis immunization is contraindicated, additional doses of DT should be administered until a total of 5 doses of diphtheria and tetanus toxoids are received by the time of school entry. The fourth dose is administered 6 to 12 months after the third dose. The preschool (fifth) dose is omitted if the fourth dose was given after the fourth birthday.

Other recommendations for tetanus immunization, including recommendations for older children, are as follows:

- For catch-up immunization for children 7 through 10 years of age, Tdap vaccine should be substituted for a single dose of Td in the catch-up series (see Fig 1.3, p 31).[1]
- Adolescents 10 or 11 through 18 years of age should receive a single dose of Tdap instead of Td for booster immunization against tetanus, diphtheria, and pertussis if they have completed the recommended childhood DTP/DTaP immunization series and have not received Td or Tdap.[1] The preferred age for Tdap immunization is 11 through 12 years of age. Adolescents 11 through 18 years of age who received Td but not Tdap are encouraged to receive a single dose of Tdap to provide protection against pertussis if they have completed the recommended childhood DTP/DTaP immunization series. Tdap should be administered regardless of interval since last tetanus- or diphtheria-containing vaccine.
- If more than 5 years have elapsed since the last dose, a booster dose of a tetanus-containing vaccine should be considered for people at risk of occupational exposure in locations where tetanus boosters may not be available readily. Tdap is preferred over Td if the person has not received Tdap previously.
- Prevention of neonatal tetanus can be accomplished by prenatal immunization of the previously unimmunized women and those for whom 10 years have passed since their previous tetanus-containing vaccine.
- Pregnant women who have not completed their primary series should do so before delivery, if time permits. If there is insufficient time, 2 doses of Td should be administered at least 4 weeks apart, and the second dose should be given at least 2 weeks before delivery. Tdap should be substituted for the first Td dose if Tdap has not been administered previously. Immunization with Tdap is recommended during pregnancy, preferably at 20 weeks' gestation or later, if Tdap has not been administered previously (see Pertussis, p 553).
- Active immunization against tetanus always should be undertaken during convalescence from tetanus, because this exotoxin-mediated disease usually does not confer immunity.

Adverse Events, Precautions, and Contraindications. Severe anaphylactic reactions, Guillain-Barré syndrome (GBS), and brachial neuritis attributable to tetanus toxoid have been reported but are rare. No increased risk of GBS has been observed with use of

---

[1] American Academy of Pediatrics, Committee on Infectious Diseases. Additional recommendations for use of tetanus toxoid, reduced-content diphtheria toxoid, and acellular pertussis vaccine (Tdap). *Pediatrics.* 2011;128(4):809–812

DTaP in children, and therefore, no special precautions are recommended when immunizing children with a history of GBS.

An immediate anaphylactic reaction to tetanus and diphtheria toxoid-containing vaccines (ie, DTaP, Tdap, DT, or Td) is a contraindication to further doses unless the patient can be desensitized to these toxoids (see Pertussis, p 553). Because of uncertainty about which vaccine component (ie, diphtheria, tetanus, or pertussis) might be responsible and the importance of tetanus immunization, people who experience anaphylactic reactions may be referred to an allergist for evaluation and possible desensitization to tetanus toxoid.

People who experienced Arthus-type hypersensitivity reactions or temperature greater than 39.4°C (103°F) after a previous dose of a tetanus toxoid-containing preparation usually have very high serum tetanus antibody concentrations and should not receive even emergency doses of tetanus toxoid-containing preparation more frequently than every 10 years, even if they have a wound that is neither clean nor minor.

Other Control Measures. Sterilization of hospital supplies will prevent the rare instances of tetanus that may occur in a hospital from contaminated sutures, instruments, or plaster casts.

For prevention of neonatal tetanus, preventive measures (in addition to maternal immunization) include community immunization programs for adolescent girls and women of childbearing age and appropriate training of midwives in recommendations for immunization and sterile technique.

Tinea Capitis
(Ringworm of the Scalp)

CLINICAL MANIFESTATIONS: Fungal infection of the scalp may manifest as one of the following distinct clinical syndromes:
- Patchy areas of dandruff-like scaling, with subtle or extensive hair loss, which may be confused with dandruff, seborrheic dermatitis, or atopic dermatitis; head/neck lymphadenopathy often is present;
- Discrete areas of hair loss studded by stubs of broken hairs, which is referred to as *black-dot ringworm;*
- Numerous discrete pustules or excoriations with little hair loss or scaling; or
- Kerion, a boggy inflammatory mass surrounded by follicular pustules, which is a hypersensitivity reaction to the fungal infection; may be accompanied by fever and local lymphadenopathy and commonly is misdiagnosed as impetigo, cellulitis, or an abscess of the scalp.
- A pruritic, fine, papulovesicular eruption (dermatophytid or id reaction) involving the trunk, extremities, and/or face caused by a hypersensitivity response to the infecting fungus.

Tinea capitis may be confused with many other diseases, including seborrheic dermatitis, atopic dermatitis, psoriasis, alopecia areata, trichotillomania, folliculitis, impetigo, head lice, and lupus erythematosus.

ETIOLOGY: *Trichophyton tonsurans* is the cause of tinea capitis in more than 90% of cases in North and Central America. *Microsporum canis, Microsporum audouinii, Trichophyton violaceum,* and *Trichophyton mentagrophytes* are less common. Causative agents may vary in different geographic areas.

EPIDEMIOLOGY: Infection of the scalp with *T tonsurans* is thought to result primarily from person-to-person transmission. The organism remains viable on combs, hairbrushes, and other fomites for long periods of time, and the role of fomites in transmission is a concern but has not been defined. *T tonsurans* often is cultured from the scalp of family members or asymptomatic children in close contact with an index case. Asymptomatic carriers are thought to have a significant role as reservoirs for infection and reinfection within families, schools, and communities. Tinea capitis attributable to *T tonsurans* occurs most commonly in children between 3 and 9 years of age and appears to be more common in black children. Cases in young infants have been documented.

M canis infection results primarily from animal-to-human transmission, although person-to-person transmission can occur. Infection often is the result of contact with household cats or dogs.

The **incubation period** is unknown but is thought to be 1 to 3 weeks; infections have occurred in infants within the first week of life.

DIAGNOSTIC TESTS: Potassium hydroxide wet mount and cultures may be used to confirm the diagnosis before treatment. Wood's light examination is helpful if the pathogen is *Microsporum* species. Hairs and scale obtained by gentle scraping of a moistened area of the scalp with a blunt scalpel, toothbrush, brush, tweezers, or a moistened cotton swab are used for potassium hydroxide wet mount examination and culture. In cases of *T tonsurans* infection, microscopic examination of a potassium hydroxide wet mount preparation will disclose numerous arthroconidia within the hair shaft. In *Microsporum* infection, spores surround the hair shaft. Use of dermatophyte test medium also is a reliable, simple, and inexpensive method of diagnosing tinea capitis. Skin scrapings, brushings, or hairs from lesions are inoculated directly onto culture medium and incubated at room temperature. After 1 to 2 weeks, a phenol red indicator in the agar will turn from yellow to red in the area surrounding a dermatophyte colony. When necessary, diagnosis also may be confirmed by culture on Sabouraud dextrose agar by direct plating technique or by samples collected on cotton-tipped applicators and transported to reference laboratories. Periodic acid-Schiff staining of histopathologic specimens and polymerase chain reaction evaluation are possible in academic centers but are expensive and rarely required for confirmation.

Examination of hair of patients with *Microsporum* infection under Wood light results in brilliant green fluorescence. However, because *T tonsurans* does not fluoresce under Wood light, this diagnostic test is not helpful for most patients with tinea capitis.

TREATMENT: Because topical antifungal medications are not effective for treatment of tinea capitis, systemic antifungal therapy is required. Microsize griseofulvin, 20 mg/kg per day (maximum, 1 g), or ultramicrosize griseofulvin, 10 to 15 mg/kg per day (maximum, 750 mg), is administered orally, once daily. Optimally, griseofulvin is given after a meal containing fat (eg, peanut butter or ice cream). Treatment typically is necessary for 4 to 6 weeks and should be continued for 2 weeks beyond clinical resolution. Some children may require higher doses to achieve clinical cure. Griseofulvin is approved for children older than 2 years of age. Children who have no history or clinical evidence of liver disease are not required to have serum hepatic enzyme values tested either before or during a standard course of therapy lasting up to 8 weeks. Prolonged therapy may be associated with a greater risk of hepatotoxicity, and enzyme testing every 8 weeks during treatment should be considered. A 6-week course of terbinafine in the form of oral granules has been shown to be as effective as a 6-week course of griseofulvin for treatment of tinea capitis, and terbinafine is approved by the US Food and Drug Administration for use in children 4 years of age and older. Terbinafine dosage is based on body weight, and a pediatric granule formulation is available in 125-mg and 187.5-mg packets. Dosing for this formulation is 125 mg for children weighing <25 kg; 187.5 mg for children weighing 25 to 35 kg, and 250 mg for children weighing >35 kg, taken once a day with food for 6 weeks. Baseline serum transaminase (alanine transaminase and aspartate transaminase) testing is advised. Terbinafine tablets, used off-label for tinea capitis, often are dosed on a weight-based sliding scale (67.5 mg/day for patients weighing <20 kg; 125 mg/day for patients weighing 20–40 kg; and 250 mg for patients weighing >40 kg). In addition, off-label treatment with oral itraconazole or fluconazole may be effective for tinea capitis; itraconazole is not approved for use in children. *Microsporum* infections are more likely to respond to griseofulvin, and *Trichophyton* infections are more likely to respond to terbin-afine. Selenium sulfide shampoo, either 1% or 2.5%, used twice a week, decreases fungal shedding and may help curb spread of infection.

Kerion can be treated with griseofulvin; terbinafine may be used if a *Trichophyton* species is the pathogen. Corticosteroid therapy consisting of prednisone or predniso-lone administered orally in dosages of 1.5 to 2 mg/kg per day (maximum, 20 mg/day) occasionally is needed for optimal therapeutic response. Treatment with a corticosteroid should be continued for approximately 2 weeks, with tapering doses toward the end of therapy. Antibacterial agents generally are not needed, except if there is suspected sec-ondary infection. Surgery is not indicated.

ISOLATION OF THE HOSPITALIZED PATIENT: Standard precautions are recommended.

CONTROL MEASURES: Early treatment of infected people is indicated, as is examina-tion of siblings and other household contacts for evidence of tinea capitis. Sharing of ribbons, combs, and hairbrushes should be discouraged. Families should be queried regarding other symptomatic members, and examination performed on such individu-als. People with tinea capitis should not return to wrestling for 14 days after commencing systemic therapy.

Children receiving treatment for tinea capitis may attend school once they start ther-apy with griseofulvin, terbinafine, or other effective systemic agent, with or without the addition of selenium sulfide shampoo. Haircuts, shaving of the head, or wearing a cap during treatment are unnecessary.

Tinea Corporis
(Ringworm of the Body)

CLINICAL MANIFESTATIONS: Superficial tinea infections of the nonhairy (glabrous) skin termed tinea corporis involve the face, trunk, or limbs. The lesion often is ring-shaped or circular (hence, the term "ringworm"), slightly erythematous, and well demarcated with a scaly, vesicular, or pustular border. Small confluent plaques or papules as well as multiple lesions can occur, particularly in wrestlers (tinea gladiatorum). Lesions can be mistaken for psoriasis, pityriasis rosea, or atopic, seborrheic, or contact dermatitis. A frequent source of confusion is an alteration in the appearance of lesions as a result of application of a topical corticosteroid preparation, termed tinea incognito. Such patients may also develop Majocchi granuloma, a follicular fungal infection associated with a granuloma-tous dermal reaction. In patients with diminished T-lymphocyte function (eg, human immunodeficiency virus infection), skin lesions may appear as grouped papules or pustules unaccompanied by scaling or erythema.

A pruritic, fine, papulovesicular eruption (dermatophytic or id reaction) involving the trunk, hands, or face, caused by a hypersensitivity response to infecting fungus, may accompany skin lesions. Tinea corporis can occur in association with tinea capitis, and examination of the scalp should be performed, particularly in affected wrestlers and people who have lesions on the neck and face.

ETIOLOGY: The prime causes of the disease are fungi of the genus *Trichophyton,* especially *Trichophyton tonsurans, Trichophyton rubrum,* and *Trichophyton mentagrophytes;* the genus *Microsporum,* especially *Microsporum* canis; and *Epidermophyton floccosum. Microsporum gypseum* also occasionally can cause infection.

EPIDEMIOLOGY: These causative fungi occur worldwide and are transmissible by direct contact with infected humans, animals, soil or fomites. Fungi in lesions are communicable.

The incubation period is thought to be 1 to 3 weeks but can be shorter, as documented infections have occurred at 6 days of life in infants with unaffected mothers.

DIAGNOSTIC TESTS: Fungi responsible for tinea corporis can be detected by microscopic examination of a potassium hydroxide wet mount of skin scrapings. Use of dermatophyte test medium also is a reliable, simple, and inexpensive method of diagnosis. Skin scrapings from lesions are inoculated directly onto culture medium and incubated at room temperature. After 1 to 2 weeks, a phenol red indicator in the agar will turn from yellow to red in the area surrounding a dermatophyte colony. When necessary, the diagnosis also can be confirmed by culture on Sabouraud dextrose agar. Histopathologic diagnosis using periodic acid-Schiff staining and polymerase chain reaction diagnostic tools are available but are expensive and generally unnecessary.

TREATMENT: Topical application of a miconazole, clotrimazole, terbinafine (12 years of age and older), tolnaftate, naftifine, or ciclopirox (10 years of age and older) preparation twice a day or of a ketoconazole, econazole, oxiconazole, butenafine (12 years of age and older), or sulconazole preparation once a day is recommended (see Topical Drugs for Superficial Fungal Infections, p 836). Topical econazole, ketoconazole, naftifine, and sulconazole are not approved by the US Food and Drug Administration for use as antifungal agents in children. Although clinical resolution may be evident within 2 weeks of therapy, continuing therapy for another 2 to 4 weeks generally is recommended. If significant clinical improvement is not seen after 4 to 6 weeks of treatment, an alternate diagnosis should be considered. Topical preparations of antifungal medication mixed with high-potency corticosteroids should not be used, because these often are less effective and can lead to a more deep-seated follicular infection (Majocchi granuloma); in addition, local and systemic adverse events from the corticosteroids can occur.

If lesions are extensive or unresponsive to topical therapy, griseofulvin is administered orally for 4 weeks (see Tinea Capitis, p 712). Oral itraconazole, fluconazole, and terbinafine are alternative effective options for more severe cases; these agents are not approved by the FDA for this purpose in children and have a much different benefit-to-risk profile.

ISOLATION OF THE HOSPITALIZED PATIENT: Standard precautions are recommended. People with corporis tinea should not return to wrestling for 72 hours after commencement of topical therapy.

CONTROL MEASURES: Direct contact with known or suspected sources of infection should be avoided. Periodic inspections of contacts for early lesions and prompt therapy are recommended. Wrestling mats and equipment should be cleaned frequently, and actively infected wrestlers must be excluded from competitions.

Tinea Cruris
(Jock Itch)

CLINICAL MANIFESTATIONS: Tinea cruris is a common superficial fungal disorder of the groin and upper thighs. The eruption usually is bilaterally symmetric and sharply marginated, often with polycyclic borders. Involved skin is erythematous and scaly and varies from red to brown; occasionally, the eruption is accompanied by central clearing and a vesiculopapular border. In chronic infections, the margin may be subtle, and lichenification may be present. Tinea cruris skin lesions may be extremely pruritic. These lesions should be differentiated from candidiasis, intertrigo, seborrheic dermatitis, psoriasis, atopic dermatitis, irritant or allergic contact dermatitis (generally caused by therapeutic agents applied to the area), and erythrasma. The latter is a superficial bacterial infection of the skin caused by *Corynebacterium minutissimum*.

ETIOLOGY: The fungi *Epidermophyton floccosum*, *Trichophyton rubrum*, and *Trichophyton mentagrophytes* are the most common causes. *Trichophyton tonsurans* also has been identified.

EPIDEMIOLOGY: Tinea cruris occurs predominantly in adolescent and adult males, mainly via indirect contact from desquamated epithelium or hair. Moisture, close-fitting garments, friction, and obesity are predisposing factors. Direct or indirect person-to-person transmission may occur. This infection commonly occurs in association with tinea pedis, and all infected patients should be evaluated for this possibility, with careful evaluation of the interdigital web spaces. Onychomycosis also is a possible association, particularly in adolescents and adults.

The **incubation period** is unknown but is thought to be approximately 1 to 3 weeks.

DIAGNOSTIC TESTS: Fungi responsible for tinea cruris may be detected by microscopic examination of a potassium hydroxide wet mount of scales. Use of dermatophyte test medium also is a reliable, simple, and inexpensive method of diagnosing tinea cruris. Skin scrapings from lesions are inoculated directly onto culture medium and incubated at room temperature. After 1 to 2 weeks, a phenol red indicator in the agar will turn from yellow to red in the area surrounding a dermatophyte colony. When necessary, the diagnosis also can be confirmed by culture on Sabouraud dextrose agar. Polymerase chain reaction assay is a more expensive diagnostic tool that generally is not required. A characteristic coral-red fluorescence under Wood light can identify the presence of erythrasma (an eruption of reddish brown patches attributable to the presence of *Corynebacterium minutissimum*) and, thus, exclude tinea cruris.

TREATMENT: Twice-daily topical application for 4 to 6 weeks of a clotrimazole, miconazole, terbinafine (12 years of age and older), tolnaftate, or ciclopirox (10 years of age and older) preparation rubbed or sprayed onto the affected areas and surrounding skin is effective. Once-daily therapy with topical econazole, ketoconazole, naftifine, oxiconazole, butenafine (12 years of age and older), or sulconazole preparation also is effective (see Topical Drugs for Superficial Fungal Infections, p 836). Topical econazole, ketoconazole, naftifine, and sulconazole are not approved by the US Food and Drug Administration for use as antifungal agents in children. Tinea pedis, if present, should be treated concurrently (see Tinea Pedis, p 717).

Topical preparations of antifungal medication mixed with high-potency corticosteroids should be avoided because of the potential for prolonged infections and local and systemic adverse corticosteroid-induced events. Loose-fitting, washed cotton underclothes to decrease chafing as well as the use of an absorbent powder can be helpful adjuvants to therapy. Griseofulvin, given orally for 2 to 6 weeks, may be effective in unresponsive cases (see Tinea Capitis, p 712). Oral itraconazole, fluconazole, and terbinafine are more effective therapies in adults but have a much different benefit-to-risk profile. Because many conditions mimic tinea cruris, a differential diagnosis should be considered if primary treatments fail.

ISOLATION OF THE HOSPITALIZED PATIENT: Standard precautions are recommended.

CONTROL MEASURES: Infections should be treated promptly. Potentially involved areas should be kept dry, and loose undergarments should be worn. Patients should be advised to dry the groin area before drying their feet to avoid inoculating dermatophytes of tinea pedis into the groin area.

Tinea Pedis and Tinea Unguium
(Athlete's Foot, Ringworm of the Feet)

CLINICAL MANIFESTATIONS: Tinea pedis manifests as a fine scaly or vesiculopustular eruption that commonly is pruritic. Lesions can involve all areas of the foot but usually are patchy in distribution, with a predisposition to fissures and scaling between toes, particularly in the third and fourth interdigital spaces or distributed around the sides of the feet. Toenails may be infected and can be dystrophic (tinea unguium). Tinea pedis must be differentiated from dyshidrotic eczema, atopic dermatitis, contact dermatitis, juvenile plantar dermatosis, palmoplantar keratoderma, and erythrasma (an eruption of reddish brown patches caused by *Corynebacterium minutissimum*). Tinea pedis commonly occurs in association with tinea cruris and onychomycosis (tinea unguium), a nail infection by any fungus. Dermatophyte infections commonly affect otherwise healthy people, but immunocompromised people have increased susceptibility.

Tinea pedis and many other fungal infections can be accompanied by a hypersensitivity reaction to the fungi (the dermatophytid or id reaction), with resulting papular or papulovesicular eruptions on the palms and the sides of fingers and, occasionally, by an erythematous vesicular eruption on the extremities and trunk.

ETIOLOGY: The fungi *Trichophyton rubrum*, *Trichophyton mentagrophytes*, and *Epidermophyton floccosum* are the most common causes of tinea pedis.

EPIDEMIOLOGY: Tinea pedis is a common infection worldwide in adolescents and adults but is less common in young children. Fungi are acquired by contact with skin scales containing fungi or with fungi in damp areas, such as swimming pools, locker rooms, and showers. Tinea pedis can spread throughout the household among family members and is communicable for as long as infection is present.

The **incubation period** is unknown.

DIAGNOSTIC TESTS: Tinea pedis usually is diagnosed by clinical manifestations and may be confirmed by microscopic examination of a potassium hydroxide wet mount of the cutaneous scrapings. Use of dermatophyte test medium is a reliable, simple, and inexpensive method of diagnosis in complicated or unresponsive cases but must be interpreted by an experienced observer. Skin scrapings are inoculated directly onto the culture medium and incubated at room temperature. After 1 to 2 weeks, a phenol red indicator in the agar will turn from yellow to red in the area surrounding a dermatophyte colony. When necessary, the diagnosis also can be confirmed by culture on Sabouraud dextrose agar. Infection of the nail can be verified by direct microscopic examination with potassium hydroxide, fungal culture of desquamated subungual material, or fungal stain of a nail clipping fixed in formalin.

TREATMENT: Topical application of terbinafine, twice daily; ciclopirox; or an azole agent (clotrimazole, miconazole, econazole, oxiconazole, sertaconazole, ketoconazole), once or twice daily, usually is adequate for milder cases. Acute vesicular lesions may be treated with intermittent use of open wet compresses (eg, with Burrow solution, 1:80). Dermatophyte infections in other locations, if present, should be treated concurrently (see Tinea Cruris, p 716).

Tinea pedis that is severe, chronic, or refractory to topical treatment may be treated with oral therapy. Oral itraconazole or terbinafine is the most effective, with griseofulvin next and fluconazole least effective. None are approved by the US Food and Drug Administration (FDA) for treatment of tinea pedis. Id (hypersensitivity response) reactions are treated by wet compresses, topical corticosteroids, occasionally systemic corticosteroids, and eradication of the primary source of infection.

Recurrence is prevented by proper foot hygiene, which includes keeping the feet dry and cool, gentle cleaning, drying between the toes, use of absorbent antifungal foot powder, frequent airing of affected areas, and avoidance of occlusive footwear and nylon socks or other fabrics that interfere with dissipation of moisture.

In people with onychomycosis (tinea unguium), topical therapy should be used only when the infection is confined to the distal ends of the nail; however, even topical therapy for 48 weeks typically has a cure rate less than 50%. Topical ciclopirox (8% [approved by the FDA for people 12 years of age and older]) may be applied to affected toenail(s) once daily in combination with a comprehensive nail management program. Studies in adults have demonstrated the best cure rates after therapy with oral itraconazole or terbinafine; however, safety and effectiveness in children has not been established. Terbinafine is approved by the FDA as 250 mg, daily, for 12 weeks in adults for toenail infection and 250 mg, daily, for 6 weeks for fingernail infection. However, preferred treatment in adults is pulse therapy with terbinafine, 500 mg, daily, for 1 week each month for 2 months (fingernails) to 4 months (toenails). Guidelines for dosing of terbinafine for children are based on studies for tinea capitis and are weight based: children weighing 12 to 20 kg, 62.5 mg/day, orally; children weighing 20 to 40 kg, 125 mg/day, orally; and children weighing >40 kg, 250 mg/day, orally. The duration of therapy is the same as in adults. Pediatric dosing of itraconazole is less well established. Recurrences are common. Removal of the nail plate followed by use of oral therapy during the period of regrowth can help to affect a cure in resistant cases.

ISOLATION OF THE HOSPITALIZED PATIENT: Standard precautions are recommended.

CONTROL MEASURES: Treatment of patients with active infections should decrease transmission. Public areas conducive to transmission (eg, swimming pools) should not be used by people with active infection. Chemical foot baths are of no value and can facilitate spread of infection. Because recurrence after treatment is common, proper foot hygiene is important (as described in Treatment). People should be advised to dry the groin area before drying their feet to avoid inoculating tinea pedis dermatophytes into the groin area.

Toxocariasis
(Visceral Larva Migrans, Ocular Larva Migrans)

CLINICAL MANIFESTATIONS: The severity of symptoms depends on the number of larvae ingested and the degree of allergic response. Most people who are infected lightly are asymptomatic. Toxocariasis may manifest only as asymptomatic eosinophilia or pulmonary wheezing. Characteristic manifestations of visceral toxocariasis include fever, leukocytosis, eosinophilia, hypergammaglobulinemia, and hepatomegaly. Other manifestations include malaise, anemia, cough, and in rare instances, pneumonia, myocarditis, and encephalitis. When ocular invasion (resulting in endophthalmitis or retinal granulomas) occurs, other evidence of infection usually is lacking, suggesting that the visceral and ocular manifestations are distinct syndromes. Atypical manifestations include hemorrhagic rash and seizures.

ETIOLOGY: Toxocariasis is caused by *Toxocara* species, which are common roundworms of dogs and cats (especially puppies or kittens), specifically *Toxocara canis* and *Toxocara cati* in the United States; most cases are caused by *T canis*. Other nematodes of animals also can cause this syndrome, although rarely.

EPIDEMIOLOGY: On the basis of a nationally representative survey, 14% of the US population has serologic evidence of *Toxocara* infection, and the rate is concentrated among the poor. Visceral toxocariasis typically occurs in children 2 to 7 years of age often with a history of pica but can occur in older children and adults. Ocular larva migrans usually occurs in older children and adolescents. Humans are infected by ingestion of soil containing infective eggs of the parasite. Eggs may be found wherever dogs and cats defecate, often in sandboxes and playgrounds. Direct contact with dogs is of secondary importance, because eggs are not infective immediately when shed in the feces. Infection risk is highest in hot, humid regions where eggs persist in soil.

The **incubation period** cannot be accurately determined.

DIAGNOSTIC TESTS: Hypereosinophilia and hypergammaglobulinemia associated with increased titers of isohemagglutinin to the A and B blood group antigens are presumptive evidence of infection. Microscopic identification of larvae in a liver biopsy specimen is diagnostic, but this finding is rare. A liver biopsy negative for larvae, therefore, does not exclude the diagnosis. An enzyme immunoassay for *Toxocara* antibodies in serum, available at the Centers for Disease Control and Prevention and some commercial laboratories, can provide confirmatory evidence of toxocariasis but does not distinguish between past and current, active infection. This assay is specific and sensitive for diagnosis of visceral larva migrans but is less sensitive for diagnosis of ocular larva migrans.

TREATMENT: Albendazole is the recommended drug for treatment of toxocariasis (see Drugs for Parasitic Infections, p 848). The drug has been approved by the US Food and Drug Administration, but not for this indication. In severe cases with myocarditis or involvement of the central nervous system, corticosteroid therapy is indicated. Correcting the underlying causes of pica helps prevent reinfection.

Antiparasitic treatment of ocular larva migrans may not be effective. Inflammation may be decreased by topical or systemic corticosteroids, and secondary damage decreased with surgery.

ISOLATION OF THE HOSPITALIZED PATIENT: Standard precautions are recommended.

CONTROL MEASURES: Proper disposal of cat and dog feces is essential. Regular treatment of dogs and cats, and especially puppies and kittens, with anthelmintics at 2, 4, 6, and 8 weeks of age prevents excretion of eggs by worms acquired from the environment, transplacentally, or through mother's milk. Covering sandboxes when not in use is helpful. No specific management of exposed people is recommended.

Toxoplasma gondii Infections
(Toxoplasmosis)

CLINICAL MANIFESTATIONS: Infants with congenital infection are asymptomatic at birth in 70% to 90% of cases, although visual or hearing impairment, learning disabilities, or mental retardation will become apparent in a large proportion of children several months to years later. Signs of congenital toxoplasmosis at birth can include a maculopapular rash, generalized lymphadenopathy, hepatomegaly, splenomegaly, jaundice, pneumonitis, diarrhea, hypothermia, petechiae, and thrombocytopenia. As a consequence of intrauterine infection, meningoencephalitis, cerebrospinal fluid (CSF) abnormalities, hydrocephalus, microcephaly, chorioretinitis, seizures, and deafness can develop. Some severely affected fetuses/infants die in utero or within a few days of birth. Cerebral calcifications can be demonstrated by plain films, ultrasonography, or computed tomography (CT) of the head. However, CT is the radiologic technique of choice, because it is the most sensitive for calcifications and can reveal brain abnormalities when plain radiographic and/or ultrasonographic studies are normal. The classical triad of cerebral calcifications, chorioretinitis, and hydrocephalus is rare but it is highly suggestive of congenital toxoplasmosis, and it is seen primarily in babies whose mothers were not treated for toxoplasmosis during gestation.

Toxoplasma gondii infection acquired after birth may be asymptomatic, except in immunocompromised people. When symptoms develop, they are nonspecific and include malaise, fever, headache, sore throat, arthralgia, and myalgia. Lymphadenopathy, frequently cervical, is the most common sign. Occasionally, patients may have a mononucleosis-like illness associated with a macular rash and hepatosplenomegaly. The clinical course usually is benign and self-limited. Myocarditis, myositis, hepatitis, pericarditis, pneumonia, and skin lesions are rare complications in the United States and Europe. However, these manifestations and more aggressive disease, including brain abscesses, life-threatening syndromes, and death, have been observed in immunocompetent people infected in certain tropical countries in South America, such as French Guiana, Brazil, and Colombia.

Isolated ocular toxoplasmosis commonly results from reactivation of congenital infection but also occurs in people with acquired infection. In Brazil and Canada, up to 17% of patients diagnosed with postnatally acquired toxoplasmosis have been found to have toxoplasmic chorioretinitis. Characteristic retinal lesions (chorioretinitis) develop in up to 85% of young adults after untreated congenital infection. Acute ocular involvement manifests as blurred vision, eye pain, decreased visual acuity, floaters, scotoma, photophobia, or epiphora. The most common late finding is chorioretinitis, which can result in unilateral vision loss. Ocular disease can become reactivated years after the initial infection in healthy and immunocompromised people.

In chronically infected immunodeficient patients, including people with human immunodeficiency virus (HIV) infection, reactivation of *T gondii* can result in life-threatening encephalitis, pneumonitis, fever of unknown origin, or disseminated toxoplasmosis. In patients with acquired immunodeficiency syndrome (AIDS), toxoplasmic encephalitis (TE) is the most common syndrome and typically presents with acute to subacute neurologic or psychiatric symptoms and multiple ring-enhancing brain lesions. In these patients, a clear improvement in their symptoms and signs within 7 to 10 days of beginning empiric antitoxoplasma drugs is considered diagnostic of TE. However, immunocompromised patients without AIDS (eg, transplant or cancer patients, patients taking immunosuppressive drugs) who are chronically infected with *T gondii* and who present with multiple ring-enhancing brain lesions should undergo an immediate brain biopsy rather than receiving empiric treatment only. In this latter group of patients, the differential diagnosis should be widened to other pathogens, such as molds and nocardia. TE also can present as single brain lesion by magnetic resonance imaging (MRI) or as a diffuse and rapidly progressive process in the setting of apparently negative brain MRI studies. MRI is superior to CT for the diagnosis of toxoplasmic encephalitis and can detect lesions not revealed by CT.

Seropositive hematopoietic stem cell and solid organ transplant patients are at risk of their latent *T gondii* infection being reactivated. In these patients, toxoplasmosis may manifest as pneumonia, unexplained fever, myocarditis, hepatosplenomegaly, lymphadenopathy, or skin lesions in addition to brain abscesses and diffuse encephalitis. *T gondii*-seropositive solid organ donors (D+) can transmit the parasite via the allograft to seronegative recipients (R-). Thirty percent of D+/R- heart transplant recipients develop toxoplasmosis in the absence of anti-*T gondii* prophylaxis.

The term *T gondii* infection is reserved for the asymptomatic presence of the parasite in the setting of an acute or chronic infection. In contrast, the term toxoplasmosis should be used when the parasite causes symptoms and/or signs during the acute infection or reactivation of chronic infection in immunosuppressed patients.

ETIOLOGY: *T gondii* is a protozoan and obligate intracellular parasite. *T gondii* organisms exist in nature in 3 primary clonal lineages (types I, II, and III) and several infectious forms (tachyzoite, tissue cysts containing bradyzoites, and oocysts containing sporozoites). The tachyzoite and the host immune response are responsible for symptoms observed during the acute infection in humans or during the reactivation of a latent infection in immunocompromised patients. The tissue cyst is responsible for latent infection and usually is present in skeletal muscle, cardiac tissue, brain, and eyes of humans and other vertebrate animals. It is the tissue cyst form that is transmitted through undercooked or raw meat. The oocyst is present in the small intestine of cats and other members of the feline family; it is responsible for transmission through soil, water, or food contaminated with infected cat feces.

EPIDEMIOLOGY: *T gondii* is worldwide in distribution and infects most species of warm-blooded animals. The seroprevalence of *T gondii* infection (a reflection of the chronic infection and measured by the presence of *T gondii*-specific IgG antibodies) varies by geographic locale and the socioeconomic strata of the population. The age-adjusted seroprevalence of the parasite in the United States has been estimated at 11%. Members of the feline family are definitive hosts. Cats generally acquire the infection by feeding on infected animals (eg, mice), uncooked household meats, or water or food contaminated with their own oocysts. The parasite replicates sexually in the feline small intestine. Cats may begin to excrete millions of oocysts in their stools 3 to 30 days after primary infection and may shed oocysts for 7 to 14 days. After excretion, oocysts require a maturation phase (sporulation) of 24 to 48 hours in temperate climates before they are infective by the oral route. Sporulated oocysts survive for long periods under most ordinary environmental conditions and can survive in moist soil, for example, for months and even years. Intermediate hosts (including sheep, pigs, and cattle) can have tissue cysts in the brain, myocardium, skeletal muscle, and other organs. These cysts remain viable for the lifetime of the host. Humans usually become infected by consumption of raw or undercooked meat that contains cysts or by accidental ingestion of sporulated oocysts from soil or in contaminated food or water. A large outbreak linked epidemiologically to contamination of a municipal water supply also has been reported. A recent epidemiologic study revealed the following risk factors associated with acute infection in the United States: eating raw ground beef; eating rare lamb; eating locally produced cured, dried, or smoked meat; working with meat; drinking unpasteurized goat milk; and having 3 or more kittens. In this study, eating raw oysters, clams, or mussels also was identified as novel risk factor. Untreated water also was found to have a trend towards increased risk for acute infection in the United States. Although the risk factors for acute infection have been reported in studies from Europe, South America, and the United States, up to 50% of acutely infected people do not have identifiable risk factors or symptoms. Thus, *T gondii* infection and toxoplasmosis may occur even in patients without a suggestive epidemiologic history or illness. Only appropriate laboratory testing can establish or rule out the diagnosis of *T gondii* infection or toxoplasmosis.

Transmission of *T gondii* has been documented to result from solid organ (eg, heart, kidney, liver) or hematopoietic stem cell transplantation from a seropositive donor with latent infection to a seronegative recipient. Rarely, infection has occurred as a result of a laboratory accident or from blood or blood product transfusion. In most cases, congenital transmission occurs as a result of primary maternal infection during gestation. Rarely, in utero infection may occur as a result of reactivated parasitemia during pregnancy in chronically infected immunocompromised women. There is no evidence of any other type of human-to-human transmission. The incidence of congenital toxoplasmosis in the United States has been estimated to be 1 in 1000 to 1 in 10 000 live births.

The **incubation period** of acquired infection, on the basis of a well-studied outbreak, is estimated to be approximately 7 days, with a range of 4 to 21 days.

DIAGNOSTIC TESTS: Serologic tests are the primary means of diagnosing primary and latent infection. Polymerase chain reaction (PCR) assays of body fluids and staining of a biopsy specimen with *T gondii*-specific immunoperoxidase are valuable for confirming the diagnosis of toxoplasmosis. Isolation of the parasite occasionally is attempted for the purpose of genotyping the infecting strain. Correlation of genotype with clinical manifestations may be attempted, but results must be interpreted carefully in the context of each clinical scenario. Laboratories with special expertise in *Toxoplasma* serologic assays and their interpretation, such as the Palo Alto Medical Foundation Toxoplasma Serology Laboratory (PAMF-TSL; Palo Alto, CA; **www.pamf.org/serology/**; +1-650-853-4828; e-mail toxolab@pamf.org), are useful to clinicians and nonreference laboratories.

Immunoglobulin (Ig) G-specific antibodies achieve a peak concentration 1 to 2 months after infection and remain positive indefinitely. To determine the approximate time of infection in IgG-positive adults, specific IgM antibody determinations should be performed. The lack of *T gondii*-specific IgM antibodies in a person with low titers of IgG antibodies (eg, a Dye test at PAMF-TSL ≤512) indicates infection of at least 6 months' duration. The presence of *T gondii*-specific IgM antibodies can indicate recent infection, can be detected in chronically infected people, or can result from a false-positive reaction. Sera with positive *T gondii*-specific IgM test results may be sent to PAMF-TSL for confirmatory testing and to establish whether the patient has an acute or a chronic infection. Enzyme immunoassays (EIAs) are the most sensitive tests for IgM, and indirect fluorescent antibody tests are the least sensitive tests for detecting IgM. IgM-specific antibodies can be detected 2 weeks after infection (IgG-specific antibodies usually are negative during this period), achieve peak concentrations in 1 month, decrease thereafter, and usually become undetectable within 6 to 9 months. However, in some people, a positive IgM test result may persist for years and without an apparent clinical significance. In adults, a positive IgM test should be followed by confirmatory testing at a laboratory with special expertise in *Toxoplasma* serology when determining the timing of infection is important clinically (eg, in a pregnant woman).

Laboratory tests that have been found to be helpful in determining timing of infection include an IgG avidity test, the AC/HS or differential agglutination test, and IgA- and IgE-specific antibody tests. The presence of high-avidity IgG antibodies indicates that infection occurred at least 12 to 16 weeks prior. However, the presence of low-avidity antibodies is not a reliable indication of recent infection, and treatment may affect the maturation of IgG avidity and prolong the presence of low-avidity antibodies. A nonacute pattern in the AC/HS test usually is indicative of an infection that was acquired at least 12 months before serum was obtained. Tests to detect IgA and IgE antibodies, which decrease to undetectable concentrations sooner than IgM antibodies do, are useful for diagnosis of congenital infections and infections in pregnant women, for whom more precise information about the duration of infection is needed. *T gondii*-specific IgA and IgE antibody tests are available in *Toxoplasma* reference laboratories but generally not in other laboratories. Diagnosis of *Toxoplasma* infection during pregnancy should be made on the basis of results of serologic assays performed in a reference laboratory.

PCR and *T gondii*-specific immunoperoxidase staining can be attempted in virtually any body fluid or tissue, depending on the clinical scenario. Specimens on which PCR can be performed include vitreous fluid, aqueous humor, CSF, bronchoalveolar lavage fluid, peritoneal fluid, ascitic fluid, pleural fluid, peripheral blood, amniotic fluid, bone marrow, and urine. A positive test result for presence of *T gondii* DNA in any body fluid is diagnostic of toxoplasmosis. Essentially any tissue can be stained with *T gondii*-specific immunoperoxidase; the presence of extracellular antigens and a surrounding inflammatory response are diagnostic of toxoplasmosis.

Special Situations.

Prenatal. A definitive diagnosis of congenital toxoplasmosis can be made prenatally by detecting parasite DNA by PCR in amniotic fluid. Isolation of the parasite by mouse or tissue culture inoculation also can be attempted from amniotic fluid. Serial fetal ultrasonographic examinations can be performed in cases of suspected congenital infection to detect any increase in size of the lateral ventricles of the central nervous system or other signs of fetal infection, such as brain, hepatic, or splenic calcifications.

Postnatal. Infants who are born to women suspected of having or who have been diagnosed with primary *T gondii* infection during gestation should be assessed for congenital toxoplasmosis. Women infected shortly before conception (eg, within 3 months of conception) also may be at risk. In addition, infants born to immunocompromised women (HIV-infected or otherwise) with serologic evidence of past infection with *T gondii* should be evaluated for the possibility of congenital toxoplasmosis.

If an infant's *Toxoplasma* infection status is unclear at the time of delivery, *Toxoplasma*-specific laboratory tests for IgG, IgM (by the ISAGA method), and IgA in newborn serum samples should be performed at a laboratory with special expertise in *Toxoplasma* serologic assays. Detection of *Toxoplasma*-specific IgA antibodies is more sensitive than IgM detection in congenitally infected infants. None of the current commercial assays offered in the United States have been cleared by the Food and Drug Administration for in vitro diagnostic use for infants. IgA testing is not offered by the Centers for Disease Control and Prevention. Infected newborn infants may be IgM and IgA positive, IgM positive but IgA negative, IgM negative but IgA positive, or IgM and IgA negative. A maternal serum sample also should be tested for IgG, IgM, and AC/HS. Peripheral blood white blood cells, CSF, urine, and amniotic fluid specimens should be assayed for *T gondii* by PCR assay in a reference laboratory. Evaluation of the infant should include ophthalmologic, auditory, and neurologic examinations; lumbar puncture; and CT of the head. An attempt may be made to isolate *T gondii* by mouse inoculation from placenta, umbilical cord, CSF, urine, or blood specimens.

Congenital infection is confirmed serologically by persistently positive IgG titers beyond the first 12 months of life. Before 12 months of age, a persistently positive or increasing IgG antibody concentration in the infant compared with the mother and/or a positive *Toxoplasma*-specific IgM or IgA assay in the infant indicate congenital infection. Although placental leak occasionally can lead to false-positive IgM or IgA reactions in the newborn infant, repeat testing after approximately 10 days of life can help confirm the diagnosis, because the half-life of these immunoglobulins is short and the titers in an infant who is not infected should decrease rapidly. The sensitivity of *T gondii*-specific IgM by an immunosorbent agglutination assay (ISAGA) is 87% in newborn infants born to mothers not treated during gestation; sensitivity for IgA antibodies is 77%; and when both are taken into consideration, the sensitivity increases to 93%. The indirect fluorescent assay or EIA for IgM should not be relied on to diagnose congenital infection. In an uninfected infant, a continuous decrease in IgG titer without detection of IgM or IgA antibodies will occur. Transplacentally transmitted IgG antibody usually will become undetectable by 6 to 12 months of age.

Immunocompromised patients. Immunocompromised patients (eg, patients with AIDS, solid organ transplant recipients, patients with cancer, or people taking immunosuppressive drugs) who are infected latently with *T gondii* have variable titers of IgG antibody to *T gondii* but rarely have IgM antibody. Immunocompromised patients should be tested for *T gondii*-specific IgG before commencing immunosuppressive therapy or as soon as their status of immunosuppression is diagnosed to determine whether they are chronically infected with *T gondii* and at risk of reactivation of latent infection. Active disease in immunosuppressed patients may or may not result in seroconversion and a fourfold increase in IgG antibody titers; consequently, serologic diagnosis in these patients often is difficult. Previously seropositive patients may have changes in their IgG titers in any direction (increase, decrease, or no change) without any clinical relevance. In these patients, PCR testing, histologic examination, and attempts to isolate the parasite become the laboratory methods of choice to diagnose toxoplasmosis.

In HIV-infected patients who are seropositive for *T gondii* IgG, reactivation of their latent infection usually is manifested by TE. TE can be diagnosed presumptively on the basis of characteristic clinical and radiographic findings. MRI usually reveals the presence of multiple brain-occupying and ring-enhancing lesions. If there is no clinical response within 10 days to an empiric trial of anti-*T gondii* therapy, demonstration of *T gondii* organisms, antigen, or DNA in specimens such as blood, CSF, or bronchoalveolar fluid may be necessary to confirm the diagnosis. TE also can present as diffuse encephalitis without space-occupying lesions on brain MRI. Prompt recognition of this syndrome and confirmation of the diagnosis by PCR testing in CSF is crucial, because these patients usually exhibit a rapidly progressive and fatal clinical course.

Diagnosis of TE in immunocompromised patients other than HIV-infected people requires confirmation by brain biopsy or PCR testing of CSF. In this group of patients, other organisms, such as invasive mold infections and nocardia, should be considered before beginning an empiric trial of anti-*T gondii* therapy.

Infants born to women who are infected simultaneously with HIV and *T gondii* should be evaluated for congenital toxoplasmosis because of an increased likelihood of maternal reactivation and congenital transmission in this setting. Expert advice is available at the PAMF-TSL (**http://www.pamf.org/serology/**; telephone [650] 853-4828; e-mail toxolab@pamf.org) and the National Collaborative Chicago-Based Congenital Toxoplasmosis Study (NCCCTS; Chicago, IL; **http://www.uchospitals.edu/specialties/infectious-diseases/toxoplasmosis/;** telephone [773] 834-4131; e-mail rmcleod@midway.uchicago.edu).

Ocular toxoplasmosis. Toxoplasmic chorioretinitis usually is diagnosed on the basis of characteristic retinal lesions in conjunction with serum *T gondii*-specific IgG. Confirmatory testing for IgM may yield positive results in situations in which eye lesions are the result of a concomitant acute *T gondii* infection rather than reactivation of a chronic infection. Patients who have atypical retinal lesions or who fail to respond to anti-*T gondii* therapy should undergo examination of vitreous fluid or aqueous humor by PCR, and immune load (Goldmann-Witmer coefficient) should be considered.

TREATMENT: Most cases of acquired infection in an immunocompetent host do not require specific antimicrobial therapy unless infection occurs during pregnancy or symptoms are severe or persistent. When indicated (eg, chorioretinitis or significant organ damage), the combination of pyrimethamine and sulfadiazine,[1] with supplemental leucovorin (folinic acid) to minimize pyrimethamine-associated hematologic toxicity, is the regimen most widely accepted for children and adults with acute symptomatic disease (see Drugs for Parasitic Infections, p 848). Trimethoprim-sulfamethoxazole (TMP-SMX),

---

[1] Available from Sandoz Inc, Princeton, NJ (800-526-0225).

also available in the intravenous form, has been reported to be equivalent to pyrimethamine/sulfadiazine in the treatment of patients with toxoplasmic chorioretinitis. In addition, pyrimethamine can be used in combination with clindamycin, atovaquone, or azithromycin if the patient does not tolerate sulfonamide compounds. Corticosteroids appear to be useful in management of ocular complications, central nervous system disease (CSF protein >1000 mg/dL), and focal lesions with substantial mass effects in certain patients.

HIV-infected adolescents and children 6 years of age or older who have completed initial therapy (at least 6 weeks and clinical response) for toxoplasmic encephalitis should receive suppressive therapy (secondary prophylaxis; see Table 3.74, p 727) to prevent recurrence until their CD4+ T-lymphocyte count recovers above 200 cells/μL and their HIV viral load is nondetectable for at least 6 months. HIV-infected children 1 through 5 years of age also should receive suppressive therapy after completion of initial therapy; discontinuation may be considered after they have been on stable antiretroviral therapy (ART) for longer than 6 months, are asymptomatic, and have demonstrated an increase in CD4+ T-lymphocyte percentage above 15% for more than 3 consecutive months. Prophylaxis should be reinstituted whenever these parameters are not met. Regimens for primary treatment also are effective for suppressive therapy.

Secondary prophylaxis with TMP-SMX or atovaquone also is recommended for previously seropositive patients who undergo allogeneic hematopoietic stem cell or bone marrow transplantation. In addition, D+/R- heart transplant recipients also must receive primary prophylaxis with TMP-SMX, atovaquone, or pyrimethamine. For immunocompromised patients without HIV infection, suppressive therapy should be continued lifelong or until the patient no longer is significantly immunosuppressed.

Primary prophylaxis to prevent the first episode of toxoplasmosis generally is recommended for HIV-infected adolescents and children 6 years of age or older who are *T gondii*-seropositive and have CD4+ T-lymphocyte counts less than 100/μL (see Table 3.74, p 727). HIV-infected children 1 through 5 years of age should initiate primary prophylaxis when CD4+ T-lymphocyte percentage falls below 15%. Alternative regimens and recommendations for discontinuation of prophylaxis after CD4+ T-lymphocyte count recovers in association with (ART) are available.[1] TMP-SMX, when administered for *Pneumocystis jirovecii* pneumonia (PCP) prophylaxis, also provides prophylaxis against toxoplasmosis. Atovaquone or dapsone also may provide protection. Children older than 12 months of age who qualify for PCP prophylaxis and who are receiving an agent other than TMP-SMX or atovaquone should have serologic testing for *Toxoplasma* antibodies, because alternative drugs for PCP prophylaxis might not be effective against *Toxoplasma* species. Severely immunosuppressed children who are not receiving TMP-SMX or atovaquone and who are found to be seropositive for *Toxoplasma* infection should receive prophylaxis for both PCP and toxoplasmosis (ie, dapsone plus pyrimethamine).

For symptomatic and asymptomatic congenital infections, pyrimethamine combined with sulfadiazine (supplemented with folinic acid) is recommended as initial therapy. Duration of therapy is prolonged and often is 1 year. However, the optimal dosage and

---

[1] Centers for Disease Control and Prevention. Guidelines for prevention and treatment of opportunistic infections in HIV-infected children and adolescents. Recommendations from the CDC, the National Institutes of Health, and the HIV Medicine Association of the Infectious Diseases Society of America. *MMWR Recomm Rep.* 2009;58(RR-4):1–207

Table 3.74. Prophylaxis to Prevent First Episode and Recurrence of Toxoplasmosis in Children

First episode of toxoplasmosis[a]	Severe immuno-suppression and presence of immunoglobulin G antibody to *Toxoplasma*	Trimethoprim-sulfamethoxazole, 150–750 mg/m^2/day in 2 divided doses, orally, every day	Dapsone (children 1 mo of age or older), 2 mg/kg or 15 mg/m^2 (max 25 mg), orally, every day; **PLUS** pyrimethamine, 1 mg/kg, orally every day (max 25 mg); **PLUS** leucovorin, 5 mg, orally, every 3 days Atovaquone, children 1 through 3 mo or older than 24 mo of age; 30 mg/kg, orally, every day; children 4–24 mo of age: 45 mg/kg, orally, every day
Recurrence of toxoplasmosis[b]	Prior to toxoplasmic encephalitis	Sulfadiazine, 85–120 mg/kg/day (max 2–4 g) in 2–4 divided doses, orally, every day, **PLUS** pyrimeth-amine, 1 mg/kg or 15 mg/m^2 (maximum, 25 mg), orally, every day; **PLUS** leucovorin, 5 mg, orally, every 3 days	Clindamycin, 20–30 mg/kg/day in 3–4 divided doses, orally, every day, **PLUS** pyrimethamine 1 mg/kg, orally, every day (max 25 mg); **PLUS** leucovorin, 5 mg, orally, every 3 days Atovaquone, children 1 through 3 mo or older than 24 mo of age; 30 mg/kg, orally, every day; children 4–24 mo of age: 45 mg/kg, orally, every day

[a]Protection against toxoplasmosis is provided by the preferred antipneumocystis regimen (TMP-SMX) and possibly by atovaquone but not by pentamidine. Atovaquone may be used with or without pyrimethamine. Pyrimethamine alone provides little, if any, protection (for information about severe immunosuppression, see Table 3.52, p 585).
[b]Only pyrimethamine plus sulfadiazine confers protection against *Pneumocystis jirovecii* pneumonia as well as toxoplasmosis. Although the clindamycin plus pyrimethamine regimen is recommended in adults, this regimen has not been tested in children and has been found to have high rates of relapses in adults. However, these drugs are safe and are used for other infections.

duration are not established definitively and should be determined in consultation with an infectious diseases specialist. For children who have mild congenital toxoplasmosis, some experts alternate pyrimethamine/sulfadiazine/folinic acid monthly with spiramycin during months 7 through 12 of treatment. Children with moderate or severe congenital toxoplasmosis should receive pyrimethamine/sulfadiazine for the full 12 months.

Treatment of primary *T gondii* infection in pregnant women, including women with HIV infection, is recommended. Appropriate specialists should be consulted for management. Spiramycin treatment of primary infection during gestation is used in an attempt to decrease transmission of *T gondii* from the mother to the fetus. Spiramycin treatment in pregnant women may reduce congenital transmission but does not treat the fetus if in utero infection has already occurred. Maternal therapy may decrease the severity of sequelae in the fetus once congenital toxoplasmosis has occurred. Spiramycin is available only as an investigational drug in the United States. Spiramycin may be obtained from the manufacturer, at no cost, following the advice of PAMF-TSL and with authorization from the US Food and Drug Administration.[1] If fetal infection is confirmed at or after 18 weeks of gestation or if the mother acquires infection during the third trimester, consideration should be given to starting therapy with pyrimethamine and sulfadiazine.

ISOLATION OF THE HOSPITALIZED PATIENT: Standard precautions are recommended.

CONTROL MEASURES: Pregnant women whose serostatus for *T gondii* is negative or unknown should avoid activities that potentially expose them to cat feces (such as changing litter boxes, gardening, and landscaping), or they should wear gloves and wash their hands if such activities are unavoidable. Daily changing of cat litter will decrease the chance of infection, because oocysts are not infective during the first 1 to 2 days after passage. Domestic cats can be protected from infection by feeding them commercially prepared cat food and preventing them from eating undercooked meat and hunting wild rodents and birds.

Oral ingestion of viable *T gondii* can be avoided by: (1) avoiding consumption of raw or undercooked meat and cooking meat—particularly pork, lamb, and venison—to an internal temperature of 65.5°C to 76.6°C (150°F–170°F [no longer pink]) before consumption (smoked meat and meat cured in brine are not considered safe); (2) freezing meat to −12°C (10°F) for 24 hours; (3) washing fruits and vegetables; (4) washing hands and cleaning kitchen surfaces after handling fruits, vegetables, and raw meat; (5) washing hands after gardening or other contact with soil; (6) preventing contamination of food with raw or undercooked meat or soil; (7) avoiding eating raw shellfish such as oysters, clams, and mussels; and (8) avoiding ingestion of untreated water, particularly in developing countries. All HIV-infected people and pregnant women should be counseled about the various sources of toxoplasmic infection. There currently is no vaccine available for prevention of *T gondii* infection or toxoplasmosis. Additional resources for health care personnel may be found at **www.cdc.gov/parasites/toxocariasis/health_ professionals/index.html.**

Trichinellosis
(Trichinella spiralis)

CLINICAL MANIFESTATIONS: The clinical spectrum of infection ranges from inapparent to fulminant and fatal illness, but most infections are asymptomatic. The severity of disease is proportional to the infective dose. During the first week after ingesting infected meat, a person may experience abdominal discomfort, nausea, vomiting, and/or diarrhea as excysted larvae infect the intestine. Two to 8 weeks later, as progeny larvae migrate into tissues, fever (54%), myalgia (70%), periorbital edema (25%), urticarial rash, and conjunctival and subungual hemorrhages may develop. In severe infections, myocarditis, neurologic involvement, and pneumonitis can follow in 1 or 2 months. Larvae may remain viable in tissues for years; calcification of some larvae in skeletal muscle usually occurs within 6 to 24 months and may be detected on radiographs.

---

[1] US Food and Drug Administration, Division of Special Pathogens and Transplant Drug Products. Telephone: (301) 796-1600; fax: (301) 796-9882

ETIOLOGY: Infection is caused by nematodes (roundworms) of the genus *Trichinella*. At least 5 species capable of infecting only warm-blooded animals have been identified. Worldwide, *Trichinella spiralis* is the most common cause of human infection. The number of cases in the United States has decreased in recent years.

EPIDEMIOLOGY: Infection is enzootic worldwide in carnivores and omnivores, especially scavengers. Infection occurs as a result of ingestion of raw or insufficiently cooked meat containing encysted larvae of *Trichinella* species. Commercial and home-raised pork remain a source of human infections, but meats other than pork, such as venison, horse meat, and particularly meats from wild carnivorous or omnivorous game (bear, boar, seal, and walrus) now are common sources of infection. The disease is not transmitted from person to person.

The **incubation period** usually is less than 1 month.

DIAGNOSTIC TESTS: Eosinophilia approaching 70%, in conjunction with compatible symptoms and dietary history, suggests the diagnosis. Increases in concentrations of muscle enzymes, such as creatinine phosphokinase and lactic dehydrogenase, occur. Identification of larvae in suspect meat can be the most rapid source of diagnostic information. Encapsulated larvae in a skeletal muscle biopsy specimen (particularly deltoid and gastrocnemius) can be visualized microscopically beginning 2 weeks after infection by examining hematoxylin-eosin stained slides or sediment from digested muscle tissue. Serologic tests are available through commercial and state laboratories and the Centers for Disease Control and Prevention. Serum antibody titers rarely become positive before the second week of illness. Testing paired acute and convalescent serum specimens usually is diagnostic.

TREATMENT: Albendazole and mebendazole have comparable efficacy for treatment of trichinellosis (see Drugs for Parasitic Infections, p 848). However, albendazole and mebendazole are less effective for *Trichinella* larvae already in the muscles, and neither drug is approved by the US Food and Drug Administration for trichinellosis. Coadministration of corticosteroids with mebendazole or albendazole often is recommended when systemic symptoms are severe. Corticosteroids can be lifesaving when the central nervous system or heart is involved.

ISOLATION OF THE HOSPITALIZED PATIENT: Standard precautions are recommended.

CONTROL MEASURES: Transmission to pigs can be prevented by not feeding pigs garbage, by preventing cannibalism among animals, and by effective rat control. The public should be educated about the necessity of cooking pork and meat of wild animals thoroughly (>160°F [71°C] internal temperature). Freezing pork less than 6 inches thick at 5°F (−15°C) for 20 days kills *T spiralis*. However, *Trichinella* organisms in wild animals, such as bears and raccoons, are resistant to freezing. People known to have ingested contaminated meat recently should be treated with albendazole (or mebendazole).

Trichomonas vaginalis Infections
(Trichomoniasis)

CLINICAL MANIFESTATIONS: *Trichomonas vaginalis* infection is asymptomatic in up to 90% of infected men and 85% of infected women. Clinical manifestations in symptomatic pubertal or postpubertal female patients consist of a diffuse vaginal discharge, odor, and vulvovaginal pruritus and irritation. Dysuria and, less often, lower abdominal pain can occur. Vaginal discharge usually is yellow-green in color and may have a disagreeable odor. The vulva and vaginal mucosa can be erythematous and even edematous. The cervix can appear inflamed and sometimes is covered with numerous punctate cervical hemorrhages and swollen papillae, referred to as "strawberry" cervix. Clinical manifestations in symptomatic men include urethritis and, more rarely, epididymitis or prostatitis. Reinfection is common, and resistance to treatment is rare but possible. *T vaginalis* infection can increase both the acquisition and transmission of human immunodeficiency virus (HIV).

ETIOLOGY: *T vaginalis* is a flagellated protozoan that is the size of a leukocyte. It requires adherence to host cells for survival. The genome of *T vaginalis* has been sequenced.

EPIDEMIOLOGY: *T vaginalis* infection is the most common "curable" sexually transmitted infection (STI) in the United States and globally and commonly coexists with other conditions, particularly with *Neisseria gonorrhoeae* and *Chlamydia trachomatis* infections and bacterial vaginosis. The presence of *T vaginalis* in a child or preadolescent should raise suspicion of sexual abuse. *T vaginalis* acquired during birth by female newborn infants can cause vaginal discharge during the first weeks of life but usually resolves as maternal hormones are metabolized.

The **incubation period** averages 1 week but ranges from 5 to 28 days.

DIAGNOSTIC TESTS: Diagnosis in a symptomatic female usually is established by careful and immediate examination of a wet-mount preparation of vaginal discharge. The jerky motility of the protozoan and the movement of the flagella are distinctive. Microscopy has 60% to 70% sensitivity for diagnosis of *T vaginalis* in vaginal secretions of a symptomatic female but is less sensitive if she is asymptomatic. The presence of symptoms and the identification of the organism are related directly to the number of organisms. Apart from polymerase chain reaction (not yet approved by the US Food and Drug Administration), culture of the organism is the most sensitive and specific method of diagnosis in females but demonstrates low sensitivity in males. Two point-of-care tests are available when no microscope is available: an immunochromatographic capillary flow dipstick and a nucleic acid probe test. These tests are reported to be more sensitive (79%–83% when compared with culture) than microscopy, but because of specificity of 97% to 99%, these tests may result in more false-positive results in populations with a low prevalence of disease (ie, adolescents). They have not been approved for use in men.

TREATMENT: Treatment of adults with metronidazole (2 g, orally, in a single dose) results in cure rates of approximately 90% to 95%. Treatment with tinidazole (2 g, orally, in a single dose) appears to be similar or even superior to metronidazole. Both drugs are approved for this indication in adults and adolescents, and metronidazole also is approved in children (see Drugs for Parasitic Infections, p 848). Topical vaginal preparations should not be used, because they do not achieve therapeutic concentrations in the urethra or perivaginal glands. Sexual partners should be treated concurrently, even if asymptomatic, because reinfection is a major factor in treatment failures. *T vaginalis* strains with decreased susceptibility to metronidazole have been reported. If treatment failure occurs with metronidazole and reinfection is excluded, either metronidazole (either 250 mg, 3 times daily for 7 days, or 375 mg, 2 times daily for 7 days) or tinidazole (2 g, orally, in a single dose) can be used. If treatment failure occurs with either of these regimens, then either metronidazole (2 g, daily for 5 days) or tinidazole (2 g, daily for 5 days) can be used. In the event of continued treatment failure, consultation with an expert in STIs is advised. Consultation is available from the Centers for Disease Control and Prevention at **www.cdc.gov/std.**

Current recommendations do not include "broader" screening for pregnant women, and if *T vaginalis* infection is diagnosed in asymptomatic pregnant women, some experts recommend waiting to treat until after 37 weeks' gestation. If the pregnant woman is symptomatic, treatment should be considered regardless of week of gestation. Use of metronidazole (2 g, in a single dose) may be used at any stage of pregnancy. Metronidazole is a pregnancy category B drug (animal studies have revealed no evidence of harm to the fetus, but no adequate and well-controlled studies in pregnant women have been conducted). Tinidazole is a pregnancy category C drug (animal studies have demonstrated an adverse effect, and no adequate and well-controlled studies in pregnant women have been conducted), and its safety in pregnant women has not been well evaluated. In lactating women to whom metronidazole is administered, withholding breastfeeding during treatment and for 12 to 24 hours after the last dose will reduce the exposure of metronidazole to the infant. While using tinidazole, interruption of breastfeeding is recommended during treatment and for 3 days after the last dose.

People infected with *T vaginalis* should be evaluated for other STIs, including syphilis, gonorrhea, chlamydia, and HIV infection. For newborn infants, infection with *T vaginalis* acquired maternally is self-limited, and treatment generally is not recommended.

ISOLATION OF THE HOSPITALIZED PATIENT: Standard precautions are recommended.

CONTROL MEASURES: Measures to prevent STIs, particularly the consistent and correct use of condoms, are indicated. Patients should be instructed to avoid sexual activity until they and their sexual partners are treated and asymptomatic. In states where it is allowed, patient-delivered partner treatment should be offered (**www.cdc.gov/std/ept/**).

Trichuriasis
(Whipworm Infection)

CLINICAL MANIFESTATIONS: Disease is proportional to the intensity of the infection. Most infected children are asymptomatic. Children with heavy infestations can develop *Trichuris trichiura* colitis that mimics inflammatory bowel disease and leads to anemia, physical growth restriction, and clubbing. *T trichiura* dysentery syndrome is more intense and consists of abdominal pain, tenesmus, and bloody diarrhea with mucus; it can be associated with rectal prolapse.

ETIOLOGY: *T trichiura*, the human whipworm, is the causative agent. Adult worms are 30 to 50 mm long with a large, thread-like anterior end that is embedded in the mucosa of the large intestine.

EPIDEMIOLOGY: The parasite is the second most common soil-transmitted helminth in the world and is more common in the tropics and in areas of poor sanitation. It is coendemic with ascaris and hookworm species. Humans are the natural reservoir. In the United States, trichuriasis no longer is a public health problem, although migrants from tropical areas may be infected. Eggs require a minimum of 10 days of incubation in the soil before they are infectious. The disease is not communicable from person to person.

The **incubation period** is approximately 12 weeks.

DIAGNOSTIC TESTS: Eggs may be found on direct examination of stool or, preferably, by using concentration techniques.

TREATMENT: Mebendazole, albendazole, or ivermectin administered for 3 days provide moderate rates of cure, with mebendazole being the treatment of choice. In mass treatment efforts involving entire communities, a single dose of either mebendazole (500 mg) or albendazole (400 mg) will reduce worm burdens (see Drugs for Parasitic Infections, p 848). In 1-year-old children, the World Health Organization recommends reducing the albendazole dose to half of that given to older children and adults for single-dose and 3-day treatment. Albendazole and ivermectin are not approved by the US Food and Drug Administration for treatment of trichuriasis. Reexamination of stool specimens 2 weeks after therapy to determine whether the worms have been eliminated is helpful for assessing therapy.

ISOLATION OF THE HOSPITALIZED PATIENT: Only standard precautions are recommended, because there is no direct person-to-person transmission.

CONTROL MEASURES: Proper disposal of fecal material is indicated. Mass treatment of infected school-aged populations can reduce whipworm transmission in communities with endemic infection.

African Trypanosomiasis
(African Sleeping Sickness)

CLINICAL MANIFESTATIONS: The disease appears in 2 stages: the first is the hemolymphatic stage, and the second is the meningoencephalitis stage, which is characterized by invasion of the central nervous system. The rapidity and severity of clinical manifestations vary with the infecting subspecies. With *Trypanosoma brucei gambiense* (West African) infection, a cutaneous nodule or chancre may appear at the site of parasite inoculation within a few days of a bite by an infected tsetse fly. Systemic illness is chronic, occurring months to years later, and is characterized by intermittent fever, posterior cervical lymphadenopathy (Winterbottom sign), and multiple nonspecific complaints, including malaise, weight loss, arthralgia, rash, pruritus, and edema. If the central nervous system (CNS) is involved, chronic meningoencephalitis with behavioral changes, cachexia, headache, hallucinations, delusions, and somnolence can occur. In contrast, *Trypanosoma brucei rhodesiense* (East African) infection is an acute, generalized illness that develops days to weeks after parasite inoculation, with manifestations including high fever, thrombocytopenia, hepatitis, cutaneous chancre, anemia, myocarditis, and rarely, laboratory evidence of disseminated intravascular coagulopathy. Clinical meningoencephalitis can develop as early as 3 weeks after onset of the untreated systemic illness. Both forms of African trypanosomiasis have high fatality rates; without treatment, infected patients usually die within weeks to months after clinical onset of disease caused by *T brucei rhodesiense* and within a few years from disease caused by *T brucei gambiense*.

ETIOLOGY: Human African trypanosomiasis (sleeping sickness) occurs in sub-Saharan Africa. It is caused by the protozoan parasite *Trypanosoma brucei*, transmitted by blood-feeding tsetse flies. The west and central African (Gambian) form is endemic and is caused by *T brucei gambiense*. The east and southern African (Rhodesian) form is more acute and is caused by *T brucei rhodesiense*. Both are extracellular protozoan hemoflagellates that live in blood and tissue of the human host. The genome of *T brucei* has been sequenced.

EPIDEMIOLOGY: Approximately 10 000 human cases are reported annually worldwide, although only a few cases, which are acquired in Africa, are reported every year in the United States. Transmission is confined to an area in Africa between the latitudes of 15° north and 20° south, corresponding precisely with the distribution of the tsetse fly vector (*Glossina* species). In East Africa, wild animals, such as antelope, bush buck, and hartebeest, constitute the major reservoirs for sporadic infections with *T brucei rhodesiense*, although cattle serve as reservoir hosts in local outbreaks. Domestic pigs and dogs have been found as incidental reservoirs of *T brucei gambiense;* however, humans are the only important reservoir in West and Central Africa.

The **incubation period** for *T brucei rhodesiense* infection is 3 to 21 days and usually is 5 to 14 days; for *T brucei gambiense* infection, the incubation period usually is longer but is not well defined.

DIAGNOSTIC TESTS: Diagnosis is made by identification of trypomastigotes in specimens of blood, cerebrospinal fluid (CSF), or fluid aspirated from a chancre or lymph node or by inoculation of susceptible laboratory animals (mice) with heparinized blood. Examination of CSF is critical to management and should be performed using the double-centrifugation technique. Concentration and Giemsa staining of the buffy coat layer of peripheral blood also can be helpful and is easier for *T brucei rhodesiense*, because the density of organisms in blood circulating is higher than for *T brucei gambiense*. *T brucei gambiense* is more likely to be found in lymph node aspirates. Although an increased concentration of immunoglobulin M in serum or CSF is considered characteristic of African trypanosomiasis, polyclonal hyperglobulinemia is common. There is no serologic screening test for *T brucei rhodesiense*.

TREATMENT: When no evidence of CNS involvement is present (including absence of trypanosomes and CSF pleocytosis), the drug of choice for the acute hemolymphatic stage of infection is pentamidine for *T brucei gambiense* infection and suramin for *T brucei rhodesiense* infection. For treatment of infection with CNS involvement, the drug of choice is eflornithine for *T brucei gambiense* infection and melarsoprol for *T brucei rhodesiense* infection. Suramin, eflornithine, and melarsoprol can be obtained from the Centers for Disease Control and Prevention Drug Service (404-639-3670). For specific dosing recommendations, see Drugs for Parasitic Infections (p 848). Because of the risk of relapse, patients who have had CNS involvement should undergo repeated CSF examinations every 6 months for 2 years.

ISOLATION OF THE HOSPITALIZED PATIENT: Standard precautions are recommended.

CONTROL MEASURES: Travelers to areas with endemic infection should avoid known foci of sleeping sickness and tsetse fly infestation and minimize fly bites by the use of protective clothing. Infected patients should not breastfeed or donate blood. Elimination of this disease might be possible with national vector-control programs to reduce the number of tsetse flies in existing foci.

American Trypanosomiasis
(Chagas Disease)

CLINICAL MANIFESTATIONS: The acute phase of *Trypanosoma cruzi* infection lasts 2 to 3 months, followed by the chronic phase, which, in the absence of successful antiparasitic treatment, lasts life-long. The acute phase commonly is asymptomatic or characterized by mild, nonspecific symptoms. Young children are more likely to exhibit symptoms than are adults. In some patients, a red, indurated nodule known as a *chagoma* develops at the site of the original inoculation, usually on the face or arms. Unilateral edema of the eyelids, known as the Romaña sign, may occur if the portal of entry was the conjunctiva; it is not always present. The edematous skin may be violaceous and associated with conjunctivitis and enlargement of the ipsilateral preauricular lymph node. Fever, malaise, generalized lymphadenopathy, and hepatosplenomegaly may develop. In rare instances, acute myocarditis and/or meningoencephalitis can occur. The symptoms of acute Chagas disease resolve without treatment within 3 months, and patients pass into the chronic phase of the infection. Most people with chronic *T cruzi* infection have no signs or symptoms and are said to have the indeterminate form. In 20% to 30% of cases, serious progressive sequelae affecting the heart and/or gastrointestinal tract develop years to decades after the initial infection (sometimes called determinate forms of chronic *T cruzi* infection). Chagas cardiomyopathy is characterized by conduction system abnormalities, especially right bundle branch block, and ventricular arrhythmias and may progress to dilated cardiomyopathy and congestive heart failure. Patients with Chagas cardiomyopathy may die suddenly from ventricular arrhythmias, complete heart block, or emboli phenomena; death also may occur from intractable congestive heart failure. Congenital Chagas disease may be characterized by low birth weight, hepatosplenomegaly, myocarditis, and/or meningoencephalitis with seizures and tremors, but most infants with congenital *T cruzi* infection have no signs or symptoms of disease. Reactivation of chronic *T cruzi* infection may occur in immunocompromised people, including people infected with human immunodeficiency virus and those who are immunosuppressed after transplantation.

ETIOLOGY: *T cruzi*, a protozoan hemoflagellate, is the cause.

EPIDEMIOLOGY: Parasites are transmitted in feces of infected triatomine insects (sometimes called "kissing bugs"; local Spanish names include *vinchuca, chinche picuda*). The bugs defecate during or after taking blood. The bitten person is inoculated through inadvertently rubbing the insect feces containing the parasite into the site of the bite or mucous membranes of the eye or the mouth. The parasite also can be transmitted congenitally, during solid organ transplantation, through blood transfusion, and by ingestion of food or drink contaminated by the vector's excreta. Accidental laboratory infections can result from handling parasite cultures or blood from infected people or laboratory animals, usually through needlestick injuries. Vectorborne transmission of the disease is limited to the Western hemisphere, predominantly Mexico and Central and South America. The southern United States has established enzootic cycles of *T cruzi* involving several triatomine vector species and mammalian hosts, such as raccoons, opossums, rodents, and domestic dogs. Nevertheless, most *T cruzi*-infected individuals in the United States are immigrants from areas of Latin America with endemic infection.

Several transfusion- and transplantation-associated cases have been documented in the United States. The disease is an important cause of morbidity and death in Latin America, where an estimated 8 to 10 million people are infected, of whom 30% to 40% either have or will develop cardiomyopathy.

The **incubation period** for the acute phase of disease is 1 to 2 weeks or longer. Chronic manifestations do not appear for years to decades.

DIAGNOSTIC TESTS: During the acute phase of disease, the parasite is demonstrable in blood specimens by Giemsa staining after a concentration technique or in direct wet-mount or buffy coat preparations. Molecular techniques and hemoculture in special media (available at the Centers for Disease Control and Prevention [CDC]) also have high sensitivity in the acute phase. The chronic phase of *T cruzi* infection is characterized by low-level parasitemia; the sensitivity of culture and polymerase chain reaction (PCR) generally is less than 50%. Diagnosis in the chronic phase relies on serologic tests to demonstrate immunoglobulin (Ig) G antibodies against *T cruzi*. Serologic tests to detect anti-*T cruzi* IgG antibodies include indirect immunofluorescent and enzyme immunosorbent assays. The Pan American Health Organization and the World Health Organization recommend that samples be tested in 2 assays based on different formats before diagnostic decisions are made. Two blood donor screening assays (Ortho *T cruzi* test system and the Abbott Prism Chagas assay) have been approved by the US Food and Drug Administration for blood donor screening. Confirmation of positive serologic test by Radioimmune Precipitation Assay (Chagas RIPA) or an in vitro enzyme strip assay (Abbott ESA Chagas [*T cruzi* {*E coli* recombinant} antigen]) is recommended.

The diagnosis of congenital Chagas disease can be made during the first 3 months of life by identification of motile trypomastigotes by direct microscopy of fresh anticoagulated blood specimens. PCR assay has higher sensitivity than microscopy. All infants born to seropositive mothers should be screened using conventional serologic testing after 9 months of age, when IgG measurements reflect infant response. Diagnostic testing and consultation are available from the CDC Division of Parasitic Diseases and Malaria (phone: 770-488-7775; e-mail: parasites@cdc.gov; CDC Emergency Operator [after business hours and on weekends]: 770-488-7100).

TREATMENT: Antitrypanosomal treatment is recommended for all cases of acute and congenital Chagas disease, reactivated infection, and chronic *T cruzi*-infection in children younger than 18 years of age. Treatment of chronic *T cruzi* infection in adults without advanced cardiomyopathy also generally is recommended. The only drugs with proven efficacy are benznidazole and nifurtimox (see Drugs for Parasitic Infections, p 848). Both drugs can be obtained from the CDC Drug Service (404-639-3670).

ISOLATION OF THE HOSPITALIZED PATIENT: Standard precautions should be followed.

CONTROL MEASURES: Risk to travelers is low. Travelers to areas with endemic infection should avoid contact with triatomine bugs by avoiding habitation in buildings vulnerable to infestation, particularly those constructed of mud, palm thatch, or adobe brick. The use of insecticide-impregnated bed nets also may be beneficial. Camping or sleeping outdoors in areas with endemic transmission is not recommended. Diagnostic testing should be performed on members of households with an infected patient if they have had exposure to the vector similar to that of the patient. All children of women with *T cruzi* infection should be tested for Chagas disease.

Education about the mode of spread and methods of prevention is warranted in areas with endemic infection. Homes should be examined for the presence of the vectors, and if found, measures to eliminate the vector should be taken.

Since 2006, the FDA has approved 2 tests to detect antibodies to *T cruzi* in donated blood. The American Red Cross and Blood Systems Inc voluntarily began screening all blood donations in January 2007. In December 2010, the FDA issued final guidance recommending appropriate use of serologic tests to reduce the risk of transfusion-transmitted *T cruzi* infection (**www.fda.gov/BiologicsBloodVaccines/GuidanceCompliance RegulatoryInformation/Guidances/Blood/ucm235855.htm**).

Tuberculosis

CLINICAL MANIFESTATIONS: Tuberculosis disease is caused by infection with organisms of the *Mycobacterium tuberculosis* complex, which includes *M tuberculosis, Mycobacterium bovis,* and *Mycobacterium africanum. M africanum* is rare in the United States, and clinical laboratories do not distinguish it routinely. *M bovis* can be distinguished routinely from *M tuberculosis,* and although the spectrum of illness that is caused by *M bovis* is similar to that of *M tuberculosis,* the epidemiology, treatment, and prevention are distinct. Most infections caused by *M tuberculosis* complex in children and adolescents are asymptomatic. When tuberculosis disease does occur, clinical manifestations most often appear 1 to 6 months after infection and include fever, weight loss, or poor weight gain and possibly growth delay, cough, night sweats, and chills. Chest radiographic findings after infection range from normal to diverse abnormalities, such as lymphadenopathy of the hilar, subcarinal, paratracheal, or mediastinal nodes; atelectasis or infiltrate of a segment or lobe; pleural effusion; cavitary lesions; or miliary disease. Extrapulmonary manifestations include meningitis and granulomatous inflammation of the lymph nodes, bones, joints, skin, and middle ear and mastoid. Gastrointestinal tuberculosis can mimic inflammatory bowel disease. Renal tuberculosis and progression to disease from latent tuberculosis infection ("adult-type pulmonary tuberculosis") are unusual in younger children but can occur in adolescents. In addition, chronic abdominal pain with intermittent partial intestinal obstruction can be present in disease caused by *M bovis.* Clinical findings in patients with drug-resistant tuberculosis disease are indistinguishable from manifestations in patients with drug-susceptible disease.

ETIOLOGY: The agent is *M tuberculosis* complex, a group of closely related acid-fast bacilli (AFB): *M tuberculosis, M bovis,* and *M africanum.*

Definitions:

- **Positive tuberculin skin test (TST).** A positive TST result (see Table 3.75, p 737) indicates possible infection with *M tuberculosis* complex. Tuberculin reactivity appears 2 to 10 weeks after initial infection; the median interval is 3 to 4 weeks (see Tuberculin Testing, p 740).
- **Positive interferon-gamma release assay (IGRA).** A positive IGRA result indicates possible infection with *M tuberculosis* complex.
- **Exposed person** refers to a person who has had recent contact with another person with suspected or confirmed contagious pulmonary tuberculosis disease and who has a negative TST or IGRA result, normal physical examination findings, and chest radiographic findings that are not compatible with tuberculosis. Some exposed people

Table 3.75. Definitions of Positive Tuberculin Skin Test (TST) Results in Infants, Children, and Adolescents[a]

Induration 5 mm or greater

Children in close contact with known or suspected contagious people with tuberculosis disease

Children suspected to have tuberculosis disease:
- Findings on chest radiograph consistent with active or previous tuberculosis disease
- Clinical evidence of tuberculosis disease[b]

Children receiving immunosuppressive therapy[c] or with immunosuppressive conditions, including human immunodeficiency (HIV) infection

Induration 10 mm or greater

Children at increased risk of disseminated tuberculosis disease:
- Children younger than 4 years of age
- Children with other medical conditions, including Hodgkin disease, lymphoma, diabetes mellitus, chronic renal failure, or malnutrition (see Table 3.76, p 740)

Children with likelihood of increased exposure to tuberculosis disease:
- Children born in high-prevalence regions of the world
- Children who travel to high-prevalence regions of the world
- Children frequently exposed to adults who are HIV infected, homeless, users of illicit drugs, residents of nursing homes, incarcerated or institutionalized

Induration 15 mm or greater

Children age 4 years or older without any risk factors

[a] These definitions apply regardless of previous bacille Calmette-Guérin (BCG) immunization (see also Interpretation of TST Results in Previous Recipients of BCG Vaccine, p 742); erythema alone at TST site does not indicate a positive test result. Tests should be read at 48 to 72 hours after placement.

[b] Evidence by physical examination or laboratory assessment that would include tuberculosis in the working differential diagnosis (eg, meningitis).

[c] Including immunosuppressive doses of corticosteroids (see Corticosteroids, p 752) or tumor necrosis factor-alpha antagonists (see Biologic Response Modifiers, p 82).

become infected (and subsequently, develop a positive TST or IGRA result); others do not become infected after exposure; the 2 groups cannot be distinguished initially.

- **Source case** is defined as the person who has transmitted infection with *M tuberculosis* complex to another person who subsequently has either latent tuberculosis infection (LTBI) or tuberculosis disease.
- **LTBI** is defined as *M tuberculosis* complex infection in a person who has a positive TST or IGRA result, no physical findings of disease, and chest radiograph findings that are normal or reveal evidence of healed infection (eg, calcification in the lung, hilar lymph nodes, or both).
- **Tuberculosis disease** is defined as disease in a person with infection in whom symptoms, signs, or radiographic manifestations caused by *M tuberculosis* complex are apparent; disease may be pulmonary, extrapulmonary, or both. Infectious tuberculosis refers to tuberculosis disease of the lungs or larynx in a person who has the potential to transmit the infection to other people.
- **Directly observed therapy (DOT)** is defined as an intervention by which medication is administered directly to the patient by a health care professional or trained third party (not a relative or friend) who observes and documents that the patient ingests each dose of medication.

- **Multiply drug-resistant (MDR) tuberculosis** is defined as tuberculosis infection or disease caused by a strain of *M tuberculosis* complex that is resistant to at least isoniazid and rifampin, the 2 first-line drugs with greatest efficacy.
- **Extensively drug-resistant (XDR) tuberculosis** is a subset of MDR tuberculosis. It is defined as infection or disease caused by a strain of *M tuberculosis* complex that is resistant to isoniazid and rifampin, at least 1 fluoroquinolone, and at least 1 of the following parenteral drugs: amikacin, kanamycin, or capreomycin.
- **Bacille Calmette-Guérin (BCG)** is an attenuated live vaccine strain of *M bovis*. BCG vaccine rarely is administered to children in the United States but probably is one of the most widely used vaccines in the world. An isolate of BCG can be distinguished from wild-type *M bovis* only in a reference laboratory.

EPIDEMIOLOGY: Case rates of tuberculosis for all ages are higher in urban, low-income areas and in nonwhite racial and ethnic groups; 80% of reported cases in the United States occur in Hispanic and nonwhite people. In recent years, foreign-born children have accounted for more than one quarter of newly diagnosed cases in children age 14 years or younger. Specific groups with greater LTBI and disease rates include immigrants, international adoptees, and refugees from or travelers to high-prevalence regions (eg, Asia, Africa, Latin America, and countries of the former Soviet Union); homeless people; and residents of correctional facilities.

Infants and postpubertal adolescents are at increased risk of progression of LTBI to tuberculosis disease. Other predictive factors for development of disease include recent infection (within the past 2 years); immunodeficiency, especially from human immunodeficiency virus (HIV) infection; use of immunosuppressive drugs, such as prolonged or high-dose corticosteroid therapy or chemotherapy; intravenous drug use; and certain diseases or medical conditions, including Hodgkin disease, lymphoma, diabetes mellitus, chronic renal failure, and malnutrition. There have been reports of tuberculosis disease in adolescents and adults being treated for arthritis, inflammatory bowel disease, and other conditions with tumor necrosis factor-alpha (TNF-alpha) antagonists, such as infliximab and etanercept. Before use of TNF-alpha antagonists, patients should be screened for risk factors for *M tuberculosis* complex infection and have a TST or IGRA performed before the initiation of systemic steroids, antimetabolite agents, or these monoclonal antibodies.

A diagnosis of LTBI or tuberculosis disease in a young child is a public health sentinel event usually representing recent transmission. Transmission of *M tuberculosis* complex is airborne, with inhalation of droplet nuclei usually produced by an adult or adolescent with contagious pulmonary or laryngeal tuberculosis disease. *M bovis* is transmitted most often by unpasteurized dairy products, but airborne transmission can occur. The duration of contagiousness of an adult receiving effective treatment depends on drug susceptibilities of the organism, the number of organisms in sputum, and frequency of cough. Although contagiousness usually lasts only a few days to weeks after initiation of effective drug therapy, it can last longer, especially when the adult patient has cavitary disease, does not adhere to medical therapy, or is infected with a drug-resistant strain. If the sputum smear is negative for AFB organisms on 3 separate specimens at least 8 hours apart and the patient has improved clinically with resolution of cough, the treated person can be considered at low risk of disease transmission. Children younger than age 10 years of age with pulmonary tuberculosis rarely are contagious, because their pulmonary lesions are small (paucibacillary disease), cough is nonproductive, and few or no bacilli are expelled. Unusual cases of adult-form pulmonary disease in young children and cases of congenital tuberculosis can be highly contagious.

The **incubation period** from infection to development of a positive TST or IGRA result is 2 to 10 weeks. The risk of developing tuberculosis disease is highest during the 6 months after infection and remains high for 2 years; however, many years can elapse between initial tuberculosis infection and tuberculosis disease.

DIAGNOSTIC TESTS: Laboratory isolation of *M tuberculosis* complex by culture from specimens of gastric aspirates, sputum, bronchial washings, pleural fluid, cerebrospinal fluid (CSF), urine, or other body fluids or a tissue biopsy specimen establishes the diagnosis. Children older than 5 years of age and adolescents frequently can produce sputum spontaneously or by induction with aerosolized hypertonic saline. Studies have demonstrated successful collections of induced sputum from infants with pulmonary tuberculosis, but this requires special expertise. The best specimen for diagnosis of pulmonary tuberculosis in any child or adolescent in whom the cough is absent or nonproductive and sputum cannot be induced is an early-morning gastric aspirate. Gastric aspirate specimens should be obtained with a nasogastric tube on awakening the child and before ambulation or feeding.[1] Aspirates collected on 3 separate days should be submitted for testing. Results of AFB smears of gastric aspirates usually are negative, and false-positive smear results caused by the presence of nontuberculous mycobacteria can occur. Gastric aspirates have the highest culture yield in young children on the first day of collection. Fluorescent staining methods for gastric aspirate smears are more sensitive than AFB smears and, if available, are preferred. The overall diagnostic yield of gastric aspirates is less than 50%. Histologic examination for and demonstration of AFB and granulomas in biopsy specimens from lymph node, pleura, mesentery, liver, bone marrow, or other tissues can be useful, but *M tuberculosis* complex organisms cannot be distinguished reliably from other mycobacteria in stained specimens. Regardless of results of the AFB smears, each specimen should be cultured.

Because *M tuberculosis* complex organisms are slow growing, detection of these organisms may take as long as 10 weeks using solid media; use of liquid media allows detection within 1 to 6 weeks and usually within 3 weeks. Even with optimal culture techniques, *M tuberculosis* complex organisms are isolated from fewer than 50% of children and 75% of infants with pulmonary tuberculosis diagnosed by other clinical criteria. Species identification of isolates from culture can be more rapid if a DNA probe or high-pressure liquid chromatography is used. The differentiation between *M tuberculosis* and *M bovis* usually is based on pyrazinamide resistance, which is characteristic of almost all *M bovis* isolates.

One nucleic acid amplification test (NAAT) for rapid diagnosis is approved by the Food and Drug Administration (FDA) for acid-fast stain positive respiratory tract specimens only, and another NAAT is approved for any respiratory tract specimens. These NAATs have decreased sensitivity for gastric aspirate, CSF, and tissue specimens, with false-negative and false-positive results reported. Further research is needed before NAATs can be recommended for the diagnosis of extrapulmonary tuberculosis or pulmonary tuberculosis in children who cannot produce sputum.

---

[1] **www.nationaltbcenter.ucsf.edu/catalogue/epub/index.cfm?tableName=GAP**

Identification of the culture-positive source case supports the child's presumptive diagnosis and provides the likely drug susceptibility of the child's organism. Culture material should be collected from children with evidence of tuberculosis disease, especially when (1) an isolate from a source case is not available; (2) the presumed source case has drug-resistant tuberculosis; (3) the child is immunocompromised (eg, HIV infection); or (4) the child has extrapulmonary disease. Drug resistance cannot be confirmed without a bacterial isolate.

Testing for M tuberculosis ***Infection.*** The TST is the most common method for diagnosing LTBI in asymptomatic people. The Mantoux method consists of 5 tuberculin units of purified protein derivative (0.1 mL) injected intradermally using a 27-gauge needle and a 1.0-mL syringe into the volar aspect of the forearm. Creation of a palpable induration 6 to 10 mm in diameter is crucial to accurate testing. Multiple puncture tests are not recommended, because they lack adequate sensitivity and specificity.

A TST should be performed in children who are at increased risk of infection with *M tuberculosis* (see Table 3.76). Routine TST performance, including programs based at schools, child care centers, and camps that include populations at low risk, is discouraged, because it results in either a low yield of positive results or a large proportion of false-positive results, leading to an inefficient use of health care resources. Simple questionnaires

Table 3.76. Tuberculin Skin Test (TST) Recommendations for Infants, Children, and Adolescents[a]

Children for whom immediate TST or IGRA is indicated[b]:
- Contacts of people with confirmed or suspected contagious tuberculosis (contact investigation)
- Children with radiographic or clinical findings suggesting tuberculosis disease
- Children immigrating from countries with endemic infection (eg, Asia, Middle East, Africa, Latin America, countries of the former Soviet Union), including international adoptees
- Children with travel histories to countries with endemic infection and substantial contact with indigenous people from such countries[c]

Children who should have annual TST or IGRA:
- Children infected with HIV infection (TST only)

Children at increased risk of progression of LTBI to tuberculosis disease: Children with other medical conditions, including diabetes mellitus, chronic renal failure, malnutrition, congenital or acquired immunodeficiencies, and children receiving tumor necrosis factor (TNF) antagonists deserve special consideration. Without recent exposure, these people are not at increased risk of acquiring tuberculosis infection. Underlying immune deficiencies associated with these conditions theoretically would enhance the possibility for progression to severe disease. Initial histories of potential exposure to tuberculosis should be included for all of these patients. If these histories or local epidemiologic factors suggest a possibility of exposure, immediate and periodic TST or IGRA should be considered. **An initial TST or IGRA should be performed before initiation of immunosuppressive therapy, including prolonged steroid administration, use of TNF-alpha antagonists, or other immunosuppressive therapy in any child requiring these treatments.**

IGRA indicates interferon-gamma release assay; HIV, human immunodeficiency virus; LTBI, latent tuberculosis infection.
[a] Bacille Calmette-Guérin immunization is not a contraindication to a TST.
[b] Beginning as early as 3 months of age.
[c] If the child is well and has no history of exposure, the TST or IGRA should be delayed for up to 10 weeks after return.

can identify children with risk factors for LTBI who then should have a TST performed (see Table 3.77, p 741). Risk assessment for tuberculosis should be performed at first contact with a child and every 6 months thereafter for the first year of life (eg, 2 weeks and 6 and 12 months of age). If, at any time, tuberculosis disease is suspected, a TST should be performed, although a negative result should be considered as especially unreliable in infants younger than 3 months of age. After 1 year of age, risk assessment for tuberculosis should be performed annually, if possible.

Recommendations for use of the TST are independent of those for immunization. Tuberculin testing at any age is not required before administration of live-virus vaccines. Measles vaccine temporarily can suppress tuberculin reactivity for at least 4 to 6 weeks. A TST can be applied at the same visit during which these vaccines are administered. The effect of live-virus varicella, yellow fever, and live-attenuated influenza vaccines on TST reactivity and IGRA results is not known. In the absence of data, the same TST spacing recommendation should be applied to these vaccines as described for measles-mumps-rubella (MMR) vaccine. There is no evidence that inactivated vaccines, polysaccharide vaccines, or recombinant or subunit vaccines or toxoids interfere with immune response to TST.

Administration of TSTs and interpretation of results should be performed by experienced health care professionals who have been trained in the proper methods, because administration and interpretation by unskilled people and family members are unreliable. The recommended time for assessing the TST result is 48 to 72 hours after administration. However, induration that develops at the site of administration more than 72 hours later should be measured, and some experts advise that this should be considered the result. The diameter of induration in millimeters is measured transversely to the long axis of the forearm. Positive TST results, as defined in Table 3.75, can persist for several weeks.

A negative TST result does not exclude LTBI or tuberculosis disease. Approximately 10% to 40% of immunocompetent children with culture-documented tuberculosis disease do not react initially to a TST. Host factors, such as young age, poor nutrition, immunosuppression, other viral infections (especially measles, varicella, and influenza), recent tuberculosis infection, and disseminated tuberculosis disease can decrease TST reactivity. Many children and adults coinfected with HIV and *M tuberculosis* complex do not react to a TST. Control skin tests to assess cutaneous anergy are not recommended routinely.

Interpretation of TST Results (see Table 3.75, p 737). Classification of TST results is based on epidemiologic and clinical factors. The size of induration (mm) for a positive result varies with the person's risk of LTBI and progression to tuberculosis disease.

Table 3.77. Validated Questions for Determining Risk of LTBI in Children in the United States

- Has a family member or contact had tuberculosis disease?
- Has a family member had a positive tuberculin skin test result?
- Was your child born in a high-risk country (countries other than the United States, Canada, Australia, New Zealand, or Western and North European countries)?
- Has your child traveled (had contact with resident populations) to a high-risk country for more than 1 week?

LTBI indicates latent tuberculosis infection.

Interpretation is aided by knowledge of the child's risk factors for LTBI and tuberculosis disease and is summarized in Table 3.75 (p 737). Current guidelines from the Centers for Disease Control and Prevention (CDC), American Thoracic Society, and American Academy of Pediatrics accept 15 mm or greater of induration as a positive TST result for any person who has not received BCG vaccine. Prompt clinical and radiographic evaluation of all children and adolescents with a positive TST reaction is recommended.

Interpretation of TST Results in Previous Recipients of BCG Vaccine. Generally, interpretation of TST results in BCG recipients who are known contacts of a person with tuberculosis disease or at high risk for tuberculosis disease is the same as for people who have not received BCG vaccine. After BCG immunization, distinguishing between a positive TST result caused by pathogenic *M tuberculosis* complex infection and that caused by BCG is difficult. Reactivity of the TST after receipt of BCG vaccine does not occur in some patients. The size of the TST reaction (ie, mm of induration) attributable to BCG immunization depends on many factors, including age at BCG immunization, quality and strain of BCG vaccine used, number of doses of BCG vaccine received, nutritional and immunologic status of the vaccine recipient, frequency of TST administration, and time lapse between immunization and TST. Because IGRAs do not cross-react with BGC, an IGRA is the preferred test by many experts for the diagnosis of LTBI in a BCG-immunized child older than 4 years of age.

Tuberculosis disease should be suspected strongly in any symptomatic person regardless of a TST or IGRA result and history of BCG immunization. When evaluating an asymptomatic child who has a positive TST result and who possibly received BCG vaccine, certain factors, such as documented receipt of multiple BCG immunizations (as evidenced by BCG scars), decrease the likelihood that the positive TST result is attributable to LTBI. Evidence that increases the probability that a positive TST result is attributable to LTBI includes known contact with a person with contagious tuberculosis, a family history of tuberculosis disease, a long interval (more than 5 years) since neonatal BCG immunization, and a TST reaction 15 mm or greater.

Prompt clinical and radiographic evaluation of all children with a positive TST reaction is recommended. Chest radiographic findings of a granuloma, calcification, or adenopathy can be caused by infection with *M tuberculosis* complex but not by BCG immunization. BCG can cause suppurative lymphadenitis in the regional lymph node drainage of the infectious site of a healthy child and can cause disseminated disease in children with some forms of immunodeficiency.

Recommendations for TST Use. The most reliable strategies for preventing LTBI and tuberculosis disease in children are based on thorough and expedient contact investigations rather than nonselective skin testing of large populations. Contact investigations are public-health interventions that should be coordinated through the local public health department. Specific recommendations for TST use are given in Table 3.76 (p 740). All children need routine health care evaluations that include an assessment of their risk of exposure to tuberculosis. Only children deemed to have increased risk of contact with people with contagious tuberculosis or children with suspected tuberculosis disease should be considered for a TST. Household investigation is indicated whenever a TST result of a household member converts from negative to positive (indicating recent infection).

Immunologic-Based Testing.[1] QuantiFERON-TB Gold, T-SPOT.TB, and Gold In-Tube are IGRAs and are the preferred tests in asymptomatic children older than 4 years of age who have been immunized against BCG. These FDA-approved tests measure ex vivo interferon-gamma production from T lymphocytes in response to stimulation with antigens that are fairly specific to *M tuberculosis* complex. As with TSTs, IGRAs cannot distinguish between latent infection and disease, and a negative result from these tests cannot exclude the possibility of tuberculosis disease in a patient with findings that raise suspicion for these conditions. The sensitivity of these blood IGRA tests is similar to that of TSTs for detecting infection in adults and children who have untreated culture-confirmed tuberculosis. The specificity of IGRAs is higher than that for TSTs, because the antigens used are not found in BCG or most pathogenic nontuberculous mycobacteria (eg, are not found in *M avium* complex but are found in *Mycobacterium kansasii*, *Mycobacterium szulgai*, and *Mycobacterium marinum*). IGRAs are recommended by the CDC, and some experts prefer IGRAs for use in adults in all circumstances in which a TST would have been used. The published experience testing children with IGRAs is less extensive than for adults, but a number of studies have demonstrated that IGRAs perform well in children 5 years of age and older. Some children who received BCG vaccine can have a false-positive TST result, and LTBI is overestimated by use of the TST in these circumstances. The negative predictive value of IGRAs is not clear, but in general, if the IGRA result is negative and the TST result is positive in an asymptomatic child, the diagnosis of LTBI is unlikely.

At this time, neither an IGRA nor the TST can be considered a "gold standard" for diagnosis of LTBI. Current recommendations for use of IGRAs in children are in Table 3.78:

- Children with a positive result from an IGRA should be considered infected with *M tuberculosis* complex. A negative IGRA result cannot be interpreted universally as absence of infection.
- Indeterminate IGRA results do not exclude tuberculosis infection and may necessitate repeat testing and should not be used to make clinical decisions.

Serologic tests for tuberculosis disease are not recommended; although they are used in some Asian and African countries, they have unsatisfactory sensitivity and specificity, and none of them have been approved for use in the United States.

HIV Infection. Children with HIV infection are considered at high risk of tuberculosis, and an annual TST beginning at 3 through 12 months of age is recommended or, if older, when HIV infection is diagnosed. Children who have tuberculosis disease should be tested for HIV infection.

TREATMENT (SEE TABLE 3.79, P 745):

Specific Drugs. Antituberculosis drugs kill *M tuberculosis* complex organisms or inhibit multiplication of the organism, thereby arresting progression of LTBI and preventing most complications of early tuberculosis disease. Chemotherapy does not cause rapid disappearance of already caseous or granulomatous lesions (eg, mediastinal lymphadenitis). Dosage recommendations and the more commonly reported adverse reactions of major antituberculosis drugs are summarized in Tables 3.79 (p 745) and 3.80 (p 746). For treatment of tuberculosis disease, these drugs always must be used in recommended combination

---

[1] Centers for Disease Control and Prevention. Updated guidelines for using interferon gamma release assays to detect *Mycobacterium tuberculosis* infection—United States. *MMWR Recomm Rep.* 2010;59(RR-5):1–26

Table 3.78. Recommendations for Use of the Tuberculin Skin Test (TST) and an Interferon-Gamma Release Assay (IGRA) in Children

TST preferred, IGRA acceptable
- Children <5 y of age[a]

IGRA preferred, TST acceptable
- Children ≥5 y of age who have received BCG vaccine
- Children ≥5 y of age who are unlikely to return for TST reading

TST and IGRA should be considered when:
- The initial and repeat IGRA are indeterminate
- The initial test (TST or IGRA) is *negative* and:
  - Clinical suspicion for TB disease is moderate to high[b]
  - Risk of progression and poor outcome is high[b]
- The initial TST is *positive* and:
  - >5 y of age and history of BCG vaccination
  - Additional evidence needed to increase compliance
  - Nontuberculous mycobacterial disease is suspected

[a]Positive result of either test is considered significant in these groups.

[b]IGRAs should not be used in children <2 years of age unless tuberculosis disease is suspected. In children 2 through 4 years of age, there are limited data about the usefulness of IGRAs in determining tuberculosis infection, but IGRA testing can be performed if tuberculosis disease is suspected.

given as single doses to minimize emergence of drug-resistant strains. Use of nonstandard regimens for any reason (eg, drug allergy or drug resistance) should be undertaken only in consultation with an expert in treating tuberculosis.

Isoniazid is bactericidal, rapidly absorbed, and well tolerated and penetrates into body fluids, including cerebrospinal fluid (CSF). Isoniazid is metabolized in the liver and excreted primarily through the kidneys. Hepatotoxic effects are rare in children but can be life threatening. In children and adolescents given recommended doses, peripheral neuritis or seizures caused by inhibition of pyridoxine metabolism are rare, and most do not need pyridoxine supplements. Pyridoxine supplementation is recommended for exclusively breastfed infants and for children and adolescents on meat- and milk-deficient diets; children with nutritional deficiencies, including all symptomatic HIV-infected children; and pregnant adolescents and women. For infants and young children, isoniazid tablets can be pulverized or made into a suspension by a pharmacy.

Rifampin is a bactericidal agent in the rifamycin class of drugs that is absorbed rapidly and penetrates into body fluids, including CSF. Other drugs in this class approved for treating tuberculosis are rifabutin and rifapentine. Rifampin is metabolized by the liver and can alter the pharmacokinetics and serum concentrations of many other drugs. Rare adverse effects include hepatotoxicity, influenza-like symptoms, and pruritus. Rifampin is excreted in bile and urine and can cause orange urine, sweat, and tears and discoloration of soft contact lenses. Rifampin can make oral contraceptives ineffective, so other birth-control methods should be adopted when rifampin is administered to sexually active female adolescents and adults. For infants and young children, the contents of the capsules can be suspended in wild cherry-flavored syrup or sprinkled on semisoft foods (eg, pudding). *M tuberculosis* complex isolates that are resistant to rifampin are uncommon in the United States. Rifabutin is a suitable alternative to rifampin in children with

Table 3.79. Recommended Treatment Regimens for Drug-Susceptible Tuberculosis in Infants, Children, and Adolescents

Infection or Disease Category	Regimen	Remarks
Latent tuberculosis infection (positive TST or IGRA result, no disease)		
• Isoniazid susceptible	9 mo of isoniazid, once a day	If daily therapy is not possible, DOT twice a week can be used for 9 mo.
• Isoniazid resistant	6 mo of rifampin, once a day	If daily therapy is not possible, DOT twice a week can be used for 6 mo.
• Isoniazid-rifampin resistant[a]	Consult a tuberculosis specialist	
Pulmonary and extrapulmonary (except meningitis)	2 mo of isoniazid, rifampin, pyrazinamide, and ethambutol daily or twice weekly, followed by 4 mo of isoniazid and rifampin[b] by DOT[c] for drug-susceptible *Mycobacterium tuberculosis* 9 to 12 mo of isoniazid and rifampin for drug-susceptible *Mycobacterium bovis*	If possible drug resistance is a concern (see text), some experts recommend a 3-drug initial regimen (isoniazid, rifampin, and pyrazinamide) if the risk of drug resistance is low. DOT is highly desirable. If hilar adenopathy only, a 6-mo course of isoniazid and rifampin is sufficient. Drugs can be given 2 or 3 times/wk under DOT in the initial phase if nonadherence is likely.
Meningitis	2 mo of isoniazid, rifampin, pyrazinamide, and an aminoglycoside or ethambutol or ethionamide, once a day, followed by 7–10 mo of isoniazid and rifampin, once a day or twice a week (9–12 mo total) for drug-susceptible *M tuberculosis* At least 12 mo of therapy without pyrazinamide for drug-susceptible *M bovis*	For patients who may have acquired tuberculosis in geographic areas where resistance to streptomycin is common, kanamycin, amikacin, or capreomycin can be used instead of streptomycin.

TST indicates tuberculin skin test; IGRA, interferon-gamma release assay; HIV, human immunodeficiency virus; DOT, directly observed therapy.

[a] Duration of therapy is longer for human immunodeficiency virus (HIV)-infected people, and additional drugs may be indicated (see Tuberculosis Disease and HIV Infection, p 753).

[b] Medications should be administered daily for the first 2 weeks to 2 months of treatment and then can be administered 2 to 3 times per week by DOT.

[c] If initial chest radiograph shows cavitary lesions and sputum after 2 months of therapy remains positive, duration of therapy is extended to 9 months.

Table 3.80. Commonly Used Drugs for Treatment of Tuberculosis in Infants, Children, and Adolescents

Drugs	Dosage Forms	Daily Dosage, mg/kg	Twice a Week Dosage, mg/kg per Dose	Maximum Dose	Adverse Reactions
Ethambutol	Tablets 100 mg 400 mg	20	50	2.5 g	Optic neuritis (usually reversible), decreased red-green color discrimination, gastrointestinal tract disturbances, hypersensitivity
Isoniazid[a]	Scored tablets 100 mg 300 mg Syrup 10 mg/mL	10–15[b]	20–30	Daily, 300 mg Twice a week, 900 mg	Mild hepatic enzyme elevation, hepatitis,[b] peripheral neuritis, hypersensitivity Diarrhea and gastric irritation caused by vehicle in the syrup
Pyrazinamide[a]	Scored tablets 500 mg	30–40	50	2 g	Hepatotoxic effects, hyperuricemia, arthralgia, gastrointestinal tract upset
Rifampin[a]	Capsules 150 mg 300 mg Syrup formulated capsules	10–20	10–20	600 mg	Orange discoloration of secretions or urine, staining of contact lenses, vomiting, hepatitis, influenza-like reaction, thrombocytopenia, pruritus; oral contraceptives may be ineffective

[a]Rifamate is a capsule containing 150 mg of isoniazid and 300 mg of rifampin. Two capsules provide the usual adult (greater than 50 kg) daily doses of each drug. Rifater, in the United States, is a capsule containing 50 mg of isoniazid, 120 mg of rifampin, and 300 mg of pyrazinamide. Isoniazid and rifampin also are available for parenteral administration.

[b]When isoniazid in a dosage exceeding 10 mg/kg/day is used in combination with rifampin, the incidence of hepatotoxic effects may be increased.

HIV infection receiving antiretroviral therapy that proscribes the use of rifampin; however, experience in children is limited. Major toxicities of rifabutin include leukopenia, gastrointestinal tract upset, polyarthralgia, rash, increased transaminase concentrations, and skin and secretion discoloration (pseudojaundice). Anterior uveitis has been reported among children receiving rifabutin as prophylaxis or as part of a combination regimen for treatment, usually when administered at high doses. Rifabutin also increases hepatic metabolism of many drugs but is a less potent inducer of cytochrome P450 enzymes than rifampin and has fewer problematic drug interactions than rifampin. However, adjustments in doses of rifabutin and coadministered antiretroviral drugs may be necessary for certain combinations. Rifapentine is a long-acting rifamycin that permits weekly dosing in selected adults and adolescents, but its evaluation in younger pediatric patients has been limited.

Pyrazinamide attains therapeutic CSF concentrations, is detectable in macrophages, is administered orally, and is metabolized by the liver. Administration of pyrazinamide for the first 2 months with isoniazid and rifampin allows for 6-month regimens in immunocompetent patients with drug-susceptible tuberculosis. Almost all isolates of *M bovis* are resistant to pyrazinamide, precluding 6-month therapy for this pathogen. In daily doses of 40 mg/kg per day or less, pyrazinamide seldom has hepatotoxic effects and is well tolerated by children. Some adolescents and many adults develop arthralgia and hyperuricemia because of inhibition of uric acid excretion. Pyrazinamide must be used with caution in people with underlying liver disease; when administered with rifampin, pyrazinamide is associated with somewhat higher rates of hepatotoxicity.

Ethambutol is well absorbed after oral administration, diffuses well into tissues, and is excreted in urine. However, concentrations in CSF are low. At 20 mg/kg per day, ethambutol is bacteriostatic, and its primary therapeutic role is to prevent emergence of drug resistance. Ethambutol can cause reversible or irreversible optic neuritis, but reports in children with normal renal function are rare. Children who are receiving ethambutol should be monitored monthly for visual acuity and red-green color discrimination if they are old enough to cooperate. Use of ethambutol in young children whose visual acuity cannot be monitored requires consideration of risks and benefits, but should be used routinely to treat tuberculosis disease in infants and children unless otherwise contraindicated.

Streptomycin is regarded as a "second-line" drug and is available only on a limited basis. It is administered intramuscularly. When streptomycin is not available, kanamycin, amikacin, or capreomycin are alternatives that can be prescribed by intravenous administration for the initial 4 to 8 weeks of therapy. Patients who receive any of these drugs should be monitored for otic, vestibular, and renal toxicity.

The less commonly used (eg, "second-line") antituberculosis drugs, their doses, and adverse effects are listed in Table 3.81 (p 748). These drugs have limited usefulness because of decreased effectiveness and greater toxicity and should be used only in consultation with a specialist familiar with childhood tuberculosis. Ethionamide is an orally administered antituberculosis drug that is well tolerated by children, achieves therapeutic CSF concentrations, and may be useful for treatment of people with meningitis or drug-resistant tuberculosis. Fluoroquinolones have antituberculosis activity and can be used in special circumstances including drug resistant organisms but are not FDA approved for this indication. Because some fluoroquinolones are approved by the FDA for use only in people 18 years of age and older, their use in younger patients necessitates careful

Table 3.81. Less Commonly Used Drugs for Treatment of Drug-Resistant Tuberculosis in Infants, Children, and Adolescents[a]

Drugs	Dosage, Forms	Daily Dosage, mg/kg	Maximum Dose	Adverse Reactions
Amikacin[b]	Vials, 500 mg and 1 g	15–30 mg/kg (intravenous or intramuscular administration)	1 g	Auditory and vestibular toxic effects, nephrotoxic effects
Capreomycin[b]	Vials, 1 g	15–30 mg/kg (intramuscular administration)	1 g	Auditory and vestibular toxicity and nephrotoxic effects
Cycloserine	Capsules, 250 mg	10–20 mg/kg, given in 2 divided doses	1 g	Psychosis, personality changes, seizures, rash
Ethionamide	Tablets, 250 mg	15–20 mg/kg, given in 2–3 divided doses	1 g	Gastrointestinal tract disturbances, hepatotoxic effects, hypersensitivity reactions, hypothyroid
Kanamycin	Vials 75 mg/2 mL 500 mg/2 mL 1 g/3 mL	15–30 mg/kg (intramuscular or intravenous administration)	1 g	Auditory and vestibular toxic effects, nephrotoxic effects
Levofloxacin[c]	Tablets 250 mg 500 mg 750 mg Vials 25 mg/mL	Adults 750–1000 mg (once daily) Children: not routinely recommended	1 g	Theoretical effect on growing cartilage, gastrointestinal tract disturbances, rash, headache, restlessness, confusion
Ofloxacin	Tablets 200 mg 300 mg 400 mg Vials 20 mg/mL 40 mg/mL	Adults and adolescents: 800 mg Children: 15–20 mg/kg daily	800 mg	Arthropathy, arthritis

Table 3.81. Less Commonly Used Drugs for Treatment of Drug-Resistant Tuberculosis in Infants, Children, and Adolescents,[a] continued

Drugs	Dosage, Forms	Daily Dosage, mg/kg	Maximum Dose	Adverse Reactions
Moxifloxacin	Tablets 400 mg Intravenous solution 400 mg/250 mL in 0.8% saline	Adults and adolescents: 400 mg Children: 7.5–10 mg/kg daily	400 mg	Arthropathy, arthritis
Para-aminosalicylic acid (PAS)	Packets, 3 g	200–300 mg/kg (2–4 times a day)	10 g	Gastrointestinal tract disturbances, hypersensitivity, hepatotoxic effects
Streptomycin[b]	Vials 1 g 4 g	20–40 mg/kg (intramuscular administration)	1 g	Auditory and vestibular toxic effects, nephrotoxic effects, rash

[a] These drugs should be used in consultation with a specialist in tuberculosis.

[b] Dose adjustment in renal insufficiency.

[c] Levofloxacin is not approved for use in children younger than 18 years of age; its use in younger children necessitates assessment of the potential risks and benefits (see Antimicrobial Agents and Related Therapy, p 799).

assessment of the potential risks and benefits (see Antimicrobial Agents and Related Therapy, p 799).

Occasionally, a patient cannot tolerate oral medications. Isoniazid, rifampin, strepto-mycin and related drugs, and fluoroquinolones can be administered parenterally.

Isoniazid Therapy for LTBI. Isoniazid given to adults who have LTBI (ie, no clinical or radiographic abnormalities suggesting tuberculosis disease) provides substantial protec-tion (54%–88%) against development of tuberculosis disease for at least 20 years. Among children, efficacy approaches 100% with adherence to therapy. All infants, children, and adolescents who have a positive TST or IGRA result but no evidence of tuberculosis disease and who never have received antituberculosis therapy should be considered for isoniazid unless resistance to isoniazid is suspected (ie, known exposure to a person with isoniazid-resistant tuberculosis) or a specific contraindication exists. Isoniazid, in this cir-cumstance, is therapeutic and prevents development of disease. A physical examination and chest radiograph should be performed at the time isoniazid therapy is initiated to exclude tuberculosis disease; if the radiograph is normal, the child remains asymptomatic, and treatment is completed, radiography need not be repeated.

Duration of Isoniazid Therapy for LTBI. For infants, children, and adolescents, includ-ing those with HIV infection or other immunocompromising conditions, the recom-mended duration of isoniazid therapy is 9 months. Isoniazid is given daily in a single dose. Physicians who treat LTBI should educate patients and their families about the adverse effects of isoniazid, provide written information about adverse drug effects, and prescribe it in monthly allocations, with clinic visits scheduled for periodic face-to-face monitoring. Successful completion of therapy is based on total number of doses taken. When adherence with daily therapy with isoniazid cannot be ensured, twice-a-week DOT can be considered. The twice-weekly regimen should not be prescribed unless each dose is documented by DOT. Routine determination of serum transaminase values during the 9 months of therapy for LTBI is not indicated. If therapy is completed suc-cessfully, there is no need to perform additional tests or chest radiographs unless a new exposure to tuberculosis is documented or the child develops a clinical illness consistent with tuberculosis.

Isoniazid-Rifapentine Therapy for LTBI.[1] In 2011, on the basis of a large clinical trial, the CDC recommended a 12-week, once-weekly dose of isoniazid and rifapentine, **given under DOT by a health department,** as an alternative regimen for treating LTBI in people 12 years of age and older. This regimen was shown to be at least as effective as 9 months of isoniazid given by self-supervision. Although children between 2 and 12 years of age were enrolled in the trial, data for safety, tolerability, and efficacy of this regimen in this group currently are not available, and the regimen is not recommended for children younger than 12 years of age.

Therapy for Contacts of Patients With Isoniazid-Resistant M tuberculosis. The incidence of isoniazid resistance among *M tuberculosis* complex isolates from US patients is approxi-mately 9%. Risk factors for drug resistance are listed in Table 3.82, p 751. However, most experts recommend that isoniazid be used to treat LTBI in children unless the child has had contact with a person known to have isoniazid-resistant tuberculosis. If the source case is found to have isoniazid-resistant, rifampin-susceptible organisms, isoniazid should

---

[1] Centers for Disease Control and Prevention. Recommendations for use of an isoniazid-rifapentine regi-men with direct observation to treat latent *Mycobacterium tuberculosis* infection. *MMWR Morb Mortal Wkly Rep.* 2011;60(48):1650–1653

Table 3.82. People at Increased Risk of Drug-Resistant Tuberculosis Infection or Disease

- People with a history of treatment for tuberculosis disease (or whose source case for the contact received such treatment)
- Contacts of a patient with drug-resistant contagious tuberculosis disease
- People from countries with high prevalence of drug-resistant tuberculosis
- Infected people whose source case has positive smears for acid-fast bacilli or cultures after 2 months of appropriate antituberculosis therapy and patients who do not respond to a standard treatment regimen
- Residence in geographic area with a high percentage of drug-resistant isolates

be discontinued and rifampin should be given for a total course of 6 months. Optimal therapy for children with LTBI caused by organisms with resistance to isoniazid and rifampin (ie, MDR) is not known. In these circumstances, multidrug regimens have been used. Drugs to consider include pyrazinamide, a fluoroquinolone, and ethambutol, depending on susceptibility of the isolate. Consultation with a tuberculosis specialist is indicated.

Treatment of Tuberculosis Disease. The goal of treatment is to achieve killing of replicating organisms in the tuberculous lesion in the shortest possible time. Achievement of this goal minimizes the possibility of development of resistant organisms. The major problem limiting successful treatment is poor adherence to prescribed treatment regimens. The use of DOT decreases the rates of relapse, treatment failures, and drug resistance; therefore, DOT is recommended strongly for treatment of all children and adolescents with tuberculosis disease in the United States.

For tuberculosis disease, a 6-month, 4-drug regimen consisting of isoniazid, rifampin, pyrazinamide, and ethambutol for the first 2 months and isoniazid and rifampin for the remaining 4 months is recommended for treatment of pulmonary disease, pulmonary disease with hilar adenopathy, and hilar adenopathy disease in infants, children, and adolescents when an MDR case is not suspected as the source of infection or when drug-susceptibility results are available. Some experts would administer 3 drugs (isoniazid, rifampin, and pyrazinamide) as the initial regimen if a source case has been identified with known pansusceptible *M tuberculosis*, if the presumed source case has no risk factors for drug-resistant *M tuberculosis*, or if the source case is unknown but the child resides in an area with low rates of isoniazid resistance. If the chest radiograph shows one or more cavitary lesions and sputum culture remains positive after 2 months of therapy, the duration of therapy should be extended to 9 months. For children with hilar adenopathy in whom drug resistance is not a consideration, a 6-month regimen of only isoniazid and rifampin is considered adequate by some experts.

In the 6-month regimen with 4-drug therapy, isoniazid, rifampin, pyrazinamide, and ethambutol are given once a day for at least the first 2 weeks by daily (at least 5 days per week) DOT. An alternative to daily dosing between 2 weeks and 2 months of treatment is to give these drugs twice or 3 times a week by DOT. After the initial 2-month period, a DOT regimen of isoniazid and rifampin given 2 or 3 times a week is acceptable (see Table 3.79, p 745, for doses). Several alternative regimens with differing durations of daily therapy and total therapy have been used successfully in adults and children. These alternative regimens should be prescribed and managed by a specialist in tuberculosis.

When **drug resistance** is possible (see Table 3.82, p 751), initial therapy should be adjusted by adding at least 2 drugs to match the presumed drug susceptibility pattern until drug susceptibility results are available. If an isolate from the pediatric case under treatment is not available, drug susceptibilities can be inferred by the drug susceptibility pattern of isolates from the adult source case. Data for guiding drug selection may not be available for foreign-born children or in circumstances of international travel. If this information is not available, a 4-drug initial regimen is recommended with close monitoring for clinical response.

Therapy for Drug-Resistant Tuberculosis Disease. Drug resistance is most common in the following: (1) people previously treated for tuberculosis disease; (2) people born in areas such as Russia and the former Soviet Union, Asia, Africa, and Latin America; and (3) contacts, especially children, with tuberculosis disease whose source case is a person from one of these groups (see also Table 3.82, p 751). Most cases of pulmonary tuberculosis in children that are caused by an isoniazid-resistant but rifampin- and pyrazinamide-susceptible strain of *M tuberculosis* complex can be treated with a 6-month regimen of rifampin, pyrazinamide, and ethambutol. For cases of MDR tuberculosis disease, the treatment regimen needed for cure should include at least 4 antituberculosis drugs to which the organism is susceptible administered for 12 to 24 months of therapy from the time of culture conversion. Regimens in which drugs are administered 2 or 3 times per week are not recommended for drug-resistant disease; daily DOT is critical to prevent emergence of further resistance.

Extrapulmonary M tuberculosis Tuberculosis Disease. In general, extrapulmonary tuberculosis—with the exception of meningitis—can be treated with the same regimens as used for pulmonary tuberculosis. For suspected drug-susceptible tuberculous meningitis, daily treatment with isoniazid, rifampin, pyrazinamide, and ethambutol or ethionamide, if possible, or an aminoglycoside should be initiated. When susceptibility to all drugs is established, the ethambutol, ethionamide, or aminoglycoside can be discontinued. Pyrazinamide is given for a total of 2 months, and isoniazid and rifampin are given for a total of 9 to 12 months. Isoniazid and rifampin can be given daily or 2 or 3 times per week after the first 2 months of treatment.

Corticosteroids. The evidence supporting adjuvant treatment with corticosteroids for children with tuberculosis disease is incomplete. Corticosteroids are indicated for children with tuberculous meningitis, because corticosteroids decrease rates of mortality and long-term neurologic impairment. Corticosteroids can be considered for children with pleural and pericardial effusions (to hasten reabsorption of fluid), severe miliary disease (to mitigate alveolocapillary block), endobronchial disease (to relieve obstruction and atelectasis), and abdominal tuberculosis (to decrease the risk of strictures). Corticosteroids should be given only when accompanied by appropriate antituberculosis therapy. Most experts consider 2 mg/kg per day of prednisone (maximum, 60 mg/day) or its equivalent for 4 to 6 weeks followed by tapering to be adequate.

Tuberculosis Disease and HIV Infection.[1] Adults and children with HIV infection have an increased incidence of tuberculosis disease. Hence, *HIV testing is indicated for all patients with tuberculosis disease.* The clinical manifestations and radiographic appearance of tuberculosis disease in children with HIV infection tend to be similar to those in immunocompetent children, but manifestations in these children can be more severe and unusual and can include extrapulmonary involvement of multiple organs. In HIV-infected patients, a TST result of 5-mm induration or more is considered positive (see Table 3.75, p 737); however, a negative TST result attributable to HIV-related immunosuppression also can occur. Specimens for culture should be obtained from all HIV-infected children with suspected tuberculosis.

Most HIV-infected adults with drug-susceptible tuberculosis respond well to antituberculosis drugs when appropriate therapy is initiated early. However, optimal therapy for tuberculosis in children with HIV infection has not been established. Treating tuberculosis in an HIV-infected child is complicated by antiretroviral drug interactions with the rifamycins and overlapping toxicities caused by antiretroviral drugs and medications used to treat tuberculosis. Therapy always should include at least 4 drugs initially; should be administered daily, and should be continued for at least 6 months. Isoniazid, rifampin, and pyrazinamide, usually with ethambutol or an aminoglycoside, should be given for at least the first 2 months. Ethambutol can be discontinued once drug-resistant tuberculosis disease is excluded. Rifampin may be contraindicated in people who are receiving antiretroviral therapy. Rifabutin can be substituted for rifampin in some circumstances. Consultation with a specialist who has experience in managing HIV-infected patients with tuberculosis strongly is advised.

Evaluation and Monitoring of Therapy in Children and Adolescents. Careful monthly monitoring of clinical and bacteriologic responses to therapy is important. With DOT, clinical evaluation is an integral component of each visit for drug administration. For patients with pulmonary tuberculosis, chest radiographs should be obtained after 2 months of therapy to evaluate response. Even with successful 6-month regimens, hilar adenopathy can persist for 2 to 3 years; normal radiographic findings are not necessary to discontinue therapy. Follow-up chest radiography beyond termination of successful therapy usually is not necessary unless clinical deterioration occurs.

If therapy has been interrupted, the date of completion should be extended. Although guidelines cannot be provided for every situation, factors to consider when establishing the date of completion include the following: (1) length of interruption of therapy; (2) time during therapy (early or late) when interruption occurred; and (3) the patient's clinical, radiographic, and bacteriologic status before, during, and after interruption of therapy. The total doses administered by DOT should be calculated to guide the duration of therapy. Consultation with a specialist in tuberculosis is advised.

Untoward effects of isoniazid therapy, including severe hepatitis in otherwise healthy infants, children, and adolescents, are rare. Routine determination of serum transaminase concentrations is not recommended. However, for children with severe tuberculosis disease, especially children with meningitis or disseminated disease, transaminase concentrations should be monitored approximately monthly during the first several months

---

[1] Centers for Disease Control and Prevention. Guidelines for prevention and treatment of opportunistic infections in HIV-infected adults and adolescents. Recommendations from CDC, the National Institutes of Health, and the HIV Medicine Association of the Infectious Diseases Society of America. *MMWR Recomm Rep.* 2009;58(RR-4):1–207. Available at: **http://www.cdc.gov/mmwr/pdf/rr/rr58e324.pdf**

of treatment. Other indications for testing include the following: (1) having concurrent or recent liver or biliary disease; (2) being pregnant or in the first 6 weeks postpartum; (3) having clinical evidence of hepatotoxic effects; or (4) concurrently using other hepatotoxic drugs (eg, anticonvulsant or HIV agents). In most other circumstances, monthly clinical evaluations to observe for signs or symptoms of hepatitis and other adverse effects of drug therapy without routine monitoring of transaminase concentrations is appropriate follow-up. In all cases, regular physician-patient contact to assess drug adherence, efficacy, and adverse effects is an important aspect of management. Patients should be given written instructions and advised to call a physician immediately if signs of adverse events, in particular hepatotoxicity (eg, vomiting, abdominal pain, jaundice), develop.

Immunizations. Patients who are receiving treatment for tuberculosis can be given measles and other age-appropriate attenuated live-virus vaccines unless they are receiving high-dose corticosteroids, are severely ill, or have other specific contraindications to immunization.

Tuberculosis During Pregnancy and Breastfeeding. Tuberculosis treatment during pregnancy varies because of the complexity of management decisions. During pregnancy, if tuberculosis disease is diagnosed, a regimen of isoniazid, rifampin, and ethambutol is recommended. Pyrazinamide commonly is used in a 3- or 4-drug regimen, but safety during pregnancy has not been established. At least 6 months of therapy is indicated for drug-susceptible tuberculosis disease if pyrazinamide is used; at least 9 months of therapy is indicated if pyrazinamide is not used. Prompt initiation of therapy is mandatory to protect mother and fetus.

Asymptomatic pregnant women with a positive TST or IGRA result, normal chest radiographic findings, and recent contact with a contagious person should be considered for isoniazid therapy. The recommended duration of therapy is 9 months. Therapy in these circumstances should begin after the first trimester. Pyridoxine supplementation is indicated for all pregnant and breastfeeding women receiving isoniazid.

Isoniazid, ethambutol, and rifampin are relatively safe for the fetus. The benefit of ethambutol and rifampin for therapy of tuberculosis disease in the mother outweighs the risk to the infant. Because streptomycin can cause ototoxic effects in the fetus, it should not be used unless administration is essential for effective treatment. The effects of other second-line drugs on the fetus are unknown, and ethionamide has been demonstrated to be teratogenic, so its use during pregnancy is contraindicated.

Although isoniazid is secreted in human milk, no adverse effects of isoniazid on nursing infants have been demonstrated (see Human Milk, p 126). Breastfed infants do not require pyridoxine supplementation unless they are receiving isoniazid.

Congenital Tuberculosis. Women who have only pulmonary tuberculosis are not likely to infect the fetus but can infect their infant after delivery. Congenital tuberculosis is rare, but in utero infections can occur after maternal bacillemia.

If a newborn infant is suspected of having congenital tuberculosis, a TST, chest radiography, lumbar puncture, and appropriate cultures should be performed promptly. The TST result usually is negative in newborn infants with congenital or perinatally acquired infection. Hence, regardless of the TST or IGRA results, treatment of the infant should be initiated promptly with isoniazid, rifampin, pyrazinamide, and an aminoglycoside (eg, amikacin). The placenta should be examined histologically for granulomata and AFB, and a specimen should be cultured for *M tuberculosis* complex. The mother should be evaluated for presence of pulmonary or extrapulmonary disease, including uterine tuberculosis disease. If the physical examination and chest radiographic findings support the diagnosis of tuberculosis disease, the newborn infant should be treated with regimens recommended for tuberculosis disease. If meningitis is confirmed, corticosteroids should be added (see Corticosteroids, p 752). Drug susceptibility testing of the organism recovered from the mother or household contact, infant, or both should be performed.

Management of the Newborn Infant Whose Mother (or Other Household Contact) Has LTBI or Tuberculosis Disease. Management of the newborn infant is based on categorization of the maternal (or household contact) infection. Although protection of the infant from exposure and infection is of paramount importance, contact between infant and mother should be allowed when possible. Differing circumstances and resulting recommendations are as follows:

- *Mother (or household contact) has a positive TST or IGRA result and normal chest radiographic findings.* If the mother (or household contact) is asymptomatic, no separation is required. The mother usually is a candidate for treatment of LTBI after the initial postpartum period. The newborn infant needs no special evaluation or therapy. Because the positive TST or IGRA result could be a marker of an unrecognized case of contagious tuberculosis within the household, other household members should have a TST or IGRA and further evaluation, but this should not delay the infant's discharge from the hospital. These mothers can breastfeed their infants.

- *Mother (or household contact) has clinical signs and symptoms or abnormal findings on chest radiograph consistent with tuberculosis disease.* Cases of suspected or proven tuberculosis disease in mothers (or household contacts) should be reported immediately to the local health department, and investigation of all household members should start within 7 days. If the mother has tuberculosis disease, the infant should be evaluated for congenital tuberculosis (see Congenital Tuberculosis), and the mother should be tested for HIV infection. The mother (or household contact) and the infant should be separated until the mother (or household contact) has been evaluated and, if tuberculosis disease is suspected, until the mother (or household contact) and infant are receiving appropriate antituberculosis therapy, the mother wears a mask, and the mother understands and is willing to adhere to infection-control measures. Once the infant is receiving isoniazid, separation is not necessary unless the mother (or household contact) has possible MDR tuberculosis disease or has poor adherence to treatment and DOT is not possible. In this circumstance, the infant should be separated from the mother (or household contact), and BCG immunization should be considered for the infant if HIV infection is not present. If the mother is suspected of having MDR tuberculosis disease, an expert in tuberculosis disease treatment should be consulted. Women with tuberculosis disease who have been treated appropriately for 2 or more weeks and who are not considered contagious can breastfeed.

If congenital tuberculosis is excluded, isoniazid is given until the infant is 3 or 4 months of age, when a TST should be performed. If the TST result is positive, the infant should be reassessed for tuberculosis disease. If tuberculosis disease is excluded, isoniazid should be continued for a total of 9 months. The infant should be evaluated at monthly intervals during treatment. If the TST result is negative at 3 to 4 months of age and the mother (or household contact) has good adherence and response to treatment and no longer is contagious, isoniazid is discontinued.

- ***Mother (or household contact) has abnormal findings on chest radiography but no evidence of tuberculosis disease.*** If the chest radiograph of the mother (or household contact) appears abnormal but is not suggestive of tuberculosis disease and the history, physical examination, and sputum smear indicate no evidence of tuberculosis disease, the infant can be assumed to be at low risk of tuberculosis infection and need not be separated from the mother (or household contact). The mother and her infant should receive follow-up care and the mother should be treated for LTBI. Other household members should have a TST or IGRA and further evaluation.

ISOLATION OF THE HOSPITALIZED PATIENT: Most children with tuberculosis disease, especially children younger than 10 years of age, are not contagious. Exceptions are the following: (1) children with cavitary pulmonary tuberculosis; (2) children with positive sputum AFB smears; (3) children with laryngeal involvement; (4) children with extensive pulmonary infection; or (5) children with congenital tuberculosis undergoing procedures that involve the oropharyngeal airway (eg, endotracheal intubation). In these instances, isolation for tuberculosis or AFB is indicated until effective therapy has been initiated, sputum smears demonstrate a diminishing number of organisms, and cough is abating. Children with no cough and negative sputum AFB smears can be hospitalized in an open ward. Infection-control measures for hospital personnel exposed to contagious patients should include the use of personally "fitted" and "sealed" particulate respirators for all patient contacts (see Infection Control for Hospitalized Children, p 160). The contagious patient should be placed in an airborne infection isolation room in the hospital.

The major concern in infection control relates to adult household members and contacts who can be the source of infection. Visitation should be limited to people who have been evaluated medically. Household members and contacts should be managed with tuberculosis precautions when visiting until they are demonstrated not to have contagious tuberculosis. Nonadherent household contacts should be excluded from hospital visitation until evaluation is complete and tuberculosis disease is excluded or treatment has rendered source cases noncontagious.

TUBERCULOSIS CAUSED BY *M BOVIS*: Infections with *M bovis* account for approximately 1% to 2% of tuberculosis cases in the United States. Children who come from countries where *M bovis* is prevalent in cattle or whose parents come from those countries are more likely to be infected. Most infections in humans are transmitted from cattle by unpasteurized milk and its products, such as fresh cheese, although human-to-human transmission by the airborne route has been documented. In children, *M bovis* more commonly causes cervical lymphadenitis, intestinal tuberculosis disease, and meningitis. In adults, latent *M bovis* infection can progress to advanced pulmonary disease, with a risk of transmission to others.

An IGRA or TST typically is positive in a person infected with *M bovis*. However, the definitive diagnosis requires a culture isolate. The commonly used methods for identifying *M tuberculosis* complex do not distinguish *M bovis* from *M tuberculosis, M africanum,* and BCG; *M bovis* is identified in clinical laboratories routinely by its resistance to pyrazinamide. This approach can be unreliable, and species confirmation at a reference laboratory should be requested when *M bovis* is suspected. Molecular genotyping through the state health department may assist in identifying *M bovis*. Resistance to first-line drugs in addition to pyrazinamide has been reported. BCG rarely is isolated from pediatric clinical specimens; however, it should be suspected from the characteristic lesions or localized

BCG suppuration or draining lymphadenitis in children who have received BCG vaccine. Only a reference laboratory can distinguish an isolate of BCG from an isolate of *M bovis*.

Therapy for M bovis *Disease*. Controlled clinical trials for treatment of *M bovis* disease have not been conducted, and treatment recommendations for *M bovis* disease in adults and children are based on results from treatment trials for *M tuberculosis* disease. Although most strains of *M bovis* are pyrazinamide-resistant and resistance to other first-line drugs has been reported, MDR strains are rare. Initial therapy should include 3 or 4 drugs besides pyrazinamide that would be used to treat disease from *M tuberculosis* infection. For isoniazid- and rifampin-susceptible strains, a total treatment course of at least 9 to 12 months is recommended.

Parents should be counseled about the many infectious diseases transmitted by unpasteurized milk and its products, and parents who might import traditional dairy products from countries where *M bovis* infection is prevalent in cattle should be advised against giving those products to their children. When people are exposed to an adult who has pulmonary disease caused by *M bovis* infection, they should be evaluated by the same methods as other contacts to contagious tuberculosis.

CONTROL MEASURES[1]: Control of tuberculosis disease in the United States requires collaboration between health care professionals and health department personnel, obtaining a thorough history of exposure(s) to people with infectious tuberculosis, timely and effective contact investigations, proper interpretation of TST or IGRA results, and appropriate antituberculosis therapy, including DOT services. A plan to control and prevent extensively drug-resistant tuberculosis has been published.[2] Eliminating ingestion of unpasteurized dairy products will prevent most *M bovis* infection.

Management of Contacts, Including Epidemiologic Investigation.[3] Children with a positive TST or IGRA result or tuberculosis disease should be the starting point for epidemiologic investigation by the local health department. Close contacts of a TST- or IGRA-positive child should have a TST or IGRA, and people with a positive TST or IGRA result or symptoms consistent with tuberculosis disease should be investigated further. Because children with tuberculosis usually are not contagious unless they have an adult-type multibacillary form of pulmonary or laryngeal disease, their contacts are not likely to be infected unless they also have been in contact with an adult source case. After the presumptive adult source of the child's tuberculosis is identified, other contacts of that adult should be evaluated.

Therapy for Contacts. Children and adolescents exposed to a contagious case of tuberculosis disease should have a TST or IGRA and an evaluation for tuberculosis disease (chest radiography and physical examination). For exposed contacts with impaired immunity (eg, HIV infection) and all contacts younger than 4 years of age, isoniazid therapy should be initiated, even if the TST result is negative, once tuberculosis disease is excluded (see Therapy for LTBI, p 750). Infected people can have a negative TST or IGRA

---

[1] American Thoracic Society, Centers for Disease Control and Prevention, and Infectious Diseases Society of America. Controlling tuberculosis in the United States. Recommendations from the American Thoracic Society, CDC, and the Infectious Diseases Society of America. *MMWR Recomm Rep.* 2005;54(RR-12):1–81

[2] Centers for Disease Control and Prevention. Plan to combat extensively drug-resistant tuberculosis: recommendations of the Federal Tuberculosis Task Force. *MMWR Recomm Rep.* 2009;58(RR-3):1–43

[3] National Tuberculosis Controllers Association and Centers for Disease Control and Prevention. Guidelines for the investigation of contacts of persons with infectious tuberculosis. Recommendations from the National Tuberculosis Controllers Association and CDC. *MMWR Recomm Rep.* 2005;54(RR-15):1–47

result because a cellular immune response has not yet developed or because of cutaneous anergy. People with a negative TST or IGRA result should be retested 8 to 10 weeks after the last exposure to a source of infection. If the TST or IGRA result still is negative in an immunocompetent person, isoniazid is discontinued. If the contact is immunocompromised and LTBI cannot be excluded, treatment should be continued for 9 months. If a TST or IGRA result of a contact becomes positive, isoniazid should be continued for 9 months.

Child Care and Schools. Children with tuberculosis disease can attend school or child care if they are receiving therapy (see Children in Out-of-Home Child Care, p 133). They can return to regular activities as soon as effective therapy has been instituted, adherence to therapy has been documented, and clinical symptoms have diminished. Children with LTBI can participate in all activities whether they are receiving treatment or not.

BCG Vaccines. BCG vaccine is a live vaccine originally prepared from attenuated strains of *M bovis*. Use of BCG vaccine[1] is recommended by the Expanded Programme on Immunization of the World Health Organization for administration at birth (see Table 1.5, p 13) and is used in more than 100 countries. BCG vaccine is used to reduce the incidence of disseminated and other life-threatening manifestations of tuberculosis in infants and young children. Although BCG immunization appears to decrease the risk of serious complications of tuberculosis disease in children, the various BCG vaccines used throughout the world differ in composition and efficacy.

Two meta-analyses of published clinical trials and case-control studies concerning the efficacy of BCG vaccines concluded that BCG vaccine has relatively high protective efficacy (approximately 80%) against meningeal and miliary tuberculosis in children. The protective efficacy against pulmonary tuberculosis differed significantly among the studies, precluding a specific conclusion. Protection afforded by BCG vaccine in 1 meta-analysis was estimated to be 50%. Two BCG vaccines, one manufactured by Merck/Schering-Plough and the other by Sanofi Pasteur, are licensed in the United States. Comparative evaluations of these and other BCG vaccines have not been performed.

Indications. In the United States, administration of BCG vaccine should be considered only in limited and select circumstances, such as unavoidable risk of exposure to tuberculosis and failure or unfeasibility of other control methods. Recommendations for use of BCG vaccine for control of tuberculosis among children and health care personnel have been published by the Advisory Committee on Immunization Practices of the CDC and the Advisory Council for the Elimination of Tuberculosis.[2] For infants and children, BCG immunization should be considered only for people with a negative TST result who are not infected with HIV in the following circumstances:

- The child is exposed continually to a person or people with contagious pulmonary tuberculosis resistant to isoniazid and rifampin, and the child cannot be removed from this exposure.
- The child is exposed continually to a person or people with untreated or ineffectively treated contagious pulmonary tuberculosis, and the child cannot be removed from such exposure or given antituberculosis therapy.

---

[1] **www.bcgatlas.org**

[2] Centers for Disease Control and Prevention. The role of BCG vaccine in the prevention and control of tuberculosis in the United States: a joint statement by the Advisory Committee for the Elimination of Tuberculosis and the Advisory Committee on Immunization Practices. *MMWR Recomm Rep.* 1996;45(RR-4):1–18

Careful assessment of the potential risks and benefits of BCG vaccine and consultation with personnel in local tuberculosis control programs are recommended strongly before use of BCG vaccine.

Healthy infants from birth to 2 months of age may be given BCG vaccine without a TST unless congenital infection is suspected; thereafter, BCG vaccine should be given only to children with a negative TST result.

Adverse Reactions. Uncommonly (1%–2% of immunizations), BCG vaccine can result in local adverse reactions, such as subcutaneous abscess and regional lymphadenopathy, which generally are not serious. One rare complication, osteitis affecting the epiphysis of long bones, can occur as long as several years after BCG immunization. Disseminated fatal infection occurs rarely (approximately 2 per 1 million people), primarily in people who are immunocompromised severely. Antituberculosis therapy is recommended to treat osteitis and disseminated disease caused by BCG vaccine. Pyrazinamide is not believed to be effective against BCG and should not be included in treatment regimens. Most experts do not recommend treatment of draining skin lesions or chronic suppurative lymphadenitis caused by BCG vaccine, because spontaneous resolution occurs in most cases. Large-needle aspiration of suppurative lymph nodes can hasten resolution. People with complications caused by BCG vaccine should be referred for management, if possible, to a tuberculosis expert.

Contraindications. People with burns, skin infections, and primary or secondary immunodeficiencies, including HIV infection, should not receive BCG vaccine. Because an increasing number of cases of localized and disseminated BCG have been described in infants and children with HIV infection, the World Health Organization no longer recommends BCG in healthy, HIV-infected children. Use of BCG vaccine is contraindicated for people receiving immunosuppressive medications, including high-dose corticosteroids (see Corticosteroids, p 752). Although no untoward effects of BCG vaccine on the fetus have been observed, immunization during pregnancy is not recommended.

Reporting of Cases. Reporting of suspected and confirmed cases of tuberculosis disease is mandated by law in all states. A diagnosis of LTBI or tuberculosis disease in a child is a sentinel event representing recent transmission of *M tuberculosis* in the community. Physicians should assist local health department personnel in the search for a source case and others infected by the source case. Members of the household, such as relatives, babysitters, au pairs, boarders, domestic workers, and frequent visitors or other adults, such as child care providers and teachers with whom the child has frequent contact, potentially are source cases.

Diseases Caused by Nontuberculous Mycobacteria
(Atypical Mycobacteria, Mycobacteria Other Than *Mycobacterium tuberculosis*)

CLINICAL MANIFESTATIONS: Several syndromes are caused by nontuberculous mycobacteria (NTM). In children, the most common of these syndromes is cervical lymphadenitis. Less common syndromes include soft tissue infection, osteomyelitis, otitis media, central line catheter-associated bloodstream infections, and pulmonary infection, especially in adolescents with cystic fibrosis. NTM, especially *Mycobacterium avium* complex (MAC [including *M avium* and *Mycobacterium avium-intracellulare*]) and *Mycobacterium abscessus*, can be recovered from sputum in 10% to 20% of adolescents and young adults with cystic fibrosis and can be associated with fever and declining clinical status. Disseminated infections almost always are associated with impaired cell-mediated immunity, as found in children with congenital immune defects (eg, interleukin-12 deficiency, NF-kappa-B essential modulator [NEMO] mutation and related disorders, and interferon-gamma receptor defects), hematopoietic stem cell transplants, or advanced human immunodeficiency virus (HIV) infection. Disseminated MAC is rare in HIV-infected children during the first year of life. The frequency of disseminated MAC increases with increasing age and declining CD4+ T-lymphocyte counts, typically less than 50 cells/μL, in children older than 6 years of age. Manifestations of disseminated NTM infections depend on the species and route of infection but include fever, night sweats, weight loss, abdominal pain, fatigue, diarrhea, and anemia. In HIV-infected patients developing immune restoration with initiation of antiretroviral therapy (ART), local MAC symptoms can worsen. This immune reconstitution syndrome usually occurs 2 to 4 weeks after initiation of ART. Symptoms can include worsening fever, swollen lymph nodes, local pain, and laboratory abnormalities.

ETIOLOGY: Of the more than 130 species of NTM that have been identified, only a few account for most human infections. The species most commonly infecting children in the United States are MAC, *Mycobacterium fortuitum, M abscessus,* and *Mycobacterium marinum* (see Table 3.83, 761). Several new species that can be detected by nucleic acid amplification testing but cannot be grown by routine culture methods have been identified in lymph nodes of children with cervical adenitis. NTM disease in patients with HIV infection usually is caused by MAC. *M fortuitum, Mycobacterium chelonae,* and *M abscessus* commonly are referred to as "rapidly growing" mycobacteria, because sufficient growth and identification can be achieved in the laboratory within 3 to 7 days, whereas other NTM and *Mycobacterium tuberculosis* usually require several weeks before sufficient growth occurs for identification. Rapidly growing mycobacteria have been implicated in wound, soft tissue, bone, pulmonary, central venous catheter, and middle-ear infections. Other mycobacterial species that usually are not pathogenic have caused infections in immunocompromised hosts or have been associated with the presence of a foreign body.

EPIDEMIOLOGY: Many NTM species are ubiquitous in nature and are found in soil, food, water, and animals. Tap water is the major reservoir for *Mycobacterium kansasii, Mycobacterium lenteflavum, Mycobacterium xenopi, Mycobacterium simiae,* and health care-associated infections attributable to the rapidly growing mycobacteria *M abscessus* and *M fortuitum.* For *M marinum,* water in a fish tank or aquarium or an injury in a salt-water environment are the major sources of infection. The environmental reservoir for *M abscessus* and MAC causing pulmonary infection is unknown. Although many people are exposed to NTM, it is unknown why some exposures result in acute or chronic infection. Usual portals of entry for NTM infection are believed to be abrasions in the skin (eg, cutaneous lesions caused by *M marinum*), penetrating trauma (needles and organic material most often associated with *M abscessus* and *M fortuitum*), surgical sites (especially for central vascular catheters), oropharyngeal mucosa (the presumed portal of entry for cervical lymphadenitis), gastrointestinal or respiratory tract for disseminated MAC, and respiratory tract (including tympanostomy tubes for otitis media). Pulmonary disease and rare cases of mediastinal adenitis and endobronchial disease do occur. NTM can be an important pathogen in patients with cystic fibrosis. Most infections remain localized at the portal of entry or in regional lymph nodes. Dissemination to distal sites primarily occurs in immunocompromised hosts. No definitive evidence of person-to-person transmission

Table 3.83. Diseases Caused by Nontuberculous *Mycobacterium* Species

Clinical Disease	Common Species	Less Common Species in the United States
Cutaneous infection	*M chelonae, M fortuitum, M abscessus, M marinum*	*M ulcerans*[a]
Lymphadenitis	MAC; *M haemophilum; M lenteflavum*	*M kansasii, M fortuitum, M malmoense*[b]
Otologic infection	*M abscessus*	*M fortuitum*
Pulmonary infection	MAC, *M kansasii, M abscessus*	*M xenopi, M malmoense,*[b] *M szulgai, M fortuitum, M simiae*
Catheter-associated infection	*M chelonae, M fortuitum*	*M abscessus*
Skeletal infection	MAC, *M kansasii, M fortuitum*	*M chelonae, M marinum, M abscessus, M ulcerans*[a]
Disseminated	MAC	*M kansasii, M genavense, M haemophilum, M chelonae*

MAC indicates *Mycobacterium avium* complex.
[a] Not endemic in the United States.
[b] Found primarily in Northern Europe.

of NTM exists. Outbreaks of otitis media caused by *M abscessus* have been associated with polyethylene ear tubes and use of contaminated equipment or water. A waterborne route of transmission has been implicated for MAC infection in some immunodeficient hosts. Buruli ulcer disease is a skin and bone infection caused by *Mycobacterium ulcerans,* an emerging disease causing significant morbidity and disability in tropical areas such as Africa, Asia, South America, Australia, and the western Pacific.

The **incubation periods** are variable.

DIAGNOSTIC TESTS: Definitive diagnosis of NTM disease requires isolation of the organism. Consultation with the laboratory should occur to ensure that culture specimens are handled correctly. For example, isolation of *Mycobacterium haemophilum* requires that the culture be maintained at 25°C. Because these organisms commonly are found in the environment, contamination of cultures or transient colonization can occur. Caution must be exercised in interpretation of cultures obtained from nonsterile sites, such as gastric washing specimens, endoscopy material, a single expectorated sputum sample, or urine specimens and if the species cultured usually is nonpathogenic (eg, *Mycobacterium terrae* complex or *Mycobacterium gordonae*). An acid-fast bacilli smear-positive sample or repeated isolation of a single species on culture media is more likely to indicate disease than are culture contamination or transient colonization. Diagnostic criteria for NTM lung disease in adults include 2 or more separate sputum samples that grow NTM or 1 bronchial alveolar lavage specimen that grows NTM.[1] These criteria have not been validated in children and apply best to MAC, *M kansasii,* and *M abscessus.* Unlike other bacteria, NTM isolates from draining sinus tracts or wounds almost always are significant clinically. Recovery of

[1] American Thoracic Society and Infectious Disease Society of America. An official ATS/IDSA statement: diagnosis, treatment, and prevention of nontuberculous mycobacterial diseases. *Am J Respir Crit Care Med.* 2007;175(4):367–416

NTM from sites that usually are sterile, such as cerebrospinal fluid, pleural fluid, bone marrow, blood, lymph node aspirates, middle ear or mastoid aspirates, or surgically excised tissue, is the most reliable diagnostic test. With radiometric or nonradiometric broth techniques, blood cultures are highly sensitive in recovery of disseminated MAC and other bloodborne NTM species. Disseminated MAC disease should prompt a search for underlying immunodeficiency.

Patients with NTM infection, such as *M marinum* or MAC cervical lymphadenitis, can have a positive tuberculin skin test (TST) result, because the purified protein derivative preparation, derived from *M tuberculosis*, shares a number of antigens with NTM species. These TST reactions usually measure less than 10 mm of induration but can measure more than 15 mm (see Tuberculosis, p 736). The interferon-gamma release assays use 2 or 3 antigens to detect infection with *M tuberculosis*. Although these antigens are not found on *M avium-intracellulare*, cross reactions can occur with infection caused by *M kansasii*, *M marinum*, and *Mycobacterium szulgai* (See Tuberculosis, p 736).

TREATMENT: Many NTM relatively are resistant in vitro to antituberculosis drugs. In vitro resistance to these agents, however, does not necessarily correlate with clinical response, especially with MAC infections. Only limited controlled trials of antituberculous drugs have been performed in patients with NTM infections. The approach to therapy should be directed by the following: (1) the species causing the infection; (2) the results of drug-susceptibility testing; (3) the site(s) of infection; (4) the patient's immune status; and (5) the need to treat a patient presumptively for tuberculosis while awaiting culture reports that subsequently reveal NTM.

For NTM lymphadenitis in otherwise healthy children, especially when the disease is caused by MAC, complete surgical excision is curative. Antimicrobial therapy has been shown in a randomized, controlled trial to provide no additional benefit. Therapy with clarithromycin or azithromycin combined with ethambutol or rifampin or rifabutin may be beneficial for children in whom surgical excision is incomplete or for children with recurrent disease (see Table 3.84, p 763).

Isolates of rapidly growing mycobacteria (*M fortuitum*, *M abscessus*, and *M chelonae*) should be tested in vitro against drugs to which they commonly are susceptible and that have been used with some therapeutic success (eg, amikacin, imipenem, sulfamethoxazole or trimethoprim-sulfamethoxazole, cefoxitin, ciprofloxacin, clarithromycin, linezolid, and doxycycline).[1] Clarithromycin and at least one other agent is the treatment of choice for cutaneous (disseminated) infections attributable to *M chelonae* or *M abscessus*. Indwelling foreign bodies should be removed, and surgical débridement for serious localized disease is optimal. The choice of drugs, dosages, and duration should be reviewed with a consultant experienced in the management of NTM infections.

For patients with cystic fibrosis and isolation of MAC species, treatment is suggested only for those with clinical symptoms not attributable to other causes, worsening lung function, and chest radiographic progression. The decision to embark on therapy should take into consideration susceptibility testing results and involve consultation with an expert in cystic fibrosis care. *M abscessus* is difficult to treat, and the role of therapy in clinical benefit is unknown.

---

[1] American Thoracic Society and Infectious Disease Society of America. An official ATS/IDSA statement: diagnosis, treatment, and prevention of nontuberculous mycobacterial diseases. *Am J Respir Crit Care Med.* 2007;175(4):367–416

Table 3.84. Treatment of Nontuberculous Mycobacteria Infections in Children

Organism	Disease	Initial Treatment
Slowly Growing Species		
Mycobacterium avium complex (MAC); *Mycobacterium haemophilum*; *Mycobacterium lentiflavum*	Lymphadenitis	Complete excision of lymph nodes; if excision incomplete or disease recurs, clarithromycin or azithromycin plus ethambutol and/or rifampin (or rifabutin).
	Pulmonary infection	Clarithromycin or azithromycin plus ethambutol with rifampin or rifabutin (pulmonary resection in some patients who fail to respond to drug therapy). For severe disease, an initial course of amikacin or streptomycin often is included. Clinical data in adults support that 3-times-weekly therapy is as effective as daily therapy, with less toxicity for adult patients with mild to moderate disease. For patients with advanced or cavitary disease, drugs should be given daily.
	Disseminated	See text.
Mycobacterium kansasii	Pulmonary infection	Rifampin plus ethambutol with isoniazid daily. If rifampin-resistance is detected, a 3-drug regimen based on drug susceptibility testing should be used.
	Osteomyelitis	Surgical débridement and prolonged antimicrobial therapy using rifampin plus ethambutol with isoniazid.
Mycobacterium marinum	Cutaneous infection	None, if minor; rifampin, trimethoprim-sulfamethoxazole, clarithromycin, or doxycycline[a] for moderate disease; extensive lesions may require surgical débridement. Susceptibility testing not routinely required.
Mycobacterium ulcerans	Cutaneous and bone infections	Daily intramuscular streptomycin and oral rifampin for 8 weeks; excision to remove necrotic tissue, if present; disability prevention

Table 3.84. Treatment of Nontuberculous Mycobacteria Infections in Children, continued

Organism	Disease	Initial Treatment
Rapidly Growing Species		
Mycobacterium fortuitum group	Cutaneous infection	Initial therapy for serious disease is amikacin plus meropenem, IV, followed by clarithromycin, doxycycline,[a] or trimethoprim-sulfamethoxazole or ciprofloxacin, orally, on the basis of in vitro susceptibility testing; may require surgical excision. Up to 50% of isolates are resistant to cefoxitin.
	Catheter infection	Catheter removal and amikacin plus meropenem, IV; clarithromycin, trimethoprim-sulfamethoxazole, or ciprofloxacin, orally, on the basis of in vitro susceptibility testing.
Mycobacterium abscessus	Otitis media; cutaneous infection	There is no reliable antimicrobial regimen because of variability in drug susceptibility. Clarithromycin plus initial course of amikacin plus cefoxitin or meropenem; may require surgical débridement on the basis of in vitro susceptibility testing (50% are amikacin resistant).
	Pulmonary infection (in cystic fibrosis)	Serious disease, clarithromycin, amikacin, and cefoxitin or meropenem on the basis of susceptibility testing; may require surgical resection.
Mycobacterium chelonae	Catheter infection	Catheter removal and tobramycin (initially) plus clarithromycin.
	Disseminated cutaneous infection	Tobramycin and meropenem or linezolid (initially) plus clarithromycin.

IV indicates intravenously.

[a]Doxycycline should not be given to children younger than 8 years of age unless no other therapeutic options are available (see Tetracyclines, p 801).

Only 50% of isolates of *M marinum* are susceptible to doxycycline.

In patients with acquired immunodeficiency syndrome (AIDS) and in other immuno-compromised people with disseminated MAC infection, multidrug therapy is recommended. Clinical isolates of MAC usually are resistant to many of the approved antituberculosis drugs, including isoniazid, but are susceptible to clarithromycin and azithromycin and often are susceptible to combinations of ethambutol, rifabutin or rifampin, and amikacin or streptomycin. Susceptibility testing to these agents has not been standardized and, thus, is not recommended routinely. The optimal regimen is yet to be determined. Treatment of disseminated MAC infection should be undertaken in consultation with an expert. In addition, the following treatment guidelines should be considered:

- Susceptibility testing to drugs other than the macrolides is not predictive of in vivo response and should not be used to guide therapy.
- Unless there is clinical or laboratory evidence of macrolide resistance, treatment regimens should contain clarithromycin (preferred) or azithromycin, combined with ethambutol. This 2-drug regimen is the foundation for any MAC treatment.
- Many clinicians have added a third agent (rifampin or rifabutin), especially for pulmonary disease and, in some situations, a fourth agent (amikacin or streptomycin).
- Drug-drug interactions can occur between medications used to treat disseminated MAC and HIV infections. Protease inhibitors (PIs) can increase and efavirenz can decrease clarithromycin concentrations. Available data are not adequate to make recommendations for clarithromycin dose adjustments in these circumstances. Azithromycin is not metabolized by the cytochrome P450 (CYP 450) system, and drug-drug interactions with PIs and efavirenz is not a concern. Rifampin and rifabutin increase CYP 450 activity and lead to more rapid clearance of PIs and efavirenz and increase toxicity. Rifampin and rifabutin should be avoided in HIV-infected children receiving PIs or efavirenz.[1]
- The optimal time to initiate ART in a child in whom HIV and disseminated MAC are diagnosed newly is not established. Many experts would provide treatment of disseminated MAC for 2 weeks before initiating ART in an attempt to minimize occurrence of the immune reconstitution syndrome and minimize confusion relating to the cause of drug-associated toxicity.
- Clofazimine is ineffective for treatment of MAC infection and should not be used.
- Patients receiving therapy should be monitored. Considerations are as follows:
  - Most patients who respond ultimately show substantial clinical improvement in the first 4 to 6 weeks of therapy. Elimination of the organisms from blood cultures can take longer, often up to 12 weeks.
  - Patients receiving clarithromycin plus rifabutin or high-dose rifabutin (with another drug) should be observed for the rifabutin-related development of leukopenia, uveitis, polyarthralgias, and pseudojaundice.

The duration of therapy for NTM infections will depend on host status, site(s) of involvement, and severity. Most experts recommend a minimum of 3 to 6 months or longer.

---

[1] Centers for Disease Control and Prevention. Guidelines for the prevention and treatment of opportunistic infections among HIV-exposed and HIV-infected children: recommendations from the CDC, the National Institutes of Health, the HIV Medicine Association of the Infectious Diseases Society of America, the Pediatric Infectious Diseases Society, and the American Academy of Pediatrics. *MMWR Recomm Rep.* 2009;58(RR-11):1–166

Chemoprophylaxis. The most effective way to prevent disseminated MAC in HIV-infected children is to preserve their immune function through use of effective ART. HIV infected children with advanced immunosuppression should be offered prophylaxis against disseminated MAC with azithromycin or clarithromycin.[1] Age-related advanced immunosuppression is defined according to the following CD4+ T-lymphocyte thresholds:

- 6 years of age or older: <50 cells/μL;
- 2 through 5 years of age: <75 cells/μL;
- 1 through 2 years of age: <500 cells/μL; and
- younger than 1 year of age: <750 cells/μL.

Rifabutin is a less effective alternative agent but should not be used until tuberculosis disease has been excluded. Disseminated MAC should be excluded by a negative blood culture result before prophylaxis is initiated.

Oral suspensions of clarithromycin and azithromycin are available in the United States. Appropriate doses would be: clarithromycin, 7.5 mg/kg (maximum, 500 mg), orally, twice daily; azithromycin, 20 mg/kg (maximum, 1200 mg), orally, weekly; or azithromycin, 5 mg/kg (maximum, 250 mg), orally, daily. No pediatric formulation of rifabutin is available, but a dosage of 5 mg/kg per day (maximum, 300 mg) seems appropriate. Rifabutin should be used only for children older than 6 years of age. Prophylaxis can be discontinued in some HIV-infected children after immune reconstitution (see Table 3.85).

ISOLATION OF THE HOSPITALIZED PATIENT: Standard precautions are recommended.

CONTROL MEASURES: Control measures include chemoprophylaxis for high-risk patients with HIV infection (see Treatment, p 762), avoidance of tap water contamination of central venous catheters, surgical wounds, skin antisepsis, or endoscopic equipment, and use of sterile equipment for middle-ear instrumentation, including otoscopic equipment, for prevention of *M abscessus* otitis media. Because MAC and *M abscessus* are common in environmental sources, current information does not support specific recommendations about avoidance of exposure for HIV-infected people (MAC) or adolescents with cystic fibrosis (MAC or *M abscessus*).

---

[1] Centers for Disease Control and Prevention. Guidelines for the prevention and treatment of opportunistic infections among HIV-exposed and HIV-infected children: recommendations from the CDC, the National Institutes of Health, the HIV Medicine Association of the Infectious Diseases Society of America, the Pediatric Infectious Diseases Society, and the American Academy of Pediatrics. *MMWR Recomm Rep.* 2009;58(RR-11):1–166

Table 3.85. Criteria for Discontinuing and Restarting MAC Prophylaxis in HIV-Infected Children

Age	Criteria for Discontinuing Primary Prophylaxis	Criteria for Restarting Primary Prophylaxis	Criteria for Discontinuing Secondary Prophylaxis	Criteria for Restarting Secondary Prophylaxis
Younger than 2 y	Do not discontinue	...	Do not discontinue	...
2 through 5 y	ART 6 mo or more CD4+ T-lymphocyte count greater than 200 cells/mm³ for more than 3 consecutive mo	CD4+ T-lymphocyte count less than 200/mm³	ART 6 mo or more More than 12 mo MAC therapy Asymptomatic CD4+ T-lymphocyte count greater than 200/mm³ for 6 mo or more	CD4+ T-lymphocyte count less than 200/mm³
6 y or older	ART 6 mo or longer CD4+ T-lymphocyte count greater than 200 cells/mm³ for more than 3 consecutive mo	CD4+ T-lymphocyte count less than 100/mm³	ART 6 mo or more More than 12 mo MAC therapy Asymptomatic CD4+ T-lymphocyte count less than 100/mm³ for 6 mo or more	CD4+ T-lymphocyte count less than 100/mm³

MAC indicates *Mycobacterium avium* complex; HIV, human immunodeficiency virus; ART, antiretroviral therapy.

Tularemia

CLINICAL MANIFESTATIONS: Most patients with tularemia have abrupt onset of fever, chills, myalgia, and headache. Illness usually conforms to one of several tularemic syndromes. Most common is the ulceroglandular syndrome, characterized by a maculopapular lesion at the entry site, with subsequent ulceration and slow healing associated with painful, acutely inflamed regional lymph nodes, which can drain spontaneously. The glandular syndrome (regional lymphadenopathy with no ulcer) also is common. Less common disease syndromes are: oculoglandular (severe conjunctivitis and preauricular lymphadenopathy), oropharyngeal (severe exudative stomatitis, pharyngitis, or tonsillitis and cervical lymphadenopathy), vesicular skin lesions that can be mistaken for herpes simplex virus or varicella zoster virus, typhoidal (high fever, hepatomegaly, and splenomegaly), intestinal (intestinal pain, vomiting, and diarrhea), and pneumonic. Pneumonic tularemia, characterized by fever, dry cough, chest pain, and hilar adenopathy, would be the typical syndrome after intentional aerosol release of organisms.

ETIOLOGY: *Francisella tularensis* is a small, weakly-staining, gram-negative pleomorphic coccobacillus. Two subspecies cause human infection in North America, *F tularensis* subspecies tularensis (type A), and *F tularensis* subspecies holartica (type B).

EPIDEMIOLOGY: *F tularensis* can infect more than 100 animal species; vertebrates considered most important in enzootic cycles are rabbits, hares, and rodents, especially muskrats, voles, and beavers. In the United States, human infection usually is associated with direct contact with one of these species, the bite of an infected domestic cat, or the bite of arthropod vectors ticks and deer flies. Infection has been reported in commercially traded hamsters and in a child bitten by a pet hamster. Infection also can be acquired following ingestion of contaminated water or inadequately cooked meat, inhalation of contaminated aerosols generated during lawn mowing, brush cutting, or piling contaminated hay. At-risk people have occupational or recreational exposure to infected animals or their habitats, such as rabbit hunters and trappers, people exposed to certain ticks or biting insects, and laboratory technicians working with *F tularensis*, which is highly infectious and aerosolized easily when grown in culture. In the United States, most cases occur during June to October. Approximately two thirds of cases occur in males, and one quarter of cases occur in children 1 to 14 years of age. Since 2000, when tularemia was redesignated a nationally notifiable disease, there have been 90 to 154 cases reported per year. Organisms can be present in blood during the first 2 weeks of disease and in cutaneous lesions for as long as 1 month if untreated. Person-to-person transmission does not occur.

The **incubation period** usually is 3 to 5 days, with a range of 1 to 21 days.

DIAGNOSTIC TESTS: Diagnosis is established most often by serologic testing. Most patients do not develop antibodies until the second week of illness. A single serum antibody titer of 1:128 or greater determined by microagglutination (MA) or of 1:160 or greater determined by tube agglutination (TA) is consistent with recent or past infection and constitutes a presumptive diagnosis. Confirmation by serologic testing requires a fourfold or greater titer change between serum samples obtained at least 2 weeks apart, with 1 of the specimens having a minimum titer of 1:128 or greater by MA or 1:160 or greater by TA. Nonspecific cross-reactions can occur with specimens containing hetero-phile antibodies or antibodies to *Brucella* species, *Legionella* species, or other gram-negative bacteria. However, cross-reactions rarely result in MA or TA titers that are diagnostic. Some clinical laboratories presumptively can identify *F tularensis* in ulcer exudate or aspirate material by polymerase chain reaction (PCR) or direct fluorescent antibody assays. Immunohistochemical staining is specific for detection of *F tularensis* in fixed tissues; however, this method is not available in most clinical laboratories. Isolation of *F tularensis* from specimens of blood, skin, ulcers, lymph node drainage, gastric washings, or respiratory tract secretions is best achieved by inoculation of cysteine-enriched media. Suspect growth on culture can be identified presumptively by PCR or direct fluorescent antibody assays. Because of its propensity for causing laboratory-acquired infections, laboratory personnel should be alerted when *F tularensis* infection is suspected.

TREATMENT: Streptomycin or gentamicin is recommended for treatment of tularemia. Duration of therapy usually is 10 days. A longer course is required for more severe illness. Ciprofloxacin is an alternative for mild disease, but ciprofloxacin is not recommended for this indication in patients younger than 18 years of age. Doxycycline is another alternative agent. Treatment with doxycycline should be continued for at least 14 days because of a higher rate of relapses when compared with other therapies. Doxycycline should not be given to children younger than 8 years of age unless the benefits of therapy are greater than the risks of dental staining (see Tetracyclines, p 801). Suppuration of lymph nodes can occur despite antimicrobial therapy. *F tularensis* is resistant to beta-lactam drugs and carbapenems.

ISOLATION OF THE HOSPITALIZED PATIENT: Standard precautions are recommended.

CONTROL MEASURES:
- People should protect themselves against arthropod bites by wearing protective clothing, by frequent inspection for and removal of ticks from the skin and scalp, and by using insect repellents (see Prevention of Tickborne Infections, p 207).
- Children should be instructed not to handle sick or dead animals.
- Rubber gloves should be worn by hunters, trappers, and food preparers when handling the carcasses of wild rabbits and other potentially infected animals.
- Game meats should be cooked thoroughly.
- Face masks and rubber gloves should be worn by laboratory personnel handling cultures or infective material, and the work should be performed in a biologic safety cabinet.
- Standard precautions should be used for handling clinical materials.
- A 14-day course of doxycycline or ciprofloxacin (which is only approved for specific indications in patients younger than 18 years of age) is recommended for children and adults after exposure to an intentional release of tularemia.
- A live-attenuated vaccine derived from *F tularensis* subspecies holarctica (type B) strain used to protect people routinely working with *F tularensis* in the laboratory is not available.

Endemic Typhus
(Murine Typhus)

CLINICAL MANIFESTATIONS: Endemic typhus resembles epidemic (louseborne) typhus but usually has a less abrupt onset with less severe systemic symptoms. In young children, the disease can be mild. Fever, present in almost all patients, can be accompanied by a persistent, usually severe, headache and myalgia. Nausea and vomiting also develop in approximately half of patients. A rash typically appears on day 4 to 7 of illness, is macular or maculopapular, lasts 4 to 8 days, and tends to remain discrete, with sparse lesions and no hemorrhage. Rash is present in approximately 50% of patients. Illness seldom lasts longer than 2 weeks; visceral involvement is uncommon. Fatal outcome is rare except in untreated severe disease.

ETIOLOGY: Endemic typhus is caused by *Rickettsia typhi*.

EPIDEMIOLOGY: Rats, in which infection is unapparent, are the natural reservoirs for *Rickettsia typhi*. The primary vector for transmission among rats and to humans is the rat flea, *Xenopsylla cheopis*, although other fleas and mites have been implicated. Cat fleas and opossums have been implicated as the source of some cases of endemic typhus caused by *Rickettsia felis*. Infected flea feces are rubbed into broken skin or mucous membranes or inhaled. The disease is worldwide in distribution and tends to occur most commonly in adults, in males, and during the months of April to October; in children, males and females are affected equally. Exposure to rats and their fleas is the major risk factor for infection, although a history of such exposure often is absent. Endemic typhus is rare in the United States, with most cases occurring in southern California, southern Texas, the southeastern Gulf Coast, and Hawaii.

The **incubation period** is 6 to 14 days.

DIAGNOSTIC TESTS: Antibody titers determined with *R typhi* antigen by an indirect fluorescent antibody (IFA) assay, enzyme immunoassay, or latex agglutination test peak around 4 weeks after infection, but these test results often are negative up to 10 days after illness onset. A fourfold immunoglobulin (Ig) G titer change between acute and convalescent serum specimens taken 2 to 3 weeks apart is diagnostic. Although more prone to false-positive results, immunoassays demonstrating rises in specific IgM antibody can aid in distinguishing clinical illness from previous exposure if interpreted with a concurrent IgG test; use of IgM assays alone is not recommended. Serologic tests may not differentiate murine typhus from epidemic (louseborne) typhus, *Rickettsia felis* infection, or infection with spotted fever rickettsiosis such as *R rickettsii* without antibody cross-absorption for IFA or western blotting analyses, which are not available routinely. Isolation of the organism in cell culture potentially is hazardous and is best performed by specialized laboratories, such as the Centers for Disease Control and Prevention (CDC). Routine hospital blood cultures are not suitable for culture of *R typhi*. Molecular diagnostic assays on infected whole blood and skin biopsies can distinguish endemic and epidemic typhus and other rickettsioses and are performed at the CDC. Immunohistochemical procedures on formalin-fixed skin biopsy tissues can be performed at the CDC.

TREATMENT: Doxycycline is the treatment of choice for endemic typhus, regardless of patient age. The recommended dosage of doxycycline is 4 mg/kg per day, divided every 12 hours, intravenously or orally (maximum 100 mg/dose; see Tetracyclines, p 801). Doxycycline has not been demonstrated to cause cosmetic staining of developing permanent teeth when used in the dose and duration recommended to treat rickettsial diseases. Treatment should be continued for at least 3 days after defervescence and evidence of clinical improvement is documented, usually for 7 to 14 days. Fluoroquinolones or chloramphenicol are alternative medications but may not be as effective; fluoroquinolones are not approved for this use in children younger than 18 years of age (see Fluoroquinolones, p 800).

ISOLATION OF THE HOSPITALIZED PATIENT: Standard precautions are recommended.

CONTROL MEASURES: Fleas should be controlled by appropriate insecticides before use of rodenticides, because fleas will seek alternative hosts, including humans. Suspected animal populations should be controlled by animal-appropriate means. No prophylaxis is recommended for exposed people. The disease should be reported to local or state public health departments.

Epidemic Typhus
(Louseborne or Sylvatic Typhus)

CLINICAL MANIFESTATIONS: Epidemic louseborne typhus usually is characterized by the abrupt onset of high fever, chills, and myalgia accompanied by severe headache and malaise. A rash appears 4 to 7 days after illness onset, beginning on the trunk and spreading to the limbs. A concentrated eruption can be present in the axillae. The rash typically is maculopapular, becomes petechial or hemorrhagic, and then develops into brownish pigmented areas. The face, palms, and soles usually are not affected. There is no eschar, as often is present in many other rickettsial diseases. Changes in mental status are common, and delirium or coma can occur. Myocardial and renal failure can occur when the disease is severe. The fatality rate in untreated people is as high as 30%. Mortality is less common in children, and the rate increases with advancing age. Untreated patients who recover typically have an illness lasting 2 weeks. Brill-Zinsser disease is a relapse of epidemic louseborne typhus that can occur years after the initial episode. Factors that reactivate the rickettsiae are unknown, but relapse often is more mild and of shorter duration.

ETIOLOGY: Epidemic typhus is caused by *Rickettsia prowazekii.*

EPIDEMIOLOGY: Humans are the primary reservoir of the organism, which is transmitted from person to person by the human body louse, *Pediculus humanus corporis.* Infected louse feces are rubbed into broken skin or mucous membranes or inhaled. All ages are affected. Poverty, crowding, poor sanitary conditions, and poor personal hygiene contribute to the spread of body lice and, hence, the disease. Cases of epidemic louseborne typhus are rare in the United States but have occurred throughout the world, including Asia, Africa, some parts of Europe, and Central and South America. Epidemic typhus is most common during winter, when conditions favor person-to-person transmission of the vector, the body louse. Rickettsiae are present in the blood and tissues of patients during the early febrile phase but are not found in secretions. Direct person-to-person spread of the disease does not occur in the absence of the louse vector. In the United States, sporadic human cases associated with close contact with infected flying squirrels, their nests or their ectoparasites occasionally are reported in the eastern United States. Flying squirrel-associated disease, called sylvatic typhus, typically presents as a milder illness than body louse transmitted infection. *Amblyomma* ticks in the Americas and in Ethiopia have been shown to carry *R prowazekii,* but their vector potential is unknown.

The **incubation period** is 1 to 2 weeks.

DIAGNOSTIC TESTS: *R prowazekii* can be isolated from acute blood specimens by animal passage or through tissue culture but can be hazardous. Definitive diagnosis requires immunohistochemical visualization of rickettsiae in tissues, isolation of the organism, detection of rickettsial DNA by polymerase chain reaction assay, or a fourfold change in antibody titer between acute and convalescent serum specimens obtained 2 to 3 weeks apart. The indirect fluorescent antibody test is the preferred serologic assay, but enzyme immunoassay and dot immunoassay tests also are available. Specific molecular assays, isolation, and an immunohistochemical assay for typhus group rickettsiae in formalin-fixed tissue specimens are available at the Centers for Disease Control and Prevention.

TREATMENT: Doxycycline is the drug of choice to treat epidemic typhus, regardless of patient age. The recommended dosage of doxycycline is 4 mg/kg per day, divided every 12 hours, intravenously or orally (maximum 100 mg/dose; see Tetracyclines, p 801). Doxycycline has not been demonstrated to cause cosmetic staining of developing permanent teeth when used in the dose and duration recommended to treat rickettsial diseases. Treatment should be continued for at least 3 days after defervescence and evidence of clinical improvement is documented, usually for 7 to 14 days. Ciprofloxacin is not recommended, because treatment failures have occurred. Chloramphenicol is an acceptable alternative drug. To halt the spread of disease to other people, louse-infested patients should be treated with cream or gel pediculicides containing pyrethrins or permethrin; malathion is prescribed most often when pyrethroids fail. In epidemic situations in which antimicrobial agents may be limited (eg, refugee camps), a single dose of doxycycline may provide effective treatment (100 mg for children; 200 mg for adults).

ISOLATION OF THE HOSPITALIZED PATIENT: Standard precautions are recommended. Precautions should be taken to delouse hospitalized patients with louse infestations.

CONTROL MEASURES: Thorough delousing in epidemic situations, particularly among exposed contacts of cases, is recommended. Several applications of pediculicides may be needed, because lice eggs are resistant to most insecticides. Washing clothes in hot water kills lice and eggs. During epidemics, insecticides dusted onto clothes of louse-infested populations are effective. Prevention and control of flying squirrel-associated typhus requires application of insecticides and precautions to prevent contact with these animals and their ectoparasites and to exclude them from human dwellings. No prophylaxis is recommended for people exposed to flying squirrels. Cases should be reported to local or state public health departments.

Ureaplasma urealyticum Infections

CLINICAL MANIFESTATIONS: There has been an inconsistent association with *Ureaplasma urealyticum* infections and nongonococcal urethritis (NGU). Although 15% to 55% of cases of NGU are caused by *Chlamydia trachomatis, U urealyticum* has been implicated as an etiologic agent in some cases. Without treatment, the disease usually resolves within 1 to 6 months, although asymptomatic infection may persist. There also has been an inconsistent relationship with *U urealyticum* infection and prostatitis and epididymitis in men and salpingitis, endometritis, and chorioamnionitis in women. Some reports also describe an association between infection and infectivity and recurrent pregnancy loss. The association of *U urealyticum* as a cofactor with human papillomavirus in the development of cervical cancer has been described.

U urealyticum has been isolated from the lower respiratory tract and from lung biopsy specimens of preterm infants and contributes to intrauterine pneumonia and chronic lung disease of prematurity. Although the organism also has been recovered from respiratory tract secretions of infants 3 months of age or younger with pneumonia, its role in development of lower respiratory tract disease in otherwise healthy young infants is controversial. *U urealyticum* has been isolated from cerebrospinal fluid of newborn infants with meningitis, intraventricular hemorrhage, and hydrocephalus. The contribution of *U urealyticum* to the outcome of these newborn infants is unclear given the confounding effects of preterm birth and intraventricular hemorrhage.

Isolated cases of *U urealyticum* arthritis, osteomyelitis, pneumonia, pericarditis, meningitis, and progressive sinopulmonary disease in immunocompromised patients have been reported.

ETIOLOGY: *Ureaplasma* and *Mycoplasma* are genera in the Mycoplasmataceae family. *Ureaplasma* organisms are small pleomorphic bacteria that lack a cell wall. The genus *Ureaplasma* contains 2 species capable of causing human infection, *U urealyticum* and *Ureaplasma parvum*. At least 14 serotypes have been described.

EPIDEMIOLOGY: The principal reservoir of human *U urealyticum* is the genital tract of sexually active adults. Colonization occurs in approximately half of sexually active women; the incidence in sexually active men is lower. Colonization is uncommon in prepubertal children and adolescents who are not sexually active, but a positive genital tract culture is not clearly definitive of sexual abuse. Transmission during delivery is likely from an asymptomatic colonized mother to her newborn infant. *U urealyticum* may colonize the throat, eyes, umbilicus, and perineum of newborn infants and may persist for several months after birth.

Because *U urealyticum* commonly is isolated from the female lower genital tract and neonatal respiratory tract in the absence of disease, a positive culture does not establish its causative role in acute infection. However, recovery from an upper genital tract or lower respiratory tract specimen is much more indicative of infection.

The **incubation period** after sexual transmission is 10 to 20 days.

DIAGNOSTIC TESTS: Specimens for culture require specific *Ureaplasma* transport media with refrigeration at 4°C (39°F). Dacron or calcium alginate swabs should be used; cotton swabs should be avoided. Several rapid, sensitive polymerase chain reaction assays for detection of *U urealyticum* have been developed and have greater sensitivity than culture but are not available routinely. *U urealyticum* can be cultured in urea-containing broth in 1 to 2 days. Serologic testing for *U urealyticum* antibodies is of limited value and should not be used for routine diagnosis.

TREATMENT: A positive culture does not indicate need for therapy if the patient is asymptomatic. Mycoplasmas generally are susceptible to tetracyclines (eg, minocycline, doxycycline) and quinolones, but because they lack a cell wall, mycoplasmas are not susceptible to penicillins or cephalosporins. For symptomatic older children, adolescents, and adults, doxycycline is the drug of choice. Persistent urethritis after doxycycline treatment can occur by doxycycline-resistant *U urealyticum* or *Mycoplasma genitalium*. Recurrences are common. Azithromycin is the preferred antimicrobial agent for children younger than 8 years of age, people who are allergic to tetracycline, and people with infections caused by tetracycline-resistant strains. Studies in adult men with NGU indicate that single-dose azithromycin (1 g, orally) is effective. Antimicrobial treatment with erythromycin has failed both in small randomized trials and in reports of cohort studies in pregnant women to prevent preterm delivery and in preterm infants to prevent pulmonary disease. Although better in vitro efficacy is observed with clarithromycin and newer quinolones, adequate efficacy trials that control for confounding attributable to concurrent infections or concomitant medications, such as anti-inflammatory agents, have not yet been completed. Neither clarithromycin nor ciprofloxacin are approved by the US Food and Drug Administration for the treatment of *Ureaplasma* infections, although both are approved for other indications in pediatric patients. Clarithromycin and ciprofloxacin cannot be recommended for *Ureaplasma* infection in preterm infants. Similarly, definitive evidence of efficacy of antimicrobial agents in treatment of central nervous system infections in infants and children is lacking.

ISOLATION OF THE HOSPITALIZED PATIENT: Standard precautions are recommended.

CONTROL MEASURES: Partners of patients with NGU attributable to *U urealyticum* should be offered treatment.

Varicella-Zoster Infections

CLINICAL MANIFESTATIONS: Primary infection results in varicella (chickenpox), manifesting as a generalized, pruritic, vesicular rash typically consisting of 250 to 500 lesions in varying stages of development and resolution (crusting), low-grade fever, and other systemic symptoms. Complications include bacterial superinfection of skin lesions, pneumonia, central nervous system involvement (acute cerebellar ataxia, encephalitis), thrombocytopenia, and other rare complications, such as glomerulonephritis, arthritis, and hepatitis. Varicella tends to be more severe in infants, adolescents, and adults than in young children. Breakthrough chickenpox cases usually are mild and clinically modified and occur in immunized children as described later in Active Immunization (p 783). Reye syndrome can follow cases of chickenpox, although Reye syndrome currently is rare because of decreased use of salicylates during varicella. In immunocompromised children, progressive, severe varicella characterized by continuing eruption of lesions and high fever persisting into the second week of illness as well as encephalitis, hepatitis, and pneumonia can develop. Hemorrhagic varicella is much more common among immunocompromised patients than among immunocompetent hosts. Pneumonia is relatively less common among immunocompetent children but is the most common complication in adults. In children with human immunodeficiency virus (HIV) infection, recurrent varicella or disseminated herpes zoster can develop. Severe and even fatal varicella has been reported in otherwise healthy children receiving intermittent courses of high-dose corticosteroids (greater than 2 mg/kg of prednisone or equivalent) for treatment of asthma and other illnesses. The risk especially is high when corticosteroids are given during the incubation period for chickenpox.

Varicella-zoster virus (VZV) establishes latency in the dorsal root ganglia during primary infection and/or breakthrough varicella that may develop despite immunization. Reactivation results in herpes zoster ("shingles"), characterized by grouped vesicular lesions in the distribution of 1 to 3 sensory dermatomes, sometimes accompanied by pain and/or itching localized to the area. *Postherpetic neuralgia,* which may last for weeks to months, is defined as pain that persists after resolution of the zoster rash. Zoster occasionally can become disseminated in immunocompromised patients, with lesions appearing outside the primary dermatomes and with visceral complications. Childhood zoster tends to be milder than disease in adults and is less frequently associated with postherpetic neuralgia. The attenuated VZV in the varicella vaccine can also establish latent infection and reactivate as herpes zoster. However, data from immunocompromised children indicate that the risk of developing zoster is lower among vaccine recipients than among children who have experienced natural varicella. Postlicensure data also suggest a lower risk of herpes zoster among healthy vaccinees.

Fetal infection after maternal varicella during the first or early second trimester of pregnancy occasionally results in fetal death or varicella embryopathy, characterized by limb hypoplasia, cutaneous scarring, eye abnormalities, and damage to the central nervous system (congenital varicella syndrome). The incidence of congenital varicella syndrome among infants born to mothers with varicella is approximately 1% to 2% when infection occurs before 20 weeks of gestation. Two cases of congenital varicella syndrome have been reported in infants of women infected after 20 weeks of pregnancy, the latest occurring at 28 weeks. Children exposed to VZV in utero also can develop inapparent varicella and subsequent zoster early in life without having had extrauterine varicella. Varicella infection has a higher case-fatality rate in infants when the mother develops varicella from 5 days before to 2 days after delivery, because there is little opportunity for development and transfer of antibody from mother to infant and the infant's cellular immune system is immature. When varicella develops in a mother more than 5 days before delivery and gestational age is 28 weeks or more, the severity of disease in the newborn infant is modified by transplacental transfer of VZV-specific maternal immunoglobulin (Ig) G antibody.

ETIOLOGY: VZV (also known as human herpesvirus 3) is a member of the herpesvirus family, the alphaherpes subfamily, and the varicellovirus genus.

EPIDEMIOLOGY: Humans are the only source of infection for this highly contagious virus. Humans are infected when the virus comes in contact with the mucosa of the upper respiratory tract or the conjunctiva. Person-to-person transmission occurs by the airborne route from direct contact with patients with vesicular VZV lesions (varicella and herpes zoster); vesicles contain infectious virus that can be aerosolized. Transmission also may occur from infected respiratory tract secretions. There is no evidence of VZV spread from fomites, because the virus is extremely labile and is unable to survive long periods in the environment. In utero infection occurs as a result of transplacental passage of virus during maternal varicella infection. VZV infection in a household member usually results in infection of almost all susceptible people in that household. Children who acquire their infection at home (secondary family cases) often have more skin lesions than the index case. Health care-associated transmission is well documented in pediatric units, but transmission is rare in newborn nurseries.

In temperate climates in the prevaccine era, varicella was a childhood disease with a marked seasonal distribution, with peak incidence during late winter and early spring. In tropical climates, the epidemiology of varicella is different; acquisition of disease occurs at later ages, resulting in a higher proportion of adults being susceptible to varicella compared with adults in temperate climates. In the prevaccine era, most cases of varicella in the United States occurred in children younger than 10 years of age. Following implementation of universal immunization in the United States in 1995, varicella disease has declined in all age groups, with evidence of herd protection. The age of peak varicella incidence is shifting from children younger than 10 years of age to children 10 through 14 years of age, although the incidence in this and all age groups is lower than in the prevaccine era. Immunity generally is lifelong. Cellular immunity is more important than humoral immunity for limiting the extent of primary infection with VZV and for preventing reactivation of virus with herpes zoster. Symptomatic reinfection is uncommon in immunocompetent people; asymptomatic reinfection is more frequent. Asymptomatic primary infection is unusual.

Since 2007, coverage with 1 dose of varicella vaccine among 19- through 35-month-old children in the United States has been 90%. As vaccine coverage increases and the incidence of wild-type varicella decreases, a greater proportion of varicella cases are occurring in immunized people as breakthrough disease. This should not be confused as an increasing rate of breakthrough disease or as evidence of increasing vaccine failure. In the surveillance areas with high vaccine coverage, the rate of varicella disease decreased by approximately 90% from 1995 to 2005 with use of varicella vaccine. Since recommendation of a routine second dose of vaccine in 2006, the incidence of varicella has declined further in children.

Immunocompromised people with primary (varicella) or recurrent (herpes zoster) infection are at increased risk of severe disease. Severe varicella and disseminated zoster are more likely to develop in children with congenital T-lymphocyte defects or acquired immunodeficiency syndrome than in people with B-lymphocyte abnormalities. Other groups of pediatric patients who may experience more severe or complicated disease include infants, adolescents, patients with chronic cutaneous or pulmonary disorders, and patients receiving systemic corticosteroids, other immunosuppressive therapy, or long-term salicylate therapy.

Patients are contagious from 1 to 2 days before onset of the rash until all lesions have crusted.

The **incubation period** usually is 14 to 16 days and occasionally is as short as 10 or as long as 21 days after exposure to rash. The incubation period may be prolonged for as long as 28 days after receipt of Varicella-Zoster Immune Globulin or Immune Globulin Intravenous (IGIV) and shortened in immunocompromised patients. Varicella can develop between 2 and 16 days after birth in infants born to mothers with active varicella around the time of delivery; the usual interval from onset of rash in a mother to onset in her neonate is 9 to 15 days.

DIAGNOSTIC TESTS: Diagnostic tests for VZV are summarized in Table 3.86, p 777. Vesicular fluid or a scab can be used to identify VZV using a polymerase chain reaction (PCR) test. This testing also can be used to distinguish between wild-type and vaccine-strain VZV (genotyping), which may especially be desirable and informative in immunized children who develop herpes zoster. PCR assay currently is the diagnostic method of choice. During the acute phase of the illness, VZV also can be identified by PCR assay of saliva or buccal swabs, from both unimmunized and immunized patients. VZV also can be demonstrated by direct fluorescent antibody (DFA) assay or isolated in cell culture, using scrapings of a vesicle base during the first 3 to 4 days of the eruption. Viral culture and DFA assay both are less sensitive than PCR assay, and neither test has the capacity to distinguish vaccine strain from wild-type viruses. Genotyping is available free of charge through the specialized reference laboratory at the Centers for Disease Control and

Table 3.86. Diagnostic Tests for Varicella-Zoster Virus (VZV) Infection

Test	Specimen	Comments
Tissue culture	Vesicular fluid, CSF, biopsy tissue	Distinguishes VZV from HSV. Cost, limited availability, requires up to a week for result.
PCR	Vesicular swabs or scrapings, scabs from crusted lesions, biopsy tissue, CSF	Very sensitive method. Specific for VZV. Real-time methods (not widely available) have been designed that distinguish vaccine strain from wild-type (rapid, within 3 hours).
DFA	Vesicle scraping, swab of lesion base (must include cells)	Specific for VZV. More rapid and more sensitive than culture, less sensitive than PCR.
Tzanck smear	Vesicle scraping, swab of lesion base (must include cells)	Observe multinucleated giant cells with inclusions. Not specific for VZV. Less sensitive and accurate than DFA.
Serology (IgG)	Acute and convalescent serum specimens for IgG	Specific for VZV. Commercial assays generally have low sensitivity to reliably detect vaccine-induced immunity. gpELISA and FAMA are the only IgG methods that can readily detect vaccine seroconversion, but these tests are not commercially available.
Capture IgM	Acute serum specimens for IgM	Specific for VZV. IgM inconsistently detected. Not reliable method for routine confirmation but positive result indicates current/recent VZV activity. Requires special equipment.

CSF indicates cerebrospinal fluid; HSV, herpes simplex virus; PCR, polymerase chain reaction; DFA, direct fluorescent antibody; IgG, immunoglobulin G; gpELISA, glycoprotein enzyme-linked immunoassay; FAMA, fluorescent antibody to membrane antigen (assay); IgM, immunoglobulin M.

Prevention (CDC [404-639-0066]) and also through a safety research program sponsored by Merck & Co (1-800-672-6372). A significant increase in serum varicella IgG antibody between acute and convalescent samples by any standard serologic assay can confirm a diagnosis retrospectively. These antibody tests are reliable for diagnosing natural infection in healthy hosts but may not be reliable in immunocompromised people (see Care of Exposed People, p 779). Commercially available enzyme immunoassay (EIA) tests are not sufficiently sensitive to demonstrate reliably a vaccine-induced antibody response. IgM tests are not reliable for routine confirmation or ruling out of acute infection, but positive results indicate current or recent VZV infection or reactivation.

TREATMENT: The decision to use antiviral therapy and the route and duration of therapy should be determined by specific host factors, extent of infection, and initial response to therapy. Antiviral drugs have a limited window of opportunity to affect the outcome of VZV infection. In immunocompetent hosts, most virus replication has stopped by 72 hours after onset of rash; the duration of replication may be extended in immunocompromised hosts. Oral acyclovir or valacyclovir are not recommended for routine use in otherwise healthy children with varicella. Administration within 24 hours of onset of rash results in only a modest decrease in symptoms. Oral acyclovir or valacyclovir should be considered for otherwise healthy people at increased risk of moderate to severe varicella, such as unvaccinated people older than 12 years of age, people with chronic cutaneous or pulmonary disorders, people receiving long-term salicylate therapy, and people receiving short, intermittent, or aerosolized courses of corticosteroids. Some experts also recommend use of oral acyclovir or valacyclovir for secondary household cases in which the disease usually is more severe than in the primary case. For recommendations on dosage and duration of therapy, see Antiviral Drugs (p 841).

Acyclovir is a category B drug based on US Food and Drug Administration (FDA) Drug Risk Classification in pregnancy. Some experts recommend oral acyclovir or valacyclovir for pregnant women with varicella, especially during the second and third trimesters. Intravenous acyclovir is recommended for the pregnant patient with serious complications of varicella.

Intravenous acyclovir therapy is recommended for immunocompromised patients, including patients being treated with chronic corticosteroids. Therapy initiated early in the course of the illness, especially within 24 hours of rash onset, maximizes efficacy. Oral acyclovir should not be used to treat immunocompromised children with varicella because of poor oral bioavailability. In 2008, valacyclovir (20 mg/kg per dose, with a maximum dose of 1000 mg, administered 3 times daily for 5 days) was licensed for treatment of chickenpox in children 2 to <18 years of age. Some experts have used valacyclovir, with its improved bioavailability compared with oral acyclovir, in selected immunocompromised patients perceived to be at lower risk of developing severe varicella, such as HIV-infected patients with relatively normal concentrations of CD4+ T-lymphocytes and children with leukemia in whom careful follow-up is ensured. Although the antiviral drug famciclovir is available for treatment of VZV infections in adults, its efficacy and safety have not been established for children. Although Varicella-Zoster Immune Globulin or, if not available, IGIV given shortly after exposure can prevent or modify the course of disease, Immune Globulin preparations are not effective once disease is established (see Care of Exposed People, p 779).

Infections caused by acyclovir-resistant VZV strains, which generally are limited to immunocompromised hosts, should be treated with parenteral foscarnet.

Children with varicella should not receive salicylates or salicylate-containing products, because administration of salicylates to such children increases the risk of Reye syndrome. Salicylate therapy should be stopped in a child who is exposed to varicella.

ISOLATION OF THE HOSPITALIZED PATIENT: In addition to standard precautions, airborne and contact precautions are recommended for patients with varicella for a minimum of 5 days after onset of rash and until all lesions are crusted, which, in immunocompromised patients, can be a week or longer. For immunized patients with breakthrough varicella with only maculopapular lesions, isolation is recommended until no new lesions appear within a 24 hour period; lesions do not have to be completely resolved. For exposed patients without evidence of immunity (see Evidence of Immunity to Varicella, p 785), airborne and contact precautions from 8 until 21 days after exposure to the index patient also are indicated; these precautions should be maintained until 28 days after exposure for those who received Varicella-Zoster Immune Globulin or IGIV.

Airborne and contact precautions are recommended for neonates born to mothers with varicella and, if still hospitalized, should be continued until 21 or 28 days of age if they received Varicella-Zoster Immune Globulin or IGIV. Infants with varicella embryopathy do not require isolation if they do not have active lesions.

Immunocompromised patients who have zoster (localized or disseminated) and immunocompetent patients with disseminated zoster require airborne and contact precautions for the duration of illness. For immunocompetent patients with localized zoster, contact precautions are indicated until all lesions are crusted.

CONTROL MEASURES:

Child Care and School. Children with uncomplicated chickenpox who have been excluded from school or child care may return when the rash has crusted or, in immunized people without crusts, until no new lesions appear within a 24-hour period.

Exclusion of children with zoster whose lesions cannot be covered is based on similar criteria. Children who are excluded may return after the lesions have crusted. Lesions that are covered pose little risk to susceptible people, although transmission has been reported.

CARE OF EXPOSED PEOPLE: Potential interventions for people without evidence of immunity exposed to a person with varicella include either varicella vaccine, administered ideally within 3 days but up to 5 days after exposure (followed by a second dose of vaccine at the age-appropriate interval after the first dose) or, when indicated, Varicella-Zoster Immune Globulin. In 2012, the FDA extended the period for administration of Varicella-Zoster Immune Globulin from 96 hours to 10 days after exposure.[1] If Varicella-Zoster Immune Globulin is not available, IGIV can be used (see Unavailability of Varicella-Zoster Immune Globulin, p 782).[2] Prophylactic administration of oral acyclovir beginning 7 days after exposure also may prevent or attenuate varicella disease in healthy children. There is little information on whether prophylactic oral acyclovir is protective for immunocompromised people.

Hospital Exposure. If an inadvertent exposure occurs in the hospital to an infected person by a health care professional, or visitor, the following control measures are recommended:

- Health care professionals, patients, and visitors who have been exposed (see Table 3.87, p 780) and who lack evidence of immunity to varicella should be identified.
- Varicella immunization is recommended for people without evidence of immunity, provided there are no contraindications to vaccine use.
- Varicella-Zoster Immune Globulin should be administered to appropriate candidates (see Table 3.88, p 780). If Varicella-Zoster Immune Globulin is not available, IGIV should be considered as an alternative (see "Unavailability of VariZIG," p 782).
- All exposed patients without evidence of immunity should be discharged as soon as possible.
- All exposed patients without evidence of immunity who cannot be discharged should be placed in isolation from day 8 to day 21 after exposure to the index patient. For people who received Varicella-Zoster Immune Globulin or IGIV, isolation should continue until day 28.
- Health care professionals who have received 2 doses of vaccine and who are exposed to VZV should be monitored daily during days 10 through 21 after exposure through the employee health program or by an infection-control nurse to determine clinical status. They should be placed on sick leave immediately if symptoms occur.

---

[1] Centers for Disease Control and Prevention. FDA approval of an extended period for administering VariZIG for postexposure prophylaxis of varicella. *MMWR Morb Mortal Wkly Rep.* 2012;61(12):212–214

[2] Centers for Disease Control and Prevention. A new product (VariZIG) for postexposure prophylaxis of varicella available under an investigational new drug application expanded access protocol. *MMWR Morb Mortal Wkly Rep.* 2006;55(8):209–210

Table 3.87. Types of Exposure to Varicella or Zoster for Which Varicella-Zoster Immune Globulin Is Indicated for People Without Evidence of Immunity[a]

- Household: residing in the same household
- Playmate: face-to-face[b] indoor play
- Hospital:
  Varicella: In same 2- to 4-bed room or adjacent beds in a large ward, face-to-face[b] contact with an infectious staff member or patient, or visit by a person deemed contagious.
  Zoster: Intimate contact (eg, touching or hugging) with a person deemed contagious.
  Newborn infant: onset of varicella in the mother 5 days or less before delivery or within 48 h after delivery; Varicella-Zoster Immune Globulin or IGIV is not indicated if the mother has zoster.

IGIV indicates Immune Globulin Intravenous.

[a] Patients should meet criteria of both significant exposure and candidacy for receiving Varicella-Zoster Immune Globulin, as given in Table 3.88. Varicella-Zoster Immune Globulin should be administered as soon as possible and no later than 10 days after exposure.

[b] Experts differ in opinion about the duration of face-to-face contact that warrants administration of Varicella-Zoster Immune Globulin. However, the contact should be nontransient. Some experts suggest a contact of 5 or more minutes as constituting significant exposure for this purpose; others define close contact as more than 1 hour.

Table 3.88. Candidates for Varicella-Zoster Immune Globulin, Provided Significant Exposure Has Occurred[a]

- Immunocompromised children[b] without evidence of immunity[c]
- Pregnant women without evidence of immunity[d]
- Newborn infant whose mother had onset of chickenpox within 5 days before delivery or within 48 h after delivery
- Hospitalized preterm infant (28 wk or more of gestation) whose mother lacks evidence of immunity against varicella
- Hospitalized preterm infants (less than 28 wk of gestation or birth weight 1000 g or less), regardless of maternal immunity

[a] See text and Table 3.87, for additional discussion.

[b] Includes children who are infected with human immunodeficiency virus.

[c] Immunocompromised adolescents and adults without evidence of immunity also should receive Varicella-Zoster Immune Globulin.

[d] If Varicella-Zoster Immune Globulin is not available, clinicians may choose to administer Immune Globulin Intravenous (IGIV) or closely monitor the pregnant woman for signs and symptoms of varicella and institute treatment with acyclovir if disease develops.

- Health care professionals who have received only 1 dose of vaccine and who are exposed to VZV should receive the second dose with a single-antigen varicella vaccine, provided 4 weeks have elapsed after the first dose. After immunization, management is similar to that of 2-dose vaccine recipients. For more information, see the recommendations of the CDC.[1]

---

[1] Centers for Disease Control and Prevention. Prevention of varicella: recommendations of the Advisory Committee on Immunization Practices (ACIP). *MMWR Recomm Rep.* 2007;56(RR-4):1–40

- Immunized health care professionals who develop breakthrough infection should be considered infectious until vesicular lesions have crusted or, if they had maculopapular lesions, until no new lesions appear within a 24-hour period.

Postexposure Immunization. Administration of varicella vaccine to people without evidence of immunity 12 months of age or older, including adults, as soon as possible within 72 hours and possibly up to 120 hours after varicella exposure may prevent or modify disease and should be considered in these circumstances if there are no contra-indications to vaccine use. A second dose should be given at the age-appropriate interval after the first dose. Physicians should advise parents and their children that the vaccine may not protect against disease in all cases, because some children may have been exposed at the same time as the index case. However, if exposure to varicella does not cause infection, postexposure immunization with varicella vaccine will result in protection against subsequent exposure. There is no evidence that administration of varicella vaccine during the presymptomatic or prodromal stage of illness increases the risk of vaccine-associated adverse events or more severe natural disease.

Passive Immunoprophylaxis. The decision to administer Varicella-Zoster Immune Globulin depends on 3 factors: (1) the likelihood that the exposed person has no evidence of immunity to varicella; (2) the probability that a given exposure to varicella or zoster will result in infection; and (3) the likelihood that complications of varicella will develop if the person is infected.

Data are unavailable regarding the sensitivity and specificity of serologic tests in immunocompromised patients. However, no test is 100% sensitive or specific and, consequently, false-positive results can occur. Therefore, regardless of serologic test results, careful questioning of children's parents about potential past exposure to disease or clinical description of disease can be helpful in determining immunity. Administration of Varicella-Zoster Immune Globulin or IGIV as soon as possible within 10 days to immunocompromised children who are exposed with no history of varicella and/or unknown or negative serologic test results is recommended. The degree and type of immunosuppression should be considered in making this decision. Varicella-Zoster Immune Globulin is given intramuscularly at the recommended dose of 125 units/10 kg, up to a maximum of 625 units (ie, 5 vials). IGIV is given intravenously at the dose of 400 mg/kg.

Patients receiving monthly high-dose IGIV (400 mg/kg or greater) at regular intervals are likely to be protected if the last dose of IGIV was given 3 weeks or less before exposure.

Where to Obtain Varicella-Zoster Immune Globulin. Varicella-Zoster Immune Globulin is available under an investigational new drug (IND) protocol and can be requested by calling the 24-hour telephone number of FFF Enterprises (800-843-7477).

Suggested Use of Varicella-Zoster Immune Globulin. Tables 3.87 (p 780) and 3.88 (p 780) indicate people without evidence of immunity who should receive Varicella-Zoster Immune Globulin if exposed, including immunocompromised people, pregnant women, and certain newborn infants.

For healthy term infants exposed postnatally to varicella, including infants whose mother's rash developed more than 48 hours after delivery, Varicella-Zoster Immune Globulin is not indicated. However, some experts advise use of Varicella-Zoster Immune

Globulin for exposed newborn infants within the first 2 weeks of life whose mothers do not have evidence of immunity to VZV.

Subsequent exposures and follow-up of Varicella-Zoster Immune Globulin recipients. Because administration of Varicella-Zoster Immune Globulin can cause varicella infection to be asymptomatic, testing of recipients 2 months or later after administration of Varicella-Zoster Immune Globulin to ascertain their immune status may be helpful in the event of subsequent exposure. Most experts, however, would advise Varicella-Zoster Immune Globulin administration after subsequent exposures regardless of serologic results because of the unreliability of serologic test results in immunocompromised people and the uncertainty about whether asymptomatic infection after Varicella-Zoster Immune Globulin administration confers lasting protection.

Any patient to whom Varicella-Zoster Immune Globulin is administered to prevent varicella subsequently should receive age-appropriate varicella vaccine, provided that receipt of live vaccines is not contraindicated. Varicella immunization should be delayed until 5 months after Varicella-Zoster Immune Globulin administration. Varicella vaccine is not needed if the patient develops varicella after administration of Varicella-Zoster Immune Globulin.

Unavailability of Varicella-Zoster Immune Globulin. If Varicella-Zoster Immune Globulin is not available, IGIV can be used. The recommendation for use of IGIV is based on "best judgment of experts" and is supported by reports comparing VZV IgG antibody titers measured in both IGIV and Varicella-Zoster Immune Globulin preparations and patients given IGIV and Varicella-Zoster Immune Globulin. Although licensed IGIV preparations contain antivaricella antibodies, the titer of any specific lot of IGIV is uncertain, because IGIV is not tested routinely for antivaricella antibodies. No clinical data demonstrating effectiveness of IGIV for postexposure prophylaxis of varicella are available. The recommended IGIV dose for postexposure prophylaxis of varicella is 400 mg/kg, intravenously administered once.

Chemoprophylaxis. If Varicella-Zoster Immune Globulin is not available or more than 96 hours have passed since exposure, some experts recommend prophylaxis with acyclovir (20 mg/kg per dose, administered 4 times per day, with a maximum daily dose of 3200 mg) or valacyclovir (20 mg/kg per dose, administered 3 times per day, with a maximum daily dose of 3000 mg) beginning 7 to 10 days after exposure and continuing for 7 days for immunocompromised patients without evidence of immunity who have been exposed to varicella. A 7-day course of acyclovir or valacyclovir also may be given to adults without evidence of immunity if vaccine is contraindicated. Limited data on acyclovir as postexposure prophylaxis are available for healthy children, and no studies have been performed for adults or immunocompromised people. However, limited clinical experience supports use of acyclovir or valacyclovir as postexposure prophylaxis, and clinicians may choose this option if active or passive immunization is not possible. Most adults born before 1980 with no history or an uncertain history of chickenpox are immune if they were raised in the continental United States or Canada.

Active Immunization.[1,2]

Vaccine. Varicella vaccine is a live-attenuated preparation of the serially propagated and attenuated wild Oka strain. The product contains gelatin and trace amounts of neomycin. The monovalent vaccine was licensed in March 1995 by the FDA for use in healthy people 12 months of age or older who have not had varicella illness. Quadrivalent measles-mumps-rubella-varicella (MMRV) vaccine was licensed in September 2005 by the FDA for use in healthy children 12 months through 12 years of age.

Dose and Administration. The recommended dose of vaccine is 0.5 mL, administered subcutaneously.

Immunogenicity. Approximately 76% to 85% of immunized healthy children older than 12 months of age develop humoral immune response to VZV at levels associated with protection (using ≥5 glycoprotein enzyme-linked immunosorbent assay [gpELISA] units/mL or fluorescent antibody to membrane antigen [FAMA] ≥1:4) after a single dose of varicella vaccine. Seroprotection rates are significantly higher (approaching 100% for ≥ 5gpELISA units/mL) after 2 doses. Cell-mediated immune response is also higher after 2 doses.

Effectiveness. The efficacy of 1 dose of varicella vaccine in open-label studies ranged from 70% to 90% against infection and 95% against severe disease. In general, postlicensure effectiveness studies have reported a similar range for prevention against infection (median 85%), with a few studies yielding lower or higher values. The vaccine is highly effective (97% or greater) in preventing severe varicella in postlicensure evaluations. Recipients of 2 doses of varicella vaccine are 3.3-fold less likely to have breakthrough varicella as compared with recipients of 1 dose during the first 10 years after immunization. A study evaluating postlicensure effectiveness of the current 2-dose varicella vaccine schedule demonstrated 98% effectiveness for 2 doses, compared with 86% for 1 dose.

Simultaneous Administration With Other Vaccines or Antiviral Agents. Varicella-containing vaccines may be given simultaneously with other childhood immunizations recommended for children 12 through 15 months of age and 4 through 6 years of age (see Fig 1.1, p 27–28). If not administered at the same visit or as MMRV vaccine, the interval between administration of a varicella-containing vaccine and measles-mumps-rubella (MMR) vaccine should be at least 28 days. Because of susceptibility of vaccine virus to acyclovir, valacyclovir, or famciclovir, these antiviral agents usually should be avoided from 1 day before to 21 days after receipt of a varicella-containing vaccine.

Adverse Events. Varicella vaccine is safe; reactions generally are mild and occur with an overall frequency of approximately 5% to 35%. Approximately 20% to 25% of immunized people will experience minor injection site reactions (eg, pain, redness, swelling). In approximately 1% to 3% of immunized children, a localized rash develops, and in an additional 3% to 5%, a generalized varicella-like rash develops. These rashes typically consist of 2 to 5 lesions and may be maculopapular rather than vesicular; lesions usually appear 5 to 26 days after immunization. However, not all observed postimmunization rashes can be attributable to vaccine. In the early stages of the immunization program, many generalized varicelliform rashes that occurred within the first 2 weeks after varicella

---

[1] Centers for Disease Control and Prevention. Prevention of varicella: recommendations of the Advisory Committee on Immunization Practices (ACIP). *MMWR Recomm Rep.* 2007;56(RR-4):1–40

[2] American Academy of Pediatrics, Committee on Infectious Diseases. Prevention of varicella: update of recommendations for use of quadrivalent and monovalent varicella vaccines in children, including a recommendation for a routine 2-dose varicella immunization schedule. *Pediatrics.* 2011;128(3):630–632

immunization were attributable to wild-type VZV infection and were not an adverse effect of the vaccine. As varicella has continued to decline, rashes in the interval of 0 to 42 days after immunization are less commonly caused by wild-type VZV. In a 2-dose regimen of monovalent vaccine separated by 3 months, injection site complaints were slightly higher after the second dose. After 1 dose, recipients of MMRV are more likely than are recipients of monovalent varicella vaccine and MMR given at separate injection sites to have fever (22% vs 15%, respectively) and a measles-like rash (3% vs 2%, respectively). Both fever and measles-like rash usually occurred within 5 to 12 days of immunization, were of short duration, and resolved without long-term sequelae.

A slightly increased risk of febrile seizures is associated with the higher likelihood of fever following the first dose of MMRV compared with MMR and monovalent varicella. After dose 1 of MMRV vaccine, 1 additional febrile seizure is expected to occur per approximately 2300 to 2600 children immunized, compared with MMR and monovalent varicella. After the second dose, there were no differences in incidence of fever, rash, or febrile seizures among recipients of MMRV vaccine compared with recipients of simultaneous MMR and varicella vaccines.[1]

Serious adverse events, such as anaphylaxis, meningitis, herpes zoster requiring hospitalization (see section below), encephalitis, ataxia, erythema multiforme, Stevens-Johnson syndrome, pneumonia, thrombocytopenia, seizures, neuropathy, Guillain-Barré syndrome, secondary bacterial infections, and death have been reported rarely in temporal association with varicella vaccine. In rare instances, a causal relationship between varicella vaccine and some of these serious adverse events has been established, most often in children with immunocompromising conditions, although the frequency of serious adverse events is much lower than after natural infection. In most cases, data are insufficient to determine a causal association.

Breakthrough Disease. Breakthrough disease is defined as a case of infection with wild-type VZV occurring more than 42 days after immunization. Varicella in vaccine recipients usually is milder than that occurring in unimmunized children, with rash frequently atypical, predominantly maculopapular with a median of fewer than 50 lesions; lower rate of fever; and faster recovery. In contrast, the median number of lesions in unimmunized children with varicella is more than 250. At times, the breakthrough varicella disease is so mild that it is not recognizable easily as varicella, because skin lesions may resemble insect bites. Vaccine recipients with mild breakthrough disease are approximately one third as contagious as unimmunized children. Nonetheless, transmission from mild breakthrough disease has been documented.

Herpes Zoster After Immunization. Varicella vaccine virus has been associated with development of herpes zoster in immunocompetent and immunocompromised people. However, data from postlicensure surveillance indicate that the clinical severity may be milder and the age-specific risk of herpes zoster is lower among immunocompetent children immunized with varicella vaccine than among children who have had natural varicella infection. Wild-type VZV has been identified in vesicles in people with herpes zoster after immunization, indicating that herpes zoster in immunized people also may result from natural varicella infection that occurred before or after immunization. Therefore, it is important that physicians obtain event-appropriate clinical specimens for

---

[1] Centers for Disease Control and Prevention. Use of combination measles, mumps, rubella, and varicella vaccine: recommendations of the Advisory Committee on Immunization Practices (ACIP). *MMWR Recomm Rep.* 2010;59(RR-3):1–12

strain identification when a vaccine adverse event (eg, herpes zoster, meningitis, encephalitis) is suspected. Rare cases of vaccine-strain meningitis or encephalitis with herpes zoster have been documented; all patients recovered fully. A zoster vaccine for adults has been licensed by the FDA in the United States for use in people 50 years of age and older and currently is recommended by CDC for administration to healthy people 60 years of age and older for prevention of herpes zoster.[1,2] Among zoster vaccinees who develop zoster, postherpetic neuralgia is reduced by two thirds in vaccine recipients, compared with placebo recipients.

Transmission of Vaccine-Associated Virus. Vaccine-associated virus transmission to contacts is rare (documented in only 7 immunized people, resulting in 8 secondary cases), and the documented risk of transmission exists only if the immunized person develops a rash. One case of possible transmission without rash is being investigated.

Postexposure prophylaxis with Varicella-Zoster Immune Globulin, IGIV, acyclovir, or valacyclovir in high-risk people exposed to immunized people with lesions has not been studied. However, some experts believe that immunocompromised people in whom skin lesions develop, possibly related to vaccine virus, should receive acyclovir or valacyclovir treatment. Attempts to confirm the presence of VZV by laboratory means should be made in these patients.

Storage. The lyophilized vaccine should be stored in a frost-free freezer at an average temperature of $-15°C$ $(+5°F)$ or colder. The diluent used for reconstitution should be stored separately in a refrigerator or at room temperature. Once the vaccine has been reconstituted, it should be injected as soon as possible and discarded if not used within 30 minutes.

Evidence of Immunity to Varicella. Evidence of immunity to varicella includes any of the following:

1. Documentation of age-appropriate immunization.
   - Preschool-aged children (ie, ≥12 months of age): 1 dose
   - School-aged children, adolescents, and adults: 2 doses
   Postimmunization serologic testing is neither necessary nor recommended following immunization, including in health care personnel.
2. Laboratory evidence of immunity or laboratory confirmation of disease.
3. Varicella diagnosed by a physician or verification of history of varicella disease.
   - For people reporting or presenting with typical disease, verification can be performed by any health care professional (eg, school or occupational clinic nurse, nurse practitioner, physician assistant, physician).
   - For people reporting or presenting with atypical and/or mild cases, assessment by a physician or physician's designee is recommended, and one of the following should be sought: (a) an epidemiologic link to a typical varicella case or to a laboratory-confirmed case; or (b) evidence of laboratory confirmation, if it was performed at the time of acute disease. When such documentation is lacking, people should not be considered as having a valid history of disease, because other diseases may mimic mild atypical varicella.
4. History of herpes zoster diagnosed by a physician.

---

[1] Centers for Disease Control and Prevention. Prevention of herpes zoster: recommendations of the Advisory Committee on Immunization Practices (ACIP). *MMWR Recomm Rep.* 2008;57(RR-5):1–30

[2] Centers for Disease Control and Prevention. Update on herpes zoster vaccine: licensure for persons aged 50 through 59 years. *MMWR Morb Mortal Wkly Rep.* 2011;60(44):1528

5. Birth in the United States before 1980. However, for health care professionals, pregnant women, and immunocompromised people, birth before 1980 should not be considered evidence of immunity.

Recommendations for Immunization.

Children 12 Months Through 12 Years of Age. Both monovalent varicella vaccine and MMRV have been licensed for use for healthy children 12 months through 12 years of age.[1] Children in this age group should receive two 0.5-mL doses of varicella vaccine administered subcutaneously, separated by at least 3 months. The recommendation for at least a 3-month interval between doses is based on the design of the studies evaluating 2 doses in this age group; if the second dose inadvertently is administered between 28 days and 3 months after the first dose, the second dose does not need to be repeated.

All healthy children routinely should receive the first dose of varicella-containing vaccine at 12 through 15 months of age. The second dose of vaccine is recommended routinely when children are 4 through 6 years of age (ie, before a child enters kindergarten or first grade) but can be administered at an earlier age. Because of the minimal potential for increased febrile seizures after the first dose of MMRV vaccine in children 12 through 15 months of age, the American Academy of Pediatrics recommends a choice of either MMR plus monovalent varicella vaccine or MMRV for toddlers receiving their first immunization of this kind.[2] Parents should be counseled about the rare possibility of their child developing a febrile seizure 1 to 2 weeks after immunization with MMRV for the first immunizing dose. For the second dose at 4 through 6 years of age, MMRV generally is preferred over MMR plus monovalent varicella to minimize the number of injections. Varicella vaccine should be administered to all children in this age range unless there is evidence of immunity to varicella or a contraindication to administration of the vaccine. A catch-up second dose of varicella vaccine should be offered to all children 7 years of age and older who have received only 1 dose. A routine health maintenance visit at 11 through 12 years of age is recommended for all adolescents to evaluate immunization status and administer necessary vaccines, including the varicella vaccine.

People 13 Years of Age or Older. People 13 years of age or older without evidence of immunity should receive two 0.5-mL doses of varicella vaccine, separated by at least 28 days. The recommendation for at least a 28-day interval between doses is based on the design of the studies evaluating 2 doses in this age group. For people who previously received only 1 dose of varicella vaccine, a second dose is necessary. Only monovalent varicella vaccine is licensed for use in this age group.

Contraindications and Precautions.

Intercurrent Illness. As with other vaccines, varicella vaccine should not be administered to people who have moderate or severe illnesses, with or without fever (see Vaccine Safety, p 41).

---

[1] Centers for Disease Control and Prevention. Use of combination measles, mumps, rubella, and varicella vaccine: recommendations of the Advisory Committee on Immunization Practices (ACIP). *MMWR Recomm Rep.* 2010;59(RR-3):1–12

[2] American Academy of Pediatrics, Committee on Infectious Diseases. Prevention of varicella: update of recommendations for use of quadrivalent and monovalent varicella vaccines in children, including a recommendation for a routine 2-dose varicella immunization schedule. *Pediatrics.* 2011;128(3):630–632

Immunization of Immunocompromised Patients.

General recommendations. Varicella vaccine should not be administered routinely to children who have congenital or acquired T-lymphocyte immunodeficiency, including people with leukemia, lymphoma, and other malignant neoplasms affecting the bone marrow or lymphatic systems, as well as children receiving long-term immunosuppressive therapy. An exception includes certain children infected with HIV, as discussed below. Children with impaired humoral immunity may be immunized.

Immunodeficiency should be excluded before immunization in children with a family history of hereditary immunodeficiency. The presence of an immunodeficient or HIV-seropositive household family member does not contraindicate vaccine use in other family members.

In people with possible altered immunity, immunization against chickenpox should utilize only monovalent varicella vaccine. The Oka vaccine strain remains susceptible to acyclovir, and if a high-risk patient develops vaccine-related varicella, then acyclovir should be used as treatment.

Acute lymphocytic leukemia. Before routine immunization of healthy children against varicella was instituted in the United States in 1995, many young children with leukemia were susceptible to chickenpox. Considering the variability in intensity of chemotherapy regimens and the current decreasing incidence of varicella in the United States, these high-risk children should not be immunized routinely. Immunization of leukemic children, if susceptible, without evidence of immunity in remission should be undertaken only with expert guidance and with availability of antiviral therapy, should complications occur.

Live-virus vaccines usually are withheld for an interval of at least 3 months after immunosuppressive cancer chemotherapy has been discontinued. However, the interval until immune reconstruction varies with the intensity and type of immunosuppressive therapy, radiation therapy, underlying disease, and other factors. Therefore, it often is not possible to make a definitive recommendation for an interval after cessation of immunosuppressive therapy when live-virus vaccines can be administered safely and effectively.

HIV infection.[1] Screening for HIV infection is not indicated before routine VZV immunization. Varicella vaccine should be considered for nonimmune HIV-infected children with a CD4+ T-lymphocyte percentage of 15% or greater, especially if they are receiving antiretroviral therapy (ART). Eligible children should receive 2 doses of monovalent varicella vaccine with a 3-month interval between doses and return for evaluation if they experience a postimmunization varicella-like rash. Hundreds of such HIV-infected children have now been safely immunized in the United States, and the vaccine is tolerated much as it is in healthy immunized children. Varicella vaccine has been shown to protect these children not only against varicella but also against developing herpes zoster by preventing infection with wild-type VZV.

Children receiving corticosteroids. Varicella vaccine should not be administered to people who are receiving high doses of systemic corticosteroids (2 mg/kg per day or more of prednisone or its equivalent or 20 mg/day of prednisone or its equivalent) for 14 days or more. The recommended interval between discontinuation of corticosteroid therapy and

---

[1] Centers for Disease Control and Prevention. Guidelines for the Prevention and Treatment of Opportunistic Infections Among HIV-Exposed and HIV-Infected Children. Recommendations from CDC, the National Institutes of Health, the HIV Medicine Association of the Infectious Diseases Society of America, the Pediatric Infectious Diseases Society, and the American Academy of Pediatrics. *MMWR Recomm Rep.* 2009;58(RR-11):1–166

immunization with varicella vaccine is at least 1 month. Varicella vaccine may be administered to people receiving inhaled, nasal, and topical steroids.

Children with nephrotic syndrome. The results of one small study indicate that 2 doses of the varicella vaccine in 29 children between 12 months and 18 years of age generally were well tolerated and immunogenic, including children receiving low-dose, alternate-day prednisone.

Households with potential contact with immunocompromised people. Household contacts of immunocompromised people should be immunized if they have no evidence of immunity to decrease the likelihood that wild-type VZV will be introduced in the household. Transmission of vaccine-strain VZV from healthy people has been documented in 7 instances, resulting in 8 secondary cases. Even in families with immunocompromised people, including people with HIV infection, no precautions are needed after immunization of healthy children in whom a rash does not develop. Immunized people in whom a rash develops should avoid direct contact with immunocompromised hosts without evidence of immunity for the duration of the rash.

Pregnancy and Lactation. Varicella vaccine should not be administered to pregnant women, because the possible effects on fetal development are unknown, although no cases of congenital varicella syndrome or patterns of malformation have been identified after inadvertent immunization of pregnant women. When postpubertal females are immunized, pregnancy should be avoided for at least 1 month after immunization. A pregnant mother or other household member is not a contraindication for immunization of a child in the household. Reporting of instances of inadvertent immunization with a varicella-zoster–containing vaccine during pregnancy by telephone is encouraged (1-800-986-8999). (See Pregnancy, p 71–72, and **www.merckpregnancyregistries. com/varivax.html.**)

A study of nursing mothers and their infants showed no evidence of excretion of vaccine strain in human milk or of transmission to infants who are breastfeeding. Varicella vaccine should be administered to nursing mothers who lack evidence of immunity.

Immune Globulin. Whether Immune Globulin (IG) can interfere with varicella vaccine-induced immunity is unknown, although IG can interfere with immunity induction by measles vaccine. Pending additional data, varicella vaccine should be withheld for the same intervals after receipt of any form of IG or other blood product as measles vaccine (see Measles, p 489). Conversely, IG should be withheld for at least 2 weeks after receipt of varicella vaccine. Transplacental antibodies to VZV do not interfere with the immunogenicity of varicella vaccine administered at 12 months of age or older.

Salicylates. Whether Reye syndrome results from administration of salicylates after immunization for varicella in children is unknown. No cases have been reported. However, because of the association among Reye syndrome, natural varicella infection, and salicylates, the vaccine manufacturer recommends that salicylates be avoided for 6 weeks after administration of varicella vaccine. Physicians need to weigh the theoretical risks associated with varicella vaccine against the known risks of wild-type virus in children receiving long-term salicylate therapy.

Allergy to Vaccine Components. Varicella vaccine should not be administered to people who have had an anaphylactic-type reaction to any component of the vaccine, including gelatin and neomycin. Most people with allergy to neomycin have resulting contact dermatitis, a reaction that is not a contraindication to immunization. Monovalent varicella vaccine does not contain preservatives or egg protein, and although the measles and mumps vaccines included in MMRV vaccine are produced in chick embryo culture, the amounts of egg cross-reacting proteins are not significant. Therefore, children with egg allergy routinely may be given MMRV without previous skin testing.

VIBRIO INFECTIONS

Cholera
(Vibrio cholerae)

CLINICAL MANIFESTATIONS: Cholera is characterized by painless, voluminous watery diarrhea without abdominal cramps or fever. Severe dehydration, hypokalemia, metabolic acidosis, and occasionally, hypovolemic shock can occur within 4 to 12 hours if fluid losses are not replaced. Coma, seizures, hypoglycemia, and death also can occur, particularly in children. Stools are colorless, with small flecks of mucus ("rice-water") , and contain high concentrations of sodium, potassium, chloride, and bicarbonate. Most infected people with toxigenic *Vibrio cholerae* O1 have no symptoms, and some have only mild to moderate diarrhea lasting 3 to 7 days.

ETIOLOGY: *V cholerae* is a gram-negative, curved or comma shaped rod that is motile. There are more than 200 *V cholerae* serogroups, some of which carry the cholera toxin (CT) gene. Although those serogroups with the CT gene and others without the CT gene can cause acute watery diarrhea, only toxin-producing serogroups O1 and O139 cause epidemic clinical cholera, with O1 causing more than 98% of cases of cholera. There are 3 serotypes of *V cholerae* O1: Inaba, Ogawa, and Hikojima. The 2 biotypes of *V cholerae* are classical and El Tor. El Tor is present globally, and the classical biotype is limited to Bangladesh. Both El Tor and classical biotypes can be further classified into 2 serotypes: Ogawa and Inaba. Since 1992, toxigenic *V cholerae* serogroup O139 has been recognized as a cause of cholera in Asia. Nontoxigenic strains of *V cholerae* O1 and some toxigenic non-O1 serogroups (eg, 0141) can cause sporadic diarrheal illness, but they have not caused epidemics.

EPIDEMIOLOGY: Since the early 1800s, there have been 7 cholera pandemics. During the last 5 decades, *V cholerae* O1 biotype El Tor has spread from India and Southeast Asia to Africa, the Middle East, Southern Europe, and the Western Pacific Islands (Oceania). In 1991, epidemic cholera caused by toxigenic *V cholerae* O1, serotype Inaba, biotype El Tor, appeared in Peru and spread to most countries in South, Central, and North America. After causing more than 1 million cases, the cholera epidemic in the Americas largely has subsided, with very few cases reported in the past decade. In the United States, cases resulting from travel to or ingestion of contaminated food transported from Latin America or Asia have been reported. In addition, the Gulf Coast of Louisiana and Texas has an endemic focus of a unique strain of toxigenic *V cholerae* O1. Most cases of disease from this strain have resulted from consumption of raw or undercooked shellfish. In 2010, an outbreak of *V cholerae* serogroup O1, serotype Ogawa, biotype El Tor, began in Haiti.[1]

---

[1] Centers for Disease Control and Prevention. Update: cholera outbreak—Haiti, 2010. *MMWR Morb Morbid Wkly Rep.* 2010;59(45):1473–1479

Humans are the only documented natural host, but free-living *V cholerae* organisms can exist in the aquatic environment. The usual mode of infection is ingestion of large numbers of organisms from contaminated water or food (particularly raw or undercooked shellfish, raw or partially dried fish, or moist grains or vegetables held at ambient temperature). Direct person-to-person spread has not been documented. People with low gastric acidity and with blood group O are at increased risk of severe cholera infection.

The **incubation period** usually is 1 to 3 days, with a range of a few hours to 5 days.

DIAGNOSTIC TESTS: *V cholerae* can be cultured from fecal specimens (preferred) or vomitus plated on thiosulfate citrate bile salts sucrose agar. Because most laboratories in the United States do not culture routinely for *V cholerae* or other *Vibrio* organisms, clinicians should request appropriate cultures for clinically suspected cases. Isolates of *V cholerae* should be sent to a state health department laboratory for serogrouping; all isolates of serogroup O1 or O139 should be sent through the state health department to the Centers for Disease Control and Prevention (CDC) for confirmation, antimicrobial susceptibility testing, and detection of the cholera toxin gene. Other tests, such as the vibriocidal assay and/or an anticholera toxin enzyme linked immunoassay, can be performed under certain circumstances. Both require the submission of acute and convalescent serum specimens. A fourfold increase in vibriocidal or anticholera toxin antibody titers between acute and convalescent serum can confirm the diagnosis.

TREATMENT: Oral or parenteral rehydration therapy to correct dehydration and electrolyte abnormalities is the most important therapeutic intervention and should be initiated as soon as the diagnosis is suspected.[1] Oral rehydration is preferred unless the patient is in shock, is obtunded, or has intestinal ileus. The World Health Organization's reduced-osmolality oral rehydration solution (ORS) has been the standard, but data suggest that rice-based ORS or amylase-resistant starch ORS is more effective.

Antimicrobial therapy results in prompt eradication of vibrios, decreases the duration of diarrhea, and decreases fluid losses. Antimicrobial therapy should be considered for people who are moderately to severely ill. Oral doxycycline or azithromycin as a single dose or tetracycline for 3 days is recommended for cholera treatment. If strains are resistant to tetracyclines, then ciprofloxacin, ofloxacin, furazolidone, or trimethoprim-sulfamethoxazole can be used. Antimicrobial susceptibility testing of newly isolated organisms should be performed.

ISOLATION OF THE HOSPITALIZED PATIENT: In addition to standard precautions, contact precautions are indicated for diapered or incontinent children for the duration of illness.

CONTROL MEASURES:

Hygiene. Disinfection, through chlorination, or boiling of drinking water prevents waterborne transmission of *V cholerae*. Thoroughly cooking crabs, oysters, and other shellfish from the Gulf Coast before eating is recommended to decrease the likelihood of transmission. Foods such as fish, rice, or grain gruels should be refrigerated promptly after meals and thoroughly reheated before eating. Appropriate hand hygiene after defecating and before preparing or eating food is important for preventing transmission.

Treatment of Contacts. The administration of doxycycline, tetracycline, ciprofloxacin, ofloxacin, or trimethoprim-sulfamethoxazole within 24 hours of identification of the index case may prevent coprimary cases of cholera among household contacts. However,

---

[1] Centers for Disease Control and Prevention. Managing acute gastroenteritis among children: oral rehydration, maintenance, and nutritional therapy. *MMWR Recomm Rep.* 2003;52(RR-16):1–16

because secondary transmission of cholera is rare, chemoprophylaxis of contacts is not recommended by the World Health Organization, except in special circumstances in which the probability of fecal exposure is high and medication can be delivered rapidly.

Vaccine. No cholera vaccines are available in the United States. Two inactivated oral vaccines are available in other countries. Dukoral (Crucell, The Netherlands), licensed in 1992, is a monovalent vaccine based on heat-killed whole cells of serogroup O1 plus recombinant cholera toxin B subunit. The second vaccine, licensed in 2009 as mORCVAX in Vietnam and Shanchol in India, is a bivalent (O1 and O139) vaccine. Cholera immunization is not required for travelers entering the United States from cholera-affected areas, and the World Health Organization no longer recommends immunization for travel to or from areas with cholera infection. No country requires cholera vaccine for entry.

Reporting. Confirmed cases of cholera must be reported to health authorities in any country in which they occur and were contracted. Local and state health departments should be notified immediately of presumed or known cases of cholera attributable to *V cholerae* O1 or O139.

Other *Vibrio* Infections

CLINICAL MANIFESTATIONS: Several nontoxigenic *Vibrio* species (ie, those that do not cause cholera) can cause a variety of clinical syndromes, including gastroenteritis, wound infection, and bacteremia. Gastroenteritis is the most common syndrome and is characterized by acute onset of watery stools and crampy abdominal pain. Approximately half of those afflicted will have low-grade fever, headache, and chills; approximately 30% will have vomiting. Spontaneous recovery follows in 2 to 5 days. Primary septicemia is uncommon but can develop in immunocompromised people with preceding gastroenteritis or wound infection. Wound infections can be severe in people with liver disease or who are immunocompromised. Septicemia and hemorrhagic bullous or necrotic skin lesions can be seen in people with infections caused by *Vibrio vulnificus*, with associated high morbidity and mortality rates.

ETIOLOGY: *Vibrio* organisms are facultatively anaerobic, motile, gram-negative bacilli that are tolerant of salt. The most commonly reported nontoxigenic *Vibrio* species associated with diarrhea are *Vibrio parahaemolyticus* and *Vibrio cholerae* non-O1/non-O139. *V vulnificus* typically causes primary septicemia and severe wound infections; the other species can also cause these syndromes. *Vibrio alginolyticus* typically causes wound infections.

EPIDEMIOLOGY: Noncholera *Vibrio* species are natural inhabitants of marine and estuarine environments. Most infections occur during summer and fall months, when *Vibrio* populations in seawater are highest. Gastroenteritis usually follows ingestion of undercooked seafood, especially oysters, crabs, and shrimp. Wound infections can result from exposure of a preexisting wound to contaminated seawater or from punctures resulting from handling of contaminated shellfish. Exposure to contaminated water during natural disasters such as hurricanes has resulted in wound infections. Transmission of infection person to person has not been reported. People with liver disease, low gastric acidity, and immunodeficiency have increased susceptibility to infection with *Vibrio* species. Infections associated with noncholera *Vibrio* organisms became nationally notifiable in January 2007.

The **incubation period** for gastroenteritis is 23 hours, with a range of 5 to 92 hours.

DIAGNOSTIC TESTS: *Vibrio* organisms can be isolated from stool of patients with gastro-enteritis, from blood specimens, and from wound exudates. Because identification of the organism in stool requires special techniques, laboratory personnel should be notified when infection with *Vibrio* species is suspected.

TREATMENT: Most episodes of diarrhea are mild and self-limited and do not require treatment other than oral rehydration. Antimicrobial therapy can benefit people with severe diarrhea, wound infection, or septicemia. Septicemia with or without hemorrhagic bullae should be treated with a third-generation cephalosporin plus doxycycline (see Tetracyclines, p 801). In younger children, a combination of trimethoprim-sulfamethoxazole and an aminoglycoside is an alternative regimen. Wound infections require surgical débridement of necrotic tissue, if present.

ISOLATION OF THE HOSPITALIZED PATIENT: In addition to standard precautions, contact precautions are recommended for diapered or incontinent children.

CONTROL MEASURES: Seafood should be cooked adequately and, if not ingested imme-diately, should be refrigerated. Cross-contamination of cooked seafood by contact with surfaces and containers contaminated by raw seafood should be avoided. Uncooked mollusks and crustaceans should be handled with care and gloves can be worn during preparation. Abrasions suffered by ocean bathers should be rinsed with clean fresh water. All children, immunocompromised people, and people with chronic liver disease should avoid eating raw oysters or clams and should be advised of risks associated with seawater exposure if a wound is present or likely to occur. Vibriosis is a nationally notifiable dis-ease, and cases should be reported to local or state health departments.

West Nile Virus

CLINICAL MANIFESTATIONS: Approximately 80% of human West Nile virus (WNV) infections are asymptomatic. Most symptomatic people experience an acute systemic febrile illness that often includes headache, myalgia, or arthralgia; gastrointestinal tract symptoms and a transient maculopapular rash also are commonly reported. Fewer than 1% of infected people develop neuroinvasive disease, which typically manifests as meningitis, encephalitis, or acute flaccid paralysis. WNV meningitis is indistinguish-able clinically from aseptic meningitis caused by most other viruses. Patients with WNV encephalitis usually present with seizures, mental status changes, focal neurologic deficits, or movement disorders. WNV acute flaccid paralysis often is clinically and pathologically identical to poliovirus-associated poliomyelitis, with damage of anterior horn cells, and may progress to respiratory paralysis requiring mechanical ventilation. WNV-associated Guillain-Barré syndrome has also been reported and can be distinguished from WNV poliomyelitis by clinical manifestations and electrophysiologic testing. Cardiac dysrhyth-mias, myocarditis, rhabdomyolysis, optic neuritis, uveitis, chorioretinitis, orchitis, pan-creatitis, and hepatitis have been described rarely after WNV infection.

Routine clinical laboratory results are generally nonspecific in WNV infections. In patients with neuroinvasive disease, cerebrospinal fluid (CSF) examination generally shows lymphocytic pleocytosis, but neutrophils may predominate early in the illness. Brain magnetic resonance imaging frequently is normal, but signal abnormalities may be seen in the basal ganglia, thalamus, and brainstem with WNV encephalitis and in the spinal cord with WNV poliomyelitis.

Most patients with WNV nonneuroinvasive disease or meningitis recover completely, but fatigue, malaise, and weakness can linger for weeks or months. Patients who recover from WNV encephalitis or poliomyelitis often have residual neurologic deficits. Among patients with neuroinvasive disease, the overall case-fatality rate is approximately 10% but significantly is higher in WNV encephalitis and poliomyelitis than in WNV meningitis.

Most women known to have been infected with WNV during pregnancy have delivered infants without evidence of infection or clinical abnormalities. In the single known instance of confirmed congenital WNV infection, the mother developed WNV encephalitis during week 27 of gestation, and the infant was born with cystic destruction of cerebral tissue and chorioretinitis. If WNV disease is diagnosed during pregnancy, a detailed examination of the fetus and of the newborn infant should be performed.[1]

ETIOLOGY: WNV is an RNA flavivirus which is related antigenically to St. Louis encephalitis and Japanese encephalitis viruses.

EPIDEMIOLOGY:

WNV is an <u>arthropod</u><u>borne</u> <u>virus</u> (arbovirus) that is transmitted in an enzootic cycle between mosquitoes and amplifying vertebrate hosts, primarily birds. WNV is transmitted to humans primarily through bites of infected *Culex* mosquitoes. Humans usually do not develop a level or duration of viremia sufficient to infect mosquitoes. Therefore, humans are dead-end hosts. However, person-to-person WNV transmission can occur through blood transfusion and solid organ transplantation. Intrauterine and probable breastfeeding transmission also have been described rarely. Percutaneous and aerosol transmission have occurred in laboratory workers, and an outbreak among turkey handlers suggested WNV transmission via aerosol.

WNV transmission has been documented on every continent except Antarctica. Since the 1990s, the largest outbreaks of WNV neuroinvasive disease have occurred in the Middle East, Europe, and North America. WNV first was detected in the Western Hemisphere in New York City in 1999 and subsequently spread across the continental United States and Canada. From 1999 through 2009, 12 208 cases of WNV neuroinvasive disease were reported in the United States, including 481 (4%) cases among children younger than 18 years of age. Neuroinvasive disease occurs more commonly in people older than 50 years of age. A map of the distribution of WNV neuroinvasive disease across the United States can be found at **www.cdc.gov/ncidod/dvbid/westnile/ Mapsincidence/surv&control09IncidMaps.htm.**

In temperate and subtropical regions, most human WNV infections occur in summer or early fall. Although all age groups and both sexes are equally susceptible to WNV infection, the incidence of encephalitis and death are highest among older adults. History of solid organ transplantation, other immunocompromising conditions, diabetes, and hypertension are other reported risk factors for WNV neuroinvasive disease.

The **incubation period** usually is 2 to 6 days but ranges from 2 to 14 days and can be up to 21 days in immunocompromised people.

---

[1] Centers for Disease Control and Prevention. Interim guidelines for the evaluation of infants born to mothers infected with West Nile virus during pregnancy. MMWR *Morb Mortal Wkly Rep.* 2004;53(7):154–157. Available at: **www.cdc.gov/mmwr/preview/mmwrhtml/mm5307a4.htm**

DIAGNOSTIC TESTS: Anti-WNV immunoglobulin (Ig) M antibodies in serum or CSF are the preferred tests for diagnosis of WNV infection. The presence of anti-WNV IgM usually is good evidence of recent WNV infection but may indicate infection with another closely related flavivirus. Because anti-WNV IgM can persist in some patients for longer than 1 year, a positive test result occasionally may reflect past infection. Serum collected within 10 days of illness onset may lack detectable IgM, and the test should be repeated on a convalescent-phase sample. IgG antibody generally is detectable shortly after IgM and persists for years. Plaque-reduction neutralization tests can be performed to measure virus-specific neutralizing antibodies. A fourfold or greater increase in virus-specific neutralizing antibodies between acute- and convalescent-phase serum specimens collected 2 to 3 weeks apart may be used to confirm recent WNV infection and to discriminate between cross-reacting antibodies from closely related flaviviruses.

Viral culture and WNV nucleic acid amplification tests can be performed on acute-phase serum, CSF, or tissue specimens. However, by the time most immunocompetent patients present with clinical symptoms, WNV RNA no longer is detectable; the sensitivity of these tests is likely higher in immunocompromised patients. Immunohistochemical staining can detect WNV antigens in fixed tissue, but negative results are not definitive.

WNV disease should be considered in the differential diagnosis of febrile or acute neurologic illnesses associated with recent exposure to mosquitoes, blood transfusion, or solid organ transplantation and of illnesses in neonates whose mothers were infected with WNV during pregnancy or while breastfeeding. In addition to other more common causes of aseptic meningitis and encephalitis (eg, herpes simplex virus and enteroviruses), other arboviruses should also be considered in the differential diagnosis (see Arboviruses, p 232).

TREATMENT: Management of WNV disease is supportive. Although various therapies have been evaluated or used for WNV disease, none has shown specific benefit thus far. Information regarding ongoing clinical trials for treating WNV disease can be found at **http://clinicaltrials.gov/ct2/home.**

ISOLATION OF THE HOSPITALIZED PATIENT: Standard precautions are recommended.

CONTROL MEASURES: Candidate WNV vaccines are being evaluated, but none are licensed for use in humans. In the absence of a vaccine, prevention of WNV disease depends on community-level mosquito control programs to reduce vector densities, personal protective measures to decrease exposure to infected mosquitoes, and screening of blood and organ donors. Personal protective measures include use of mosquito repellents, wearing long-sleeved shirts and long pants, and limiting outdoor exposure from dusk to dawn (see Prevention of Mosquitoborne Infections, p 209). Using air conditioning, installing window and door screens, and reducing peridomestic mosquito breeding sites can further decrease the risk of WNV exposure. Blood donations in the United States are screened for WNV infection, but physicians should remain vigilant for the possible transmission of WNV through blood transfusion or organ transplantation. Any suspected WNV infections temporally associated with blood transfusion or organ transplantation should be reported promptly to the appropriate state health department.

Pregnant women should take aforementioned precautions to avoid mosquito bites. Products containing N,N-diethyl-meta-toluamide (DEET) can be used in pregnancy without adverse effects. Pregnant women who develop meningitis, encephalitis, flaccid paralysis, or unexplained fever in areas of ongoing WNV transmission should be tested for WNV infection. Confirmed WNV infections should be reported to the local or state health department, and women should be followed to determine the outcomes of their pregnancies. Although WNV probably has been transmitted through human milk, such transmission appears rare and no adverse effects on infants have been described. Because the benefits of breastfeeding outweigh the risk of WNV disease in breastfeeding infants, mothers should be encouraged to breastfeed even in areas on ongoing WNV transmission.

Yersinia enterocolitica and *Yersinia pseudotuberculosis* Infections
(Enteritis and Other Illnesses)

CLINICAL MANIFESTATIONS: *Yersinia enterocolitica* causes several age-specific syndromes and a variety of other less common clinical illnesses. Infection with *Y enterocolitica* typically manifests as fever and diarrhea in young children; stool often contains leukocytes, blood, and mucus. Relapsing disease and, rarely, necrotizing enterocolitis also have been described. In older children and adults, a pseudoappendicitis syndrome (fever, abdominal pain, tenderness in the right lower quadrant of the abdomen, and leukocytosis) predominates. Bacteremia with *Y enterocolitica* most often occurs in children younger than 1 year of age and in older children with predisposing conditions, such as excessive iron storage (eg, desferrioxamine use, sickle cell disease, and beta-thalassemia) and immunosuppressive states. Focal manifestations of *Y enterocolitica* are uncommon and include pharyngitis, meningitis, osteomyelitis, pyomyositis, conjunctivitis, pneumonia, empyema, endocarditis, acute peritonitis, abscesses of the liver and spleen, and primary cutaneous infection. Postinfectious sequelae with *Y enterocolitica* infection include erythema nodosum, reactive arthritis, and proliferative glomerulonephritis. These sequelae occur most often in older children and adults, particularly people with HLA-B27 antigen.

Major manifestations of *Yersinia pseudotuberculosis* infection are fever, scarlatiniform rash, and abdominal symptoms. Acute pseudoappendiceal abdominal pain is common, resulting from ileocecal mesenteric adenitis, or terminal ileitis. Other findings include diarrhea, erythema nodosum, septicemia, and sterile pleural and joint effusions. Clinical features can mimic those of Kawasaki disease; in Hiroshima, Japan, nearly 10% of children with a diagnosis of Kawasaki disease have serologic or culture evidence of *Y pseudotuberculosis* infection.

ETIOLOGY: The genus *Yersinia* consists of 11 species of gram-negative bacilli. *Y enterocolitica, Y pseudotuberculosis,* and *Yersinia pestis* are the 3 recognized human pathogens. Fifteen pathogenic O groups of *Y enterocolitica* are recognized. Differences in virulence exist among various O groups of *Y enterocolitica;* serotype O:3 now predominates as the most common type in the United States.

EPIDEMIOLOGY: *Y enterocolitica* infections are uncommon in the United States. According to the Foodborne Disease Active Surveillance Network, during the years 1996 through 2009, 3.5 laboratory-confirmed infections per 1 million people were reported to surveillance sites. The median age of reported people was 6 years; 30% were hospitalized, and 1% died. Most isolates were recovered from stool. In contrast, the average annual incidence of *Y pseudotuberculosis* was 0.04 cases per 1 million people; the median age was 47 years, 72% were hospitalized, and 11% died. Two-thirds of *Y pseudotuberculosis* isolates were recovered from blood.

The principal reservoir of *Y enterocolitica* is swine; feral *Y pseudotuberculosis* has been isolated from ungulates (deer, elk, goats, sheep, cattle), rodents (rats, squirrels, beaver), rabbits, and many bird species. Infection with *Y enterocolitica* is believed to be transmitted by ingestion of contaminated food (raw or incompletely cooked pork products, tofu, and unpasteurized or inadequately pasteurized milk), by contaminated surface or well water, by direct or indirect contact with animals, by transfusion with contaminated packed red blood cells, and rarely, by person-to-person transmission. Cross-contamination can lead to infection in infants if their caregivers handle raw pork intestines (chitterlings) and do not cleanse their hands adequately before handling the infant or the infant's toys, bottles, or pacifiers. *Y enterocolitica* and *Y pseudotuberculosis* are isolated most often during the cool months of temperate climates. Recent outbreaks of *Y pseudotuberculosis* infection in Finland have been associated with eating fresh produce, presumably contaminated by wild animals carrying the organism.

The **incubation period** typically is 4 to 6 days, with a range of 1 to 14 days. Organisms are excreted for a mean of 42 days, and prolonged asymptomatic carriage is possible.

DIAGNOSTIC TESTS: *Y enterocolitica* and *Y pseudotuberculosis* can be recovered from stool, throat swabs, mesenteric lymph nodes, peritoneal fluid, and blood. *Y enterocolitica* also has been isolated from synovial fluid, bile, urine, cerebrospinal fluid, sputum, pleural fluid, and wounds. Stool cultures generally yield bacteria during the first 2 weeks of illness, regardless of the nature of gastrointestinal tract manifestations. Because of the relatively low incidence of *Yersinia* infection in the United States, *Yersinia* organisms are not sought routinely in stool specimens by most laboratories. Consequently, laboratory personnel should be notified when *Yersinia* infection is suspected so that stool can be cultured on suitable media (eg, CIN agar). Biotyping and serotyping for further identification of pathogenic strains are available through public health reference laboratories. Infection also can be confirmed by demonstrating increases in serum antibody titer after infection, but these tests generally are available only in reference or research laboratories. Cross-reactions of these antibodies with *Brucella, Vibrio, Salmonella,* and *Rickettsia* organisms and *Escherichia coli* lead to false-positive *Y enterocolitica* and *Y pseudotuberculosis* titers. In patients with thyroid disease, persistently increased *Y enterocolitica* antibody titers can result from antigenic similarity of the organism with antigens of the thyroid epithelial cell membrane. Characteristic ultrasonographic features demonstrating edema of the wall of the terminal ileum and cecum help to distinguish pseudoappendicitis from appendicitis and can help avoid exploratory surgery.

TREATMENT: Patients with septicemia or sites of infection other than the gastrointestinal tract and immunocompromised hosts with enterocolitis should receive antimicrobial therapy. Other than decreasing the duration of fecal excretion of *Y enterocolitica* and *Y pseudotuberculosis,* a clinical benefit of antimicrobial therapy for immunocompetent patients with enterocolitis, pseudoappendicitis syndrome, or mesenteric adenitis has not been established. *Y enterocolitica* and *Y pseudotuberculosis* usually are susceptible to trimethoprim-sulfamethoxazole, aminoglycosides, cefotaxime, fluoroquinolones (for patients 18 years of age and older; see Fluoroquinolones, p 800), tetracycline or doxycycline (for children 8 years of age and older; see Tetracyclines, p 801), and chloramphenicol. *Y enterocolitica* isolates usually are resistant to first-generation cephalosporins and most penicillin.

ISOLATION OF THE HOSPITALIZED PATIENT: In addition to standard precautions, contact precautions are indicated for diapered or incontinent children for the duration of diarrheal illness.

CONTROL MEASURES: Ingestion of uncooked or undercooked meat, unpasteurized milk, or contaminated water should be avoided. People who handle raw pork products should minimize contact with young children and their possessions while handling raw products. Meticulous hand hygiene should be practiced before and after handling and preparation of uncooked products.

Antimicrobial Agents and Related Therapy

....
INTRODUCTION

The product label (package insert) approved by the US Food and Drug Administration (FDA) for a given antimicrobial drug provides information on indications based on clinical trial data reviewed by the FDA. Virtually all current antimicrobial product labels are available at **http://dailymed.nlm.nih.gov/dailymed/about.cfm**. The FDA also maintains a general Web site (**www.accessdata.fda.gov/scripts/cder/ob/default.cfm**) of approved drug products with therapeutic equivalence evaluations that can be searched by active ingredient or proprietary names.

An FDA-approved indication means that statistically adequate and well-controlled studies were conducted, reviewed, and approved by the FDA. However, accepted medical practice (ie, when to use which antimicrobial agent for a specific infection) often includes use of drugs for indications that are not reflected in approved drug labeling. These additional indications are based on studies conducted by clinical investigators. These studies may not have been presented formally to the FDA for review. Lack of FDA approval for an indication, therefore, does not necessarily mean lack of effectiveness but signifies that either FDA-required studies have not been performed or have not been submitted to the FDA for approval for that specific indication. Therefore, unapproved use does not imply improper use, provided that reasonable medical evidence supports such an indication and that use of the drug is deemed to be in the best interest of the patient. The decision to prescribe a drug is the responsibility of the physician, who must weigh risks and benefits of using the drug for the specific indication.

In addition, occasional drug shortages can occur, at which time a pharmaceutical company may share information about the shortage with the FDA (**www.fda.gov/cder/drug/shortages/default.htm**). Alternative, nonstandard therapy can be required when drug shortages occur.

Some antimicrobial agents with proven therapeutic benefit in adults are not approved by the FDA for use in pediatric patients or, more rarely, are considered contraindicated in children because of possible toxicity. Drugs such as fluoroquinolones (in people younger than 18 years of age), tetracyclines (in children younger than 8 years of age), and other agents approved for use in adults may be used in special circumstances after careful assessment of risks and benefits. The following information delineates general principles for use of fluoroquinolones, tetracyclines, and other agents that are approved for adults with serious bacterial infections.

Fluoroquinolones

Use of fluoroquinolones (eg, ciprofloxacin, levofloxacin, gemifloxacin, moxifloxacin) in children younger than 18 years of age generally is discouraged, as specified in the FDA-approved product labeling, because fluoroquinolones have been shown to cause cartilage damage in juvenile animals. For some fluoroquinolones, cartilage damage in animal models occurs at doses that approximate therapeutic doses in humans. The mechanism of damage remains speculative. Fluoroquinolones are associated with an increased risk of tendon rupture in people who have received renal, heart, or lung transplants, and with concurrent use of corticosteroids. In some pediatric studies, an increased incidence of reversible adverse events involving joints or surrounding tissues has been observed. However, to date, no child treated with fluoroquinolone agents has developed physician-documented, drug-attributable bone or joint toxicity. Current information on the safety of fluoroquinolones for children was reviewed and published by the American Academy of Pediatrics.[1]

Ciprofloxacin and levofloxacin are the fluoroquinolones that have been used most extensively in children and adolescents. On the basis of past experience, these drugs appear to be well tolerated, do not appear to cause arthropathy, and are effective as oral agents for treating a number of diseases in children that otherwise would require parenteral therapy. (**www.fda.gov/Drugs/DrugSafety/PostmarketDrugSafety InformationforPatientsandProviders/ucm126085.htm**). Circumstances in which use of systemic fluoroquinolones may be justified in children include the following: (1) parenteral therapy is not practical and no other safe and effective oral agent is available; and (2) infection is caused by a multidrug-resistant pathogen, such as certain *Pseudomonas* or *Mycobacterium* strains, for which there is no other effective intravenous or oral agent available. The only indications for which a fluoroquinolone is approved by the FDA for use in patients younger than 18 years of age are complicated urinary tract infection or pyelonephritis (ciprofloxacin) and postexposure prophylaxis for inhalation anthrax (ciprofloxacin, levofloxacin). Potential uses, accordingly, include the following[1]:

- Urinary tract infections caused by *Pseudomonas aeruginosa* or other multidrug-resistant, gram-negative bacteria.
- Chronic suppurative otitis media or malignant otitis externa caused by *P aeruginosa*.
- Chronic or acute osteomyelitis or osteochondritis caused by *P aeruginosa*, or other multi-drug-resistant, gram-negative bacterial infection caused by isolates known to be susceptible to fluoroquinolones but resistant to standard, nonfluoroquinolone agents.
- Gram-negative bacterial infections in immunocompromised hosts in which oral therapy is desired or resistance to alternative agents is present.
- Gastrointestinal tract infection caused by suspected or documented multidrug-resistant *Shigella* species, *Salmonella* species, *Vibrio cholerae, Campylobacter jejuni,* or *Campylobacter coli.*
- Serious infections attributable to fluoroquinolone-susceptible pathogen(s) in children with severe allergy to alternative agents.
- Topical fluoroquinolone-containing agents are preferred as safer alternatives to amino-glycoside-containing agents for treatment of otorrhea associated with tympanic membrane perforation, and tympanostomy tube otorrhea.

---

[1] American Academy of Pediatrics, Committee on Infectious Diseases. The use of systemic and topical fluoroquinolones. *Pediatrics* 2011;128(4):e1034–e1045

If use of a fluoroquinolone is recommended for a patient younger than 18 years of age, the risks and benefits should be explained to the patient and parents. Inappropriate overuse of fluoroquinolones in children and adults is likely to be associated with increasing resistance to these agents.

Tetracyclines

Use of tetracyclines in pediatric patients has been limited, because these drugs can cause permanent dental discoloration in children younger than 8 years of age. Studies have documented that tetracyclines and their colored degradation products are incorporated in enamel. The period of odontogenesis to completion of formation of enamel in permanent teeth appears to be the critical time for effects of these drugs and virtually ends by 8 years of age, at which time the drug can be given without concern for dental staining. The degree of staining appears to depend on dosage, duration of therapy, and which drug in the tetracycline class is used. In addition to dental discoloration, tetracyclines can cause enamel hypoplasia and reversible delay in rate of bone growth. These possible adverse events have resulted in use of alternative, equally effective antimicrobial agents in most circumstances in young children in which tetracyclines are likely to be effective.

Even with these constraints, in some cases, the benefits of therapy with a tetracycline can exceed the risks, particularly if alternative drugs provide less effective therapy for serious infections or if pathogens are only susceptible to tetracyclines. In these cases, use of tetracyclines for a single therapeutic course in young children is justified. Examples include life-threatening infections caused by pathogens in the *Rickettsia/Ehrlichia/Anaplasma* group, including Rocky Mountain spotted fever (see p 623) and ehrlichiosis (see p 312), cholera (see p 789), and anthrax (see p 228). Doxycycline usually is the agent of choice in children with these infections, because doxycycline has not been demonstrated to cause cosmetic staining of developing permanent teeth when used in the dose and duration recommended to treat these serious infections.

Other Agents

Other antimicrobial agents in a variety of classes have been studied and approved by the FDA for use in adults for certain indications but still are under investigation for pharmacokinetics, safety, and efficacy in children. These agents include but are not limited to ceftaroline, daptomycin, doripenem, and tigecycline. These drugs should be used in children only when no other safe and effective agents that are FDA approved for use in children are available and when benefits are expected to exceed risks for that patient. For these agents with poorly defined safety and efficacy in pediatrics, consultation with an expert in pediatric infectious diseases should be considered.

....

ANTIMICROBIAL STEWARDSHIP: APPROPRIATE AND JUDICIOUS USE OF ANTIMICROBIAL AGENTS[1]

The primary goal of antimicrobial stewardship is to optimize antimicrobial use, with the aim of decreasing inappropriate use that leads to unwarranted toxicity and to selection and spread of resistant organisms. Core members of an antimicrobial stewardship program include infectious diseases specialists, clinical pharmacists, clinical microbiologists, and hospital epidemiologists.[1,2]

The increasing incidence of infection caused by antimicrobial-resistant pathogens in adults and children is a major concern. Highly resistant gram-negative (*Pseudomonas aeruginosa, Acinetobacter* species, carbapenemase-producing *Klebsiella pneumoniae,* and *Burkholderia cepacia*) and gram-positive (methicillin-resistant *Staphylococcus aureus,* NAP1 strains of *Clostridium difficile,* and *Enterococcus* organisms resistant to ampicillin and vancomycin) pathogens increasingly are associated with invasive infections. The presence of resistant pathogens complicates patient management, increases morbidity and mortality, and increases medical expenses for patients and the health care system.

Overuse of antimicrobial agents, inappropriate antimicrobial selection of an antimicrobial agent for a specific pathogen at a specific tissue site, and unnecessarily prolonged administration of antimicrobial agents place increased and unnecessary antimicrobial pressure on bacteria. Not only are resistant organisms selected, but also, overgrowth of pathogens is facilitated by eradication of normal flora. The principles for appropriate use of antimicrobial agents, combined with infection-control programs, have become a central focus of measures to combat development and spread of resistant organisms.[1,2] Health care organizations that provide care for both inpatients and outpatients are encouraged to support these programs.

Additional information for health care professionals and parents on judicious use of antimicrobial agents (The Get Smart Campaign) and antimicrobial resistance is available on the Centers for Disease Control and Prevention Web sites: **www.cdc.gov/getsmart/** and **www.cdc.gov/drugresistance.**

Principles of Appropriate Use for Upper Respiratory Tract Infections

More than half of all outpatient prescriptions for antimicrobial agents for children are given for 5 conditions: otitis media, sinusitis, cough illness/bronchitis, pharyngitis, and nonspecific upper respiratory tract infection (the common cold). Antimicrobial agents often are prescribed, even though many of these illnesses are caused by viruses and are unresponsive to antimicrobial therapy. Children treated with an antimicrobial agent for respiratory tract infections are at increased risk of becoming colonized by resistant

---

[1] Dellit TH, Owens RC, McGowan JE Jr, et al. Infectious Diseases Society of America and the Society for Healthcare Epidemiology of America guidelines for developing an institutional program to enhance antimicrobial stewardship. *Clin Infect Dis.* 2007;44(2):159–177

[2] Antimicrobial stewardship for the community hospital: practical tools and techniques for implementation. *Clin Infect Dis.* 2011;53(Suppl 1):S1–S29

respiratory tract flora, including *Streptococcus pneumoniae* and *Haemophilus influenzae.* Children who subsequently develop respiratory tract infections are more likely to experience failure of antimicrobial therapy and are likely to spread resistant bacteria to close contacts, both children and adults. The following principles, with supporting evidence, were published by the American Academy of Pediatrics, American Academy of Family Physicians, and CDC to identify clinical conditions for which antimicrobial therapy could be curtailed without compromising patient care (**www.cdc.gov/getsmart/**).

OTITIS MEDIA

* Antimicrobial agents are indicated for treatment of acute otitis media (AOM) but not for middle ear effusions (ie, otitis media with effusion [OME]). Diagnosis of AOM requires a history of acute onset, evidence of middle ear effusion, and signs or symptoms of inflammation of the middle ear.
* Observation without use of an antimicrobial agent in a child with uncomplicated AOM is an option for selected children on the basis of diagnostic certainty, age, illness severity, and assurance of follow-up.[1]
* When antimicrobial agents are used for AOM, a narrow-spectrum antimicrobial agent (eg, amoxicillin, 80–90 mg/kg per day) in 2 divided doses for 5 to 7 days should be used for episodes in most children 2 years of age or older. Microbiologic and clinical failure with high-dose amoxicillin has been associated with highly penicillin-resistant pneumococci (uncommon currently with widespread use of the 13-valent pneumococcal conjugate vaccine [PCV13]), and beta-lactamase–producing *Haemophilus* species and *Moraxella* species, an increasing problem as the proportion of cases of AOM caused by pneumococci decreases.
* Younger children and children with underlying medical conditions, craniofacial abnormalities, chronic or recurrent otitis media, or perforation of the tympanic membrane represent a more complicated and diverse population. Initial therapy with a 10-day course of an antimicrobial agent is likely to be more effective than shorter courses for many of these children.[2]
* Persistent middle ear effusion (OME) for 2 to 3 months after therapy for AOM is expected and does not require routine retreatment; treatment for 10 to 14 days may be considered an option if effusions persist for 3 months, especially if hearing is impaired. Repetitive or prolonged courses of antimicrobial agents are not recommended. Management with tympanic membrane ventilation tubes may be preferred to repetitive courses of antibiotics for children with persistent effusions and recurrent acute bacterial otitis media.

---

[1] American Academy of Pediatrics, Subcommittee on Management of Acute Otitis Media; American Academy of Family Physicians. Clinical practice guideline: diagnosis and management of acute otitis media. *Pediatrics.* 2004;113(5):1451–1465

[2] American Academy of Family Physicians; American Academy of Otolaryngology-Head and Neck Surgery; and American Academy of Pediatrics, Subcommittee on Otitis Media With Effusion. Clinical practice guideline: otitis media with effusion. *Pediatrics.* 2004;113(5):1412–1429

ACUTE SINUSITIS

- Clinical diagnosis of acute bacterial sinusitis requires the presence of nasal or post-nasal discharge (of any quality) without evidence of clinical improvement for 10 to 14 days, with or without daytime cough (cough may be worse at night); or temperature of ≥39°C (102°F) or higher and purulent nasal discharge or facial pain present concurrently for at least 3 consecutive days in a child who seems ill.
- Findings on sinus radiographs correlate poorly with disease and should not be used. Computed tomography of sinuses may be indicated when symptoms of sinusitis are persistent or recurrent or when complications are suspected.
- Initial antimicrobial treatment of acute sinusitis should be with a narrow-spectrum agent (eg, amoxicillin, 80–90 mg/kg per day in 2 divided doses) for most children, with the same considerations for antimicrobial resistance associated with amoxicillin treatment failure as outlined previously for AOM.
- Guidelines from the Infectious Diseases Society of America address the inability of existing clinical criteria to differentiate accurately bacterial from viral acute rhinosinusitis, gaps in knowledge and quality of evidence regarding empiric recommendations, changing prevalence and antimicrobial susceptibility profiles of bacterial associated isolates, and the impact of PCV7/PCV13 on pneumococcal organisms associated with sinusitis.[1]

COUGH ILLNESS/BRONCHITIS

- Nonspecific cough illness/bronchitis in children, regardless of duration, does not warrant antimicrobial treatment.
- Prolonged cough (10–14 days or more) may be caused by *Bordetella pertussis, Bordetella parapertussis, Mycoplasma pneumoniae,* or *Chlamydophila pneumoniae.* When infection caused by one of these organisms is suspected clinically or is confirmed, appropriate antimicrobial therapy is indicated (see Pertussis, p 553, *Mycoplasma pneumoniae* Infections, p 518, and Chlamydial Infections, p 272).

PHARYNGITIS

(See Group A Streptococcal Infections, p 668)
- Diagnosis of group A streptococcal pharyngitis should be made on the basis of results of appropriate laboratory tests in conjunction with clinical and epidemiologic findings.
- Most cases of pharyngitis are viral in origin. Antimicrobial therapy should not be given to a child with pharyngitis in the absence of identified group A streptococci. Rarely, other bacteria may cause pharyngitis (eg, *Corynebacterium diphtheriae, Francisella tularensis,* groups G and C hemolytic streptococci, *Neisseria gonorrhoeae, Arcanobacterium haemolyticum*), and treatment should be provided according to recommendations in disease-specific chapters in Section 3.
- Penicillin remains the drug of choice for treating group A streptococcal pharyngitis. Amoxicillin and other oral antimicrobial agents may be better tolerated and have improved efficacy of microbiologic eradication of group A streptococci from the pharynx, but this potential advantage must be considered against the disadvantage of increased antimicrobial pressure from use of more broad-spectrum antimicrobial agents.

---

[1] Chow AW, Benninger MS, Brook I, et al. IDSA clinical practice guideline for acute bacterial rhinosinusitis in children and adults. *Clin Infect Dis.* 2012;54(8):e72–e112

THE COMMON COLD

- Antimicrobial agents should not be given for the common cold.
- Mucopurulent rhinitis (thick, opaque, or discolored nasal discharge that begins a few days into a viral upper respiratory tract infection) commonly accompanies the common cold and is not an indication for antimicrobial treatment unless it persists without signs of improvement for 10 to 14 days, suggesting possible acute bacterial sinusitis.

Principles of Appropriate Use of Vancomycin[1]

The use of vancomycin is responsible for the emergence of vancomycin-resistant gram-positive organisms, most commonly *Enterococcus* species, leading to colonization and subsequent infection. Increasingly, the development of vancomycin-heteroresistant strains of *Staphylococcus aureus* have been documented during vancomycin therapy, resulting in treatment failure. Of even greater concern is the emergence of vancomycin-resistant strains of *S aureus*. Risk occurs particularly among patients receiving hematology-oncology, nephrology, neonatology, cardiac surgery, and neurosurgery services. Prevention of further emergence and spread of vancomycin resistance will depend on more limited and focused use of vancomycin for treatment and prophylaxis. With most vancomycin use in pediatrics targeting methicillin-resistant *Staphylococcus aureus* (MRSA), FDA approval of agents for adults that are considered safer and equally effective, compared with vancomycin, including the approval of ceftaroline, the first cephalosporin with activity against MRSA, soon may allow decreased use of vancomycin in children if pediatric clinical trials support published data on safety and efficacy for adults.

SITUATIONS IN WHICH USE OF VANCOMYCIN IS APPROPRIATE INCLUDE THE FOLLOWING:

- Treatment of serious infections attributable to methicillin-resistant, gram-positive organisms.
- Treatment of infections attributable to gram-positive microorganisms in patients with serious allergy to beta-lactam agents.
- Antimicrobial-associated colitis that fails to respond to metronidazole therapy or colitis that is severe and potentially life threatening (see *Clostridium difficile*, p 285).
- Prophylaxis, as recommended by the 2007 American Heart Association guidelines (**http://circ.ahajournals.org/cgi/content/full/116/15/1736**), for endocarditis after certain procedures in patients at high risk of endocarditis caused by methicillin-resistant *S aureus* (MRSA), or in people intolerant of beta-lactam agents (see Prevention of Bacterial Endocarditis, p 879).
- Prophylaxis for major surgical procedures involving implantation of prosthetic materials or devices at institutions with a high rate of infections attributable to MRSA or methicillin-resistant coagulase-negative staphylococci.

---

[1] Centers for Disease Control and Prevention. Recommendations for preventing the spread of vancomycin resistance: recommendations of the Hospital Infection Control Practices Advisory Committee. *MMWR Recomm Rep.* 1995;44(RR-12):1–13

SITUATIONS IN WHICH USE OF VANCOMYCIN IS DISCOURAGED INCLUDE THE FOLLOWING:

- Routine prophylaxis for the following:
  - Surgical patients other than patients with a life-threatening allergy to beta-lactam antimicrobial agents or in a setting delineated previously;
  - Infants with very low birth weight;
  - Patients receiving continuous ambulatory peritoneal dialysis or hemodialysis; or
  - Preventing infection or colonization of indwelling central or peripheral intravascular catheters (either systemic or antimicrobial lock).
- Prolonged vancomycin therapy for a patient with neutropenia and fever in the absence of positive culture results, unless strong evidence indicates an infection attributable to gram-positive microorganisms that are only susceptible to vancomycin.
- Treatment in response to a single positive result of a blood culture for coagulase-negative staphylococcus that is likely to be a contaminant, if other blood culture results obtained in the same period prior to starting antimicrobial therapy are negative.
- Continued empiric use for presumed infections in patients whose culture results are negative for methicillin-resistant, gram-positive microorganisms.
- Selective decontamination of the digestive tract.
- Attempted eradication of MRSA colonization.
- Primary treatment of nonlife-threatening antimicrobial-associated colitis (see *Clostridium difficile*, p 285).
- Treatment of infections attributable to methicillin-susceptible gram-positive micro-organisms, including vancomycin given for dosing convenience in patients with renal failure.
- Topical application or irrigation.

When vancomycin is started for empiric therapy its use should be discontinued when reliable cultures reveal that alternate antimicrobial agents are available (eg, nafcillin to treat methicillin-susceptible *S aureus*) or if appropriate and reliable cultures fail to provide evidence that vancomycin is needed (eg, lack of beta-lactam resistant gram-positive organisms).

DRUG INTERACTIONS

Use of multiple drugs for therapy of seriously ill patients increases the probability of drug-drug interactions. Drug-drug interactions can be considered as producing either changes in drug concentrations (pharmacokinetics) or changes in the drug effect/toxicity profile (pharmacodynamics). Pharmacokinetic interactions result from alterations in the absorption, distribution, metabolism, or elimination of a drug and thereby result in a change in concentration in the body. Pharmacodynamic drug-drug interactions may produce synergistic, additive, or antagonistic drug effects or toxicities. Many of the serious adverse interactions between drugs are attributable to inhibition (some macrolides, quinolones, and azole agents) or induction (rifabutin, rifampin) of hepatic intestinal cytochrome P450 (CYP) isoenzymes, especially CYP3A, which is thought to be involved in metabolism of more than 50% of prescribed drugs. Drug interactions related to inhibition of transporter proteins increasingly are being recognized. P-glycoprotein probably is the best understood of these transport proteins. Examples of transporter-based effects include interactions of penicillin with probenecid and digoxin with quinidine.

Complete drug interaction software programs are used by most hospital and health care system pharmacies. The scope and cost of these programs usually is beyond the needs of most physicians. Labels for individual drugs often include information about clinically significant drug interactions. Drug labels can be found online through the DailyMed (**http://dailymed.nlm.nih.gov/dailymed/about.cfm**) or Drugs@FDA (**www.accessdata.fda.gov/scripts/cder/drugsatfda/**) Web sites.

TABLES OF ANTIBACTERIAL DRUG DOSAGES

Recommended dosages for antibacterial agents commonly used for neonates (see Table 4.1, p 808) and for infants and children (see Table 4.2, p 810) are provided separately because of differences in drug disposition and elimination in neonates and resulting differences in pharmacokinetics and tissue site drug exposure. The table for neonates is divided by postnatal age and weight because of age and weight differences in pharmacokinetics.

Recommended dosages are not absolute and are intended only as a guide. Clinical judgment about the disease, alterations in renal or hepatic function, coadministration of other drugs, and other factors affecting pharmacokinetics, patient response, and laboratory results may dictate modifications of these recommendations in an individual patient. In some cases, monitoring of serum drug concentrations is recommended to avoid toxicity and to ensure therapeutic efficacy.

Product label information or a pediatric pharmacist should be consulted for details, such as the appropriate diluent for reconstitution of injectable preparations, measures to be taken to avoid incompatibilities, drug interactions, and other precautions. Drug labels can be found online through the DailyMed (**http://dailymed.nlm.nih.gov/ dailymed/about.cfm**) or Drugs@FDA (**www.accessdata.fda.gov/scripts/cder/ drugsatfda/**) Web sites.

Table 4.1 Antibacterial Drugs for Neonates (≤28 Postnatal Days of Age)[a]

Drug	Route	Dose per kg and Frequency of Administration			
		Body Weight ≤2 kg		Body Weight >2 kg	
		≤7 days of age	8–28 days of age[b]	≤7 days of age	8–28 days of age
Aminoglycosides[c,d]					
Amikacin	IV, IM	15 mg every 48 h	15 mg every 24–48 h	15 mg every 24 h	15 mg every 12–24 h
Gentamicin	IV, IM	5 mg every 48 h	4–5 mg every 24–48 h	4 mg every 24 h	4 mg every 12–24 h
Tobramycin	IV, IM	5 mg every 48 h	4–5 mg every 24–48 h	4 mg every 24 h	4 mg every 12–24 h
Carbapenems					
Imipenem/cilastatin[e]	IV	20 mg every 12 h	25 mg every 12 h	25 mg every 12 h	25 mg every 8 h
Meropenem[f]	IV	20 mg every 12 h	20 mg every 8 h	20 mg every 8 h	20 mg every 8 h
Cephalosporins[f]					
Cefepime[g]	IV, IM	30 mg every 12 h	30 mg every 12 h	30 mg every 12 h	30 mg every 12 h
Cefotaxime	IV, IM	50 mg every 12 h	50 mg every 8–12 h	50 mg every 12 h	50 mg every 8 h
Cefazolin	IV, IM	25 mg every 12 h	25 mg every 12 h	25 mg every 12 h	25 mg every 8 h
Ceftazidime	IV, IM	50 mg every 12 h	50 mg every 8–12 h	50 mg every 12 h	50 mg every 8 h
Ceftriaxone[h]	IV, IM	50 mg every 24 h	50 mg every 24 h	50 mg every 24 h	50 mg every 24 h
Cefuroxime	IV, IM	50 mg every 12 h	50 mg every 8–12 h	50 mg every 12 h	50 mg every 8 h
Penicillins					
Ampicillin[f,i]	IV, IM	50 mg every 12 h[j]	50 mg every 8 h	50 mg every 8 h[j]	50 mg every 6 h
Nafcillin, oxacillin[f]	IV, IM	25 mg every 12 h	25 mg every 8 h	25 mg every 8 h	25 mg every 6 h
Penicillin G crystalline[f]	IV, IM	25 000–50 000 U every 12 h	25 000–50 000 U every 8 h	25 000–50 000 U every 12 h	25 000–50 000 U every 8 h
Penicillin G procaine	IM only	50 000 U every 24 h	50 000 U every 24 h	50 000 U every 24 h	50 000 U every 24 h
Piperacillin-tazobactam	IV	100 mg every 12 h	100 mg every 8 h	100 mg every 12 h	100 mg every 8 h

Table 4.1 Antibacterial Drugs for Neonates (≤28 Postnatal Days of Age),[a] continued

Drug	Route	Dose per kg and Frequency of Administration			
		Body Weight ≤2 kg		Body Weight >2 kg	
		≤7 days of age	8–28 days of age[b]	≤7 days of age	8–28 days of age
Ticarcillin-clavulanate	IV	75 mg every 12 h	75 mg every 8 h	75 mg every 12 h	75 mg every 8 h
Other agents					
Azithromycin	PO	10–20 mg every 24 h	10–20 mg every 24 h	10–20 mg every 24 h	10–20 mg every 24 h
	IV	10 mg every 24 h	10 mg every 24 h	10 mg every 24 h	10 mg every 24 h
Aztreonam[g]	IV, IM	30 mg every 12 h	30 mg every 8–12 h	30 mg every 8 h	30 mg every 6 h
Clindamycin	IV, IM, PO	5 mg every 12 h	5 mg every 8 h	5 mg every 8 h	5 mg every 6 h
Erythromycin	IV, PO	10 mg every 12 h	10 mg every 8 h	10 mg every 12 h	10 mg every 8 h
Linezolid	IV	10 mg every 12 h	10 mg every 8 h	10 mg every 8 h	10 mg every 8 h
Metronidazole	IV	7.5 mg every 24–48 h[k]	15 mg every 24 h	15 mg every 24 h	15 mg every 12 h
Vancomycin	IV	See comment[l]			

IV indicates intravenous; IM, intramuscular; PO, oral.

[a] Adapted from American Academy of Pediatrics. *2012–2013 Nelson's Pediatric Antimicrobial Therapy*. Bradley JS, Nelson JD, eds. 19th ed. Elk Grove Village, IL: American Academy of Pediatrics; 2012.

[b] May use the longer dosing interval in extremely low birth weight (less than 1000 g) neonates until 2 weeks of life.

[c] Dosages for aminoglycosides may differ from those recommended by the manufacturer and approved by the US Food and Drug Administration.

[d] Optimal, individualized dosage should be based on determination of serum concentrations.

[e] Accumulation of cilastatin may occur in neonates with multiple doses.

[f] Higher doses than those listed may be required for meningitis.

[g] 50 mg/kg/dose may be required for *Pseudomonas* infections.

[h] Neonates should not receive ceftriaxone intravenously if they also are receiving, or are expected to receive, intravenous calcium in any form, including parenteral nutrition. See Bradley JS, Wassel RT, Lee L, Nambiar S. Intravenous ceftriaxone and calcium in the neonate: assessing the risk for cardiopulmonary adverse events. *Pediatrics.* 2009;123(4):e609–e613.

[i] Some experts recommend 75 mg/kg/dose every 6 h for group B streptococcal meningitis for all weight groups.

[j] 100 mg/kg/dose every 12 hours also is acceptable for treatment of presumed early-onset group B streptococcal septicemia.

[k] May begin therapy with a 15 mg/kg loading dose, then use the longer dosing interval for extremely low birth weight (less than 1000 g) neonates.

[l] Dosing algorithm for vancomycin is based on serum creatinine concentration; if <0.7 mg/dL, then 15 mg/kg every 12 h; if 0.7–0.9 mg/dL, then 20 mg/kg every 24 h; if 1–1.2 mg/dL, then 15 mg/kg every 24 h; if 1.3–1.6 mg/dL, then 10 mg/kg every 24 h; if >1.6 mg/dL, then 15 mg/kg every 48h. Add 0.2 to serum creatinine concentration when using algorithm in neonates ≤28 weeks' gestational age.

Table 4.2. Antibacterial Drugs for Pediatric Patients Beyond the Newborn Period[a]

Drug Generic (Trade Name)	Route	Dosage per kg per Day		Comments
		Mild to Moderate Infections	Severe Infections	
Aminoglycosides[b]				
Amikacin (Amikin)	IV, IM	Inappropriate	15–22.5 mg in 3 doses	Individualize dose and frequency based on analysis of serum concentrations.[b]
Gentamicin	IV, IM	Inappropriate	3–7.5 mg in 3 doses	
Kanamycin (Kantrex)	IV, IM	Inappropriate	15–30 mg in 3 doses	
Neomycin	PO only	100 mg in 4 doses	100 mg in 4 doses	For some enteric infections.
Tobramycin (Nebcin)	IV, IM	Inappropriate	3–7.5 mg in 3 doses	Higher doses (8–10 mg) are appropriate for pulmonary exacerbations in patients with cystic fibrosis.
Carbapenems[c]				
Doripenem (Doribax)	IV	Inappropriate	Adults 1500 mg per day in 3 doses	FDA approved for adults in 2008.
Imipenem/cilastatin (Primaxin)	IV, IM	Inappropriate	60–100 mg in 4 doses (daily adult dose, 1–4 g)	IM form not approved for children <12 y. IM form contains lidocaine. Caution in use for treatment of meningitis because of possible seizures. Higher doses for more severe infections or *Pseudomonas aeruginosa* infections.
Meropenem (Merrem)	IV	Inappropriate	30–60 mg in 3 doses (daily adult dose, 1.5–6 g)	Higher dose (120 mg in 3 doses) used for treatment of meningitis.
Ertapenem (Invanz)	IV/IM	Inappropriate	30 mg in 2 doses (adult dose, 1 g, once daily)	Poor activity against *Pseudomonas* and *Acinetobacter* species.

Table 4.2. Antibacterial Drugs for Pediatric Patients Beyond the Newborn Period,[a] continued

Drug Generic (Trade Name)	Route	Dosage per kg per Day		Comments
		Mild to Moderate Infections	Severe Infections	
Cephalosporins[c]				The generation of each agent is listed as a rough guide to antimicrobial spectrum.
Cefaclor (Ceclor)	PO	20–40 mg in 2 or 3 doses (daily adult dose, 750 mg–1.5 g)	Inappropriate	Second-generation.
Cefadroxil (Duricef)	PO	30 mg in 2 doses (daily adult dose, 1–2 g)	Inappropriate	First-generation.
Cefazolin (Ancef)	IV, IM	25–50 mg in 3 doses (daily adult dose, 3 g)	100–150 mg in 3 doses (daily adult dose, 4–6 g)	First-generation. Limited data on dosages above 100 mg/kg/day.
Cefdinir (Omnicef)	PO	14 mg in 1 or 2 doses (max, 600 mg/day)	Inappropriate	Extended-spectrum. Inadequate activity against penicillin-resistant pneumococci.
Cefditoren (Spectracef[d])	PO	400–800 mg total daily dose (not per kg) in 2 doses	Inappropriate	Extended-spectrum. Contraindicated for patients with carnitine deficiency states, because pivoxil causes renal excretion of carnitine. Only available in tablet form.
Cefepime (Maxipime)	IV, IM	100 mg in 2 doses (daily adult dose, 2–4 g)	100–150 mg in 2–3 doses (daily adult dose, 4–6 g)	Extended-spectrum. Higher dose (150 mg in 3 doses) used for febrile neutropenia.
Cefixime (Suprax)	PO	8 mg in 1 or 2 doses (daily adult dose, 400 mg)	Inappropriate	Extended-spectrum. Inadequate activity against penicillin-resistant pneumococci. Single-dose treatment for gonorrhea (400 mg × 1 in children ≥45 kg).
Cefotaxime (Claforan)	IV, IM	50–180 mg in 3 or 4 doses (daily adult dose, 3–6 g)	200–225 mg in 4 or 6 doses (daily adult dose, 8–12 g)	Extended-spectrum. Up to 300 mg in 4 or 6 doses for meningitis.

Table 4.2. Antibacterial Drugs for Pediatric Patients Beyond the Newborn Period,[a] continued

Drug Generic (Trade Name)	Route	Dosage per kg per Day		Comments
		Mild to Moderate Infections	Severe Infections	
Cefotetan (Cefotan)	IV, IM	60 mg in 2 doses (daily adult dose, 2–4 g)	100 mg in 2 doses (daily adult dose, 4–6 g)	Second-generation. A cephamycin, with enhanced anaerobic activity. Not FDA approved for use in children.
Cefoxitin (Mefoxin)	IV, IM	80 mg in 3–4 doses (daily adult dose, 3–4 g)	160 mg in 4 doses (daily adult dose, 6–12 g)	Second-generation. A cephamycin, with enhanced anaerobic activity. Active against *Bacteroides fragilis*.
Cefpodoxime (Vantin)	PO	10 mg in 2 doses (daily adult dose, 200–400 mg, 800 mg for SSTIs)	Inappropriate	Extended-spectrum.
Cefprozil (Cefzil)	PO	15–30 mg in 2 doses (daily adult dose, 0.5–1 g)	Inappropriate	Second-generation.
Ceftaroline (Teflaro)	IV	Inappropriate	Adults, 1200 mg per day in 2 doses	FDA approved for adults in 2010. Active against MRSA.
Ceftazidime (Fortaz)	IV, IM	90–150 mg in 3 doses (daily adult dose, 3 g)	200–300 mg in 3 doses (daily adult dose, 6 g)	Extended-spectrum. Anti-*Pseudomonas* activity.
Ceftibuten (Cedax)	PO	9 mg once daily (daily adult dose, 400 mg)	Inappropriate	Extended-spectrum. Inadequate activity against penicillin-resistant pneumococci.
Ceftizoxime (Cefizox)	IV, IM	150 mg in 3 doses (daily adult dose, 3–4 g)	150–200 mg in 3 or 4 doses (daily adult dose, 6–12 g)	Extended-spectrum.
Ceftriaxone (Rocephin)	IV, IM	50–75 mg once daily (daily adult dose, 1 g)	100 mg in 1 or 2 doses (daily adult dose, 2–4 g)	Extended-spectrum. Larger dosage (up to that used for meningitis) appropriate for penicillin-resistant pneumococcal pneumonia. 50 mg/kg, IM, ×1–3 days for AOM (up to 1g).[e]

Table 4.2. Antibacterial Drugs for Pediatric Patients Beyond the Newborn Period,[a] continued

Drug Generic (Trade Name)	Route	Dosage per kg per Day			Comments
		Mild to Moderate Infections	Severe Infections		
Cefuroxime (Zinacef)	IV, IM	75–100 mg in 3 doses (daily adult dose, 2.25–4.5 g)	100–200 mg in 3–4 doses (daily adult dose, 3–6 g)		Second-generation. Less active than parenteral third-generation cephalosporins against penicillin-resistant pneumococcus.
Cefuroxime (Ceftin)	PO	20–30 mg in 2 doses (daily adult dose, 0.5–1 g)	Inappropriate		Second-generation. Limited activity against penicillin-resistant pneumococcus.
Cephalexin (Keflex)	PO	25–50 mg in 2 or 4 doses (daily adult dose, 1–2 g)	75–100 mg in 3–4 doses (daily adult dose, 2–4 g)		First-generation. The 100 mg/kg/day dosage has been studied for osteoarticular infections.
Chloramphenicol (Chloromycetin)	IV	Inappropriate	50–100 mg in 4 doses (daily adult dose, 2–4 g)		Individualize dose and frequency based on analysis of serum concentrations. Usually reserved for serious infections due to rare risk of aplastic anemia.
Clindamycin (Cleocin)	IM, IV	20 mg in 3 doses (daily adult dose, 0.9–1.8 g)	40 mg in 3–4 doses (daily adult dose, 1.8–2.7 g)		Active against anaerobes, especially *Bacteroides* species. Active against many multidrug-resistant pneumococci and MRSA
	PO	10–25 mg in 3 doses (daily adult dose, 600 mg–1.8 g)	30–40 mg in 3–4 doses (daily adult dose, 1.2–1.8 g)		The 30–40 mg dosage recommended for AOM,[e] community-associated MRSA.
Daptomycin (Cubicin)	IV	Inappropriate	4–6 mg, once daily for children ≥12 years; 7 mg in one dose for children between 6 and 12 years of age; and 8–10 mg in one dose for children 2–6 years of age (daily adult dose, 4–6 mg/kg of total body weight)		Not FDA-approved for <18 y of age.

Table 4.2. Antibacterial Drugs for Pediatric Patients Beyond the Newborn Period,[a] continued

Drug Generic (Trade Name)	Route	Dosage per kg per Day		Comments
		Mild to Moderate Infections	Severe Infections	
Fluoroquinolones[f]				
Ciprofloxacin (Cipro)	PO	20 mg in 2 doses (daily adult dose, 0.5–1 g)	30–40 mg in 2 doses (daily adult dose, 1–1.5 g)	Also see p 800.
	IV	Inappropriate	20–30 mg in 2 or 3 doses (daily adult dose, 0.8–1.2 g)	
Levofloxacin (Leva-quin)	IV, PO	Inappropriate	20 mg in 2 doses if <5 y; 10 mg once daily if ≥5 y (daily adult dose, 500 mg)	Also see p 800.
Macrolides				
Azithromycin (Zithro-max, Zmax)	PO	5–12 mg once daily (adult single or total course dose, 1.5–2 g)	Inappropriate	All doses once daily: AOM[e]: 10 mg/kg/day × 3 days or 30 mg/kg × 1 day or 10 mg/kg/day × 1 day, then 5 mg/kg/day × 4 days Pharyngitis: 12 mg/kg/day (maximum 500 mg) on day 1, then 6 mg/kg/day (maximum 250 mg) on days 2–5 Sinusitis: 10 mg/kg/day × 3 days or 10 mg/kg/day × 1 day, then 5 mg/kg/day × 4 days CAP: 10 mg/kg × 1 day, then 5 mg/kg/day × 4 days or 60 mg/kg × 1 day of Zmax suspension for infants and children >6 months of age. Shigellosis: 12 mg/kg × 1 day, 6 mg/kg/d × 4 days.
	IV	Inappropriate	10 mg/kg, once daily	
Clarithromycin (Biaxin)	PO	15 mg in 2 doses (daily adult dose, 0.5–1 g)	Inappropriate	Similar to erythromycin; more activity against *Mycobacterium avium* and *Helicobacter pylori.*

Table 4.2. Antibacterial Drugs for Pediatric Patients Beyond the Newborn Period,[a] continued

Drug Generic (Trade Name)	Route	Dosage per kg per Day		Comments
		Mild to Moderate Infections	Severe Infections	
Erythromycins (numerous)	PO	50 mg in 3–4 doses (daily adult dose, 1–2 g)	Inappropriate	Available in base, stearate, and ethylsuccinate preparations.
	IV	Inappropriate	20 mg in 4 doses (daily adult dose, 2–4 g)	Administer over at least 60 minutes potentially to prevent cardiac arrhythmias.
Metronidazole (Flagyl)	PO	30–50 mg in 3 doses (daily adult dose, 0.75–2.25 g)	Same	
	IV	22.5–40 mg in 3 doses (daily adult dose, 1.5 g)	Same	
Monobactam				
Aztreonam[c] (Azactam)	IV, IM	90 mg in 3 doses (daily adult dose, 3 g)	90–120 mg in 3 or 4 doses (maximum daily adult dose, 8 g)	…
Nitrofurantoin (Furadantin)	PO	5–7 mg in 4 doses (daily adult dose, 200–400 mg)	Inappropriate	UTI prophylaxis: 1–2 mg once daily.
Oxazolidinones				
Linezolid (Zyvox)	PO, IV	For children <12 y of age: 30 mg in 3 doses For adolescents ≥12 y and adults: 1200 mg per day in 2 doses	Same	Myelosuppression increases with duration of therapy over 10 days.

Table 4.2. Antibacterial Drugs for Pediatric Patients Beyond the Newborn Period,[a] continued

Drug Generic (Trade Name)	Route	Dosage per kg per Day		Comments
		Mild to Moderate Infections	Severe Infections	
PENICILLINS[c]				
Broad-spectrum penicillins				
Amoxicillin (Amoxil)	PO	25–50 mg in 3 doses (daily adult dose, 750 mg–1.5 g)	High dosage for oral step-down therapy of invasive, non-AOM infections: 80–100 mg in 3 doses	90 mg/kg in 2 doses recommended for initial therapy of AOM.[e]
Amoxicillin-clavulanic acid (Augmentin)	PO	14:1 Formulation: 90 mg amoxicillin component in 2 doses (<40 kg) for recurrent AOM, treatment failures[e] 7:1 Formulation: 25–45 mg amoxicillin component in 2 doses (daily adult dose, 1750 mg) 4:1 Formulation: 20–40 mg amoxicillin component in 3 doses (daily adult dose, 1500 mg)	Inappropriate	
Ampicillin	IV, IM	100–150 mg in 4 doses (daily adult dose, 2–4 g)	200–400 mg in 4 doses (daily adult dose, 6–12 g)	
	PO	50–100 mg in 4 doses (daily adult dose, 2–4 g)	Inappropriate	

Table 4.2. Antibacterial Drugs for Pediatric Patients Beyond the Newborn Period,[a] continued

| Drug Generic (Trade Name) | Route | Dosage per kg per Day | | Comments |
		Mild to Moderate Infections	Severe Infections	
Ampicillin-sulbactam (Unasyn)	IV	100–200 mg of ampicillin component in 4 doses (daily adult dose, 4 g)	200 mg ampicillin component in 4 doses (daily adult dose, 8 g)	
Piperacillin[d,g]	IV, IM	200 mg in 3–4 doses (daily adult dose, 6–12 g)	300–400 mg in 4–6 doses (daily adult dose, 12–24 g)	
Piperacillin-tazobactam[g] (Zosyn)	IV	Inappropriate	300 mg piperacillin component in 3 doses (daily adult dose, 9–16 g)	Lower dose (240 mg piperacillin component in 3 doses) recommended for patients 2–9 mo of age.
Ticarcillin-clavulanate (Timentin)	IV	Inappropriate	200–300 mg ticarcillin component in 4–6 doses (daily adult dose, 12–18 g)	
Penicillin[c,g]				
Penicillin G, crystalline potassium or sodium	IV, IM	100 000–150 000 U in 4 doses (daily adult dose, 4–8 million U)	200 000–300 000 U in 6 doses (daily adult dose, 12–24 million U)	
Penicillin G procaine	IM	50 000 U in 1–2 doses (daily adult dose, 300 000–1.2 million U)	Inappropriate	Not safe for IV administration.
Penicillin G benzathine (Bicillin LA)	IM	<27 kg (60 lb) 300 000–600 000 U (not per kg) one time ≥27 kg (60 lb) 900 000 U (not per kg) one time	Inappropriate	Not safe for IV administration. 50 000 U/kg for newborns and infants. Major use is treatment of rheumatic fever prophylaxis and treponemal infections.

Table 4.2. Antibacterial Drugs for Pediatric Patients Beyond the Newborn Period,[a] continued

Drug Generic (Trade Name)	Route	Dosage per kg per Day		Comments
		Mild to Moderate Infections	Severe Infections	
Penicillin G benzathine/procaine (Bicillin CR)	IM	<14 kg (30 lb) 600 000 U[h] (not per kg) one time 14–27 kg (30–60 lb) 900 000–1 200 000 U (not per kg) one time ≥27 kg (60 lb) 2 400 000 U (not per kg) one time		Not safe for IV administration. Major use is treatment of group A streptococcal infections.
Penicillin V	PO	25–50 mg in 3 or 4 doses (daily adult dose, 1–2 g)	Inappropriate	
Penicillinase-resistant penicillins[c]				Methicillin (oxacillin)-resistant staphylococci usually are resistant to all semisynthetic antistaphylococcal penicillins and cephalosporins except ceftaroline.
Oxacillin (Bactocill)	IV, IM	100–150 mg in 4 doses (daily adult dose, 4 g)	150–200 mg in 4–6 doses (daily adult dose, 6–12 g)	…
Nafcillin (Nallpen)	IV, IM	100–150 mg in 4 doses (daily adult dose, 4 g)	150–200 mg in 4–6 doses (daily adult dose, 6–12 g)	
Dicloxacillin (Dynapen)	PO	12–25 mg in 4 doses (daily adult dose, 0.5–1 g)	100 mg in 4 divided doses (for step-down therapy of osteo-articular infections)	
Rifamycins				
Rifampin (Rifadin)	IV, PO	10–20 mg in 1–2 doses (daily adult dose, 600 mg)	20 mg in 2 doses (daily adult dose, 600 mg)	Should not be used routinely as monotherapy because of rapid emergence of resistance. See p 745–746 for *M tuberculosis* dosing.

Table 4.2. Antibacterial Drugs for Pediatric Patients Beyond the Newborn Period,[a] continued

| Drug Generic (Trade Name) | Route | Dosage per kg per Day | | Comments |
		Mild to Moderate Infections	Severe Infections	
Rifaximin[e] (Xifaxan)	PO	≥12 y of age: 600 mg/day (not per kg) in 3 doses	Inappropriate	Treatment of traveler's diarrhea caused by nonentero-invasive *Escherichia coli*; should not be used for bloody diarrhea with risk of bacteremia.
Streptogramin				
Quinupristin/ dalfopristin (Syn-ercid)	IV	Inappropriate	15–22.5 mg in 2–3 doses (daily adult dose, same)	Moderate activity against vancomycin-resistant *E faecium* (but not *Enterococcus faecalis*) as well as *Staphylococcus aureus*. Limited experience in children.
Sulfonamides				
Sulfadiazine	PO	120–150 mg in 4–6 doses (daily adult dose, 4–6 g)	120–150 mg in 4–6 doses (daily adult dose, 4–6 g)	...
Sulfisoxazole (Gantrisin)	PO	120–150 mg in 4–6 doses (daily adult dose, 2–4 g)		10–20 mg in 2 doses for UTI prophylaxis.
Trimethoprim (TMP)-sulfamethoxazole (SMX) (Bactrim, Septra)	PO, IV	8–12 mg of TMP com-ponent in 2 doses (daily adult dose, 320 mg TMP)	same	2 mg of TMP component once daily for UTI prophylaxis. See p 583 for *Pneumocystis jiroveci* dosing.
Tetracyclines				
Tetracycline (Sumycin)	PO	25–50 mg in 4 doses (daily adult dose, 1–2 g)	For Rickettsia or *Ehrlichia* disease (Rocky Mountain Spotted Fever)	Responsible for staining of developing teeth; routine use only in children 8 y of age or older. Exceptions for circumstances in which the benefits of therapy exceed the risks and alternative drugs are less effec-tive or more toxic (see p 801).

Table 4.2. Antibacterial Drugs for Pediatric Patients Beyond the Newborn Period,[a] continued

Drug Generic (Trade Name)	Route	Dosage per kg per Day		Comments
		Mild to Moderate Infections	Severe Infections	
Doxycycline (Vibramycin)	PO, IV	2–4 mg in 1–2 doses (daily adult dose, 100–200 mg)	For Rickettsia or *Ehrlichia* disease (Rocky Mountain Spotted Fever)	Adverse effects similar to those of other tetracycline products except that risk of dental staining in children younger than 8 y of age with doxycycline is unlikely at the dose and duration recommended to treat serious infections.
Vancomycin (Vancocin)	IV	40–45 mg in 3–4 doses (daily adult dose, 1–2 g)[i]	45–60 mg in 3–4 doses (daily adult dose, 2–4 g)[i]	Individualize dose and frequency based on analysis of serum concentrations.

IV, indicates intravenous; IM, intramuscular; PO, oral; FDA, US Food and Drug Administration; SSTI, skin and soft tissue infection; MRSA, methicillin-resistant *Staphylococcus aureus*; AOM, acute otitis media; CAP, community acquired pneumonia; UTI, urinary tract infection.

[a] Adapted from American Academy of Pediatrics. *2012–2013 Nelson's Pediatric Antimicrobial Therapy*. Bradley JS, Nelson JD, eds. 19th ed. Elk Grove Village, IL: American Academy of Pediatrics; 2012.

[b] Once-daily aminoglycoside dosing (amikacin 15–20 mg/kg; gentamicin/tobramycin 4.5–7.5 mg/kg) may provide equal efficacy with reduced toxicity and may be used as an alternative or multiple daily dosing. See Contopoulos-Ioannidis DG, Giotis ND, Baliatsa DV, Ioannidis JP. Extended-inverval aminoglycoside administration for children: a meta-analysis. *Pediatrics*. 2004;114(1):e111–e118.

[c] In patients with history of allergy to penicillin or one of its many congeners, alternative drugs are recommended. In some circumstances, a cephalosporin or other beta-lactam–class drug may be acceptable. However, these drugs should not be used in patients with an immediate hypersensitivity (anaphylaxis) to penicillin, because approximately 5% to 15% of penicillin-allergic patients also will be allergic to cephalosporins.

[d] Not FDA approved for use in patients younger than 12 years of age.

[e] American Academy of Pediatrics, Subcommittee on Management of Acute Otitis Media. Diagnosis and management of acute otitis media. *Pediatrics*. 2004;113(5):1451–1465

[f] Ciprofloxacin only licensed for use in patients younger than 18 years of age for complicated urinary tract infections and postexposure inhalation anthrax. Levofloxacin has been studied in children and adolescents for treatment of AOM, community acquired pneumonia (see Fluoroquinolones, p 800).

[g] Patients with a history of allergy to penicillin G or penicillin V should be considered for subsequent skin testing where available. Many such patients can be treated safely with penicillin; only 10% of children with such history are proven allergic when skin tested.

[h] As 300 000 U benzathine + 300 000 U procaine/mL in 2-mL syringe size.

[i] Higher dosages may be needed based on therapeutic monitoring of trough concentrations.

SEXUALLY TRANSMITTED INFECTIONS

Table 4.3. Guidelines for Treatment of Sexually Transmitted Infections in Children and Adolescents According to Syndrome

Preferred regimens are listed. For further information concerning other acceptable regimens and diseases not included, see recommendations in disease-specific chapters in Section 3. In addition, revised recommendations on treatment of sexually transmitted infections have been issued by the Centers for Disease Control and Prevention in 2010[a]; updates are posted at **www.cdc.gov/std/treatment.**

Syndrome	Organisms/Diagnoses	Treatment of Adolescent[a]	Treatment of Infant/Child
Urethritis and cervicitis Urethritis: Inflammation of urethra with erythema and/or mucoid, mucopurulent, or purulent discharge Cervicitis: Inflammation of cervix with erythema, friability and/or mucopurulent or purulent cervical discharge. Cervicitis occurs rarely in prepubertal girls (see Prepubertal vaginitis)	*Neisseria gonorrhoeae,* *Chlamydia trachomatis* Other causes of urethritis and cervicitis include *Mycoplasma genitalium,* possibly *Ureaplasma urealyticum,* and sometimes *Trichomonas vaginalis* and herpes simplex virus (HSV)	Ceftriaxone, 250 mg, IM, in a single dose[b] **OR** Cefixime, 400 mg, orally, in a single dose[b] **PLUS EITHER** Azithromycin, 1 g, orally, in a single dose **OR** Doxycycline, 100 mg, orally, twice a day for 7 days	*Children <45 kg:* Ceftriaxone, 125 mg, IM, in a single dose **OR** Cefixime, 8 mg/kg (maximum 400 mg, orally, in a single dose) **PLUS** *Children ≤45 kg and <8 y of age:* Erythromycin base or ethylsuccinate, 50 mg/kg per day, orally, in 4 divided doses (maximum 2 g/day) for 14 days *Children ≥45 kg but <8 y of age:* Azithromycin, 1 g, orally, in a single dose *Children ≥45 kg and ≥8 y of age:* Azithromycin, 1 g, orally, in a single dose **OR** Doxycycline, 100 mg, orally, twice a day for 7 days

Table 4.3. Guidelines for Treatment of Sexually Transmitted Infections in Children and Adolescents According to Syndrome, continued

Syndrome	Organisms/Diagnoses	Treatment of Adolescent	Treatment of Infant/Child
Prepubertal vaginitis (STI related):	*N gonorrhoeae*[a]	…	***Children <45 kg:*** Ceftriaxone, 125 mg, in a single dose
	C trachomatis[a]	…	***Children <45 kg and <8 y of age:*** Erythromycin base or ethylsuccinate, 50 mg/kg per day, orally, in 4 divided doses (maximum 2 g/day) for 14 days ***Children ≥45 kg but <8 y of age:*** Azithromycin, 1 g, orally, in a single dose ***Children ≥45 kg and ≥8 y of age:*** Azithromycin, 1 g, orally, in a single dose **OR** Doxycycline, 100 mg, orally, twice a day for 7 days
	T vaginalis	…	***Children <45 kg:*** Metronidazole, 15 mg/kg per day, orally, in 3 divided doses (maximum 2 g/day) for 7 days

Table 4.3. Guidelines for Treatment of Sexually Transmitted Infections in Children and Adolescents According to Syndrome, continued

Syndrome	Organisms/Diagnoses	Treatment of Adolescent	Treatment of Infant/Child
	Bacterial vaginosis	...	**Children <45 kg:** Metronidazole, 15 mg/kg per day, orally, in 2 divided doses (maximum 1 g/day) for 7 days
	HSV—primary infection	Acyclovir, 400 mg, orally, 3 times/day for 7–10 days **OR** Acyclovir, 200 mg, orally, 5 times/day for 7–10 days **OR** Famciclovir (250 mg, orally, 3 times/day) for 7–10 days **OR** Valacyclovir (1 g, orally, twice daily) for 7–10 days	**Children <45 kg:** Acyclovir, 80 mg/kg per day, orally, in 3–4 divided doses (maximum 1.2 g/day) for 7–10 days / Valacyclovir, 40 mg/kg per day, orally, in 2 divided doses for 7–10 days
Adolescent vulvovaginitis	*T vaginalis*	Metronidazole, 2 g, orally, in a single dose **OR** Tinidazole, 2 g, orally, in a single dose	...
	Bacterial vaginosis	Metronidazole, 500 mg, orally, twice daily for 7 days **OR** Metronidazole gel 0.75%, 1 full applicator (5 g), intravaginally, once a day for 5 days **OR** Clindamycin cream 2%, 1 full applicator (5 g), intravaginally at bedtime, for 7 days	...
	Candida species	See Table 4.4, Recommended Regimens for Vulvovaginal Candidiasis (p 827)	...

Table 4.3. Guidelines for Treatment of Sexually Transmitted Infections in Children and Adolescents According to Syndrome, continued

Syndrome	Organisms/Diagnoses	Treatment of Adolescent	Treatment of Infant/Child
	HSV—primary infection	Acyclovir, 400 mg, orally, 3 times/day for 7–10 days **OR** Famciclovir, 250 mg, orally, 3 times/day for 7–10 days **OR** Valcyclovir, 1 g, orally twice/day for 7–10 days	…
Pelvic inflammatory disease (PID)	*N gonorrhoeae, C trachomatis,* anaerobes, coliform bacteria, and *Streptococcus* species	See Pelvic Inflammatory Disease (Table 3.43, p 552)	PID occurs rarely, if at all, in prepubertal girls
Syphilis	*Treponema pallidum*	See Syphilis, p 690	*Children <45 kg:* Same as for congenital syphilis (see p 697 and Fig 3.7, p 695)
Genital ulcer disease	*T pallidum*	Same as for syphilis	*Children <45 kg:* Same as for congenital syphilis (see p 697 and Fig 3.7, p 695)
	HSV—primary infection	See prepubertal vaginitis	*Children <45 kg:* See prepubertal vaginitis

Table 4.3. Guidelines for Treatment of Sexually Transmitted Infections in Children and Adolescents According to Syndrome, continued

Syndrome	Organisms/ Diagnoses	Treatment of Adolescent	Treatment of Infant/Child
	Haemophilus ducreyi (chancroid)	Azithromycin, 1 g, orally, in a single dose **OR** Ceftriaxone, 250 mg, IM, in a single dose **OR** Ciprofloxacin, 500 mg, orally, twice daily for 3 days[e] **OR** Erythromycin base, 500 mg, orally, 3 times/day for 7 days	***Children <45 kg:*** Ceftriaxone, 50 mg/kg, IM, in a single dose (maximum 250 mg) **OR** ***Children <45 kg:*** Azithromycin, 20 mg/kg, orally, in a single dose (maximum 1 g)
	Klebsiella granulomatis (granuloma inguinale [Donovanosis])[d]	Doxycycline, 100 mg, orally, twice a day for at least 3 wk and until all lesions have healed completely **OR** Azithromycin, 1 g, orally, once/wk for at least 3 wk and until all lesions have healed completely **OR** Ciprofloxacin, 750 mg, orally, twice a day for at least 3 wk and until all lesions have healed completely **OR** Erythromycin base, 500 mg, orally, 4 times/day for at least 3 wk and until all lesions have healed completely **OR** Trimethoprim-sulfamethoxazole, 1 double-strength (160 g/800 mg) tablet, orally; twice a day for at least 3 wk and until all lesions have healed completely	
Sexually acquired epididymitis	*C trachomatis, N gonorrhoeae*	Ceftriaxone, 250 mg, IM, in a single dose **PLUS** Doxycycline, 100 mg, orally, twice daily for 10 days	…

Table 4.3. Guidelines for Treatment of Sexually Transmitted Infections in Children and Adolescents According to Syndrome, continued

Syndrome	Organisms/Diagnoses	Treatment of Adolescent	Treatment of Infant/Child
	Enteric organisms (for patients allergic to cephalosporins and/or tetracycline)	Levofloxacin, 500 mg, orally, once daily for 10 days **OR** Ofloxacin, 300 mg, orally, twice a day for 10 days	...
Gonococcal infections of the pharynx	*N gonorrhoeae*	Ceftriaxone, 250 mg, IM, in a single dose	Ceftriaxone, 125 mg, IM, in a single dose ***Children <45 kg:*** Same as for adolescents
Anogenital warts	Human papillomavirus	*Patient-applied:* Podofilox 0.5% solution or gel[c] **OR** Imiquimod 5% cream **OR** Sinecatechins 15% ointment *Provider-administered:* Cryotherapy **OR** Podophyllin resin 10%–25%[c] **OR** Trichloroacetic acid **OR** Bichloroacetic acid **OR** Surgical removal	

IM indicates intramuscularly; STI, sexually transmitted infection.

[a] For additional information and recommendations, see Centers for Disease Control and Prevention. Sexually transmitted diseases treatment guidelines, 2010. *MMWR Morb Mortal Wkly Rep.* 2010;59(RR-12);1–110 (see **www.cdc.gov/std/treatment**). Some regimens are not indicated for pregnant adolescents.

[b] Fluoroquinolones no longer are recommended for treatment of gonococcal infections because of increasing prevalence of resistant organisms (Centers for Disease Control and Prevention. Update to CDC's sexually transmitted diseases treatment guidelines, 2006: fluoroquinolones no longer recommended for treatment of gonococcal infections. *MMWR Morb Mortal Wkly Rep.* 2007;56[14]:332–336).

[c] Not tested for safety in children and contraindicated in pregnancy.

[d] For infections that do not respond to therapy within several days, consider the addition of intravenous gentamicin.

Table 4.4. Recommended Regimens for Vulvovaginal Candidiasis

Intravaginal agents:

Butoconazole, 2% cream, 5 g, intravaginally, for 3 days[a,b]

OR

Butoconazole, 2% cream (sustained release), 5 g, single dose intravaginal application for 1 day

OR

Clotrimazole, 1% cream, 5 g, intravaginally, for 7–14 days[a,b]

OR

Clotrimazole 2% cream, 5 g, intravaginally, for 3 days[a,b]

OR

Miconazole, 2% cream, 5 g, intravaginally, for 7 days[a,b]

OR

Miconazole, 4% cream, 5 g, intravaginally, for 3 days[a,b]

OR

Miconazole, 100-mg vaginal suppository, 1 suppository for 7 days[a,b]

OR

Miconazole, 200-mg vaginal suppository, 1 suppository for 3 days[a,b]

OR

Miconazole, 1200 mg vaginal suppository, 1 suppository for 1 day[a,b]

OR

Nystatin, 100 000-U vaginal tablet, 1 tablet for 14 days

OR

Tioconazole, 6.5% ointment, 5 g, intravaginally, in a single application[a,b]

OR

Terconazole, 0.4% cream, 5 g, intravaginally, for 7 days[a]

OR

Terconazole, 0.8% cream, 5 g, intravaginally, for 3 days[a]

OR

Terconazole, 80-mg vaginal suppository, 1 suppository for 3 days[a]

Oral agent:

Fluconazole, 150-mg oral tablet, 1 tablet in single dose

---

[a] These creams and suppositories are oil-based and might weaken latex condoms and diaphragms. Refer to condom or diaphragm product labeling for additional information.
[b] Over-the-counter preparations.

ANTIFUNGAL DRUGS FOR SYSTEMIC FUNGAL INFECTIONS

Polyenes

Amphotericin B is the drug of choice for several disseminated, potentially life-threatening fungal infections. Amphotericin B is a fungicidal agent that is effective against a broad array of fungal species. Amphotericin B, especially the deoxycholate formulation, can cause adverse reactions, particularly renal toxicity, so its use is limited in certain patients. Lipid-associated formulations of amphotericin B, especially liposomal amphotericin B, limit renal toxicity but also can cause adverse effects and cannot achieve optimal concentrations in some sites of infection (eg, kidney).

Amphotericin B deoxycholate is the preferred formulation for treatment of neonates and young infants because of penetration into the central nervous system, urinary tract, and eye, which often are involved in *Candida* species infections; lipid-associated formulations do not penetrate as well into these body sites. Amphotericin B deoxycholate is given intravenously in a single daily dose of 1 to 1.5 mg/kg (maximum, 1.5 mg/kg/day). Amphotericin B is administered in 5% dextrose in water at a concentration of 0.1 mg/mL and delivered through a central or peripheral venous catheter (see Table 4.5, p 831). Infusion times of 1 to 2 hours have been shown to be well tolerated in adults and older children and theoretically increase the blood-to-tissue gradient, thereby improving drug delivery. After completing 1 week of daily therapy, adequate serum concentrations of the drug usually can be maintained by administering double the daily dose (maximum, 1.5 mg/kg) on alternate days. The duration of therapy depends on the type and extent of the specific fungal infection.

Amphotericin B deoxycholate is eliminated by a renal mechanism for approximately 2 weeks after therapy is discontinued. No adjustment in dose is required for neonates or for children with impaired renal function, because serum concentrations are not increased significantly in these patients. If renal toxicity occurs, alternate-day dosing is preferred to a decrease in daily dose. Neither hemodialysis nor peritoneal dialysis significantly decreases serum concentrations of the drug.

Infusion-related reactions to amphotericin B deoxycholate include fever, chills, and sometimes nausea, vomiting, headache, generalized malaise, hypotension, and arrhythmias; these reactions are rare in neonates. Onset usually is within 1 to 3 hours after starting the infusion; duration typically is less than an hour. Hypotension and arrhythmias are idiosyncratic reactions that are unlikely to occur if not observed after the initial dose but also can occur in association with rapid infusion. Multiple regimens have been used to prevent infusion-related reactions, but few have been studied in controlled clinical trials. Pretreatment with acetaminophen, alone or combined with diphenhydramine, may alleviate febrile reactions; these reactions appear to be less common in children than in adults. Hydrocortisone (25–50 mg in adults and older children) also can be added to the infusion to decrease febrile and other systemic reactions. Tolerance to febrile reactions develops with time, allowing tapering and eventual discontinuation of the hydrocortisone and often diphenhydramine and antipyretic agents.

Meperidine and ibuprofen have been effective in preventing or treating fever and chills in some patients who are refractory to the conventional premedication regimen. Toxicity from amphotericin B deoxycholate can include nephrotoxicity, hepatotoxicity, anemia, or neurotoxicity. Nephrotoxicity is caused by decreased renal blood flow and can be prevented or ameliorated by hydration, saline solution loading (0.9% saline solution over 30 minutes) before infusion of amphotericin B, and avoiding diuretic drugs. Hypokalemia is common and can be exacerbated by sodium loading. Renal tubular acidosis can occur but usually is mild. Permanent nephrotoxicity is related to cumulative dose. Nephrotoxicity can be enhanced by concomitant administration of amphotericin B and aminoglycosides, cyclosporine, tacrolimus, cisplatin, nitrogen mustard compounds, and acetazolamide. Anemia is secondary to inhibition of erythropoietin production. Neurotoxicity occurs rarely and can manifest as confusion, delirium, obtundation, psychotic behavior, seizures, blurred vision, or hearing loss.

Lipid-associated and liposomal formulations of amphotericin B have a role in children who are intolerant of or refractory to amphotericin B deoxycholate or who have renal insufficiency or at risk of significant renal toxicity from concomitant medications (see Table 4.5, p 831). In adults, none of the lipid-associated formulations have been demonstrated to be more effective than has conventional amphotericin B deoxycholate. Amphotericin B lipid formulations approved by the US Food and Drug Administration (FDA) for treatment of invasive fungal infections in children and adults who are refractory to or intolerant of amphotericin B deoxycholate therapy are amphotericin B lipid complex (ABLC, Abelcet), and liposomal amphotericin B (L-AmB, AmBisome). Compared with amphotericin B deoxycholate, acute infusion-related reactions occur with both formulations but are less frequent with AmBisome. Nephrotoxicity is less common with lipid-associated products than with amphotericin B deoxycholate. Liver toxicity, which generally is not associated with amphotericin B deoxycholate, has been reported with the lipid formulations.

Pyrimidines

Among pyrimidine antifungal agents, only flucytosine (5-fluorocytosine) is approved by the FDA for use in children. Flucytosine has a limited spectrum of activity against fungi and has potential for toxicity (see Table 4.5, p 831), and when flucytosine is used as a single agent, resistance often emerges rapidly. Flucytosine can be used in combination with amphotericin B for cryptococcal meningitis. It is important to monitor serum concentrations of flucytosine to avoid bone marrow toxicity.

Azoles

Five oral azoles are available in the United States and include ketoconazole, fluconazole, itraconazole, voriconazole, and posaconazole. All have relatively broad activity against common fungi but differ in their in vitro activity, bioavailability, adverse effects, and potential for drug interactions (see Table 4.5, p 831). Fewer data are available regarding the safety and efficacy of azoles in pediatric than in adult patients, and trials comparing these agents to amphotericin B have been limited. Azoles are easy to administer and have little toxicity, but their use can be limited by the frequency of their interactions with coadministered drugs. These drug interactions can result in decreased serum concentrations of the azole (ie, poor therapeutic activity) or unexpected toxicity from the coadministered drug (ie, increased serum concentrations of the coadministered drug). When considering use of azoles, the patient's concurrent medications should be reviewed to avoid potential adverse clinical outcomes. Another potential limitation of azoles is emergence of resistant fungi, especially *Candida* species resistant to fluconazole. *Candida krusei* intrinsically are resistant to fluconazole and strains of *Candida glabrata* are becoming increasing resistance to fluconazole and voriconazole. Itraconazole is approved by the FDA for treatment of blastomycosis, histoplasmosis (nonmeningeal), and aspergillosis in patients who are intolerant to amphotericin B and for empiric therapy of febrile neutropenic patients with suspected fungal infection. Itraconazole does not cross the blood-brain barrier and should not be used for infections of the central nervous system. Voriconazole has been approved by the FDA for primary treatment of invasive *Aspergillus* species, for candidemia in nonneutropenic patients, for esophageal candidiasis, and for refractory infection with some *Scedosporium* species, such as *Scedosporium apiospermum*, and *Fusarium* species. Therapeutic monitoring of voriconazole with measurement of serum trough concentrations is important in patients with serious infections. Limited data are available regarding use of voriconazole in children. Posaconazole is approved for use in adults for prophylaxis of invasive aspergillosis and candidiasis and treatment of oropharyngeal candidiasis. Ketoconazole seldom is used, because other azoles have fewer adverse effects and generally are preferred.

Echinocandins

Caspofungin, micafungin, and anidulafungin are the only echinocandins approved by the FDA. Caspofungin is approved for treatment of pediatric patients 3 months and older with esophageal candidiasis, empiric therapy for presumed fungal infections in febrile neutropenic patients, invasive candidiasis, and aspergillosis in adults who are refractory to or intolerant of other antifungal drugs. Clinical trials have demonstrated safety and efficacy in pediatric patients down to 3 months of age; noncomparative anecdotal experience in neonatal infections also is reported. Micafungin is approved by the FDA for intravenous treatment of esophageal candidiasis and prophylaxis of invasive *Candida* infections in patients undergoing hematopoietic stem cell transplantation. Anidulafungin is approved by the FDA for intravenous treatment of candidemia, *Candida* infections, and esophageal candidiasis. Table 4.6 (p 835) provides recommendations for treatment of serious fungal infections with amphotericin B, flucytosine, azoles, echinocandins, and other antifungal agents.

RECOMMENDED DOSES OF PARENTERAL AND ORAL ANTIFUNGAL DRUGS

Table 4.5. Recommended Doses of Parenteral and Oral Antifungal Drugs

Drug	Route	Dose (per day)	Adverse Reactions[a,b]
Amphotericin B deoxycholate (see Antifungal Drugs for Systemic Fungal Infections, p 828, for detailed information)	IV	1.0–1.5 mg/kg; infuse as a single dose over 2 h	Fever, chills, gastrointestinal tract symptoms, headache, hypotension, renal dysfunction, hypokalemia, anemia, cardiac arrhythmias, neurotoxicity; anaphylaxis
	IT	0.025 mg, increase to 0.5 mg, twice a week	Headache, gastrointestinal tract symptoms, arachnoiditis/radiculitis
Amphotericin B lipid complex (Abelcet)[c,d]	IV	5 mg/kg, infused over 2 h	Fever, chills, other reactions associated with amphotericin B deoxycholate, but less nephrotoxicity; hepatotoxicity has been reported with lipid complex
Anidulafungin[c,d]	IV	Adults: 100–200 mg loading dose, then 50–100 mg once daily (higher dose for candidemia) Children: load with 1.5 to 3 mg/kg once, then 0.75–1.5 mg/kg per day	Fever, headache, nausea, vomiting, diarrhea, leukopenia, hepatic enzyme elevations, and phlebitis
Liposomal amphotericin B (AmBisome)[c,d]	IV	3–5 mg/kg, infused over 1–2 h	Fever, chills, other reactions associated with amphotericin B, but less nephrotoxicity; hepatotoxicity has been reported
Caspofungin[c,d]	IV	Adults: 70 mg loading dose, then 50 mg once daily Children: 70 mg/m² loading dose, then 50 mg/m² once daily	Fever, rash, pruritus, phlebitis, headache, gastrointestinal tract symptoms, anemia; concomitant use with cyclosporine is not recommended unless potential benefits outweigh potential risks
Clotrimazole	PO	10-mg tablet, 5 times per day (dissolved slowly in mouth)	Gastrointestinal tract symptoms, hepatotoxicity

Table 4.5. Recommended Doses of Parenteral and Oral Antifungal Drugs, continued

Drug	Route	Dose (per day)	Adverse Reactions[a,b]
Fluconazole[b,d]	IV	Children: 3–6 mg/kg per day, single dose (up to 12 mg/kg per day for serious infections)	Rash, gastrointestinal tract symptoms, hepatotoxicity, Stevens-Johnson syndrome, anaphylaxis
	PO	Children: 6 mg/kg once, then 3 mg/kg per day for oropharyngeal or esophageal candidiasis; 6–12 mg/kg per day for invasive fungal infections; 6 mg/kg per day for suppressive therapy in HIV-infected children with cryptococcal meningitis Adults: 200 mg once, followed by 100 mg/day for oropharyngeal or esophageal candidiasis; 400–800 mg/day for other invasive fungal infections; 400 mg/day for suppressive therapy in HIV-infected patients with cryptococcal meningitis	
Flucytosine	PO	50–150 mg/kg per day in 4 doses at 6-h intervals (adjust dose if renal dysfunction); follow trough levels closely	Bone marrow suppression, renal dysfunction, gastrointestinal tract symptoms, rash, neuropathy, hepatotoxicity, confusion, hallucinations
Griseofulvin	PO	Ultramicrosize: 5–15 mg/kg, single dose; maximum dose, 750 mg Microsize: 10–20 mg/kg per day divided in 2 doses; maximum dose, 1000 mg	Rash, paresthesias, leukopenia, gastrointestinal tract symptoms, proteinuria, hepatotoxicity, mental confusion, headache
Itraconazole[b,d]	IV, PO	Children: 5–10 mg/kg per day divided into 2 doses Adults: 200–400 mg/day once or twice a day; 200 mg, once a day, for suppressive therapy in HIV-infected patients with histoplasmosis	Gastrointestinal tract symptoms, rash, edema, headache, hypokalemia, hepatotoxicity, thrombocytopenia, leukopenia; cardiac toxicity is possible in patients also taking terfenadine or astemizole

Table 4.5. Recommended Doses of Parenteral and Oral Antifungal Drugs, continued

Drug	Route	Dose (per day)	Adverse Reactions[a,b]
Ketoconazole[b,d]	PO	Children[e]: 3.3–6.6 mg/kg per day, single dose Adults: 200 mg, twice a day for 4 doses, then 200 mg, once a day	Hepatotoxicity, gastrointestinal tract symptoms, rash, anaphylaxis, thrombocytopenia, hemolytic anemia, gynecomastia, adrenal insufficiency; cardiac toxicity is possible in patients also taking terfenadine or astemizole
Micafungin[c,d]	IV	Adults: 50–150 mg once daily Children: 4–12 mg/kg per day once daily (higher dose needed for patients <8 y of age)	Fever, headache, nausea, vomiting, diarrhea, leukopenia, hepatic enzyme elevations, and phlebitis
Nystatin	PO	Infants: 200 000 U, 4 times a day, after meals Children and adults: 400 000–600 000 U, 3 times a day, after meals	Gastrointestinal tract symptoms, rash
Posaconazole[c,d]	PO	Adults: 400 mg 2 times a day with fatty meals (or liquid nutritional supplement) for treatment, 200 mg, 3 times a day (prophylaxis) Children: Not known	Gastrointestinal tract symptoms, rash, edema, headache, anemia, neutropenia, thrombocytopenia, fatigue, arthralgia, myalgia, fever
Terbinafine[c]	PO	Adults: 250 mg, once a day Children: <20 kg: 67.5 mg/day; 20–40 kg: 125 mg/day; >40 kg: 250 mg/day	Gastrointestinal tract symptoms, rash, taste abnormalities, cholestatic hepatitis

Table 4.5. Recommended Doses of Parenteral and Oral Antifungal Drugs, continued

Drug	Route	Dose (per day)	Adverse Reactions[a,b]
Voriconazole[d]	IV	Children 2–12 years: 9 mg/kg, IV, every 12 h for 1 day, then 9 mg/kg, IV, every 12 h (maximum dose, 350 mg, every 12 h) Adults and children ≥12 years: 6 mg/kg, every 12 h for 1 day (loading dose), then 4 mg/kg, every 12 h	Visual disturbance, photosensitive rash, increased liver function tests
	PO	Children 2–12 years: 9 mg/kg, every 12 h Adults: <40 kg: 200 mg, every 12 h for 1 day, then 100 mg, every 12 h; >40 kg: 400 mg, every 12 h for 1 day, then 200 mg, every 12 h	

IV indicates intravenous; IT, intrathecal; PO, oral; HIV, human immunodeficiency virus.

[a] See package insert or listing in current edition of the *Physicians' Desk Reference* or **www.pdr.net** (for registered users only).

[b] Interactions with other drugs are common. Consult **www.fda.gov/Drugs/DevelopmentApprovalProcess/DevelopmentResources/DrugInteractionsLabeling/default.htm?utm_campaign=Google2&utm_source=fdaSearch&utm_medium=website&utm_term=drug%20interactions&utm_content=1** and the *Physicians' Desk Reference* (a drug interaction reference or database) or a pharmacist before prescribing these medications.

[c] Experience with drug in children is limited.

[d] Limited or no information about use in newborn infants is available.

[e] For children 2 years of age and younger, the daily dose has not been established.

DRUGS FOR INVASIVE AND OTHER SERIOUS FUNGAL INFECTIONS IN CHILDREN

Table 4.6. Drugs for Invasive and Other Serious Fungal Infections

Disease	Intravenous		Oral	Intravenous or Oral			
	Amphotericin B	Caspofungin,a Micafungin,a,b or Anidulafungina,b	Flucytosine	Itra-conazolea	Flu-conazolea	Vori-conazolea	Posa-conazolea
Aspergillosis	A	A	…	M	…	P	…
Blastomycosis	P	…	…	M	M	…	…
Candidiasis: Chronic, mucocutaneous							A
Oropharyngeal	A	A	…	A	P	A	A
esophageal	P (severe cases)	P	…	A	P	A	
Systemic	Pc	P	S	…	P, M	A	
Coccidioidomycosis	P	…	…	P, M	P, M	…	…
Cryptococcosis	P, S	…	S	…	A, M	…	…
Fusariosis	A	…	…	…	…	P	…
Histoplasmosis	P	…	…	P, A	A, M	…	…
Mucormycosis (zygomycosis)	P	…	…	…	…	…	…
Paracoccidioidomycosis	Pd	…	…	P, M	…	…	…
Pseudallescheriasis	…	…	…	M	…	P	…
Sporotrichosis	P	…	…	M	…	…	…

P indicates preferred treatment in most cases; A, efficacy less well established or alternative drug; M, for mild and moderately severe cases; S, combination recommended if infection is severe or central nervous system is involved.

a Approved by the Food and Drug Administration for adults.

b Efficacy has not been established for children.

c Preferred treatment in neonates; alternate treatment for children and adults.

d Usually in combination with itraconazole or a sulfonamide.

TOPICAL DRUGS FOR SUPERFICIAL FUNGAL INFECTIONS

Table 4.7. Topical Drugs for Superficial Fungal Infections

Drug	Strength	Formulation	Trade Name Examples	Application(s) per Day	Adverse Reactions/Notes
Amorolfine (OTC)	5%	NL	Loceryl	1–2 weekly (mild onychomycosis)	Well tolerated; minor local.
Basic fuchsin, resorcinol, and acetone (Rx)		S	Castellani Paint Modified	1	Excellent for intertriginous areas. Stains everything. Also available as a colorless solution with alcohol and without basic fuchsin. This is an alternative if the patient cannot tolerate other topical antifungals.
Butenafine (Rx)	1%	C	Mentax	1	Safety and efficacy in patients younger than 12 y of age have not been established. Do not occlude. Sensitivity to allylamines.
Ciclopirox olamine (Rx)	1%; 8%	C, L, S, P, G	Loprox; Penlac nail lacquer	2	Irritant dermatitis, hair discoloration; shake lotion vigorously before application; safety and efficacy in children younger than 10 y of age have not been established. Precautions: diabetes mellitus; immune compromise; seizures.
Clioquinol (Rx)		C, O (F available in Canada)	Iodo Plain	2–3/day for up to 1 week	Not recommended in children younger than 2 years of age. Can stain skin, hair, nails, and clothing yellow in color.
Clotrimazole (Rx and OTC)	1%	C, L, S, P, Com, SpP, SpL; check with pharmacist	Topical solution (more than 10 preparations); Lotrimin, Mycelex, Desenex	1 (Rx) 2 (OTC)	Irritant dermatitis. Avoid topical steroid combinations.[a]

Table 4.7. Topical Drugs for Superficial Fungal Infections, continued

Drug	Strength	Formulation	Trade Name Examples	Application(s) per Day	Adverse Reactions/Notes
Clotrimazole and betamethasone dipropionate (Rx)		C, L	Lotrisone[b]	2[a]	Irritant dermatitis: safety and efficacy in children have been established. Beware of topical steroid combinations,[a] especially when applied to the diaper area, because high systemic steroid exposure can occur. Contraindication: varicella.
Econazole nitrate (Rx)	1%	C, L, P, S, F	Spectazole, Pevaryl-Ecreme	1 (dermatophyte) 2 (candidiasis)	Irritant dermatitis; safety and efficacy in children have not been established.
Iodoquinol and 2% hydrocortisone acetate (Rx)	1%	G	Alcortin A	3–4	Burning/itching sensation. Local allergic reaction. Can stain skin and clothes. Can interfere with results of thyroid function tests. Not to be used under occlusion in the diaper area.
Iodoquinol and 1% aloe polysaccharides (Rx)	1.25%	G	Aloquin	3–4	Can interfere with thyroid function tests. False-positive ferric chloride test (used for PKU) if present in the diaper or urine. Discoloration of skin, hair, and fabric, which can be removed with normal cleansing.
Ketoconazole (Rx and OTC)	1, 2%	C, Sh, G, F	Nizoral, Nizoral AD, Sebizol, Xolegel, Extina	1 (tinea dermatophyte) 2 (candidiasis)	Potential sulfite reaction with anaphylactic or asthmatic reaction; shampoo can cause dry or oily hair and increase hair loss; irritant dermatitis. May interfere with permanent waving or changes in hair texture.

Table 4.7. Topical Drugs for Superficial Fungal Infections, continued

Drug	Strength	Formulation	Trade Name Examples	Application(s) per Day	Adverse Reactions/Notes
Miconazole (Rx and OTC)	2%	O, C, P, S, SpP, SpL; check with pharmacist[c]	More than 10 preparations; Monistat-Derm, Zeasorb AF, Micatin, Daktarin tincture	2 (seborrhea), apply 2–3 times/day for several months 2 (C, L) 2 (P, L)	Irritant and allergic contact dermatitis.
Miconazole nitrate and 15% Zinc oxide (Rx)	0.25%	O	Vusion	Every diaper change for 1 week	Skin irritation. Can be used in children age 4 weeks and older.
Naftifine HC (Rx)	1%	C, G	Naftin	1 (C) 2 (Gel)	Burning/stinging, irritant dermatitis, safety and efficacy in children have not been established.
Nystatin (Rx and OTC)	100 000 U/mL or 100 000 U/g	C, P, O, Com	Nystatin, Nystop powder; Pedi-Dri powder; Mycostatin	2 (C) 2–3 (P)	Nontoxic except with topical steroid combinations.[d]
Nystatin and triamcinolone acetonide (Rx)		C, O	Mytrex cream, Mytrex ointment, Mycolog-II	2	Contraindications: varicella or vaccinia. Do not occlude. Use lowest effective dose.
Oxiconazole (Rx)	1%	C, L	Oxistat	1–2 (tinea dermatophyte)	Pruritus, burning, irritant dermatitis.
Sertaconazole (Rx)	2%	C	Ertaczo	2	Dry skin, skin tenderness, contact dermatitis, local hypersensitivity; safety and efficacy in children have not been established.

Table 4.7. Topical Drugs for Superficial Fungal Infections, continued

Drug	Strength	Formulation	Trade Name Examples	Application(s) per Day	Adverse Reactions/Notes
Sulconazole (Rx)	1%	C, S	Exelderm	1–2 (tinea vesicular)	Irritant dermatitis; safety and efficacy in children have not been established.
Terbinafine (Rx and OTC)	1%	C, G, S, Sp	Lamisil, Lamisil AT	1–2	Irritant dermatitis; avoid use of occlusive clothing or dressings. Do not apply spray to face. Safety and efficacy in children have not been established.
Tolnaftate (OTC)	1%	C, P, S, G, SpP, SpL Check with pharmacist[e]	>10 preparations; Tinactin, Zeasorb AF, Fungicure	2	Irritant and allergic contact dermatitis. Not recommended if younger than 2 y of age.
Triacetin (Rx)	% varies	S, C, Sp	Fungoid tincture, Fungoid cream only-clean nail	3 (C, S)	Irritant dermatitis; active ingredient is miconazole 2%.
Undecylenic acid and derivatives (OTC)	8%–25%	C, O, S, F, SpP, P, soap	See pharmacist for formulations and applications[e]	2 (tincture); spray 1–2 sec	Irritant dermatitis.
Undecylenic acid and chloroxylenol	25% 3%	S	Gordochom solution	2 for 4 wk	Local hypersensitivity.
Other Remedies					
Benzoic acid and 6% salicylic acid (OTC)	12%	O	Whitfields Ointment, Bensal HP	2	Warm, burning sensation. Avoid eyes, mouth and, nose. Keep out of the reach of children.
Gentian violet (OTC)	2%	S	…	2	Staining.

Table 4.7. Topical Drugs for Superficial Fungal Infections, continued

Drug	Strength	Formulation	Trade Name Examples	Application(s) per Day	Adverse Reactions/Notes
Selenium sulfide (OTC)	2.5%	Sh	Selsun 2.5%	Use twice weekly for 2 wk	Irritant dermatitis and ulceration. For tinea capitis, to decrease spore formation and to decrease the potential spread of the dermatophyte.
	1%	Sh	Head & Shoulders, Selsun Blue	Use twice weekly for 2 wk	For tinea capitis, to decrease spore formation and to decrease the potential spread of the dermatophyte.
Sodium thiosulfate		L	Versiclear Lotion	2	Safety and effectiveness in children has not been established. Use with extreme caution in children.

OTC indicates over the counter; NL, nail lacquer; Rx, prescription; S, solution; C, cream; L, lotion; P, powder G, gel; O, ointment; F, foam; Com, combinations; SpP, spray powder; SpL, spray lotion; PKU, phenylketonuria; Sh, shampoo.

[a] Topical steroids must be used with caution in young children and in areas of thin skin (eg, diaper area). In these circumstances, high systemic exposure may occur, resulting in endogenous synthesis suppression with the potential for serious adverse effects. Potential adverse effects include irritant dermatitis, folliculitis, hypertrichosis, acneiform eruptions, hypopigmentation, perioral dermatitis, allergic contact dermatitis, maceration, secondary infection, skin atrophy, striae, and miliaria.

[b] Lotrisone cream no longer is available; lotion is available. Also available are Lotrim and Fungizid spray.

[c] Pharmacists are the best resource to verify formulations that are available and new (they use *Facts and Comparisons* reference products).

[d] Any topical preparation has the potential to irritate the skin and cause itching, burning, stinging, erythema, edema, vesicles, and blister formation.

For more information on individual drugs, see *Physician's Desk Reference* or **www.pdr.net** (for registered users only).

ANTIVIRAL DRUGS

Table 4.8. Antiviral Drugs[a]

Generic (Trade Name)	Indication	Route	Age	Usually Recommended Dosage
Acyclovir[b,c,d] (Zovirax)	Neonatal herpes simplex virus (HSV) infection	IV	Birth to 3 mo	60 mg/kg per day in 3 divided doses for 14–21 days.
	HSV encephalitis	IV	≥3 mo to 12 y	30–45 mg/kg per day in 3 divided doses for 14–21 days; FDA-approved dose for this indication and age range is 60 mg/kg per day in 3 divided doses, but nephrotoxicity may be increased at this higher dose.[e]
		IV	≥12 y	30 mg/kg per day in 3 divided doses for 14–21 days.
	Varicella in immunocompetent host[f]	Oral	≥2 y	80 mg/kg per day in 4 divided doses for 5 days; maximum dose, 3200 mg/day.
	Varicella in immunocompetent host requiring hospitalization	IV	≥2 y	≤40 kg: 80 mg/kg per day in 4 divided doses; maximum dose, 3200 mg/day. >40 kg: 3200 mg in 4 divided doses
	Varicella in immuno-compromised host	IV	<1 y	30 mg/kg per day in 3 divided doses for 7–10 days.
		IV	≥1 y	1500 mg/m² per day in 3 doses for 7–10 days; some experts recommend the 30 mg/kg per day dose.
	Zoster in immunocompetent host	IV (if requiring hospitalization)	All ages	Same as for varicella in immunocompromised host.
		Oral	≥12 y	4000 mg/day in 5 divided doses for 5–7 days.
	Zoster in immunocompromised host	IV	<12 y	30 mg/kg per day in 3 divided doses, for 7–10 days.
		IV	≥12 y	30 mg/kg per day in 3 divided doses, for 7–10 days.

Table 4.8. Antiviral Drugs, continued

Generic (Trade Name)	Indication	Route	Age	Usually Recommended Dosage
Acyclovir[b,c,d] (Zovirax), continued	HSV infection in immunocompromised host (localized, progressive, or disseminated)	IV	All ages	30 mg/kg per day in 3 divided doses for 7–14 days.
		Oral	≥2 y	1000 mg/day in 3–5 divided doses for 7–14 days.
	Prophylaxis of HSV in immunocompromised hosts who are HSV seropositive	Oral	≥2 y	600–1000 mg/day in 3–5 divided doses during period of risk.
		IV	All ages	15 mg/kg in 3 divided doses during period of risk.
	Genital HSV infection: first episode	Oral	≥12 y	1000–1200 mg/day in 3–5 divided doses for 7–10 days. Oral pediatric dose: 40–80 mg/kg per day divided in 3–4 doses for 5–10 days (maximum 1.0 g/day).
		IV	≥12 y	15 mg/kg per day in 3 divided doses for 5–7 days.
	Genital HSV infection: recurrence	Oral	≥12 y	1000 mg in 5 divided doses for 5 days, or 1600 mg in 2 divided doses for 5 days, or 2400 mg in 3 divided doses for 2 days.
	Chronic suppressive therapy for recurrent genital and cutaneous (ocular) HSV episodes	Oral	≥12 y	800 mg/day in 2 divided doses for as long as 12 continuous mo.
Adefovir (Hepsera)	Chronic hepatitis B	Oral	≥12 y	10 mg once daily in patients with adequate renal function; optimal duration of therapy unknown.
Amantadine (Symmetrel)[g]	Influenza A: treatment and prophylaxis (see Influenza, p 439)[g]	Oral	1–9 y	Treatment or prophylaxis: 5 mg/kg per day, maximum 150 mg/day, in 2 divided doses.

Table 4.8. Antiviral Drugs, continued

Generic (Trade Name)	Indication	Route	Age	Usually Recommended Dosage
Amantadine (Symmetrel),[g] continued		Oral	≥10 y	Treatment or prophylaxis: <40 kg: 5 mg/kg per day, in 2 divided doses; ≥40 kg: 200 mg/day in 2 divided doses.
		Oral	Dose by weight, not age	Alternative prophylactic dose for children >20 kg and adults: 100 mg/day.
Cidofovir (Vistide)	Cytomegalovirus (CMV) retinitis	IV	Adult dose[h]	Induction: 5 mg/kg once weekly × 2 doses with probenecid and hydration. Maintenance: 5 mg/kg once every 2 weeks with probenecid and hydration.
Entecavir (Baraclude)	Chronic hepatitis B	Oral	≥16 y[h]	0.5 mg once daily in patients who have not received prior nucleoside therapy; 1 mg once daily in patients who are previously treated (not first choice in this setting); optimum duration of therapy unknown.
Famciclovir (Famvir)	Genital HSV infection, episodic recurrent episodes	Oral	Adult dose[h]	Immunocompetent: 2000 mg/day in 2 divided doses for 1 day. HIV-infected patients: 1000 mg in 2 divided doses for 7 days.
	Daily suppressive therapy	Oral	Adult dose[h]	Immunocompetent: 500 mg/day in 2 divided doses for 1 y, then reassess for recurrence of HSV infection.
	Recurrent herpes labialis	Oral	Adult dose[h]	Immunocompetent: 1500 mg as a single dose. HIV-infected patients: 1000 mg/day in 2 divided doses for 7 days.
	Herpes zoster	Oral	Adult dose[h]	1500 mg/day in 3 divided doses for 7 days.

Table 4.8. Antiviral Drugs, continued

Generic (Trade Name)	Indication	Route	Age	Usually Recommended Dosage
Foscarnet[b] (Foscavir)	CMV retinitis in patients with acquired immunodeficiency syndrome	IV	Adult dose[h]	180 mg/kg per day in 2–3 divided doses for 14–21 days, then 90–120 mg/kg once a day as maintenance dose.
	HSV infection resistant to acyclovir in immunocompromised host	IV	Adult dose[h]	80–120 mg/kg per day in 2–3 divided doses until infection resolves.
	VZV infection resistant to acyclovir	IV	Adult dose[h]	120 mg/kg/day; divided every 8 h, up to 3 weeks.
Ganciclovir[b] (Cytovene)	Acquired CMV retinitis in immunocompromised host[i]	IV	Adult dose[h]	Treatment: 10 mg/kg per day in 2 divided doses for 14–21 days; Long-term suppression; 5 mg/kg per day for 7 days/wk or 6 mg/kg per day for 5 days/wk.
	Prophylaxis of CMV in high-risk host	IV	Adult dose[h]	10 mg/kg per day in 2 divided doses for 1–2 wk, then 5 mg/kg per day in 1 dose for 100 days or 6 mg/kg per day for 5 days/wk.
Interferon alfa-2b (Intron A)	Chronic hepatitis B	SC	1–18 y	6 million IU/m² 3 times/wk for 16–24 weeks.
			>18 y	5 million IU/day; or 10 million IU 3 times/wk for 16 weeks.
	Chronic hepatitis C	SC; IM	>18 y[h]	3 million IU, 3 times/wk, for 24–48 wk, depending on HCV genotype. Note: pegylated interferon preferred over interferon alfa-2b.
Lamivudine (Epivir-HBV)	Treatment of chronic hepatitis B	Oral	≥2 y	3 mg/kg once a day (maximum 100 mg/day) (children coinfected with HIV and hepatitis B should use the approved dose for HIV).
Oseltamivir[j] (Tamiflu)	Influenza A and B: treatment (see Influenza, p 439)	Oral[j]	Birth to <12 mo	3 mg/kg/dose twice daily.

Table 4.8. Antiviral Drugs, continued

Generic (Trade Name)	Indication	Route	Age	Usually Recommended Dosage
Oseltamivir[j] (Tamiflu), continued		Oral	1–12 y	≤15 kg: 30 mg, twice daily; 16–23 kg: 45 mg, twice daily; 24–40 kg: 60 mg, twice daily; >40 kg: 75 mg, twice daily.
		Oral	≥13 y	75 mg, twice daily for treatment.
	Influenza A and B: prophylaxis	Oral	1–12 y	Same as treatment for patients 1–12 y of age, except dose given once daily.
		Oral	≥13 y	75 mg once daily.
Pegylated interferon alfa-2a	Chronic hepatitis B	SC	>18 y[h]	180 μg once weekly for 48 wk.
	Chronic hepatitis C	SC	>18 y[h]	180 μg once weekly for 24–48 wk, depending on HCV genotype.
Pegylated interferon-alfa-2b	Chronic hepatitis C	SC	>18 y	1.5 mg/kg once weekly for 24–48 weeks, depending on HCV genotype.
			>3 to 17 y	60 μg/m² once weekly for 24–48 weeks, depending on HCV genotype.
Ribavirin (Rebetol or Copegus)	Treatment of hepatitis C in combination with an alfa interferon	Oral/capsule	≥3 y (Note: capsule doses recommended for use with pegylated interferon alfa-2a and alfa-2b are different)	Fixed dose by weight is suggested: 25–36 kg: 200 mg AM and PM; >36–49 kg: 200 mg AM and 400 mg PM; >49–61 kg: 400 mg AM and PM; >61–75 kg: 400 mg AM and 600 mg PM; >75 kg: 600 mg AM and PM.
		Oral/solution	≥3 y (<25 kg)	15 mg/kg per day in 2 divided doses.

Table 4.8. Antiviral Drugs, continued

Generic (Trade Name)	Indication	Route	Age	Usually Recommended Dosage
Rimantadine (Flumadine)[g]	Influenza A: treatment[i]	Oral	≥13 y	200 mg/day in 2 divided doses.
	Influenza A: prophylaxis (see Influenza, p 439)[g]	Oral	≥1 y	1–9 y of age: 5 mg/kg per day, maximum 150 mg/day, once daily. ≥10 y of age, <40 kg: 5 mg/kg per day, in 2 divided doses; ≥40 kg: 200 mg/day in 2 divided doses.
Telbivudine (Tyzeka)	Chronic hepatitis B	Oral	Adult dose[h]	600 mg once daily.
Tenofovir	Chronic hepatitis B	Oral	Adult and adolescent dose	300 mg once daily.
			2–8 y old (for HIV)	8 mg/kg once daily.
Valacyclovir (Valtrex)	Chickenpox	Oral	2 to <18 y	20 mg/kg per dose 3 times daily for 5 days, not to exceed 1 g per dose 3 times daily.
	Genital HSV infection, first episode	Oral	Adult dose[h]	2 g/day in 2 divided doses for 10 days.
	Episodic recurrent genital HSV infection	Oral	Adult dose[h]	1 g/day in 2 divided doses for 3 days.
	Daily suppressive therapy for recurrent genital HSV infection	Oral	Adult dose[h]	1000 mg, once daily for 1 year, then reassess for recurrences.
	Recurrent herpes labialis	Oral	>12 y	4 g/day in 2 divided doses for 1 day.
	Herpes zoster	Oral	Adult dose[h]	3 g/day in 3 divided doses for 7 days.
Valganciclovir (Valcyte)	Acquired CMV retinitis in immunocompromised host	Oral	Adult dose[h]	Treatment: 900 mg twice daily for 3 weeks Long-term suppression: 900 mg once daily.

Table 4.8. Antiviral Drugs, continued

Generic (Trade Name)	Indication	Route	Age	Usually Recommended Dosage
Valganciclovir (Valcyte), continued	Prevention of CMV disease in kidney or heart transplant patients	Oral	4 mo–16 y	Dose once a day within 10 days of transplantation until 100 days post-transplantation according to dosage algorithm based on body surface area and creatinine clearance. Dose (mg) = 7 × body surface area × creatinine clearance (see drug package insert).
Zanamivir (Relenza)	Influenza A and B: treatment (see Influenza, p 439)	Inhalation	≥7 y (treatment)	10 mg, twice daily for 5 days.
	Influenza A and B: prophylaxis	Inhalation	≥5 y (prophylaxis)	10 mg, once daily for as long as 28 days (community outbreaks) or 10 days (household setting).

IV indicates intravenous; FDA, US Food and Drug Administration; VZV, varicella-zoster virus; SC, subcutaneous; IM, intramuscular; HCV, hepatitis C virus; HIV, human immunodeficiency virus.

a Drugs for human immunodeficiency virus infection are not included. See **http://aidsinfo.nih.gov** for current information on HIV drugs and treatment recommendations.

b Dose should be decreased in patients with impaired renal function.

c Oral dosage of acyclovir in children should not exceed 80 mg/kg per day (3200 mg/day).

d Acyclovir doses listed in this table are based on clinical trials and clinical experience and may not be identical to doses approved by the US Food and Drug Administration.

e Monitor for nephrotoxicity and neurologic irritation. Consider involving an infectious diseases or pharmacology specialist if weight-based dosing exceeds 800 mg per dose or if being administered with other nephrotoxic medications.

f Selective indications; see Varicella-Zoster Infections (p 774).

g Since 2005–2006, most influenza A (H3N2) strains and 2009 pandemic H1N1 strains tested have been resistant to adamantanes. See Influenza (p 439) for specific recommendations.

h There are not sufficient clinical data to identify the appropriate dose for use in children.

i Some experts use ganciclovir in immunocompromised hosts with CMV gastrointestinal tract disease and CMV pneumonitis (with or without CMV Immune Globulin Intravenous).

j See Influenza (p 439) and **www.cdc.gov/flu/professionals/antivirals/index.htm** for specific recommendations, which may vary on the basis of most recent influenza virus susceptibility patterns.

For more information on individual drugs, see *Physician's Desk Reference* or **www.pdr.net** (for registered users only).

DRUGS FOR PARASITIC INFECTIONS

The following tables (4.9, 4.10, 4.11, and 4.12) are reproduced from *The Medical Letter*.[1] These tables provide recommendations that are likely to be consistent in many cases with those of the American Academy of Pediatrics (AAP), as provided in the disease-specific chapters in Section 3. However, because *The Medical Letter* recommendations are developed independently, these recommendations occasionally may differ from recommendations of the AAP. Accordingly, both should be consulted. The AAP appreciates the consideration of *The Medical Letter* in allowing this information to be reprinted.

In Table 4.9 (p 849), first-choice and alternative drugs with recommended adult and pediatric dosages for most parasitic infections are provided. In each case, the need for treatment must be weighed against the toxic effects of the drug. A decision to withhold therapy often may be correct, particularly when the drugs are associated with severe adverse events. When the first-choice drug initially is ineffective and the alternative is more hazardous, a second course of treatment with the first drug before giving the alternative may be prudent.

Several drugs recommended in Table 4.9 (p 849) have not been approved by the US Food and Drug Administration and, thus, are investigational (see footnotes). When prescribing an unlicensed drug, the physician should inform the patient or parents of the investigational status and adverse effects of the drug. In the absence of approved package insert labeling for specific use, treatment with commercially available drugs for specific infections is considered off-label use.

These recommendations periodically (usually every other year) are updated by *The Medical Letter* (**www.medicalletter.com**) and, thus, likely are to be superseded by new ones before the next edition of the *Red Book* is published.

---

[1] Reprinted with permission from Drugs for Parasitic Infections. *Treatment Guidelines from the Medical Letter.* 2010; 2nd ed.

Table 4.9. Drugs for Parasitic Infections

With increasing travel, immigration, use of immunosuppressive drugs and the spread of AIDS, physicians anywhere may see infections caused by parasites. The table below lists first-choice and alternative drugs for most parasitic infections. Table 4.10 (p 862) summarizes the principal adverse effects of antiparasitic drugs, and Table 4.11 (p 866) summarizes the known prenatal risks of antiparasitic drugs. The brand names and manufacturers of the drugs are listed in Table 4.12, p 868.

Infection		Drug	Adult dosage	Pediatric dosage
ACANTHAMOEBA keratitis				
Drug of choice:		See footnote 1		
AMEBIASIS *(Entamoeba histolytica)*				
asymptomatic				
Drug of choice:		Iodoquinol[2]	650 mg PO tid x 20d	30-40 mg/kg/d (max. 2g) PO in 3 doses x 20d
	OR	Paromomycin[3]	25-35 mg/kg/d PO in 3 doses x 7d	25-35 mg/kg/d PO in 3 doses x 7d
	OR	Diloxanide furoate[4]*	500 mg PO tid x 10d	20 mg/kg/d PO in 3 doses x 10d
mild to moderate intestinal disease				
Drug of choice:[5]		Metronidazole	500-750 mg PO tid x 7-10d	35-50 mg/kg/d PO in 3 doses x 7-10d
	OR	Tinidazole[6]	2 g once PO daily x 3d	≥3yrs: 50 mg/kg/d (max. 2g) PO in 1 dose x 3d
		either followed by		
		Iodoquinol[2]	650 mg PO tid x 20d	30-40 mg/kg/d (max. 2g) PO in 3 doses x 20d
	OR	Paromomycin[3]*	25-35 mg/kg/d PO in 3 doses x 7d	25-35 mg/kg/d PO in 3 doses x 7d
severe intestinal and extraintestinal disease				
Drug of choice:		Metronidazole	750 mg PO tid x 7-10d	35-50 mg/kg/d PO in 3 doses x 7-10d
	OR	Tinidazole[6]	2 g once PO daily x 5d	≥3yrs: 50 mg/kg/d (max. 2g) PO in 1 dose x 5d
		either followed by		
		Iodoquinol[2]	650 mg PO tid x 20d	30-40 mg/kg/d (max. 2g) PO in 3 doses x 20d
	OR	Paromomycin[3]*	25-35 mg/kg/d PO in 3 doses x 7d	25-35 mg/kg/d PO in 3 doses x 7d
AMEBIC MENINGOENCEPHALITIS, primary and granulomatous				
Naegleria fowleri				
Drug of choice:		Amphotericin B[7,8]	1.5 mg/kg/d IV in 2 doses x 3d, then 1 mg/kg/d x 6d plus 1.5 mg/d intrathecally x 2d, then 1 mg/d every other day x 8d	1.5 mg/kg/d IV in 2 doses x 3d, then 1 mg/kg/d x 6d plus 1.5 mg/d intrathecally x 2d, then 1 mg/d every other day x 8d
***Acanthamoeba* spp.**				
Drug of choice:		See footnote 9		

* Availability problems.
1. Keratitis is typically associated with contact lens use (FR Carvalho et al, Cornea 2009; 28:516). Topical 0.02% chlorhexidine and polyhexamethylene biguanide (PHMB, 0.02%), either alone or in combination, have been used successfully in a large number of patients. Treatment with either chlorhexidine or PHMB is often combined with propamidine isethionate *(Brolene)* or hexamidine *(Desmodine)*. None of these drugs is commercially available or approved for use in the US, but they can be obtained from compounding pharmacies (see footnote 4). Leiter's Park Avenue Pharmacy, San Jose, CA (800-292-6773; www.leiterrx.com) is a compounding pharmacy that specializes in ophthalmic drugs. Propamidine is available over the counter in the UK and Australia. Hexamidine is available in France. The combination of chlorhexidine, natamycin (pimaricin) and debridement also has been successful (K Kitagawa et al, Jpn J Ophthalmol 2003; 47:616), as has 0.1% sodium diclofenac (AL Agahan et al, Ann Acad Med Singapore 2009; 38: 175) in a small series of 3 patients. Debridement is most useful during the stage of corneal epithelial infection; keratoplasty in medically unresponsive keratitis was successful in 31 patients (AS Kitzmann et al, Ophthalmology 2009; 116: 864). Most cysts are resistant to neomycin; its use is no longer recommended. Azole antifungal drugs (ketoconazole, itraconazole) have been used as oral or topical adjuncts. Use of corticosteroids is controversial. Prolonged therapy (≥6 months) may be necessary (JK Dart et al, Am J Ophthalmol 2009; 148:487).
2. Iodoquinol should be taken after meals.
3. Paromomycin should be taken with a meal.
4. Not available commercially. It may be obtained through compounding pharmacies such as Expert Compounding Pharmacy, 6744 Balboa Blvd, Lake Balboa, CA 91406 (800-247-9767) or Medical Center Pharmacy, New Haven, CT (203-688-7064). Other compounding pharmacies may be found through the National Association of Compounding Pharmacies (800-687-7850) or the Professional Compounding Centers of America (800-331-2498, www.pccarx.com).
5. Nitazoxanide may be effective against a variety of protozoan and helminth infections (DA Bobak, Curr Infect Dis Rep 2006; 8:91; E Diaz et al, Am J Trop Med Hyg 2003; 68:384). It is effective against mild to moderate amebiasis, 500 mg bid x 3d (JF Rossignol et al, Trans R Soc Trop Med Hyg 2007; 101:1025; AE Escobedo et al, Arch Dis Child 2009; 94:478). It is FDA-approved only for treatment of diarrhea caused by *Giardia* or *Cryptosporidium* (Med Lett Drugs Ther 2003; 45:29). Nitazoxanide is available in 500-mg tablets and an oral suspension; it should be taken with food.
6. A nitroimidazole similar to metronidazole, tinidazole appears to be as effective as metronidazole and better tolerated (Med Lett Drugs Ther 2004; 46:70). It should be taken with food to minimize GI adverse effects. For children and patients unable to take tablets, a pharmacist can crush the tablets and mix them with cherry syrup (Humco, and others). The syrup suspension is good for 7 days at room temperature and must be shaken before use (HB Fung and TL Doan, Clin Ther 2005; 27:1859). Ornidazole, a similar drug, is also used outside the US.
7. Not FDA-approved for this indication.

Table 4.9. Drugs for Parasitic Infections, continued

Infection	Drug	Adult dosage	Pediatric dosage
AMEBIC MENINGOENCEPHALITIS (continued)			
Balamuthia mandrillaris			
Drug of choice:	See footnote 10		
Sappinia diploidea			
Drug of choice:	See footnote 11		
ANCYLOSTOMA caninum (Eosinophilic enterocolitis)			
Drug of choice:	Albendazole[7,12]	400 mg PO once	400 mg PO once
OR	Mebendazole	100 mg PO bid x 3d	100 mg PO bid x 3d
OR	Endoscopic removal		
Ancylostoma duodenale, see HOOKWORM			
ANGIOSTRONGYLIASIS *(Angiostrongylus cantonensis, Angiostrongylus costaricensis)*			
Drug of choice:	See footnote 13		
ANISAKIASIS (*Anisakis* spp.)			
Treatment of choice:[14]	Surgical or endoscopic removal		
ASCARIASIS (*Ascaris lumbricoides,* roundworm)			
Drug of choice:[5]	Albendazole[7,12]	400 mg PO once	400 mg PO once
OR	Mebendazole	100 mg bid PO x 3d or 500 mg once	100 mg PO bid x 3d or 500 mg once
OR	Ivermectin[7,15]	150-200 mcg/kg PO once	150-200 mcg/kg PO once
BABESIOSIS			
Drug of choice:[16]	Atovaquone[7,17]	750 mg PO bid x 7-10d	40 mg/kg/d PO in 2 doses x 7-10d
	plus azithromycin[7]	500-1000 mg PO on d1, then 250-1000 mg PO on d2-10	10 mg/kg (max 500 mg/dose) PO on d 1, then 5 mg/kg/d (max 250 mg dose) PO on d 2-10
OR	Clindamycin[7,18]	300-600 mg IV qid or 600 mg PO tid x 7-10d	20-40 mg/kg/d PO in 3 doses x 7-10d
	plus quinine[7,19]	650 mg PO tid x 7-10d	30 mg/kg/d PO in 3 doses x 7-10d
Balamuthia mandrillaris, see AMEBIC MENINGOENCEPHALITIS, PRIMARY			
BALANTIDIASIS *(Balantidium coli)*			
Drug of choice:	Tetracycline[7,20]	500 mg PO qid x 10d	40 mg/kg/d (max. 2 g) PO in 4 doses x 10d
Alternative:	Metronidazole[7]	500-750 mg PO tid x 5d	35-50 mg/kg/d PO in 3 doses x 5d
OR	Iodoquinol[2,7]	650 mg PO tid x 20d	30-40 mg/kg/d (max 2 g) PO in 3 doses x 20d

* Availability problems.

8. A *Naegleria fowleri* infection was treated successfully in a 9-year old girl with combination of amphotericin B and miconazole (both drugs given intravenously and intrathecally) plus oral rifampin (JS Seidel et al NEJM 1982; 306:346). While amphotericin B and miconazole appear to have a synergistic effect, Medical Letter consultants believe the rifampin probably had no additional effect (GS Visvesvara et al, FEMS Immunol Med Microbiol 2007; 50:1). Parenteral miconazole is no longer available in the US. Azithromycin (changed to clarithromycin during therapy because of toxicity concerns and for better CNS penetration) has been used in multidrug combination regimens to treat *Balamuthia* infection. *In vitro,* azithromycin is more active than clarithromycin against *Naegleria,* so may be a better choice combined with amphotericin B for treatment of *Naegleria* (TR Deetz et al, Clin Infect Dis 2003; 37:1304; FL Schuster and GS Visvesvara, Drug Resistance Updates 2004; 7:41). Combinations of amphotericin B, ornidazole and rifampin (R Jain et al, Neurol India 2002; 50:470), amphotericin B, fluconazole (IV and PO) and rifampin (J Vargas-Zepeda et al, Arch Med Research 2005;36:83) and amphotericin B, chloramphicol and rifampacin have also been used (R Rai et al, Indian Pediatr 2008; 45:1004). Case reports of other successful therapy have been described (FL Schuster and GS Visvesvara, Int J Parasitol 2004; 34:1001).

9. Several patients with granulomatous amebic encephalitis (GAE) have been successfully treated with combinations of pentamidine, sulfadiazine, flucytosine, and either fluconazole or itraconazole (GS Visvesvara et al, FEMS Immunol Med Microbiol 2007; 50:1). GAE in an AIDS patient was treated successfully with sulfadiazine, pyrimethamine and fluconazole combined with surgical resection of the CNS lesion (M Seijo Martinez et al, J Clin Microbiol 2000; 38:3892). Chronic *Acanthamoeba* meningitis was successfully treated in 2 children with a combination of oral trimethoprim/sulfamethoxazole, rifampin and ketoconazole (T Singhal et al, Pediatr Infect Dis J 2001; 20:623). Disseminated cutaneous infection in an immunocompromised patient was treated successfully (FL Schuster and GS Visvesvara, Drug Resistance Updates 2004; 7:41; AC Aichelburg et al, Emerg Infect Dis 2008; 14:1743). Susceptibility testing of *Acanthamoeba* isolates has shown differences in drug sensitivity between species and even among strains of a single species; antimicrobial susceptibility testing is advisable (FL Schuster and GS Visvesvara, Int J Parasitol 2004; 34:1001).

9a. *B. mandrillaris* is a free-living ameba that causes subacute to fatal granulomatous amebic encephalitis (GAE) and cutaneous disease (MMWR 2008; 57:768; FL Schuster et al, Clin Infect Dis 2009; 48:879). These cases of *Balamuthia* encephalitis have been successfully treated with pentamidine, flucytosine, fluconazole and sulfadiazine plus either azithromycin or clarithromycin combined with surgical resection of the CNS lesion; in two cases flucytosine was given as well. Clarithromycin may have less toxicity and better penetration into CSF than azithromycin (TR Deetz et al, Clin Infect Dis 2003; 37:1304; S Jung et al, Arch Pathol Lab Med 2004; 128:466).

11. A free-living ameba that may rarely be pathogenic to humans (GS Visvesvara et al, FEMS Immunol Med Microbiol 2007; 50:1; F Marciano-Cabral, J Infect Dis 2009; 199: 1104). *S. diploidea* has been successfully treated with azithromycin, pentamidine, itraconazole and flucytosine combined with surgical resection of the CNS lesion (BB Gelman et al, J Neuropathol Exp Neurol 2003; 62:990).

12. Albendazole must be taken with food; a fatty meal increases oral bioavailability.

13. *A. cantonensis* causes predominantly neurotropic disease (QP Wang et al, Lancet Infect Dis 2008; 8:621). *A. costaricensis* causes gastrointestinal disease. Most patients infected with either species have a self-limited course and recover completely. Analgesics, corticosteroids and periodic removal of CSF can relieve symptoms from increased intracranial pressure (L Ramirez-Avila et al, Clin Infect Dis 2009; 48:322). Treatment of *A. cantonensis* is controversial and varies across endemic areas. No antihelminthic drug is proven to be effective and some patients have worsened with therapy. Mebendazole or albendazole used alone or with-out a corticosteroid appear to shorten the course of infection (K Sawanyawisuth and K Sawanyawisuth, Trans R Soc Trop Med Hyg 2008; 102:990; V Chotmongkol et al, Am J Trop Med Hyg 2009; 81:443).

14. Gastric anisakiasis can usually be diagnosed and treated by endoscopic removal of the worm. Enteric anisakiasis is more difficult to diagnose; it can be managed without worm removal as the worms eventually die. Surgery may be needed in the event of intestinal obstruction or peritonitis (A Repiso Ortega et al, Gastroenterol Hepatol 2003; 26:341; K Nakaji, Intern Med 2009; 48:573). Successful treatment of anisakiasis with albendazole 400 mg PO bid x 3-5d has been reported, but diagnosis was presumptive (DA Moore et al, Lancet 2002; 360:54; E Pacios et al, Clin Infect Dis 2005; 41:1825).

15. Safety of ivermectin in young children (<15 kg) and pregnant women remains to be established. Ivermectin should be taken on an empty stomach with water (NM Fox, Curr Opin Infect Dis 2006; 19:588).

16. E Vannier et al, Infect Dis Clin North Am 2008; 22:469; GP Wormser et al, Clin Infect Dis 2006; 43:1089. *B. microti* is most common in the US. Most disease in Europe is attributed to *B. divergens* and is generally more severe. Several cases caused by various *B. divergens*-like agents have also been documented in the US (BL Herwaldt et al, Emerg Infect Dis 2004; 10:622). Exchange transfusion has been used in combination with drug treatment in severely ill patients and those with high (>10%) parasitemia. In non-immunosuppressed patients infected with *B. microti* who were not severely ill, combination therapy with atovaquone and azithromycin was as effective as clindamycin and quinine and better tolerated (PJ Krause et al, N Engl J Med 2000; 343:1454). Immunosuppressed patients and those with asplenia should be treated a minimum of 6 weeks and at least 2 weeks past the last positive smear. Resistance to azithromycin-atovaquone treatment has been reported in immunocompromised patients (GP Wormser et al, Clin Infect Dis 2010; 50:381). Some patients may be co-infected with the etiologic agents of Lyme disease and human granulocytic anaplasmosis.

17. Atovaquone is available in an oral suspension that should be taken with a meal to increase absorption.

18. Oral clindamycin should be taken with a full glass of water to minimize esophageal ulceration.

Table 4.9. Drugs for Parasitic Infections, continued

Infection	Drug	Adult dosage	Pediatric dosage
BAYLISASCARIASIS *(Baylisascaris procyonis)*			
Drug of choice:	See footnote 21		
BLASTOCYSTIS spp. infection			
Drug of choice:	See footnote 22		
CAPILLARIASIS *(Capillaria philippinensis)*			
Drug of choice:	Mebendazole[7]	200 mg PO bid x 20d	200 mg PO bid x 20d
Alternative:	Albendazole[7,12]	400 mg PO daily x 10d	400 mg PO daily x 10d
Chagas' disease, see TRYPANOSOMIASIS			
Clonorchis sinensis, see FLUKE infection			
CRYPTOSPORIDIOSIS *(Cryptosporidium)* **Non-HIV infected**			
Drug of choice:	Nitazoxanide[5]	500 mg PO bid x 3d	1-3yrs: 100 mg PO bid x 3d 4-11yrs: 200 mg PO bid x 3d >12yrs: 500 mg PO bid x 3d
HIV infected			
Drug of choice:	See footnote 23		
CUTANEOUS LARVA MIGRANS (creeping eruption, dog and cat hookworm)			
Drug of choice:[24]	Albendazole[7,12]	400 mg PO daily x 3d	400 mg PO daily x 3d
OR	Ivermectin[7,15]	200 mcg/kg PO daily x 1-2d	200 mcg/kg PO daily x 1-2d
CYCLOSPORIASIS *(Cyclospora cayetanensis)*			
Drug of choice:[25]	Trimethoprim/ sulfamethoxazole[7]	TMP 160 mg/SMX 800 mg (1 DS tab) PO bid x 7-10d	TMP 10 mg/kg/SMX 50 mg/kg/d PO in 2 doses x 7-10d
Alternative:	Ciprofloxacin[7]	500 mg PO bid x 7d	—
CYSTICERCOSIS, see TAPEWORM infection			
CYSTOISOSPORIASIS *(Cystoisospora belli,* formerly known as *Isospora)*			
Drug of choice:[26]	Trimethoprim- sulfamethoxazole[7]	TMP 160 mg/SMX 800 mg (1 DS tab) PO bid x 10d	TMP 10 mg/kg/d/SMX 50 mg/kg/d PO in 2 doses x 10d
DIENTAMOEBA fragilis infection[27]			
Drug of choice:[28]	Iodoquinol[2,7]	650 mg PO tid x 20d	30-40 mg/kg/d (max. 2g) PO in 3 doses x 20d
OR	Paromomycin[3,7*]	25-35 mg/kg/d PO in 3 doses x 7d	25-35 mg/kg/d PO in 3 doses x 7d
OR	Metronidazole[7]	500-750 mg PO tid x 10d	35-50 mg/kg/d PO in 3 doses x 10d
Diphyllobothrium latum, see TAPEWORM infection			
DRACUNCULUS medinensis (guinea worm) infection			
Drug of choice:	See footnote 29		
Echinococcus, see TAPEWORM infection			
Entamoeba histolytica, see AMEBIASIS			
ENTEROBIUS vermicularis (pinworm) infection			
Drug of choice:[30]	Albendazole[7,12]	400 mg PO once; repeat in 2wks	400 mg PO once; repeat in 2wks
OR	Mebendazole	100 mg PO once; repeat in 2wks	100 mg PO once; repeat in 2wks
OR	Pyrantel pamoate[31*]	11 mg/kg base PO once (max. 1 g); repeat in 2wks	11 mg/kg base PO once (max. 1 g); repeat in 2wks
Fasciola hepatica, see FLUKE infection			
FILARIASIS[32, 33]			
Wuchereria bancrofti, Brugia malayi, Brugia timori			
Drug of choice:[34]	Diethylcarbamazine*	6 mg/kg/d PO in 3 doses x 12d[35,36]	6 mg/kg/d PO in 3 doses x 12d[35,36]
Loa loa			
Drug of choice:[37]	Diethylcarbamazine*	9 mg/kg/d PO in 3 doses x 12d[35,36]	9 mg/kg/d PO in 3 doses x 12d[35,36]

* Availability problems.

19. Quinine should be taken with or after a meal to decrease gastrointestinal adverse effects.
20. Use of tetracyclines is contraindicated in pregnancy and in children <8 years old. Tetracycline should be taken 1 hour before or 2 hours after meals and/or dairy products.
21. No drug has been demonstrated to be effective. Albendazole 25 mg/kg/d PO x 20d started as soon as possible (up to 3d after possible infection) might prevent clinical disease and is recommended for children with known exposure (ingestion of raccoon stool or contaminated soil) (WJ Murray and KR Kazacos, Clin Infect Dis 2004; 39:1484). Mebendazole, levamisole or ivermectin could be tried if albendazole is not available. Steroid therapy may be helpful, especially in eye and CNS infections (PJ Gavin et al, Clin Microbiol Rev 2005; 18:703). Ocular baylisascariasis has been treated successfully using laser photocoagulation therapy to destroy the intraretinal larvae (CA Garcia et al, Eye (Lond) 2004; 18:624).
22. Blastocystis has been reclassified as a fungus. Clinical significance of these organisms is controversial; metronidazole 750 mg PO tid x 10d, iodoquinol 650 mg PO tid x 20d or trimethoprim/sulfamethoxazole 1 DS tab PO bid x 7d have been reported to be effective (KS Tan, Clin Microbiol Rev 2008; 21:639). Metronidazole resistance may be common in some areas (J Yakoob et al, Br J Biomed Sci 2004; 61:75). Nitazoxanide has been effective in clearing organisms and improving symptoms (E Diaz et al, Am J Trop Med Hyg 2003; 68:384; JF Rossignol, Clin Gastroenterol Hepatol 2005; 3:987).
23. No drug has proven efficacy against cryptosporidiosis in advanced AIDS (I Abubakar et al, Cochrane Database Syst Rev 2007; 1:CD004932). Potent antiretroviral therapy (ART) is the mainstay of treatment. Nitazoxanide, paromomycin, or a combination of paromomycin and azithromycin may be tried to decrease diarrhea and recalcitrant malabsorption of antimicrobial drugs, which can occur with chronic cryptosporidiosis (B Pantenburg et al, Expert Rev Anti Infect Ther 2009; 7:385).
24. J Heukelbach and H Feldmeier, Lancet Infect Dis 2008; 8:302.
25. CA Warren, Curr Infect Dis Rep 2009; 11:108. In one study of HIV-infected patients with *Cyclospora* infection, ciprofloxacin treatment led to resolution in 87% of patients compared to 100% with TMP/SMX (RI Verdier et al, Ann Intern Med 2000; 132:885). HIV-infected patients may need higher dosage and long-term maintenance. Nitazoxanide (see also footnote 5) has also been used in a few patients (SM Zimmer et al, Clin Infect Dis 2007; 44:466; E Diaz et al, Am J Trop Med Hyg 2003; 68:384)
26. *Isospora belli* has been renamed and included the *Cystoisospora* genus. Usually a self-limited illness in immunocompetent patients. Immunosuppressed patients may need higher doses and longer duration (TMP/SMX qid for up to 3 to 4 weeks (Morbid Mortal Wkly Rep 2009; 58 RR4:1). They may require secondary prophylaxis (TMP/SMX DS tiw). In sulfa-allergic patients, pyrimethamine 50-75 mg daily in divided doses (plus leucovorin 10-25 mg/d) has been effective.
27. DJ Stark et al, Trends Parasitol 2006; 22:92; O Vandenberg et al, Pediatr Infect Dis J 2007; 26:88.
28. In one study, single-dose ornidazole, a nitroimidazole similar to metronidazole that is available in Europe, was effective and better tolerated than 5 days of metronidazole (O Kurt, Clin Microbiol Infect 2008; 14:601).
29. No drug is curative against *Dracunculus*. A program for monitoring local sources of drinking water to eliminate transmission has dramatically decreased the number of cases worldwide. The treatment of choice is slow extraction of worm combined with wound care and pain management (Morbid Mortal Wkly Rep 2009; 58:1123).
30. Since family members are usually infected, treatment of the entire household is recommended; retreatment after 14-21d may be needed.
31. Pyrantel pamoate suspension can be mixed with milk or fruit juice.

Table 4.9. Drugs for Parasitic Infections, continued

Infection	Drug	Adult dosage	Pediatric dosage
FILARIASIS (continued)[32,33]			
Mansonella ozzardi			
Drug of choice:	See footnote 38		
Mansonella perstans			
Drug of choice[39]	Albendazole[7,12]	400 mg PO bid x 10d	400 mg PO bid x 10d
OR	Mebendazole[7]	100 mg PO bid x 30d	100 mg PO bid x 30d
Mansonella streptocerca			
Drug of choice:[40]	Diethylcarba-mazine*	6 mg/kg/d PO in 3 doses x 12d[36]	6 mg/kg/d PO in 3 doses x 12d[36]
OR	Ivermectin[7,15]	150 mcg/kg PO once	150 mcg/kg PO once
Tropical Pulmonary Eosinophilia (TPE)[41]			
Drug of choice:	Diethylcarba-mazine*	6 mg/kg/d in 3 doses x 12-21d[36]	6 mg/kg/d in 3 doses x 12-21d[36]
Onchocerca volvulus (River blindness)			
Drug of choice:	Ivermectin[15,42]	150 mcg/kg PO once, repeated every 6-12mos until asymptomatic	150 mcg/kg PO once, repeated every 6-12mos until asymptomatic
FLUKE, hermaphroditic, infection			
Clonorchis sinensis (Chinese liver fluke)[43]			
Drug of choice:	Praziquantel[44]	75 mg/kg/d PO in 3 doses x 2d	75 mg/kg/d PO in 3 doses x 2d
OR	Albendazole[7,12]	10 mg/kg/d PO x 7d	10 mg/kg/d PO x 7d
Fasciola hepatica (sheep liver fluke)[43]			
Drug of choice:[45]	Triclabendazole*	10 mg/kg PO once or twice	10 mg/kg PO once or twice
Alternative:	Bithionol*	30-50 mg/kg on alternate days x 10-15 doses	30-50 mg/kg on alternate days x 10-15 doses
OR	Nitazoxanide[5,7]	500 mg PO bid x 7d	1-3yrs: 100 mg PO bid x 7d 4-11yrs: 200 mg PO bid x 7d >12yrs: 500 mg PO bid x 7d
Fasciolopsis buski, Heterophyes heterophyes, Metagonimus yokogawai (intestinal flukes)			
Drug of choice:	Praziquantel[7,44]	75 mg/kg/d PO in 3 doses x 1d	75 mg/kg/d PO in 3 doses x 1d
Metorchis conjunctus (North American liver fluke)			
Drug of choice:	Praziquantel[7,44]	75 mg/kg/d PO in 3 doses x 1d	75 mg/kg/d PO in 3 doses x 1d
Nanophyetus salmincola			
Drug of choice:	Praziquantel[7,44]	60 mg/kg/d PO in 3 doses x 1d	60 mg/kg/d PO in 3 doses x 1d
Opisthorchis viverrini (Southeast Asian liver fluke)[43]			
Drug of choice:	Praziquantel[44]	75 mg/kg/d PO in 3 doses x 2d	75 mg/kg/d PO in 3 doses x 2d
Paragonimiasis (*P. westermani, P. miyazaki, P. skrjabini, P. hueitungensis, P. heterotrema, P. utcerobilaterus, P. Africanus, P. Mexicanus, P. Kellicotti,*) (lung fluke)			
Drug of choice:	Praziquantel[7,44]	75 mg/kg/d PO in 3 doses x 2d	75 mg/kg/d PO in 3 doses x 2d
Alternative:	Triclabendazole[46]*	10 mg/kg PO once or twice	10 mg/kg PO once or twice
	Bithionol*	30-50 mg/kg on alternate days x 10-15 doses	30-50 mg/kg on alternate days x 10-15 doses

* Availability problems.

32. Antihistamines or corticosteroids may be required to decrease allergic reactions to components of disintegrating microfilariae that result from treatment, especially in infection caused by *Loa loa*.

33. Endosymbiotic *Wolbachia* bacteria, which are present in most human filariae except *Loa loa*, are essential to filarial growth, development, embryogenesis and survival and represent an additional target for therapy. Doxycycline 100 or 200 mg/d PO x 6-8wks in lymphatic filariasis, onchocerciasis, and *Mansonella perstans* has resulted in substantial loss of *Wolbachia* and decrease in both micro- and macrofilariae (MJ Bockarie et al, Expert Rev Anti Infect Ther 2009; 7:595; A Hoerauf Curr Opin Infect Dis 2008; 21:673; YI Coulibaly et al, N Engl J Med 2009; 361:1448). Use of tetracyclines is contraindicated in pregnancy and in children <8 yrs old.

34. Most symptoms are caused by adult worm. A single-dose combination of albendazole (400 mg PO) with either ivermectin (200 mcg/kg PO) or diethylcarbamazine (6 mg/kg PO) is effective for reduction or suppression of *W. bancrofti* microfilaria; none of these drug combinations kills all the adult worms (D Addiss et al, Cochrane Database Syst Rev 2004; CD003753).

35. For patients with microfilaria in the blood, Medical Letter consultants start with a lower dosage and scale up: d1: 50 mg; d2: 50 mg tid; d3: 100 mg tid; d4-14: 6 mg/kg/d in 3 doses (for *Loa Loa* d4-14: 9 mg/kg/d in 3 doses). Multi-dose regimens have been shown to provide more rapid reduction in microfilaria than single-dose diethylcarbamazine, but microfilaria levels are similar 6-12 months after treatment (LD Andrade et al, Trans R Soc Trop Med Hyg 1995; 89:319; PE Simonsen et al, Am J Trop Med Hyg 1995; 53:267). A single dose of 6 mg/kg is used in endemic areas for mass treatment, but there are no studies directly comparing the efficacy of the single-dose regimen to a 12-day course. It should be used cautiously in geographic regions where *O. volvulus* coexists with other filariae. One review concluded that the 12-day regimen did not have a higher macrofilaricidal effect than single dose (A Hoerauf, Curr Opin Infect Dis 2008; 21: 673; J Figueredo-Silva et al, Trans R Soc Trop Med Hyg 1996; 90:192; J Noroes et al, Trans R Soc Trop Med Hyg 1997; 91:78).

36. Diethylcarbamazine should not be used for treatment of *Onchocerca volvulus* due to the risk of increased ocular side effects (including blindness) associated with rapid killing of the worms. It should be used cautiously in geographic regions where *O. volvulus* coexists with other filariae. Diethylcarbamazine is contraindicated during pregnancy. See also footnote 42.

37. In heavy infections with *Loa loa*, rapid killing of microfilariae can provoke encephalopathy. Apheresis has been reported to be effective in lowering microfilarial counts in patients heavily infected with *Loa loa* (EA Ottesen, Infect Dis Clin North Am 1993; 7:619). Albendazole may be useful for treatment of loiasis when diethylcarbamazine is ineffective or cannot be used, but repeated courses may be necessary (AD Klion et al, Clin Infect Dis 1999; 29:680; TE Tabi et al, Am J Trop Med Hyg 2004; 71:211). Ivermectin has also been used to reduce microfilaremia, but albendazole is preferred because of its slower onset of action and lower risk of precipitating encephalopathy (AD Klion et al, J Infect Dis 1993; 168:202; M Kombila et al, Am J Trop Med Hyg 1998; 58:458). Diethylcarbamazine, 300 mg PO once/wk, has been recommended for prevention of loiasis (TB Nutman et al, N Engl J Med 1988; 319:752).

38. Diethylcarbamazine has no effect. A single dose of ivermectin 200 mcg/kg PO reduces microfilaria densities and provides both short- and long-term reductions in *M. ozzardi* microfilaremia (AA Gonzalez et al, W Indian Med J 1999; 48:231).

39. One small study compared single-dose ivermectin to albendazole alone or the two together although the combination reduced microfilaremia 1 and 3 months post treatment, the effect was not significant at 6 and 12 months (SM Asio et al, Ann Trop Med Parasitol 2009; 103:31).

40. Diethylcarbamazine is potentially curative due to activity against both adult worms and microfilariae. Ivermectin is active only against microfilariae.

41. VK Vijayan, Curr Opin Pulm Med 2007; 13:428. Relapses occur and can be treated with a repeated course of diethylcarbamazine.

42. Diethylcarbamazine should not be used for treatment of this disease because rapid killing of the worms can lead to blindness. Periodic treatment with ivermectin (every 3-12 months), 150 mcg/kg PO, can prevent blindness due to ocular onchocerciasis (DN Udall, Clin Infect Dis 2007; 44:53). Skin reactions after ivermectin treatment are often reported in persons with high microfilarial skin densities. Ivermectin has been inadvertently given to pregnant women during mass treatment pro-

Table 4.9. Drugs for Parasitic Infections, continued

Infection		Drug	Adult dosage	Pediatric dosage
GIARDIASIS *(Giardia duodenalis)*				
Drug of choice:		Metronidazole[7]	250 mg PO tid x 5-7d	15 mg/kg/d PO in 3 doses x 5-7d
	OR	Tinidazole[6]	2 g PO once	≥3yrs: 50 mg/kg PO once (max. 2 g)
	OR	Nitazoxanide[5]	500 mg PO bid x 3d	1-3yrs: 100 mg PO bid x 3d
				4-11yrs: 200 mg PO bid x 3d
				>12yrs: 500 mg PO bid x 3d
Alternative:[47]		Paromomycin[3,7,48]*	25-35 mg/kg/d PO in 3 doses x 5-10d	25-35 mg/kg/d PO in 3 doses x 5-10d
	OR	Furazolidone*	100 mg PO qid x 7-10d	6 mg/kg/d PO in 4 doses x 7-10d
	OR	Quinacrine[4,49]*	100 mg PO tid x 5d	6 mg/kg/d PO in 3 doses x 5d (max 300 mg/d)
GNATHOSTOMIASIS *(Gnathostoma spinigerum)* [50]				
Treatment of choice:		Albendazole[7,12]	400 mg PO bid x 21d	400 mg PO bid x 21d
	OR	Ivermectin[7,15]	200 mcg/kg/d PO x 2d	200 mcg/kg/d PO x 2d
		either		
	±	Surgical removal		
GONGYLONEMIASIS *(Gongylonema sp.)* [51]				
Treatment of choice:		Surgical removal		
	OR	Albendazole[7,12]	400 mg/d PO x 3d	400 mg/d PO x 3d
HOOKWORM infection *(Ancylostoma duodenale, Necator americanus)*				
Drug of choice:		Albendazole[7,12]	400 mg PO once	400 mg PO once
	OR	Mebendazole	100 mg PO bid x 3d or 500 mg once	100 mg PO bid x 3d or 500 mg once
	OR	Pyrantel pamoate[7,31]*	11 mg/kg (max. 1g) PO daily x 3d	11 mg/kg (max. 1g) PO daily x 3d
Hydatid cyst, see TAPEWORM infection				
Hymenolepis nana, see TAPEWORM infection				
Isospora belli, see *Cystoisospora*				
LEISHMANIASIS				
Visceral[52,53]				
Drug of choice:		Liposomal amphotericin B[54]	3 mg/kg/d IV d 1-5, 14 and 21[55]	3 mg/kg/d IV d 1-5, 14 and 21[55]
	OR	Sodium stibo-gluconate*	20 mg Sb/kg/d IV or IM x 28d	20 mg Sb/kg/d IV or IM x 28d
	OR	Meglumine antimonate*	20 mg Sb/kg/d IV or IM x 28d	20 mg Sb/kg/d IV or IM x 28d
	OR	Miltefosine[56,57]*	2.5 mg/kg/d PO (max 150 mg/d) x 28d	2.5 mg/kg/d PO (max 150 mg/d) x 28d
Alternative:	OR	Amphotericin B[7]	1 mg/kg IV daily x 15-20d or every second day for up to 8 wks (total usually 15-20 mg/kg)	1 mg/kg IV daily x 15-20d or every second day for up to 8 wks (total usually 15-20 mg/kg)
	OR	Paromomycin[3,7,58]* sulfate	15 mg/kg/d IM x 21d	15 mg/kg/d IM x 21d

* Availability problems.

grams; the rates of congenital abnormalities were similar in treated and untreated women. Because of the high risk of blindness from onchocerciasis, the use of ivermectin after the first trimester is considered acceptable according to the WHO. Addition of 6-8 weeks of doxycycline to ivermectin is increasingly common. Doxycycline (100 mg/day PO for 6 weeks), followed by a single 150 mcg/kg PO dose of ivermectin, resulted in up to 19 months of amicrofilaridermia and 100% elimination of *Wolbachia* species (A Hoerauf et al, Lancet 2001; 357:1415).

43. LA Marcos, Curr Opin Infect Dis 2008; 21:523.

44. Praziquantel should be taken with liquids during a meal.

45. Unlike infections with other flukes, *Fasciola hepatica* infections may not respond to praziquantel. Triclabendazole *(Egaten* - Novartis) appears to be safe and effective, but data are limited (J Keiser et al, Expert Opin Investig Drugs 2005; 14:1513). It is available from Victoria Pharmacy, Zurich, Switzerland (www.pharmaworld.com; 011-4143-344-60-60) and should be given with food for better absorption. Nitazoxanide also appears to have efficacy in treating fascioliasis in adults and in children (L Favennec et al, Aliment Pharmacol Ther 2003; 17:265; JF Rossignol et al, Trans R Soc Trop Med Hyg 1998; 92:103; SM Kabil et al, Curr Ther Res 2000; 61:339).

46. J Keiser et al, Expert Opin Investig Drugs 2005; 14:1513. See footnote 45 for availability.

47. Additional option: albendazole (400 mg/d PO x 5d in adults and 10 mg/kg/d PO x 5d in children) (K Yereli et al, Clin Microbiol Infect 2004; 10:527; O Karabay et al, World J Gastroenterol 2004; 10:1215). Refractory disease: standard doses of metronidazole plus quinacrine x 3wks (TE Nash et al, Clin Infect Dis 2001; 33:22). In one study, nitazoxanide was used successfully in high doses (1.5 g PO bid x 30d) to treat a case of *Giardia* resistant to metronidazole and albendazole (P Abboud et al, Clin Infect Dis 2001; 32:1792).

48. Poorly absorbed; may be useful for treatment of giardiasis in pregnancy.

49. Quinacrine should be taken with liquids after a meal. It is not available in the US but can be compounded by Gallipot Pharmacy (www.gallipot.com; 800-423-6967).

50. All patients should be treated with medication whether surgery is attempted or not. JS Herman and PL Chiodini, Clin Microbiol Rev 2009; 22:484; L Ramirez-Avila et al, Clin Infect Dis 2009; 48:322.

51. S Pasuralertsakul et al, Am Trop Med Parasitol 2008; 102:455; G Molavi et al, J Helminth 2006; 80:425.

52. To maximize effectiveness and minimize toxicity, the choice of drug, dosage and duration of therapy should be individualized based on the region of disease acquisition, likely infecting species, and host factors such as immune status (BL Herwaldt, Lancet 1999; 354:1191). Some of the listed drugs and regimens are effective only against certain *Leishmania* species/strains and only in certain areas of the world (J Arevalo et al, J Infect Dis 2007; 195:1846). Medical Letter consultants recommend consultation with physicians experienced in management of this disease.

53. Visceral infection is most commonly due to the Old World species *L. donovani* (kala-azar) and *L. infantum* (referred to as *L. chagasi* in the New World).

54. Liposomal amphotericin B *(AmBisome)* is the only lipid formulation of amphotericin B FDA-approved for treatment of visceral leishmania, largely based on clinical trials in patients infected with *L. infantum* (A Meyerhoff, Clin Infect Dis 1999; 28:42). In one open-label study one 10 mg/kg dose of liposomal amphotericin B was as effective as 15 infusions of amphotericin B (1 mg/kg/d) on alternate days (S Sundar et al, N Engl J Med 2010; 362:504). It is the drug of choice for visceral leishmania in pregnancy. Two other amphotericin B lipid formulations, amphotericin B lipid complex *(Abelcet)* and amphotericin B cholesteryl sulfate *(Amphotec)* have been used, but are considered investigational for this condition and may not be as effective (C Bern et al, Clin Infect Dis 2006; 43:917).

55. The FDA-approved dosage regimen for immunocompromised patients (e.g., HIV infected) is 4 mg/kg/d IV on days 1-5, 10, 17, 24, 31 and 38. The relapse rate is high; maintenance therapy (secondary prevention) may be indicated, but there is no consensus as to dosage or duration.

56. Miltefosine *(Impavido)* is manufactured in 10- or 50-mg capsules by Paladin (Montreal, Canada) and is not available in the US. The drug is contraindicated in pregnancy; a negative pregnancy test before drug initiation and effective contraception during and for 2 months after treatment is recommended (HW Murray et al, Lancet 2005; 366:1561).

57. Miltefosine is effective for both antimony-sensitive and -resistant *L. donovani* (Indian).

Table 4.9. Drugs for Parasitic Infections, continued

Infection	Drug	Adult dosage	Pediatric dosage
LEISHMANIASIS (continued)			
Cutaneous[52,59]			
Drugs of choice:	Sodium stibogluconate*	20 mg Sb/kg/d IV or IM x 20d	20 mg Sb/kg/d IV or IM x 20d
OR	Meglumine antimonate*	20 mg Sb/kg/d IV or IM x 20d	20 mg Sb/kg/d IV or IM x 20d
OR	Miltefosine[56,60]*	2.5 mg/kg/d PO (max 150 mg/d) x 28d	2.5 mg/kg/d PO (max 150 mg/d) x 28d
Alternative:[61]	Paromomycin[3,7,58]*	Topically 2x/d x 10-20d	Topically 2x/d x 10-20d
OR	Pentamidine[7]	2-3 mg/kg IV or IM daily or every second day x 4-7 doses[62]	2-3 mg/kg IV or IM daily or every second day x 4-7 doses[62]
Mucosal[52,63]			
Drug of choice:	Sodium stibogluconate*	20 mg Sb/kg/d IV or IM x 28d	20 mg Sb/kg/d IV or IM x 28d
OR	Meglumine antimonate*	20 mg Sb/kg/d IV or IM x 28d	20 mg Sb/kg/d IV or IM x 28d
OR	Amphotericin B[7]	0.5-1 mg/kg IV daily or every second day for up to 8wks	0.5-1 mg/kg IV daily or every second day for up to 8wks
OR	Miltefosine[56,64]*	2.5 mg/kg/d PO (max 150 mg/d) x 28d	2.5 mg/kg/d PO (max 150 mg/d) x 28d
LICE infestation *(Pediculus humanus, P. capitis, Phthirus pubis)* [65]			
Drug of choice:	Pyrethrins with piperonyl butoxide[66]	Topically, 2 x at least 7d apart	Topically, 2 x at least 7d apart
OR	1% Permethrin[66]	Topically, 2 x at least 7d apart	Topically, 2 x at least 7d apart
OR	5% Benzyl alcohol lotion[67]	Topically, 2 x at least 7d apart	Topically, 2 x at least 7d apart
OR	0.5% Malathion[68]	Topically, 2 x at least 7d apart	Topically, 2 x at least 7d apart
Alternative:	Ivermectin[7,15,69]	200 or 400 mcg/kg PO	≥15kg: 200 or 400 mcg/kg PO
Loa loa, see FILARIASIS			
MALARIA, Treatment of *(Plasmodium falciparum,*[70] *P. vivax,*[71] *P. ovale, P. malariae*[72] and *P. knowlesi*[73])			
ORAL (Uncomplicated or mild infection)[74]			
P. falciparum or unidentified species[75] acquired in areas of chloroquine-resistant *P. falciparum*[70]			
Drug of choice:	Atovaquone/ proguanil[76]	4 adult tabs PO once/d or 2 adult tabs PO bid[77] x 3d	<5kg: not indicated 5-8kg: 2 peds tabs PO once/d x 3d 9-10kg: 3 peds tabs PO once/d x 3d 11-20kg: 1 adult tab PO once/d x 3d 21-30kg: 2 adult tabs PO once/d x 3d 31-40kg: 3 adult tabs PO once/d x 3d >40kg: 4 adult tabs PO once/d x 3d[77]
OR	Artemether/ lumefantrine[78,79]	6 doses over 3d (4 tabs/dose at 0, 8, 24, 36, 48 and 60 hours)	6 doses over 3d at same intervals as adults; 5-15kg: 1 tab/dose ≥15-25kg: 2 tabs/dose ≥25-35kg: 3 tabs/dose ≥35kg: 4 tabs/dose

* Availability problems.

58. Paromomycin IM has been effective against *Leishmania* in India; it has not yet been tested in South America or the Mediterranean and there are insufficient data to support its use in pregnancy (S Sundar et al, N Engl J Med 2007; 356:2571; S Sundar and J Chakravarty, Expert Opin Investig Drugs 2008; 17:787). One study in India used a 14-day course of paromomycin (S Sundar et al, Clin Infect Dis 2009; 49:914). Topical paromomycin should be used only in geographic regions where cutaneous leishmaniasis species have low potential for mucosal spread. A formulation of 15% paromomycin/12% methylbenzethonium chloride (*Leshcutan*) in soft white paraffin for topical use has been reported to be partially effective against cutaneous leishmaniasis due to *L. major* in Israel and *L. mexicana* and *L. (V.) braziliensis* in Guatemala, where mucosal spread is very rare (BA Arana et al, Am J Trop Med Hyg 2001; 65:466; DH Kim et al, PLoS Negl Trop Dis 2009; 3:e381). The methylbenzethonium is irritating to the skin; lesions may worsen before they improve.

59. Cutaneous infection is most commonly due to the Old World species *L. major* and *L. tropica* and the New World species *L. mexicana, L. (Vianna) braziliensis, L. (V.) panamensis* and others.

60. In a placebo-controlled trial in patients ≥12 years old, miltefosine was effective for treatment of cutaneous leishmaniasis due to *L.(V.) panamensis* in Colombia, but not *L.(V.) braziliensis* or *L. mexicana* in Guatemala (J Soto et al, Clin Infect Dis 2004; 38:1266). For forms of disease that require long periods of treatment, such as diffuse cutaneous leishmaniasis and post kala-azar dermal leishmaniasis, miltefosine might be a useful treatment (JJ Berman, Expert Opin Drug Metab Toxicol 2008; 4:1209).

61. Although azole drugs (fluconazole, ketoconazole, itraconazole) have been used to treat cutaneous disease, they are not reliably effective and have very limited if any efficacy against mucosal disease (JA Blum and CS Hatz, J Travel Med 2009; 16:123). For treatment of *L. major* cutaneous lesions, a study in Saudi Arabia found that oral fluconazole, 200 mg once/d x 6wks appeared to modestly accelerate the healing process (AA Alrajhi et al, N Engl J Med 2002; 346:891). Thermotherapy may be an option for some cases of cutaneous *L. tropica* infection (R Reithinger et al, Clin Infect Dis 2005; 40:1148). A device that generates focused and controlled heating of the skin is being marketed (*ThermoMed* – ThermoSurgery Technologies Inc., Phoenix, AZ, 602-264-7300; www.thermosurgery.com). In one small study after 12 months of followup localized thermal heat was as effective as 10 doses of sodium stibogluconate with less toxicity (NE Aronson et al, PLOS Negl Trop Dis 2010; 4:e628).

62. At this dosage pentamidine has been effective in Colombia predominantly against *L. (V.) panamensis* (J Soto-Mancipe et al, Clin Infect Dis 1993; 16:417; J Soto et al, Am J Trop Med Hyg 1994; 50:107). Activity against other species is not well established.

63. Mucosal infection (espundia) is most commonly due to New World species *L. (V.) braziliensis, L. (V.) panamensis,* or *L. (V.) guyanensis*.

64. Miltefosine has been effective for mucosal leishmania due to *L.(V.) braziliensis* in Bolivia (J Soto et al, Clin Infect Dis 2007; 44:350; J Soto et al, Am J Trop Med Hyg 2009; 81:387).

65. Pediculocides should not be used for infestations of the eyelashes. Such infestations are treated with petrolatum ointment applied 2-4x/d x 8-10d. Oral TMP/SMX has also been used (TL Meinking and D Taplin, Curr Probl Dermatol 1996; 24:157). For pubic lice, treat with 5% permethrin or ivermectin as for scabies (see page 10). TMP/SMX has also been effective when used together with permethrin for head lice (RB Hipolito et al, Pediatrics 2001; 107:E30).

66. Permethrin and pyrethrin are pediculocidal; retreatment in 7-10d is needed to eradicate the infestation. Some lice are resistant to pyrethrins and permethrin (TL Meinking et al, Arch Dermatol 2002; 138:220). Medical Letter consultants prefer pyrethrin products with a benzyl alcohol vehicle.

Table 4.9. Drugs for Parasitic Infections, continued

Infection		Drug	Adult dosage	Pediatric dosage
MALARIA, Treatment of (continued)				
ORAL (continued)				
P. falciparum (continued)				
	OR	Quinine sulfate **plus**	650 mg PO q8h x 3 **or** 7d[80]	30 mg/kg/d PO in 3 doses x 3 **or** 7d[80]
		doxycycline[7,20,81] **or plus**	100 mg PO bid x 7d	4 mg/kg/d PO in 2 doses x 7d
		tetracycline[7,20] **or plus**	250 mg PO qid x 7d	25 mg/kg/d PO in 4 doses x 7d
		clindamycin[7,18,82]	20 mg/kg/d PO in 3 doses x 7d[83]	20 mg/kg/d PO in 3 doses x 7d[83]
Alternative:		Mefloquine[84,85]	750 mg PO followed 12 hrs later by 500 mg	15 mg/kg PO followed 12 hrs later by 10 mg/kg
	OR	Artesunate[78]* **plus** see footnote 86	4 mg/kg/d PO x 3d	4 mg/kg/d PO x 3d
P. vivax acquired in areas of chloroquine-resistant *P. vivax*[71]				
Drug of choice:		Artemether/ lumefantrine[78,79]	6 doses over 3d (4 tabs/dose at 0, 8, 24, 36, 48 and 60 hours)	6 doses over 3d at same intervals as adults; 5-15kg: 1 tab/dose ≥15-25kg: 2 tabs/dose ≥25-35kg: 3 tabs/dose ≥35kg: 4 tabs/dose
	OR	Atovaquone/ proguanil[76]	4 adult tabs PO once/d or 2 adult tabs bid[77] x 3d	<5kg: not indicated 5-8kg: 2 peds tabs PO once/d x 3d 9-10kg: 3 peds tabs PO once/d x 3d 11-20kg: 1 adult tab PO once/d x 3d 21-30kg: 2 adult tabs PO once/d x 3d 31-40kg: 3 adult tabs PO once/d x 3d >40kg: 4 adult tabs PO once/d x 3d[77]
	OR	Quinine sulfate **plus**	650 mg PO q8h x 3-7d[80]	30 mg/kg/d PO in 3 doses x 3-7d[80]
		doxycycline[7,20,81]	100 mg PO bid x 7d	4 mg/kg/d PO in 2 doses x 7d
	ALL PLUS	primaquine phosphate[75,87]	30 mg base/d PO x 14d	0.5 mg/kg/d PO x 14d
Alternative:		Mefloquine[84]	750 mg PO followed 12 hrs later by 500 mg	15 mg/kg PO followed 12 hrs later by 10 mg/kg
		Chloroquine phosphate[88,89] **plus**	25 mg base/kg PO in 3 doses over 48 hrs	25 mg base/kg PO in 3 doses over 48 hrs
		doxycycline[7,20,81]	100 mg PO bid x 7d	4 mg/kg/d PO in 2 doses x 7d
	ALL PLUS	primaquine phosphate[75,87]	30 mg base/d PO x 14d	0.5 mg/kg/d PO x 14d
All *Plasmodium* species except chloroquine-resistant *P. falciparum*[70] and chloroquine-resistant *P. vivax*[71]				
Drug of choice:[75]		Chloroquine phosphate[88]	1 g (600 mg base) PO, then 500 mg (300 mg base) 6 hrs later, then 500mg (300 mg base) at 24 and 48 hrs	10 mg base/kg (max. 600 mg base) PO, then 5 mg base/kg 6 hrs later, then 5 mg base/kg at 24 and 48 hrs

* Availability problems.
67. FDA-approved to treat head lice in 2009, benzyl alcohol prevents lice from closing their respiratory spiracles and the lotion vehicle then obstructs their airway causing them to asphyxiate. It is not ovicidal. Two applications at least 7d apart are needed. Resistance, which is a problem with other drugs, is unlikely to develop (Med Lett Drugs Ther 2009; 51:57).
68. Malathion is both ovicidal and pediculocidal; 2 applications at least 7d apart are generally necessary to kill all lice and nits.
69. Ivermectin is pediculocidal, but not ovicidal; more than one dose is generally necessary to eradicate the infestation (KN Jones and JC English 3rd, Clin Infect Dis 2003; 36:1355). The number of doses and interval between doses has not been established. In one study for treatment of head lice, 2 doses of ivermectin (400 mcg/kg) 7 days apart was more effective than treatment with topical malathion (O Chosidow et al, N Engl J Med 2010; 362:896). In one study for treatment of body lice, 3 doses of ivermectin (12 mg each) administered at 7d intervals were effective (C Fouault et al, J Infect Dis 2006; 193:474).
70. Chloroquine-resistant *P. falciparum* occurs in all malarious areas except Central America (including Panama north and west of the Canal Zone), Mexico, Haiti, the Dominican Republic, Paraguay, northern Argentina, North and South Korea, Georgia, Armenia, most of rural China and some countries in the Middle East (chloroquine resistance has been reported in Yemen, Saudi Arabia and Iran). For treatment of multiple-drug-resistant *P. falciparum* in Southeast Asia, especially Thailand, where mefloquine resistance is frequent, atovaquone/proguanil, quinine plus either doxycycline or clindamycin, or artemether/lumefantrine may be used.
71. *P. vivax* with decreased susceptibility to chloroquine is a significant problem in Papua-New Guinea and Indonesia. There are also reports of resistance from Myanmar, Vietnam, Korea, India, the Solomon Islands, Vanuatu, Indonesia, Guyana, Brazil, Colombia and Peru (JK Baird, Clin Microbiol Rev 2009; 22:508).
72. Chloroquine-resistant *P. malariae* has been reported from Sumatra (JD Maguire et al, Lancet 2002; 360:58).
73. Human infection with the simian species, *P. knowlesi* has been reported in Malaysia where it was initially misdiagnosed as *P. malariae*. Additional cases have been reported from Thailand, Myanmar, Singapore, the Thai-Burma border, and the Philippines (J Cox-Singh et al, Clin Infect Dis 2008; 46:165; MMWR 2009; 58:229). Treatment with the usual antimalarials, such as chloroquine and atovaquone/proguanil appear to be effective.
74. Uncomplicated or mild malaria may be treated with oral drugs. Severe malaria (e.g. impaired consciousness, parasitemia >5%, shock, etc.) should be treated with parenteral drugs (KS Griffin et al, JAMA 2007; 297:2264).
75. Primaquine is given as part of primary treatment to prevent relapse after infection with *P. vivax* or *P. ovale*. Some experts also prescribe primaquine phosphate 30 mg base/d (0.6 mg base/kg/d for children) for 14d after departure from areas where these species are endemic (Presumptive Anti-Relapse Therapy [PART], "terminal prophylaxis"). Since this is not always effective as prophylaxis (E Schwartz et al, N Engl J Med 2003; 349:1510), others prefer to rely on surveillance to detect cases when they occur, particularly when exposure was limited or doubtful. See also footnote 87.
76. Atovaquone/proguanil is available as a fixed-dose combination tablet: adult tablets (*Malarone*; atovaquone 250 mg/proguanil 100 mg) and pediatric tablets (*Malarone Pediatric*; atovaquone 62.5 mg/proguanil 25 mg). To enhance absorption and reduce nausea and vomiting, it should be taken with food or a milky drink. Safety in pregnancy is unknown; in a few small studies; outcomes were normal in women treated with the combination in the 2nd and 3rd trimester (AK Boggild et al, Am J Trop Med Hyg 2007; 76:208). The drug should not be given to patients with severe renal impairment (creatinine clearance <30mL/min). There have been isolated case reports of resistance in *P. falciparum* in Africa, but Medical Letter consultants do not believe there is a high risk for acquisition of *Malarone*-resistant disease (E Schwartz et al, Clin Infect Dis 2003; 37:450; A Farnert et al, BMJ 2003; 326:628; S Kuhn et al, Am J Trop Med Hyg 2005; 72:407; CT Happi et al, Malaria Journal 2006; 5:82).

Table 4.9. Drugs for Parasitic Infections, continued

Infection	Drug	Adult dosage	Pediatric dosage
PARENTERAL (severe infection)[74]			
All *Plasmodium* species (Chloroquine-sensitive and resistant)			
Drug of choice:[75,90]	Quinidine gluconate[91]	10 mg/kg IV loading dose (max. 600 mg) in normal saline over 1-2 hrs, followed by continuous infusion of 0.02 mg/kg/min until PO therapy can be started	10 mg/kg IV loading dose (max. 600 mg) in normal saline over 1-2 hrs, followed by continuous infusion of 0.02 mg/kg/min until PO therapy can be started
OR	Quinine dihydro-chloride[91]*	20 mg/kg IV loading dose in 5% dextrose over 4 hrs, followed by 10 mg/kg over 2-4 hrs q8h (max. 1800 mg/d) until PO therapy can be started	20 mg/kg IV loading dose in 5% dextrose over 4 hrs, followed by 10 mg/kg over 2-4 hrs q8h (max. 1800 mg/d) until PO therapy can be started
OR	Artesunate[78]*	2.4 mg/kg/dose IV x 3d at 0, 12, 24, 48 and 72 hrs	2.4 mg/kg/dose IV x 3d at 0, 12, 24, 48 and 72 hrs
plus see footnote 86			
MALARIA, Prevention of[92]			
All *Plasmodium* species in chloroquine-resistant areas[70-73]			
Drug of choice:[75]	Atovaquone/ proguanil[76]	1 adult tab/d[93]	5-8kg: ½ peds tab/d[76,93] 9-10kg: ¾ peds tab/d[76,93] 11-20kg: 1 peds tab/d[76,93] 21-30kg: 2 peds tabs/d[76,93] 31-40kg: 3 peds tabs/d[76,93] >40kg: 1 adult tab/d[76,93]
OR	Doxycycline[20,81]	100 mg PO daily[94]	2 mg/kg/d PO, up to 100 mg/d[94]
OR	Mefloquine[85,95]	250 mg PO once/wk[96]	≤ 9kg: 5 mg/kg salt once/wk[96] 9-19kg: ¼ tab once/wk[96] >19-30kg: ½ tab once/wk[96] >31-45kg: ¾ tab once/wk[96] >45kg: 1 tab once/wk[96]
Alternative:[97]	Primaquine[7,87] phosphate	30 mg base PO daily[98]	0.5 mg/kg base PO daily[98]
All *Plasmodium* species in chloroquine-sensitive areas[70-73]			
Drug of choice:[75,99]	Chloroquine phosphate[88,100]	500 mg (300 mg base) PO once/wk[101]	5 mg/kg base PO once/wk, up to adult dose of 300 mg base[101]

*   Availability problems.

77. Although approved for once-daily dosing, Medical Letter consultants usually divide the dose in two to decrease nausea and vomiting.

78. The artemisinin-derivatives, artemether and artesunate, are both frequently used globally in combination regimens to treat malaria. Both are available in oral, parenteral and rectal formulations, but manufacturing standards are not consistent (HA Karunajeewa et al, JAMA 2007; 297:2381; EA Ashley and NJ White, Curr Opin Infect Dis 2005; 18:531). Oral artesunate is not available in the US; the IV formulation is available through the CDC Malaria branch (M-F, 8am-4:30pm ET, 770-488-7788, or after hours, 770-488-7100) under an IND for patients with severe disease who do not have timely access, cannot tolerate, or fail to respond to IV quinidine (Med Lett Drugs Ther 2008; 50:37). To avoid development of resistance, monotherapy should be avoided (PE Duffy and CH Sibley, Lancet 2005; 366:1908). Reduced susceptibility to artesunate characterized by slow parasitic clearance has been reported in Cambodia (WO Rogers et al, Malaria J 2009; 8:10; AM Dundorp et al, N Engl J Med 2009; 361:455). Based on the few studies available, artemisin have been relatively safe during pregnancy (I Adam et al, Am Trop Med Parisito 2009; 103; 205), but some experts will not prescribe them in the 1st trimester (RL Clark, Reprod Toxicol 2009; 28:285).

79. Artemether/lumefantrine is available as a fixed-dose combination tablet (*Coartem* in the US and in countries with endemic malaria, *Riamet* in Europe and countries without endemic malaria); each tablet contains artemether 20 mg and lumefantrine 120 mg. It is FDA-approved for treatment of uncomplicated malaria and should not be used for severe infection or for prophylaxis. It is contraindicated during the 1st trimester of pregnancy; safety during the 2nd and 3rd trimester is not known. The tablets should be taken with fatty food (tablets may be crushed and mixed with 1-2 tsp water, and taken with milk). Artemether/lumefantrine should not be used in patients with cardiac arrhythmias, bradycardia, severe cardiac disease or QT prolongation. Concomitant use of drugs that prolong the QT interval or are metabolized by CYP2D6 is contraindicated (Med Lett Drugs Ther 2009; 51:75).

80. Available in the US in a 324-mg capsule; 2 capsules suffice for adult dosage. In Southeast Asia, relative resistance to quinine has increased and treatment should be continued for 7d. Quinine should be taken with or after meals to decrease gastrointestinal adverse effects. It is generally considered safe in pregnancy.

81. Doxycycline should be taken with adequate water to avoid esophageal irritation. It can be taken with food to minimize gastrointestinal adverse effects.

82. For use in pregnancy and in children <8 yrs.

83. B Lell and PG Kremsner, Antimicrob Agents Chemother 2002; 46:2315; M Ramharter et al, Clin Infect Dis 2005; 40:1777.

84. At this dosage, adverse effects include nausea, vomiting, diarrhea and dizziness. Disturbed sense of balance, toxic psychosis and seizures can also occur. Mefloquine should not be used for treatment of malaria in pregnancy unless there is not another treatment option (F Nosten et al, Curr Drug Saf 2006; 1:1). It should be avoided for treatment of malaria in persons with active depression or with a history of psychosis or seizures and should be used with caution in persons with any psychiatric illness. Mefloquine should not be used in patients with conduction abnormalities; it can be given to patients taking β-blockers if they do not have an underlying arrhythmia. Mefloquine should not be given together with quinine or quinidine, and caution is required in using quinine or quinidine to treat patients with malaria who have taken mefloquine for prophylaxis. Mefloquine should not be taken on an empty stomach; it should be taken with at least 8 oz of water.

85. *P. falciparum* with resistance to mefloquine is a significant problem in the malarious areas of Thailand and in areas of Myanmar and Cambodia that border on Thailand. It has also been reported on the borders between Myanmar and China, Laos and Myanmar, and in Southern Vietnam. In the US, a 250-mg tablet of mefloquine contains 228 mg mefloquine base. Outside the US, each 275-mg tablet contains 250 mg base.

86. Adults treated with artesunate should also receive oral treatment doses of either atovaquone/proguanil, doxycycline, clindamycin or mefloquine; children should take either atovaquone/proguanil, clindamycin or mefloquine (F Nosten et al, Lancet 2000; 356:297; M van Vugt, Clin Infect Dis 2002; 35:1498; F Smithuis et al, Trans R Soc Trop Med Hyg 2004; 98:182). If artesunate is given IV, oral medication should be started when the patient is able to tolerate it (SEAQUAMAT group, Lancet 2005; 366:717).

87. Primaquine phosphate can cause hemolytic anemia, especially in patients whose red cells are deficient in G-6-PD. This deficiency is most common in African, Asian and Mediterranean peoples. Patients should be screened for G-6-PD deficiency before treatment. Primaquine should not be used during pregnancy. It should be taken with food to minimize nausea and abdominal pain. Primaquine-tolerant *P. vivax* can be found globally. Relapses of primaquine-resistant strains may be retreated with 30 mg (base) x 28d.

88. Chloroquine should be taken with food to decrease gastrointestinal adverse effects. If chloroquine phosphate is not available, hydroxychloroquine sulfate is as effective; 400 mg of hydroxychloroquine sulfate is equivalent to 500 mg of chloroquine phosphate.

89. Chloroquine combined with primaquine was effective in 85% of patients with *P. vivax* resistant to chloroquine and could be a reasonable choice in areas where other alternatives are not available (JK Baird et al, J Infect Dis 1995; 171:1678).

90. Exchange transfusion is controversial, but has been helpful for some patients with high-density (>10%) parasitemia, altered mental status, pulmonary edema or renal complications (PJ Van Genderen et al, Transfusion 2009; Nov 20 epub).

91. Continuous EKG, blood pressure and glucose monitoring are recommended. Quinine IV is not available in the US. Quinidine may have greater antimalarial activity than quinine. The loading dose should be decreased or omitted in patients who have received quinine or mefloquine. If more than 48 hours of parenteral treat-

Table 4.9. Drugs for Parasitic Infections, continued

Infection		Drug	Adult dosage	Pediatric dosage
MALARIA, Prevention of relapses: _P. vivax_ and _P. ovale_[75]				
Drug of choice:		Primaquine phosphate[87]	30 mg base/d PO x 14d	0.5 mg base/kg/d PO x 14d
MALARIA, Self-Presumptive Treatment[102]				
Drug of Choice:		Atovaquone/ proguanil[7,76]	4 adult tabs once/d or 2 adult tabs bid x 3d[77]	<5kg: not indicated 5-8kg: 2 peds tabs once/d x 3d 9-10kg: 3 peds tabs once/d x 3d 11-20kg: 1 adult tab once/d x 3d 21-30kg: 2 adult tabs once/d x 3d 31-40kg: 3 adult tabs once/d x 3d >40kg: 4 adult tabs once/d x 3d[77]
	OR	Artemether/ lumefantrine[7,78,79]	6 doses over 3d (4 tabs/dose at 0, 8, 24, 36, 48 and 60 hours)	6 doses over 3d at same intervals as adults; 5-15kg: 1 tab/dose 15-25kg: 2 tabs/dose 25-35kg: 3 tabs/dose >35kg: 4 tabs/dose
	OR	Quinine sulfate **plus**	650 mg PO q8h x 3 or 7d[70]	30 mg/kg/d PO in 3 doses x 3 or 7d[70]
		doxycycline[7,20,81]	100 mg PO bid x 7d	4 mg/kg/d PO in 2 doses x 7d
	OR	Artesunate[78]* **plus** see footnote 86	4 mg/kg/d PO x 3d	4 mg/kg/d PO x 3d
MICROSPORIDIOSIS				
Ocular _(Encephalitozoon hellem, E. cuniculi, Vittaforma [Nosema] corneae)_				
Drug of choice:		Fumagillin[103]* **plus**		
		albendazole[7,12]	400 mg PO bid	15 mg/kg/d in 2 doses (max 400 mg/dose)
Intestinal _(E. bieneusi, E. [Septata] intestinalis)_				
E. bieneusi				
Drug of choice:		Fumagillin[104]*	20 mg PO tid x 14d	
E. intestinalis				
Drug of choice:		Albendazole[7,12]	400 mg PO bid x 21d	15 mg/kg/d in 2 doses (max 400 mg/dose)
Disseminated _(E. hellem, E. cuniculi, E. intestinalis, Pleistophora sp., Trachipleistophora sp. and Anncaliia [Brachiola] vesicularum)_				
Drug of choice:[105]		Albendazole[7,12]	400 mg PO bid	15 mg/kg/d in 2 doses (max 400 mg/dose)
Mites, see SCABIES				
MONILIFORMIS _moniliformis_ infection				
Drug of choice:		Pyrantel pamoate[7,31]*	11 mg/kg PO once, repeat twice, 2wks apart	11 mg/kg PO once, repeat twice, 2wks apart

* Availability problems.

    ment is required, the quinine or quinidine dose should be reduced by 30-50%. Intraretcal quinine has been tried for the treatment of cerebral malaria in children (J Achan et al, Clin Infect Dis 2007; 45:1446).

92. No drug guarantees protection against malaria. Travelers should be advised to seek medical attention if fever develops after they return. Insect repellents, insecticide-impregnated bed nets and proper clothing are important adjuncts for malaria prophylaxis (Treat Guidel Med Lett 2009; 7:83). Malaria in pregnancy is particularly serious for both mother and fetus; prophylaxis is indicated if exposure cannot be avoided.

93. Beginning 1-2 d before travel and continuing for the duration of stay and for 1wk after leaving malarious zone. In one study of malaria prophylaxis, atovaquone/proguanil was better tolerated than mefloquine in nonimmune travelers (D Overbosch et al, Clin Infect Dis 2001; 33:1015). The protective efficacy of _Malarone_ against _P. vivax_ is variable ranging from 84% in Indonesian New Guinea (J Ling et al, Clin Infect Dis 2002; 35:825) to 100% in Colombia (J Soto et al, Am J Trop Med Hyg 2006; 75:430). Some Medical Letter consultants prefer alternate drugs if traveling to areas where _P. vivax_ predominates.

94. Beginning 1-2 d before travel and continuing for the duration of stay and for 4wks after leaving malarious zone. Doxycycline can cause gastrointestinal disturbances, vaginal moniliasis and photosensitivity reactions.

95. Mefloquine has not been approved for use during pregnancy. However, it has been reported to be safe for prophylactic use during the second and third trimester of pregnancy and possibly during early pregnancy as well (CDC Health Information for International Travel, 2010, page 141). Not recommended for use in travelers with active depression or with a history of psychosis or seizures and should be used with caution in persons with psychiatric illness. Mefloquine should not be used in patients with conduction abnormalities; it can be given to patients taking β-blockers if they do not have an underlying arrhythmia.

96. Beginning 1-2 wks before travel and continuing weekly for the duration of stay and for 4wks after leaving malarious zone. Most adverse events occur within 3 doses. Some Medical Letter consultants favor starting mefloquine 3 weeks prior to travel and monitoring the patient for adverse events, this allows time to change to an alternative regimen if mefloquine is not tolerated. Mefloquine should not be taken on an empty stomach; it should be taken with at least 8 oz of water. For pediatric doses <½ tablet, it is advisable to have a pharmacist crush the tablet, estimate doses by weighing, and package them in gelatin capsules. There is no data for use in children <5 kg, but based on dosages in other weight groups, a dose of 5 mg/kg can be used.

97. The combination of weekly chloroquine (300 mg base) and daily proguanil (200 mg) is recommended by the World Health Organization (www.WHO.int) for use in selected areas; this combination is no longer recommended by the CDC. Proguanil (_Paludrine_ – AstraZeneca, United Kingdom) is not available alone in the US but is widely available in Canada and Europe. Prophylaxis is recommended during exposure and for 4 weeks afterwards. Proguanil has been used in pregnancy without evidence of toxicity (PA Phillips-Howard and D Wood, Drug Saf 1996; 14:131).

98. Studies have shown that daily primaquine beginning 1d before departure and continued until 3-7 d after leaving the malarious area provides effective prophylaxis against chloroquine-resistant _P. falciparum_ (DR Hill et al, Am J Trop Med Hyg 2006; 75:402). Nausea and abdominal pain can be diminished by taking with food.

99. Alternatives for patients who are unable to take chloroquine include atovaquone/proguanil, mefloquine, doxycycline or primaquine dosed as for chloroquine-resistant areas.

100. Has been used extensively and safely for prophylaxis in pregnancy.

101. Beginning 1-2wks before travel and continuing weekly for the duration of stay and for 4 wks after leaving malarious zone.

102. Travelers can be given a supply of medication for presumptive self-treatment of febrile illness. The drug given for self-treatment should be different from that used for prophylaxis. This approach should be used only in very rare circumstances when a traveler would not be able to get medical care promptly.

103. CM Chan et al, Ophthalmology 2003; 110:1420. Ocular lesions due to _E. hellem_ in HIV-infected patients have responded to fumagillin eyedrops prepared from _Fumidil-B_ (bicyclohexyl ammonium fumagillin) used to control a microsporidial disease of honey bees (MJ Garvey et al, Ann Pharmacother 1995; 29:872), available from Leiter's Park Avenue Pharmacy (see footnote 1). For lesions due to _V. corneae_, topical therapy is generally not effective and keratoplasty may be required (RM Davis et al, Ophthalmology 1990; 97:953).

104. Oral fumagillin (_Flisint_ – Sanofi-Aventis, France) has been effective in treating _E. bieneusi_ in patients with HIV or solid organ transplants (J-M Molina et al, N Engl J Med 2002; 346:1963; F Lanternier et al, Transpl Infect Dis 2009; 11:83), but has been associated with thrombocytopenia and neutropenia. Potent anti

Table 4.9. Drugs for Parasitic Infections, continued

Infection	Drug	Adult dosage	Pediatric dosage
Naegleria species, see AMEBIC MENINGOENCEPHALITIS, PRIMARY			
Necator americanus, see HOOKWORM infection			
OESOPHAGOSTOMUM _bifurcum_			
Drug of choice:	See footnote 106		
Onchocerca volvulus, see FILARIASIS			
Opisthorchis viverrini, see FLUKE infection			
Paragonimus westermani, see FLUKE infection			
Pediculus capitis, humanus, Phthirus pubis, see LICE			
Pinworm, see ENTEROBIUS			
PNEUMOCYSTIS JIROVECII (formerly _carinii_) pneumonia (PCP)[107]			
Moderate to severe disease[108]			
Drug of choice:	Trimethoprim/ sulfamethoxazole	TMP 15-20 mg/kg/d SMX 75-100 mg/kg/d PO or IV in 3 or 4 doses (change to PO after clinical improvement) x 21d	TMP 15-20 mg/kg/d SMX 75-100 mg/kg/d PO or IV in 3 or 4 doses (change to PO after clinical improvement) x 21d
Alternative:	Pentamidine	3-4 mg/kg IV daily x 21d	3-4 mg/kg IV daily x 21d
OR	Primaquine[7,87]	30 mg base PO daily x 21d	0.3 mg/kg base PO (max. 30 mg) daily x 21d
	plus clindamycin[7,18]	600-900 mg IV tid or qid x 21d, or 300-450 mg PO tid or qid x 21d (change to PO after clinical improvement)	15-25 mg/kg IV tid or qid (max 600 mg/dose) x 21 d, or 10 mg/kg PO tid or qid (max 300-450 mg/dose)x 21d (change to PO after clinical improvement)
Mild to moderate disease			
Drug of Choice:	Trimethoprim/ sulfamethoxazole	2 DS tablets (160 mg/800 mg) PO tid x 21d	TMP 15-20 mg/kg/SMX 75-100 mg/kg/d PO in 3 or 4 doses x 21d
Alternative:	Dapsone[7] **plus**	100 mg PO daily x 21d	2 mg/kg/d (max. 100 mg) PO x 21d
	Trimethoprim[7]	15 mg/kg/d PO in 3 doses	15 mg/kg/d PO in 3 doses
OR	Primaquine[7,87]	30 mg base PO daily x 21d	0.3 mg/kg base PO daily (max. 30 mg) x 21d
	plus clindamycin[7,18]	300-450 mg PO tid or qid x 21 d	10 mg/kg PO tid or qid (max 300-450 mg/dose) x 21d
OR	Atovaquone[17]	750 mg PO bid x 21d	1-3 mos: 30 mg/kg/d PO x 21d 4-24 mos: 45 mg/kg/d PO x 21d >24 mos: 30 mg/kg/d PO x 21d
Primary and secondary prophylaxis[109]			
Drug of Choice:	Trimethoprim/ sulfamethox-azole	1 tab (SS or DS) daily or 1 DS tab PO 3d/wk	TMP 150 mg/SMX 750 mg/m^2/d PO in 2 doses 3d/wk
Alternative:	Dapsone[7]	50 mg PO bid or 100 mg PO daily	≥ 1 mos: 2 mg/kg/d (max. 100 mg) PO or 4 mg/kg (max. 200 mg) PO each wk
OR	Dapsone[7] **plus** pyrimeth-amine[110]	50 mg PO daily or 200 mg PO each wk 50 mg PO daily or 75 mg PO each wk	
OR	Atovaquone[7,17]	1500 mg/d PO in 1 or 2 doses	1-3mos: 30 mg/kg/d PO 4-24mos: 45 mg/kg/d PO >24mos: 30 mg/kg/d PO
OR	Pentamidine	300 mg aerosol inhaled monthly via _Respirgard II_ nebulizer	≥5yrs: 300 mg inhaled monthly via _Respirgard II_ nebulizer
River Blindness, see FILARIASIS			
Roundworm, see ASCARIASIS			
Sappinia diploidea, See AMEBIC MENINGOENCEPHALITIS, PRIMARY			
SARCOCYSTIS spp. (intestinal and muscular), see footnote 111			
SCABIES (_Sarcoptes scabiei_)[112]			
Drug of choice:	5% Permethrin	Topically, 2x at least 7 d apart	Topically, 2x at least 7 d apart
Alternative:[113]	Ivermectin[7,15]	200 mcg/kg PO 2x at least 7 d apart[114]	200 mcg/kg PO, 2x at least 7 d apart[114]
	10% Crotamiton	Topically overnight on days 1, 2, 3, 8	Topically overnight on days 1, 2, 3, 8

* Availability problems.
retroviral therapy (ART) may lead to microbiologic and clinical response in HIV-infected patients with microsporidial diarrhea. Octreotide _(Sandostatin)_ has provided symptomatic relief in some patients with large-volume diarrhea.

105. J-M Molina et al, J Infect Dis 1995; 171:245. There is no established treatment for _Pleistophora_. For disseminated disease due to _Trachipleistophora_ or _Anncaliia_, itraconazole 400 mg PO once/d plus albendazole may also be tried (CM Coyle et al, N Engl J Med 2004; 351:42).
106. Albendazole or pyrantel pamoate may be effective (JB Ziem et al, Ann Trop Med Parasitol 2004; 98:385).
107. Pneumocystis has been reclassified as a fungus.

Table 4.9. Drugs for Parasitic Infections, continued

Infection	Drug	Adult dosage	Pediatric dosage
SCHISTOSOMIASIS *(Bilharziasis)*			
S. haematobium			
Drug of choice:	Praziquantel[44,115]	40 mg/kg/d PO in 1 or 2 doses x 1d	40 mg/kg/d PO in 2 doses x 1d
***S. intercalatum*[116]**			
Drug of Choice:	Praziquantel[44,115]	40 mg/kg/d PO in 1 or 2 doses x 1d	40 mg/kg/d PO x 1d
S. japonicum			
Drug of choice:	Praziquantel[44,115]	60 mg/kg/d PO in 2 or 3 doses x 1d	60 mg/kg/d PO in 3 doses x 1d
S. mansoni			
Drug of choice:	Praziquantel[44,115]	40 mg/kg/d PO in 1 or 2 doses x 1d	40 mg/kg/d PO in 2 doses x 1d
Alternative:	Oxamniquine[117]*	15 mg/kg PO once[118]	20 mg/kg/d PO in 2 doses x 1d[118]
S. mekongi			
Drug of choice:	Praziquantel[44,115]	60 mg/kg/d PO in 2 or 3 doses x 1d	60 mg/kg/d PO in 3 doses x 1d
Sleeping sickness, see TRYPANOSOMIASIS			
STRONGYLOIDIASIS *(Strongyloides stercoralis)*			
Drug of choice:[119]	Ivermectin[15]	200 mcg/kg/d PO x 2d	200 mcg/kg/d PO x 2d
Alternative:	Albendazole[7,12]	400 mg PO bid x 7d	400 mg PO bid x 7d
TAPEWORM infection			
— Adult (intestinal stage)			
***Diphyllobothrium latum* (fish), *Taenia saginata* (beef), *Taenia solium* (pork), *Dipylidium caninum* (dog)**			
Drug of choice:	Praziquantel[7,44]	5-10 mg/kg PO once	5-10 mg/kg PO once
Alternative:	Niclosamide[120]*	2 g PO once	50 mg/kg PO once
***Hymenolepis nana* (dwarf tapeworm)**			
Drug of choice:	Praziquantel[7,44]	25 mg/kg PO once	25 mg/kg PO once
Alternative:[121]	Niclosamide[120]*	2 g PO daily x 7 d	11-34 kg: 1 g PO on d 1 then 500 mg/d PO x 6 days > 34 kg: 1.5 g PO on d 1 then 1 g/d PO x 6 days
— Larval (tissue stage)			
***Echinococcus granulosus* (hydatid cyst)**			
Drug of choice:[122]	Albendazole[12]	400 mg PO bid x 1-6mos	15 mg/kg/d (max. 800 mg) PO in 2 doses x 1-6mos
Echinococcus multilocularis			
Treatment of choice:	See footnote 123		
***Taenia solium* (Cysticercosis)**			
Treatment of choice:	See footnote 124		
Alternative:	Albendazole[12]	400 mg PO bid x 8-30d; can be repeated as necessary	15 mg/kg/d (max. 800 mg) PO in 2 doses x 8-30d; can be repeated as necessary
OR	Praziquantel[7,44]	100 mg/kg/d PO in 3 doses x 1 day then 50 mg/kg/d in 3 doses x 29 days	100 mg/kg/d PO in 3 doses x 1 day then 50 mg/kg/d in 3 doses x 29 days

* Availability problems.

108. In severe disease with room air $PO_2 \leq 70$ mmHg or Aa gradient ≥ 35 mmHg, prednisone or its IV equivalent should also be used. For adults: d 1-5: 40 mg PO bid; d 6-10: 40 mg PO daily; d 11-21: 20 mg PO daily. For children: d 1-5: 2 mg/kg/d PO in 2 doses; d 6-10: 1 mg/kg/d PO in 2 doses; d 11-21: 0.5 mg/kg/d PO daily (ML Ferrari et al, Morbid Mortal Wkly Rep 2009; 58(RR04):1; Morbid Mortal Wkly Rep 2009; 58(RR11):1).

109. Primary/secondary prophylaxis in patients with HIV can be discontinued after CD4 count increases to >200 x 10^6/L for >3mos.

110. Plus leucovorin 25 mg with each dose of pyrimethamine. Pyrimethamine should be taken with food to minimize gastrointestinal adverse effects.

111. Sarcocystis in humans is acquired by ingesting sporocysts in infected meat, infections characterized by nausea, abdominal pain and diarrhea. Muscular infections are usually mild or subclinical (R Fayer, Clin Microbiol Rev 2004; 17:894). Albendazole was reported to be efficacious (MK Arness et al, Am J Trop Med Hyg 1999; 61:548).

112. TL Meinking et al, Infestations in LA Schachner and RA Hansen, eds. *Pediatric Dermatology.* 3rd ed. St Louis: Mosby; 2003, page 1291.

113. Lindane (γ-benzene hexachloride) should be reserved for treatment of patients who fail to respond to other drugs. The FDA has recommended it not be used for immunocompromised patients, young children, the elderly, pregnant and breast-feeding women, and patients weighing <50 kg.

114. BJ Currie and JS McCarthy, N Engl J Med 2010; 362:717. A second ivermectin dose taken 2 weeks later increased the cure rate to 95%, which is equivalent to that of 5% permethrin (V Usha et al, J Am Acad Dermatol 2000; 42:236). Ivermectin, either alone or in combination with a topical scabicide, is the drug of choice for crusted scabies in immunocompromised patients (P del Giudice, Curr Opin Infect Dis 2004; 15:123).

115. MJ Doenhoff et al, Curr Opin Infect Dis 2008; 21:659.

116. Geographically restricted to Central Western Africa and the island of São Tomé. Usually a disease of the lower GI tract; there are also case reports of complications including central nervous system, liver and cardiopulmonary involvement (A Murinello et al, GE - J Port Gastrenterol 2006; 13:97).

117. Oxamniquine, which is not available in the US, is generally not as effective as praziquantel. It has been useful, however, in some areas in which praziquantel is less effective (ML Ferrari et al, Bull World Health Organ 2003; 81:190; A Harder, Parasitol Res 2002; 88:395). Oxamniquine is contraindicated in pregnancy. It should be taken after food.

118. In East Africa, the dose should be increased to 30 mg/kg, PO, and in Egypt and South Africa to 30 mg/kg/d PO x 2d. Some experts recommend 40-60 mg/kg PO over 2-3d in all of Africa (KC Shekhar, Drugs 1991; 42:379).

119. In immunocompromised patients or disseminated disease, it may be necessary to prolong or repeat therapy, or to use other agents. Veterinary parenteral and enema formulations of ivermectin have been used in severely ill patients with hyperinfection who were unable to take or reliably absorb oral medications (FM Marty et al, Clin Infect Dis 2005; 41:e5; P Lichtenberger et al, Transpl Infect Dis 2009; 11:137). In disseminated strongyloidiasis, combination therapy with albendazole and ivermectin has been suggested (M Seqarra, Ann Pharmacother 2007; 41:1992).

120. Niclosamide must be thoroughly chewed or crushed and swallowed with a small amount of water.

121. Nitazoxanide may be an alternative (JJ Ortiz et al, Trans R Soc Trop Med Hyg 2002; 96:193; JC Chero et al, Trans R Soc Trop Med Hyg 2007; 101:203; E Diaz et al, Am J Trop Med Hyg 2003; 68:384).

122. Patients may benefit from surgical resection or percutaneous drainage of cysts. Praziquantel is useful preoperatively or in case of spillage of cyst contents during surgery. Percutaneous aspiration-injection-reaspiration (PAIR) with ultrasound guidance plus albendazole therapy has been effective for management of hepatic hydatid cyst disease (P Moro and PM Schantz, Int J Infect Dis 2009; 13:125.).

123. Surgical excision is the only reliable means of cure. Reports have suggested that in nonresectable cases use of albendazole (400 mg bid) can stabilize and sometimes cure infection (P Moro and PM Schantz, Int J Infect Dis 2009; 13:125).

124. Advances in neuroimaging using CT and MRI have facilitated the ability to make an accurate diagnosis (AC White Jr, J Infect Dis 2009; 199:1261). Initial therapy for patients with inflamed parenchymal cysticercosis should focus on symptomatic treatment with anti-seizure medication (S Sinha and BS Sharma, J Clin Neurosci 2009; 16:867). Patients with live parenchymal cysts who have seizures should be treated with albendazole together with steroids and an anti-seizure

Table 4.9. Drugs for Parasitic Infections, continued

Infection	Drug	Adult dosage	Pediatric dosage
Toxocariasis, see VISCERAL LARVA MIGRANS			
TOXOPLASMOSIS *(Toxoplasma gondii)*			
CNS disease[125]			
Drug of choice:	Pyrimethamine[126]	200 mg PO x 1 then 50-75 mg/d PO x 3-6 wks	2 mg/kg/d PO x 2d, then 1 mg/kg/d (max. 25 mg/d) x 3-6 wks
	plus		
	sulfadiazine[127]	1-1.5 g PO qid x 3-6 wks	100-200 mg/kg/d PO x 3-6 wks
OR	**plus**		
	clindamycin[7,128]	1.8-2.4 g/d IV or PO in 3 or 4 doses	5-7.5 mg/kg/d IV or PO in 3 or 4 doses (max 600 mg/dose)
OR	**plus**		
	atovaquone[7,17,128]	1500 mg PO bid	1500 mg PO bid
Alternative:	Trimethoprim/ sulfamethox- azole[7]	15-20 mg/kg/SMX 75-100 mg/kg/d PO or IV in 3 or 4 doses	15-20 mg/kg/SMX 75-100 mg/kg/d PO or IV in 3 or 4 doses
Primary infection in pregnancy			
Treatment of choice:	See footnote 129		
TRICHINELLOSIS *(Trichinella spiralis)*			
Drug of choice:[130]	Steroids for severe symptoms, e.g.	prednisone 30-60 mg PO daily x10-15 d	
	plus		
	Albendazole[7,12]	400 mg PO bid x 8-14d	400 mg PO bid x 8-14d
Alternative:	Mebendazole[7]	200-400 mg PO tid x 3d, then 400-500 mg tid x 10d	200-400 mg PO tid x 3d, then 400-500 mg tid x 10d
TRICHOMONIASIS *(Trichomonas vaginalis)*			
Drug of choice:[131]	Metronidazole	2 g PO once	15 mg/kg/d PO in 3 doses x 7d
OR	Tinidazole[6]	2 g PO once	50 mg/kg once (max. 2 g)
TRICHOSTRONGYLUS infection			
Drug of choice:	Pyrantel pamoate[7,31]*	11 mg/kg base PO once (max. 1 g)	11 mg/kg PO once (max. 1 g)
Alternative:	Mebendazole[7]	100 mg PO bid x 3d	100 mg PO bid x 3d
OR	Albendazole[7,12]	400 mg PO once	400 mg PO once
TRICHURIASIS *(Trichuris trichiura, whipworm)*			
Drug of choice:	Albendazole[7,12]	400 mg PO x 3d	400 mg PO x 3d
Alternative:	Mebendazole	100 mg PO bid x 3d	100 mg PO bid x 3d
OR	Ivermectin[7,15]	200 mcg/kg/d PO x 3d	200 mcg/kg/d PO x 3d
TRYPANOSOMIASIS			
T. cruzi (American trypanosomiasis, Chagas' disease)[132]			
Drug of choice:	Nifurtimox*	8-10 mg/kg/d PO in 3-4 doses x 90-120d	1-10yrs: 15-20 mg/kg/d PO in 4 doses x 90-120d 11-16yrs: 12.5-15 mg/kg/d PO in 4 doses x 90-120d
OR	Benznidazole[133]*	5-7 mg/kg/d PO in 2 doses x 60-90d	≤12yrs: 10 mg/kg/d PO in 2 doses x 60-90d >12 yrs: 5-7 mg/kg/d PO in 2 doses x 60-90d
T. brucei gambiense (West African trypanosomiasis, sleeping sickness)[134]			
Hemolymphatic stage			
Drug of choice:[135]	Pentamidine[7]	4 mg/kg/d IM x 7d	4 mg/kg/d IM x 7d
Alternative:	Suramin*	100-200 mg (test dose) IV, then 1 g IV on days 1,3,7,14 and 21	20 mg/kg on d 1,3,7,14 and 21
Late disease with CNS involvement			
Drug of Choice:[136]	Eflornithine[137]*	400 mg/kg/d IV in 4 doses x 14d	400 mg/kg/d IV in 4 doses x 14d
OR	Eflornithine[137]*	400 mg/kg IV in 2 doses x 7d	
	plus		
	Nitfurtimox	15 mg/kg/d PO in 3 doses x 10d	
OR	Melarsoprol[138]	2.2 mg/kg/d IV x 10d	2.2 mg/kg/d IV x 10d

*   Availability problems.

medication (HH Garcia et al, N Engl J Med 2004; 350:249). Patients with subarachnoid cysts or giant cysts in the fissures should be treated for at least 30d (JV Proaño et al, N Engl J Med 2001; 345:879). Surgical intervention (especially neuroendoscopic removal) or CSF diversion followed by albendazole and steroids is indicated for obstructive hydocephalus. Arachnoiditis, vasculitis or cerebral edema is treated with albendazole or praziquantel plus prednisone (60 mg/d) or dexamethasone (4-6 mg/d). Any cysticercocidal drug may cause irreparable damage when used to treat ocular or spinal cysts, even when corticosteroids are used. An ophthalmic exam should always precede treatment to rule out intraocular cysts.

125. Treatment is followed by chronic suppression with lower dosage regimens of the same drugs. For primary prophylaxis in HIV patients with CD4 <100 x 10^6 cells/L, either trimethoprim-sulfamethoxazole, pyrimethamine with dapsone, or atovaquone with or without pyrimethamine can be used. Primary or secondary prophylaxis may be discontinued when the CD4 count increases to >200 x 10^6 cells/L for >3mos (MMWR Morb Mortal Wkly Rep 2009; 58 [RR4]:1). In ocular toxoplasmosis with macular involvement, corticosteroids are recommended in addition to antiparasitic therapy (JG Montoya and O Liesenfeld, Lancet 2004; 363:1965).

126. Plus leucovorin 10-25 mg with each dose of pyrimethamine. Pyrimethamine should be taken with food to minimize gastrointestinal adverse effects.

127. Sulfadiazine should be taken on an empty stomach with adequate water.

128. Clindamycin has been used in combination with pyrimethamine to treat CNS toxoplasmosis in HIV infected patients who developed sulfonamide sensitivity while on sulfadiazine (G Beraud et al, Am J Trop Med Hygiene 2009; 80:583). Atovaquone has also been used to treat sulfonamide-intolerant patients (K Chirgwin et al, Clin Infect Dis 2002; 34:1243).

129. Women who develop toxoplasmosis during the first trimester of pregnancy should be treated with spiramycin (3-4 g/d). After the first trimester, if there is no documented transmission to the fetus, spiramycin can be continued until term. Spiramycin is not currently available in the US but can be obtained at no cost

Table 4.9. Drugs for Parasitic Infections, continued

Infection	Drug	Adult dosage	Pediatric dosage
TRYPANOSOMIASIS (continued)			
T. b. rhodesiense (East African trypanosomiasis, sleeping sickness)[134]			
Hemolymphatic stage			
Drug of choice:	Suramin*	100-200 mg (test dose) IV, then 1 g IV on days 1,3,7,14 and 21	20 mg/kg IV on d 1,3,7,14 and 21
Late disease with CNS involvement			
Drug of choice:	Melarsoprol[138]	2-3.6 mg/kg/d IV x 3d; after 7d 3.6 mg/kg/d x 3d; repeat again after 7d	2-3.6 mg/kg/d IV x 3d; after 7d 3.6 mg/kg/d x 3d; repeat again after 7d
VISCERAL LARVA MIGRANS[139] *(Toxocariasis)*			
Drug of choice:	Albendazole[7,12]	400 mg PO bid x 5d	400 mg PO bid x 5d
OR	Mebendazole[7]	100-200 mg PO bid x 5d	100-200 mg PO bid x 5d
Whipworm, see TRICHURIASIS			
Wuchereria bancrofti, see FILARIASIS			

*   Availability problems.
      from Palo Alto Medical Foundation Toxoplasma Serology Laboratory (PAMF-TSL, 650-853-4828), US National Collaborative Treatment Trials Study (773-834-4152), or the FDA (301-796-1600). If transmission has occurred *in utero*, therapy with pyrimethamine and sulfadiazine should be started. Pyrimethamine is a potential teratogen and should be used only after the first trimester (JG Montoya and JS Remington, Clin Infect Dis 2008; 47:554). Congenitally infected new borns should be treated with pyrimethamine every 2 or 3 days and a sulfonamide daily for about one year (JS Remington and G Desmonts in JS Remington and JO Klein, eds, *Infectious Disease of the Fetus and Newborn Infant*, 6th ed, Philadelphia:Saunders, 2006, page 1038).

130.   B Gottstein et al. Clin Microbiol Rev 2009; 22:127.

131.   Sexual partners should be treated simultaneously with same dosage. If treatment failure occurs and reinfection is excluded, treat with metronidazole 500 mg PO bid x7d, or tinidazole 2 g PO once (MMWR Morb Mortal Wkly Rep 2006; 55 [RR11]:1).

132.   Treatment of chronic or indeterminate Chagas' disease with benznidazole has been associated with reduced progression and increased negative seroconversion (C Bern et al, JAMA 2007; 298:2171; JA Perez-Molina et al, J Antimicrob Chemother 2009; 64:1139).

133.   Benznidazole should be taken with meals to minimize gastrointestinal adverse effects. It is contraindicated during pregnancy.

134.   PG Kennedy, Ann Neurol 2008; 64:116.

135.   Pentamidine and suramin have equal efficacy, but pentamidine is better tolerated.

136.   In one study eflornithine for 7 days combined with nifurtimox x 10 d was more effective and less toxic than eflornithine x 14 d (G Priotto et al, Lancet 2009; 374:56).

137.   Eflornithine is highly effective in *T.b. gambiense*, but not in *T.b. rhodesiense* infections. In one study of treatment of CNS disease due to *T.b. gambiense*, there were fewer serious complications with eflornithine than with melarsoprol (PG Kennedy, Ann Neurol 2008; 64:116). Eflornithine is available in limited supply only from the WHO. It is contraindicated during pregnancy.

138.   E Schmid et al, J Infect Dis 2005; 191:1922. Corticosteroids have been used to prevent arsenical encephalopathy (J Pepin et al, Trans R Soc Trop Med Hyg 1995; 89:92). Up to 20% of patients with *T.b.gambiense* fail to respond to melarsoprol (MP Barrett, Lancet 1999; 353:1113). In one study, a combination of low-dose melarsoprol (1.2 mg/kg/d IV) and nifurtimox (7.5 mg/kg PO bid) x 10 d was more effective than standard-dose melarsoprol alone (S Bisser et al, J Infect Dis 2007; 195:322).

139.   Optimum duration of therapy is not known; some Medical Letter consultants would treat x 20 d. For severe symptoms or eye involvement, corticosteroids can be used in addition (D Despommier, Clin Microbiol Rev 2003; 16:265).

Table 4.10. Principal Adverse Effects of Antiparasitic Drugs

Adverse effects of antiparasitic drugs vary with dosage, duration of administration, concomitant therapy, renal and hepatic function, immune competence, and the age of the patient. The principal adverse effects of antiparasitic agents are listed in the following table. The designation of adverse effects as "frequent," "occasional" or "rare" is based on published reports and on the experience of Medical Letter consultants. Information about adverse interactions between drugs, including probable mechanisms and recommendations for clinical management, are available in the Medical Letter Adverse Drug Interactions Program.

ALBENDAZOLE *(Albenza)*
Occasional: abdominal pain; reversible alopecia; increased serum transaminases
Rare: leukopenia; rash; renal toxicity

AMPHOTERICIN B DEOXYCHOLATE *(Fungizone, and others)*
Frequent: renal damage; hypokalemia; thrombophlebitis at site of peripheral vein infusion; anorexia; headache; nausea; weight loss; bone marrow suppression with reversible decline in hematocrit; chills, fever, vomiting during infusion, possibly with delirium, hypotension or hypertension, wheezing, and hypoxemia, especially in cardiac or pulmonary diease
Occasional: hypomagnesemia; normocytic, normochromic anemia
Rare: hemorrhagic gastroenteritis; blood dyscrasias; rash; blurred vision; peripheral neuropathy; convulsions; anaphylaxis; arrhythmias; acute liver failure; reversible nephrogenic diabetes insipidus; hearing loss; acute pulmonary edema; spinal cord damage with intrathecal use

AMPHOTERICIN B LIPID FORMULATIONS *(AmBisone, Abelcet, Amphotec)*
Similar to amphotericin B but generally better tolerated. Nephrotoxicity is less common and less severe with the lipid-based formulations. Acute infusion reactions are worse with *Amphotec,* less with *Abelcet* and least with *AmBisome.* Liver toxicity has been reported.

ARTEMETHER *(Artenam)*
Occasional: neurological toxicity; possible increase in length of coma; increased convulsions; prolongation of QTc interval

ARTEMETHER/LUMEFANTRINE *(Coatem, Riamet)*
Frequent: abdominal pain; anorexia; headache; dizziness; diarrhea; vomiting; nausea; palpitations; arthralgia; myalgia; asthenia; fatigue; pruritus; rash; sleep disorder; cough
Occasional: somnolence; involuntary muscle contractions; paresthesia; hypoesthesia; abnormal gait; ataxia
Rare: Hypersensitivity

ARTESUNATE
Occasional: ataxia; slurred speech; neurological toxicity; possible increase in length of coma; increased convulsions; prolongation of QTc interval

ATOVAQUONE *(Mepron, Malarone* [with *proguanil*])
Frequent: rash; nausea
Occasional: diarrhea; increased amino-transferases; cholestasis

AZITHROMYCIN *(Zithromax, and others)*
Occasional: nausea; diarrhea; abdominal pain; headache; dizziness; vaginitis
Rare: angioedema; cholestatic jaundice; photosensitivity; reversible dose-related hearing loss

BENZNIDAZOLE *(Rochagan)*
Frequent: allergic rash; dose-dependent polyneuropathy; GI disturbance; psychic disturbances

BENZYL ALCOHOL *(Ulesfia Lotion)*
Frequent: eye irritation; contact dermatitis

BITHIONOL *(Bitin)*
Frequent: photosensitivity reactions; vomiting; diarrhea; abdominal pain; urticaria
Rare: leukopenia; toxic hepatitis

CHLOROQUINE HCL and **CHLOROQUINE PHOSPHATE** *(Aralen, and others)*
Occasional: pruritus; vomiting; headache; confusion; depigmentation of hair; skin eruptions; corneal opacity; weight loss; partial alopecia; extraocular muscle palsies; exacerbation of psoriasis, eczema, and other exfoliative dermatoses; myalgias; photophobia
Rare: irreversible retinal injury (especially when total dosage exceeds 100 grams); discoloration of nails and mucus membranes; nerve-type deafness; peripheral neuropathy and myopathy; heart block; blood dyscrasias; hematemesis

CLARITHROMYCIN *(Biaxin, and others)*
Occasional: nausea; diarrhea; abdominal pain; abnormal taste; headache; dizziness
Rare: reversible dose-related hearing loss; pseudomembranous colitis; pancreatitis; torsades de pointes

CLINDAMYCIN *(Cleocin, and others)*
Frequent: diarrhea; allergic reactions
Occasional: pseudomembranous colitis, sometimes severe, can occur even with topical use
Rare: blood dyscrasias; esophageal ulceration; hepatotoxicity; arrhythmia due to QTc prolongation

CROTAMITON *(Eurax)*
Occasional: rash

DAPSONE
Frequent: rash; transient headache; GI irritation; anorexia; infectious mononucleosis-like syndrome
Occasional: cyanosis due to methemoglobinemia and sulfhemoglobinemia; other blood dyscrasias, including hemolytic anemia; nephrotic syndrome; liver damage; peripheral neuropathy; hypersensitivity reactions; increased risk of lepra reactions; insomnia; irritability; uncoordinated speech; agitation; acute psychosis
Rare: renal papillary necrosis; severe hypoalbuminemia; epidermal necrolysis; optic atrophy; agranulocytosis; neonatal hyperbilirubinemia after use in pregnancy

Table 4.10. Principal Adverse Effects of Antiparasitic Drugs, continued

DIETHYLCARBAMAZINE CITRATE *(Hetrazan)*
Frequent: allergic or febrile reactions, which may be severe, in patients with microfilaria in the blood or the skin; GI disturbance
Rare: encephalopathy

DILOXANIDE FUROATE *(Furamide)*
Frequent: flatulence
Occasional: nausea; vomiting; diarrhea
Rare: diplopia; dizziness; urticaria; pruritus

EFLORNITHINE (Difluoromethylornithine, DFMO, *Ornidyl*)
Frequent: anemia; leukopenia
Occasional: diarrhea; thrombocytopenia; seizures
Rare: hearing loss

FLUCONAZOLE *(Diflucan,* and others)
Occasional: nausea; vomiting; diarrhea; abdominal pain; headache; rash; increased aminotransferases
Rare: severe hepatic toxicity; exfoliative dermatitis; anaphylaxis; Stevens-Johnson syndrome; toxic epidermal necrolysis; hair loss

FLUCYTOSINE *(Ancobon)*
Frequent: blood dyscrasias, including pancytopenia and fatal agranulocytosis; GI disturbance, including severe diarrhea and ulcerative colitis; rash; hepatic dysfunction
Occasional: confusion; hallucinations
Rare: anaphylaxis

FURAZOLIDONE *(Furoxone)*
Frequent: nausea; vomiting
Occasional: allergic reactions, including pulmonary infiltration; hypotension; urticaria; fever; vesicular rash; hypoglycemia; headache
Rare: hemolytic anemia in G-6-PD deficiency and neonates; disulfiram-like reaction with alcohol; MAO-inhibitor interactions; polyneuritis

IODOQUINOL *(Yodoxin,* and others)
Occasional: rash; acne; slight enlargement of the thyroid gland; nausea; diarrhea; cramps; anal pruritus
Rare: optic neuritis, atrophy and loss of vision; peripheral neuropathy after prolonged use in high dosage (for months); iodine sensitivity

ITRACONAZOLE *(Sporanox,* and others)
Occasional: nausea; epigastric pain; headache; dizziness; edema; hypokalemia; rash; hepatic toxicity
Rare: congestive heart failure

IVERMECTIN *(Stromectol)*
Occasional: Mazzotti-type reaction seen in onchocerciasis, including fever; pruritus; tender lymph nodes; headache; and joint and bone pain
Rare: hypotension

KETOCONAZOLE *(Nizoral,* and others)
Frequent: nausea; vomiting
Occasional: decreased testosterone synthesis; gynecomastia; oligospermia and impotence in men; abdomina pain; rash; hepatitis; pruritus; dizziness; constipation; diarrhea; fever and chills; photophobia; headache
Rare: fatal hepatic necrosis; liver injury with jaundice; transient elevated transaminase; severe epigastric burning and pain; may interfere with adrenal function; anaphylaxis

MALATHION *(Ovide)*
Occasional: local irritation

MEBENDAZOLE *(Vermox)*
Occasional: diarrhea; abdominal pain
Rare: leukopenia; agranulocytosis; hypospermia

MEFLOQUINE *(Lariam)*
Frequent: vertigo; lightheadedness; nausea; other GI disturbances; nightmares; visual disturbances; headache; insomnia
Occasional: confusion
Rare: psychosis; hypotension; convulsions; coma; paresthesias

MEGLUMINE ANTIMONIATE *(Glucantime)*
— Similar to sodium stibogluconate

MELARSOPROL *(Mel B)*
Frequent: myocardial damage; albuminuria; hypertension; colic; Herxheimer-type reaction; encephalopathy; vomiting; peripheral neuropathy
Rare: shock

METRONIDAZOLE *(Flagyl,* and others)
Frequent: nausea; headache; anorexia; metallic taste
Occasional: vomiting; diarrhea; insomnia; weakness; dry mouth; stomatitis; vertigo; tinnitus; paresthesias; rash; dark urine; urethral burning; disulfiram-like reaction with alcohol; candidiasis
Rare: pseudomembranous colitis; leukopenia; pancreatitis; seizures; peripheral neuropathy; encephalopathy; cerebellar syndrome with ataxia, dysarthria and MRI abnormalities

MICONAZOLE *(Monistat i.v.)*
Occasional: phlebitis; thrombocytosis; chills; intense, persistent pruritus; rash; vomiting; hyperlipidemia; dizziness; blurred vision; local burning and irritation with topical use
Rare: anemia; thrombocytopenia; hyponatremia; renal insufficiency; anaphylaxis; cardiac and respiratory arrest with initial dose

MILTEFOSINE *(Impavido)*
Frequent: nausea; vomiting; diarrhea; motion sickness; increased creatinine

NICLOSAMIDE *(Niclocide)*
Occasional: nausea; abdominal pain

Table 4.10. Principal Adverse Effects of Antiparasitic Drugs, continued

NITAZOXANIDE *(Alinia)*
Occasional: GI disturbance; headache
Rare: yellow discoloration of sclera; allergic reactions; increased creatinine; dizziness; flatulence; malaise; salivary gland enlargement; discolored urine; anemia; leukoytosis

ORNIDAZOLE *(Tiberal)*
Occasional: dizziness; headache; GI disturbance
Rare: reversible peripheral neuropathy

OXAMNIQUINE *(Vansil)*
Occasional: headache; fever; dizziness; somnolence and insomnia; nausea; diarrhea; rash; increased aminotransferases; ECG changes; EEG changes; orange-red discoloration of urine
Rare: seizures; neuropsychiatric disturbances

PAROMOMYCIN (aminosidine; *Humatin*)
Frequent: GI disturbance with oral use
Rare: eighth-nerve damage (mainly auditory) and renal damage when aminosidine is given IV; vertigo; pancreatitis

PENTAMIDINE ISETHIONATE *(Pentam 300, NebuPent,* and others)
Frequent: hypotension; hypoglycemia often followed by diabetes mellitus; vomiting; blood dyscrasias; renal damage; pain at injection site; GI disturbance
Occasional: may aggravate diabetes; shock; hypocalcemia; liver damage; cardiotoxicity; delirium; rash
Rare: Herxheimer-type reaction; anaphylaxis; acute pancreatitis; hyperkalemia

PERMETHRIN (*Nix,* and others)
Occasional: burning; stinging; numbness; increased pruritus; pain; edema; erythema; rash

PRAZIQUANTEL *(Biltricide)*
Frequent: abdominal pain; diarrhea; malaise; headache; dizziness
Occasional: sedation; fever; sweating; nausea; eosinophilia
Rare: pruritus; rash; edema; hiccups

PRIMAQUINE PHOSPHATE
Frequent: hemolytic anemia in G-6-PD deficiency
Occasional: neutropenia; GI disturbance; methemoglobinemia
Rare: CNS symptoms; hypertension; arrhythmias

PROGUANIL *(Paludrine; Malarone* [with atovaquone])
Occasional: oral ulceration; hair loss; scaling of palms and soles; urticaria
Rare: hematuria (with large doses); vomiting; abdominal pain; diarrhea (with large doses); thrombocytopenia

PYRANTEL PAMOATE *(Antiminth,* and others)
Occasional: GI disturbance; headache; dizziness; rash; fever

PYRETHRINS with PIPERONYL BUTOXIDE *(A-200,* and others)
Occasional: allergic reactions

PYRIMETHAMINE *(Daraprim)*
Occasional: blood dyscrasias; folic acid deficiency
Rare: rash; vomiting; convulsions; shock; possibly pulmonary eosinophilia; fatal cutaneous reactions with pyrimethamine-sulfadoxine *(Fansidar)*

QUINACRINE
Frequent: disulfiram-like reaction with alcohol; nausea and vomiting; colors skin and urine yellow
Occasional: headache; dizziness
Rare: rash; fever; psychosis; extensive exfoliative dermatitis in patients with psoriasis

QUININE DIHYDROCHLORIDE and QUININE SULFATE
Frequent: cinchonism (tinnitus, headache, nausea, abdominal pain, visual disturbance)
Occasional: deafness; hemolytic anemia; other blood dyscrasias; photosensitivity reactions; hypoglycemia; arrhythmias; hypotension; fever
Rare: blindness; sudden death if injected too rapidly; hypersensitivity reaction with TTP-HUS

SODIUM STIBOGLUCONATE *(Pentostam)*
Frequent: myalgia and arthralgia (typically, large joint, may or may not br symmetric); malaise, fatigue and weakness; headache; anorexia; nausea; increased aminotransferases; increased amylase and lipase; T-wave flattening or inversion
Occasional: abdominal pain; liver damage; bradycardia; leukopenia; thrombocytopenia; rash; vomiting
Rare: diarrhea; pruritus; myocardial damage; hemolytic anemia; renal damage; shock; sudden death

SPIRAMYCIN *(Rovamycine)*
Occasional: GI disturbance
Rare: allergic reactions

SULFONAMIDES
Frequent: allergic reactions (rash, photosensitivity, drug fever)
Occasional: kernicterus in newborn; renal damage; liver damage; Stevens-Johnson syndrome (particularly with long-acting sulfonamides); hemolytic anemia; other blood dyscrasias; vasculitis
Rare: transient acute myopia; pseudomembranous colitis; reversible infertility in men with sulfasalazine; CNS toxicity with trimethoprim-sulfamethoxazole in patients with AIDS

SURAMIN SODIUM
Frequent: vomiting; pruritus; urticaria; paresthesias; hyperesthesia of hands and feet; peripheral neuropathy; photophobia
Occasional: kidney damage; blood dyscrasias; shock; optic atrophy

TETRACYCLINES
(doxycycline – *Vibramycin,* and others; tetracycline hydrochloride – *Sumycin,* and others)
Frequent: GI disturbance; bone lesions and staining and deformity of teeth in children up to 8 years old, and in the newborn when given to pregnant women after the fourth month of pregnancy

Table 4.10. Principal Adverse Effects of Antiparasitic Drugs, continued

Occasional: malabsorption; enterocolitis; photosensitivity reactions; increased azotemia with renal insufficiency (except doxycycline, but exacerbation of renal failure with doxycycline has been reported); hepatic injury; parenteral doses may cause serious liver damage, especially in pregnant women and patients with renal disease receiving 1 gram or more daily; esophageal ulcerations; cutaneous and mucosal hyperpigmentation
Rare: allergic reactions, including serum sickness and anaphylaxis; pseudomembranous colitis; blood dyscrasias; drug-induced lupus; autoimmune hepatitis; increased intracranial pressure; fixed-drug eruptions; transient acute myopia; blurred vision; diplopia; papilledema; photoonycholysis and onycholysis; aggravation of myasthenic symptoms with IV injection, reversed with calcium; possibly transient neuropathy; hemolytic anemia

TINIDAZOLE *(Tindamax)*
Occasional: metallic taste; GI symptoms; rash
Rare: weakness

TRIMETHOPRIM *(Proloprim*, and others)
Frequent: nausea and vomiting with high doses
Occasional: megaloblastic anemia; thrombocytopenia; neutropenia; rash; fixed drug eruption
Rare: pancytopenia; hyperkalemia

TRIMETHOPRIM/SULFAMETHOXAZOLE *(Bactrim, Septra*, and others)
Frequent: rash; fever; nausea and vomiting
Occasional: hemolysis in G-6-PD deficiency; acute megaloblastic anemia; granulocytopenia; thrombocytopenia; pseudomembranous colitis; kernicterus in newborn; hyperkalemia
Rare: agranulocytosis; aplastic anemia; hepatotoxicity; Stevens-Johnson syndrome; aseptic meningitis; fever; confusion; depression; hallucinations; deterioration in renal disease; intrahepatic cholestasis; methemoglobinemia; pancreatitis; ataxia; CNS toxicity in patients with AIDS; renal tubular acidosis; hyperkalemia

4.11. Safety of Antiparasitic Drugs in Pregnancy

Drug	Toxicity in Pregnancy	Recommendations	FDA
Albendazole (Albenza)	Teratogenic and embryotoxic in animals	Caution*	C
Amphotericin B (Fungizone, and others)	None known	Caution*	B
Amphotericin B liposomal (AmBisome)	None known	Caution*	B
Artemether/lumefantrine (Coartem, Riamet)[1]	Unknown	Contraindicated during 1st trimester; caution 2nd and 3rd trimesters*	C
Artesunate[2]	Embryocidal and teratogenic in rats	Contraindicated during 1st trimester; caution 2nd and 3rd trimesters*	N/A
Atovaquone (Mepron)	Maternal and fetal toxicity in animals	Caution*	C
Atovaquone/proguanil (Malarone)[3]	Maternal and fetal toxicity in animals	Caution*	C
Azithromycin (Zithromax, and others)	None known	Probably safe	B
Benznidazole (Rochagan)	Unknown	Contraindicated	N/A
Benzyl alcohol lotion (Ulesfia Lotion)	Unknown	Probably safe	B
Chloroquine (Aralen, and others)	None known with doses recommended for malaria prophylaxis	Probably safe in low doses	C
Clarithromycin (Biaxin, and others)	Teratogenic in animals	Contraindicated	C
Clindamycin (Cleocin, and others)[4]	None known	Caution*	B
Crotamiton (Eurax)	Unknown	Caution*	C
Dapsone	None known; carcinogenic in rats and mice; hemolytic reactions in neonates	Caution*, especially at term	C
Diethylcarbamazine (DEC; Hetrazan)	Not known; abortifacient in one study in rabbits	Contraindicated	N/A
Diloxanide (Furamide)	Safety not established	Caution*	N/A
Doxycycline (Vibramycin, and others)	Tooth discoloration and dysplasia inhibition of bone growth in fetus; hepatic toxicity and azotemia with IV use in pregnant patients with decreased renal function or with overdosage	Contraindicated	D
Eflornithine (Ornidyl)	Embryocidal in animals	Contraindicated	C
Fluconazole (Diflucan, and others)	Teratogenic	Contraindicated for high dose; caution* for single dose	C
Flucytosine (Ancoban)	Teratogenic in rats	Contraindicated	C
Furazolidone (Furoxone)	None known; carcinogenic in rodents; hemolysis with G-6-PD deficiency in newborn	Caution*; contraindicated at term	N/A
Hydroxychloroquine (Plaquenil)	None known with doses recommended for malaria prophylaxis	Probably safe in low doses	C
Itraconazole (Sporanox, and others)	Teratogenic and embryotoxic in rats	Caution*	C
Iodoquinol (Yodoxin, and others)	Unknown	Caution*	C
Ivermectin (Stromectol)[5]	Teratogenic in animals	Contraindicated	C
Ketoconazole (Nizoral, and others)	Teratogenic and embryotoxic in rats	Contraindicated; topical probably safe	C
Lindane	Absorbed from the skin; potential CNS toxicity in fetus	Contraindicated	C
Malathion, topical	None known	Probably safe	B
Mebendazole (Vermox)	Teratogenic and embryotoxic in rats	Caution*	C
Mefloquine[6]	Teratogenic in animals	Caution*	C
Meglumine (Glucantine)	Not known	Caution*	N/A
Metronidazole (Flagyl, and others)	None known – carcinogenic in rats and mice	Caution*	B
Miconazole (Monistat i.v.)	None known	Caution*	C

4.11. Safety of Antiparasitic Drugs in Pregnancy, continued

Miltefosine *(Impavido)*	Teratogenic in rats and induces abortions inanimals	Contraindicated; effective contraception must be used for 2 months after the last dose	N/A
Niclosamide *(Niclocide)*	Not absorbed; no known toxicity in fetus	Probably safe	B
Nitazoxanide *(Alinia)*	None known	Probably safe	B
Oxamniquine *(Vansil)*	Embryocidal in animals	Contraindicated	N/A
Paromomycin	Poorly absorbed; toxicity in fetus unknown	Oral capsules probably safe	C
Pentamidine (*Pentam 300, NebuPent,* and others)	Safety not established	Caution*	C
Permethrin (*Nix,* and others)	Poorly absorbed; no known toxicity in fetus	Probably safe	B
Praziquantel *(Biltricide)*	None known	Caution	B
Primaquine	Hemolysis in G-6-PD deficiency	Contraindicated	C
Pyrantel pamoate (*Antiminth,* and others)	Absorbed in small amounts; no known toxicity in fetus	Probably safe	C
Pyrethrins and piperonyl butoxide (*A-200,* and others)	Poorly absorbed; no known toxicity in fetus	Probably safe	C
Pyrimethamine *(Daraprim)*[7]	Teratogenic in animals	Caution*; contraindicated during 1st trimester	C
Quinacrine *(Atabrine)*	Safety not established	Caution*	N/A
Quinidine	Large doses can cause abortion	Probably safe	C
Quinine *(Qualaquin)*	Large doses can cause abortion; auditory nerve hypoplasia, deafness in fetus; visual changes, limb anomalies, visceral defects also reported	Caution*	C
Sodium stibogluconate *(Pentostam)*	Not known	Caution*	N/A
Spiramycin *(Rovamycine)*[7]	None known	Probably safe	N/A
Sulfonamides	Teratogenic in some animal studies;hemolysis in newborn with G-6-PD deficiency; increased risk of kernicterus in newborn	Caution*; contraindicated at term	C
Suramin sodium *(Germanin)*	Teratogenic in mice	Caution*	N/A
Tetracycline (*Sumycin,* and others)	Tooth discoloration and dysplasia, inhibition of bone growth in fetus; hepatic toxicity and azotemia with IV use in pregnant patients with decreased renal function or with overdosage	Contraindicated	D
Tinidazole *(Tindamax)*	Increased fetal mortality in rats	Caution*	C
Trimethoprim	Folate antagonism; teratogenic in rats	Caution*	C
Trimethoprim-sulfamethoxazole (*Bactrim,* and others)	Same as sulfonamides and trimethoprim	Caution*; contraindicated at term	C

N/A= FDA pregnancy category not available

*Use only for strong clinical indication in absence of suitable alternative.
1. See also footnotes 78 and 79 in Table 4.9.
2. See also footnote 78 in Table 4.9.
3. See also footnote 76 in Table 4.9.
4. See also footnote 82 in Table 4.9.
5. See also footnote 42 in Table 4.9.
6. See also footnotes 84 and 95 in Table 4.9.
7. See also footnote 129 in Table 4.9.

4.12. Manufacturers of Drugs Used to Treat Parasitic Infections

A-200 (Hogil) – pyrethrins and piperonyl butoxide
albendazole – *Albenza* (GlaxoSmithKline)
Albenza (GlaxoSmithKline) – albendazole
Alinia (Romark) – nitazoxanide
AmBisome (Gilead) – amphotericin B, liposomal
amphotericin B – *Fungizone* (Apothecon), others
amphotericin B, liposomal – *AmBisome* (Gilead)
Ancobon (Valeant) – flucytosine
§ *Antiminth* (Pfizer) – pyrantel pamoate
• *Aralen* (sanofi-aventis) – chloroquine HCl and chloroquine phosphate
§ artemether – *Artenam* (Arenco, Belgium)
artemether/lumefantrine – *Coartem, Riamet* (Novartis)
§ *Artenam* (Arenco, Belgium) – artemether
• † artesunate – (Guilin No. 1 Factory, People's Republic of China)
atovaquone – *Mepron* (GlaxoSmithKline)
atovaquone/proguanil – *Malarone* (GlaxoSmithKline)
azithromycin – *Zithromax* (Pfizer), others
• *Bactrim* (AR Scientific) – TMP/Sulfa
Benzyl alcohol lotion – *Ulesfia* (Sciele)
§ benznidazole – *Rochagan* (Brazil)
• *Biaxin* (Abbott) – clarithromycin
Biltricide (Bayer) – praziquantel
† bithionol – *Bitin* (Tanabe, Japan)
† *Bitin* (Tanabe, Japan) – bithionol
§ *Brolene* (Aventis, Canada) – propamidine isethionate
chloroquine HCl and chloroquine phosphate – *Aralen* (sanofi-aventis), others
• clarithromycin – *Biaxin* (Abbott), others
• *Cleocin* (Pfizer) – clindamycin
clindamycin – *Cleocin* (Pfizer), others
Coartem (Novartis) – artemether/lumefantrine
crotamiton – *Eurax* (Ranbaxy)
dapsone – (Jacobus)
§ *Daraprim* (GlaxoSmithKline) – pyrimethamine USP
† diethylcarbamazine citrate (DEC) – *Hetrazan*
• *Diflucan* (Pfizer) – fluconazole
§ diloxanide furoate – *Furamide*
doxycycline – *Vibramycin* (Pfizer), others
§ eflornithine (Difluoromethylornithine, DFMO) – *Ornidyl* (Aventis)
§ *Egaten* (Novartis) – triclabendazole
Elimite (Allergan) – permethrin
Eurax (Ranbaxy) – crotamiton
• *Flagyl* (Pfizer) – metronidazole
§ *Flisint* (Sanofi-Aventis, France) – fumagillin
fluconazole – *Diflucan* (Pfizer), others
flucytosine – *Ancobon* (Valeant)
§ fumagillin – *Flisint* (Sanofi-Aventis, France)
• *Fungizone* (Apothecon) – amphotericin
§ *Furamide* – diloxanide furoate
§ furazolidone – *Furoxone* (Roberts)
§ *Furoxone* (Roberts) – furazolidone
† *Germanin* (Bayer, Germany) – suramin sodium
§ *Glucantime* (Aventis, France) – meglumine antimonate
† *Hetrazan* – diethylcarbamazine citrate (DEC)
§ *Impavido* (Paladin, Montreal, Canada) – miltefosine
iodoquinol – *Yodoxin* (Glenwood), others
itraconazole – *Sporanox* (Ortho-McNeil-Janssen), others
ivermectin – *Stromectol* (Merck)
ketoconazole – *Nizoral* (Janssen), others
† *Lampit* (Bayer, Germany) – nifurtimox
§ *Leshcutan* (Teva, Israel) – topical paromomycin
lumefantrine/artemether – *Coartem, Riamet* (Novartis)
Malarone (GlaxoSmithKline) – atovaquone/proguanil
malathion – *Ovide* (Taro)
mebendazole
mefloquine
§ meglumine antimonate – *Glucantime* (Aventis, France)

† melarsoprol – *Mel-B*
† *Mel-B* – melarsoprol
Mepron (GlaxoSmithKline) – atovaquone
metronidazole – *Flagyl* (Pfizer), others
§ miconazole – *Monistat i.v.*
§ miltefosine – *Impavido* (Paladin, Montreal, Canada)
§ *Monistat i.v.* – miconazole
NebuPent (Fujisawa) – pentamidine isethionate
Neutrexin (US Bioscience) – trimetrexate
§ niclosamide – *Yomesan* (Bayer, Germany)
† nifurtimox – *Lampit* (Bayer, Germany)
nitazoxanide – *Alinia* (Romark)
• *Nizoral* (Janssen) – ketoconazole
Nix (GlaxoSmithKline) – permethrin
§ ornidazole – *Tiberal* (Roche, France)
Ornidyl (Aventis) – eflornithine (Difluoromethylornithine, DFMO)
Ovide (Taro) – malathion
§ oxamniquine – *Vansil* (Pfizer)
§ *Paludrine* (AstraZeneca, United Kingdom) – proguanil
§ paromomycin – Oral generics; *Leshcutan* (Teva, Israel; (topical formulation not available in US)
Pentam 300 (Fujisawa) – pentamidine isethionate
pentamidine isethionate – *Pentam 300* (Fujisawa), *NebuPent* (Fujisawa)
† *Pentostam* (GlaxoSmithKline, United Kingdom) – sodium stibogluconate
permethrin – *Nix* (GlaxoSmithKline), *Elimite* (Allergan)
praziquantel – *Biltricide* (Bayer)
primaquine phosphate USP
§ proguanil – *Paludrine* (AstraZeneca, United Kingdom)
proguanil/atovaquone – *Malarone* (GlaxoSmithKline)
§ propamidine isethionate – *Brolene* (Aventis, Canada)
§ pyrantel pamoate – *Antiminth* (Pfizer)
pyrethrins and piperonyl butoxide – *A-200* (Hogil), others
§ pyrimethamine USP – *Daraprim* (GlaxoSmithKline)
Qualaquin (AR Scientific) – quinine sulfate
quinidine gluconate
§ quinine dihydrochloride
quinine sulfate – *Qualaquin* (AR Scientific)
Riamet (Novartis) – artemether/lumefantrine
• *Rifadin* (sanofi-aventis) – rifampin
rifampin – *Rifadin* (sanofi-aventis), others
§ *Rochagan* (Brazil) – benznidazole
* *Rovamycine* (Aventis) – spiramycin
§ sodium stibogluconate – *Pentostam* (GlaxoSmithKline, United Kingdom)
* spiramycin – *Rovamycine* (Aventis)
• *Sporanox* (Ortho-McNeil-Janssen) – itraconazole
Stromectol (Merck) – ivermectin
sulfadiazine
† suramin sodium – *Germanin* (Bayer, Germany)
§ *Tiberal* (Roche, France) – ornidazole
Tindamax (Mission) – tinidazole
tinidazole – *Tindamax* (Mission)
TMP/Sulfa – *Bactrim* (AR Scientific), others
§ triclabendazole – *Egaten* (Novartis)
trimetrexate – *Neutrexin* (US Bioscience)
Ulesfia – benzyl alcohol
§ *Vansil* (Pfizer) – oxamniquine
• *Vibramycin* (Pfizer) – doxycycline
• *Yodoxin* (Glenwood) – iodoquinol
§ *Yomesan* (Bayer, Germany) – niclosamide
• *Zithromax* (Pfizer) – azithromycin

---

§ Not available in the US; may be available through a compounding pharmacy (see footnote 4 in Table 4.9).
† Available from the CDC Drug Service, Centers for Disease Control and Prevention, Atlanta, Georgia 30333; 404-639-3670 (evenings, weekends, or holidays: 770-488-7100).
• Also available generically.

....

MEDWATCH–THE FDA SAFETY INFORMATION AND ADVERSE EVENT-REPORTING PROGRAM

MedWatch, the Food and Drug Administration (FDA) Safety Information and Adverse Event Reporting Program, is an outreach program for the health care system, including physicians, nurses, pharmacists, patients, and manufacturers, to enhance the effectiveness of the FDA's risk management activities for all regulated clinical medical products. These products include prescription and over-the-counter drugs, biologic products, medical and radiation-emitting devices, and special nutritional products (eg, dietary supplements, infant formulas).

The MedWatch program has 2 goals: (1) to provide clinically useful and timely safety information about safety alerts, recalls, and withdrawals to physicians and their patients (**www.fda.gov/medwatch/**); and (2) to encourage and facilitate reporting of serious adverse events, which include events that are reported as fatal, disabling, life-threatening, requiring hospital admission, prolonging a hospital stay, resulting in a congenital anomaly, or requiring medical intervention to prevent such an outcome. Reports are used by the FDA as a data source to identify and evaluate new safety concerns with drugs and devices after they are approved and more widely used in clinical practice. Many prelicensure clinical trials are not large enough to reveal rare adverse events. With information from postmarketing safety surveillance, the FDA can develop, with the manufacturer, a modified product, revised and strengthened professional labeling and patient instructions, and a modified use strategy that will lead to a safer product.

Physicians as well as other health care personnel and consumers are encouraged to report problems and adverse events. The MedWatch voluntary form for adverse events related to products other than vaccines is a 1-page, postage-paid form (see Fig 4.1, p 870). An outline version that can be completed and submitted immediately to the FDA is available at the MedWatch Web site (**www.fda.gov/medwatch**). This form then can be returned by fax (800-FDA-0178) or mail. A toll-free number (800-FDA-1088) is available to report by phone or request blank forms with instructions.

Vaccine-related adverse events are not reported to MedWatch but should be reported to the Vaccine Adverse Event Reporting System (**http://vaers.hhs.gov/**) (see Reporting of Adverse Events, p 44).

Fig 4.1 MedWatch Reporting Form

Available for download at **http://www.fda.gov/downloads/Safety/MedWatch/ HowToReport/DownloadForms/UCM082725.pdf.**

U.S. Department of Health and Human Services

MedWatch

The FDA Safety Information and
Adverse Event Reporting Program

For VOLUNTARY reporting of
adverse events, product problems and
product use errors

Page ____ of ____

Form Approved: OMB No. 0910-0291, Expires: 10/31/08
See OMB statement on reverse.

FDA USE ONLY

Triage unit
sequence #

PLEASE TYPE OR USE BLACK INK

A. PATIENT INFORMATION

1. Patient Identifier	2. Age at Time of Event, or Date of Birth:	3. Sex	4. Weight
In confidence		☐ Female ☐ Male	____ lb or ____ kg

B. ADVERSE EVENT, PRODUCT PROBLEM OR ERROR

Check all that apply:

1. ☐ Adverse Event　☐ Product Problem (e.g. defects/malfunctions)
☐ Product Use Error　☐ Problem with Different Manufacturer of Same Medicine

2. Outcomes Attributed to Adverse Event
(Check all that apply)

☐ Death: ____ (mm/dd/yyyy)
☐ Life-threatening
☐ Hospitalization - initial or prolonged
☐ Required Intervention to Prevent Permanent Impairment/Damage (Devices)
☐ Disability or Permanent Damage
☐ Congenital Anomaly/Birth Defect
☐ Other Serious (Important Medical Events)

3. Date of Event (mm/dd/yyyy)　4. Date of this Report (mm/dd/yyyy)

5. Describe Event, Problem or Product Use Error

6. Relevant Tests/Laboratory Data, Including Dates

7. Other Relevant History, Including Preexisting Medical Conditions (e.g., allergies, race, pregnancy, smoking and alcohol use, liver/kidney problems, etc.)

C. PRODUCT AVAILABILITY

Product Available for Evaluation? (Do not send product to FDA)

☐ Yes　☐ No　☐ Returned to Manufacturer on: ____ (mm/dd/yyyy)

D. SUSPECT PRODUCT(S)

1. Name, Strength, Manufacturer (from product label)
#1
#2

2. Dose or Amount　　Frequency　　Route
#1
#2

3. Dates of Use (if unknown, give duration) from/to (or best estimate)
#1
#2

5. Event Abated After Use Stopped or Dose Reduced?
#1 ☐ Yes ☐ No ☐ Doesn't Apply
#2 ☐ Yes ☐ No ☐ Doesn't Apply

4. Diagnosis or Reason for Use (Indication)
#1
#2

6. Event Reappeared After Reintroduction?
#1 ☐ Yes ☐ No ☐ Doesn't Apply
#2 ☐ Yes ☐ No ☐ Doesn't Apply

6. Lot #　　7. Expiration Date
#1　　#1
#2　　#2

9. NDC # or Unique ID

E. SUSPECT MEDICAL DEVICE

1. Brand Name

2. Common Device Name

3. Manufacturer Name, City and State

4. Model #　　Lot #
Catalog #　　Expiration Date (mm/dd/yyyy)
Serial #　　Other #

5. Operator of Device
☐ Health Professional
☐ Lay User/Patient
☐ Other:

6. If Implanted, Give Date (mm/dd/yyyy)　7. If Explanted, Give Date (mm/dd/yyyy)

8. Is this a Single-use Device that was Reprocessed and Reused on a Patient?
☐ Yes　☐ No

9. If Yes to Item No. 8, Enter Name and Address of Reprocessor

F. OTHER (CONCOMITANT) MEDICAL PRODUCTS

Product names and therapy dates (exclude treatment of event)

G. REPORTER (See confidentiality section on back)

1. Name and Address

Phone #　　E-mail

2. Health Professional?　3. Occupation　4. Also Reported to:
☐ Yes　☐ No
☐ Manufacturer
☐ User Facility
☐ Distributor/Importer

5. If you do NOT want your identity disclosed to the manufacturer, place an "X" in this box: ☐

FORM FDA 3500 (10/05)　Submission of a report does not constitute an admission that medical personnel or the product caused or contributed to the event.

Antimicrobial Prophylaxis

ANTIMICROBIAL PROPHYLAXIS

Antimicrobial agents commonly are prescribed to prevent infections in infants and children. The efficacy of prophylactic antimicrobial agents has been documented for some conditions but is unsubstantiated for many. *Prophylaxis* is defined as the use of antimicrobial drugs in the absence of suspected or documented infection to prevent development of an infection.

Effective chemoprophylaxis should be directed at specific pathogens, for infection-prone body sites, in vulnerable hosts. Examples are shown in Table 5.1 (p 872). In any situation in which prophylactic antimicrobial therapy is being considered, the risk of emergence of resistant organisms and the possibility of an adverse event must be weighed against potential benefits. Prophylactic agents should have as narrow a spectrum of antimicrobial activity as possible and should be used for as brief a period of time as possible. Uses of antimicrobial agents in doses or routes of administration other than oral, intramuscular, or intravenous, such as "antibiotic solutions" for irrigation or instillation, should not be considered prophylaxis and generally are unproven as efficacious for prevention of infection.

Infection-Prone Body Sites

Prevention of infection of vulnerable body sites is most likely to be successful if (1) the period of risk is defined and brief; (2) the expected pathogens have predictable antimicrobial susceptibility; and (3) the site is accessible to adequate antimicrobial concentrations.

Acute Otitis Media. Acute otitis media recurs less frequently in otitis-prone children treated prophylactically with antimicrobial agents. Studies have demonstrated that amoxicillin, sulfisoxazole, and trimethoprim-sulfamethoxazole are effective. However, antimicrobial prophylaxis may alter the nasopharyngeal flora and foster colonization with resistant organisms, compromising long-term efficacy of the prophylactic drug. Continuous orally administered antimicrobial prophylaxis should be reserved for control of recurrent acute otitis media, only when defined as 3 or more distinct and well-documented episodes during a period of 6 months or 4 or more episodes during a period of 12 months. Although prophylactic administration of an antimicrobial agent limited to a period of time when a person is at high risk of otitis media, such as during acute viral respiratory tract infection, has been suggested, this method has not been evaluated critically. The risks and benefits of other methods of preventing recurrent otitis media in high risk children, such as placement of tympanostomy tubes, should be compared with the risks and benefits of antimicrobial prophylaxis.

Table 5.1. Antimicrobial Chemoprophylaxis[a]

Site-Related Infections	Exposed Host	Vulnerable Host (Pathogen)
Otitis media Urinary tract infection Endocarditis	*Bordetella pertussis* exposure	Oncology patients (*Pneumocystis jirovecii*, fungi)
	Neisseria meningitidis exposure	
	Traveler's diarrhea (*Escherichia coli, Shigella* species, *Salmonella* species)	HIV-infected children; (*P jirovecii*; polysaccharide encapsulated bacteria)
	Perinatal group B *Streptococcus* (mother/infant) exposure	Preterm neonates (*Candida* species)
	Bite wound (human, animal, reptile)	Anatomic or functional asplenia (polysaccharide-encapsulated bacteria)
	Infants born to HIV-infected mothers, to decrease the risk of HIV infection.	Chronic granulomatous disease (*Staphylococcus aureus* and certain other catalase-positive bacteria and fungi)
	Influenza virus, following close family exposure in those unimmunized	
	Susceptible contacts of index cases of invasive *Haemophilus influenzae* type b disease	Congenital immune deficiencies (various pathogens)
	Exposure to aerosolized spores of *Bacillus anthracis*	Rheumatic fever (group A streptococcus)

HIV indicates human immunodeficiency virus.

[a] Prophylactic regimens for exposed hosts and vulnerable hosts (pathogens) are described in each pathogen or disease-specific chapter in Section 3.

Urinary Tract Infection.[1] The role of chemoprophylaxis for urinary tract infection has come under increasing scrutiny. The effectiveness of therapy depends on the rate of emergence of antimicrobial resistance in the gastrointestinal tract flora, which is the usual source of bacteria causing urinary tract infection. Resistance ultimately will develop to any agent used for prophylaxis. Careful consideration of the anatomic abnormalities of the urinary tract, the consequences of recurrent infection, the risks of infection caused by a resistant pathogen, and the anticipated duration of prophylaxis need to be assessed for each child. Data do not support use of antimicrobial prophylaxis to prevent febrile recurrent UTI in infants without vesicoureteral reflux (VUR) or with grade I to IV VUR.[1]

Exposure to Specific Pathogens

Prophylaxis may be appropriate or indicated if an increased risk of serious infection with a specific pathogen exists and a specific antimicrobial agent has been demonstrated to decrease the risk of infection by that pathogen. It is assumed that the benefit of prevention of infection is greater than the risk of adverse effects of the antimicrobial agent or the risk of subsequent infection by antimicrobial-resistant organisms. For some pathogens, such as *Neisseria meningitidis,* that colonize the upper respiratory tract, elimination of the carrier state can be difficult and may require use of a particular antimicrobial agent, such as rifampin, which achieves microbiologically effective concentrations in nasopharyngeal secretions, a property often lacking among antimicrobial agents ordinarily used to treat meningococcal infections.

[1] American Academy of Pediatrics, Subcommittee on Urinary Tract Infections, Steering Committee on Quality Improvement and Management. Urinary tract infection: clinical practice guideline for the diagnosis and management of the initial UTI in febrile infants and children 2 to 24 months. *Pediatrics.* 2011;128(3):595–610

Vulnerable Hosts

Attempts to prevent serious infections in vulnerable patients with antimicrobial prophylaxis have been successful in carefully defined populations that are known to be at risk of infection caused by defined pathogens. In some situations, such as prophylaxis of pneumococcal bacteremia in asplenic children, resistance to beta-lactam agents may lead to decreased effectiveness of continuous prophylaxis. In other situations, such as prophylaxis of *Pneumocystis* infection in immune-compromised children, anti-infective resistance has not appeared to develop despite years of continuous prophylaxis.

....

ANTIMICROBIAL PROPHYLAXIS IN PEDIATRIC SURGICAL PATIENTS

A major use of antimicrobial agents in hospitalized children is for prevention of postoperative wound infections through perioperative prophylaxis, generally for procedures with moderate or high infection rates, such as appendectomy for ruptured appendix, and procedures in which the consequences of infection are likely to be serious, such as procedures involving implantation of prosthetic material. Because of this frequent use, consensus recommendations for prevention of surgical site infections in adults and children have been developed. Although few data exist specifically for pediatric surgical prophylaxis, the principles of antimicrobial agent selection and exposure at the surgical site in adults should apply to children. Consequences of inappropriate prophylactic use of antimicrobial agents include increased costs as a result of unnecessary drug use, potential emergence of resistant organisms, and unnecessary adverse events.

Guidelines for Appropriate Use

Guidelines for prevention of surgical site infections have been published.[1] General principles are presented with the understanding that future studies in children or application to settings unique to infants and children may justify modification of these recommendations.

Indications for Prophylaxis

Systemic prophylaxis is indicated when the probability of postoperative infection is moderate or high, the morbidity of infection is expected to be substantial (including infection of surgically placed prosthetic material), and the benefits of preventing wound infection outweigh potential risks from adverse drug reactions or emergence of resistant organisms. The latter poses a potential risk not only to the recipient but also to other hospitalized patients in whom a health care-associated infection caused by resistant organisms can develop. Major determinants of postoperative surgical site infection include number of microorganisms in the wound during the procedure, virulence of the microorganisms, presence of foreign material in the wound, and host risk factors. The classification of surgical procedures is based on an estimation of bacterial contamination and, thus, risk of subsequent infection. The 4 classes are: (1) clean wounds; (2) clean-contaminated wounds; (3) contaminated wounds; and (4) dirty and infected

---

[1] Antimicrobial prophylaxis for surgery. *Treat Guidel Med Lett.* 2009;7(82):47–52

wounds. Additional independent factors include site of operation, duration of procedure, and patient's preoperative health status. A patient risk index, which incorporates the American Society of Anesthesiologists preoperative physical status assessment score and the duration of the operation, in addition to the aforementioned wound classification, has been demonstrated to be a good predictor of postoperative surgical site infection.[1]

CLEAN WOUNDS

Clean wounds are uninfected operative wounds in which no inflammation is encountered and the respiratory, alimentary, and genitourinary tracts or oropharyngeal cavity is not entered. The operative procedures are elective, and wounds are closed primarily and, if necessary, drained with closed drainage. No break in aseptic technique occurs. Operative incisional wounds that follow nonpenetrating (blunt) abdominal trauma should be included in this category, provided that the surgical procedure does not entail entry into the gastrointestinal or genitourinary tracts. The benefits of systemic antimicrobial prophylaxis do not justify the potential risks associated with antimicrobial use in most clean wound procedures, because the risk of infection is low (1%–2%). Some exceptions exist in which either the risks or consequences of infection are high. Examples are implantation of intravascular prosthetic material (eg, insertion of a prosthetic heart valve) or a prosthetic joint, open-heart surgery for repair of structural defects, body cavity exploration in neonates, and most neurosurgical operations. Prophylaxis generally is given in these circumstances.

CLEAN-CONTAMINATED WOUNDS

In clean-contaminated operative wounds, the respiratory, alimentary, or genitourinary tracts are entered under controlled conditions without significant contamination. Operations involving the gastrointestinal tract, the biliary tract, appendix, vagina, or oropharynx and urgent or emergency surgery in an otherwise clean procedure are included in this category, provided that no evidence of infection is encountered and no major break in aseptic technique occurs. Prophylaxis is limited to procedures in which a substantial amount of wound contamination is expected. The overall risk of infection for the surgical site is 3% to 15%. On the basis of data from adults, procedures for which prophylaxis is indicated for pediatric patients include the following: (1) all gastrointestinal tract procedures in which there is obstruction, when the patient is receiving H_2 receptor antagonists or proton pump blockers, or when the patient has a permanent foreign body; (2) selected biliary tract operations (eg, when there is obstruction from common bile duct stones); and (3) urinary tract surgery or instrumentation in the presence of bacteriuria or obstructive uropathy.

CONTAMINATED WOUNDS

Contaminated wounds are previously sterile tissue sites that are likely to be heavily contaminated with bacteria, and include open, fresh, accidental wounds; operative wounds in the setting of major breaks in aseptic technique or gross spillage from the gastrointestinal tract; exposed viscera at birth from congenital anomalies; penetrating trauma of fewer

[1] Gaynes RP, Culver DH, Horan TC, Edwards JR, Richards C, Tolson JS. Surgical site infection (SSI) rates in the United States, 1992–1998: the National Nosocomial Surveillance System basic SSI risk index. *Clin Infect Dis.* 2001;33(suppl2):S69–S77

than 4 hours duration; and incisions in which acute nonpurulent inflammation is encountered. The estimated rate of infection for the surgical site is 15%. In contaminated wound procedures, antimicrobial prophylaxis is appropriate for some patients with acute nonpurulent inflammation isolated to and contained within an inflamed viscus (such as acute nonperforated appendicitis or cholecystitis). For wounds in which contaminating bacteria have had an opportunity to establish inflammation and ongoing infection, antimicrobial therapy should be considered treatment rather than prophylaxis.

DIRTY AND INFECTED WOUNDS

Dirty and infected wounds include penetrating trauma of more than 4 hours' duration, wounds with retained devitalized tissue, and wounds involving existing clinical infection or perforated viscera. This definition suggests that the organisms causing postoperative infection were present in the operative field before surgery. The estimated rate of infection for the surgical site is 40%. In dirty and infected wound procedures, such as procedures for a perforated abdominal viscus (eg, ruptured appendix), a compound fracture, a laceration attributable to an animal or human bite, or major break in sterile technique, antimicrobial agents are given as treatment rather than prophylaxis.

Timing of Administration of Prophylactic Antimicrobial Agents

Effective prophylaxis occurs only when adequate drug concentrations in tissues are present when bacterial contamination occurs intraoperatively. Administration of an antimicrobial agent within 1 hour or 2 hours (vancomycin) before surgery has been demonstrated to decrease the risk of wound infection. Accordingly, administration of the prophylactic agent is recommended at least 60 minutes before surgical incision to ensure adequate tissue concentrations at the start of the procedure, although with antimicrobial agents requiring longer administration times, such as glycopeptides and aminoglycosides, administration is recommended 120 minutes before the surgery begins.

Duration of Administration of Antimicrobial Agents

A single dose of an antimicrobial agent that provides adequate tissue concentrations throughout the surgical procedure is sufficient. When surgery is prolonged (more than 3 hours), major blood loss occurs, or an antimicrobial agent with a short half-life is used, redosing every 1 to 2 half-lives of the drug should provide adequate antimicrobial concentrations during the procedure. For example, during spinal rod placement, cefazolin may be administered every 3 to 4 hours because of large-volume blood loss. Postoperative doses after closure generally are not recommended.

Recommended Antimicrobial Agents

An antimicrobial agent is chosen on the basis of bacterial pathogens most likely to cause infectious complications after the specific procedure, the antimicrobial susceptibility pattern of these pathogens, and the safety and efficacy of the drug. New, more broad-spectrum and more costly antimicrobial agents generally are not recommended unless prophylactic efficacy has been proven to be superior to drugs of established benefit or there is a shift in organisms causing surgical site infections or in their antimicrobial resistance patterns. Antimicrobial agents administered prophylactically do not have to be active in vitro against every potential organism to be effective, because it is unlikely that all potential organisms are actually contaminating the wound. Doses and routes of administration are determined on the basis of the need to achieve therapeutic blood and tissue concentrations throughout the procedure. Antimicrobial prophylaxis for most surgical procedures (including gastric, biliary, thoracic [noncardiac], vascular, neurosurgical, and orthopedic operations) can be achieved effectively using an agent such as a first-generation cephalosporin (eg, cefazolin) unless the risk for methicillin-resistant *Staphylococcus aureus* (MRSA) infection is high, in which case vancomycin may be indicated. For colorectal surgery or appendectomy, effective prophylaxis requires antimicrobial agents that are active against aerobic and anaerobic intestinal flora. Table 5.2 (p 878) provides recommendations for drugs, including preoperative doses, to be used in children undergoing surgical manipulation or invasive procedures. Physicians should be aware of potential interactions and adverse effects associated with prophylactic antimicrobial agents and other medications the patient may be receiving. Routine use of extended-spectrum cephalosporins for surgical prophylaxis generally is not recommended.

Routine use of vancomycin for prophylaxis is not recommended, although for children known to be colonized or previously infected by MRSA or for children living in a community with a high rate of MRSA infections, vancomycin prophylaxis may be considered.

Special considerations should be given to the patient with congenital heart disease who undergoes surgery. Recommendations are found in Prevention of Bacterial Endocarditis, p 879.

Table 5.2. Recommendations for Preoperative Antimicrobial Prophylaxis[a]

Operation	Likely Pathogens	Recommended Drugs	Preoperative Dose
Neonatal (≤72 h of age)— all major procedures	Group B streptococci, enteric gram-negative bacilli, enterococci	Ampicillin **PLUS**	50 mg/kg
		gentamicin	2.5–3 mg/kg
Neonatal (>72 h of age)— all major procedures	Prophylaxis targeted to colonizing organisms, nosocomial organisms, and operative site		
Cardiac (prosthetic valve or pacemaker)	*Staphylococcus epidermidis, Staphylococcus aureus, Corynebacterium* species, enteric gram-negative bacilli	Cefazolin **OR,**	25 mg/kg
		if MRSA[a] or MRSE is likely, vancomycin	15 mg/kg
Gastrointestinal			
Esophageal and gastroduodenal	Enteric gram-negative bacilli, gram-positive cocci	Cefazolin (high risk only[b])	25 mg/kg
Biliary tract	Enteric gram-negative bacilli, enterococci, clostridia	Cefazolin[c]	25 mg/kg
Colorectal or appendectomy (nonperforated)	Enteric gram-negative bacilli, enterococci, anaerobes	Cefoxitin;	40 mg/kg
		if high risk, gentamicin **PLUS**	2 mg/kg
		clindamycin or	10 mg/kg
		metronidazole ±	10 mg/kg
		ampicillin, **OR**	50 mg/kg
		meropenem	20 mg/kg
Ruptured viscus	Enteric gram-negative bacilli, anaerobes, enterococci	Cefoxitin ±	40 mg/kg
		gentamicin **OR**	2 mg/kg
		gentamicin **PLUS**	2 mg/kg
		clindamycin **OR**	10 mg/kg
		meropenem	20 mg/kg
Genitourinary	Enteric gram-negative bacilli,[d] enterococci	Ampicillin **PLUS**	50 mg/kg
		gentamicin	2 mg/kg

Table 5.2. Recommendations for Preoperative Antimicrobial Prophylaxis,[a] continued

Operation	Likely Pathogens	Recommended Drugs	Preoperative Dose
Head and neck surgery (incision through oral or pharyngeal mucosa)	Anaerobes, enteric gram-negative bacilli, *S aureus*	Gentamicin **PLUS** clindamycin **OR** cefazolin	2 mg/kg 10 mg/kg 25 mg/kg
Neurosurgery (craniotomy, ventricular shunt placement)	*S epidermidis, S aureus*	Cefazolin **OR,** if MRSA or MRSE is likely, vancomycin	25 mg/kg 15 mg/kg
Ophthalmic	*S epidermidis, S aureus, streptococci,* enteric gram-negative bacilli, *Pseudomonas* species	Gentamicin, ciprofloxacin, ofloxacin, moxifloxacin, tobramycin, **OR** neomycin-gramicidin-polymyxin B, **OR** cefazolin	Multiple drops topically for 2–24 h before procedure 100 mg, subconjunctivally
Orthopedic (internal fixation of fractures or prosthetic joints)	*S epidermidis, S aureus*	Cefazolin **OR,** if MRSA or MRSE is likely, vancomycin	25 mg/kg 15 mg/kg
Thoracic (noncardiac)	*S epidermidis, S aureus,* streptococci, gram-negative enteric bacilli[d]	Cefazolin **OR,** if MRSA or MRSE is likely, vancomycin	25 mg/kg 15 mg/kg
Traumatic wound (nonbites)	*S aureus,* group A streptococci, *Clostridium* species	Cefazolin	25 mg/kg

[a]MRSA indicates methicillin-resistant *Staphylococcus aureus;* MRSE indicates methicillin-resistant *S epidermidis.*
[b]Esophageal obstruction, decreased gastric acidity or gastrointestinal motility; morbid obesity.
[c]Acute cholecystitis, nonfunctioning gallbladder, obstructive jaundice, common duct stones.
[d]Selection should be based on the institutional and patient colonization/infection isolate susceptibility patterns.

PREVENTION OF BACTERIAL ENDOCARDITIS

The Committee on Rheumatic Fever, Endocarditis, and Kawasaki Disease of the American Heart Association periodically issues detailed recommendations on the rationale, indications, and antimicrobial regimens for prevention of bacterial endocarditis for people at increased risk. The most recent recommendations were published in 2007.[1] The committee noted that data have cast doubt on benefits of dental prophylaxis, because bacteremia associated with most dental procedures represents only a fraction of bacteremia episodes that occur with daily living, such as brushing teeth, chewing, and other oral hygiene measures. The committee has restricted recommendations for prophylaxis to a narrower group of people who have cardiac abnormalities and for fewer procedures than in the past. Although previous recommendations stressed prophylaxis for people undergoing procedures most likely to produce bacteremia, this revision stresses cardiac conditions in which an episode of infective endocarditis would have high risk of adverse outcome. Furthermore, prophylaxis is recommended only for certain dental procedures. Prophylaxis no longer is recommended solely to prevent endocarditis for procedures involving the gastrointestinal and genitourinary tracts. The cardiac conditions and procedures for which endocarditis prophylaxis is recommended are shown below, and specific prophylactic regimens are shown in Table 5.3 (p 880). Antibiotic prophylaxis is reasonable for these patients who undergo an invasive procedure of the respiratory tract that involves incision of the respiratory tract mucosa. Physicians should consult the published recommendations for further details (**http://circ.ahajournals.org/cgi/content/full/116/15/1736**).

Cardiac conditions associated with the highest risk of adverse outcome from endocarditis for which prophylaxis with dental procedures is reasonable include the following[2]:
- Prosthetic cardiac valve or prosthetic material used for repair of valve.
- Previous infective endocarditis.
- Congenital heart disease (CHD)[2]:
  - Unrepaired cyanotic CHD, including palliative shunts and conduits.
  - Completely repaired congenital heart defect with prosthetic material or device, whether placed by surgery or by catheter intervention, during the first 6 months after the procedure.[3]
  - Repaired CHD with residual defect(s) at the site or adjacent to the site of a prosthetic patch or prosthetic device (which inhibit endothelialization).
- Cardiac transplantation with subsequent cardiac valvulopathy.

Dental procedures for which endocarditis prophylaxis is reasonable for patients listed above include the following:

---

[1] Wilson W, Taubert KA, Gewitz M, et al. Prevention of Infective Endocarditis. Guidelines from the American Heart Association. A Guideline From the American Heart Association Rheumatic Fever, Endocarditis, and Kawasaki Diseases Committee, Council on Cardiovascular Disease in the Young, and the Council on Clinical Cardiology, Council on Cardiovascular Surgery and Anesthesia, and the Quality of Care and Outcomes Research Interdisciplinary Working Group. *Circulation.* 2007;116(15):1736–1754

[2] Except for the conditions listed, antimicrobial prophylaxis no longer is recommended for any other form of CHD.

[3] Prophylaxis is recommended, because endothelialization of prosthetic material occurs within 6 months after the procedure.

Table 5.3. Regimens for Antimicrobial Prophylaxis for a Dental Procedure

| Situation | Agent | Regimen: Single Dose 30 to 60 min Before Procedure | |
		Children	Adults
Oral	Amoxicillin	50 mg/kg	2 g
Unable to take oral medication	Ampicillin	50 mg/kg, IM or IV	2 g, IM or IV
	OR		
	Cefazolin or ceftriaxone	50 mg/kg, IM or IV	1 g, IM or IV
Allergic to penicillins or oral ampicillin	Cephalexin[a,b]	50 mg/kg	2 g
	OR		
	Clindamycin	20 mg/kg	600 mg
	OR		
	Azithromycin or clarithromycin	15 mg/kg	500 mg
Allergic to penicillins or ampicillin and unable to take oral medication	Cefazolin or ceftriaxone[b]	50 mg/kg, IM or IV	1 g, IM or IV
	OR		
	Clindamycin	20 mg/kg, IM or IV	6700 mg, IM or IV

IM, indicates intramuscular; IV, intravenous.
[a] Or other first- or second-generation oral cephalosporin in equivalent pediatric or adult dosage.
[b] Cephalosporins should not be used in a person with a history of anaphylaxis, angioedema, or urticaria with penicillins or ampicillin.

- All dental procedures that involve manipulation of gingival tissue or the periapical region of teeth or perforation of the oral mucosa. The following procedures and events do not require prophylaxis: routine anesthetic injections through noninfected tissue, taking dental radiographs, placement of removable prosthodontic or orthodontic appliances, adjustment of orthodontic appliances, placement of orthodontic brackets, shedding of deciduous teeth, and bleeding from trauma to the lips or oral mucosa.

PREVENTION OF NEONATAL OPHTHALMIA

Ophthalmia neonatorum is defined as conjunctivitis occurring within the first 4 weeks of life. Routine prophylaxis is mandated in most jurisdictions in Canada and the United States. The causes of ophthalmia neonatorum are presented in Table 5.4 (p 881). Neonates with ophthalmia neonatorum require clinical evaluation with appropriate laboratory testing and prompt initiation of therapy. Screening of pregnant women for infection with *Chlamydia trachomatis* and *Neisseria gonorrhoeae* followed by appropriate treatment and follow-up of infected women and their partner(s) is the optimal approach to minimize risk of

Table 5.4. Major and Minor Etiologies in Ophthalmia Neonatorum

Etiology of Ophthalmia Neonatorum	Proportion of Cases	Incubation Period (Days)	Severity of Conjunctivitis[a]	Associated Problems
Chlamydia trachomatis	2%–40%	5–14	+	Pneumonitis 3 wk–3 mo (see Chlamydial Infections, p 272)
Neisseria gonorrhoeae	Less than 1%	2–7	+++	Disseminated infection (see Gonococcal Infections, p 336)
Other bacterial microbes[b]	30%–50%	5–14	+	Variable
Herpes simplex virus	Less than 1%	6–14	+	Disseminated infection, meningoencephalitis (see Herpes Simplex, p 398); keratitis and ulceration also possible
Chemical	Varies with silver nitrate use	1	+	...

[a]+ indicates mild; +++, severe.
[b]Includes skin, respiratory, vaginal and gastrointestinal tract pathogens such as *Staphylococcus aureus*; *Streptococcus pneumoniae*; *Haemophilus influenzae*, nontypeable; group A and B streptococci; *Corynebacterium* species; *Moraxella catarrhalis*; *Escherichia coli*; *Klebsiella pneumoniae*; *Pseudomonas aeruginosa*.

intrapartum transmission of these agents (see Chlamydial Infections, p 272, and Gonococcal Infections, p 336). In addition, a prophylactic agent should be in instilled into the eyes of all newborn infants, including infants born by cesarean delivery. Although infections usually are transmitted during passage through the birth canal; ascending infection can occur.

Three agents are licensed for neonatal ocular prophylaxis in the United States: 1% silver nitrate solution, 0.5% erythromycin ointment, and 1% tetracycline ophthalmic ointment or suspension. However, only 0.5% erythromycin ointment is available commercially in the United States. Although all 3 agents are effective against gonococcus, none prevents transmission of *C trachomatis* from mother to infant.

Gonococcal Ophthalmia

For newborn infants, 0.5% erythromycin ointment or 1% tetracycline ophthalmic ointment, if administered properly, are considered equally effective for prophylaxis of ocular gonorrheal infection. The single-dose formulation is recommended. Povidone-iodine in a 2.5% solution also can be useful, but a product for this purpose is not available in the United States. Healthy infants born to women with untreated gonococcal infection should receive 1 dose of ceftriaxone (25–50 mg/kg, intravenously [IV] or intramuscularly [IM], not to exceed 125 mg) or 1 dose of cefotaxime (100 mg/kg, IV or IM). Topical antimicrobial therapy alone is inadequate for *N gonorrhoeae*-exposed or infected infants and is not necessary when systemic antimicrobial therapy is administered. Infants who have gonococcal ophthalmia should be hospitalized, evaluated for disseminated infection, and treated (see Gonococcal Infections, p 336). Frequent eye irrigations with saline solution should be performed until resolution of the discharge.

Chlamydial Ophthalmia

Neonatal ophthalmia attributable to *Chlamydia trachomatis* is not as clinically severe as gonococcal conjunctivitis. Chlamydial conjunctivitis in the neonate is characterized by a mucopurulent discharge, eyelid swelling, a propensity to form membranes on the palpebral conjunctiva, and lack of a follicular response. Treatment is 14 days of oral antimicrobial agent (see Chlamydial Infections, p 272). Topical therapy is unnecessary and does not prevent development of chlamydial pneumonia (see Chlamydial Infections, p 272).

Nongonococcal, Nonchlamydial Ophthalmia

Neonatal ophthalmia can be caused by many different bacterial pathogens (see Table 5.4, p 881). Silver nitrate, povidone-iodine, and erythromycin are effective for preventing nongonococcal, nonchlamydial conjunctivitis during the first 2 weeks of life.

Administration of Neonatal Ophthalmic Prophylaxis

Before administering local prophylaxis, each eyelid should be wiped gently with sterile cotton. Two drops of a 1% silver nitrate solution or a 1-cm ribbon of antimicrobial ointment (0.5% erythromycin or 1% tetracycline) is placed in each lower conjunctival sac. The eyelids then should be massaged gently to spread the ointment. After 1 minute, ointment may be wiped away with sterile cotton. None of the prophylactic agents should be flushed from the eyes after instillation, because flushing can decrease efficacy.

Prophylaxis should be given shortly after birth. Efficacy is unlikely to be influenced by delaying prophylaxis for as long as 1 hour to facilitate parent-infant bonding. Longer delays have not been studied for efficacy. Hospitals should establish a process to ensure that infants are given prophylaxis appropriately.

....
APPENDIX I

Directory of Resources[a]

Organization	Telephone/Fax Number	Website
AIDSinfo PO Box 6303 Rockville, MD 20849-6303 USA	1-800-HIV-0440 (1-800-448-0440, USA and Canada) 1-301-519-0459 (International) TTY: 1-888-480-3739 Fax: 1-301-315-2818; Outside United States: 1-301-315-2816	www.aidsinfo.nih.gov
American Academy of Pediatrics (AAP) 141 Northwest Point Blvd Elk Grove Village, IL 60007-1098 USA	1-847-434-4000 or 1-800-433-9016 Fax: 1-847-434-8000 Publications/Customer Service: 1-866-THEAAP1 (1-866-843-2271)	www.aap.org
American Social Health Association	1-800-227-8922	www.ashastd.org
Canadian Paediatric Society (CPS) 2305 St Laurent Blvd Ottawa, Ontario K1G 4J8 Canada	1-613-526-9397 Fax: 1-613-526-3332	www.cps.ca
Centers for Disease Control and Prevention (CDC)[b] 1600 Clifton Rd Atlanta, GA 30333	1-404-639-3311	www.cdc.gov
• **24-Hour Service**		
• Advisory Committee on Immunization Practices	1-404-639-2888	www.cdc.gov/vaccines/recs/ACIP
• Botulism case consultation and antitoxin	1-404-639-8836	
• Division of Foodborne, Waterborne, and Environmental Diseases	1-770-488-7100 1-404-639-1603	www.cdc.gov/ncezid/dfwed/
• Division of Parasitic Diseases	1-770-488-7775 OR 1-770-488-7760	www.cdc.gov/parasites
• Division of Tuberculosis Elimination	1-404-639-8120	www.cdc.gov/tb

Directory of Resources,[a] continued

Organization	Telephone/Fax Number	Website
Centers for Disease Control and Prevention (CDC),[b] continued		
• Division of Vector-Borne Infectious Diseases	1-970-221-6400	www.cdc.gov/ncidod/dvbid/index.htm
• Division of Viral Hepatitis	1-888-4-HEP-CDC (1-888-443-7232)	www.cdc.gov/ncidod/diseases/hepatitis
• Division of High-Consequence Pathogens and Pathology	1-404-639-3574	www.cdc.gov/ncezid/dhcpp/
• Contact Center	1-800-CDC-INFO (1-800-232-4636)	www.cdc.gov/netinfo.htm
• Drug Service (weekdays, 8 AM to 4:30 PM ET)	1-404-639-3670	www.cdc.gov/ncezid/dsr/office-director. html#drugservice
• Drug Service (weekends, nights, holidays)	1-404-639-2888	www.cdc.gov/ncezid/dsr/office-director. html#drugservice
• Immunization, Infectious Diseases, and Other Health Information—Voice Information System	1-800-232-SHOT (1-800-232-7468)	
• Vaccines and Immunizations Web Site		www.cdc.gov/vaccines
• Influenza (seasonal) materials		www.cdc.gov/flu
• Malaria Hotline	1-770-488-7788	www.cdc.gov/malaria
• National Center for Immunization and Respiratory Diseases	1-404-639-8200 English Hotline: 1-800-232-4636 Spanish Hotline: 1-800-232-0233 Fax: 1-888-CDC-FAXX (1-888-232-3299)	www.cdc.gov/ncird/index.html
• National Prevention Information Network	1-800-458-5231	www.cdcnpin.org
• Public Inquiries	1-404-639-3534	
• Publications	1-800-232-2522 Fax: 1-404-639-8828	www.cdc.gov/publications.htm#pubs
• Traveler's Health Hotline and Fax	1-877-FYI-TRIP (877-394-8747) Fax (toll free): 1-888-232-3299	www.cdc.gov/travel
• Vaccine Information Statements		www.cdc.gov/vaccines/pubs/vis/default.htm

Directory of Resources,[a] continued

Organization	Telephone/Fax Number	Website
Centers for Disease Control and Prevention (CDC),[b] continued		
• VFC Operations Guide		www.cdc.gov/vaccines/programs/vfc/operations-guide.htm
• Voice/Fax Information Service (including international travel and immunization)	1-404-332-4555 Fax: 1-404-332-4565	www.cdc.gov/travel
Food and Drug Administration (FDA) 5600 Fishers Ln Rockville, MD 20857-0001	1-888-463-6332	www.fda.gov
• Center for Biologics Evaluation and Research	1-301-827-2000 or 1-800-835-4709	www.fda.gov/cber
• Center for Drug Evaluation and Research	1-301-827-4570	www.fda.gov/cder
• Division of Special Pathogen and Immunologic Drug Products	1-301-796-1600 Fax: 1-301-827-2475	
• HIV/AIDS Office of Special Health Issues	1-301-827-4460	www.fda.gov/oashi/aids/hiv.html
• Vaccines, Blood, and Biologics		www.fda.gov/BiologicsBloodVaccines/default.htm
• MedWatch	1-800-FDA-1088 (1-800-332-1088) Fax: 1-800-FDA-0178 (1-800-332-0178)	www.fda.gov/medwatch
• Vaccine Adverse Event Reporting System (VAERS)	1-800-822-7967	www.fda.gov/cber/vaers/vaers.htm
Immunization Action Coalition (IAC) 1573 Selby Ave, Ste 234 St Paul, MN 5510	1-651-647-9009 Fax: 1-651-647-9131	www.immunize.org

Directory of Resources,[a] continued

Organization	Telephone/Fax Number	Website
Infectious Diseases Society of America (IDSA) 1300 Wilson Blvd, Suite 300 Alexandria, VA 22209	1-703-299-0200 Fax: 1-703-299-0204	www.idsociety.org
Institute of Medicine (IOM) The National Academies 500 Fifth St, NW Washington, DC 20001	1-202-334-2352	www.iom.edu
National Institutes of Health (NIH) 9000 Rockville Pike Bethesda, MD 20892	1-301-496-4000	www.nih.gov
• National Institute of Allergy and Infectious Diseases (NIAID)	1-301-496-5717 or toll-free: 1-866-284-4107	www.niaid.nih.gov
• AIDS Therapies Research Guide	1-205-934-5316	www.niaid.nih.gov/daids/pdatguide/casg.htm
National Library of Medicine 8600 Rockville Pike Bethesda, MD 20894	1-888-346-3656	www.nlm.nih.gov
National Network for Immunization Information (NNii) 301 University Blvd Galveston, TX 77555-0350	1-703-299-0789 Fax: 1-409-772-5208	www.immunizationinfo.org
National Vaccine Injury Compensation Program (for information on filing claims)	1-800-338-2382	www.hrsa.gov/vaccinecompensation/index.html
National Vaccine Program Office (NVPO) Room 715-H 200 Independence Avenue, SW Washington, DC 20201	1-202-690-5566	www.hhs.gov/nvpo/

Directory of Resources,[a] continued

Organization	Telephone/Fax Number	Website
Pediatric Branch, National Cancer Institute	1-301-496-4345	http://pediatrics.cancer.gov
Pediatric Infectious Diseases Society 1300 Wilson Blvd, Suite 300 Arlington, VA 22209	1-703-299-6764 Fax: 1-703-299-0473	www.pids.org
Women, Children, and HIV		www.womenchildrenhiv.org/
World Health Organization (WHO) Avenue Appia 20 1211 Geneva 27 Switzerland	(+41 22) 791 21 11 Fax: (+41 22) 791 31 11	www.who.int

[a] Internet addresses and telephone/fax numbers are current at the time of publication.
[b] See Appendix XIII for services of the CDC or visit **www.cdc.gov.**

APPENDIX II

FDA Licensure Dates of Selected Vaccines in the United States[a]

Vaccine	Year Licensed
Diphtheria and tetanus toxoids and acellular pertussis (DTaP)	1991
Diphtheria and tetanus toxoids and whole-cell pertussis (DTP)	1970
Diphtheria and tetanus toxoids for children 7 y of age or older and adults (Td)	1953
Diphtheria and tetanus toxoids for children younger than 7 y of age (DT)	1970
DTaP-HepB-IPV (Pediarix)	2002
DTaP/Hib (TriHIBit)	1996
DTaP-IPV (Kinrix)	2008
DTaP-IPV/Hib (Pentacel)	2008
Haemophilus influenzae type b (Hib)	
Polysaccharide	1985
Conjugate (15 mo of age or older)	1987
Conjugate (6 wk of age or older)	1990
Hepatitis A (HepA)	1995
Hepatitis B (HepB)	
Plasma-derived	1981
Recombinant	1986
HepA-HepB (Twinrix)	2001
Hib/HepB (Comvax)	1996
Human papillomavirus (HPV4) (Gardasil)	2006
Human papillomavirus (HPV2) (Cervarix)	2009
Influenza	
Inactivated (TIV)[b]	1945
Live, intranasal (LAIV)	2003
High dose	2010
Intradermal	2011
LAIV, quadrivalent	2012
Meningococcal	
Polysaccharide (quadrivalent) (MPSV4)	1978
Conjugate (quadrivalent) (MCV4-D)	2005
Conjugate (quadrivalent) (MCV4-CRM)	2010
Measles-mumps-rubella (MMR)	1971
Measles-mumps-rubella-varicella (MMRV) (ProQuad)	2005
Pneumococcal	
Polysaccharide (14-valent)	1977
Polysaccharide (23-valent) (PPSV23)	1983
Conjugate (13-valent) (PCV13)	2010

FDA Licensure Dates of Selected Vaccines in the United States,[a] continued

Vaccine	Year Licensed
Poliomyelitis	
Inactivated (IPV)	1987
Oral (trivalent) (OPV)	1963
Rabies	1980
Rotavirus (RV5) (RotaTeq)	2006
Rotavirus (RV1) (Rotarix)	2008
Tetanus toxoid, reduced diphtheria toxoid, and acellular pertussis (Tdap)	
Boostrix	2005
Adacel	2005
Tetanus (TT)	1943
Varicella (VAR)	1995
Zoster (ZOS)	2006

[a]The US Food and Drug Administration (FDA) maintains and updates a Web site listing vaccines licensed for immunization in the United States (**www.fda.gov/cber/vaccine/licvacc.htm**).
[b]Additional vaccines licensed subsequently.

ICD-9-CM Codes for Commonly Administered Pediatric Vaccines/Toxoids and Immune Globulins

Immune Globulin	Separately report the administration with code 96372	Manufacturer	Brand	ICD-9-CM[a]
90375	Rabies immune globulin (RIG), human, for intramuscular and/or subcutaneous use	Novartis	HyperRAB S/D	V04.5[b]
90376	Rabies immune globulin, heat treated (RIG-HT), human, for intramuscular and/or subcutaneous use	Sanofi Pasteur	IMOGAM Rabies-HT	V04.5[b]
90378	Respiratory syncytial virus immune globulin (RSV-IGIM), for intramuscular use, 50 mg, each	MedImmune	Synagis	V04.82

Vaccine	Separately report the administration with codes 90460–90461 or 90471–90474 [Please see table below]	Manufacturer	Brand	ICD-9-CM[a]	Number of Vaccine Components
90633	Hepatitis A vaccine, pediatric/adolescent dosage, 2 doses, for intramuscular use	GlaxoSmithKline Merck	HAVRIX VAQTA	V05.3	1
90634	Hepatitis A vaccine, pediatric/adolescent dosage, 3 doses, for intramuscular use	GlaxoSmithKline	HAVRIX	V05.3	1
90636	Hepatitis A and hepatitis B vaccine (HepA-HepB), adult dosage, for intramuscular use	GlaxoSmithKline	TWINRIX	V05.3	2
90644	Meningococcal conjugate vaccine, serogroups C & Y and *Haemophilus influenzae* type b (Hib) vaccine, tetanus toxoid conjugate (Hib-MenCY-TT), 4-dose schedule, when administered to children 2-15 months of age, for intramuscular use	GlaxoSmithKline	MenHibrix	V06.8	2
90647	*Haemophilus influenzae* type b vaccine (Hib), PRP-OMP conjugate, 3 doses, for intramuscular use	Merck	PedvaxHIB	V03.81	1
90648	*Haemophilus influenzae* type b vaccine (Hib), PRP-T conjugate, 4 doses, for intramuscular use	Sanofi Pasteur GlaxoSmithKline	ActHIB HIBERIX	V03.81	1

Commonly Administered Pediatric Vaccines/Toxoids and Immune Globulins, continued

Vaccine	Separately report the administration with codes 90460–90461 or 90471–90474 [Please see table below]	Manufacturer	Brand	ICD-9-CM[a]	Number of Vaccine Components
90649	Human papillomavirus (HPV) vaccine, types 6, 11, 16, 18 (quadrivalent), 3-dose schedule, for intramuscular use	Merck	GARDASIL	V04.89	1
90650	Human papillomavirus (HPV) vaccine, types 16 and 18, bivalent, 3-dose schedule, for intramuscular use	GlaxoSmithKline	CERVARIX	V04.89	1
90655	Influenza virus vaccine, split virus, preservative free, for children 6–35 months of age, for intramuscular use	Merck Sanofi Pasteur	AFLURIA Fluzone No Preservative Pediatric	V04.81	1
90656	Influenza virus vaccine, split virus, preservative free, when administered to 3 years of age and above, for intramuscular use	Merck Novartis Sanofi Pasteur Novatis GlaxoSmithKline	AFLURIA Agriflu Fluzone No Preservative Fluvirin FLUARIX	V04.81	1
90657	Influenza virus vaccine, split virus, 6–35 months dosage, for intramuscular use	Merck Sanofi Pasteur	AFLURIA Fluzone	V04.81	1
90658	Influenza virus vaccine, split virus, 3 years and older dosage, for intramuscular use	Merck Sanofi Pasteur Novartis	AFLURIA Fluzone Fluvirin	V04.81	1
90660	Influenza virus vaccine, live, intranasal use	MedImmune	FluMist	V04.81	1
90670	Pneumococcal conjugate vaccine, 13-valent, for intramuscular use	Pfizer	PREVNAR 13	V03.82	1
90675	Rabies vaccine, for intramuscular use	Sanofi Pasteur Novartis	IMOVAX RabAvert	V04.5[b]	1
90680	Rotavirus vaccine, pentavalent, 3-dose schedule, live, for oral use	Merck	RotaTeq	V04.89	1

Commonly Administered Pediatric Vaccines/Toxoids and Immune Globulins, continued

Vaccine	Separately report the administration with codes 90460–90461 or 90471–90474 [Please see table below]	Manufacturer	Brand	ICD-9-CM[a]	Number of Vaccine Components
90681	Rotavirus vaccine, human, attenuated, 2-dose schedule, live, for oral use	GlaxoSmithKline	ROTARIX	V04.89	1
90696	Diphtheria, tetanus toxoids, and acellular pertussis vaccine and poliovirus vaccine, inactivated (DTaP-IPV), when administered to children 4 years through 6 years of age, for intramuscular use	GlaxoSmithKline	KINRIX	V06.3	4
90698	Diphtheria, tetanus toxoids, acellular pertussis vaccine, *Haemophilus influenzae* type b (Hib), and poliovirus vaccine, inactivated (DTaP-Hib-IPV), for intramuscular use	Sanofi Pasteur	Pentacel	V06.8	5
90700	Diphtheria, tetanus toxoids, and acellular pertussis vaccine (DTaP), when administered to children younger than 7 years, for intramuscular use	Sanofi Pasteur Sanofi Pasteur GlaxoSmithKline	DAPTACEL Tripedia INFANRIX	V06.1	3
90702	Diphtheria and tetanus toxoids (DT), adsorbed when administered to children younger than 7 years, for intramuscular use	Sanofi Pasteur	Diphtheria and Tetanus Toxoids Adsorbed	V06.5	2
90707	Measles, mumps, and rubella virus vaccine (MMR), live, for subcutaneous use	Merck	M-M-R II	V06.4	3
90710	Measles, mumps, rubella, and varicella vaccine (MMRV), live, for subcutaneous use	Merck	ProQuad	V06.8	4
90713	Poliovirus vaccine (IPV), inactivated, for subcutaneous or intramuscular use	Sanofi Pasteur	IPOL	V04.0	1
90714	Tetanus and diphtheria toxoids (Td) adsorbed, preservative free, when administered to people 7 years or older, for intramuscular use	Sanofi Pasteur	DECAVAC	V06.5	2

Commonly Administered Pediatric Vaccines/Toxoids and Immune Globulins, continued

Vaccine	Separately report the administration with codes 90460–90461 or 90471–90474 [Please see table below]	Manufacturer	Brand	ICD-9-CM[a]	Number of Vaccine Components
90715	Tetanus, diphtheria toxoids and acellular pertussis vaccine (Tdap), when administered to people 7 years or older, for intramuscular use	Sanofi Pasteur GlaxoSmithKline	ADACEL BOOSTRIX	V06.1	3
90716	Varicella virus vaccine, live, for subcutaneous use	Merck	VARIVAX	V05.4	1
90718	Tetanus and diphtheria toxoids (Td) adsorbed when administered to people 7 years or older, for intramuscular use	Sanofi Pasteur	Tetanus and Diphtheria Toxoids Adsorbed for Adult Use	V06.5	2
90721	Diphtheria, tetanus toxoids, and acellular pertussis vaccine and *Haemophilus influenzae* type b (Hib) vaccine (DTaP-Hib)	Sanofi Pasteur	TriHIBit	V06.8	4
90723	Diphtheria, tetanus toxoids, acellular pertussis vaccine, Hepatitis B, and poliovirus vaccine (DTaP-Hep B-IPV), for intramuscular use	GlaxoSmithKline	PEDIARIX	V06.8	5
90732	Pneumococcal polysaccharide vaccine, 23-valent, adult or immunosuppressed patient dosage, when administered to people 2 years or older, for subcutaneous or intramuscular use	Merck	PNEUMOVAX 23	V03.82	1
90733	Meningococcal polysaccharide vaccine, for subcutaneous use	Sanofi Pasteur	Menomune	V03.89	1
90734	Meningococcal conjugate vaccine, serogroups A, C, Y and W-135 (tetravalent), for intramuscular use	Sanofi Pasteur Novartis	Menactra Menveo	V03.89	1
90740	Hepatitis B vaccine, dialysis or immunosuppressed patient dosage, 3 doses, for intramuscular use	Merck	RECOMBIVAX HB	V05.3	1
90743	Hepatitis B vaccine, adolescent, 2 doses, for intramuscular use	Merck	RECOMBIVAX HB	V05.3	1

Commonly Administered Pediatric Vaccines/Toxoids and Immune Globulins, continued

Vaccine	Separately report the administration with codes 90460–90461 or 90471–90474 [Please see table below]	Manufacturer	Brand	ICD-9-CM^a	Number of Vaccine Components
90744	Hepatitis B, pediatric/adolescent dosage, 3 doses, for intramuscular use	Merck GlaxoSmithKline	RECOMBIVAX HB ENERGIX-B	V05.3	1
90746	Hepatitis B vaccine, adult dosage, for intramuscular use	Merck GlaxoSmithKline	RECOMBIVAX HB ENERGIX-B	V05.3	1
90747	Hepatitis B vaccine, dialysis or immunosuppressed patient dosage, 4 doses, for intramuscular use	GlaxoSmithKline	ENERGIX-B	V05.3	1
90748	Hepatitis B and *Haemophilus influenzae* type b (Hib) (Hep B-Hib), for intramuscular use	Merck	COMVAX	V06.8	2
90749	Unlisted vaccine or toxoid	Please	See	ICD	Manual

Immunization Administration Codes

Immunization Administration Through Age 18 With Counseling

90460	Immunization administration through 18 years of age via any route of administration, with counseling by physician or other qualified health care professional; first vaccine/toxoid component				
90461	Immunization administration through 18 years of age via any route of administration, with counseling by physician or other qualified health care professional; each additional vaccine/toxoid component				

Immunization Administration

90471	Immunization administration, one vaccine				
90472	Immunization administration, each additional vaccine				
90473	Immunization administration by intranasal/oral route; one vaccine				
90474	Immunization administration by intranasal/oral route; each additional vaccine				

^aICD-9-CM guidelines indicate that immunizations administered as part of a routine well baby or child check should be reported with code V20.2. The codes listed above can be reported in addition to the V20.2 code if specific payers request them. Immunizations administered in encounters **other than those for a routine well baby or child check** should be reported only with the codes listed above.

^bFor rabies reporting, it is important to also include the ICD-9-CM codes to describe the injuries and the E code for the animal.

^Vaccine pending FDA approval **(http://www.ama-assn.org/ama/pub/category/10902.html).**

Developed and maintained by the American Academy of Pediatrics. For reporting purposes only.

Appendix IV. Selected Vaccine Safety Resources

Selected Vaccine Safety Resources

Resource	Description	Reference
Government		
Vaccine information statement (VIS); Centers for Disease Control and Prevention (CDC)	Patient information sheet with information about benefits and possible risks of a vaccine, and information on reporting to VAERS. The National Childhood Vaccine Injury Act (NCVIA) requires that all health care professionals give parents or patients copies of VISs before administering each dose of the vaccines covered by the Act.	Appendix I, p 883, and Appendix V, p 897 Copies of VISs are available at **www.cdc. gov/vaccines/pubs/vis/default. htm.**
CDC vaccine safety information	Web site with information about vaccine safety and vaccine safety monitoring, research, and resources	**www.cdc.gov/vaccinesafety/index. html**
CDC Advisory Committee on Immunization Practices (ACIP) statements	Recommendations on vaccine use include summary of vaccine safety for vaccines for children and adults	**www.cdc.gov/vaccines/recs/acip**
Food and Drug Administration (FDA)	FDA is responsible for ensuring the safety and efficacy of biologic products; concerns about vaccine lots should be reported to the FDA	Appendix I, p 883 **www.fda.gov/BiologicsBloodVaccines/ default.htm** 800-835-4709
Vaccine Package Insert	Vaccine package inserts are detailed documents for health care professionals, produced by vaccine manufacturers and FDA Center for Biologics Evaluation and Research (CBER)	**www.fda.gov/BiologicsBlood Vaccines/Vaccines/Approved Products/ucm093830.htm**

Selected Vaccine Safety Resources, continued

Resource	Description	Reference
Vaccine Adverse Event Reporting System (VAERS)	Voluntary national vaccine safety surveillance program, coadministered by the CDC and FDA. Health care professionals are mandated to report specific adverse events after vaccination, listed in the VAERS Table of Reportable Events. In addition, health care professionals should report any clinically significant adverse event following immunization even if they are not certain the vaccine caused the event.	See p 45–47 and **http://vaers.hhs.gov/ resources/VAERS_Table_of_ Reportable_Events_Following_ Vaccination.pdf**
National Vaccine Injury Compensation Program (VICP)	The VICP provides a forum for people found to be injured by certain vaccines. Health care professionals may refer patients who believe they have been injured by vaccines.	See Appendix V, p 897 **www.hrsa.gov/vaccinecompensation**
National Vaccine Program Office (NVPO)	The NVPO is responsible for coordinating and ensuring collaboration among the many federal agencies involved in vaccine and immunization activities. The NVPO provides leadership and coordination to carry out the national vaccine plan.	**www.hhs.gov/NVPO/**

APPENDIX V

National Childhood Vaccine Injury Act Reporting and Compensation Tables[a]

Vaccine	Adverse Event and Interval From Vaccination to Onset of Event	
	For Reporting[b]	For Compensation[c]
I. Tetanus toxoid-containing vaccines in any combination (eg, DTaP, DTaP-IPV, DTaP-IPV/Hib, DTP, DTP-Hib, Tdap, DT, Td, or TT)	A. Anaphylaxis or anaphylactic shock **(7 days)** B. Brachial neuritis **(28 days)** C. Any acute complication or sequela, including death, of above events that occurred within the time period prescribed **(No applicable time interval)** D. Events described in manufacturer's package insert as contraindications to the vaccine **(See package insert)**	A. Anaphylaxis or anaphylactic shock **(4 hours)** B. Brachial neuritis **(2–28 days)** C. Any acute complication or sequela, including death, of above events that occurred within the time period prescribed **(No applicable time interval)**
II. Pertussis antigen-containing vaccines in any combination (eg, DTaP, DTaP-IPV, DTaP-IPV/Hib, DTP, P, DTP-Hib)	A. Anaphylaxis or anaphylactic shock **(7 days)** B. Encephalopathy or encephalitis **(7 days)** C. Any acute complication or sequela, including death, of above events that occurred within the time period prescribed **(No applicable time interval)** D. Events described in manufacturer's package insert as contraindications to the vaccine **(See package insert)**	A. Anaphylaxis or anaphylactic shock **(4 hours)** B. Encephalopathy or encephalitis **(72 hours)** C. Any acute complication or sequela, including death, of above events that occurred within the time period prescribed **(No applicable time interval)**
III. Measles, mumps, and rubella virus-containing vaccines in any combination (eg, MMR, MMRV, MR, M, R)	A. Anaphylaxis or anaphylactic shock **(7 days)** B. Encephalopathy or encephalitis **(15 days)** C. Any acute complication or sequela, including death, of above events that occurred within the time period prescribed **(No applicable time interval)** D. Events described in manufacturer's package insert as contraindications to the vaccine **(See package insert)**	A. Anaphylaxis or anaphylactic shock **(4 hours)** B. Encephalopathy or encephalitis **(5–15 days)** C. Any acute complication or sequela, including death, of above events that occurred within the time period prescribed **(No applicable time interval)**

National Childhood Vaccine Injury Act Reporting and Compensation Tables,[a] continued

Vaccine	Adverse Event and Interval From Vaccination to Onset of Event	
	For Reporting[b]	For Compensation[c]
IV. Rubella virus-containing vaccines in any combination (eg, MMR, MMRV, MR, R)	A. Chronic arthritis (**42 days**) B. Any acute complication or sequela, including death, of above event that occurred within the time period prescribed (**No applicable time interval**) C. Events described in manufacturer's package insert as contraindications to the vaccine (**See package insert**)	A. Chronic arthritis (**7–42 days**) B. Any acute complication or sequela, including death, of above event that occurred within the time period prescribed (**No applicable time interval**)
V. Measles virus-containing vaccines in any combination (eg, MMR, MMRV, MR, M)	A. Thrombocytopenic purpura (**30 days**) B. Vaccine-strain measles viral infection in an immunodeficient recipient (**6 months**) C. Any acute complication or sequela, including death, of above events that occurred within the time period prescribed (**No applicable time interval**) D. Events described in manufacturer's package insert as contraindications to the vaccine (**See package insert**)	A. Thrombocytopenic purpura (**7–30 days**) B. Vaccine-strain measles viral infection in an immunodeficient recipient (**6 months**) C. Any acute complication or sequela, including death, of above events that occurred within the time period prescribed (**No applicable time interval**)

National Childhood Vaccine Injury Act Reporting and Compensation Tables,[a] continued

Vaccine	Adverse Event and Interval From Vaccination to Onset of Event	
	For Reporting[b]	For Compensation[c]
VI. Polio live virus–containing vaccines (eg, OPV)	A. Paralytic polio — in a nonimmunodeficient recipient **(30 days)** — in an immunodeficient recipient **(6 months)** — in a vaccine-associated community case **(No applicable time interval)** B. Vaccine-strain polio viral infection — in a nonimmunodeficient recipient **(30 days)** — in an immunodeficient recipient **(6 months)** — in a vaccine-associated community case **(No applicable time interval)** C. Any acute complication or sequela, including death, of above events that occurred within the time period prescribed **(No applicable time interval)** D. Events described in manufacturer's package insert as contraindications to the vaccine **(See package insert)**	A. Paralytic polio — in a nonimmunodeficient recipient **(30 days)** — in an immunodeficient recipient **(6 months)** — in a vaccine-associated community case **(No applicable time interval)** B. Vaccine-strain polio viral infection — in a nonimmunodeficient recipient **(30 days)** — in an immunodeficient recipient **(6 months)** — in a vaccine-associated community case **(No applicable time interval)** C. Any acute complication or sequela, including death, of above events that occurred within the time period prescribed **(No applicable time interval)**
VII. Polio inactivated-virus containing vaccines in any combination (eg, IPV, DTaP-IPV, DTaP-IPV/Hib)	A. Anaphylaxis or anaphylactic shock **(7 days)** B. Any acute complication or sequela, including death, of above event that occurred within the time period prescribed **(No applicable time interval)** C. Events described in manufacturer's package insert as contraindications to the vaccine **(See package insert)**	A. Anaphylaxis or anaphylactic shock **(0-4 hours)** B. Any acute complication or sequela, including death, of above event that occurred within the time period prescribed **(No applicable time interval)**

National Childhood Vaccine Injury Act Reporting and Compensation Tables,[a] continued

Vaccine	Adverse Event and Interval From Vaccination to Onset of Event	
	For Reporting[b]	For Compensation[c]
VIII. Hepatitis B antigen- containing vaccines in any combination (eg, HBV, HAV-HBV)	A. Anaphylaxis or anaphylactic shock (7 days) B. Any acute complication or sequela, including death, of above event that occurred within the time period prescribed (No applicable time interval) C. Events described in manufacturer's package insert as contraindications to the vaccine (See package insert)	A. Anaphylaxis or anaphylactic shock (0–4 hours) B. Any acute complication or sequela, including death, of above event that occurred within the time period prescribed (No applicable time interval)
IX. *Haemophilus influenzae* type b (conjugate vaccines) in any combination (eg, Hib, DTaP-IPV/Hib)	Events described in manufacturer's package insert as contraindications to the vaccine (See package insert)	No condition specified for compensation
X. Varicella vaccine in any combination (eg, VZV, MMRV)	Events described in manufacturer's package insert as contraindications to the vaccine (See package insert)	No condition specified for compensation
XI. Rotavirus vaccine	Events described in manufacturer's package insert as contraindications to the vaccine (See package insert)	No condition specified for compensation
XII. Pneumococcal conjugate vaccines (eg, PCV7, PCV13)	Events described in manufacturer's package insert as contraindications to the vaccine (See package insert)	No condition specified for compensation
XIII. Hepatitis A vaccine in any combination (eg, HAV, HAV-HBV)	Events described in manufacturer's package insert as contraindications to the vaccine (See package insert)	No condition specified for compensation
XIV. Trivalent influenza vaccine (eg, TIV, LAIV)	Events described in manufacturer's package insert as contraindications to the vaccine (See package insert)	No condition specified for compensation

National Childhood Vaccine Injury Act Reporting and Compensation Tables,ᵃ continued

Vaccine	Adverse Event and Interval From Vaccination to Onset of Event	
	For Reportingᵇ	For Compensationᶜ
XV. Meningococcal vaccine (eg, MCV4, MPSV4)	Events described in manufacturer's package insert as contraindications to the vaccine **(See package insert)**	No condition specified for compensation
XVI. Human papillomavirus vaccine (eg, HPV4, HPV2)	Events described in manufacturer's package insert as contraindications to the vaccine **(See package insert)**	No condition specified for compensation
XVII. Any new vaccine recommended by the Centers for Disease Control and Prevention for routine administration to children, after publication by Secretary, HHS of a notice of coverage.	Events described in manufacturer's package insert as contraindications to the vaccine **(See package insert)**	No condition specified for compensation

DTaP indicates diphtheria and tetanus toxoids and acellular pertussis vaccine; IPV, inactivated poliovirus vaccine; Hib, *Haemophilus influenzae* type b vaccine; DTP, diphtheria and tetanus toxoids and pertussis; Tdap, tetanus and diphtheria toxoids and pertussis vaccine for adolescent/adult use; DT, diphtheria and tetanus toxoids vaccine; Td, tetanus and diphtheria toxoids vaccine for adolescent/adult use; TT, tetanus toxoid vaccine; MMR, measles-mumps-rubella vaccine; MMRV, measles-mumps-rubella-varicella vaccine; MR, measles-rubella vaccine; M, measles vaccine; R, rubella vaccine; OPV, oral poliovirus vaccine; HBV, hepatitis B virus vaccine; HAV, hepatitis A virus vaccine; VZV, varicella-zoster virus vaccine; PCV, pneumococcal conjugate vaccine; TIV, trivalent inactivated influenza vaccine; LAIV, live-attenuated influenza vaccine; MCV, meningococcal conjugate vaccine; MPSV, meningococcal polysaccharide vaccine; HPV, quadrivalent or bivalent human papillomavirus vaccines; HHS, Health and Human Services.

ᵃ **Effective date July 22, 2011.**

ᵇ Taken from the Reportable Events Table (RET), which lists conditions reportable by law (42 USC § 300aa-25) to the Vaccine Adverse Event Reporting System (VAERS), including conditions found in the manufacturer's package insert. In addition, individuals are encouraged to report **any** clinically significant or unexpected events (even if you are not certain the vaccine caused the event) for **any** vaccine, whether or not it is listed on the RET. Manufacturers also are required by regulation (21 CFR 600.80) to report all adverse events made known to them for any vaccine. VAERS reporting forms and information can be obtained by calling 1-(800) 822-7967 or from the VAERS Web site (**http://vaers.hhs.gov**).

ᶜ Taken from the Vaccine Injury Table (VIT) used in adjudication of claims filed with the National Vaccine Injury Compensation Program (VICP) on or after July 22, 2011 (42 CFR 100.3[a]). Claims filed for a condition with onset outside the designated time intervals or a condition not included in the Table may be compensable as a non-Table injury, provided they are filed within the statute of limitations period (42 USC § 300aa-16[a]) and meet other eligibility requirements. Information on filing a claim can be obtained by calling 1-(800) 338-2382 or through the VICP Web site (**http://www.hrsa.gov/vaccinecompensation**).

....
APPENDIX VI

Nationally Notifiable Infectious Diseases in the United States

Public health officials at US state and territorial health departments and the Centers for Disease Control and Prevention (CDC) collaborate in determining which diseases should be nationally notifiable and timeframes for reporting (see Table, p 904). The Council of State and Territorial Epidemiologists, with advice from the CDC, makes recommendations annually for additions and deletions to the list of nationally notifiable diseases. A disease may be added to the list as a new pathogen emerges or may be deleted as its incidence decreases. However, reporting of nationally notifiable diseases to the CDC by the states and territories is voluntary. Reporting is only mandated (ie, by legislation or regulation) at the local, state, and territorial jurisdictional level. The list of diseases that are considered reportable, therefore, varies by jurisdiction and from year to year. Health-care professionals (eg, clinicians, hospitals, laboratories) in the United States are required to report diseases, conditions, or outbreaks as determined by local, state, or territorial law or regulation, as outlined in each jurisdiction's list of reportable conditions. Additional and specific reporting requirements should be obtained from the appropriate local, state, or territorial health departments. Staff members in the local, state, or territorial health departments implement disease-control and prevention measures as needed.

The CDC acts as a common agent for states and territories for collecting information and reporting of nationally notifiable diseases. Reports of occurrences of nationally notifiable diseases are transmitted to the CDC each week from the 50 states, 2 cities (Washington, DC, and New York, NY), and 5 territories (American Samoa, Commonwealth of Northern Mariana Islands, Guam, Puerto Rico, and the US Virgin Islands). The Council of State and Territorial Epidemiologists has established standard reporting and case classification methods for "Conditions Under National Surveillance" (campylobacteriosis, influenza-associated hospitalizations, free-living amebae, and melioidosis), but these conditions are not considered nationally notifiable.

Certain diseases should be reported within 4 or within 24 hours as follows:
1. Immediate, extremely urgent phone notification to CDC within 4 hours: paralytic polio, anthrax, botulism, plague, severe acute respiratory syndrome (SARS), smallpox, tularemia, viral hemorrhagic fevers; and
2. Intermediate, urgent phone notification to CDC within 24 hours: anthrax, naturally occurring; brucellosis; diphtheria; novel influenza A; measles; nonparalytic polio; rabies; rubella; *Vibrio cholerae*; viral hemorrhagic fevers; yellow fever.

Provisional data are published weekly in the *Morbidity and Mortality Weekly Report;* final data are published each year by the CDC in the annual "Summary of Notifiable Diseases, United States." The timeliness of the provisional weekly reports provides information that the CDC and state or local epidemiologists use to detect disease occurrence and more effectively interrupt outbreaks. Reporting provides the timely information needed to measure and demonstrate the effect of changed immunization laws or a new therapeutic modality. The finalized annual data provide information on reported disease incidence that is necessary for study of epidemiologic trends and development of disease-prevention policies. The CDC is the sole repository for these national data, which are used widely by local, state, and federal health agencies and other agencies or people concerned with the trends of reportable conditions in the United States and by schools of medicine and public health, communications media, and pharmaceutical or other companies producing health-related products. Nationally notifiable diseases or conditions meeting the criteria to be considered a potential Public Health Emergency of International Concern (PHEIC), as defined by the revised 2005 International Health Regulations (IHR),[1] are reported to the World Health Organization (cholera, plague, and yellow fever). A PHEIC is an extraordinary event that (1) constitutes a public health risk to other countries through international spread of disease; and (2) potentially requires a coordinated international response.[2,3]

[1] World Health Organization. International Health Regulations, 2005. Geneva, Switzerland: World Health Organization; 2005. Available at: **http://www.who.int/ihr/en/**

[2] Council of State and Territorial Epidemiologists. Events that may constitute a public health emergency of international concern. Position statement 07-ID-06. Atlanta, GA: Council of State and Territorial Epidemiologists; 2007. Available at: **http://www.cste.org/PS/2007ps/2007psfinal/ID/07-ID-06.pdf**

[3] US Department of Health and Human Services. *Global Health: International Health Regulations,* 2005. Washington, DC: US Department of Health and Human Services; 2005. Available at: **www.globalhealth.gov/global-health-topics/health-diplomacy/agreements-and-regulations/international-health-regulations-2005/**

Table. Infectious Diseases Designated as Notifiable at the National Level—United States, 2012[a]

Anthrax
Arboviral neuroinvasive and non-neuroinvasive diseases
  California serogroup virus disease
  Eastern equine encephalitis virus disease
  Powassan virus disease
  St. Louis encephalitis virus disease
  West Nile virus disease
  Western equine encephalitis virus disease
Babesiosis
Botulism
  Botulism, foodborne
  Botulism, infant
  Botulism, other (wound and unspecified)
Brucellosis
Campylobacteriosis
Chancroid
Chlamydia trachomatis infection
Cholera
Coccidioidomycosis
Cryptosporidiosis
Cyclosporiasis
Dengue
  Dengue fever
  Dengue hemorrhagic fever
  Dengue shock syndrome
Diphtheria
Ehrlichiosis/anaplasmosis
  Ehrlichia chaffeensis
  Ehrlichia ewingii
  Anaplasma phagocytophilum
  Undetermined
Free-living amebae (infections caused by)
Giardiasis
Gonorrhea
Haemophilus influenzae, invasive disease
Hansen disease (leprosy)
Hantavirus pulmonary syndrome

Hemolytic-uremic syndrome, postdiarrheal
Hepatitis
  Hepatitis A, acute
  Hepatitis B, acute
  Hepatitis B, chronic
  Hepatitis B virus, perinatal infection
  Hepatitis C, acute
  Hepatitis C, chronic
HIV infection[b]
  HIV infection, adult/adolescent (age ≥13 y)
  HIV infection, child (age ≥18 mo and <13 y)
  HIV infection, pediatric (age <18 mo)
Influenza-associated pediatric mortality
Legionellosis
Listeriosis
Lyme disease
Malaria
Measles
Melioidosis
Meningococcal disease
Mumps
Novel influenza A virus infections
Pertussis
Plague
Poliomyelitis, paralytic
Poliovirus infection, non-paralytic
Psittacosis
Q fever
  Acute
  Chronic
Rabies
  Rabies, animal
  Rabies, human
Rubella
Rubella, congenital syndrome
Salmonellosis
Severe acute respiratory syndrome-associated coronavirus (SARS-CoV) disease

Shiga toxin-producing *Escherichia coli* (STEC)
Shigellosis
Smallpox
Spotted fever rickettsiosis[c]
Streptococcal toxic shock syndrome
Streptococcus pneumoniae, invasive disease
Syphilis
  Syphilis, primary
  Syphilis, secondary
  Syphilis, latent
  Syphilis, early latent
  Syphilis, late latent
  Syphilis, latent, unknown duration
  Neurosyphilis
  Syphilis, late, non-neurologic
  Syphilitic stillbirth
  Syphilis, congenital
Tetanus
Toxic-shock syndrome (other than streptococcal)
Trichinellosis (trichinosis)
Tuberculosis
Tularemia
Typhoid fever
Vancomycin-intermediate *Staphylococcus aureus* (VISA)
Vancomycin-resistant *Staphylococcus aureus* (VRSA)
Varicella (morbidity)
Varicella (deaths only)
Vibriosis
Viral hemorrhagic fevers attributable to:
  Ebola virus
  Marburg virus
  Crimean-Congo hemorrhagic fever virus
  Lassa virus
  Lujo virus
  New World arenaviruses (Gunarito, Machupo, Junin, and Sabia viruses)
Yellow fever

[a] http://wwwn.cdc.gov/nndss/document/2012_Case%20Definitions.pdf
[b] AIDS has been reclassified as HIV stage III.
[c] Replaced Rocky Mountain spotted fever.

APPENDIX VII

Guide to Contraindications and Precautions to Immunizations, 2012

This information is based on recommendations of the Advisory Committee on Immunization Practices (ACIP) of the Centers for Disease Control and Prevention and the Committee on Infectious Diseases of the American Academy of Pediatrics (AAP). Sometimes, these recommendations vary from those in the manufacturers' package inserts. For more detailed information, physicians should consult published recommendations of the ACIP and AAP, manufacturers' package inserts, and **www.cdc.gov/vaccines/recs/vac-admin/contraindications.htm.** These guidelines, originally issued in 1993, have been updated to give recommendations as of 2012 (on the basis of information available as of January 2012).

Guide to Contraindications and Precautions to Immunizations, 2012

Vaccine	Contraindications	Precautions[a]	Not Contraindications (Vaccines May Be Given if Indicated)
General for all vaccines (DTaP, DT, Td, Tdap, IPV, MMR, MMRV, Hib, pneumococcal, meningococcal, hepatitis B, vari-cella, hepatitis A, influenza, zoster, rotavirus, HPV)	Anaphylactic reaction to a vaccine contraindicates further doses of that vaccine Anaphylactic reaction to a vaccine constituent contra-indicates the use of vaccines containing that substance	Moderate or severe illnesses with or without fever Latex allergy[b]	Mild to moderate local reaction (soreness, redness, swelling) after a dose of an injectable antigen. Low-grade or moderate fever after a previous vaccine dose. Mild acute illness with or without low-grade fever. Current antimicrobial therapy. Convalescent phase of illnesses. Preterm birth (same dosage and indications as for healthy, full-term infants); hepatitis B is the exception (see Hepatitis B, p 369). Recent exposure to an infectious disease. History of penicillin or other nonspecific allergies or fact that relatives have such allergies. Pregnancy of mother or household contact. Unimmunized household contact. Immunodeficient household contact. Breastfeeding (nursing infant OR lactating mother).
DTaP	Encephalopathy within 7 days of administration of previous dose of DTaP/DTP	Temperature of 40.5°C (104.8°F) within 48 h after immunization with a previous dose of DTaP/DTP Collapse or shock-like state (hypotonic-hyporesponsive epi-sode) within 48 h of receiving a previous dose of DTaP/DTP Seizures within 3 days of receiving a previous dose of DTaP/DTP[c] Persistent inconsolable crying lasting 3 h, within 48 h of receiving a previous dose of DTaP/DTP	Family history of seizures.[c] Family history of sudden infant death syndrome. Family history of an adverse event after DTaP/DTP administration.

Guide to Contraindications and Precautions to Immunizations, 2012, continued

Vaccine	Contraindications	Precautions[a]	Not Contraindications (Vaccines May Be Given if Indicated)
DTaP, continued		GBS within 6 wk after a dose[d] History of Arthus-type hypersensitivity reaction after a previous dose of a tetanus-containing vaccine (defer for 10 years after last tetanus toxoid-containing vaccine)	
DT, Td	Severe allergic reaction after a previous dose or to a vaccine component	GBS 6 wk or less after previous dose of tetanus toxoid-containing vaccine Moderate or severe acute illness with or without fever History of Arthus-type hypersensitivity reaction (see DTaP)	
IPV	Anaphylactic reactions to neomycin, streptomycin, or polymyxin B	Pregnancy	...
MCV4 and MPSV4	Severe allergic reaction to any component of the vaccine, including diphtheria toxoid, or to dry natural rubber latex		
MMR[e,f]	Pregnancy Anaphylactic reaction to neomycin or gelatin Known altered immunodeficiency (hematologic and solid tumors, congenital immunodeficiency; severe HIV infection, and long-term immunosuppressive therapy)	Recent (within 3–11 mo, depending on product and dose) Immune Globulin administration[g] (see Table 1.9, p 38) Thrombocytopenia or history of thrombocytopenic purpura[g] Tuberculosis or positive PPD test result[h]	Simultaneous tuberculin skin testing or IGRA.[i] Breastfeeding. Pregnancy of mother of recipient. Immunodeficient family member or household contact. Infection with HIV. Nonanaphylactic reactions to gelatin or neomycin.

Guide to Contraindications and Precautions to Immunizations, 2012, continued

Vaccine	Contraindications	Precautions[a]	Not Contraindications (Vaccines May Be Given if Indicated)
Hib	Severe allergic reaction after a previous dose or to a vaccine component	...	...
Hepatitis B	Severe allergic reaction after a previous dose or to a vaccine component	Preterm birth[j]	Pregnancy.
PCV13 and PPSV23	Severe allergic reaction to previous dose or vaccine component	Moderate or severe acute illness with or without fever	
Tdap	Serious allergic reaction to any vaccine component History of encephalopathy (eg, coma, prolonged seizures) within 7 days of administration of a pertussis vaccine that is not attributable to another identifiable cause	GBS 6 wk or less after previous dose of a tetanus toxoid vaccine Progressive neurologic disorder; uncontrolled epilepsy; or progressive encephalopathy until the condition has stabilized History of Arthus-type hypersensitivity reaction (see DTaP)	Temperature 105°F (40.5°C) or greater within 48 h after DTP/DTaP immunization not attributable to another cause. Collapse or shock-like state (hypotonic hyporesponsive episode) within 48 h after DTP/DTaP immunization. Persistent crying lasting 3 h or longer; occurring within 48 h after DTP/DTaP immunization. Convulsions with or without fever, occurring within 3 days after DTP/DTaP immunization. History of extensive limb swelling reaction after pediatric DTP/DTaP or Td immunization that was not an Arthus-type hypersensitivity reaction. Stable neurologic disorder, including well-controlled seizures, history of seizure disorder, and cerebral palsy. Brachial neuritis.

Guide to Contraindications and Precautions to Immunizations, 2012, continued

Vaccine	Contraindications	Precautions[a]	Not Contraindications (Vaccines May Be Given if Indicated)
Tdap, continued			Latex allergy other than anaphylactic allergies (eg, a history of contact to latex gloves). The tip and rubber plunger of the Boostrix needleless syringe contain latex. This Boostrix product should not be administered to adolescents with a history of a severe (anaphylactic) allergy to latex but may be administered to people with less severe allergies (eg, contact allergy to latex gloves). The Boostrix single-dose vial and Adacel preparations do not contain latex.
			Pregnancy.
			Breastfeeding.
			Immunosuppression, including people with human immunodeficiency virus infection (Tdap poses no known safety concern for immunosuppressed people; the immunogenicity of Tdap in people with immunosuppression has not been studied and could be suboptimal).
			Intercurrent minor illness.
			Antimicrobial use.
Varicella[e]	Pregnancy Severe allergic reaction after a previous dose or to a vaccine component (ie, neomycin or gelatin) Infection with HIV[k] Known altered immunodeficiency (hematologic and solid tumors, congenital immunodeficiency, and long-term immunosuppressive therapy)[l]	Recent Immune Globulin administration (see Table 1.9, p 38) Family history of immunodeficiency[m]	Pregnancy of mother of recipient. Immunodeficiency in a household contact. Household contact with HIV.

Guide to Contraindications and Precautions to Immunizations, 2012, continued

Vaccine	Contraindications	Precautions[a]	Not Contraindications (Vaccines May Be Given if Indicated)
Hepatitis A	Severe allergic reaction after a previous dose or to a vaccine component (ie, to 2-phenoxyethanol or alum)	Pregnancy	...
Influenza (inactivated)	Severe allergic reaction to a previous dose or vaccine component including eggs	GBS within 6 wk after a previous influenza immunization	Pregnancy. Egg allergy.
Influenza (live-attenuated)	Severe allergic reaction to a previous dose or vaccine component (including eggs); pregnancy; people with any underlying medical conditions that serve as an indication to give routine inactivated influenza immunization; children 2 through 4 years of age with health care professional or medical history documentation of wheezing within the past 12 mo; receiving aspirin; history of GBS after influenza vaccine	GBS within 6 wk after a previous influenza immunization	
Rotavirus	Severe allergic reaction after a previous dose or to a vaccine component, severe combined immune deficiency (SCID), history of previous episode of intussusception	Altered immunocompetence other than SCID Moderate to severe acute gastroenteritis Moderate to severe febrile illness Chronic gastrointestinal disease	Breastfeeding. Immunodeficient family member or household contact.

Guide to Contraindications and Precautions to Immunizations, 2012, continued

Vaccine	Contraindications	Precautions[a]	Not Contraindications (Vaccines May Be Given if Indicated)
HPV	Severe allergic reaction after a previous dose or to a vaccine component	Administration to people with moderate or severe acute illness Precaution	Administration to people with minor acute illnesses.
Zoster	Severe allergic reaction after any component of the vaccine; primary or acquired immunodeficiency disease; pregnancy	Severe acute illness	Mild acute illness.

DTaP indicates diphtheria and tetanus toxoids and acellular pertussis; DT, pediatric diphtheria-tetanus toxoid; Td, adult tetanus-diphtheria toxoid; Tdap, tetanus toxoid, reduced diphtheria toxoid, and acellular pertussis; IPV, inactivated poliovirus; MMR, measles-mumps-rubella; MMRV, measles-mumps-rubella-varicella; Hib, *Haemophilus influenzae* type b; HPV, human papillomavirus; DTP, diphtheria and tetanus toxoids and pertussis; GBS, Guillain-Barré syndrome; MCV4, tetravalent (A, C, Y, W-135) meningococcal conjugate vaccine; MPSV4, tetravalent meningococcal polysaccharide vaccine; HIV, human immunodeficiency virus; PPD, purified protein derivative (tuberculin); PCV7, pneumococcal conjugate vaccine; PCV, pneumococcal conjugate vaccine; PPSV23, pneumococcal polysaccharide vaccine.

a The events or conditions listed as precautions, although not contraindications, should be reviewed carefully. The benefits and risks of administering a specific vaccine to a person under the circumstances should be considered. If the risks are believed to outweigh the benefits, the immunization should be withheld; if the benefits are believed to outweigh the risks (eg, during an outbreak or foreign travel), the immunization should be given. Whether and when to administer DTaP to children with proven or suspected underlying neurologic disorders should be decided on an individual basis.

b If a person reports a severe (anaphylactic) allergy to latex, vaccines supplied in vials or syringes that contain natural rubber should not be administered unless the benefits of immunization outweigh the risks of an allergic reaction to the vaccine. For latex allergies other than anaphylactic allergies (eg, a history of contact allergy to latex gloves), vaccines supplied in vials or syringes that contain dry natural rubber or latex can be administered.

c Acetaminophen given before administering DTaP and thereafter every 4 hours should be considered for children with a personal or family (ie, siblings or parents) history of seizures.

d The decision to give additional doses of DTaP should be made on the basis of consideration of the benefit of further immunization versus the risk of recurrence of GBS. For example, completion of the primary series in children is justified.

e The administration of multiple live-virus vaccines within 30 days (4 weeks) of one another if not given on the same day may result in suboptimal immune response. Data substantiate this risk for MMR and possibly varicella vaccine, which should, therefore, be given on the same day or more than 4 weeks apart.

f Egg allergy is not considered a contraindication or precaution.

g The decision to immunize should be made on the basis of consideration of the benefits of immunity to measles, mumps, and rubella versus the risk of recurrence or exacerbation of thrombocytopenia after immunization or from natural infections of measles or rubella. In most instances, the benefits of immunization will be much greater than the potential risks and justify giving MMR, particularly in view of the even greater risk of thrombocytopenia after measles or rubella disease. However, if a previous episode of thrombocytopenia occurred in temporal proximity to immunization, not giving a subsequent dose may be prudent.

h A theoretical basis exists for concern that measles vaccine might exacerbate tuberculosis. Consequently, before administering MMR to people with untreated active tuberculosis, initiating antituberculosis therapy is advisable.

Guide to Contraindications and Precautions to Immunizations, 2012, continued

Vaccine	Contraindications	Precautions[a]	Not Contraindications (Vaccines May Be Given if Indicated)

[i] Measles immunization may suppress tuberculin reactivity temporarily. MMR vaccine may be given after, or on the same day as, tuberculin skin testing. If MMR has been given recently, postpone the tuberculin skin test until 4 to 6 weeks after administration of MMR. The effect of MMR on IGRA test results is unknown.

[j] For infants weighing less than 2 kg at birth and born to hepatitis B surface antigen (HBsAg)-negative mothers, initiation of immunization should be delayed until just before hospital discharge if the infant weighs 2 kg or more, or until approximately 2 months of age, when other routine immunizations are given, to improve response. All infants weighing less than 2 kg born to HBsAg-positive mothers should receive immunoprophylaxis (Hepatitis B Immune Globulin and vaccine) beginning as soon as possible after birth, followed by appropriate postimmunization testing and receipt of 3 doses of hepatitis B vaccine

[k] Varicella vaccine should be considered for asymptomatic or mildly symptomatic HIV-infected children, specifically children in Centers for Disease Control and Prevention class N1 or A1, with age-specific T-lymphocyte percentages of 15% or higher.

[l] Varicella vaccine should not be administered to people who have cellular immunodeficiencies, but people with impaired humoral immunity may be immunized.

[m] Varicella vaccine should not be administered to a person who has a family history of congenital or hereditary immunodeficiency in parents or siblings unless that person's immune competence has been substantiated clinically or verified by a laboratory.

····························
Appendix VIII

Clinical Practice Guidelines for Immunization Programs for Infants, Children, and Adolescents

In 2009, the Infectious Diseases Society of America (IDSA) issued 46 evidence-based guidelines for immunization of infants, children, adolescents, and adults.[1] A panel of experts, including people with experience in pediatric clinical and laboratory medicine, nursing, public health, and infectious diseases, developed the guidelines. The AAP was one of the collaborating organizations. Each recommendation included the quality of evidence and strength of recommendations.

The 46 guidelines are classified into 4 broad categories:
1. Vaccine recommendations for infants, children, adolescents, and adults;
2. Immunization standards, overcoming barriers to immunization, vaccine safety, misconceptions, finance, access, and strategies to improve coverage;
3. Complementary (nontraditional) immunization settings; and
4. Immunization of specific groups.

Following these guidelines[1] should lead to optimal prevention of disease through vaccination in multiple population groups while maintaining a high level of safety.

I. **Vaccine Recommendations for Infants, Children, Adolescents, and Adults**
   1. Infants, children, adolescents, and adults should receive all age-appropriate vaccines recommended by the Advisory Committee on Immunization Practices, the American Academy of Family Physicians, and the American Academy of Pediatrics (A-I).
   2. Any vaccine dose not administered at the recommended age should be administered at any subsequent medical encounter when indicated and feasible without reinitiating the series (A-III).
   3. Recommendations for the minimum interval between doses for people who have delayed immunizations or who want to accelerate their schedule should be followed (B-III).
   4. When appropriate, all indicated vaccines should be administered simultaneously (B-III).
   5. Licensed combination vaccines can be administered whenever any components of the combination are indicated, other components are not contraindicated, and if the vaccine is licensed by the US Food and Drug Administration (FDA) for that dose of the series (A-I).
   6. Immunization requirements for child care, school and college attendance, and nursing homes should be followed (A-II).
   7. Vaccine delivery should be coordinated with other preventive health care services for infants, children, adolescents, and adults (B-III).
   8. All vaccines should be stored and administered as recommended by the manufacturer and as licensed by the FDA (B-II).

---
[1] Reprinted with permission from Pickering LK, Baker CJ, Freed GL, et al. Immunization programs for infants, children, adolescents, and adults: clinical practice guidelines by the Infectious Diseases Society of America. *Clin Infect Dis.* 2009;49(6):817–840

II. Immunization Standards, Overcoming Barriers to Immunization, Vaccine Safety, Misconceptions, Finances, Access, and Strategies to Improve Coverage

9. Health care providers should determine and follow valid vaccine contraindications and precautions before administration of any vaccine (B-III).
10. Health care providers should be aware of the National Vaccine Injury Compensation Program (NVICP) and its requirements (B-III).
11. All patients or parents should receive Vaccine Information Statements (VISs) for each vaccine administered as required by law for vaccines covered by the NVICP (C-III).
12. Providers should educate their patients and parents about the benefits, safety, and risks of vaccines in a culturally appropriate and easy-to-understand language prior to each immunization (C-III).
13. Clinically significant adverse events following immunization should be reported to the Vaccine Adverse Events Reporting System (VAERS) (B-III).

Finance

14. Patient out-of-pocket immunization expenses should be minimized (A-I).
15. Vaccine-financing programs, including the Vaccines for Children (VFC) program, Section 317 of the Public Health Service Act federal grant program, state programs, and private insurance, should be optimized for each patient, as appropriate (B-II).
16. Providers who serve infants, children, and adolescents aged <19 years should be enrolled in the VFC program (B-II).
17. Providers should be aware of other government-supported and other funded programs that cover the cost of vaccines and their administration for people who do not have adequate resources (C-III).

Access to Immunizations

18. Barriers to immunizations should be identified and eliminated or as minimized as possible (B-II).
19. Immunization services should be easy to access, including express immunization services (eg, influenza immunization clinics) and expanded hours of immunization services (A-II).
20. Immunization should be integrated into routine health care services offered in offices and clinics (C-III).
21. Private providers should consider participating in programs that provide financially vulnerable adults with access to immunizations at no cost (C-III).

Strategies to Improve Immunization Coverage

22. Reminder/recall systems should be used to enhance immunization rates (A-I).
23. Information regarding administration of vaccines should be entered into immunization information systems (ie, immunization registries) (B-III).
24. Standing orders for immunizations should be established in clinics, hospitals, and nursing homes (A-I).
25. The immunization status of patients should be reviewed at each patient visit (B-II), and patients and parents should be provided with accurate immunization records at office or clinic visits (B-III).
26. All health care providers who administer vaccines should be educated properly and should receive ongoing education (A-III).

27. Regular assessments of immunization coverage rates should be conducted in provider practices (A-I).

28. Demand for adolescent and adult immunization should be increased by improving public and provider awareness of immunizations recommended for adolescents and adults (B-III).

III. Complementary (Nontraditional) Immunization Settings

29. Providers should support use of community-based settings to immunize target populations that have difficulty accessing usual immunization providers (B-III).

30. Providers should support establishment of school-based, child care-based, and hospital-based immunization programs to deliver influenza immunization to school-aged children, adolescents, and adults (B-III).

31. Immunization providers in complementary settings should adhere to quality standards, including ability to appropriately manage vaccine-related adverse events, proper storage and handling of vaccines, appropriate record keeping, regulatory issues, and provision of education regarding both risks and benefits of immunizations, as well as other preventive care measures, including adherence to hand hygiene (B-III).

32. Providers of immunizations in nontraditional settings should ensure that records of immunizations administered in these settings are sent to primary care providers and to immunization information systems (registries) and should encourage vaccinees in such settings to see their primary care providers for other preventive and therapeutic services (B-III).

IV. Immunization of Specific Groups
Health Care Professionals

33. All health care professionals should be immunized appropriately (B-II). Specifically, annual immunization with influenza vaccine and receipt of a single booster dose of tetanus toxoid, reduced diphtheria toxoid, and acellular pertussis (Tdap) should be ensured, as well as adequate immunization against measles, mumps, rubella, and varicella. People whose work anticipates that they may be exposed to blood or body fluids should be immunized against hepatitis B.

34. Hospitals, clinics, and offices should implement programs to ensure that health care professionals are immunized appropriately and that annual immunization coverage assessments are performed (B-II).

Immunocompromised Persons

35. All immunocompromised infants, children, adolescents, and adults should be appropriately immunized (B-II).

36. Providers should be aware of contraindications and precautions for vaccines in people with primary and second immunodeficiencies (B-III).

37. Providers should educate immunocompromised patients that, depending on the vaccine and their degree of immune dysfunction, the vaccines that are administered may not be fully effective (C-III).

38. Providers who care for immunocompromised patients should ensure that household contacts are immunized appropriately to reduce the risk of exposure of immunocompromised patients to vaccine-preventable diseases (B-III).

Pregnancy

39. Providers should be aware of immunizations routinely recommended for women during pregnancy, including inactivated trivalent influenza vaccine (A-II).
40. Providers should administer appropriate vaccines to pregnant women with medical or exposure indications that put them at risk of certain vaccine-preventable diseases (A-I).
41. Following delivery, women should receive all recommended vaccines that could not be or were not administered during pregnancy (A-II).
42. Providers should be aware of and follow valid contraindications and precautions for immunizing pregnant women (A-III).

International Travel

43. Providers who care for people who travel should ensure that all country-specific vaccines are administered in a time frame that ensures optimal development of protection (A-I).
44. Health care professionals should be aware of key sources of information regarding immunization of travelers at every age (B-III).

Internationally Adopted Children

45. Providers should accept only written documentation as evidence of previous immunization (B-III).
46. Providers should be aware of the various approaches that can be followed if there is concern about whether vaccines administered to an international adoptee were immunogenic (B-III).

Table. Definition of Quality of Evidence and Strength of Recommendation[a]

Assessment	Type of Evidence
Strength of Recommendation	
Grade A	Good evidence to support a recommendation for use
Grade B	Moderate evidence to support a recommendation for use
Grade C	Poor evidence to support a recommendation
Quality of Evidence	
Level I	Evidence from at least 1 properly designed randomized controlled trial
Level II	Evidence from at least 1 well-designed clinical trial, without randomization; from cohort or case controlled analytic studies (preferably from >1 center); from multiple time series; or from dramatic results of uncontrolled experiments
Level III	Evidence from opinions of respected authorities, based on clinical experience, descriptive studies, or reports of expert committees

[a]Adapted from the Canadian Task Force on the Periodic Health Examination. The periodic health examination. *Can Med Assoc J.* 1979;121(9):1193–1254

······················
APPENDIX IX

Prevention of Infectious Disease From Contaminated Food Products[1]

Foodborne diseases are associated with significant morbidity and mortality in people of all ages. The Centers for Disease Control and Prevention (CDC) estimates that there are tens of millions of cases of foodborne diseases in the United States each year, resulting in approximately hundreds of thousands of hospitalizations and thousands of deaths.[2] Young children, the elderly, and immunocompromised people are especially susceptible to illness and complications caused by many of the organisms associated with foodborne illness.

The Foodborne Disease Active Surveillance Network (FoodNet) of CDC's Emerging Infections Program conducts active, population-based surveillance in 10 states for all laboratory-confirmed infections with select enteric pathogens transmitted commonly through food. The FoodNet program conducts surveillance for illnesses attributable to *Campylobacter* species, *Listeria monocytogenes*, *Salmonella* species, Shiga-toxin producing *Escherichia coli* (STEC) including O157:H7, *Shigella* species, *Vibrio* species, and *Yersinia enterocolitica* (since 1996); *Cryptosporidium* species and *Cyclospora* species since 1997; and STEC non-O157 since 2000. FoodNet also conducts surveillance for hemolytic-uremic syndrome (HUS), a complication of STEC infection. Additional information about FoodNet can be found at **www.cdc.gov/foodnet/**.

Outbreak surveillance provides insights into the causes of foodborne illness, types of implicated foods, and settings of foodborne infections. The CDC collects data on foodborne disease outbreaks submitted from all states and territories (**www.cdc.gov/outbreaknet/**). Public health, regulatory, and agricultural professionals can use this information when creating targeted control strategies and to support efforts to promote safe food preparation practices among food industry employees and the public.

Four general rules should be followed to maintain safety of foods:
* Wash hands and surfaces thoroughly and often.
* Separate—do not cross contaminate.
* Refrigerate foods promptly.
* Cook food to the proper temperature.

The following preventive measures can be implemented to decrease the risk of infection and disease from contaminated food.

Unpasteurized milk and milk products. The American Academy of Pediatrics (AAP) endorses the use of pasteurized milk and recommends that parents be fully informed of the important risks associated with consumption of unpasteurized milk. Interstate sale of unpasteurized (raw) milk and products made from unpasteurized milk (with the exception of certain cheeses) is banned by the US Food and Drug Administration (FDA). The most vulnerable populations, such as children, pregnant women, elderly people,

---

[1] Centers for Disease Control and Prevention. Diagnosis and management of foodborne illnesses: a primer for physicians. *MMWR Recomm Rep.* 2004;53(RR-4):1–33

[2] Centers for Disease Control and Prevention. Surveillance for foodborne disease outbreaks—United States, 2008. *MMWR Morb Mortal Wkly Rep.* 2011;60(35):1197–1202

and immunocompromised people should not consume unpasteurized milk or products made from unpasteurized milk, including cheese and butter, from any species, including cows, sheep, and goats. Serious systemic infections attributable to *Salmonella* species, *Campylobacter* species, *Mycobacterium bovis*, *L monocytogenes*, *Brucella* species, *E coli* O157:H7, and *Y enterocolitica* have been linked to consumption of unpasteurized milk, including certified raw milk. In particular, many outbreaks of campylobacteriosis among children are associated with school field trips to farms that include consumption of raw milk. School officials should take precautions to prevent raw milk from being served to children during educational trips. Cheeses made from unpasteurized milk also have been associated with illness attributable to *Brucella* species, *L monocytogenes*, *Salmonella* species, *Campylobacter* species, *Shigella* species, *M bovis*, and *E coli* O157:H7.

Eggs. At-risk populations, including children, should not eat raw or undercooked eggs, unpasteurized powdered eggs, or products containing raw or undercooked eggs. Ingestion of raw or improperly cooked eggs can result in severe illness attributable to *Salmonella* species. Examples of foods that may contain raw or undercooked eggs include some homemade frostings and mayonnaise, ice cream from uncooked custard, tiramisu, eggs prepared "sunny-side up," fresh Caesar salad dressing, Hollandaise sauce, cookie dough, and cake batter.

Raw and undercooked meat. Children should not eat raw or undercooked meat or meat products, particularly hamburger. Various raw or undercooked meat products have been associated with harmful bacteria, including poultry with *Salmonella* species, *Campylobacter* species, and *Clostridium perfringens*; ground beef with *E coli* O157:H7 and other STEC and *Salmonella* species; hot dogs with *Listeria* species; pork with *Trichinella* species; and wild game with *Brucella* species, *Francisella* species, and *Trichinella* species. Ground meats should be cooked to an internal temperature of 160°F; roasts and steaks should be cooked to an internal temperature of 145°F, and poultry should be cooked to an internal temperature of 165°F. Use of a food thermometer is the only sure way of knowing that food has reached a high enough temperature to destroy bacteria. Color is not a reliable indicator that ground beef patties have been cooked to a temperature high enough to kill harmful bacteria such as *E coli* O157:H7 or other STEC. Knives, cutting boards, plates, and other utensils used for raw meats should not be used for preparation of fresh fruits or vegetables until they have been cleaned properly.

Unpasteurized juices. Children should drink only pasteurized fruit juice or juice that has been otherwise treated to control harmful bacteria. Consumption of packaged fruit juices that have not undergone pasteurization or a comparable treatment have been associated with foodborne illness attributable to *E coli* O157:H7 and *Salmonella* species. To identify a packaged juice that has not undergone pasteurization or a comparable treatment, consumers should look for a warning statement that the product has not been pasteurized.

Seed sprouts. The FDA and the CDC have reaffirmed health advisories that people who are at high risk of severe foodborne disease, including children, people with compromised immune systems, and elderly people, should avoid eating raw seed sprouts until intervention methods are implemented to improve the safety of these products.[1] Raw seed sprouts have been associated with outbreaks of illness attributable to *Salmonella* species and *E coli* O157:H7 as well as other STEC.

---

[1] For additional information, contact the FDA Food Information Line at 1-800-FDA-4010 or the US Department of Agriculture at 1-800-535-4555 or 1-202-720-2791 or visit the following Web sites: **www.usda.gov** and **www.foodsafety.gov**.

Fresh fruits and vegetables, and raw nuts. Many fresh fruits and vegetables have been associated with disease attributable to *Cryptosporidium* species, *Cyclospora* species, noroviruses, hepatitis A virus, *Giardia* species, *E coli*, *Salmonella* species, and *Shigella* species. Raw shelled nuts, commercially processed vegetable snacks, spinach, lettuce, tomatoes, melons, basil, and alfalfa sprouts all have been associated with outbreaks of salmonellosis. Nuts that have been roasted or otherwise treated can help minimize the risk of foodborne illness. Washing can decrease but not eliminate contamination of fresh fruits and vegetables. Knives, cutting boards, utensils, and plates used for raw meats should not be used for preparation of fresh fruits or vegetables until the utensils have been cleaned properly.

Raw shellfish and fish. Children should not eat raw shellfish. Raw shellfish, including mussels, clams, oysters, scallops, and other mollusks, can carry many pathogens, including norovirus, and also toxins (see Appendix X, p 921). *Vibrio* species contaminating raw shellfish may cause severe disease in people with liver disease or other conditions associated with decreased immune function. Some experts caution against children ingesting raw fish, which has been associated with transmission of parasites.

Honey. Children younger than 1 year of age should not be given honey. Honey has been shown to contain spores of *Clostridium botulinum*. Light and dark corn syrups are manufactured under sanitary conditions, and although the manufacturer cannot ensure that any product will be free of *C botulinum* spores, no cases associated with corn syrup have been documented.

Powdered infant formula. For many reasons, infants should be fed human milk rather than infant formula whenever possible. Powdered infant formula is not commercially sterile and has been associated with severe illnesses attributable to *Cronobacter* species and *Salmonella enterica*. Although such infections are rare, if infant formula must be used, caregivers can reduce the risk of infection by choosing sterile, liquid formula products rather than powdered products. This may be particularly important for those at greatest risk of severe infection, such as neonates and infants with immunocompromising conditions. Additionally, the World Health Organization (WHO) has issued guidance to improve the safety of powdered infant formula.[1] Recommendations include reconstituting powdered infant formula with water at or above 70°C (158°F), which is high enough to inactivate *Cronobacter* and other pathogens. Although some cite concerns about the risk of burns and possible loss of vitamin C associated with this procedure, health authorities in Canada and Ireland have issued guidance for powdered infant formula preparation based on the WHO recommendations.

Food irradiation.[2] No single process to eliminate all foodborne diseases exists. However, irradiation of food can be an effective tool in helping to control foodborne pathogens. Irradiation involves exposing food briefly to ionizing radiation (eg, gamma rays, x-rays, or high-voltage electrons). More than 40 countries worldwide, including the United States, have approved the use of irradiation for various types of foods. In addition, every governmental and professional organization that has reviewed the efficacy and safety of food irradiation has endorsed its use. Irradiated meat, spices, shell eggs, seeds for sprouting, and some produce items may be irradiated for sale in the United States. The risk of foodborne illness in children could be decreased significantly with the routine consumption of irradiated meat, poultry, and produce.

---

[1] **www.who.int/foodsafety/publications/micro/pif_guidelines.pdf**

[2] **www.fsis.usda.gov/Fact_Sheets/Irradiation_Resources/index.asp**

Detailed information on food safety issues and practices, including steps consumers can take to protect themselves, is available on the following Web sites:

- **www.foodsafetyworkinggroup.gov**
- **www.foodsafety.gov**
- **www.fightbac.org**
- **www.cdc.gov/foodsafety**

• •

APPENDIX X

Clinical Syndromes Associated With Foodborne Diseases[1]

Foodborne disease results from consumption of contaminated foods or beverages and causes morbidity and mortality in children and adults in developing and developed countries. The epidemiology of foodborne disease is complex and dynamic because of the large number of pathogens, the variety of disease manifestations, the increasing prevalence of immunocompromised children and adults, changes in dietary habits, and trends toward centralized food production and widespread distribution.

Consideration of a foodborne etiology is important in any patient with a gastrointestinal tract illness. A detailed history is invaluable with important questions including time of onset and duration of symptoms, history of recent travel or antibiotic use, as well as presence of blood or mucus in stool. To aid in diagnosis, foodborne disease syndromes have been categorized by incubation period, duration, causative agent, and foods commonly associated with specific etiologic agents (see Table, p 922). Diagnosis can be confirmed by laboratory testing of stool, vomitus, or blood, depending on the causative agent. An outbreak should be considered when 2 or more people who have ingested the same food develop an acute illness characterized by nausea, vomiting, diarrhea, or neurologic signs or symptoms. If an outbreak is suspected, local or state public health officials should be notified immediately so they can work with local health care professionals, coordinate laboratory testing not available locally, and conduct epidemiologic investigations to curtail the outbreak.

---

[1] Centers for Disease Control and Prevention. Surveillance for foodborne-disease outbreaks—United States, 2008. *MMWR Morb Mortal Wkly Rep.* 2011;60(35):1197–1202. Additional information can be found at **www.cdc.gov/foodsafety and www.fsis.usda.gov/home/index.asp**

Table. Clinical Syndromes Associated With Foodborne Diseases

Clinical Syndrome	Incubation Period	Causative Agents	Commonly Associated Vehicles[a]
Nausea and vomiting	<1–6 h	Staphylococcus aureus (preformed toxins, A, B, C, D, E)	Ham, poultry, cream-filled pastries, potato and egg salads, mushrooms
		Bacillus cereus (emetic toxin)	Rice, meats
		Heavy metals (copper, tin, cadmium, iron, zinc)	Acidic beverages, metallic container
Flushing, dizziness, burning of mouth and throat, headache, gastrointestinal tract symptoms, urticaria	<1 h	Histamine (scombroid)	Fish (bluefish, bonita, mackerel, mahi-mahi, marlin, tuna)
Neurologic, including paresthesias	<1–6 h	Ciguateratoxin	Fish (amberjack, barracuda, grouper, snapper)
Paresthesias, nausea, vomiting, diarrhea		Carchatoxins	Shark (particularly liver)
Gastrointestinal tract symptoms		Neurotoxic shellfish toxin (brevetoxin)	Shellfish
		Domoic acid	Mussels
		Monosodium glutamate	Asian food
Neurologic, including confusion, salivation, hallucinations; gastrointestinal tract manifestations	0–2 h	Mycotoxins (early onset)	Mushrooms
Neuromuscular weakness, gastrointestinal tract manifestations	12–48 h	Clostridium botulinum (descending paralysis)	Home-canned vegetables, fruits and fish, salted fish, meats, bottled garlic, potatoes baked in aluminum foil, cheese sauce, honey (infants)
	<30 min	Tetrodotoxin (ascending paralysis)	Puffer fish

Table. Clinical Syndromes Associated With Foodborne Diseases, continued

Clinical Syndrome	Incubation Period	Causative Agents	Commonly Associated Vehicles[a]
	0.5–3 h	Paralytic shellfish toxins (saxitoxins, etc)	Shellfish (clams, muscles, oysters, scallops, other mollusks)
Abdominal cramps and watery diarrhea, vomiting	6–24 h	*B cereus* enterotoxin	Meats, stews, gravies, vanilla sauce
	6–24 h	*Clostridium perfringens* enterotoxin	Meat, poultry, gravy, dried or precooked foods
	16–72 h	Norovirus	Shellfish, salads, ice, cookies, water, sandwiches, fruit, leafy vegetables
	1–3 days	Rotavirus	Salads, fruits
	1–4 days	Enterotoxigenic *Escherichia coli*	Fruits, vegetables, water
	1–5 days	*Vibrio cholerae* O1 and O139	Shellfish (including crabs and shrimp), fish, water
		V cholerae non-O1	Shellfish
	1–14 days	*Cyclospora* species	Raspberries, vegetables, water
	2–14 days	*Cryptosporidium* species	Vegetables, fruits, milk, water
	1–4 wk	*Giardia intestinalis*	Water, food sources
Diarrhea, fever, abdominal cramps, blood and mucus in stools	16–≥72 h	*Salmonella* species	Poultry; pork; beef; eggs; dairy products, including ice cream; vegetables (alfalfa sprouts and fresh produce); fruit, including unpasteurized juices; peanut products
	1–3 days	*Shigella* species	Water, milk, other contaminated food
	2–4 wk	Amebiasis	Fecally contaminated food or water
Bloody diarrhea, abdominal cramps	72–120 h	Shiga toxin-producing *E coli*	Beef (hamburger); raw milk; roast beef; salami; salad dressings; lettuce; unpasteurized juices, including apple cider; sprouts; water
Hepatorenal failure, watery diarrhea	6–24 h	Mushroom toxins (late onset)	Mushrooms (especially *Amanita* species)

Table. Clinical Syndromes Associated With Foodborne Diseases, continued

Clinical Syndrome	Incubation Period	Causative Agents	Commonly Associated Vehicles[a]
Gastrointestinal tract manifestations, then symmetric descending paralysis including ophthalmoplegias and other bulbar symptoms (diplopia) blurred vision, dry mouth, dysarthria	12–48 h	*Clostridium botulinum*	Home-canned vegetables, fruits and fish, salted fish, meats, bottled garlic, potatoes baked in aluminum foil, cheese sauce, honey (infants)
Chronic, urgent diarrhea	Varied	Brainerd diarrhea	Unknown vehicle, but may include unpasteurized milk, and contaminated water
Other extraintestinal manifestations	Varied	*Brucella* species	Goat cheese, queso fresco, raw milk, meats
Fever, chills, headache, pharyngitis, arthralgia		Group A streptococcus	Egg and potato salad
Fever, malaise, anorexia, jaundice		Hepatitis A virus	Shellfish, raw produce (ie, strawberries, lettuce, green onions)
Meningoencephalitis sepsis		*Listeria monocytogenes*	Cheese, raw milk, hot dogs, cole slaw, ready-to eat delicatessen meats, cantaloupe
Muscle soreness and pain		*Trichinella spiralis*	Pork, wild game, meat
Fever, lymphadenopathy, neurologic (reactivation)		*Toxoplasma gondii*	Beef, pork, lamb, venison
Sepsis, meningitis		*Cronobacter* (*Enterobacter*) *sakazakii*	Powdered infant formula
		Salmonella species	Powdered infant formula
Seizures, behavioral disturbances, and other neurologic signs and symptoms		*Taenia* species (neurocysticercosis)	Food contaminated with feces from a human carrier of adult pork tapeworm

Table. Clinical Syndromes Associated With Foodborne Diseases, continued

Clinical Syndrome	Incubation Period	Causative Agents	Commonly Associated Vehicles[a]
Epigastric discomfort, abdominal pain, cholangitis, obstructive jaundice, pancreatitis		Clonorchis sinensis	Fish
		Opisthorchis species	Fish
Guillain-Barré syndrome (ascending paralysis)	Varied	Campylobacter species	Poultry, raw milk, water
		Shigella	Egg salad, vegetables, scallions
		Enteroinvasive E coli	Vegetables, hamburger, raw milk
		Yersinia enterocolitica	Pork chitterlings, tofu, raw milk
		Vibrio parahaemolyticus	Fish, shellfish
Hemolytic-uremic syndrome (acute renal failure, hemolytic anemia, thrombocytopenia)	Varied	Shiga toxin-producing E coli (especially serotype O157:H7)	Beef (hamburger); raw milk; roast beef; salami; salad dressings; lettuce; unpasteurized juices, including apple cider; alfalfa and radish sprouts; water
		Shigella dysenteriae 1	Water, milk, other contaminated food
Reactive arthritis	Varied	Campylobacter species	Water, milk, other contaminated food
		Salmonella species	Poultry, pork, beef, eggs, dairy products, including ice cream; vegetables (alfalfa sprouts and fresh produce); fruit, including unpasteurized juices; peanut butter
		Shigella species	Poultry, raw milk, water
		Yersinia enterocolitica	Pork chitterlings, tofu, raw milk

[a] List of vehicles in several categories is not exhaustive, because any number of foods can be fecally contaminated.

·······················
APPENDIX XI

Diseases Transmitted by Animals (Zoonoses)

Important zoonoses that may be encountered in North America are listed in this Appendix and reviewed in the *Red Book* (see disease-specific chapters in Section 3 for further information). Morbidity resulting from selected zoonotic diseases in the United States is reported annually by the Centers for Disease Control and Prevention (see "Summary of Notifiable Diseases" at **www.cdc.gov/mmwr/mmwr_nd/**). Information also can be obtained via the Web site of the National Center for Emerging and Zoonotic Infectious Diseases: **www.cdc.gov/ncezid/about-ncezid.html** or through the main Centers for Disease Control and Prevention Web site: **www.cdc.gov.**

Table. Diseases Transmitted by Animals

Disease and/or Organism	Common Animal Sources/Reservoirs	Vector or Modes of Transmission
Bacterial Diseases		
Aeromonas species	Aquatic animals, especially shellfish	Wound infection, ingestion of contaminated food or water
Anthrax (*Bacillus anthracis*)	Herbivores (cattle, goats, sheep)	Direct contact with infected animals or their carcasses, or contact with products from infected animals (eg, meat, hides or hair) contaminated with *B anthracis* spores
Bartonellosis (*Bartonella* species, *Bartonella vinsonii vinsonii, B vinsonii berkhoffi, B vinsonii arupensis, Bartonella koehleri, Bartonella rochalaine, Bartonella quintana*)	Dogs, cattle, cats, body lice	Bites of arthropods suspected, but evidence is lacking in many species
Brucellosis (*Brucella* species)	Cattle, goats, sheep, swine, dogs, elk, bison, deer	Direct contact with birth products, ingestion of contaminated undercooked meat or dairy products, inhalation of aerosols, contact through mucous membranes or skin wounds
Campylobacteriosis (*Campylobacter jejuni*)	Poultry, dogs (especially puppies), kittens, ferrets, hamsters, birds	Ingestion of contaminated food, water, milk, direct contact (particularly with animals with diarrhea), person-to-person (fecal-oral)
Capnocytophaga canimorsus	Dogs, rarely cats	Bites, scratches, and prolonged contact with dogs
Cat-scratch disease (*Bartonella henselae*)	Cats, infrequently other animals (less than 10%)	Scratches, bites; fleas play a role in cat-to-cat transmission (evidence for transmission from cat fleas to humans is lacking)
Erysipelothrix rhusiopathiae	Pigs, sheep, cattle, horses, birds, fish, shellfish	Direct contact with animal or contaminated animal product
Hemolytic-uremic syndrome (eg, Shiga toxin-producing *Escherichia coli*) (STEC)	Cattle, sheep, goats, deer	Ingestion of undercooked contaminated ground beef, unpasteurized milk, or other contaminated foods or water, person-to-person contact (fecal-oral), petting zoo contact, county fairs (fecal-oral)
Leptospirosis (*Leptospira* species)	Dogs, rodents, livestock, other wild animals	Contact with or ingestion of water, food, or soil contaminated with urine or fluids from infected animals, or direct contact with infected animals

Table. Diseases Transmitted by Animals, continued

Disease and/or Organism	Common Animal Sources/Reservoirs	Vector or Modes of Transmission
Lyme disease (*Borrelia burgdorferi*)	Mice, squirrels, shrews, and other small vertebrates	Black-legged or deer tick bites (*Ixodes scapularis* or *Ixodes pacificus*)
Mycobacteriosis (*Mycobacterium marinum*, others)	Fish (and cleaning aquaria)	Skin injury or contamination of existing wound
Mycobacterium bovis and *Mycobacterium tuberculosis*	Cattle, elephants, giraffes, rhinoceroses, bison, deer, elk	*M bovis* is transmitted through ingestion of contaminated food and milk from infected cattle; *M tuberculosis* is airborne
Pasteurella multocida	Cats, dogs, other animals	Bites, scratches, licks
Plague (*Yersinia pestis*)	Rodents, cats, ground squirrels, prairie dogs	Bite of rodent fleas, (especially tropical rat fleas, *Xenopsylla cheopis*), direct contact with infected animal tissues, airborne from other human or animal (eg, cat) with pneumonic plague
Q fever (*Coxiella burnetii*)	Sheep, goats, cows, cats, dogs, wild rodents, birds	Direct contact and aerosols from birth products or animal tissues or products (Possible role of ticks not well defined)
Rat-bite fever (*Streptobacillus moniliformis*, *Spirillum minus*)	Rodents (especially rats, occasionally squirrels), cats, weasels, gerbils	Bites, secretions, and contaminated food, milk, and water
Relapsing fever (tickborne) (*Borrelia* species)	Wild rodents	Soft tick bites (*Ornithodoros* species)
Salmonellosis (*Salmonella* species)	Poultry, turtles, frogs, lizards, snakes, salamanders, iguanas, dogs, cats, hamsters, hedgehogs and other rodents, ferrets, other wild and domestic animals, Komodo dragons	Ingestion of contaminated food, milk, and water; direct contact; contact with fecally contaminated surfaces; person-to-person (fecal-oral)
Streptococcus iniae	Fish grown by aquaculture	Skin injury during handling of fish
Tetanus (*Clostridium tetani*)	Any animal, usually indirect via soil containing animal feces	Wound infection, skin injury or soft tissue injury with inoculation of bacteria (as from soil or a contaminated object), contaminated bites

Table. Diseases Transmitted by Animals, continued

Disease and/or Organism	Common Animal Sources/Reservoirs	Vector or Modes of Transmission
Tularemia (*Francisella tularensis*)	Wild rabbits, hares, voles, sheep, cattle, muskrats, moles, cats, hamsters	Wood tick bites (*Dermacentor andersoni*), dog tick bites (*D variabilis*), Lone-star tick bites (*Amblyomma americanum*), deerfly bites, direct contact with infected animal, ingestion of contaminated water, mechanical transmission from claws or teeth (cats), aerosolization of tissues or excreta
Vibrio species	Shellfish	Ingestion of contaminated food or water; skin injury or contamination of existing wound
Yersiniosis (*Yersinia enterocolitica*, *Yersinia pseudotuberculosis*)	Swine, deer, elk, horses, goats, sheep, cattle, rodents, birds, rabbits	Ingestion of contaminated food, water, or milk; rarely direct contact, person-to-person (fecal-oral)
Fungal Diseases		
Cryptococcosis (*Cryptococcus neoformans*)	Excreta of birds, particularly pigeons	Inhalation of aerosols from accumulations of bird feces
Histoplasmosis (*Histoplasma capsulatum*)	Excreta of bats, birds, particularly starlings	Inhalation of aerosols from accumulations of bat and bird feces
Ringworm/tinea corporis (*Microsporum* and *Trichophyton* species)	Cats, dogs, fowl, pigs, moles, horses, rodents, cattle, monkeys, goats	Direct contact
Parasitic Diseases		
Anisakiasis (*Anisakis* species)	Saltwater and anadromous fish	Ingestion of larvae in raw or undercooked fish (eg, sushi)
Babesiosis (several *Babesia* species)	Mice, dogs, wildlife	Tick bite (in the United States, *Babesia microti* is transmitted mainly by *Ixodes scapularis*; in Europe, *Babesia divergens* is thought to be mainly transmitted by *Ixodes ricinus*); blood transfusion (rarely)
Balantidiasis (*Balantidium coli*)	Swine	Ingestion of contaminated food or water
Baylisascariasis (*Baylisascaris procyonis*)	Raccoons	Ingestion of eggs shed in raccoon feces
Dwarf tapeworm (*Hymenolepis nana*)	Rodents	Ingestion of eggs from feces (contaminated food, water), person-to-person and animal-to-person (fecal-oral)

Table. Diseases Transmitted by Animals, continued

Disease and/or Organism	Common Animal Sources/Reservoirs	Vector or Modes of Transmission
Cryptosporidiosis (*Cryptosporidium* species)	Domestic animals (including cattle, sheep, goats, horses, pigs, dogs, cats, birds), particularly young animals	Ingestion of contaminated water or foods, person-to-person (fecal-oral)
Cutaneous larva migrans (*Ancylostoma* species)	Dogs, cats	Penetration of skin by larvae, which develop in soil contaminated with animal feces
Taeniasis/pork tapeworm (*Taenia solium*)	Swine (intermediate host)	Ingestion of larvae in raw or undercooked meat (adult tapeworm infection)
Dog tapeworm (*Dipylidium caninum*)	Dogs, cats	Ingestion of fleas infected with larvae
Echinococcosis, hydatid disease (*Echinococcus* species)	Dogs, foxes, possibly other carnivores, coyotes, wolves	Ingestion of eggs shed in animal feces
Fish tapeworm (*Diphyllobothrium latum*)	Saltwater and freshwater fish	Ingestion of larvae in raw or undercooked fish
Giardiasis (*Giardia intestinalis*)	Wild and domestic animals, including dogs, cats, cattle, pigs, beavers, muskrats, rats, pet rodents, rabbits, nonhuman primates	Ingestion of contaminated water or foods, person-to-person and animal-to-person (fecal-oral)
Taeniasis, beef (*Taenia saginata*)	Cattle	Ingestion of larvae in raw or undercooked beef
Toxoplasmosis (*Toxoplasma gondii*)	Cats, livestock	Ingestion of oocysts from cat feces, consumption of cysts in raw or undercooked meat, contact with birth products of cats
Trichinellosis (*Trichinella spiralis* and other *Trichinella* species)	Swine, horses, bears, seals, walruses	Ingestion of larvae in raw or undercooked meat
Ocular or visceral toxocariasis (ocular or visceral larva migrans) Ocular or visceral toxocariasis (*Toxocara canis* and *Toxocara cati*)	Dogs, cats	Ingestion of eggs, usually from soil contaminated by animal feces

Table. Diseases Transmitted by Animals, continued

Disease and/or Organism	Common Animal Sources/Reservoirs	Vector or Modes of Transmission
Chlamydial and Rickettsial Diseases		
Human ehrlichiosis (*Ehrlichia chaffeensis* and *Ehrlichia ewingii*)	Deer, dogs, gray foxes, goats	Tick bites (lone-star ticks, *Amblyomma americanum*)
Human anaplasmosis (*Anaplasma phagocytophilum*)	Deer, dogs, elk, wild rodents, horses, ruminants	Black-legged tick (*I scapularis*) and western black-legged tick (*I pacificus*) bites
Psittacosis (*Chlamydophila psittaci*)	Pet birds (especially psittacine birds) and poultry	Inhalation of aerosols from feces of infected birds
Rickettsialpox (*Rickettsia akari*)	House mice	Mite bites (house mouse mite, *Liponyssoides sanguineus*)
Rocky Mountain spotted fever (*Rickettsia rickettsii*)	Dogs, wild rodents, rabbits	Tick bites; rarely by direct contamination with infectious material from ticks (American dog tick, *Dermacentor variabilis*; Rocky Mountain wood tick, *Dermacentor andersoni*; and brown dog tick, *Rhipicephalus sanguineus*)
Rickettsia parkeri infection (Maculatum disease, American boutonneuse fever)	Unknown, perhaps small wild rodents	Gulf coast ticks, *Amblyomma maculatum*
Typhus, fleaborne endemic typhus (*Rickettsia typhi*)	Rats, opossums, cats, dogs	Rat flea feces scratched into abrasions; less common, other fleas (Oriental rat flea, *Xenopsylla cheopis*)
Typhus, louseborne epidemic typhus (*Rickettsia prowazekii*)	Flying squirrels	Person-to-person via body louse, contact with flying squirrels, their nests, or ectoparasites (role and species of ectoparasites undefined)
Viral Diseases		
Colorado tick fever	Wild rodents, (squirrels, chipmunks)	Tick bites (Rocky Mountain wood tick, *D andersoni*)
Encephalitis		
LaCrosse (the most common North American human-disease-causing bunyavirus in the California sero-group)	Wild rodents (squirrels, chipmunks)	Mosquito bites (Eastern tree hole mosquito, *Aedes triseriatus*)

Table. Diseases Transmitted by Animals, continued

Disease and/or Organism	Common Animal Sources/Reservoirs	Vector or Modes of Transmission
Encephalitis, continued		
Eastern equine	Wild birds, poultry, horses	Mosquito bites (*Coquillettidia* species, *Aedes* species)
Western equine	Wild birds, poultry, horses	Mosquito bites (*Culex tarsalis*)
St Louis	Wild birds, poultry	Mosquito bites (*Culex pipiens, Culex quinquefasciatus, Culex tarsalis*)
Venezuelan equine	Rodents, horses	Mosquito bites (many species in many genera)
Powassan	Rodents, rabbits	Tick bites (groundhog tick, *Ixodes cookei*)
West Nile	Wild birds, horses	Mosquito bites (*Culex pipiens, C quinquefasciatus, C tarsalis*)
Nipah virus	Bats; pigs can become infected	Close contact with bats, consumption of bat contaminated fruit/sap
Hendra virus	Flying foxes; horses become infected	Contact with body fluids of infected horses
Hantaviruses	Wild and peridomestic rodents	Inhalation of aerosols of infected secreta and excreta
Ebola hemorrhagic fever	Bats; primates may become infected	Contact with bats, contact with sick/dead primates
Marburg hemorrhagic fever	Bats	Contact with bats, entering caves or mines inhabited by bats
Rift Valley fever	Cattle, sheep, goats	Animal slaughter; mosquito bites
Crimean Congo hemorrhagic fever	Small rodents, farm animals	Animal slaughter; tick bites
Kyasanur forest disease/Alkhurma hemorrhagic fever	Camels, primates, possibly farm animals	Animal slaughter; tick bites
Omsk hemorrhagic fever	Muskrat	Slaughtering muskrat, tick bites
Lassa fever	Mastomys rodents	Inhalation of aerosols of infected secreta or excreta
South American arenaviruses (Junin, Machupo, Guanarito, Sabia, Chapare)	Rodents	Inhalation of aerosols of infected secreta or excreta

Table. Diseases Transmitted by Animals, continued

Disease and/or Organism	Common Animal Sources/Reservoirs	Vector or Modes of Transmission
B virus (formerly herpesvirus simiae)	Macaque monkeys	Bite or exposure to secretions
Lymphocytic choriomeningitis	Rodents, particularly house mice and pet hamsters	Direct contact, inhalation of aerosols, ingestion of food contaminated with rodent excreta
Rabies (Lyssavirus)	In the United States, primarily wildlife (bats, raccoons, skunks, foxes, coyotes, mongooses) or, less frequently, domestic animals (dogs, cats, cattle, horses, sheep, goats, ferrets)	Bites, rarely contact of open wounds, abrasions (including scratches), or mucous membranes with saliva or other infectious materials (eg, neural tissue)
Monkeypox	Prairie dogs, African rodents	Direct contact, bite, scratch
Influenza (H5NI)	Chickens, birds, swine	Contact with infected animals or aerosols (markets, slaughter house)
Orf (pox virus of sheep)	Sheep, goats	Contact with infected saliva
Severe acute respiratory virus (coronavirus)	Bats, civet cats, potentially other animal species	Unclear; person-to-person (respiratory, contact)

·······················
APPENDIX XII

State Immunization Requirements for School Attendance

The United States relies on child care and elementary and secondary school entry immunization requirements to achieve and sustain high levels of immunization coverage. This strategy has proven successful not only in dramatically decreasing communicable disease in settings where children gather but also in decreasing the opportunity for transmission of vaccine-preventable diseases to the unimmunized, the underimmunized, and the immunologically frail. All states require immunization of children at the time of entry into school, and most states require immunization for entry into licensed child care facilities. In addition, many states require immunization of children throughout grade school, older children in upper grades, and young adults entering college. The most up-to-date information about which vaccines are required in a specific state, permissible exemptions, and minor's consent to immunization can be obtained from the immunization program manager of each state health department, from a number of local health departments, and from **www.immunize.org/laws** and the State and Territorial Health Organization (**www.astho.org**).

The Centers for Disease Control and Prevention (CDC) collects state-specific data on current school entry laws and regulations (child care and Head Start, kindergarten, first grade, and middle school), immunization coverage levels, and exemption rates through state-based surveys. The most recent surveillance results can be accessed online through the CDC at **www.cdc.gov/vaccines/stats-surv/schoolsurv/default.htm.**

·······················
APPENDIX XIII

Services of the Centers for Disease Control and Prevention (CDC)

The Centers for Disease Control and Prevention (CDC), US Public Health Service, Department of Health and Human Services, is the federal agency charged with protecting the public health of the nation by preventing disease and other disabling conditions. The CDC administers national programs for prevention and control of the following: (1) infectious diseases; (2) vaccine-preventable diseases; (3) occupational diseases and injury; (4) chronic diseases; (5) environment-related injury and illness; and (6) birth defects and developmental disabilities. The CDC also provides consultation to other nations and participates with international agencies in the control of preventable diseases. In addition, the CDC directs and enforces foreign quarantine activities and regulations and provides consultation and assistance in upgrading the performance of clinical laboratories.

The CDC provides a number of services related to infectious disease management and control. Although the CDC principally is a resource for state and local health departments, it also offers direct and indirect services to hospitals and practicing health care professionals. The range of services includes reference laboratory diagnosis and epidemiologic consultation, both usually arranged through state health departments.

The CDC Drug Service supplies some specific prophylactic or therapeutic drugs and biologic agents. Specific immunobiologic products available include equine-derived heptavalent botulism antitoxin (HBAT), which contains antitoxin against 7 (A–G) botulism toxin types, diphtheria equine antitoxin, Vaccinia Immune Globulin (VIG), vaccinia (smallpox) vaccine, and anthrax vaccine adsorbed. In addition, several drugs for treatment of parasitic disease, which currently are not approved for use in the United States, are handled under an investigational new drug permit. These antiparasitic drugs can be found in Drugs for Parasitic Infections (p 848).

Requests for biologic products, antiparasitic drugs, and related information should be directed to the CDC Drug Service (see Appendix I, Directory of Resources, p 883). For additional information, see **www.cdc.gov/ncezid/dsr/office-director.html#drugservice.**

Index

Page numbers followed by "t" indicate a table. Page numbers followed by "f" indicate a figure.

Cyst(s)
  Acanthamoeba, 226
  Balamuthia, 226
  Balantidium coli, 250
  Entamoeba, 223–224
Cystic fibrosis
  aspergillosis in, 241, 242
  Burkholderia infections in, 256, 258
  Chlamydophila pneumoniae infections in, 272
  influenza in, 441
  influenza vaccine for, 447
  nontuberculous mycobacterial infections in,
      759–760, 762
  respiratory syncytial virus infections in, 617
Cystic Fibrosis Foundation, infection control
      standards of, 160
Cysticercosis *(Cysticercus cellulosae)*
  control measures for, 705
  in internationally adopted children, 197
  transmission of, 930t
  treatment of, 704–705, 859t
Cystitis
  from adenoviruses, 220
  from *Candida*, 267
  from *Coxiella burnetii*, 599
  from microsporidiosis, 510
  from polyomaviruses, 593–595
Cystoisosporiasis *(Cystoisospora belli)*, 453–454
  HIV infection with, 419, 419t
  treatment of, 853t
Cytochrome P450 enzymes, drug interactions and,
      806–807
Cytokine inhibitors, vaccines and, 80, 81t, 82–83, 84t
Cytology, for human papillomavirus infections, 526
Cytomegalovirus (CMV) infections, XXXV, 300–305
  breastfeeding and, 129
  chemoprophylaxis for, 305
  in child care facilities, 145, 301, 304
  clinical manifestations of, 300–301
  control measures for, 305
  diagnosis of, 302–303
  epidemiology of, 301–302
  etiology of, 301
  HIV infection with, 419, 419t–421t, 431
  hospital isolation for, 304
  in pelvic inflammatory disease, 550
  in residential institutions, 97
  from transfusions, 116t, 117–118, 124
  treatment of, 303–304, 843t–844t
  Web site, www.cdc.gov/cmv/index.html, 304
Cytotoxicity assay, for *Clostridium difficile* toxins, 286

D

D zone test, for staphylococci, 658
Dactylitis, from *Salmonella* infections, 635
DailyMed Web sites, 807
Dandruff, from tinea capitis, 712
Dapsone
  adverse events from, 862t
  for leprosy, 468
  for *Pneumocystis jirovecii* infections, 586, 858t
  safety in pregnancy, 866t
  for toxoplasmosis, 726, 727t
Daptomycin
  dosage of, beyond newborn period, 813t
  for enterococcal infections, 687
  for staphylococcal infections, 660, 664
  usage in children, 801
Darkfield microscopy
  for *Campylobacter*, 263
  for syphilis, 692
Day care centers. *See* Child care facilities
Deafness and hearing loss
  from cytomegalovirus infections, 300–301
  from meningococcal infections, 500, 501
  from mumps, 514
  from mumps vaccine, 517
  from rubella, 629
  from syphilis, 690
  from toxoplasmosis, 720
Débridement, of bite wounds, 204t
Decubitus ulcers
  Bacteroides infections of, 249
  Prevotella infections of, 249
Deer tick virus, 207t
DEET (diethyltoluamide), for disease prevention,
      210–211
  leishmaniasis, 466
  malaria, 486.489
  tickborne, 208
  West Nile virus, 794
Dehydration
  from astrovirus infections, 243
  from rotavirus infections, 626
  from staphylococcal infections, 653
  from *Vibrio cholerae* infections, 789
Dehydroemetine, for amebiasis, 224
Delirium, from typhus, 771
Delusions, from African trypanosomiasis, 732
Dementia, from prion diseases, 596
Dengue fever, 305–307
  clinical manifestations of, 232, 233t, 305
  control measures for, 307
  dengue shock syndrome in, 305–307
  diagnosis of, 306
  epidemiology of, 306
  etiology of, 306

Z

Zanamivir
    dosage of, 847t
    for influenza, 443–444, 443t, 453, 847t
Zidovudine (AZT), for HIV infection, 434–437,
            435t, 434
Zoonoses. *See* Animalborne diseases
Zoster. *See* Herpes zoster
Zoster vaccine
    contraindications to, 911t
    licensing of, 889t
    precautions for, 911t
    vaccine for, 14t
Zygomycosis, 330t, 835t